CLINICAL GLAUCOMA MANAGEMENT

CLINICAL GLAUCOMA MANAGEMENT

Critical Signs in Diagnosis and Therapy

Ronald L. Gross, MD
Professor of Ophthalmology
The Clifton R. McMichael Chair in Ophthalmology
Baylor College of Medicine
Cullen Eye Institute
Houston, Texas

W.B. Saunders Company
A Harcourt Health Sciences Company
PHILADELPHIA LONDON NEW YORK ST. LOUIS SYDNEY TORONTO

W.B. SAUNDERS COMPANY
A Harcourt Health Sciences Company

The Curtis Center
Independence Square West
Philadelphia, Pennsylvania 19106

Library of Congress Cataloging-in-Publication Data

Clinical glaucoma management: critical signs in diagnosis and therapy / [edited by] Ronald L. Gross.

p. ; cm.

ISBN 0–7216–7272–8

1. Glaucoma. I. Gross, Ronald L. [DNLM: 1. Glaucoma—diagnosis. 2. Glaucoma—therapy. WW 290 C641 2000]

RE871.C56 2000 617.7′41—dc21

99-048219

Acquisitions Editor: Richard H. Lampert
Project Manager: Agnes Hunt Byrne
Production Manager: Paul Nigel Harris
Illustration Specialist: Robert Quinn

CLINICAL GLAUCOMA MANAGEMENT: Critical Signs in Diagnosis and Therapy ISBN 0–7216–7272–8

Printed in the United States of America.

Last digit is the print number: 9 8 7 6 5 4 3 2 1

I dedicate this book to my father;
I hope he enjoys reading it.

Contributors

Howard S. Barnebey, MD
Specialty Eyecare Centre, Seattle, Washington
Medical Considerations in the Management of Glaucoma

Rommel Bautista
School of Medicine, Stanford University, Stanford, California
Combined Cataract and Glaucoma Surgery

J. Brent Bond, MD
Assistant Professor, Department of Ophthalmology, Wake Forest University Eye Center, Winston-Salem, North Carolina
Eyelids, Lacrimal Apparatus, Orbit, Motility

Bruce D. Cameron, MD
Clinical Assistant Professor of Ophthalmology, New York University School of Medicine, New York; Attending Physician, St. Vincent's Hospital, New York; Associate Adjunct Attending Physician, The New York Eye and Ear Infirmary, New York, New York
Race

David P. Campbell, MD
Private Practice, Sarasota, Florida
Cornea, Conjunctiva, and Bleb

Louis B. Cantor, MD
Professor and Director of the Glaucoma Service, Indiana University School of Medicine, Indianapolis, Indiana
Filtration Surgery and Tube Shunts

George A. Cioffi, MD
Director, Glaucoma Service, Devers Eye Institute Discoveries in Sight, Portland, Oregon
Optic Nerve: Anatomy and Physiology

Anthony Economou, DO
Adjunct Faculty, Oklahoma State University College of Osteopathic Medicine, Tulsa; Medical Director, TLC—The Laser Center, Tulsa; Private Practice in Glaucoma, Britton Vision Associates, Tulsa, Oklahoma
Glaucomas Associated With External Eye Signs

Sherif M. El-Harazi, MD
Resident, The University of Texas Health Science Center at Houston, Houston, Texas
Anterior and Posterior Chambers; Gonioscopy

Robert D. Fechtner, MD
Associate Professor, Director, Glaucoma Division, University of Medicine and Dentistry of New Jersey, New Jersey Medical School, Newark, New Jersey
Vitreous and Retina

Robert M. Feldman, MD
Clinical Assistant Professor, Deputy Chairman, Department of Ophthalmology and Visual Science, University of Texas Medical School at Houston, Houston; Director of Glaucoma Service, Hermann Hospital, Hermann Eye Center, Houston, Texas
Anterior and Posterior Chambers; Gonioscopy

Ronald Fellman, MD
Associate Clinical Professor, Department of Ophthalmology, University of Texas Southwestern Medical School, Dallas; Glaucoma Associates of Texas, Dallas, Texas
Visual Fields

Lisa S. Gamell, MD
Beth Israel Medical Center, New York, New York
Optic Nerve Assessment

Sai B. Gandham, MD
Assistant Professor, Albany Medical College, Albany, New York
Cyclodestructive Procedures

Kevin C. Greenidge, MD, MPH
Professor and Chairman, Department of Ophthalmology, State University of New York Health Science Center, Brooklyn; Chairman, Department of Ophthalmology, Long Island College Hospital, Brooklyn, New York
Race

John D. Gross, MD
Department of Ophthalmology, University of Florida, Gainesville, Florida
Cornea, Conjunctiva, and Bleb

Weldon Haw, MD
Fellow, Heed Ophthalmic Foundation, Stanford University School of Medicine, Department of Ophthalmology, Stanford, California
Combined Cataract and Glaucoma Surgery

Dale K. Heuer, MD
Professor of Ophthalmology, Medical College of Wisconsin, Milwaukee; Director, The Eye Institute of the Medical College of Wisconsin and Froedtert Hospital, Milwaukee, Wisconsin
Conjunctiva and Cornea

Henry Jampel, MD, MHS
Associate Professor of Ophthalmology, Johns Hopkins University School of Medicine, Baltimore, Maryland
Intraocular Pressure

L. Jay Katz, MD
Associate Professor, Jefferson Medical College of Thomas Jefferson University, Philadelphia, Pennsylvania
Cyclodestructive Procedures

Usha Kurumety, MD
Assistant Professor of Ophthalmology, Boston University School of Medicine, Boston; Director, Glaucoma Consultation Service, Boston Medical Center and Boston Veterans Affairs Medical Center, Boston, Massachusetts
Optic Nerve Damage and Dysfunction in Glaucoma

Paul P. Lee, MD, JD
Professor, Duke University, Durham, North Carolina; Consultant, Rand, Health Sciences Program, Santa Monica, California
Preferred Practice Patterns and Economic Implications

Mary Ann Lloyd, MD
Clinical Associate Professor of Ophthalmology, Stanford University School of Medicine, Stanford; Private Practice, Palo Alto Medical Foundation, Department of Ophthalmology, Palo Alto, California
Conjunctiva and Cornea

Andrew J. Michael, MD
Associate Clinical Professor, Medical College of Virginia, Richmond; Commonwealth Eye Care Associates, Richmond, Virginia
Trabecular Meshwork and Argon Laser Trabeculoplasty

Rebecca K. Morgan, MD
Clinical Assistant Professor, Dean A. McGee Eye Institute, University of Oklahoma College of Medicine, Oklahoma City, Oklahoma
Iris and Pupil

Kimberly A. Neely, MD, PhD
Assistant Professor, Department of Ophthalmology, Hershey Medical Center, Hershey, Pennsylvania
Retina and Vitreous

Osman Oram, MD
Associate Professor and Chairman, Department of Ophthalmology, Maltepe University School of Medicine, Istanbul; Associate Professor of Ophthalmology, Eye Clinic, American Hospital, Istanbul, Turkey
Ciliary Body

Silvia Orengo-Nania, MD
Associate Professor, Baylor College of Medicine, Houston; Chief of Ophthalmology, Veterans Affairs Medical Center, Houston, Texas
Anterior and Posterior Chambers, Iris and Pupil, and Lens

Jody R. Piltz-Seymour, MD
Associate Professor of Ophthalmology, University of Pennsylvania School of Medicine, Philadelphia; Director of Glaucoma Service, Scheie Eye Institute of the University of Pennsylvania, Philadelphia, Pennsylvania
Systemic Syndromes and Diseases and Glaucoma

Tony Realini, MD
Assistant Professor, Department of Ophthalmology, University of Arkansas for Medical Sciences, Little Rock, Arkansas
Vitreous and Retina

Joel S. Schuman, MD
Professor of Ophthalmology, Tufts University School of Medicine, Boston; Director, Glaucoma Service, New England Eye Center, New England Medical Center, Boston, Massachusetts
Optic Nerve Assessment

Mark B. Sherwood, MD
Department of Ophthalmology, University of Florida, Gainesville, Florida
Cornea, Conjunctiva, and Bleb

Karl J. Siebert, MD
Private Practice, Grand Rapids, Michigan
Crystalline Lens, Refractive Error, and Cataract Surgery

Steven T. Simmons, MD
Associate Clinical Professor, Albany Medical College, Albany, New York
Glaucomas Associated With External Eye Signs

Kuldev Singh, MD
School of Medicine, Stanford University, Stanford, California
Combined Cataract and Glaucoma Surgery

Gregory L. Skuta, MD
James P. Luton Clinical Professor, Dean A. McGee Eye Institute, University of Oklahoma College of Medicine, Oklahoma City, Oklahoma
Iris and Pupil

Rohit Varma, MD
Associate Professor, Department of Ophthalmology, Keck School of Medicine of the University of Southern California, Los Angeles; Glaucoma Specialist, USC University Hospital, Los Angeles, California
Optic Nerve Damage and Dysfunction in Glaucoma

Rebecca Walker, MD
Glaucoma Specialist, Abington Memorial Hospital, Abington, Pennsylvania
Systemic Syndromes and Diseases and Glaucoma

Martin B. Wax, MD
Associate Professor, Department of Ophthalmology and Visual Sciences, Washington University School of Medicine, St. Louis, Missouri
Normal-Pressure Glaucoma

Martha M. Wright, MD
Assistant Professor, Department of Ophthalmology, University of Minnesota, Minneapolis, Minnesota
Retina and Vitreous

Darrell WuDunn, MD, PhD
Assistant Professor of Ophthalmology, Indiana University School of Medicine, Indianapolis, Indiana
Genetics

Kathy Yang-Williams, MD
Specialty Eyecare Centre, Seattle, Washington
Medical Considerations in the Management of Glaucoma

Preface

Welcome! That may seem to be an unusual beginning to a book, but it expresses the wishes of the contributors perfectly. We conceived this book to be a useful tool in the everyday care of glaucoma patients. When you are confronted with a problem in a patient with glaucoma, this book is designed specifically to provide the information you need to correctly identify the patient's situation and then deal with it properly.

The contributors have done a superb job of organizing the important information in this unique format which necessitated a different approach to writing each subject. Whenever possible, contributors for related sections collaborated to minimize overlap. However, particularly in glaucoma, there may be multiple, varied approaches to the same problem. As a result, as many different approaches as possible are included. This has resulted in what some might see as redundancy, but preferably may be viewed as reinforcement.

The underlying premise is that glaucomas are a complex group of diseases and often the specific diagnosis cannot be immediately identified, but we can almost always recognize that key abnormality in the examination that is at least a partial manifestation of the problem. Once that identification has been accomplished, we are well on the correct management path.

As background, the initial chapters deal with *Key Concepts*; the care practices and the underlying anatomy and physiology of the group of diseases commonly referred to as glaucoma. This is not meant to be all-inclusive. Rather, the purpose is to provide an initial description of how to approach the care of the glaucoma patient and to supply basic information, important in its own right, and the basic science support that will be useful for the remainder of the book. In addition, the key methods by which the optic neuropathy we call glaucoma may be assessed are discussed.

The next section involves *Key Patient Characteristics*. What can you, as the examining physician, immediately know about your patient from the initial patient history. What do we know about the genetic basis for glaucomas? How can we take a family history to identify a possible genetic basis for this type of glaucoma? Additionally, the patient characteristics, including race, provide valuable information. The past medical history includes other syndromes and diseases that may have glaucoma as a component. Also, in a disease that for much of its history was defined by intraocular pressure, what is the implication if this finding is not present? This is information that is usually obtained prior to examination of the patient.

This book will be most useful when you observe a key finding on examination that is of concern. By identifying that key sign or symptom, it allows you to begin to determine the proper care of that patient. This book allows you to take advantage of your ability to examine the patient and directly address those specific signs that differentiate the pathologic process from normal, as well as to differentiate among the pathologic possibilities. The important first step is to identify those initial key components. The key element may be important for the diagnosis of glaucoma, or it may be related to treatment, either medical or surgical. In some instances, both can apply. The section on *Key Diagnostic Signs* provides the manifestations of glaucomas throughout all portions of the standard ophthalmic examination. You may not know the patient's correct diagnosis; but, for example, you see a cellular response in the anterior chamber. It is not immediately apparent that the patient has, in this example, herpetic uveitis. Since this is a patient who has not undergone surgery, by referring to Chapter 12, which covers the anterior chamber, you can use this unique sign to help determine the cause of the inflammation, establish a working diagnosis, and embark on the proper treatment. In this particular case, treating with topical corticosteroids alone in response to the observation of inflammation may not be appropriate.

The section on *Key Therapeutic Signs* deals with problems that may arise from, or be related to, the treatment of glaucoma. In addition, the chapters at the beginning of the section deal with the most common surgical procedures used in the treatment of glaucoma. The remaining chapters deal with specific portions of the examination to aid in the correct identification and appropriate management of a problem. For example, following glaucoma filtration surgery, there is a flat chamber. Given the large number of possible causes and their very different treatments, Chapter 23 discusses the anterior chamber and allows you to assess this particular key finding to optimize your care of the patient.

The final section covers *Key Glaucoma Measures*. The treatment of the glaucoma patient represents a synthesis of numerous factors that determine the stability of the disease process. This is often our most difficult task as physicians.

These key components are intraocular pressure; the function of the optic nerve as measured by visual field testing; and the structure of the presumed site of damage, the optic nerve. This section deals with the techniques to assess and use the findings from these observations in the treatment of the patient with glaucoma.

It is our sincere hope that this tool will enhance your ability to care for patients with glaucoma by taking often difficult problems and providing a useful approach to identification and treatment.

Ronald L. Gross, MD

Acknowledgments

This book was a collaboration of many talented physicians. First and foremost, the authors must be acknowledged for their hard work. Obviously, their contributions are the centerpiece of the entire project. Next, I would like to thank Lee Spratling, without whose help the sheer weight of paper and the number of slides and figures would have been catastrophic. She kept everything, including me, in its proper place and knew the location of that place. Richard H. Lampert from W.B. Saunders was supportive and, most importantly, patient throughout the entire process.

I would also like to thank Dan Jones for giving me the freedom to undertake this project and for introducing me early in my education to the concept of simplifying a complex problem by identifying the key elements. George Spaeth nurtured and expanded an understanding of glaucoma that this book continues.

My family deserves my thanks and an apology for the dinners ruined, games missed, and being awakened too early in the morning. Thank you Pam, Jacob, Joshua, Grace, and Gabriella for your understanding.

NOTICE

Contents

Color Section following page xvi

SECTION V

KEY GLAUCOMA MEASURES

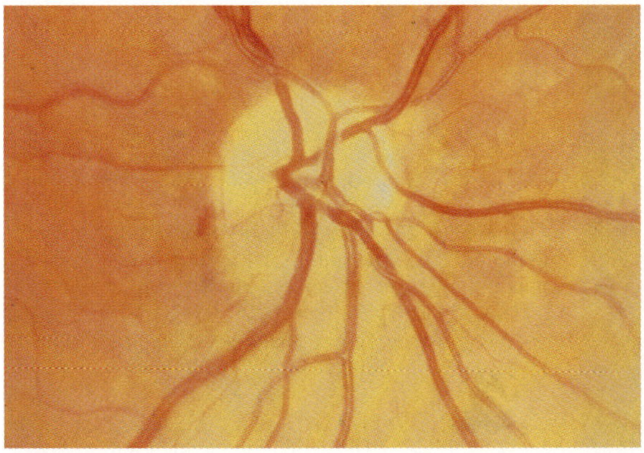

FIGURE 4–15. Photograph demonstrating marked pallor of the superior optic nerve from anterior ischemic optic neuropathy. Note that the cup is not enlarged and the central retinal vessels are not displaced.

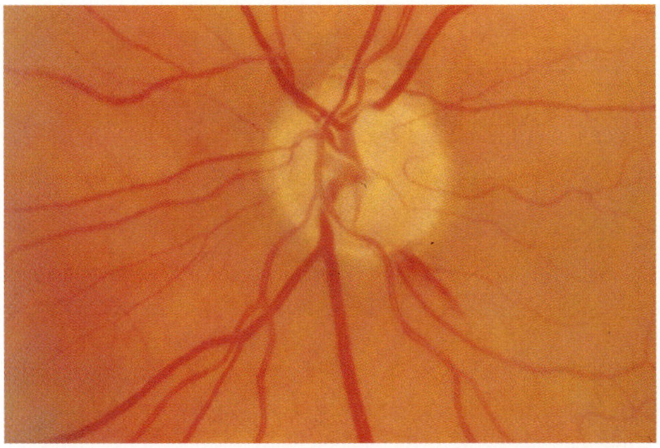

FIGURE 4–16. An optic nerve hemorrhage showing the characteristic feathery appearance of the blood within the nerve fiber layer.

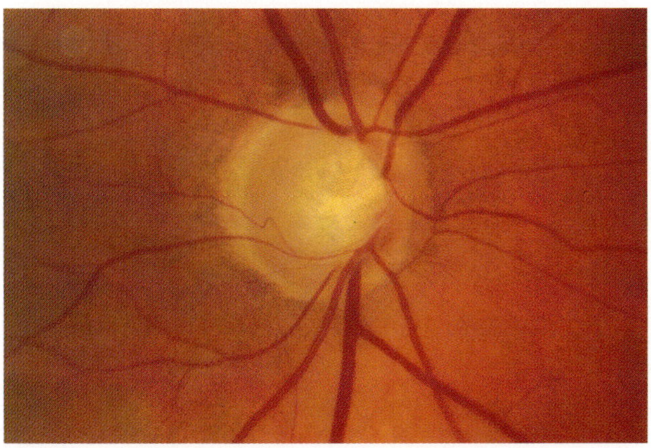

FIGURE 4–17. Photograph of a glaucomatous optic nerve with peripapillary chorioretinal atrophy. Beta-zone atrophy is immediately adjacent to the optic nerve (white crescent), and alpha-zone atrophy lies between the retina and the beta-zone (area of irregular pigmentation).

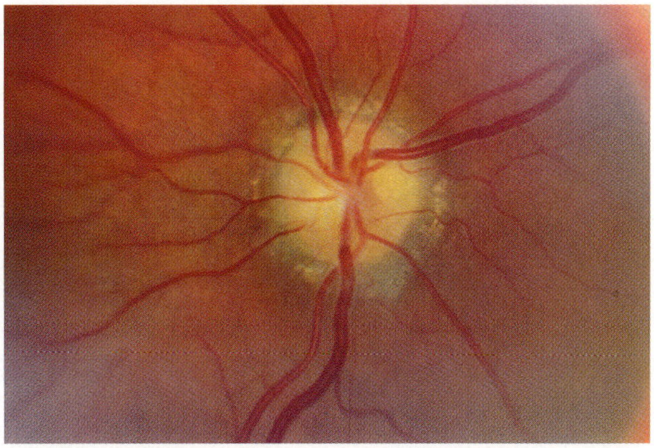

FIGURE 4–19. Photograph of an optic nerve with diffuse drusen appearing as raised irregularities of the optic nerve.

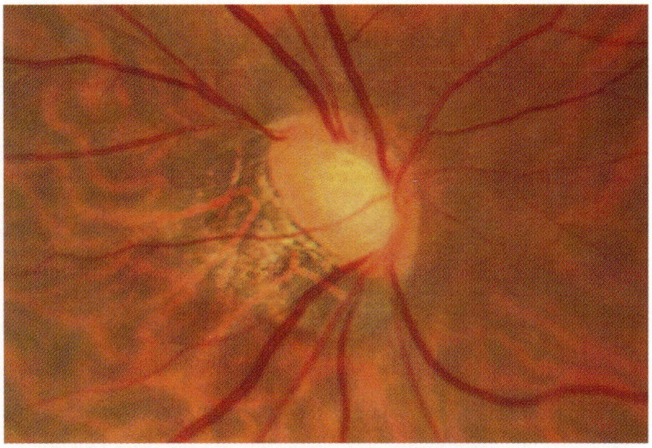

FIGURE 4–20. An optic nerve photograph of an eye with glaucoma. Note the tilted insertion of the optic nerve and a large area of visible sclera adjacent to the obliquely positioned optic nerve head.

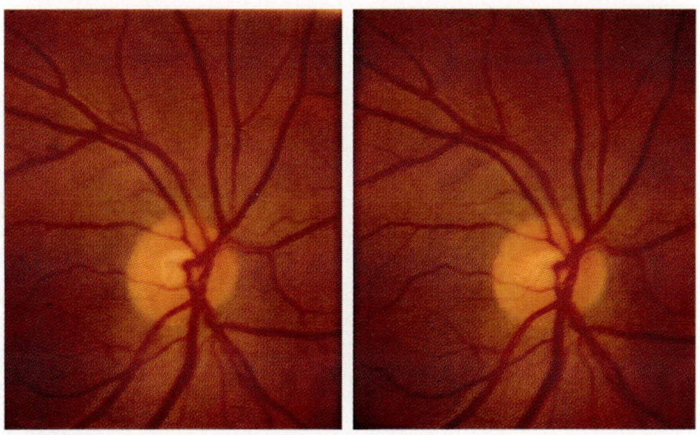

FIGURE 5–1. Healthy optic nerve head. Note the course of the vessels from the cup over the rim of the optic disc.

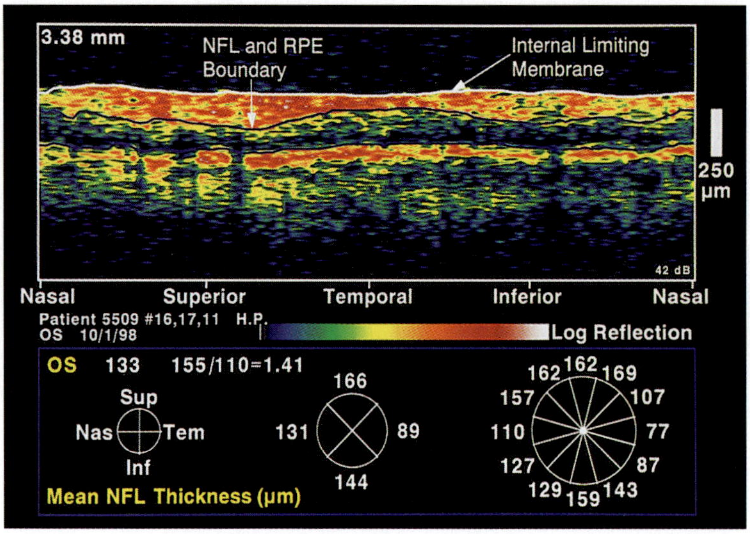

FIGURE 5–17. Optical coherence tomography scan showing the boundaries of the nerve fiber layer (NFL) and retinal pigment epithelium (RPE) (highlighted with a *blue line*), and the internal limiting membrane *(white line).* Inf, inferior; Nas, nasal; Sup, superior; Tem, temporal.

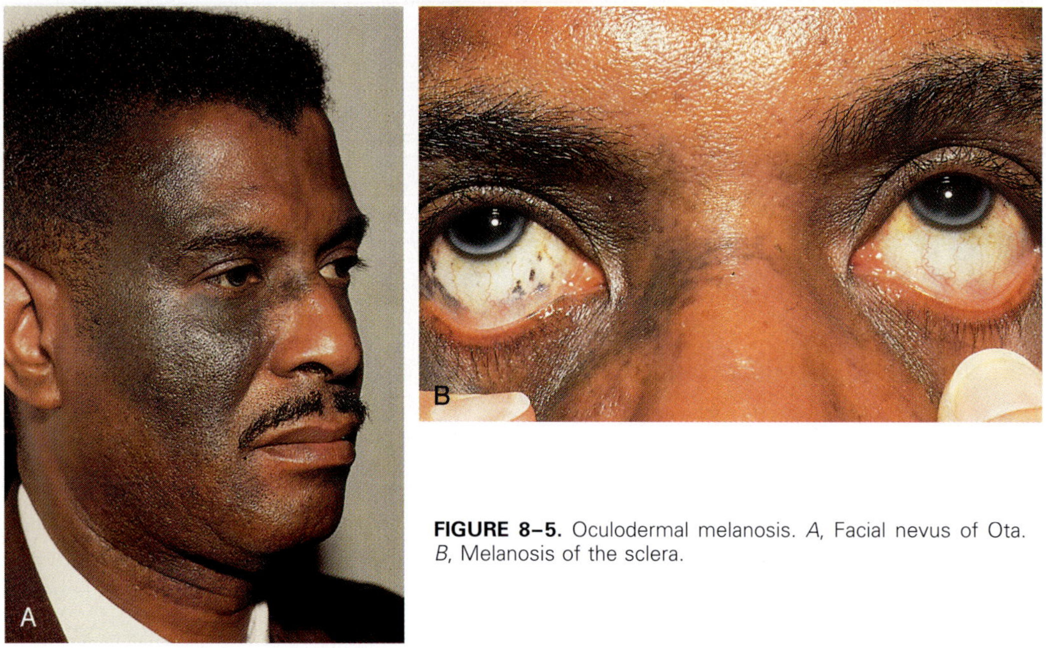

FIGURE 8–5. Oculodermal melanosis. *A*, Facial nevus of Ota. *B*, Melanosis of the sclera.

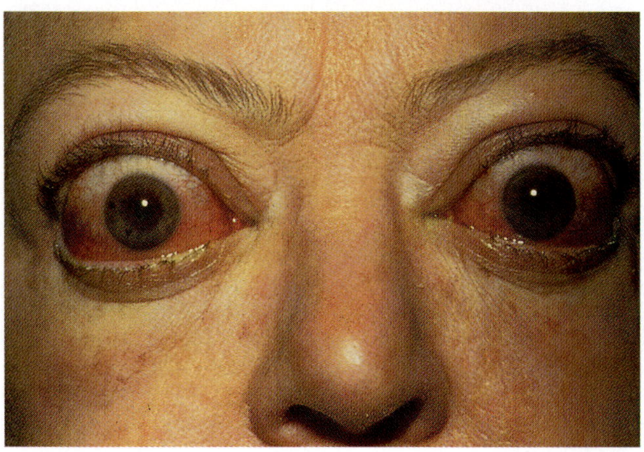

FIGURE 8–8. Bilateral exophthalmos with scleral show in thyroid ophthalmopathy. (Courtesy of S. Orlin, MD.)

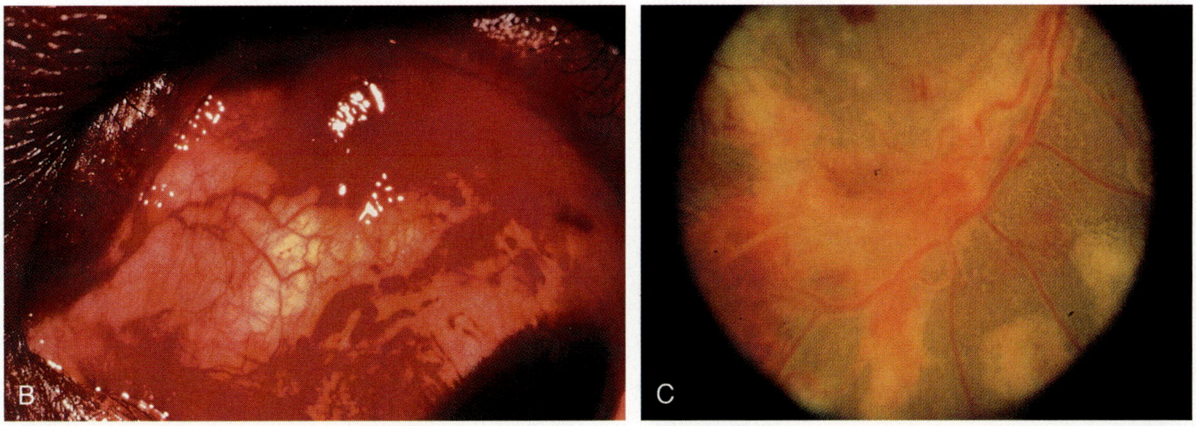

FIGURE 8–21. Clinical findings in acquired immunodeficiency syndrome (AIDS). *B*, Kaposi's sarcoma of the conjunctiva. *C*, cytomegalovirus retinitis. (Courtesy of A. Ho, MD.)

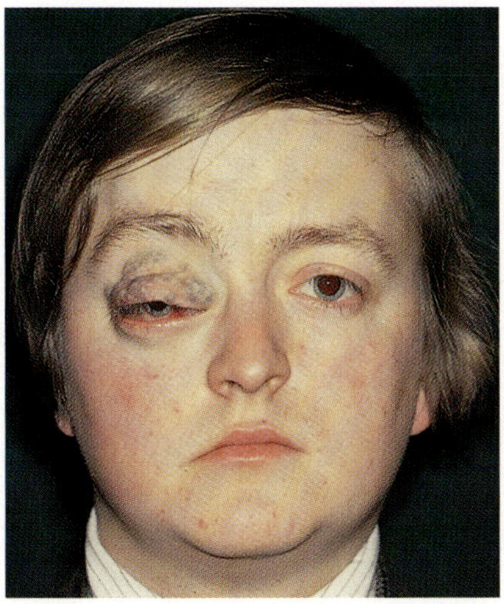

FIGURE 10–3. Unilateral proptosis with dilated veins of the eyelid and anterior orbit in a patient with an orbital varix.

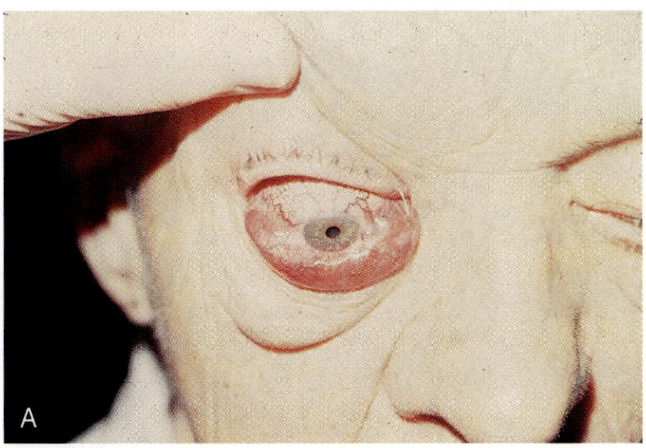

FIGURE 10–4. Proptosis and pulsatile exophthalmos with excessive inferior chemosis seen with a carotid cavernous sinus fistula *(A)*.

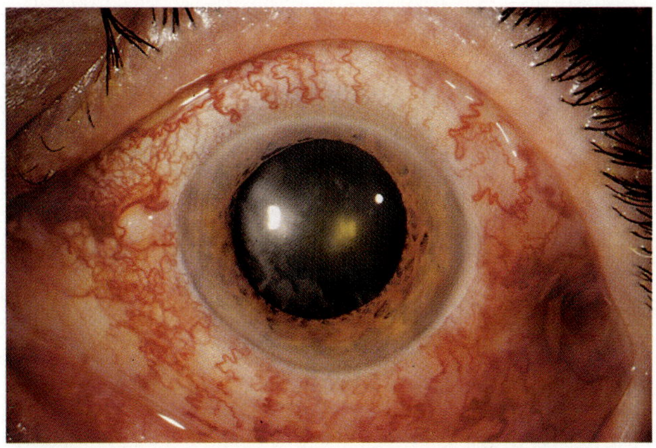

FIGURE 11–2. Conjunctival vascular engorgement due to carotid artery–cavernous sinus fistula. (Courtesy of Andrew Lee, MD.)

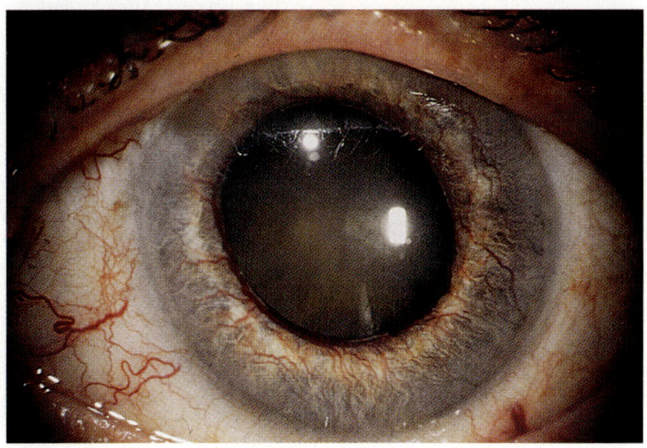

FIGURE 11–5. Rubeosis iridis.

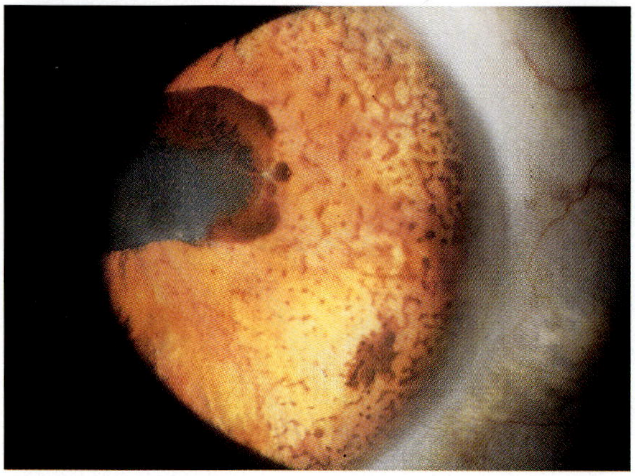

FIGURE 11–11. Cogan-Reese syndrome with pigmented iris lesions.

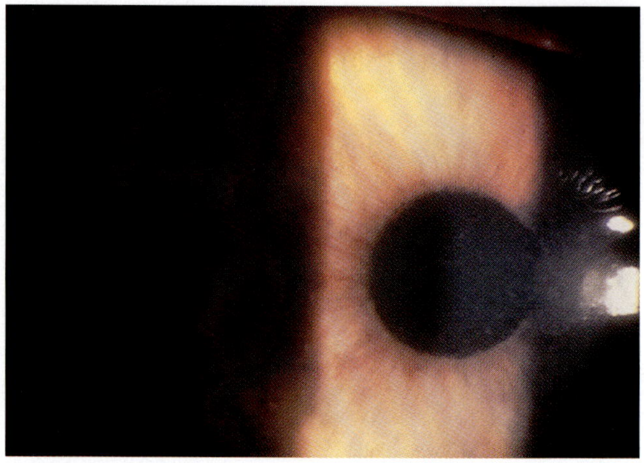

FIGURE 14–29. Normal radial iris vessels evident in thinned iris stroma of an eye with Fuchs' heterochromic iridocyclitis.

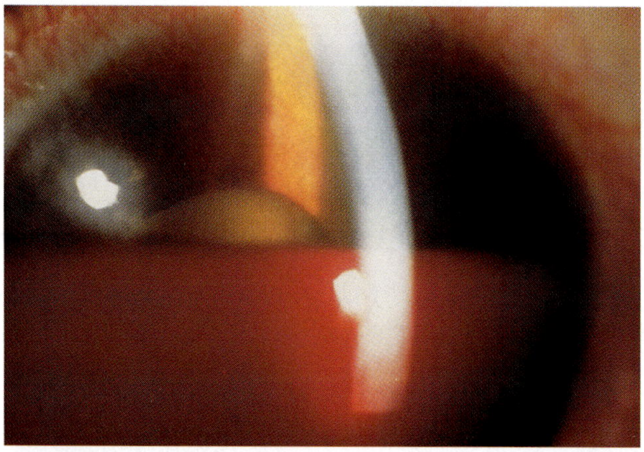

FIGURE 12–3. Slit-lamp photograph showing blood accumulation in the anterior chamber (hyphema).

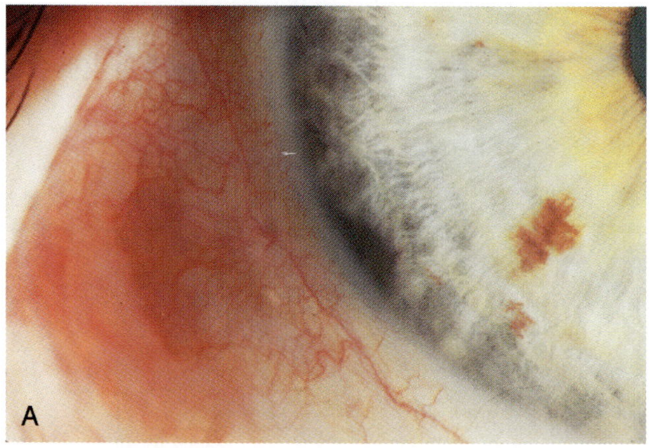

FIGURE 14–33. *A*, Slit-lamp view of suspected iris melanoma.

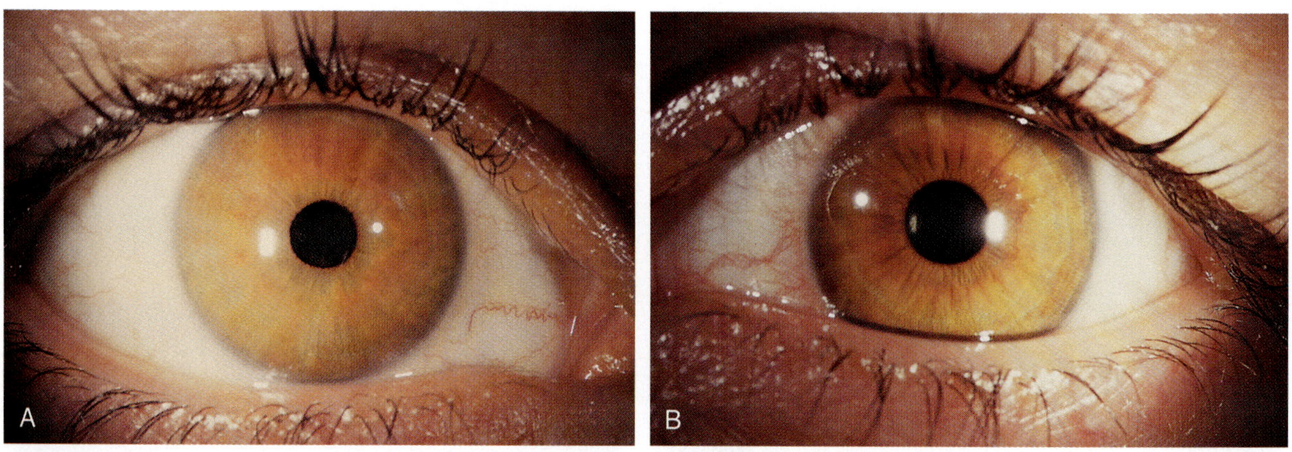

FIGURE 15–11. Fuchs' heterochromic iridocyclitis. *A* and *B*, External photographs of the eyes of a 47-year-old female patient revealing subtle iris heterochromia.

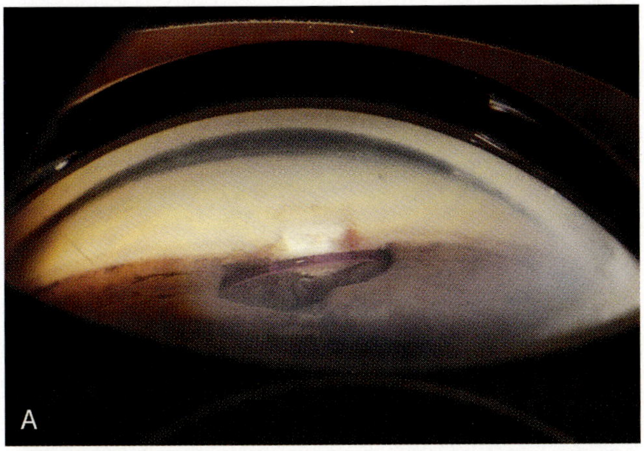

FIGURE 15–25. Neovascularization of a cataract incision. *A*, Superior gonioscopic view demonstrating neovascularization at the edge of a previous corneoscleral tunnel. (Courtesy of Dr. L. Jay Katz.)

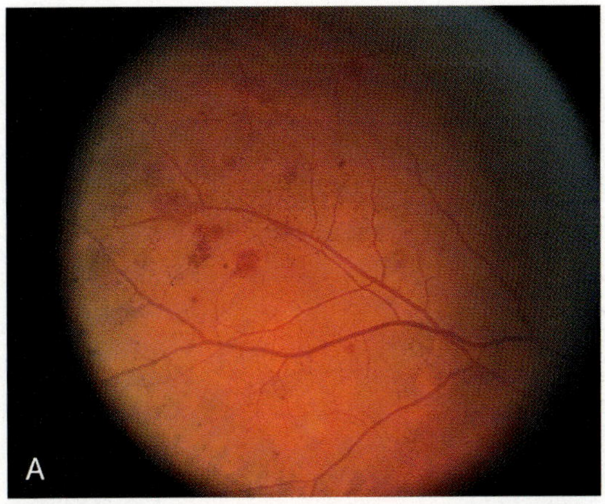

FIGURE 16–6. Carotid occlusive disease. The patient, a diabetic woman, had 100% occlusion of the right carotid artery. *A*, Funduscopic examination revealed intraretinal hemorrhages confined to the midperipheral retina.

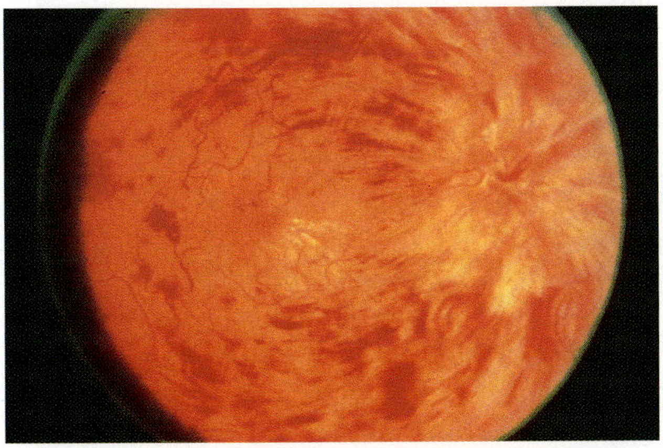

FIGURE 16–4. Central retinal vein occlusion with widely scattered hemorrhages, dilated veins, and swelling of the optic nerve.

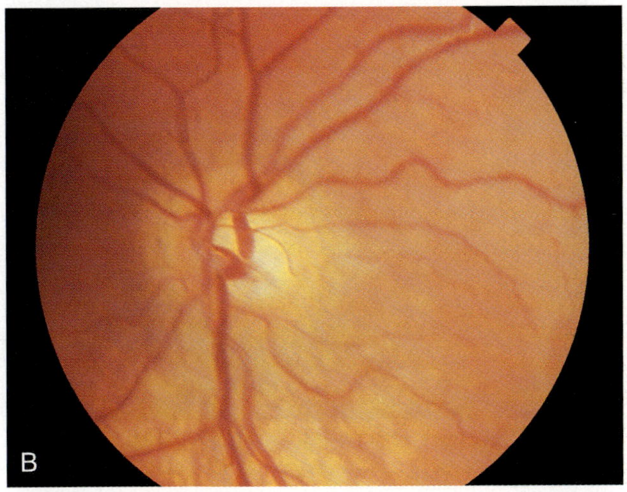

FIGURE 16–8. Sturge-Weber syndrome. *B*, With a choroidal hemangioma and increased cupping from glaucoma. (Courtesy of Dr. C. Gail Summers.)

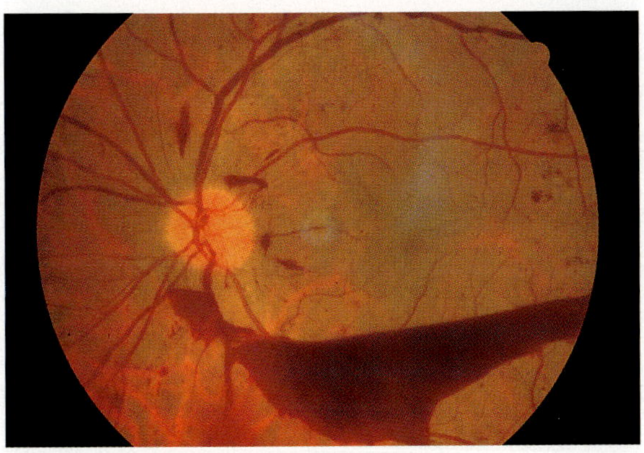

FIGURE 16–5. Proliferative diabetic retinopathy. Extensive neovascularization of the optic disc associated with preretinal hemorrhage along the inferotemporal arcade.

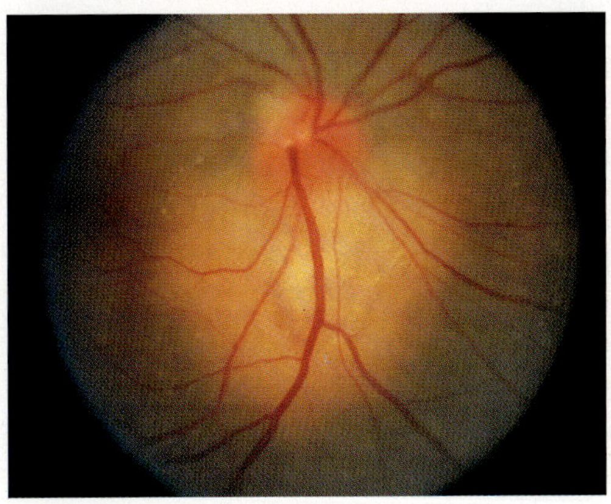

FIGURE 16–10. Peripapillary choroidal granuloma in a patient with pulmonary and ocular sarcoidosis.

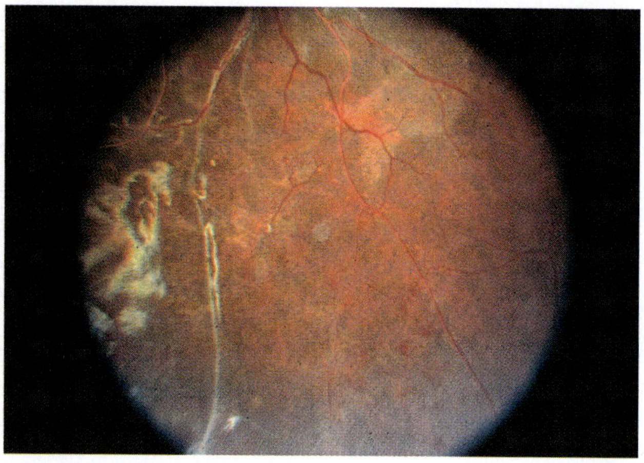

FIGURE 16–11. Retinal periphlebitis in a patient with ocular and systemic sarcoidosis.

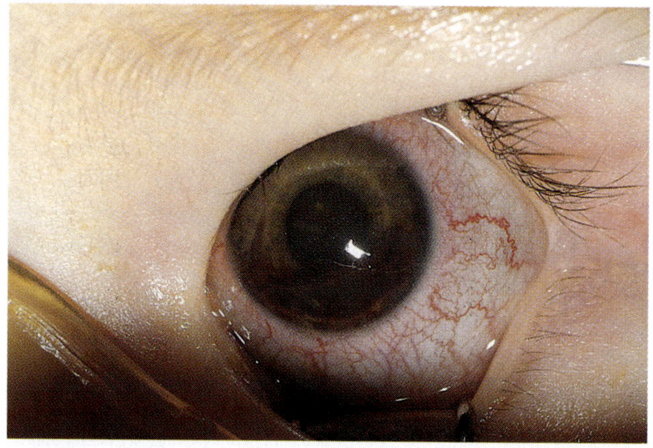

FIGURE 16–24. Juvenile xanthogranuloma. A vascular orange mass is present in the inferior iris. (Courtesy of Dr. C. Gail Summers.)

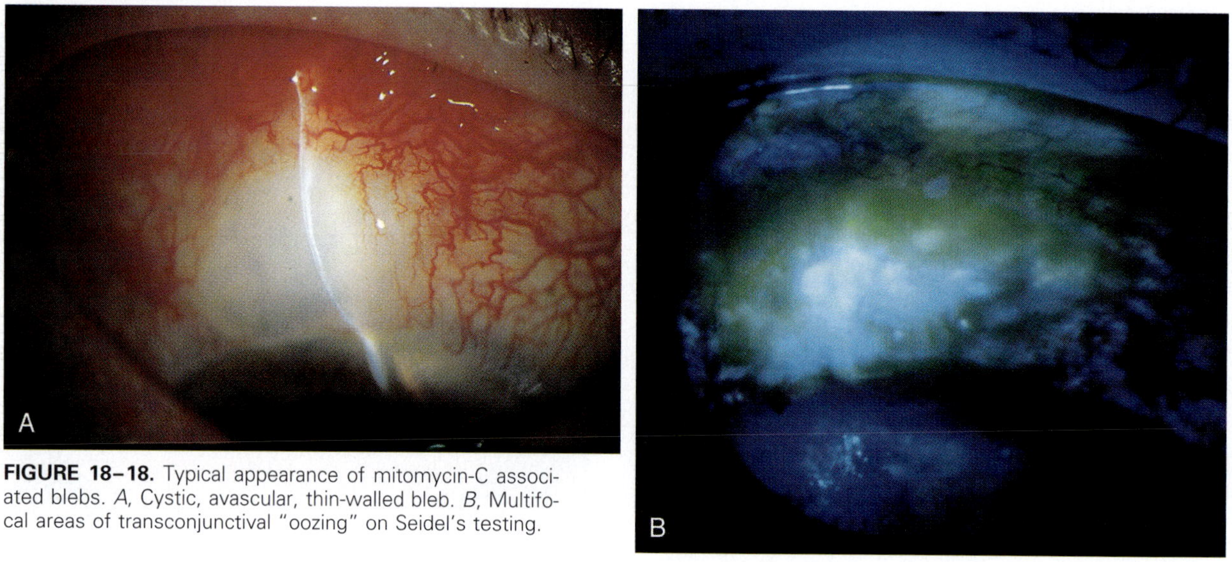

FIGURE 18–18. Typical appearance of mitomycin-C associated blebs. *A*, Cystic, avascular, thin-walled bleb. *B*, Multifocal areas of transconjunctival "oozing" on Seidel's testing.

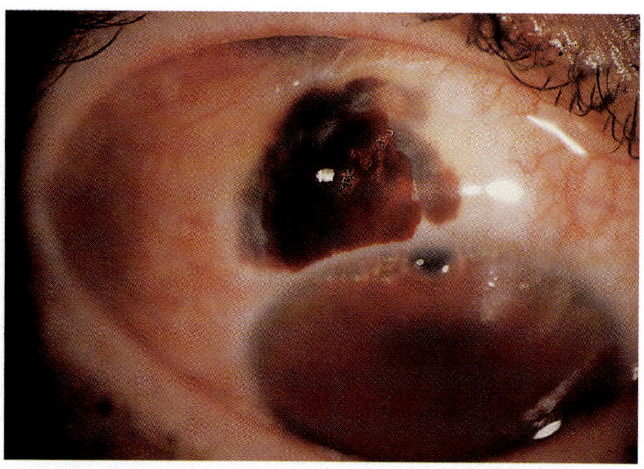

FIGURE 18–24. An autologous blood injection into an overfiltering bleb.

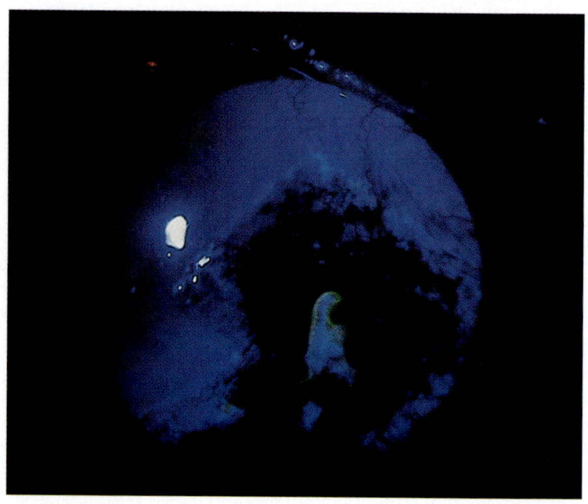

FIGURE 18–25. Clear aqueous is seen within a pool of fluorescein under cobalt-blue light in a patient with a bleb leak.

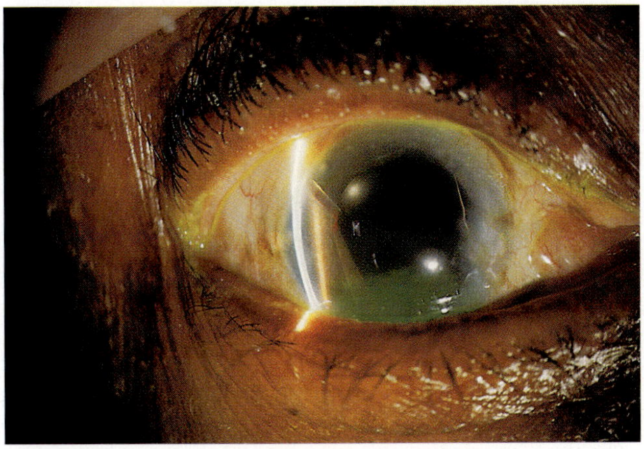

FIGURE 18–41. A blood clot within the tube of a Molteno shunt.

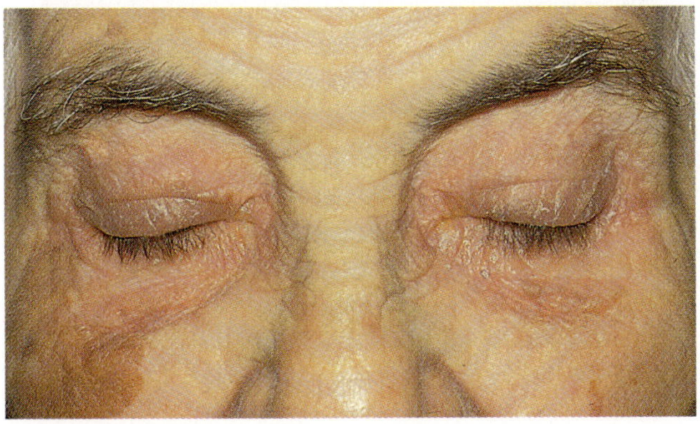

FIGURE 20–3. Allergic dermatitis, represented by erythema and scaling localized to the eyelids.

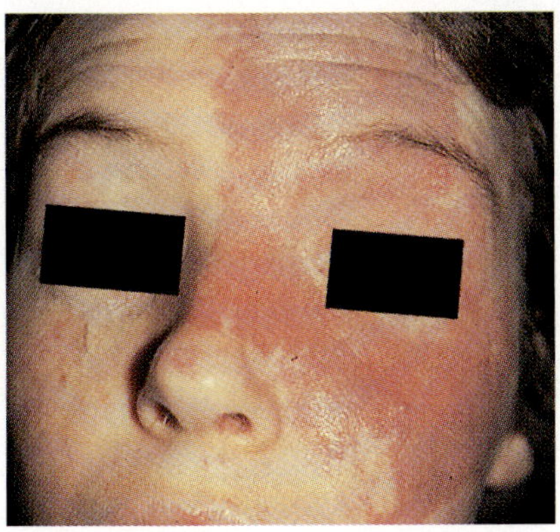

FIGURE 20–5. Unilateral nevus flammeus representative of Sturge-Weber syndrome.

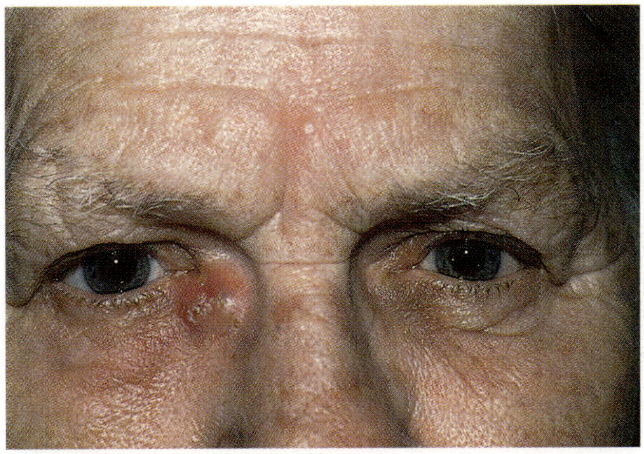

FIGURE 20–6. Focal erythematous swelling over the lacrimal sac representative of dacryocystitis in an adult. (© American Academy of Ophthalmology, San Francisco, CA.)

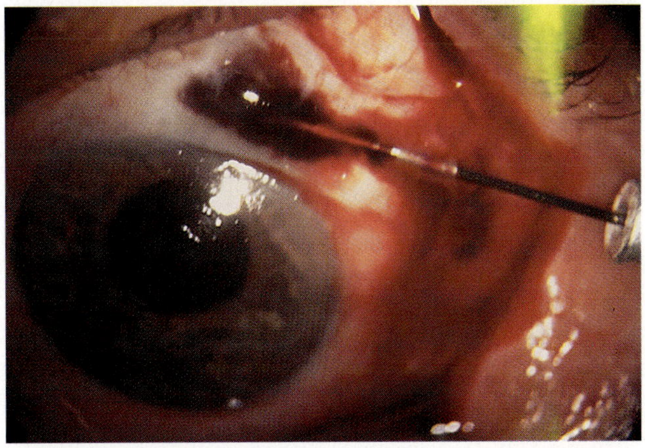

FIGURE 21–6. Injection of autologous blood into leaking bleb, and subsequent clotting.

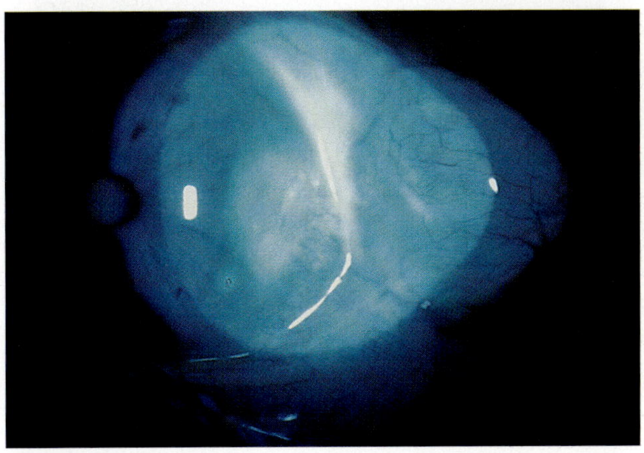

FIGURE 21–10. Dellen formed following the establishment of a filtering bleb.

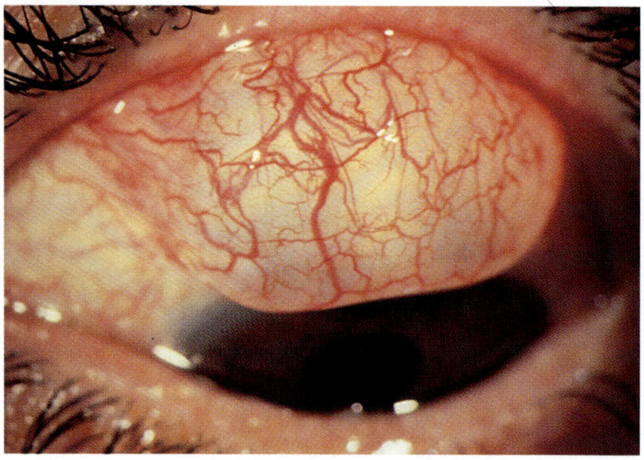

FIGURE 21–11. Tenon's cyst.

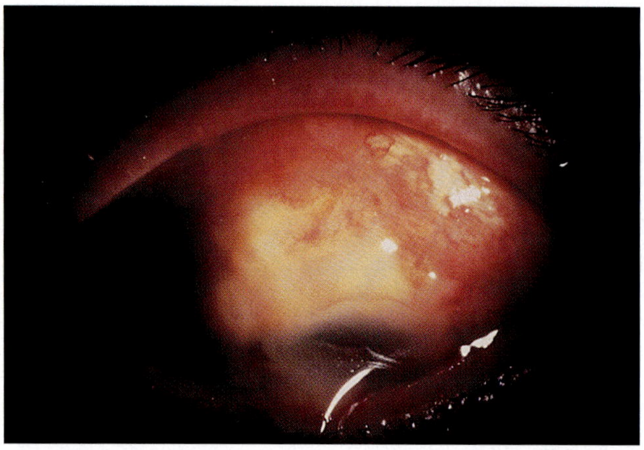

FIGURE 21–15. An infected filtering bleb.

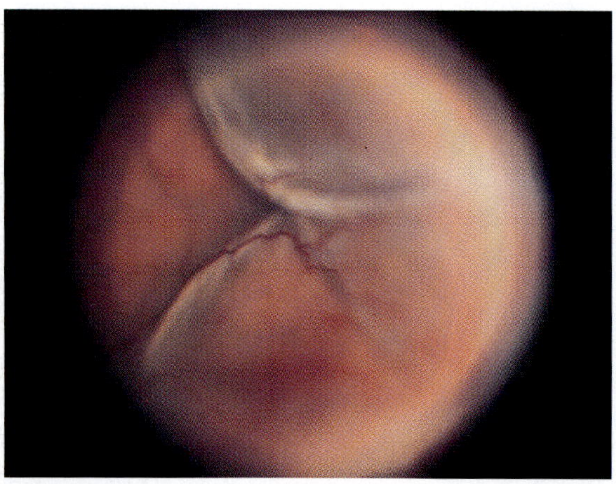

FIGURE 22–13. Choroidal detachment in a hypotonus patient.

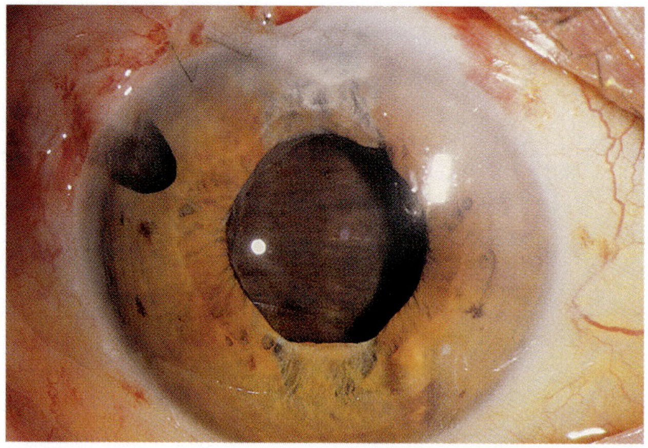

FIGURE 22–18. Hemorrhagic choroidal detachment viewed through the pupil.

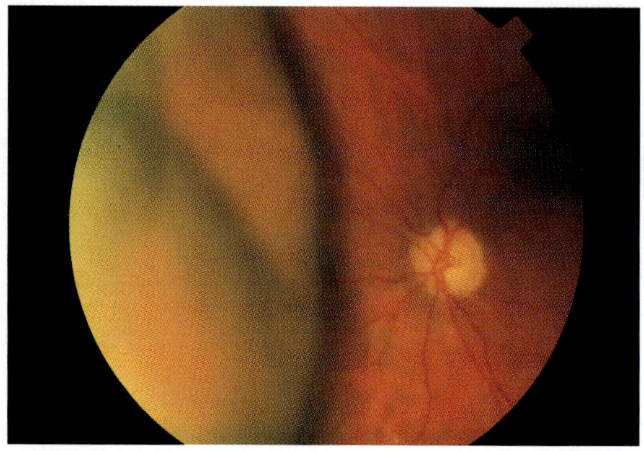

FIGURE 24–6. Postoperative choroidal effusion. (Courtesy of Lucian Del Priore, MD, PhD.)

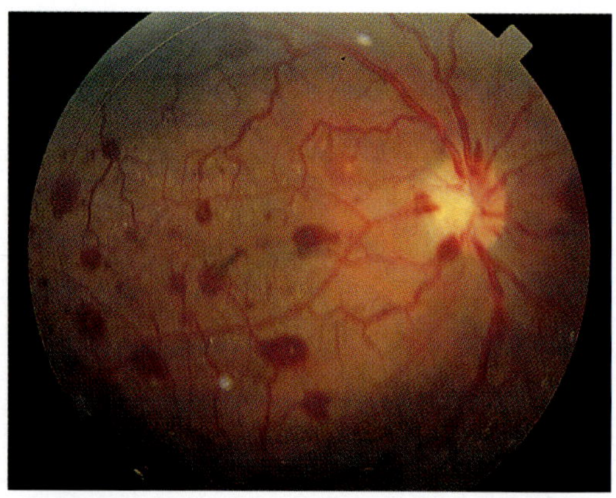

FIGURE 24–8. Multiple hemorrhages, some with white centers, are present in this eye with decompression retinopathy.

SECTION I

KEY CONCEPTS

CHAPTER 1

Preferred Practice Patterns and Economic Implications

PAUL P. LEE

This is where we begin. To what standard should you be held in caring for glaucoma patients? There are guidelines as to the accepted components of the care process. They are elucidated in the guidelines of the *Preferred Practice Patterns* (PPP) of the American Academy of Ophthalmology. In this chapter, Paul Lee explains the concept and process of the PPP and how it should be used in the everyday care of patients. He then puts this issue into perspective from an economic standpoint. This discussion sets the stage for developing and implementing your practice patterns by detailing guidelines for specific care parameters that affect the care of every patient with glaucoma. As a part of every patient interaction, you should ask yourself, "Have I done everything necessary, but not included unnecessary components in this patient's care?" Fulfilling this responsibility will facilitate optimal patient care, combining thoroughness with maximum efficiency.

The debate over whether practice guidelines should be adopted is over. The evidence in support of the benefits of the use of practice guidelines for patient care and quality of care have been demonstrated in repeated studies.[1–3] The legal system has increasingly begun to use authoritative practice guidelines as de facto legal standards of care.[4, 5] Even more significantly, as modern business principles and practices are applied to health care delivery in order to standardize care and reduce practice variation in efforts to restrain overall health care spending or to increase the value of care provided, the influence of practice guidelines will only grow over time. If patient care must meet a specific standard, it is incumbent upon physicians to make sure that the standard represents the highest feasible level.

In order to determine whether any given guideline is worthy of being used as a standard, readers can apply widely accepted and commonsense criteria to the guideline and its development. The goals of this chapter are to describe the American Academy of Ophthalmology (AAO) guideline for primary open-angle glaucoma (POAG)—the Preferred Practice Pattern (PPP),[6] and to give the reader insights into its validity, usefulness, and likely effects on health care delivery. The chapter is organized into four major sections: 1. A discussion of the attributes of a good guideline and whether the AAO PPP for POAG is one. 2. Description of the actual AAO POAG guideline and its usability in actual experience. 3. Projection of the likely effects of following the PPP on patients and on society, especially in relation to the costs of care. 4. The insights that the practicing ophthalmologist may want to consider.

Practice Guidelines and Their Development

The 2000 revision of the AAO POAG PPP was developed over 18 months by an expert panel convened by the AAO. Its members were glaucoma specialists, a patient representative, AAO staff, and a methodologist. The AAO staff, methodologist, and Panel Chair conducted a literature

No proprietary interests. The author was a member of the 1996 revision panel of the AAO guideline (see reference 6). The opinions expressed in this chapter are solely those of the author.

search from 1985 (because the original PPP covered earlier literature) in the English peer-reviewed literature and screened the resulting literature findings for review by the full panel. All relevant articles identified in the search were reviewed by the panel members. The panel made specific recommendations for care, identified the literature supporting each recommendation (if any), graded the quality of the evidence supporting each recommendation (using a three-grade system adapted from the Agency for Health Care Policy and Research's guidelines development efforts), and graded the importance of the recommendations to the care process.

The recommendations and their related attributes were then specifically identified within the body of the overall PPP document. The structure of the recommendations was intentionally chosen to follow the course of typical clinical care, starting with the history, moving to the physical examination and laboratory evaluation, and ending with the assessment and plan. Care was taken to make the recommendations as specific as possible, including definitions where needed, to make its use by clinicians as simple yet as uniform as possible. At the same time, important elements such as intervals between visits were stated in terms of ranges to allow maximum clinical flexibility within the confines of quality care. Finally, the AAO has made a commitment to review and update its PPP at least every five years.

This development process can be compared to the suggested attributes for guidelines development promulgated by the American Medical Association (AMA) and the Institute of Medicine (IOM).[7] The AMA criteria are: (1) involvement of physician organizations; (2) use of reliable methods to integrate relevant research and clinical experience; (3) being as specific and inclusive as possible; (4) reliance on up-to-date information; and (5) wide dissemination. The development of the AAO POAG PPP revision meets all five of these criteria and can thus be considered an appropriate, high-quality development from the AMA's perspective.

The IOM criteria[7, 8] are: (1) validity, (2) reliability, (3) clinical applicability, (4) clinical flexibility, (5) clarity, (6) multidisciplinary involvement, (7) documentation, and (8) ongoing review. Because the PPP panel identified critical attributes of strength of evidence, specific literature references, and importance to the care process after an exhaustive literature review, the PPP is as valid and reliable as the literature is able to support. However, because the literature fails to demonstrate that better health outcomes at specific cost levels would follow adoption of the specific interventions in question, the guideline is also deficient in some attributes of validity.

Tailoring the PPP to reflect clinical care flow, to be as specific as possible, and to retain flexibility in tailoring care to the needs and preferences of the individual patient enabled the revision also to meet the IOM criteria of clinical applicabililty, flexibility, and clarity. Where difficulty may arise is in identifying a patient as having glaucoma. Unlike past approaches that required a visual field defect, the PPP explicitly allows a patient with a normal visual field to be labeled as having glaucoma, if there are "characteristic" signs of optic neuropathy consistent with "glaucomatous" damage. Although the PPP does not define characteristic changes through illustrative findings, it does specify the nature of some of the "characteristic" changes, such as asymmetry or increased cupping. Perhaps in the next revision, the PPP will include standard photographs (as in the diabetic retinopathy studies) of defining changes as well as specific differences that would constitute "asymmetry" or "increased cupping."

Given the various attributes listed and the commitment to ongoing review and revision, the PPP also meets the IOM criteria of documentation and ongoing review. However, the process does *not* meet the criterion of multidisciplinary involvement. Overall, the PPP meets most of the IOM criteria for a high-quality practice guideline.

Given the strength of the development process for the 2000 revision, the POAG PPP will become even more of an initial de facto standard of care for patients with POAG.[5] Particularly because it is now much more specific, including numeric targets for treatment effect, it is much easier to use and thus more relevant than earlier versions of the PPP. Therefore, physicians and eye care providers who deviate from the PPP's recommended care process will face added pressures to justify their course of treatment of a patient. Although the PPP does specifically disclaim its applicability in all cases or even to any specific case and suggests that it does not take priority over the patient-physician relationship, the 2000 POAG PPP will increasingly be a starting point for discussion of the care provided.

Understanding the PPP and Its Use in Practice

The 1996 and 2000 POAG PPPs have several major structural changes from earlier versions. Perhaps the most significant is its change in the definition of *glaucoma* from one requiring visual field defects to one in which patients with early or mild cases, by definition, do not have any field defect but have only optic nerve changes consistent with "characteristic" changes of "glaucomatous optic neuropathy." Furthermore, no evidence of elevated intraocular pressure (IOP) of any kind is needed to define a case of glaucoma. With this change in definition, the number of patients in the United States with glaucoma has increased from somewhere around 2 million to well over 16 million.[9] In addition, it has rendered prior publications on the epidemiology of glaucoma—its incidence and prevalence—much more difficult to interpret. Readers now have to review such publications to look for data on optic nerve changes alone to add to those for classically defined glaucoma (IOP greater than 21 mm Hg, abnormal visual field, and optic nerve changes).

Additional changes in the PPP content were made to take advantage of the new emphasis on specificity and explicit identification of the attributes of each recommendation. Unlike the earlier versions, the 1996 and 2000 PPPs make available specific definitions of severity of glaucoma:

- Early or mild: no field defect
- Moderate: field defect in one hemisphere outside the central 10 degrees of field diameter
- Severe: field defect in both hemispheres or inside the central 10 degrees of field diameter.

The specific elements of the history and examination for

both new patients and those receiving follow-up care reflect the specificity of the older versions of the PPP, whereas the intervals for follow-up visits and follow-up optic nerve evaluations and visual field tests are explicitly stated by the 1996 and 2000 PPPs in ranges relative to specific clinical attributes present in a given patient. Thus, patients with less stable control or greater risk for progression are to be seen more often, and those with long-term stable control are to be seen less often.

Similarly, specificity is now provided for the concept of "target pressure lowering" as the explicit goal of therapy. A reduction of *at least* 20% is now the standard for determining whether the intraocular pressure has been lowered effectively, and explicit recommendations regarding adjusting the target pressure downwards (or even upwards) are provided.

Finally, and perhaps as important as any of the specific content recommendations, a patient-centered approach is built into the PPP. All care parameters require informed patient participation and the tailoring of care to the needs and preferences of the individual patient.

Table 1–1 lists the required elements of the history for new and follow-up patient evaluations. Table 1–2 lists the required elements of a physical examination for new patients (either at the initial visit or scheduled during a follow-up visit as part of the overall initial evaluation) and follow-up examination. Table 1–3 summarizes data from the only two published studies examining compliance with the AAO POAG PPP, using criteria derived from the past PPP; however, all of the elements examined in these studies were carried over into the 1996 and 2000 revisions. Thus, these figures provide estimates of compliance with these critical elements of the physical examination within the purview of the revised PPP.

Tables 1–4, 1–5, and 1–6, reprinted from the AAO PPP, provide follow-up intervals for evaluation of disease status, visual fields, and optic nerve, respectively. Because the new PPP uses a case definition of glaucoma distinct from that used by the older version, the published data from the two studies in Table 1–3 regarding compliance are not directly comparable. However, it is instructive to note that in perhaps the most critical element—the timing of follow-up evaluations based on the stability of the glaucoma control (defined similarly in the studies and in the PPP)—many patients seen in community settings with unstable or uncontrolled glaucoma were *not* seen for a follow-up visit within 4 weeks. Thus, there is a need for additional investigations in this regard.

TABLE 1–1. ELEMENTS OF HISTORY REQUIRED AT NEW AND FOLLOW-UP VISITS FOR PATIENTS WITH GLAUCOMA

Element	New Visit	Follow-up Visit
Family history	x	
Systemic history	x	x
Ocular history, including surgery	x	x
Pertinent records, when available	x	
Known intolerance for glaucoma medications	x	x
Frequency and time of last use of glaucoma medications	x	x
Severity and outcome of glaucoma in family members	x	
Impact of glaucoma on daily living and activities	x	x

TABLE 1–2. ELEMENTS OF PHYSICAL EXAMINATION REQUIRED AT NEW AND FOLLOW-UP VISITS FOR PATIENTS WITH GLAUCOMA

Element	New Visit	Follow-up Visit
Visual acuity evaluation	x	x
Pupil examination	x	
Intraocular pressure	x	x
Slit-lamp examination	x	x
Gonioscopy	x	at least every 5 years *or* for suspicion of angle closure *or* for change in miotics
Dilated, stereo evaluation of optic disc and nerve fiber layer	x	see Table 1–6
Documentation of optic nerve	x	
Evaluation of fundus	x	
Evaluation of visual field	x	see Table 1–5

TABLE 1–3. EXPERIENCE WITH PREFERRED PRACTICE PATTERNS IN ACTUAL USE

	Academic Data (%)	Community Data (%)
Severity of glaucoma in sample		
Stable moderate	8	24
Stable severe	70	57
Newly established control	8	3
Unstable	15	17
Documentation in initial examination		
Pupil	70	39
Intraocular pressure	100	100
Visual fields (inc scheduled)	92	90
Gonioscopy (inc next visit)	85	51
Disc/nerve fiber layer	98	98
Documentation of current status		
Status noted	88	44
Most recent drawing/photo of optic nerve:		
Within 6 mos of last visit	78	12
6–9 mos	12	5
9–15 mos	10	6
Not after first visit		38
Follow-up schedule		
Stable, moderate damage within 6 mos	100	100
Stable, severe damage		
Within 3 mos	100	68
Within 6 mos		98
Newly established control		
Within 3 mos	100	
Within 4 mos		83
Unstable within 4 weeks	100	63

Data from Hertzog LH, Albrecht KG, LaBree L, Lee PP: Glaucoma care and conformance with preferred practice patterns. Examination of the private, community-based ophthalmologist. Ophthalmology 1996;103:1009–1013; Albrecht KG, Lee PP: Conformance with preferred practice patterns in caring for patients with glaucoma. Ophthalmology 1994;101:1668–1671.

TABLE 1–4. RECOMMENDED GUIDELINES FOR FOLLOW-UP

Target IOP Achieved	Progression of Damage	Duration of Control (months)	Follow-up Interval
yes	no	<6	1–6 months
yes	no	>6	3–12 months
yes	yes	(n/a)	1 week–3 months
no	no	(n/a)	1 day–3 months
no	yes	(n/a)	1 day–1 month

IOP, intraocular pressure.
From American Academy of Ophthalmology: Preferred Practice Pattern: Primary Open-Angle Glaucoma. San Francisco, American Academy of Ophthalmology, 1996.

TABLE 1–6. RECOMMENDED FREQUENCY OF OPTIC NERVE EVALUATION

Target IOP Achieved	Progression of Damage	Duration of Control (months)	Follow-up Interval (months)
yes	no	<6	6–12
yes	no	>6	6–18
yes	yes	(n/a)	3–12
no	no	(n/a)	3–12
no	yes	(n/a)	3–12

IOP, intraocular pressure.
From American Academy of Ophthalmology: Preferred Practice Pattern: Primary Open-Angle Glaucoma. San Francisco, American Academy of Ophthalmology, 1996.

Economic Costs of Glaucoma Care and The Likely Impact of Practice Guidelines

Glaucoma is a costly and growing condition requiring treatment in the United States. Studies have estimated that glaucoma care costs in 1988 were $2.534 billion, representing $358 million in medication costs, $903 million in provider care, $516 million for surgical care, $164 million for supportive care, and at least $600 million in indirect costs. If simple projections are made forward in time, the aging of the American population and the escalating cost of medical care will combine to further accelerate the costs of glaucoma care in the American population (Table 1–7).[10] The restraint in growth of health care expenditures under managed care has little effect, because the component costs of glaucoma care are among the least susceptible to cost restraint. For example, although physician fees may be reduced by as much as 50% for the care of any one glaucoma patient, this change would reduce overall direct care costs by only 20%. Pharmaceutical costs may also be restrained to some degree, but this change would account for 14% of costs. The indirect costs of blindness and lost productivity cannot be controlled through managed care or other efforts at cost reduction. Indeed, to the extent that care is effective and is not being provided, these costs will increase as care is curtailed in the future.

Such cost estimates do not even take into account two significant potential occurrences that would greatly magnify the costs of glaucoma care. First, half of the people with traditionally defined glaucoma do not know that they have it and are thus not receiving treatment.[11, 12] In other words, the public health care need for glaucoma exceeds the current demand; if we as a society were to meet the public health care needs of our population with glaucoma, nearly twice the amount of care might be needed. If all patients with visual field loss were receiving treatment, the direct costs of care would almost double (but not quite, because presumably the problems of these patients are not as severe or they would have already sought care, and thus they may not need as intense a level of care).

Second, and potentially staggering in its implications, the change in definition of glaucoma means that *6 times* the current number of patients could be classified as having glaucoma. Although many such patients would not necessarily need medication or other forms of treatment, all would require some form of regular follow-up care (probably at least on an annual basis). Because such patients do not have visual field defects, they would not be as seriously affected as patients traditionally defined as having glaucoma.

One can begin to estimate the cost implications by drawing upon information from several other studies into a new, coherent picture. From the survey results of the RAND Eye Care Workforce Study,[12] we know that the average patient with POAG is seen for follow-up visits four times per year. If we assume that these new patients require less follow-up care than the average patient, we can project that they need follow-up care about half as often (which translates into two visits per year), but without requiring surgery or supportive care. The net result is that the professional fee component (excluding surgery) of their care would constitute 50% per year compared with the typical patient with glaucoma. If the typical patient with glaucoma consumes $903 per year in care, 50% of which currently goes for surgical provider fees, each of the new patients would require $451 per year in care ($451 million for medical care divided by 1 million patients). Multiplying this amount by 6 (the increase in number of patients with glaucoma) yields an increase in annual care costs of $1.35 billion in provider medical fees alone, exclusive of medication costs. This is more than half the amount we currently spend on glaucoma in total! If, on the other hand, only half of the new patients were to use such care, the increase in cost

TABLE 1–5. RECOMMENDED FREQUENCY OF VISUAL FIELD EVALUATION

Target IOP Achieved	Progression of Damage	Duration of Control (months)	Follow-up Interval (months)
yes	no	<6	6–12
yes	no	>6	6–24
yes	yes	(n/a)	2–6
no	no	(n/a)	2–6
no	yes	(n/a)	1–6

IOP, intraocular pressure.
From American Academy of Ophthalmology: Preferred Practice Pattern: Primary Open-Angle Glaucoma. San Francisco, American Academy of Ophthalmology, 1996.

TABLE 1–7. FUTURE COST PROJECTION IMPLICATIONS (IN MILLIONS OF DOLLARS)

Year	*Medication*	*Provider*	*Surgery*	*Supportive*	*Indirect*
1988	$351	$903	$516	$164	$600+
Future	1	1	1	1	1
	2	2	2		2
	3	3			
	4	4	4	4	
		5			

ELEMENTS OF FUTURE CHANGES

1. Aging of U.S. population—more patients at age with higher glaucoma.
2. Caring for all patients with glaucoma: +94%
3. Increase due to change in definition: +350%
4. Medical cost inflation
   a. 1988 to 1997: +54%
   b. 1997 onward: +3% per year
5. Decreases in provider payment:
   a. Medicare fee for service: 26% decrease
   b. Capitation contracts: 80% decrease

Data from Lee PP: Economic concerns in glaucoma management in the 21st century. J Glaucoma 1993;2:148–151; Guzman G, Javitt J, Glick H, et al: Glaucoma in the United States population: the economic burden of illness. Invest. Ophthalmol Vis Sci 1992;23 (Suppl 4):759.

would be cut in half. In either case, the new definition of POAG in the PPP has strong financial implications.

This situation is likely to be exacerbated if the care patterns proposed in the PPP were to be widely adopted. From the data obtained in Southern California regarding the severity of glaucoma seen in the study sites, the preponderance of patients seen in the community setting (which accounts for more than 95% of all patients with glaucoma) are not receiving care as often as recommended in the PPP. Whether this pattern exists or will continue to exist in the future requires further study, but it is instructive to note that the influence of managed care may be to reduce care utilization.[13] Therefore the likely influence of compliance with the PPP is to further increase service utilization and thus the costs under most systems of care.

One important caveat is the extent to which prepaid care will result in the capitation of eye care services. If physicians agree to provide all of the necessary and appropriate glaucoma care that a given population might need for a preset price, the cost is effectively capped. In such situations, the costs of glaucoma care—to the health plan and to society—would not rise as projected. Clearly, however, this would change the nature of care reimbursement for the providers holding such contracts.

Implications of the PPP

The effect of the 2000 revision of the POAG PPP is to raise the standard of care for patients. Whether this will result in better outcomes of care, expressed as better preservation of quality of life and visual functioning, is still unclear. Long-term prospective study will be needed to identify which process steps of care will result in improvement of functional and other outcomes. One should therefore be careful about thinking that following the PPP will automatically result in better care outcomes. However, to the extent that expert opinion provides a rationale for medical care, as it does in more that half of all care given today, according to the IOM, following the PPP should result in enhanced outcomes in the future. If nothing else, the specificity of follow-up and treatment goals will enhance the likelihood that deterioration will be caught earlier in many circumstances and thus be treated more aggressively at an earlier stage. Of course, whether treatment is effective in reducing or halting the rate of progression of optic nerve damage is still an open question.

If one assumes that treatment is effective, the new PPP does indeed provide more specific guidance to the ophthalmologist. At the same time, the greater specificity increases the responsibility of the practicing ophthalmologist, because it places specific actions within the purview of the health care provider. Greater specificity means that others can more easily identify what the specific care parameters for a given patient might be expected to include and thus makes it easier to assess whether an ophthalmologist has conformed to the recommended practice pattern. Thus, the new PPP will certainly heighten the applicability of the PPP itself in medicolegal actions.

Second, the new PPP also raises the responsiblity of ophthalmologists practicing in a managed care setting. Regardless of what the managed care organization believes is a reasonable interval for follow-up care or diagnostic tests, the PPP lays out what the AAO Panel considers to be reasonable intervals. Deviation from the recommendations will need to be justified or at least a sound rationale provided. To the extent that actual practice does not fulfill the recommendations of the PPP, the ophthalmologist in question faces the same medicolegal issues noted earlier. With a probable increase in service utilization to meet the care patterns for already existing patients with glaucoma, not to mention the potential six-fold increase due to the new definition, capitation rates may need to be reconsidered.

The net effect of the PPP revision is to increase the pressures on the ophthalmologist. Because, most likely, while reimbursements may be falling their services will be utilized more. Ophthalmologists may increasingly find themselves to be between the proverbial rock and a hard place. To survive, physicians will need to remember the first two dictums of medicine: First, do no harm; second, be the patient's advocate. To do any differently will be to increasingly court disaster.

REFERENCES

1. Mittman BS, Siu AL: Changing provider behavior: Applying research on outcomes and effectiveness in health care. In Shortell SM, Reinhardt U (eds): Improving Health Policy and Management: Nine Critical Research Issues for the 1990's. Ann Arbor, MI, Health Administration Press, 1992.
2. Audet AM, Geenfield S, Field M: Medical practice guidelines: Current activities and future directions. Ann Intern Med 1990;113:709–714.
3. Brook RH: Practice guidelines and practicing medicine: Are they compatible? JAMA 1989;262:3027–3030.
4. Brennan TA: Practice guidelines and malpractice litigation: Collision or cohesion? J Health Polit Policy Law 1991;16:67–85.
5. Lee PP: The effects of preferred practice patterns on physician malpractice concerns in glaucoma. J Glaucoma 1992;1:286–289.
6. American Academy of Ophthalmology: Preferred Practice Pattern: Primary Open-Angle Glaucoma. San Francisco, American Academy of Ophthalmology, 1996.
7. Lee PP: Guidelines: Cataract surgery and beyond (editorial). Arch Ophthalmol 1993;111:597–598.
8. Lohr K: Guidelines for Clinical Practice: From Development to Use. Washington, DC, Institute of Medicine, 1992.
9. Quigley HA: Open-angle glaucoma. N Engl J Med 1993;328:1097–1106.
10. Lee PP: Economic concerns in glaucoma management in the 21st century. J Glaucoma 1993;2:148–151.
11. Guzman G, Javitt J, Glick H, et al: Glaucoma in the United States population: the economic burden of illness. Invest Ophthalmol Vis Sci 1992;33 (Suppl 4):759.
12. Lee P, Jackson C, Relles D: Eye Care Workforce. Santa Monica, CA, RAND, AAO-516, 1995.
13. Goldzweig CL, Mittman BS, Carter GM, et al: Variations in cataract extraction rates in prepaid and fee-for-service settings. JAMA 1997;277:1765–1768.

CHAPTER 2

Trabecular Meshwork and Argon Laser Trabeculoplasty

ANDREW J. MICHAEL

In any discussion concerning the group of diseases called glaucoma, the trabecular meshwork plays a central role. This is the primary method of aqueous egress in humans; in nearly all forms of glaucoma, the impact of its function must be considered. In this chapter, Andrew Michael first provides us with the basic anatomy and physiology of this structure. Additionally, he explains the clinically relevant implications of those glaucoma treatments that are directed at improving the facility of outflow of aqueous through the trabecular meshwork. These modalities include medications and surgery, specifically argon laser trabeculoplasty. The details of indications, technique, complications, and mechanism of action of laser trabeculoplasty are covered. Finally, some examples of specific glaucomas and their direct impact on outflow are described. Overall, this chapter provides the necessary information to allow a better understanding of the key role the trabecular meshwork plays in glaucoma diagnosis and therapy.

Anatomy and Physiology

In the human eye, aqueous humor is produced by the nonpigmented epithelium of the ciliary body. The aqueous enters the posterior chamber, percolates around the crystalline lens, and passes through the pupillary aperture into the anterior chamber. Aqueous exits the eye predominantly by two routes: direct (conventional) outflow through the trabecular meshwork into Schlemm's canal and indirect (unconventional or uveoscleral) outflow through the ciliary body. In the normal human eye, a small proportion of aqueous may egress via transport into iris vessels and stroma or by transcorneal evaporation.

Conventional trabecular outflow is an intraocular pressure (IOP)–dependent phenomenon. Uveoscleral outflow is independent of IOP. In the normal human eye, uveoscleral flow accounts for approximately 20% of the total aqueous outflow (Fig. 2–1).[1] The existence of two aqueous outflow pathways can have significant clinical implications. For example, in angle-closure glaucomas, as conventional trabecular flow is compromised, the role uveoscleral outflow plays in controlling IOP can become dominant. Under these circumstances, the effects that some pharmacologic agents have on uveoscleral outflow are magnified. Pilocarpine, which reduces uveoscleral flow, can induce a paradoxical pressure elevation,[2] whereas agents such as atropine, which increase uveoscleral outflow, can have a profound IOP-reducing effect.

Anatomically, the trabecular meshwork is traditionally subdivided into three regions:

- Uveal meshwork
- Corneoscleral meshwork
- Juxtacanalicular tissue

The *uveal meshwork* is the inner lining of the trabecular meshwork. It extends from the cornea anteriorly to the ciliary body and the iris root posteriorly. The uveal meshwork is an irregularly arranged network.

The *corneoscleral meshwork* extends from the cornea

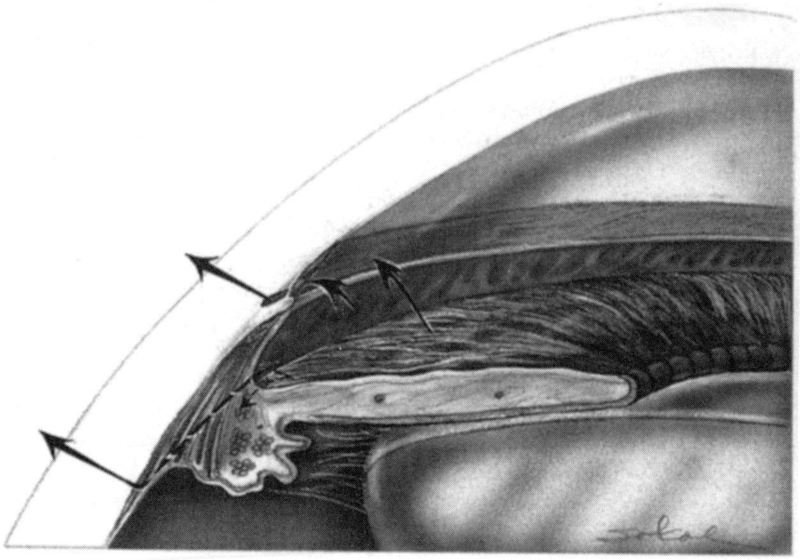

FIGURE 2–1. Key pathways of aqueous outflow in the human eye include conventional direct trabecular outflow and nonconventional uveoscleral outflow. In addition, a smaller pathway exists through iris vessels and stroma. (From Stamper RL, Lieberman MF, Drake MV: Becker-Schaffer's Diagnosis and Therapy of the Glaucomas, 7th ed. St. Louis, Mosby, 1999.)

anteriorly to the scleral spur posteriorly. The corneoscleral meshwork constitutes the bulk of the trabecular meshwork tissue. It is arranged along a much more uniform, lattice-like arrangement than the uveoscleral portion of the meshwork. Both the uveal and corneoscleral regions comprise a network of pores through a meshwork of trabecular beams. The pores measure 10 to 20 μm at the anterior chamber face of the uveal meshwork and become progressively smaller toward the external aspect of the corneoscleral meshwork near Schlemm's canal.

Just adjacent to the canal, the pores are completely replaced by the histologically distinct *juxtacanalicular tissue*, also called the *cribriform layer*. This region is composed mainly of extracellular matrix and fibroblast-like cells. The juxtacanalicular tissue does not posses the obvious open acellular spaces for bulk fluid flow present in the uveal and corneoscleral regions of the meshwork.

Functionally, the trabecular meshwork is subdivided into two regions: anterior and posterior. The *anterior* trabecular meshwork is just posterior to Schwalbe's line. Its external aspect does not contact Schlemm's canal, and thus, the anterior trabecular region has been termed the *nonfiltering* trabecular meshwork. A careful distinction should be made between "nonfiltering"—a functionally accurate term that describes the anterior trabecular meshwork—and "nonfunctional." Although the cells in this region do not appear to function in a filtration capacity, they have been hypothesized to serve regenerative and reparative functions. The *posterior* trabecular meshwork, or *filtering* portion of the trabecular meshwork, lies internal to Schlemm's canal.

Each of the trabecular beams that crisscross the uveal and corneoscleral regions of the meshwork is composed of a central core of connective tissue around which is wrapped a basal lamina that supports a monolayer of endothelium. With age, the macromolecular composition of the beams changes.[3] The extracellular matrix of the juxtacanalicular meshwork also changes with age.[4] In both regions, there appears to be an age-related increase in long-spacing collagen.[5] Hyaluronic acid decreases with age and in glaucomatous eyes.[6]

THE EXTRACELLULAR MATRIX

The extracellular matrix (ECM) of a biologic tissue is the structural and functional support of that tissue. It is the ECM that allows a group or network of cells to function as a tissue. The ECM of a given tissue may change with development, aging, disease, and other biologic stresses. Defects in a tissue's ability to regulate, remodel, degrade, and synthesize components of the ECM are often related to pathologic changes in that tissue.[7]

The most abundant macromolecules that constitute the ECM are collagens, elastins, and proteoglycans. The proteoglycans and their associated glycosaminoglycans are the most dynamic of these large molecules. They are subject to relatively rapid biologic turnover and are also known to polymerize and depolymerize rapidly. Because of the dynamic nature of proteoglycans, small alterations in synthesis or degradation can lead to changes in the functioning of the tissue in which they reside.[8] Fibronectin and laminin are the most prevalent and best-described members of a family of macromolecules known as *attachment factors*. These molecules play a role in regulation of cellular differentiation and growth. They also assist in regulation of cell migration and participate in the response to tissue injury.[9]

The cells and ECM of the trabecular meshwork function together as a one-way, sponge-like filter. In a pressure-dependent fashion, fluid in the anterior chamber passes through the trabecular meshwork and the associated juxtacanalicular tissue and then into Schlemm's canal. A hydrostatic pressure gradient exists between the anterior chamber and Schlemm's canal. Thus, there is resistance to flow of fluids through this pathway. Experimental studies demonstrate that as much as 90% of the hydrostatic resistance to flow through the trabecular meshwork resides in the juxtacanalicular tissue.[10]

A number of structural changes can be observed in trabecular meshwork in primary open-angle glaucoma. Characteristically, deposits of extracellular material are found in the juxtacanalicular tissue. This material, believed to be derived from the sheath of the elastic-like portion of the wall of Schlemm's canal, has been termed *sheath-derived plaque material* (SD-plaque).[11, 12] In normal eyes, there is a strong correlation between age and the amount of SD-plaque found in juxtacanalicular tissue. In eyes with primary open-angle glaucoma, the amount of SD-plaque is significantly greater than normal.[5] Moreover, in primary open-angle glaucoma, no age-related correlation has been found. The clinical implication of these findings is that primary open-angle glaucoma cannot be regarded as simply an age-related disorder.

CELLS OF THE TRABECULAR MESHWORK

The trabecular meshwork normally contains three main cell types (Fig. 2–2):

- □ Trabecular cell
- □ Cribriform cell
- □ Endothelial lining of Schlemm's canal

The *trabecular* endothelial cells that reside on the trabecular beams are highly phagocytic. They are capable of removing particulates, cellular debris, pigment granules, red blood cells, and bacteria from the aqueous.[13] Removed material is incorporated into intracellular phagolysosomes. It is postulated that, ultimately, the debris is removed from the trabecular meshwork entirely by either (1) migration of trabecular cells through the endothelium of Schlemm's canal and into systemic circulation or (2) re-incorporation of the debris into wandering macrophages or other cell types.[14] Experimental studies in which homologous pigment is injected into the anterior chamber of monkeys supports this hypothesis. Within days of the pigment infusion, particles were found within trabecular endothelial cells. After 6 weeks, a decrease in trabecular pigmentation was noted, although the cellularity of the trabecular meshwork was unchanged.[15]

The *cribriform* cell, found in the juxtacanalicular region of the meshwork, differs from the endothelial cells that line the trabecular beams elsewhere in the trabecular meshwork. Cribriform cells are more fibroblast-like. Unlike the trabecular cells that rest on a basal lamina, the cribriform cells appear to be dispersed throughout the ECM of the juxtacanalicular region. These cells may be responsible for the production and maintenance of the juxtacanalicular ECM.

The *endothelial lining* of Schlemm's canal is the third major type of cell found in trabecular meshwork. These cells produce their own basement membrane material but do not appear to produce the ECM of the juxtacanalicular region. This endothelium assists in transport of fluid and particulate material into the lumen of Schlemm's canal through formation of transport vacuoles and transcellular channels.[16, 17]

Therapy to Improve Outflow Facility

PHARMACOLOGIC AGENTS

Cholinergic Agents

Cholinergic drugs have been used in the treatment of glaucoma since the 19th century. The ocular cholinergic agents can be divided into two major groups, direct-acting and indirect-acting. *Direct-acting* drugs (e.g., acetylcholine, pilocarpine, carbachol) stimulate the postsynaptic muscle at neuromuscular junctions within the parasympathetic nervous system.

Indirect-acting drugs (e.g., physostigmine, echothiophate

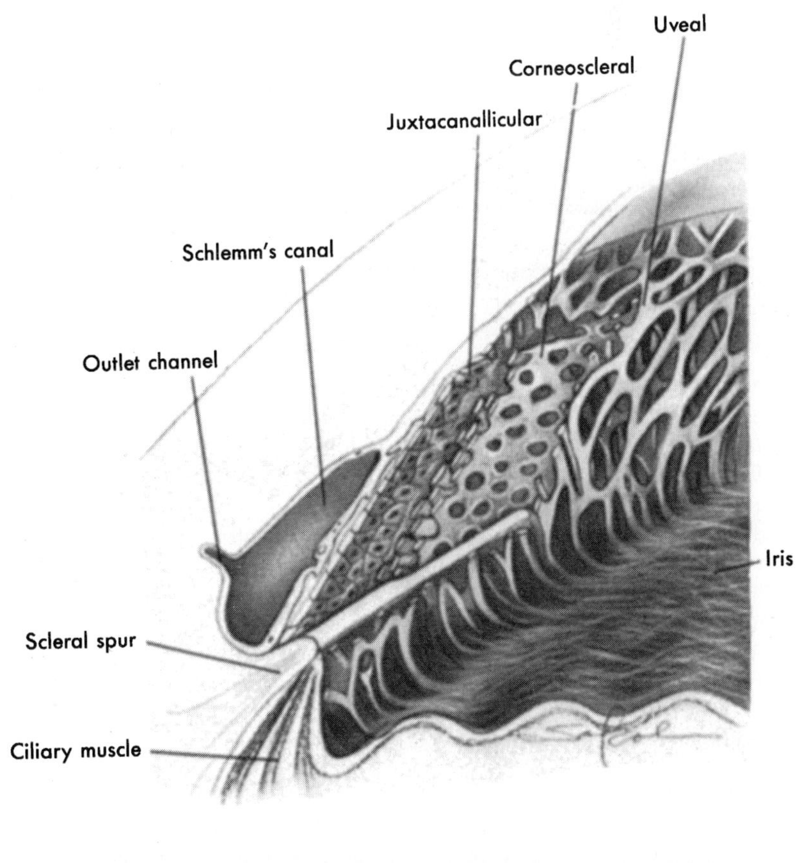

FIGURE 2–2. Cutaway diagram of layers of trabecular meshwork in aqueous outflow system. (From Hart WM Jr: Adler's Physiology of the Eye, 9th ed. St. Louis, Mosby–Year Book, 1992; modified from Shields MB: Textbook of Glaucoma. Baltimore, Williams & Wilkins, 1987.)

iodide, demecarium bromide, isoflurophate) bind acetylcholinesterase enzymes. The inhibition of these enzymes produces an increase in acetylcholine at neuromuscular junctions within the parasympathetic nervous system, thereby augmenting stimulation of the postsynaptic muscle. The indirect-acting agents can be subdivided into (1) those that reversibly bind acetylcholinesterase, such as physostigmine, and (2) those that are relatively irreversible acetylcholinesterase binders, such as echothiophate iodide and isoflurophate.

The precise site of action of the cholinergic agents varies. However, the mechanisms of action of all the members of this class appear similar. Stimulation of the parasympathetic motor junctions within the eye, by either direct or indirect means, results in constriction of the pupillary sphincter and contraction of the ciliary muscle. Because the ciliary muscle inserts anteriorly at the scleral spur, contraction of this muscle results in application of posterior tension on the scleral spur. As the scleral spur is pulled posteriorly, the trabecular meshwork is put on traction, and pores between trabecular beams are held open. With the trabecular meshwork held on traction, aqueous outflow is facilitated.

Given this mechanism of action, it is clear that the IOP-lowering effect of ocular cholinergic agents depends on ciliary muscle traction at the scleral spur. In the clinical settings of cyclodialysis, relative papillary block, angle recession, and other traumatic angle deformities, the effectiveness of cholinergic agents is reduced. Therefore, in some cases cholinergic agents can produce a paradoxical rise in IOP. These agents should be used with caution in a patient in whom anatomic deformities of the anterior chamber angle are present or suspected.

Epinephrine

Epinephrine and its pro-drug dipivefrin are nonselective α- and β-adrenergic agonists used in the treatment of glaucoma. As might be expected from agents that interact with multiple receptor classes, their mechanism of action is complex. However, studies indicate that epinephrine increases aqueous outflow facility by stimulating trabecular meshwork β-adrenergic receptors. Pretreatment with nonselective β-adrenergic agonists such as timolol blocks epinephrine's ability to increase trabecular outflow facility.

Glucocorticoids

In susceptible people, administration of glucocorticoids raises IOP. Both patients with primary open-angle glaucoma[18, 19] and their first-degree relatives[18–20] have a greater likelihood of demonstrating elevated IOP in response to corticosteroid administration.

Elevated IOP may result from administration of corticosteroids by any route, although topical administration accounts for the majority of cases. Corticosteroid-containing dermatologic preparations, periocular injections, nasal sprays, pulmonary and bronchial inhalers, and oral medications have all been reported to be responsible for increased IOP.[21–24] Hypersecretion of endogenous corticosteroids, as in Cushing's disease and adrenal hyperplasia, is also associated with elevation of IOP.[25]

The mechanism by which corticosteroids raise IOP is related to the regulatory function they have in ECM biosynthesis and turnover. For example, dexamethasone decreases collagen synthesis and increases elaboration of fibronectin. Importantly, corticosteroids alter and increase the glycosaminoglycan content of the meshwork. Because of their ability to bind water, glycosaminoglycans are believed to be important regulators of tissue hydration. Thus, glycosaminoglycans, especially those in the juxtacanalicular tissue, may be important in regulating the flow of aqueous humor through the trabecular meshwork. Morphologically, specimens from patients with steroid-induced glaucoma show amorphous and fibrillar material deposited in the juxtacanalicular tissue and in the intertrabecular spaces.[26]

ARGON LASER TRABECULOPLASTY

In the treatment of open-angle glaucomas, the role of laser trabeculoplasty has evolved since its first description by Wise and Witter[27] in 1979. Prior to that time, attempts at laser trabeculopuncture to facilitate outflow had been unsuccessful.[28] In fact, laser application to the trabecular meshwork was shown to result in elevated IOP in animals and it is used as a model for inducing glaucoma in primates.[29] Within a few years, the use of argon laser trabeculoplasty (ALT) had become widely accepted as a means to treat open-angle glaucomas.[30–32]

Indications

The use of ALT is restricted to patients with gonioscopically open angles. Under most circumstances, the diagnoses that respond best to ALT are (1) primary open-angle glaucoma, (2) glaucoma associated with the pseudoexfoliation syndrome, and (3) glaucoma associated with pigment dispersion syndrome.[33–36] This success may be related to the amount of trabecular meshwork pigmentation that is required for absorption of the laser energy.

With the exception of patients with pigmentary glaucoma, older patients show a better response to ALT than younger patients.[36] In fact, use of ALT in patients less than 40 years old (except those with pigmentary glaucoma) is usually avoided, because the procedure may increase the risk of a permanent rise in IOP.[37] In general, ALT is not effective in most other secondary forms of glaucoma, such as neovascular or uveitic glaucoma or in congenital and developmental glaucomas.[34, 35]

Initially, the timing of ALT was after maximum tolerated medical therapy and prior to filtration surgery. However, with greater experience, the procedure has been moved to an earlier place in the treatment algorithm. ALT has begun to be used even earlier, even as initial therapy.

The Glaucoma Laser Trial compared the initial use of ALT with medical therapy. At the 2-year follow-up, ALT-treated eyes had a slightly lower IOP; however, 56% of these eyes required medication during this period.[38] In the majority of the patients observed for a longer time (mean, 7 years) the ALT-treated eyes did show a slightly more than 1 mm Hg greater IOP reduction, less than 1 dB better visual field preservation, and less optic nerve change.[39] These results imply that ALT is at least as effective as, if not slightly more effective than, medications as the initial treatment for chronic open-angle glaucomas.

In spite of this study, however, most physicians do not use ALT as initial treatment for the majority of their patients. Generally, medications are tried first. If additional therapy is indicated after a reasonable attempt has been made to identify a medication that is effective and tolerated, ALT is a reasonable option at any stage of medical therapy. Currently, the use of ALT has been moved to an earlier place in the treatment regimen in appropriate patients, even being performed as initial therapy, particularly when compliance, potential medication side effects, or limited duration of effect needed make it an especially attractive alternative to medications.

The duration and magnitude of effect of ALT must be taken into account in determining whether it is a reasonable alternative for an individual patient. In general, a 2- to 5-year duration of an approximately 25% reduction of IOP is expected for a good candidate for the procedure. If these are acceptable results, ALT should be strongly considered.

Technique

ALT is a surgical procedure. Therefore, a complete discussion of risks and benefits with the patient is necessary prior to obtaining his or her consent for ALT. The laser surgery is performed with the use of topical anesthesia. After the patient (and the surgeon) are comfortably positioned at the laser, the laser lens is inserted into the interpalpebral fissure using a viscous coupling agent. Bubbles in the viscous solution should be avoided, because they can interfere with visualization and laser application. It is often useful to instruct the patient to look upward while the lower lid is gently retracted and the lens is applied to the ocular surface. This maneuver facilitates lens positioning by promoting elevation of the upper lid, widening the interpalpebral fissure, and improving access for insertion. The lenses most commonly employed are the Goldmann three-mirror lens (using the smallest parabolic mirror) and the Ritch four-mirror lens. The Goldmann lens must be rotated through the arc of treatment, whereas the Ritch lens may be left stationary because the four lenses allow visualization of the entire angle. Proper positioning of the lens affords a stable clear view of the angle.

In general it is best to begin treatment at the superior mirror, treating the inferior angle. This provides the most open angle with the greatest amount of pigmentation, facilitating proper identification of landmarks and ensuring proper treatment location.

Suggested treatment parameters are listed in Table 2–1. These parameters are guidelines only. The green wavelength is preferred, as there has been some concern that energy from the blue portion of the blue-green wavelength may damage the surgeon's macula. Other lasers, including Nd:YAG, krypton red or yellow, and diode, have been used for trabeculoplasty.[40–42] However, these have not proved superior to the argon laser.

The laser power should be individualized according to the biologic response to laser application. The proper laser power results in either mild blanching of the trabecular meshwork or the formation of a small bubble. If there is inadequate response, such as no observable tissue effect, the power should be increased. If there is too great a reaction, such as large bubble formation, the laser power can be reduced. It is often necessary to adjust the power during the procedure to optimize effects in different portions of the angle, depending on the focus and the amount of pigmentation.

TABLE 2–1. TREATMENT PARAMETERS FOR ARGON LASER TRABECULOPLASTY

Laser	Argon Green (515 nm)
Lens	Goldmann 1- or 3- mirror, Ritch trabeculoplasty
Duration	0.1 seconds
Spot size	50 μ
Number of applications	360°: 70–100 180°: 40–50
Power	0.5–0.8 W
Location	Junction of the anterior nonpigmented and posterior pigmented trabecular meshwork

It is vital to obtain precise focus of the laser. A slight amount of defocus appreciably changes the applied power of the laser. Directing the laser as perpendicularly as possible into the meshwork can assist in optimizing the focus of the laser beam. This is best accomplished by viewing the filtering angle along the plane of the iris, rather than from a vantage point at a wide angle to the plane of the iris. To achieve this view, the patient can be directed to look slightly away from the treating mirror. As the patient looks away from the treating mirror, the view of the angle may narrow, so it is important to maximize focus while still applying the laser to the proper location.

Treatment location can also be individualized. Efficacy appears equal with treatment anywhere on the meshwork. More posterior treatment increases the formation of peripheral anterior synechiae and may be more uncomfortable for the patient.[43] Anterior treatment can result in injury to the corneal endothelium and migration of the corneal endothelium over the trabecular meshwork.[44] In general, treatment should be done where there is sufficient pigmentation to allow adequate laser absorption at the lowest possible energy.

Results

The lowering of IOP by ALT is accomplished in approximately 80% to 90% of eyes treated.[27, 30, 33, 38, 45] Although some eyes may demonstrate an immediate reduction in IOP, 4 to 6 weeks are usually required for assessment of the full response. The magnitude of IOP reduction is approximately 20% to 25%; thus, in general, the patient uses antiglaucoma medications after the procedure. The mean duration of effect of ALT is 2 to 5 years. In the Glaucoma Laser Trial, 56% of eyes in which ALT was initial treatment required topical medication at 2 years.[38] Other studies found the IOP-lowering effect to be 4 to 5 years in patients receiving concomitant medical therapy. Success appears to be the same whether ALT is performed in a single treatment of 360 degrees or in two sessions of 180 degrees each.

A second ALT procedure should be considered only in

patients who experienced an excellent response to the initial procedure. The duration and success rates are both markedly reduced in second applications.[46–48] Additionally, the risk of a permanent rise in IOP is about 12% with a complete 360-degree repeat treatment.

Complications

Properly performed, ALT rarely results in severe complications. The complications that can occur can be separated into those that occur early and later in the postoperative period (Table 2–2).

By far, the most common complication of ALT is a transient rise in IOP.[49–52] The rise is usually limited to the first 24 hours. The frequency and severity are increased when greater total power is applied. This IOP rise can be markedly reduced with treatment. In patients with severe glaucomatous damage, prophylaxis should be used to minimize the risk of catastrophic visual loss from IOP elevation. In patients with mild to moderate loss, it is reasonable either to pretreat or to check the IOP 1 to 2 hours postoperatively and treat if the IOP rise occurs. α-Adrenergic agonists have been shown to be very effective for this purpose.[53, 54] Instillation of such agents immediately following the procedure is highly effective, although it is still important to check the IOP 1 to 2 hours later to ensure adequate control. With the growing use of α-adrenergic agonists for long-term therapy of glaucoma, their efficacy as treatment for acute rises in IOP after ALT may well be reduced. In these cases, an alternative agent that has not been used as long-term therapy should be considered.

Intraocular inflammation is also common, occurring to some extent in nearly half of treated patients.[55] The iritis is typically mild, lasting for only 2 to 3 days. Treatment consists of topical corticosteroid drops four times daily for 4 to 5 days. It is helpful to impress upon the patient the importance of discontinuing the corticosteroid. Longer duration of treatment can result in a rise in IOP due to a corticosteroid response. Rarely, inflammation may persist for a longer time, necessitating longer corticosteroid treatment.

Formation of peripheral anterior synechiae occurred in 34% of eyes undergoing ALT in the Glaucoma Laser Trial.[38] Their presence did not appear to affect the success of the procedure, however.

Mechanism of Action

ALT produces its effect by inducing an increase in trabecular outflow facility. Histologic studies demonstrate clearly that the laser application does not produce a hole or burn into the lumen of Schlemm's canal. The exact mechanism underlying the therapeutic effect of ALT remains controversial. Evidence suggests that multiple effects of the laser energy on the trabecular meshwork may mediate the increased facility of outflow.[56]

One hypothesis suggests that laser-induced scars produce contraction of the intervening untreated regions.[34] Thus, an overall tightening of the scleral-trabecular ring is produced. Some researchers have argued that this traction is similar to that induced by pilocarpine treatment or ciliary muscle contraction. Others have suggested that the laser energy stimulates trabecular cells or cribriform cells, producing decreased outflow resistance. The applied laser energy appears to result in a mild loss of trabecular endothelial cells with transformation of the remaining cells into a more active phagocytic, migratory, and proliferative state.[57, 58]

TABLE 2–2. POSTOPERATIVE COMPLICATIONS OF ARGON LASER TRABECULOPLASTY

Early	Immediate rise in intraocular pressure (IOP)
	Intraocular inflammation
	Corneal damage
Later	Permanent rise in IOP
	Inadequate control of IOP
	Recurrent intraocular inflammation
	Peripheral anterior synechiae

Effects of Clinical Disorders on Trabecular Outflow

CONGENITAL GLAUCOMA

Histologic and clinical evidence suggests that abnormalities of the trabecular meshwork are responsible for aqueous flow obstruction in congenital glaucoma.[59]

In the normal gestational development of the anterior chamber angle, the angle recess forms with progressive posterior sliding of the iris and ciliary muscle. In the normal newborn, the iris insertion is at the level of the scleral spur or just posterior to it. The iris and ciliary muscle continue to slide or migrate posteriorly through the first year of extrauterine life, and the angle recess is formed. In congenital glaucoma, gonioscopic examination reveals the iris insertion to be anterior to the scleral spur, often at the level of the posterior trabecular meshwork. Histologically, the trabecular beams are thickened, the uveal meshwork is thickened, and the meshwork is compressed. Of note, Schlemm's canal is open early in the course of congenital glaucoma, although it can become secondarily obstructed as the disease progresses (Fig. 2–3).[60]

COMMON SECONDARY GLAUCOMAS

Many of the secondary open-angle glaucomas are characterized by trabecular meshwork obstruction. A variety of cell types and macromolecules can induce glaucoma through this mechanism.

Glaucoma Associated with Uveitis

Multiple pathogenetic mechanisms leading to elevated IOP can converge in the setting of uveitic glaucoma, including both angle-closure and open-angle mechanisms. Angle closure can ensue from pupillary block, cyclitis with ciliary body rotation, or formation of chronic peripheral anterior synechiae. A gonioscopically open angle can harbor an obstructed trabecular meshwork or a poorly functional meshwork. Inflammatory cells and proteins can obstruct the meshwork, reducing aqueous outflow facility. Inflammatory

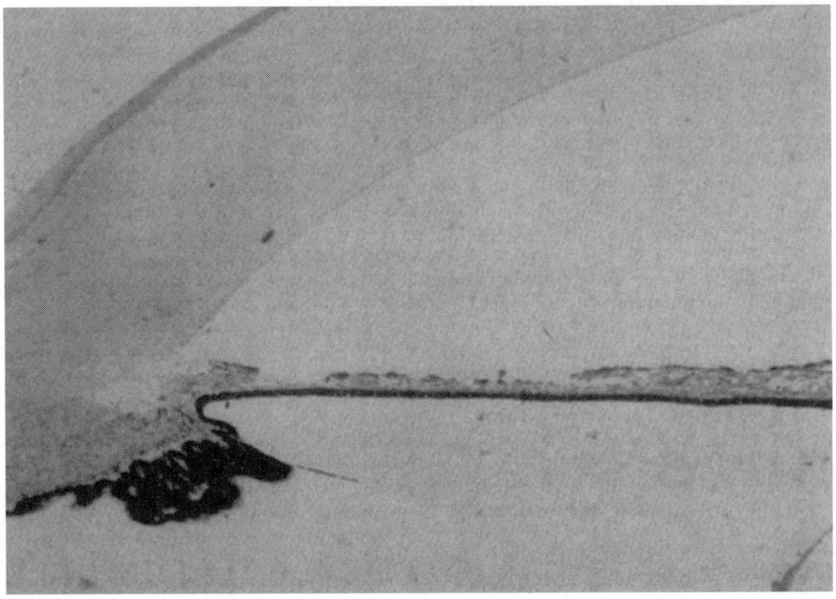

FIGURE 2–3. Primary congenital glaucoma. Note that the iris and ciliary body overlap the trabecular meshwork, with the iris insertion anterior to the scleral spur. (From Ritch R, Shields MB, Krupin T (eds): The Glaucomas, 2nd ed. St. Louis, Mosby–Year Book, 1996.)

mediators, including prostaglandins and cytokines, may directly affect trabecular outflow facility but as yet play an uncertain role in IOP regulation in uveitis.[61]

Glaucoma Associated with Pigment Dispersion Syndrome

In pigment dispersion syndrome, pigment is disrupted and liberated from the posterior surface of the iris. Aqueous flow carries the pigment to various anterior segment locations: the posterior surface of the cornea, the anterior surface of the iris, the lens equator, and angle structures, including the trabecular meshwork.

At first, the pigment that lodges in the trabecular meshwork undergoes phagocytosis by the endothelial cells that line the trabecular beams. In pigment dispersion syndrome, the trabecular endothelial cell population is heavily pigmented but not reduced in number.[62] However, when the intracellular load of pigment becomes excessive, pigment dispersion syndrome can lead to pigmentary glaucoma. An underlying abnormality of trabecular endothelial cell phagocytosis may also predispose to conversion from pigment dispersion syndrome to the associated glaucoma. Histologic studies of pigmentary glaucoma reveal trabecular cells laden with pigment that have migrated off the trabecular beams and are found in the juxtacanalicular spaces or in Schlemm's canal (Fig. 2–4).[63]

Glaucoma Associated with Exfoliation Syndrome

Exfoliation syndrome is a systemic disease characterized by elaboration of an abnormal fibrilloprotein in multiple organs and tissues throughout the body. It is currently the most commonly identified clinical finding associated with open-angle glaucoma.[64] The glaucoma associated with exfoliation syndrome probably results from obstruction of the trabecular meshwork by exfoliation material and pigment.

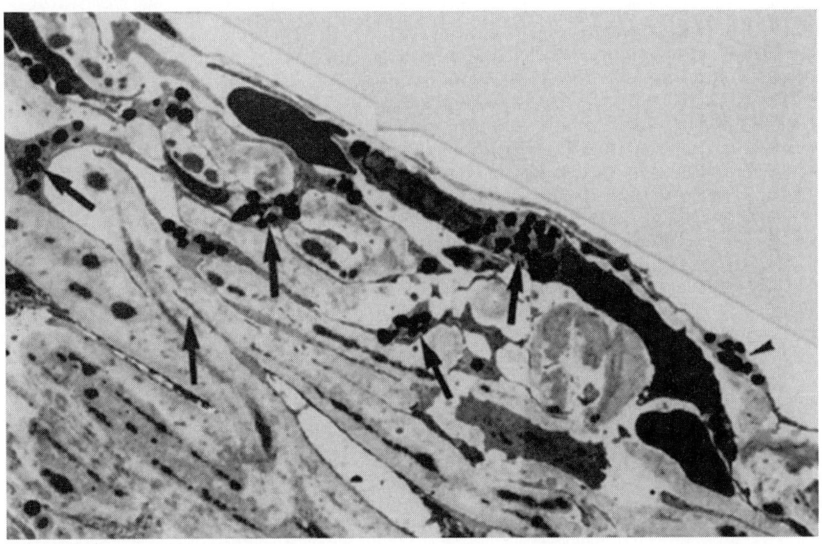

FIGURE 2–4. Electron micrograph of inner wall of Schlemm's canal in a case of glaucoma associated with pigment dispersion syndrome. Pigment granules are found within cells of the cribiform layer *(arrows)* and within the endothelium of Schlemm's canal *(arrowhead)*. (Trabeculectomy specimen; ×4800.) (From Ritch R, Shields MB, Krupin T (eds): The Glaucomas, 2nd ed. St. Louis, Mosby–Year Book, 1996.)

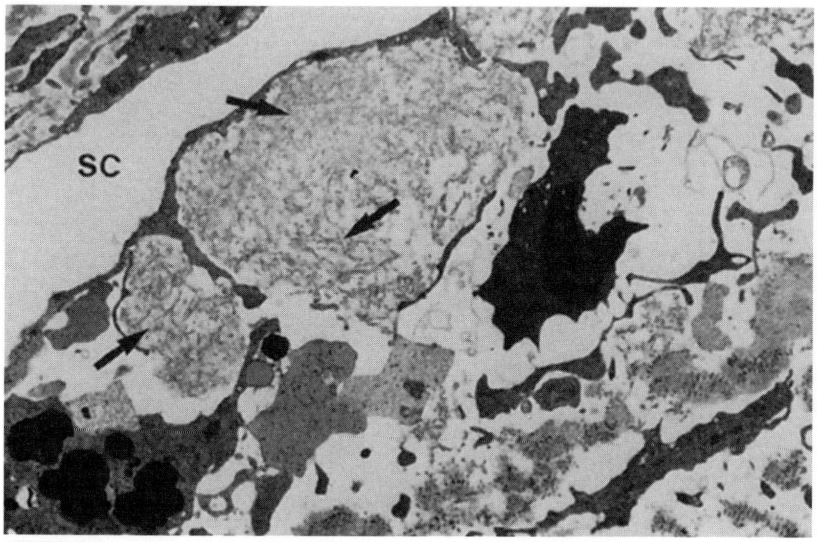

FIGURE 2–5. Electron micrographs of the trabecular meshwork in a case of glaucoma associated with pseudoexfoliation syndrome. Specimen includes cribiform layer with cluster of exfoliation fibrils *(arrows).* SC, Schlemm's canal. (Trabeculectomy specimen; ×16560.) (From Ritch R, Shields MB, Krupin T (eds): The Glaucomas, 2nd ed. St. Louis, Mosby–Year Book, 1996.)

In involved eyes, exfoliation material can be found in the intertrabecular spaces and within trabecular endothelial cells as well as further downstream in the juxtacanalicular region and beneath the endothelium of Schlemm's canal.[65] Pigment particles are deposited on or anterior to Schwalbe's line (Sampolesi's line) and are found within trabecular endothelial cells. However, the loss of endothelial cells and their migration off the trabecular beams do not appear as severe as in pigmentary glaucoma (Fig. 2–5).

REFERENCES

1. Bill A, Phillips C: Uveoscleral drainage of aqueous humor in human eyes. Exp Eye Res 1971;12:275.
2. Bleiman B, Schwartz AL: Paradoxic response to pilocarpine. Arch Ophthalmol 1979;97:1305.
3. Gong H, Trinkaus-Randall V, Freddo TF: Ultrastructural immunocytochemical localization of elastin in normal human trabecular meshwork. Curr Eye Res 1989;8:1071.
4. Babizhayev MA, Brodskaya MW: Fibronectin detection in drainage outflow system of human eyes in aging and progression of open-angle glaucoma. Mech Ageing Dev 1989;47:145.
5. Lutjen-Drecoll E, Shimizu T, Rohrbach M, et al: Quantitative analysis of "plaque material" in the inner and outer wall of Schlemm's canal in normal and glaucomatous eyes. Exp Eye Res 1986;42:443.
6. Knepper PA, Goossens W, Hvizd M, Palmberg PF: Glycosaminoglycans of the human trabecular meshwork in primary open-angle glaucoma. Invest Ophthalmol Vis Sci 1996;37:1360.
7. Hay ED (ed): Cell Biology of Extracellular Matrix, 2nd ed. New York, Plenum, 1983.
8. Spooner BS, Thompson-Pletscher HA: Matrix accumulation and the development of form: Proteoglycans and branding morphogenesis. *In* Mecham R (ed): Regulation of Matrix. San Diego, Academic Press, 1986.
9. Hynes RO: Fibronectin and its relation to cellular structure and behavior. *In* Hay ED (ed): Cell Biology of the Extracellular Matrix. New York, Plenum, 1981.
10. Maepea O, Bill A: The pressures in the episcleral veins, Schlemm's canal, and the trabecular meshwork in monkeys: Effects of changes in intraocular pressure. Exp Eye Res 1989;49:645.
11. Rohen JW, Futa R, Lutjen-Drecoll E: The fine structure of the cribriform meshwork in normal and glaucomatous eyes as seen in tangential sections. Invest Ophthalmol Vis Sci 1981;21:574.
12. Rohen JW: Why is intraocular pressure elevated in chronic simple glaucoma? Anatomical considerations. Ophthalmology 1983;90:758.
13. Rohen JW, van der Zypen E: The phagocytic activity of the trabecular meshwork endothelium: An electron microscopic study of the vervet (*Cercopithecus aethiops*). Graefes Arch Clin Exp Ophthalmol 1968;175:143.
14. Grierson I, Lee WR: Erythrocyte phagocytosis in the human trabecular meshwork. Br J Ophthalmol 1973;57:400.
15. Epstein DL, Freddo TF, Anderson PJ, et al: Experimental obstruction to aqueous outflow by pigment particles in living monkeys. Invest Ophthalmol Vis Sci 1986;27:387.
16. Inomata H, Bill A, Smelser GK: Aqueous humor pathways through the trabecular meshwork and into Schlemm's canal in the cynomolgus monkey (*Macaca irus*): An electron microscopic study. Am J Ophthalmol 1972;73:760.
17. Tripathi RC: Mechanism of aqueous outflow across the trabecular wall of Schlemm's canal. Exp Eye Res 1971;11:16.
18. Becker B, Mills DW: Corticosteroids and intraocular pressure. Arch Ophthalmol 1963;70:500.
19. Becker B, Mills DW: Elevated intraocular pressure following corticosteroid eye drops. JAMA 1963;185:884.
20. Becker B, Chevrette L: Topical corticosteroid testing in glaucoma siblings. Arch Ophthalmol 1966;76:484.
21. Cubey RB: Glaucoma following the application of corticosteroids to the skin of the eyelid. Br J Dermatol 1976;95:207.
22. Herschler J: Increased intraocular pressure induced by repository corticosteroids. Am J Ophthalmol 1976;82:90.
23. Opatowsky I, Feldman RM, Gross RL, Feldman ST: Intraocular pressure elevation associated with inhalation and nasal corticosteroids. Ophthalmology 1995;102:177.
24. Alfano JE: Changes in the intraocular pressure associated with systemic steroid therapy. Am J Ophthalmol 1963;56:245.
25. Haas JS, Nootens RH: Glaucoma secondary to benign adrenal adenoma. Am J Ophthalmol 1974;78:497.
26. Rohen JW, Linner E, Witmer R: Electron microscopic studies on the trabecular meshwork in two cases of cortisone glaucoma. Exp Eye Res 1973;17:19.
27. Wise JB, Witter SL: Argon laser therapy for open-angle glaucoma: A pilot study. Arch Ophthalmol 1979;97:319.
28. Worthen DM, Wickham MG: Argon laser trabeculectomy. Trans Am Acad Ophthalmol Otol 1974;78:371.
29. Gaasterland D, Kupfer C: Experimental glaucoma in the rhesus monkey. Invest Ophthalmol 1975;14:455.
30. Wise JB: Long-term control of adult open angle glaucoma by argon laser treatment. Ophthalmology 1981;88:197.
31. Schwartz AL, Whitten ME, Bleiman B, Martin D: Argon laser trabecular surgery in uncontrolled phakic open angle glaucoma. Ophthalmology 1981;88:203.
32. Wilensky JT, Jampol LM: Laser therapy for open angle glaucoma. Ophthalmology 1981;88:213.
33. Forbes M, Bansal RK: Argon laser goniophotocoagulation of the trabecular meshwork in open-angle glaucoma. Trans Am Ophthalmol Soc 1981;76:257.
34. Robin AL, Pollack IP: Argon laser trabeculoplasty in secondary forms of open-angle glaucoma. Arch Ophthalmol 1983;101:382.

35. Lieberman MF, Hoskins HD Jr, Hetherington J Jr: Laser trabeculoplasty and the glaucomas. Ophthalmology 1983;90:790.
36. Ritch R, Liebmann J, Robin A, et al: Argon laser trabeculoplasty in pigmentary glaucoma. Ophthalmology 1993;100:909.
37. Safran MJ, Robin AL, Pollack IP: Argon laser trabeculoplasty in younger patients with primary open-angle glaucoma. Am J Ophthalmol 1984;97:292.
38. The Glaucoma Laser Trial Research Group: The glaucoma laser trial (GLT) 2: Results of argon laser trabeculoplasty versus topical medicines. Ophthalmology 1990;97:1403.
39. Glaucoma Laser Trial Research Group: The glaucoma laser trial (GLT) and glaucoma laser trial follow-up study 7: Results. Am J Ophthalmol 1995;120:718.
40. Spurny RC, Lederer CM Jr: Krypton laser trabeculoplasty: A clinical report. Arch Ophthalmol 1984;102:1626.
41. Kwasniewska S, Fankhauser F, Larsen SE, Cruz-Orive LM: The efficacy of cw Nd:YAG laser trabeculoplasty. Ophthalmic Surg 1993;24:304.
42. Brancato R, Carassa R, Trabucchi G: Diode laser compared with argon laser for trabeculoplasty. Am J Ophthalmol 1991;112:50.
43. Traverso CE, Greenidge KC, Spaeth GL: Formation of peripheral anterior synechiae following argon laser trabeculoplasty: A prospective study to determine relationship to position of laser burns. Arch Ophthalmol 1984;102:861.
44. van der Zypen E, Fankhauser F: Ultrastructural changes of the trabecular meshwork of the monkey (*Macaca speciosa*) following irradiation with argon laser light. Graefes Arch Clin Exp Ophthalmol 1984;221:249.
45. Wise JB: Long-term control of adult open angle glaucoma by argon laser treatment. Ophthalmology 1981;88:197.
46. Spiegel D, Wegscheider E, Lund OE: Argon laser trabeculoplasty: Long-term follow-up of at least 5 years. Ger J Ophthalmol 1992;1:156.
47. Starita RJ, Fellman RL, Spaeth GL, Poryzees E: The effect of repeating full-circumference argon laser trabeculoplasty. Ophthalmic Surg 1984;15:41.
48. Feldman RM, Katz LJ, Spaeth GL, et al: Long-term efficacy of repeat argon laser trabeculoplasty. Ophthalmology 1991;98:1061.
49. Glaucoma Laser Trial Research Group: The Glaucoma Laser Trial 1: Acute effects of argon laser trabeculoplasty on intraocular pressure. Arch Ophthalmol 1989;107:1135.
50. Weinreb RN, Ruderman J, Juster R, Zweig K: Immediate intraocular pressure response to argon laser trabeculoplasty. Am J Ophthalmol 1983;95:279.
51. Hoskins HD Jr, Hetherington J Jr, Minckler DS, et al: Complications of laser trabeculoplasty. Ophthalmology 1983;90:796.
52. Krupin T, Kolker AE, Kass MA, Becker B: Intraocular pressure the day of argon laser trabeculoplasty in primary open-angle glaucoma. Ophthalmology 1984;91:361.
53. Rosenberg LF, Krupin T, Ruderman J, et al: Apraclonidine and anterior segment laser surgery: Comparison of 0.5% versus 1.0% apraclonidine for prevention of postoperative intraocular pressure rise. Ophthalmology 1995;102:1312.
54. David R, Spaeth GL, Clevenger CE, et al: Brimonidine in the prevention of intraocular pressure elevation following argon laser trabeculoplasty. Arch Ophthalmol 1993;111:1387.
55. Mermoud A, Pittet N, Herbort CP: Inflammation patterns after laser trabeculoplasty measured with the laser flare meter. Arch Ophthalmol 1992;110:368.
56. Brubaker RF, Liesegang TJ: Effect of trabecular photocoagulation on the aqueous humor dynamics of the human eye. Am J Ophthalmol 1983;96:139.
57. Alexander RA, Grierson I, Church WH: The effect of argon laser trabeculoplasty upon the normal human trabecular meshwork. Graefes Arch Clin Exp Ophthalmol 1989;227:72.
58. Bylsma SS, Samples JR, Acott TS, Van Buskirk EM: Trabecular cell division after argon laser trabeculoplasty. Arch Ophthalmol 1988;106:544.
59. Maumenee AE: The pathogenesis of congenital glaucoma. Am J Ophthalmol 1959;47:827.
60. Anderson DR: The development of the trabecular meshwork and its abnormality in primary infantile glaucoma. Trans Am Ophthalmol Soc 1981;79:458.
61. Wakefield D, Lloyd A: The role of cytokines in the pathogenesis of inflammatory eye disease. Cytokine 1992;4:1.
62. Kupfer C, Kuwabara T, Kaiser-Kupfer M: The histopathology of pigmentary dispersion syndrome with glaucoma. Am J Ophthalmol 1975;80:857.
63. Richardson TM, Hutchinson BT, Grant WM: The outflow tract in pigmentary glaucoma: A light and electron microscopic study. Arch Ophthalmol 1977;95:1015.
64. Ritch R: Exfoliation syndrome: The most common identifiable cause of open angle glaucoma. J Glaucoma 1994;3:176.
65. Ringvold A, Vegge T: Electron microscopy of the trabecular meshwork in eyes with exfoliation syndrome (pseudoexfoliation of the lens capsule). Virchows Arch A Pathol Anat Histopathol 1971;353:110.

CHAPTER 3

Ciliary Body

OSMAN ORAM

The ciliary body plays a key role in glaucoma in many ways. It is responsible for aqueous humor production, but from a clinical standpoint, both medical and surgical reduction of aqueous production are used therapeutically to lower intraocular pressure. In this chapter, Osman Oram presents the basic anatomy and physiology of the ciliary body and discusses how they pertain to aqueous humor production. He offers the reader much more, including an understandable discussion of uveoscleral outflow, the alternative mechanism of aqueous outflow that is becoming increasingly important in medical therapy. Along the lines of medical therapy, the basic mechanisms of action of all the classes of drugs used to treat glaucoma are discussed. Surgical implications are also addressed, including the potential toxic effects of antimetabolites on the ciliary body as well as cyclodestructive procedures. For more information on the surgical implications, see Chapters 18 (on filtration surgery) and 19 (cycloablation).

The ciliary body is a highly specialized structure that possesses unique morphologic features that are essential to its varied functions, including formation of aqueous humor, regulation of outflow facility, accommodation, and, possibly, secretion of vitreal hyaluronic acid.[1] In this chapter, the anatomy, ultrastructure, and physiology of the ciliary body along with its role in aqueous humor production and outflow will be explored with respect to clinical glaucoma treatment.

Anatomy

The ciliary body forms a part of the anterior uveal tract of the eye and is located circumferentially between the scleral spur anteriorly and the ora serrata posteriorly. Although its anteroposterior length varies considerably with the length of the eye, the ciliary body measures 5.6 to 6.3 mm in length temporally and 4.6 to 5.2 mm nasally.[2] The distance between the external corneoscleral limbus and the posterior border of the ciliary body is approximately 7 mm temporally and 6 mm nasally.[2,3] The shape of the ciliary body is roughly triangular in cross-section, with an anterior side forming almost a right angle with the scleral surface (Fig. 3–1). The anterior face of the ciliary body forms a part of the posterior portion of the anterior chamber angle, and the iris originates from the midportion of this anterior face, which is tightly attached at its periphery to the scleral spur and trabecular meshwork. The rest of the outer surface of the ciliary body is loosely attached to the adjacent sclera via sparse collagen fibers. The potential supraciliary space, which lies between the ciliary body and the sclera, is continuous posteriorly with the potential suprachoroidal space.

The ciliary body is divided into an anterior portion termed the *pars plicata* and a posterior portion termed the *pars plana*. The pars plicata is approximately 2 mm in anteroposterior length in the adult and has a rough surface on gross examination. It consists of 70 to 80 radially placed, 1 mm high, major ciliary processes that protrude into the posterior chamber and smaller minor ciliary processes present in the deep valleys between each pair of major processes (Fig. 3–2). These ciliary processes located in the pars plicata are responsible for the production of aqueous humor.

The pars plana is a smooth area about 4 mm long

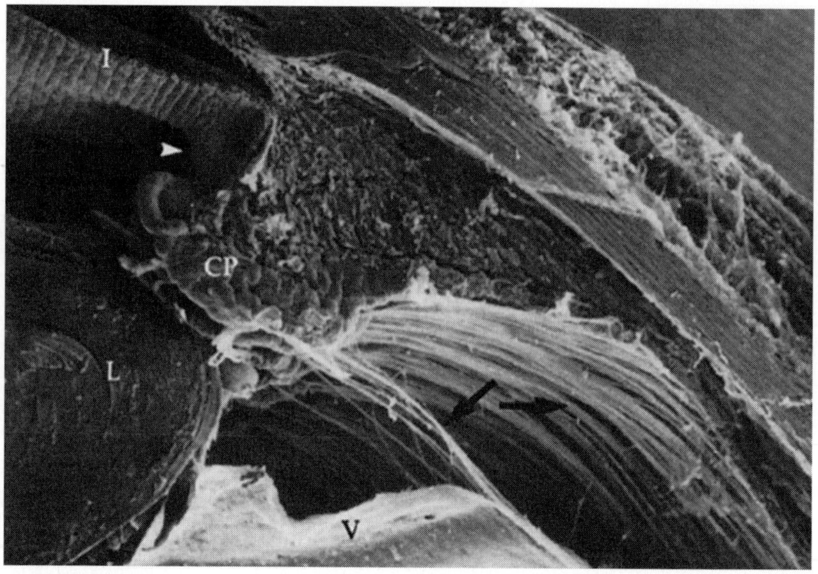

FIGURE 3–1. Scanning electron micrograph of a cross-section of human ciliary body demonstrates the ciliary body's relationship with the iris *(I)*, zonules *(arrows)*, and condensed anterior vitreous body *(V)*. Note the ciliary sulcus *(arrowhead)* between the iris and major ciliary processes *(CP)*. Shrinkage during processing of the micrograph has artifactually brought the lens *(L)* into contact with the ciliary processes. (×56.) (From Ritch R, Shields MB, Krupin T [eds]: The Glaucomas. St. Louis, Mosby–Year Book, 1996.)

temporally and 3.5 mm nasally, extending from the posterior border of the ciliary processes to the ora serrata. It features multiple narrow radial striae extending from the dentate processes of the ora serrata to the valleys between

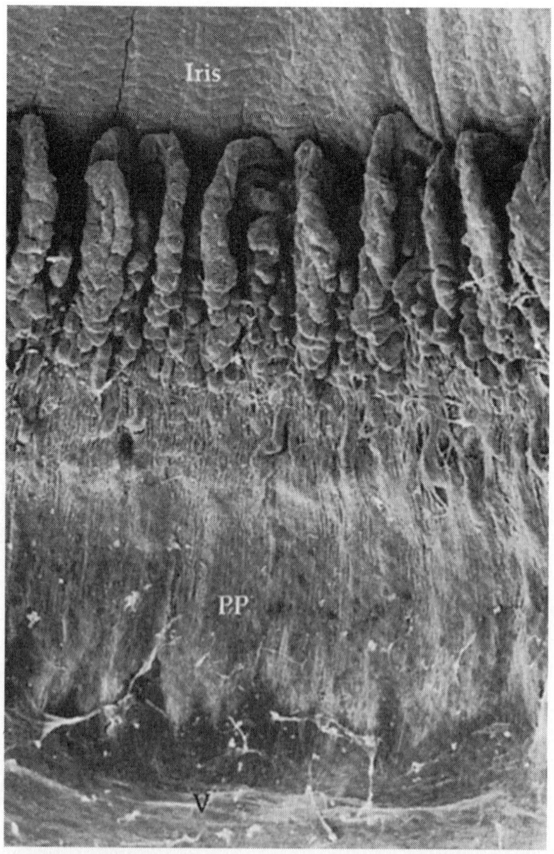

FIGURE 3–2. Scanning electron micrograph of the lateral wall of the posterior chamber with the lens and zonules removed. Major and minor ciliary processes blend posteriorly with the pars plana *(PP)*, which ends beneath the vitreous base *(V)*. (×42.) (From Ritch R, Shields MB, Krupin T [eds]: St. Louis, The Glaucomas. Mosby–Year Book, 1996.)

the ciliary processes (see Fig. 3–2). Most of the zonular fibers take origin from the pars plana approximately 1.5 mm anterior to the ora serrata, curve forward from the sides of the radial striae of the pars plana into the valleys between the ciliary processes, and then extend from the valleys to the lens capsule.[4–6] The rest of the zonules originate from between the ciliary processes to attach to the lens capsule. The posterior 1.5 to 2 mm of the pars plana also gives a dense attachment to the vitreous base that extends from its attachment to the peripheral retina just posterior to the ora serrata.

The layers of the ciliary body from the inner surface to the outer supraciliary space are (1) ciliary epithelium, (2) basal lamina, (3) ciliary body stroma, and (4) ciliary muscle. The ciliary epithelium consists of an inner nonpigmented layer (NPE) and an outer pigmented layer (PE). The apices of the cells in both layers face each other; the bases of the cells face outward, toward the posterior chamber in the NPE and toward the ciliary body stroma in the PE. The bases of both cell layers are covered by basement membrane, the internal limiting membrane in the NPE and the forward continuation of Bruch's membrane in the PE. The NPE is continuous anteriorly with the pigment epithelium of the iris and posteriorly with the neurosensory retina at the ora serrata. The PE continues anteriorly as the anterior myoepithelium of the iris and posteriorly as the retinal pigment epithelium. The NPE cells are cuboidal in the pars plicata, are nearly columnar in the pars plana, and contain numerous mitochondria as well as rough and smooth endoplasmic reticulum. The cell membrane of the NPE cells is characterized by numerous basal cytoplasmic infoldings and multiple, redundant lateral interdigitations near the posterior chamber that are most marked in the anterior half of the pars plicata.[2, 7, 8] These features greatly increase the area of the NPE cell surface, suggesting that this anterior region makes a greater contribution overall to the production of aqueous humor.[9]

Various types of intercellular junctions join the NPE and PE cells, including desmosomes, gap junctions, puncta adhaerentias, and tight junctions.[10, 11] The zonula occludens, or tight junctions, that are present at the apical portions of the NPE cells are especially important, representing the primary blood-aqueous barrier in the ciliary body. Electron micrographs demonstrate that zonula occludens are a system of continuous branching and anastomosing strands that extend around the entire circumference of each cell.[7]

The PE cells have a similar cuboidal shape in all parts of the ciliary body and contain large numbers of melanin pigment granules and free ribosomes. The mitochondria are smaller and fewer in number than in the NPE, and the rough endoplasmic reticulum is smaller in the cytoplasm of the PE cells. No tight junctions are found between the PE cells, so this layer has no barrier function. A basal lamina that splits into an outer elastic layer and an inner cuticular layer separated by a layer of avascular connective tissue is located under the PE cells.

The ciliary body stroma separates the ciliary epithelium from the ciliary muscle. This layer, which is thicker over the pars plicata and thinner over the pars plana, consists of connective tissue, a mixed cellular population comprising uveal fibroblasts, melanocytes, mast cells, lymphocytes, myelinated and unmyelinated nerves, and blood vessels. It is continuous with the iris stroma anteriorly and the stroma of the choroid posteriorly. The ciliary processes consist of a central core of highly vascularized stroma and the ciliary epithelium resting on this stromal core (Fig. 3–3). The major arterial circle of the ciliary body also lies within the ciliary body stroma anteriorly.

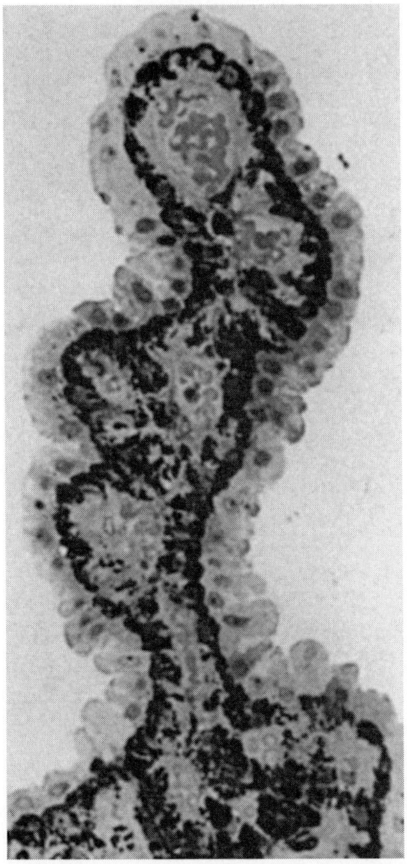

FIGURE 3–3. Ciliary process, plicated portion. In cross-section (×320), showing double cell layer and stromal capillaries. (From Albert MD, Jakobiec FA [eds]: Principles and Practice of Ophthalmology. Philadelphia, WB Saunders, 1994.)

The ciliary muscle is a ring of smooth muscle that originates from the scleral spur and trabecular beam region and inserts into the iris, the ciliary processes, and the choroid. The three divisions of the ciliary muscle are (1) the outer longitudinal or meridional portion, (2) the middle radial or oblique portion, and (3) the inner circular portion. The muscle undergoes a three-dimensional anterior and inward movement on contraction, with the interplay of all three interconnecting regions. The zonular attachments move forward and inward, the choroid is stretched forward along the sclera, and trabecular beams are pulled to increase trabecular pore size or open the lamellae during this contraction.[12, 13] The connective tissue between the muscle bundles consists of collagen fibers, fine granular ground substance, melanocytes, nerves, and blood vessels with unfenestrated capillaries. Hyaline deposition in the ciliary muscle connective tissue and lipofuscin deposition in muscle cells are seen with aging.[2]

Lying external to the outer surface of the ciliary body, the supraciliary space is composed of loose connective tissue showing a lamellar arrangement of the fibroblasts and melanocytes loosely adherent to the sclera. No intercellular tight junctions that would impede the passage of fluid have been described in the supraciliary space, and this junctional zone between the ciliary body and sclera, continuous with suprachoroidal space, may be considered a potential space with a fluid volume of approximately 10 μL.[14]

MICROVASCULATURE

The ciliary body receives its blood supply from the long posterior ciliary arteries and anterior ciliary arteries. Nasal and temporal long posterior ciliary arteries run forward in the suprachoroidal space and branch close to the posterior edge of the ciliary body. These branches interconnect with branches of the anterior ciliary arteries that are perforating the limbal sclera and arborizing within the ciliary muscle. The resulting interconnections form an anastomotic vascular ring within the ciliary muscle, the intramuscular circle, which gives off branches to supply the ciliary muscle.[15, 16] Vessels originating from the intramuscular circle ultimately form a circumferentially oriented but discontinuous major arterial circle that lies just behind the root of the iris in front of the radial portion of the ciliary muscle. The major arterial circle is the source of the extensive vascular plexus of the ciliary processes and also gives off iris arterioles and recurrent choroidal arteries.

Anterior and posterior arterioles arising from the major arterial circle supply the major and minor ciliary processes and drain into the choroidal veins (Fig. 3–4).[17] Anterior arterioles supply the anterior portion and margins of the major ciliary processes. These arterioles show localized focal constrictions as they span the ciliary sulcus and dilate into irregular, large capillaries as they enter the ciliary processes. Capillaries originating from the anterior arterioles first travel anteriorly toward the tip of the ciliary process, then turn and pass posteriorly within the internal margin of the process to empty into the choroidal veins. The anterior portion of the major ciliary processes seem to be most responsive to vasoactive agents. Posterior arteri-

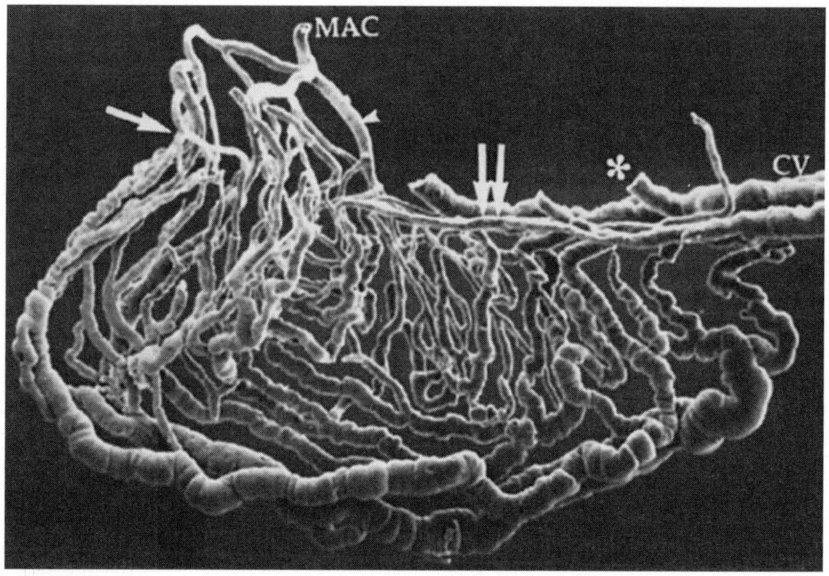

FIGURE 3–4. This profile of an individual major ciliary process casting indicates anterior *(arrow)* and posterior *(arrowhead)* ciliary process arterioles arising from the major arterial circle *(MAC)*. Irregularly dilated capillaries from the anterior arterioles pass posteriorly within the ciliary process margin to empty into choroidal veins *(CV)*. Capillaries supplied by the posterior arterioles occupy the base of the process. *Double arrow* indicates choroidal vein extending along a process base to drain the interprocess connection. Severed branches *(asterisk)* represent the drainage route of ciliary muscle capillaries (removed) into the choroidal veins. (×145.) (From Ritch R, Shields MB, Krupin T [eds]: The Glaucomas. St. Louis, Mosby–Year Book, 1996.)

oles are less constricted than the anterior arterioles and supply the inner and posterior regions of the major ciliary processes. Interprocess connections that feed minor ciliary processes on either side and the basal regions of neighboring major processes are also supplied by these arterioles. Minor ciliary process capillaries are irregularly dilated, resembling the capillaries of the major processes.

NERVE SUPPLY

The ciliary body is innervated by branches of the long posterior and short ciliary nerves and is well supplied by a plexus of myelinated and unmyelinated nerves of parasympathetic, sympathetic, and sensory type. The parasympathetic nerve fibers originate in the Edinger-Westphal nucleus, travel with the inferior division of the oculomotor nerve, and synapse in the ciliary ganglion, local ganglia within the short ciliary nerves, and the ciliary body itself. The postsynaptic parasympathetic fibers form extensive plexuses around the ciliary muscle fibers and subserve accommodation.[18]

Sympathetic fibers synapse in the superior cervical ganglion, travel with the carotid artery, join the ophthalmic division of the trigeminal nerve, and reach the ciliary body by passing through the nasociliary nerve and the long ciliary nerves. Numerous unmyelinated nerves surrounding the stromal vessels in the ciliary processes are largely nonadrenergic and probably subserve a vasomotor function.[19]

Sensory fibers originating from the ophthalmic division of the trigeminal nerve enter the ciliary body, but their distribution and function have not been well studied in the human.

Physiology

PHYSIOLOGY OF AQUEOUS HUMOR FORMATION

In an eye with an intact blood-aqueous barrier, aqueous humor is secreted from the ciliary body at a rate of 2 to 3 μL/min.[20] The production of aqueous generates an adequate intraocular pressure necessary for the structural integrity and normal optical functioning of the eye. Aqueous humor also provides nutrition for the avascular anterior segment tissues, including the cornea, lens, and trabecular meshwork, and carries the metabolic wastes away.[21] In addition, the lens removes potassium and amino acids from the aqueous, sodium is released from the lens into the aqueous, and amino acids and glucose pass from the aqueous into the vitreous.[22]

Aqueous humor formation is the result of net fluid movement across the ciliary epithelium and this movement can occur by three basic mechanisms[23]:

- *Diffusion*: the passive movement of solutes, especially lipid-soluble substances, across cell membranes from the side of greater concentration to the side of lesser concentration.
- *Ultrafiltration*: the passive movement of water and water-soluble substances across the cell membrane in response to a nonenzymatic process regulated by both the differential hydrostatic pressure in the blood and the osmotic pressure of the ciliary body.
- *Active transport*: the energy-dependent movement of solutes across the cell membrane against a concentration gradient.

Although all three processes may contribute to the formation of aqueous humor, active rather than passive forces seem to be more important. Active transport of certain solutes (especially sodium ion [Na^+]) by the ciliary epithelium followed by the osmotic flow of water into the posterior chamber is currently accepted as the major mechanism for aqueous formation. The solute transfer across the ciliary epithelium can proceed both between the cells (paracellular route) and through the cells (transcellular route).

As mentioned previously, the ciliary processes that are responsible for aqueous humor production consist of a central core of highly vascularized ciliary body stroma and the ciliary epithelium resting on the stromal core. The first step in the formation of aqueous is the development of a plasma filtrate within the stroma of the ciliary processes. The blood vessels of the ciliary processes are thin-walled and fenestrated. These vessels have a high permeability to ions and small molecules and may permit proteins as large as 150,000 daltons to enter the stromal compartment.[8] This passage of protein into the ciliary process stroma is important in the process of aqueous humor formation, influencing the transepithelial pressure relationships by way of the effective colloid osmotic pressure.

To pass into the posterior chamber, the protein-laden filtrate first has to cross the loose connective tissue of the stroma and then pass through the two-layered ciliary epithelium. The thin layer of connective tissue between the capillaries and ciliary epithelium does not hinder the movement of ions and molecules significantly. The barrier that prevents macromolecules in the plasma filtrate from entering the posterior chamber resides within the ciliary epithelium. Nonpigmented ciliary epithelial cells that are ringed with tight junctions represent a selective barrier that blocks the passage of macromolecules but still allows diffusion of water and small molecules into the posterior chamber and helps maintain the osmotic and electrical gradients across the ciliary epithelium required for the active steps in the production of aqueous humor.

Studies of the intact ciliary epithelium in the excised iris-ciliary body of the rabbit,[24] cat,[25] or toad[26] have demonstrated a spontaneous electrical potential difference between the two surfaces of the epithelium. In the presence of bicarbonate, the aqueous surface was reported to be negative relative to the contralateral surface in all these isolated preparations of vertebrate ciliary epithelia. This small electrical gradient across the ciliary epithelium provides the driving force for the positive ions in the stroma, especially for the major extracellular cation sodium to be secreted into the aqueous humor through the paracellular pathway. Because the same gradient tends to favor reabsorption of negative ions from the aqueous humor back into the stroma, it is likely that passage of chloride ion (Cl^-) into the aqueous humor is through the transcellular rather than the paracellular route.

On the basis of current studies, most of the transfer of solutes into the aqueous also occurs by the transcellular route. Because of electrical coupling among the PE and NPE cells through gap junctions, the ciliary epithelium functions as a syncytium for secretion of the aqueous humor, with solute and water entering through the PE cell and leaving through the NPE cell. Basic transport proteins thought to be present in the plasma membranes of the ciliary epithelial cells, including symports (producing cotransport of different ions in the same direction), antiports (producing counter-transport of ions in opposite directions), ion channels, and the sodium ion–potassium ion exchange (Na^+,K^+-exchange) pump, play roles in this process (Fig. 3–5).[23, 27–33]

Of the multiple symports and antiports in the ciliary epithelium presented in Figure 3–5, the $Na^+/K^+/2Cl^-$ symport is likely the most important in the formation of the aqueous humor. This symport probably provides the major route of entry for Na^+, K^+, and Cl^- from the stroma into the pigmented ciliary epithelial cells, and inhibition of the symport by bumetanide has been reported to decrease aqueous humor formation.[34] The Na^+, K^+, and Cl^- can then diffuse through gap junctions to the aqueous surface of the nonpigmented cells, from which they are extruded into the aqueous humor. At this membrane, Na^+ is extruded into the aqueous humor by the Na^+,K^+-exchange pump, whereas K^+ and Cl^- are largely secreted through parallel K^+ and Cl^- channels.[23]

The presence of a cyclic adenosine monophosphate (cAMP) activated, Cl^--selective channel and a calcium-dependent K^+ channel, which may have important roles in regulation of the rate of fluid secretion across the ciliary epithelium, has been shown in the NPE basolateral membrane.[32] The chlorine ion–bicarbonate anion (Cl^-/HCO_3^-) exchanger has been suggested as another route of Cl^- transport across the ciliary epithelia that also regulates intracellular pH.[31, 35] The $2Na^+$/ascorbate$^-$ symport is also clearly involved in transepithelial secretion.[36, 37] By coupling to the electrochemical gradient driving Na^+ into the cell, this cotransport permits intracellular ascorbate to accumulate in the ciliary epithelium. This accumulation provides the driving force for the ascorbate to exit into the aqueous humor by sodium-independent facilitated diffusion. A water channel (CHIP28) localized to the basolateral membrane of NPE cells has also been detected.[38]

As mentioned previously, besides the paracellular route, the predominant extracellular cation Na^+ is extruded into the aqueous humor by the transcellular route via the Na^+,K^+-exchange pump of the NPE cells. The molecular basis for the Na^+,K^+-exchange pump, which transports Na^+ ions out of the cell in exchange for K^+ ions into the cell, is a plasma membrane–associated protein, sodium, potassium adenosinetriphosphatase (Na^+,K^+-ATPase).[29] This membrane-bound enzyme complex is an energy-dependent active transport system that extrudes three Na^+ and accumulates two K^+ in the cell at the expense of 1 ATP. The enzyme complex is best seen predominantly on the basolateral membranes of both the pigmented and nonpigmented ciliary epithelial cells.

Experiments have shown that ouabain, which inhibits the Na^+,K^+-ATPase enzyme complex, can markedly reduce influx of Na^+ into the aqueous and decrease intraocular pressure related to the reduction of aqueous humor secretion.[39, 40] It has also been demonstrated that the transepithelial potential difference can be reduced virtually to zero by ouabain, confirming the predominance of the Na^+ pump to generate the transepithelial potential difference required for transport.[41, 42] Experiments testing possible hormonal regulation of the Na^+,K^+-exchange pump kinetics have shown that cAMP-dependent kinase can inhibit the activity of the pump.[43, 44] These studies suggest that increases in cAMP could affect the rate of Na^+ transport and thus alter aqueous formation.

Bicarbonate ion and carbonic anhydrase enzyme are crucial to the formation of aqueous humor. Carbonic anhydrase enzyme catalyzes the reaction of water (H_2O) and carbon dioxide (CO_2) in equilibrium with hydrogen ion (H^+) and HCO_3^-. The splitting of water into hydroxyl and hydrogen ions is the first step. The catalysis of hydroxyl ions and CO_2 to form the HCO_3^- is the second step, at which carbonic anhydrase enzyme comes into play.[45] In vitro and clinical observations strongly suggest that carbonic anhydrase activity and HCO_3^- significantly alter secretion of aqueous humor by the ciliary epithelium.[46–48] It is likely that carbonic anhydrase regulates aqueous humor

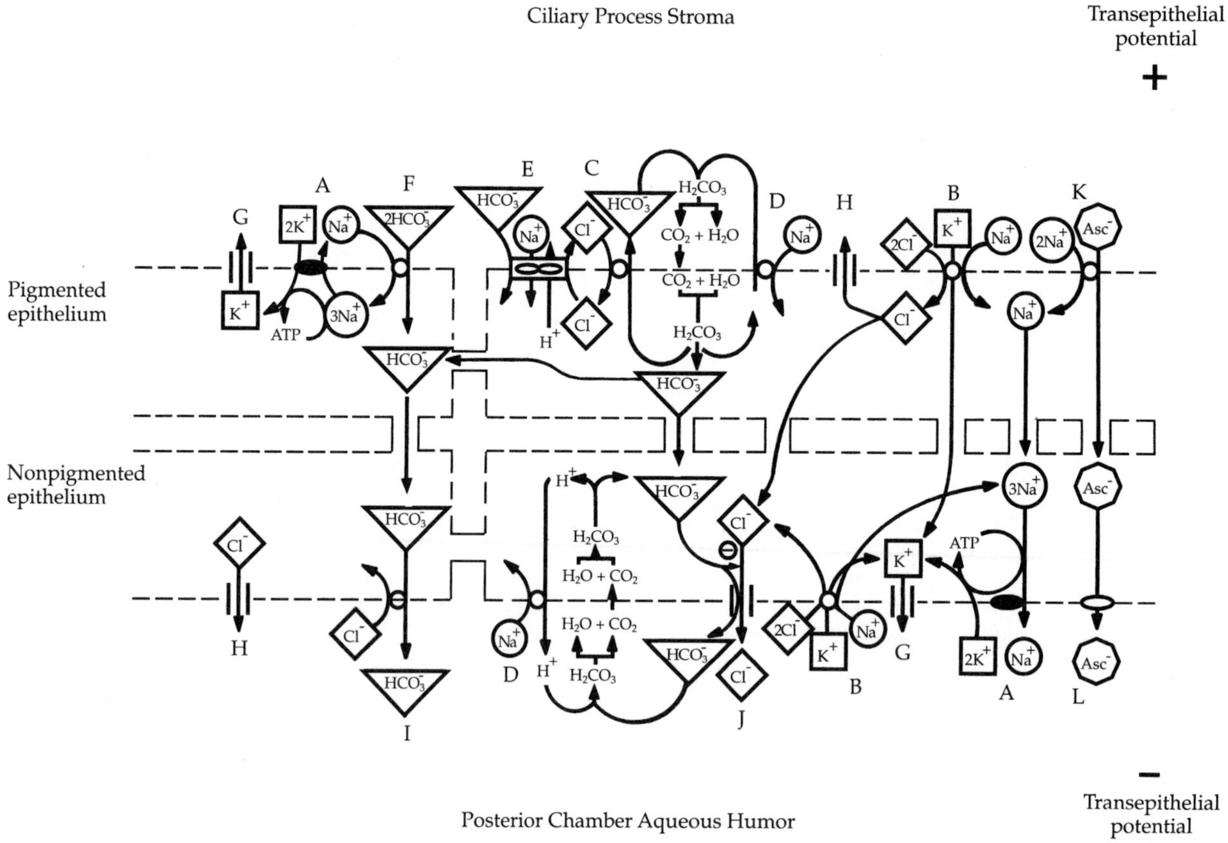

FIGURE 3–5. Diagram representing many of the transport components likely present in the plasma membranes of the pigmented (PE) and nonpigmented (NPE) ciliary epithelial cells. Because of electrical coupling among the PE and NPE cells through gap junctions, the epithelium functions as a syncytium. Tight intracellular junctions are present only between the NPE cells, so only this layer offers a complete barrier to the transepithelial movement of solutes and water. NA^+,K^+-exchange pumps *(A)* are shown on the basolateral membranes of both the PE and NPE cells. The PE cells contain: a $Na^+/K^+/2Cl^-$ symport *(B)*; an electroneutral, Na^+-independent HCO_3^-/Cl^- antiport *(C)* coupled to the Na^+/H^+ antiport *(D)*; a Na^+-dependent HCO_3^-/Cl^- antiport *(E)*; a Na^+/H^+ antiport *(D)*; and a negative $Na^+/2HCO_3^-$ symport *(F)*. These processes will affect Cl^-/Na^+-coupled transport, which in addition to the Na^+,K^+-exchange pumps, function to maintain the Cl^- electrochemical gradient. K^+ channels *(G)* are present on the PE and NPE cells, the channels on the NPE cells most likely providing the major access route of K^+ into the aqueous humor. Cl^- channels *(H)* are present on both cell layers. The NPE cells contain: a Na^+/H^+ antiport *(D)*; a $Na^+/K^+/2Cl^-$ symport *(B)*; a $H_2CO_3^-/Cl^-$ antiport *(I)*; and an anion channel that passes both Cl^- and HCO_3^- *(J)*. Also displayed are the $2Na^+$/ascorbate$^-$ symport *(K)*, subserving ascorbate uptake from the stroma, and the transporter *(L)*, which translocates ascorbate across the aqueous-side membrane. (Adapted from Ritch R, Shields MB, Krupin T [eds]: The Glaucomas. St. Louis, Mosby–Year Book, 1996.)

formation by increasing the rates of formation and breakdown of HCO_3^-.

A carbonic anhydrase enzyme inhibitor, acetazolamide, was shown to decrease intraocular pressure by reducing aqueous humor production.[49] The observation that systemic administration of acetazolamide resulted in a reduction in the entry rate of HCO_3^- into the posterior chamber appeared to lend support to the direct involvement of HCO_3^- formation and transport in the production of aqueous humor.[48, 50] In addition, a decrease in the accession rate of Na^+ into the posterior chamber was shown to occur with the use of systemic acetazolamide; this observation supports a coupling of Na^+ and HCO_3^- transport across the ciliary epithelium.[47, 48] Although the importance of HCO_3^- ion and carbonic anhydrase in regulating aqueous humor formation is known, the exact mechanisms underlying this regulation remain unclear.

CONTROL OF AQUEOUS HUMOR FORMATION

Aqueous humor formation by the ciliary epithelium is stimulated by the activation and interaction of several receptor subtypes. In 1971, a membrane-bound enzyme-receptor complex, adenylate cyclase, which is responsible for the formation of cAMP, was demonstrated in the ciliary processes of rabbits.[51] Then the presence of β-adrenergic receptors in the ciliary epithelia was shown, with a predominance of β_2-adrenergic receptors.[52, 53] Increased cAMP production was seen after β-adrenergic stimulation with isoproterenol, and the inhibition of isoproterenol-stimulated cAMP production by pretreatment with either α_2-adrenergic agonists[54, 55] or nonselective β-adrenergic blockers was described.[55]

In one study, isoproterenol, norepinephrine, epinephrine, and α_2-adrenergic agonists were used to detail the dynamic interaction between α_2-adrenergic and β-adrenergic receptors in regulating cAMP synthesis in isolated rabbit ciliary processes.[56] A biphasic dose-response curve was observed, with stimulation of cAMP production at low isoproterenol concentrations through activation of stimulatory β-adrenergic receptors, followed by inhibition of cAMP production at higher isoproterenol concentrations that activate inhibitory α_2-adrenergic receptors. The dose-response curves for the use of epinephrine or norepinephrine showed little stimulation of cAMP production, owing to the higher affinity of these catecholamines for the inhibitory α_2-adrenergic receptors than for the stimulatory β-adrenergic receptors. These results obtained with in vitro experiments, together with clinical observations of α_2-receptor–stimulated and β-receptor–mediated effects on aqueous flow and intraocular pressure, suggested the hypothesis that interactions between epithelial α_2-adrenergic and β-adrenergic receptors are important in regulating aqueous humor production.[55]

It should be noted that comparisons between expectations from in vitro experiments and in vivo measurements of aqueous humor formation are not infrequently at odds. For example, the "tone" of the system is an important factor, and it is possible that under the conditions of low tone, activation of the adenylate cyclase receptor complex stimulates aqueous humor formation, whereas at a time of high tone, either decreases (inhibition) or no effects occur after activation of the adenylate cyclase receptor complex.[57] In this connection, it was found that the nonselective β-adrenergic blocker timolol decreases aqueous humor flow in humans only during daytime conditions, when flow is relatively higher than at night.[58]

On a corresponding molecular level, inhibitory effects are a function of the receptor-mediated nucleotide-binding protein G_i (inhibitory G protein) input negatively coupled to adenylate cyclase for compounds such as α_2-agonists, α_1-adenosine agonists, and opiates, somatostatin, or neuropeptide Y.[8] Stimulatory effects of cAMP-generating systems are mediated G_s (stimulating G protein) input, by positively coupled to adenylate cyclase for epinephrine and its analogues. This duality, taken together with the circadian time at which experimentation is done, may explain the mixed effects reported for a given drug. The response of the β-adrenergic receptor to yield increased production of cAMP is modulated by endogenous mechanisms operating through G_i and the β_2 receptor. The β_2-adrenergic receptors are positively coupled to the production of cAMP through G_s, whereas α_2-receptors are associated with G_i and demonstrate an inhibitory effect on cAMP production by the ciliary epithelium. The α_2-adrenergic agonists decrease aqueous flow while decreasing cAMP production.[56] As mentioned previously, possible sites of action for cAMP to influence aqueous humor formation may be the Na^+,K^+-exchange pump, which is influenced by cAMP-dependent kinase,[44] and Cl^- transport, which is influenced by the cAMP-dependent Cl^- channel.[32]

COMPOSITION OF AQUEOUS HUMOR

Aqueous humor is normally a clear, colorless solution with an index of refraction of 1.3336 and an osmolality slightly higher than that of plasma.[59, 60] The composition of aqueous humor depends on the nature of the freshly secreted fluid, the subsequent metabolic interchanges across adjacent tissues, and its outflow rate. The chemical compositions of posterior chamber aqueous and anterior aqueous are different because of solute exchanges between aqueous and vitreous, lens, cornea, and iris.

Distribution of electrolytes and organic substances in aqueous humor varies greatly among different species. The concentrations of organic and inorganic substances in aqueous and plasma detected in some human and monkey studies are shown in Tables 3–1 and 3–2.[60–64] Although different investigators found somewhat different aqueous concentration values for many substances, most studies in human eyes have shown an apparent excess of chloride and deficit of bicarbonate in aqueous compared with plasma concentrations. The pH of aqueous is also acidic in human eyes with this excess of chloride and deficiency in bicarbonate. Most species tested have also very high concentrations of ascorbate and lactate in aqueous compared with plasma.[65, 66] Concentrations of glucose and urea are slightly lower in aqueous than in plasma. Sodium concentrations in aqueous and plasma are found to be very similar in most studies, although a few investigators have reported a slight excess of sodium in the aqueous.[62]

The concentration of proteins is markedly lower in aqueous than in plasma. The protein composition of the aqueous also differs markedly from that of the plasma, with lower-molecular-weight proteins, such as albumin and β-globulins, being more prominent; the higher-molecular-weight proteins, such as β-lipoproteins and heavy immunoglobulins, are present only in trace amounts in aqueous.[67, 68] The albumin-to-globulin ratio of the aqueous is therefore many times higher than that of plasma. Amino acids, however, frequently are at higher concentrations in aqueous than in plasma, indicating that most amino acids are secreted into the aqueous via an active process.[69]

TABLE 3–1. CONCENTRATIONS OF INORGANIC SUBSTANCES IN AQUEOUS HUMOR AND PLASMA

Substance	Aqueous Concentration	Plasma Concentration
Bicarbonate (μmol/mL)	20.2	27.5*
Sodium (μmol/mL)	152	148†
Chloride (μmol/mL)	131	107*
Potassium (μmol/mL)	3.9	4.0†
Calcium (μmol/mL)	2.5	4.9†
Magnesium (μmol/mL)	0.8	0.7†
Phosphate (μmol/mL)	0.62	1.11*
Hydrogen ion (pH)	7.21	7.40*

*Human studies.
†Monkey studies.

TABLE 3–2. CONCENTRATIONS OF ORGANIC SUBSTANCES IN AQUEOUS HUMOR AND PLASMA

Substance	Aqueous Concentration	Plasma Concentration
Ascorbate (μmol/mL)	1.06	0.04*
Glucose (μmol/mL)	2.8	5.9*
Lactate (μmol/mL)	4.5	1.9*
Protein (g/dL)	0.024	7.0*
Urea (μmol/mL)	6.1	4.9†

*Human studies.
†Monkey studies.

Anatomy and Physiology of Aqueous Humor Outflow via Ciliary Body (Uveoscleral Outflow)

Uveoscleral outflow can be defined as aqueous humor outflow from the anterior chamber, through the intermuscular spaces of the ciliary muscle, into the supraciliary-suprachoroidal space, and out through either the substance of the sclera or the perivascular spaces of the emissarial channels (Fig. 3–6).[70] Because no endothelial or epithelial layer covers the anterior surface of the anterior uvea and the intermuscular spaces of the ciliary muscle are filled with loose connective tissue and ground substance, no epithelial barrier exists between the anterior chamber and the supraciliary space. The rate of aqueous outflow from the anterior chamber into the suprachoroidal space depends on the permeability of the ciliary muscle.[71]

Once aqueous has passed from the anterior chamber into the supraciliary-suprachoroidal space, it may be osmotically absorbed by uveal vessels,[14] may leave the sclera through the emissarial channels around the blood vessels and nerves that penetrate the sclera,[72] or may flow through the narrow routes between the tightly interwoven collagen fibers of the sclera.[73] Studies in monkey eyes with different-sized particles indicate that much of the fluid enters the interstitial spaces of the ciliary muscle via the intertrabecular spaces of the uveal meshwork.[74] The fluid moves between the muscle bundles of the longitudinal part of the ciliary muscle, and even particles as large as 1 μm in diameter are rapidly carried with this flow via the interstitial spaces of the ciliary muscle into the suprachoroid and then into the perivascular spaces of the sclera. Large particles cannot pass through the scleral substance, which restricts even 10-nm particles. On its way through the uvea and the sclera, the aqueous changes in volume and composition owing to rapid exchange with the blood vessels.

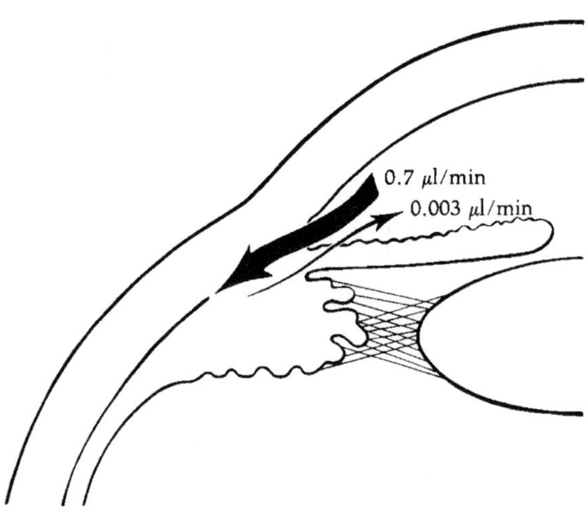

FIGURE 3–6. Unidirectional fluxes of fluorescein-isothiocyanate (FITC) dextran 70 from the anterior chamber to the suprachoroidal space and vice versa, expressed in equivalent volumes of aqueous humor. Results imply flow from the anterior chamber to the suprachoroid. (From Ritch R, Shields MB, Krupin T [eds]: The Glaucomas. St. Louis, Mosby–Year Book, 1996.)

A hydrostatic pressure gradient must exist for uveoscleral flow to proceed from the anterior chamber into the suprachoroidal space and out of the eye. In the suprachoroidal space in cats, the pressure is 2 mm Hg lower than the anterior chamber pressure.[75] In monkeys, the supraciliary pressure is 0.8 mm Hg lower, and the posterior suprachoroidal pressure 3.7 mm Hg lower, than the anterior chamber pressure.[76] This negative pressure is due to the oncotic absorptive force of the uveal vessels.

The rate of uveoscleral flow is 0.1 to 0.3 μL/min in the rabbit eye, 0.3 to 1.0 μL/min in the monkey eye, and 0.2 μL/min in the human eye.[71] Studies at different intraocular pressures have shown that the uveoscleral outflow is almost independent of the intraocular pressure.[77, 78] In these studies on monkey eyes, at intraocular pressures greater than 4 mm Hg, no significant change in the uveoscleral flow rate was observed with an increase in the intraocular pressure. However, at an intraocular pressure of 2 mm Hg, a marked decrease was noted in uveoscleral outflow. Thus, uveoscleral outflow becomes pressure-dependent at low intraocular pressures. The reason for this constancy of uveoscleral outflow in the midrange of intraocular pressure is not clear.

Expressing uveoscleral outflow as a percentage of total outflow can be misleading because of the relatively pressure-independent nature of uveoscleral outflow and the highly pressure-dependent nature of trabecular outflow. At normal intraocular pressure, however, uveoscleral flow is 15% of the total outflow. The resistance to flow through the ciliary muscle is the rate-limiting step in the pathway of uveoscleral outflow. Disorders that result in enlargement of the intramuscular spaces of the ciliary muscle, such as iridocyclitis and ciliochoroidal detachment with ciliary muscle edema, have been reported to increase uveoscleral flow.[79, 80] Cyclodialysis has also been shown to enhance uveoscleral flow, allowing free communication between the anterior chamber and the suprachoroidal space.[81, 82]

Alteration of the tone of the ciliary muscle with various drugs also has a profound effect on uveoscleral outflow. Among the drugs that are used in glaucoma treatment, α-adrenergic agonists and prostaglandins have been noted to increase uveoscleral flow, whereas pilocarpine causes a significant drop (see later). Although a significant reduction in uveoscleral outflow was shown with age in normotensive subjects and it was suggested that the reduced uveoscleral outflow may be responsible in part for the higher prevalence of ocular hypertension and chronic open-angle glaucoma with age,[83] the exact role of reduced uveoscleral outflow in the development of open-angle glaucoma is still not clear.

Significance of the Ciliary Body in Clinical Glaucoma Treatment

MEDICAL TREATMENT

Ocular Cholinergic Agents

The ocular cholinergic agents are topically used antiglaucomatous medications that can be divided into two groups according to site of action. Direct-acting cholinergic agents, such as pilocarpine, acetylcholine hydrochloride, and carbachol, bind to the parasympathetic muscarinic receptors on the ciliary muscle cell membranes and initiate ciliary muscle contraction. Indirect-acting cholinergic agents, also known as anticholinesterase agents, such as demecarium bromide, echothiophate iodide, and diisopropyl fluorophosphate, bind the enzymes acetylcholinesterase and butyrylcholinesterase, thereby preventing them from hydrolyzing the endogenously released cholinergic transmitter acetylcholine.[84] Acetylcholine then accumulates in large quantities at the neuromuscular junction, strongly stimulating the parasympathetic nerve ending. In each instance, contraction of the ciliary muscle by ocular cholinergic agents causes expansion of the trabecular meshwork and widening of the intertrabecular spaces via traction on the scleral spur.[85] Although the connective tissue spaces between the ciliary muscle bundles are also compressed and uveoscleral outflow is markedly reduced during this contraction, the enhancement of aqueous outflow via the trabecular route exceeds the obstruction via the uveoscleral route, and the intraocular pressure decreases.

Supporting evidence for this mechanism of action that linked the ability of the ocular cholinergic agents to increase the aqueous outflow facility with the traction on the trabecular meshwork by stimulation of ciliary muscle contraction was also provided by experiments in cynomolgus monkeys. These studies showed that when the ciliary muscle is completely separated from the scleral spur, the ocular cholinergic agent pilocarpine fails to increase aqueous outflow facility.[86] Although it is unlikely that cholinergic agents directly influence aqueous humor production, muscarinic cholinergic inhibition of adenylate cyclase in the rabbit ciliary body has also been shown.[87]

In addition to their aqueous humor outflow enhancement effect, the ocular cholinergic agents that are currently in use also cause accommodation of the lens and induced myopia as a result of ciliary muscle contraction. However, information about the existence of five different muscarinic receptor subtypes in the ciliary muscle and evidence that the aqueous outflow and accommodative effects of the ocular cholinergic agents can be dissociated under some experimental conditions have aroused interest in developing new selective cholinergic agents that might stimulate only certain parts of the ciliary muscle while sparing the remainder and facilitate aqueous outflow without causing significant accommodation.[88] One study has quantitatively demonstrated that among the five subtypes of muscarinic receptors (m1, m2, m3, m4, and m5), the m3 subtype is the predominant receptor in the ciliary body of the human eye.[89] The m2 and m4 subtypes are present in lower numbers, and the m1 and m5 subtypes appear to be expressed in discrete cell populations. Further studies are needed to clarify the role of muscarinic receptors in the cholinergic pharmacology of the ciliary muscle, but the extensive heterogeneity of muscarinic receptors makes it difficult to predict whether subtype-selective cholinergic agents will have improved efficacy and a better side effect profile.

Adrenergic Drugs

ADRENERGIC AGONISTS

The adrenergic agonists currently used in the glaucoma treatment can be divided into two groups: nonselective α-adrenergic and β-adrenergic agonists and selective α_2-adrenergic agonists. The intraocular pressure–lowering effect of nonselective α-adrenergic and β-adrenergic agonist epinephrine or its prodrug form dipivefrin is complex, and the mechanisms responsible for this ocular hypotensive action are not completely understood. This class of drugs affects aqueous humor flow, trabecular outflow, and uveoscleral outflow. The intraocular pressure–lowering effect is the net result of the balance between the different effects of the drugs. Nonselective adrenergic agonists cause constriction of blood vessels in the ciliary processes, reducing the pressure for ultrafiltration and, possibly, indirectly decreasing aqueous formation by α-adrenergic stimulation.[90] β-Adrenergic stimulation of the adrenoreceptors in the ciliary epithelium may cause an increase in aqueous production,[91, 92] and β_2-adrenergic stimulation may increase trabecular outflow facility by elevating cAMP levels through the adenylate cyclase–cAMP pathway.[93]

Nonselective adrenergic agonists also increase uveoscleral outflow in monkey eyes[94] and human eyes.[91, 95] Classically, this effect has been thought to be consequent to β_2-receptor–mediated relaxation of the ciliary muscle with widening of the intermuscular spaces.[94] However, some studies have indicated that if the formation of arachidonic acid metabolites is prevented, the effects of nonselective adrenergic agents on the intraocular pressure can be reduced or abolished, suggesting that the stimulation of the synthesis and release of prostaglandins by nonselective adrenergic agents may be responsible for the hypotensive action through enhancement of uveoscleral outflow.[96, 97]

Topical selective α_2-adrenergic agonists, such as apraclonidine and brimonidine, lower intraocular pressure by suppressing aqueous humor production in the ciliary body without altering the tonographically measured aqueous outflow facility.[98, 99] As mentioned earlier, ligand-binding studies showed that the postsynaptic α_2-receptors located in the ciliary body are inhibitory receptors coupled with adenylate cyclase.[54, 100] Activation of the α_2-receptors inhibits cAMP synthesis and diminishes aqueous humor formation.[54] The same effect on cAMP levels can be achieved through blockade of β-receptors, which are positively linked to adenylate cyclase.[53] This finding suggests that both α_2-adrenergic agonists and β-blockers reduce aqueous humor formation by way of a common pathway, with cAMP as a possible intracellular messenger. Despite the relative α_2-receptor selectivity of this class of drugs, decreased blood flow to the ciliary body due to α_1-receptor activity is also suggested as a potential mechanism for the pressure-lowering effect of α_2-adrenergic agonists.[101–103] Other studies also indicated a possible α_2-adrenergic agonist effect on episcleral venous pressure[104] or uveoscleral outflow.[105]

β-ADRENERGIC ANTAGONISTS

The topical β-adrenergic antagonists, or β-blockers, are currently the medications most commonly used in the treatment of glaucoma. They are classified as nonselective β_1-adrenoreceptor and β_2-adrenoreceptor antagonists and β_1-selective antagonists with respect to their actions at β-adrenoreceptor subtypes. Timolol, levobunolol, metipranolol, and carteolol are nonselective β-blockers that can block both β_1-adrenoreceptor and β_2-adrenoreceptor activity, whereas betaxolol is a selective β-blocker that predominantly blocks the β_1 subtype. Unlike the other drugs in this class, carteolol has intrinsic sympathomimetic activity, causing an early, transient agonist response at some adrenergic receptor subtypes.[90]

Fluorophotometric and tonographic studies have demonstrated that the primary mechanism of action of this class of drugs in humans is a decrease in intraocular pressure through a reduction in the rate of aqueous humor formation.[90, 106] The main site of action of the topical β-blockers is thought to be the ciliary body, and their intraocular pressure–lowering effect is believed to be due to blockade of β-adrenergic receptors on nonpigmented ciliary epithelial cells. However, the molecular mechanism by which this class of drug reduces intraocular pressure is still a subject of controversy.

It has been suggested that blocking the β-receptors that are positively linked to adenylate cyclase deactivates adenylate cyclase, thus diminishing cAMP synthesis and reducing aqueous humor formation.[53] If this is true, studies should show a synergy between the β-blockers and α_2-adrenergic agonists.[102] In several studies supporting this hypothesis, an additional decrease in intraocular pressure was shown when apraclonidine was combined with long-term nonselective β-blocker therapy.[107–109] Another study found, however, that apraclonidine combined with short-term nonselective β-blocker (timolol) treatment given during the daytime resulted in no significant additive effect compared with the use of timolol or apraclonidine alone.[110] In addition, it was reported that apraclonidine suppresses nocturnal aqueous flow, unlike timolol, which does not suppress aqueous flow during sleep.[111]

To explain the lack of synergy between acute nonselective β-blocker and α_2-adrenergic agonist treatment and the nocturnal suppression of aqueous only by α_2-adrenergic agonists, it was surmised that a basal rate of cAMP synthesis exists in the ciliary epithelium during sleep and during long-term β-blocker therapy.[107] This basal synthesis is suppressed by α_2-adrenergic agonists. Clearly, more information is required to give a sound molecular basis for the use of β-adrenergic antagonist therapy to lower intraocular pressure. In one study evaluating the effects of β-adrenergic antagonists on the ionic conductance of PE and NPE cells, Ca^{2+}-activated K^+ channels were shown to be modulated by β-adrenergic receptors, suggesting a possible role of these channels in the aqueous formation–reducing effect of β-adrenergic antagonists.[112]

Carbonic Anhydrase Inhibitors

As mentioned previously, the net effect of the carbonic anhydrase enzyme in the ciliary processes is the formation of bicarbonate ion, which is linked to secretion of sodium into the posterior chamber to form aqueous humor. The carbonic anhydrase inhibitor agents are effective in lowering intraocular pressure by inhibiting carbonic anhydrase enzyme in the ciliary body. Inhibition of the enzyme reduces the flow of bicarbonate and sodium to the posterior chamber and the production of aqueous humor.[113] Cole[114] first theorized that the action of acetazolamide was to reduce the transepithelial bioelectric potential that depends on the bicarbonate concentration and sodium transport. This action could have been related either to a reduction in intracellular pH that affected Na^+,K^+-ATPase activity or, possibly, to a reduction in the amount of Na^+ entering the cell by way of the Na^+/H^+ antiport.[114]

It has been shown that inhibiting the carbonic anhydrase enzyme lowers intraocular pressure because of a decrease in aqueous humor production of approximately 20% to 40% with little or no effect on aqueous outflow or episcleral venous pressure.[115] A critical property of carbonic anhydrase inhibitors is that in order to obtain the effect of inhibiting the enzyme, one must completely inhibit nearly 100% of the enzyme at all times.[116] For the oral carbonic anhydrase inhibitor agents that have been an important part of the medical regimen of the glaucoma treatment, obtaining the effect of maximally lowering intraocular pressure involves systemic side effects, including malaise, fatigue, anorexia, depression, loss of libido, gastrointestinal discomfort, paresthesias of the extremities, metabolic acidosis, renal calculi formation, and aplastic anemia.[116] Theoretically, a portion of the effect of systemic carbonic anhydrase inhibitors on aqueous production could also be secondary to their systemic effect on acid-base balance, because systemic acidosis decreases aqueous formation.[117] However, such a contribution would be anticipated to be small. The clinical development of topical carbonic anhydrase inhibitor agents, such as dorzolamide and brinzolamide, allows the effective lowering of intraocular pressure to be achieved without many of the undesirable systemic complications of oral carbonic anhydrase inhibitors; these agents specifically inhibit the carbonic anhydrase isoenzymes important in aqueous humor production.

Prostaglandins

On the basis of early studies in rabbits and monkeys demonstrating the ocular hypotensive effect after intracameral or topical application of certain prostaglandins (PGs), including $PGF_{2\alpha}$ and PGE_2,[118, 119] a variety of PGs, their esters, and their analogues were investigated to evaluate their possible role in the clinical treatment of glaucoma.[120] Latanoprost, a pro-drug of a 17-phenyl–substituted $PGF_{2\alpha}$ analogue, was shown to be a safe and effective agent for treating ocular hypertension and glaucoma.[121] Studies evaluating the mechanism by which PGs reduce intraocular pressure in humans demonstrated that $PGF_{2\alpha}$ and its clinically used analogue latanoprost fail to alter either aqueous humor production or trabecular outflow facility but show their effect by increasing uveoscleral outflow.[122, 123]

Although the biochemical or cellular mechanism by which PGs increase uveoscleral outflow in humans is not known clearly, it has been proposed that $PGF_{2\alpha}$ and latanoprost exert their initial short-term effect (increased uveoscleral outflow) by inducing ciliary muscle relaxation.[124–126] However, results of the studies are conflicting, and either no effect on[127] or no contractile response from[128] the ciliary muscle was also reported with the use of $PGF_{2\alpha}$. One study hypothesized that some of the effects of $PGF_{2\alpha}$ and its analogues may be mediated through the release of endogenous PGs and documented that exogenous $PGF_{2\alpha}$ and latanoprost stimulate the formation of PGE_2, PGD_2, and $PGF_{2\alpha}$ in iris and ciliary muscles isolated from cat, cow, rabbit, dog, rhesus monkey, and human eyes.[129] According to this study, relaxation of ciliary muscle by $PGF_{2\alpha}$ and its analogues via release of endogenous PGE_2, a potent activator of the adenylate cyclase system, could in part explain how these PGs may increase uveoscleral outflow and consequently lower intraocular pressure.

That PGs exert their effect on the ciliary body extracellular matrix at a biochemical level to alter uveoscleral outflow is also suggested as a possible mechanism of action for reducing intraocular pressure.[130] In cultured human ciliary muscle cells, $PGF_{2\alpha}$ has been shown to induce c-fos (a proto-oncogene), which may stimulate several matrix metalloproteinases, leading to extracellular matrix degradation.[131] Demonstration of an increase in the concentrations of metalloproteinases with the use of $PGF_{2\alpha}$ and latanoprost in another study suggested that induction of matrix metalloproteinases in situ following topical PG treatment may degrade ciliary muscle extracellular matrix and possibly contributes to increased uveoscleral outflow as well.[132] The results of an in vitro study showing that PG treatment of ciliary smooth muscle cells can reduce collagen types I and III in the adjacent extracellular matrix also support this hypothesis.[133]

SURGICAL TREATMENT

Antimetabolites

The use of antimetabolites, such as 5-fluorouracil and mitomycin C, in conjunction with glaucoma filtration surgery to limit fibroblast proliferation at the filtering site has been advocated to improve success of surgical treatment. In addition to their wound healing–retardation effects, antimetabolites may also exert an intraocular pressure–lowering effect by reducing aqueous humor production related to a direct impact on the ciliary body.

Among the currently used antimetabolites, mitomycin C seems to have toxic suppressive effects on aqueous humor production in the ciliary epithelium. Supporting evidence comes from one study in which eyes treated with mitomycin C during trabeculectomy showed a reduction of aqueous humor flow of about 56% compared with the unoperated other eye.[134] In another study, histopathologic examination revealed vacuolated cytoplasm and disruption of mitochondria in the ciliary epithelium of a patient who had died 1 week after intraoperative application of mitomycin C during trabeculectomy.[135] Severe signs of destruction were also detected in unmyelinated and myelinated nerves in rabbit ciliary bodies after application of mitomycin C on intact sclera for 5 minutes; this effect is suggested to compromise the production of aqueous humor in rabbits and possibly also in humans.[136] Changes in nonpigmented ciliary epithelium, including swollen and disrupted mitochondria, irregular endoplasmic reticulum, and an electron-dense material within the cytoplasm, have been demonstrated adjacent to and directly opposite the areas where a sponge with mitomycin C has been placed.[137] In contrast to the previously described histopathologic findings, another study found no stromal or epithelial morphologic changes of toxic origin in the ciliary processes, even in specimens adjacent to the surgical area, after the use of intraoperative mitomycin C during trabeculectomy.[138]

Cyclodestructive Procedures

The cyclodestructive procedures cyclodiathermy, cyclocryotherapy, therapeutic ultrasound, and laser cyclophotocoagulation are used in glaucoma treatment to decrease aqueous humor production by destroying the ciliary epithelium, the stroma, and the vascular supply of the ciliary body.[139] Because of their relatively high rate of complications, this group of procedures has generally been reserved for treatment of eyes with refractory glaucoma.

Cyclodiathermy was introduced in 1932 as an operation for the treatment of glaucoma; it involved the use of electrocautery to produce selective destruction of ciliary processes.[140] In this technique, heat was applied to the scleral surface through a probe and transmitted through full-thickness or partial-thickness sclera to the ciliary body. Although selective ciliary body destruction was demonstrated as the cause of the decrease in aqueous humor production in cyclodiathermy, hemorrhage and inflammation were also described as likely causes of lower intraocular pressure.[141] Demonstration of a 5% chance of useful intraocular pressure reduction and a 5% incidence of phthisis bulbi reduced the use of cyclodiathermy as the primary mode of cyclodestruction.[142] However, a 1990 report has concluded that this technique remains a clinically important therapy with results as effective and complications as limited as those of newer cyclodestructive procedures.[143]

Cyclocryotherapy was introduced in 1950[144] and, as a simple, relatively more predictable and less destructive procedure than cyclodiathermy, became the most widely used cyclodestructive technique until relatively recently. It was demonstrated histopathologically that cryotherapy destroys epithelial, vascular, and stromal elements of the ciliary processes, which were replaced by fibroblast-like cells.[145, 146] The loss of the ciliary epithelium and reduction of ciliary body blood flow[147] secondary to cryotherapy were believed to result in decreased aqueous production. However, reports from other studies suggested that hypotension may not be directly due to cyclodestruction but instead may be related to the ocular irritative response to and the extent of neuroepithelial defect caused by the procedure.[148]

The therapeutic ultrasound technique, which uses focused transscleral ultrasound radiation to produce localized ciliary body ablation, was first used in glaucoma treatment in 1985.[149] Although the mechanism by which therapeutic ultrasound lowers the intraocular pressure is not clear, the ciliary destruction, scleral thinning, and the creation of a cyclodialysis cleft seem to contribute to the final reduction in intraocular pressure.[149, 150]

In the last several years, laser cyclophotocoagulation techniques, including laser transpupillary or transscleral cyclophotocoagulation and laser endophotocoagulation, have become the treatments of choice when ciliary body destruction is indicated.[139] The particular appeal of cyclophotocoagulation is that it may selectively target the structures involved in aqueous production.[151] Laser energy is generally absorbed by melanin, which is contained within the stromal and epithelial melanophores of the ciliary body.[152] Blood also absorbs laser energy, and it is likely that cyclophotocoagulation treatments produce substantial thrombosis, which can theoretically render the ciliary body ischemic.[153] It is also quite possible that secondary inflammatory effects associated with laser cyclophotocoagulation treatments could produce substantial lowering of intraocular pressure through a variety of cellular effects upon the ciliary epithelium.[151]

Histopathologic studies of eyes treated with laser transscleral cyclophotocoagulation demonstrated destruction of both the nonpigmented and pigmented ciliary body epithelium with occlusion of the capillaries of the ciliary processes and stromal necrosis.[154–156] Hyperplasia of the pigmented and nonpigmented epithelium with fibrosis and atrophy of the ciliary processes has been shown 4 to 8 weeks after treatment.[154] Histopathologic studies of eyes treated with laser endophotocoagulation indicated partial ciliary epithelium disruption and stromal hemorrhage.[157]

REFERENCES

1. Fine BS, Zimmerman LE: Light and electron microscopic observations on the ciliary epithelium in man and rhesus monkey. Invest Ophthalmol 1963;2:105.
2. Streeten BW: Ciliary body. *In* Tasman W, Jaeger EA (eds): Duane's Foundations of Clinical Ophthalmology, vol 1. Hagerstown, MD, JB Lippincott, 1995.
3. Straatsma BR, Landers MB, Kreiger AE: The ora serrata in the adult human eye. Arch Ophthalmol 1968;80:3.
4. McCulloch C: The zonules of Zinn: Its origin, course, and insertion and its relation to neighboring structures. Trans Am Ophthalmol Soc 1954;52:525.
5. Raviola G: The fine structure of the ciliary zonule and ciliary epithelium: With special regard to the organization and insertion of the zonular fibrils. Invest Ophthalmol Vis Sci 1971;10:851.
6. Rohen J: Scanning electron microscopic studies of the zonular apparatus in human and monkey eyes. Invest Ophthalmol Vis Sci 1979;18:133.
7. Morrison JC, Freddo TF: Anatomy, microcirculation, and ultrastructure of the ciliary body. *In* Ritch R, Shields MB, Krupin T (eds): The Glaucomas, 2nd ed, vol 1. St. Louis, Mosby–Year Book, 1996, p 125.
8. Sears ML: Dynamics of ocular fluids and control of intraocular pressure: Formation of aqueous humor. *In* Albert DM, Jakobiec FA (eds): Principles and Practice of Ophthalmology: Basic Sciences. Philadelphia, WB Saunders, 1994, p 182.
9. Hara K, Lütjen-Drecoll E, Prestle H, et al: Structural differences between regions of the ciliary body in primates. Invest Ophthalmol Vis Sci 1977;6:912.
10. Raviola G: The structural basis of the blood-ocular barriers. Exp Eye Res 1977;25(suppl):27.
11. Raviola G, Raviola E: Intercellular junctions in the ciliary epithelium. Invest Ophthalmol Vis Sci 1978;17:958.
12. Araki M: Changes of the ciliary region and the ciliary zonule in accommodation. Jpn J Ophthalmol 1965;9:150.
13. Kupfer C: Relationship of ciliary body meridional muscle and corneoscleral trabecular meshwork. Arch Ophthalmol 1962;68:818.
14. Pederson JE, Gaasterland DE, MacLellan HM: Uveoscleral aqueous outflow in the rhesus monkey: Importance of uveal reabsorption. Invest Ophthalmol Vis Sci 1977;16:1008.
15. Morrison JC, Van Buskirk EM: Anterior collateral circulation in the primate eye. Ophthalmology 1983;90:707.
16. Morrison JC, Van Buskirk EM: Sequential microdissection and scanning electron microscopy of ciliary microvascular castings. Scanning Electron Microsc 1984;2:857.
17. Morrison JC, Van Buskirk EM: Ciliary process microvasculature of the primate eye. Ophthalmology 1984;97:372.
18. Westheimer G, Blair SM: The parasympathetic pathways to internal eye muscles. Invest Ophthalmol Vis Sci 1973;12:193.
19. Ehinger B: Ocular and orbital vegetative nerves. Acta Physiol Scand 1966;67:1.
20. Kinsey VE, Barany E: The rate of flow of aqueous humor: Derivation of rate of flow and its physiological significance. Am J Ophthalmol 1949;32:189.
21. Green K, Pederson JE: Aqueous humor formation. Exp Eye Res 1973;16:273.
22. Reddy DVN: Dynamics of transport systems in the eye. Invest Ophthalmol Vis Sci 1979;18:1000.
23. Krupin T, Civan MM: Physiologic basis of aqueous humor formation. *In* Ritch R, Shields MB, Krupin T (eds): The Glaucomas, 2nd ed, vol 1. St. Louis, Mosby–Year Book, 1996.
24. Kishida K, Sasabe T, Manabe R, et al: Electric characteristics of the isolated rabbit ciliary body. Jpn J Ophthalmol 1981;25:407.
25. Holland MG, Stockwell M: Sodium ion transport of ciliary body in vitro. Invest Ophthalmol 1967;6:401.
26. Watanabe T, Saito Y: Characteristics of ion transport across the isolated ciliary epithelium of the toad as studied by electrical measurements. Exp Eye Res 1978;27:215.
27. Edelman J, Sachs G, Adorante JS: Ion transport asymmetry and functional coupling in bovine pigmented and nonpigmented ciliary epithelial cells. Am J Physiol 1994;266:C1210.
28. Oh J, Krupin T, Tang L, et al: Dye coupling of rabbit ciliary epithelial cells in vitro. Invest Ophthalmol Vis Sci 1994;35:2509.
29. Levenson R: Isoforms of the Na,K-ATPase: Family membranes in search of function. Rev Physiol Pharmacol 1994;123:1.
30. Kuwahara S, Mito T, Delamere NA: Studies on Na,K-ATPase in cultured non-pigmented ciliary epithelial cells. Invest Ophthalmol Vis Sci 1996;37:S1107.
31. Wiederholt M, Helbig H, Korbmacher C: Ion transport across the ciliary epithelium: Lessons from cultured cells and proposed role of the carbonic anhydrase. *In* Botre F, Gross G, Storey BT (eds): Carbonic Anhydrase. New York, Cambridge University Press, 1991, p 232.
32. Edelman JL, Loo DDF, Sachs G: Characterization of potassium and chloride channels in the basolateral membrane of bovine nonpigmented ciliary epithelial cells. Invest Ophthalmol Vis Sci 1995;36:2706.
33. Botchkin LM, Balaev AG, Matthews G: Physiological regulation of Ca-dependent K current in rabbit ciliary body epithelial cells. Invest Ophthalmol Vis Sci 1997;38:S1042.
34. Gabelt BT, Kiland JA, Peterson JA, et al: Effects of the Na/K/2Cl co-transport inhibitor bumetanide on aqueous humor formation and outflow facility in monkeys. Invest Ophthalmol Vis Sci 1996;37:S201.
35. Helbig H, Korbmacher C, Kuhner D, et al: Characterization of Cl^-/HCO_3^- exchange in cultured pigmented ciliary epithelial cells. Curr Eye Res 1988;8:595.
36. Delamere NA, Williams RN: A comparative study on the uptake of ascorbic acid by the iris-ciliary body of the rabbit, guinea pig, and rat. Comp Biochem Physiol 1987;88:847.
37. Helbig H, Korbmacher C, Wohlfarth J, et al: Electrogenic Na^+-ascorbate cotransport in cultured bovine pigmented ciliary epithelial cells. Am J Physiol 1989;256:C44.
38. Hasegawa H, Lian SC, Finkbeiner WE, et al: Extrarenal tissue distribution of CHIP28 water channels by in situ hybridization and antibody staining. Am J Physiol 1994;266:C893.
39. Bonting SL, Becker B: Studies on sodium-potassium–activated adenosinetriphosphatase. IV: Inhibition of enzyme activity and aqueous humor flow in the rabbit eye after intravitreal injection of ouabain. Invest Ophthalmol 1964;3:523.
40. Cole DF: Secretion of the aqueous humor. Exp Eye Res 1977;25 Suppl:161.
41. Krupin T, Fritz C, Reinach PS, et al: Transepithelial electrical measurements on the isolated rabbit iris-ciliary body. Exp Eye Res 1984;38:115.
42. Sears ML, Yamada E, Cummins D, et al: The isolated ciliary epithelial bilayer is useful for in vitro studies of aqueous humor formation. Invest Ophthalmol Vis Sci 1991;32:978.
43. Delamere NA, Socci R, King KI: Alteration of sodium, potassium-adenosine triphosphatase activity in rabbit ciliary processes by cyclic adenosine monophosphate-dependent protein kinase. Invest Ophthalmol Vis Sci 1990;31:2164.
44. Delamere NA, King KI: The influence of cyclic AMP upon Na,K-ATPase activity in rabbit ciliary epithelium. Invest Ophthalmol Vis Sci 1992;33:430.
45. Maren TH: HCO_3^- formation in aqueous humor: Mechanism and relation to the treatment of glaucoma. Invest Ophthalmol 1974;13:479.
46. Becker B: The effects of carbonic anhydrase inhibitor, acetazola-

mide, on the composition of the aqueous humor. Am J Ophthalmol 1955;40:129.
47. Garg LC, Oppelt WW: The effect of ouabain and acetazolamide on transport of sodium and chloride from plasma to aqueous humor. J Pharmacol Exp Ther 1970;175:237.
48. Zimmerman TJ, Garg LC, Vogh BP, et al: The effect of acetazolamide on the movement of sodium into the posterior chamber of the dog eye. J Pharmacol Exp Ther 1976;199:510.
49. Becker B: Decrease in intraocular pressure in man by a carbonic anhydrase inhibitor, Diamox: A preliminary report. Am J Ophthalmol 1954;37:13.
50. Maren TH: Ion secretion into the posterior aqueous humor of dogs and monkeys. Exp Eye Res 1977;25(suppl):245.
51. Waitzman MB, Woods WD: Some characteristics of an adenyl cyclase preparation from rabbit ciliary process tissue. Exp Eye Res 1971;12:99.
52. Bromberg BB, Gregory DS, Sears ML: Beta adrenergic receptors in ciliary processes of the rabbit. Invest Ophthalmol Vis Sci 1980;19:203.
53. Nathanson JA: Adrenergic regulation of intraocular pressure: Identification of β_2-adrenergic-stimulated adenylate cyclase in ciliary process epithelium. Proc Natl Acad Sci U S A 1980;77:7420.
54. Mittag TW, Tormay A: Drug responses of adenylate cyclase in iris-ciliary body determined by labelling. Invest Ophthalmol Vis Sci 1985;26:396.
55. Horio B, Sears M, Mead A, et al: Regulation and bioelectrical effects of cyclic adenosine monophosphate production in the ciliary epithelial bilayer. Invest Ophthalmol Vis Sci 1996;37:607.
56. Bausher LP, Gregory DS, Sears ML: Interaction between alpha 2- and beta 2-adrenergic receptors in rabbit ciliary processes. Curr Eye Res 1987;6:497.
57. Sears ML: Regulation of aqueous flow by the adenylate cyclase receptor complex in the ciliary epithelium. Am J Ophthalmol 1985;100:194.
58. Topper JE, Brubaker RF: Effects of timolol, epinephrine, and acetazolamide on aqueous flow during sleep. Invest Ophthalmol Vis Sci 1985;26:1315.
59. Levene AZ: Osmolarity in the normal state and following acetazolamide. Arch Ophthalmol 1958;59:597.
60. Caprioli J: The ciliary epithelium and aqueous humor. *In* Moses RA, Hart WM (eds): Adler's Physiology of the Eye: Clinical Application. St. Louis, Mosby–Year Book, 1987, p 204.
61. De Berardinis E, Tieri O, Polzella A, Iuglio N: The chemical composition of the human aqueous humor in normal and pathological conditions. Exp Eye Res 1965;4:179.
62. Gaasterland DF, Pedersen JE, MacLellan HM, Reddy VN: Rhesus monkey aqueous humor composition and a primate ocular perfusate. Invest Ophthalmol Vis Sci 1979;18:1139.
63. Bito L: Intraocular fluid dynamics. I: Steady-state concentration gradients of magnesium, potassium and calcium in relation to the sites and mechanisms of ocular cation transport processes. Exp Eye Res 1970;10:102.
64. Walker AM: Comparison of the chemical composition of aqueous humor, cerebrospinal fluid, lymph, and blood from frogs, higher animals and man. J Biol Chem 1933;101:269.
65. Kinsey VE: Transfer of ascorbic acid and related compounds across the blood-aqueous barrier. Am J Ophthalmol 1947;30:1262.
66. Socci RR, Delamere NA: Characteristics of ascorbate transport in the rabbit iris-ciliary body. Exp Eye Res 1988;46:853.
67. Stjernschantz J, Uusitalo R, Palkama A: The aqueous proteins of the rat in the normal eye and after aqueous withdrawal. Exp Eye Res 1973;16:215.
68. Dernouchamps JP: The proteins of the aqueous humor. Doc Ophthalmol 1982;53:193.
69. Reddy DVN, Rosenberg C, Kinsey VE: Steady-state distribution of free amino acids in the aqueous humors, vitreous body, and plasma of the rabbit. Exp Eye Res 1961;1:175.
70. Bill A: Basic physiology of the drainage of aqueous humor. Exp Eye Res 1997;25(Suppl):291.
71. Pederson JE: Uveoscleral outflow. *In* Ritch R, Shields MB, Krupin T (eds): The Glaucomas, 2nd ed, vol 1. St. Louis, Mosby–Year Book, 1996, p 337.
72. Inomata H, Bill A: Exit sites of uveoscleral outflow aqueous humor in cynomolgus monkey eyes. Exp Eye Res 1977;25:113.
73. Kleinstein RN, Fatt I: Pressure dependency of transcleral flow. Exp Eye Res 1977;24:335.
74. Inomata H, Bill A, Smelser GK: Unconventional routes of aqueous humor outflow in cynomolgus monkeys (*Macaca irus*): An electron microscopic study. Am J Ophthalmol 1972;73:893.
75. Van Alpen GWHM: On emmetropia and ametropia. Ophthalmologica 1961;142(suppl):47.
76. Emi K, Pederson JE, Toris CB: Hydrostatic pressure of the suprachoroidal space. Invest Ophthalmol Vis Sci 1989;30:233.
77. Bill A: Conventional and uveoscleral drainage of aqueous humor in the cynomolgus monkey (*Macaca irus*) at normal and high intraocular pressures. Exp Eye Res 1966;5:45.
78. Bill A: Further studies on the influence of the intraocular pressure on aqueous humor dynamics in cynomolgus monkeys. Invest Ophthalmol Vis Sci 1967;6:364.
79. Toris CB, Gregerson DS, Pederson JE: Uveoscleral outflow using different-sized fluorescent tracers in normal and inflamed eyes. Exp Eye Res 1987;45:525.
80. Toris CB, Pederson JE: Aqueous humor dynamics in experimental iridocyclitis. Invest Ophthalmol Vis Sci 1987;28:477.
81. Suguro K, Toris CB, Pederson JE: Uveoscleral outflow following cyclodialysis in the monkey eye using a fluorescent tracer. Invest Ophthalmol Vis Sci 1985;26:810.
82. Toris CB, Pederson JE: Effect of intraocular pressure on uveoscleral outflow following cyclodialysis in the monkey eye. Invest Ophthalmol Vis Sci 1985;26:1745.
83. Toris CB, Yablonski ME, Camras CB, et al: Uveoscleral outflow decreases with age in ocular normotensive humans. Invest Ophthalmol Vis Sci 1996;37:S410.
84. Nardin GF, Zimmerman TJ: Ocular cholinergic agents. *In* Ritch R, Shields MB, Krupin T (eds): The Glaucomas, 2nd ed, vol 3. St. Louis, Mosby–Year Book, 1996, p 1399.
85. Erickson KA: Basic aspects of parasympathetic pharmacology. *In* Ritch R, Shields MB, Krupin T (eds): The Glaucomas, 2nd ed, vol 3. St. Louis, Mosby–Year Book, 1996, p 1385.
86. Kaufman PL, Barany EH: Loss of acute pilocarpine effect on outflow facility following surgical disinsertion and retrodisplacement of the ciliary muscle from the scleral spur in the cynomolgus monkey. Invest Ophthalmol 1976;15:793.
87. Jumblatt JE, North GT, Hackmiller RC: Muscarinic cholinergic inhibition of adenylate cyclase in the rabbit iris-ciliary body and ciliary epithelium. Invest Ophthalmol Vis Sci 1990;31:1103.
88. Erickson-Lamy KA, Schroeder A: Dissociation between the effect of aceclidine on outflow facility and accommodation. Exp Eye Res 1990;50:143.
89. Gil DW, Krauss HA, Bogardus AM, et al: Muscarinic receptor subtypes in human iris-ciliary body measured by immunoprecipitation. Invest Ophthalmol Vis Sci 1997;38:1434.
90. Gieser SC, Juzych M, Robin AL, et al: Clinical pharmacology of adrenergic drugs. *In* Ritch R, Shields MB, Krupin T (eds): The Glaucomas, 2nd ed, vol 3. St. Louis, Mosby–Year Book, 1996, p 1425.
91. Townsend DJ, Brubaker RF: Immediate effect of epinephrine on aqueous formation in the normal human eye as measured by fluorophotometry. Invest Ophthalmol Vis Sci 1980;19:256.
92. Higgins RG, Brubaker RF: Acute effect of epinephrine on aqueous humor formation in the timolol-treated normal eye as measured by fluorophotometry. Invest Ophthalmol Vis Sci 1980;19:420.
93. Robinson JC, Kaufman PL: Effects and interactions of epinephrine, norepinephrine, timolol, and betaxolol on outflow facility in the cynomolgus monkey. Am J Ophthalmol 1990;109:189.
94. Bill A: Early effects of epinephrine on aqueous humor dynamics in vervet monkeys (*Cercopithecus ethiops*). Exp Eye Res 1969;8:35.
95. Schenker H, Yablonski MF, Podos SM, et al: Fluorophotometric study of epinephrine and timolol in human subjects. Arch Ophthalmol 1981;99:1212.
96. Bhattacherjee P, Hammond BR: Effect of indomethacin on the ocular hypotensive action of adrenaline on the rabbit. Exp Eye Res 1977;24:307.
97. Camras CB, Feldman SC, Podos SM, et al: Inhibition of the epinephrine-induced reduction of intraocular pressure by systemic indomethacin in humans. Am J Ophthalmol 1985;100:169.
98. Gharagozloo NZ, Relf SJ, Brubaker RF: Aqueous flow is reduced by the alpha-adrenergic agonist, apraclonidine hydrochloride (ALO 2145). Ophthalmology 1988;95:1217.
99. Serle JB, Steidl S, Wang RF, et al: Selective α_2-adrenergic agonists B-HT 920 and UK14304-18. Effects on aqueous humor dynamics in monkeys. Arch Ophthalmol 1991;109:1158.

100. Mittag TW, Tormay A: Adrenergic receptor subtypes in rabbit iris-ciliary body membranes: Classification by radioligand studies. Exp Eye Res 1985;40:239.
101. Funk R, Rohen JW: Scanning electron microscopical and microendoscopical studies on the vasculature of human and rabbit ciliary processes. Invest Ophthalmol Vis Sci 1990;31(suppl):380.
102. Huang AS, Pollack IP: Apraclonidine and the treatment of glaucoma. Ophthalmol Clin North Am 1995;8:303-314.
103. Zhan GL, Toris CB, Gaffney MM, et al: Effects of apraclonidine and brimonidine on rabbit ocular blood flow. Invest Ophthalmol Vis Sci 1997;38:S783.
104. Abrams DL, Robin AL, Crandall AS, et al: A limited comparison of apraclonidine's dose response in subjects with normal or increased intraocular pressure. Am J Ophthalmol 1989;108:230.
105. Wang RF, Lee PY, Taniguchi T, et al: Effect of oxymetazoline on aqueous humor dynamics and ocular blood flow in monkeys and rabbits. Arch Ophthalmol 1993;111:535.
106. Dailey RA, Brubaker RF, Bourne WM: The effects of timolol maleate and acetazolamide on the rate of aqueous formation in normal human subjects. Am J Ophthalmol 1982;93:232.
107. Gharagozloo NZ, Brubaker RF: Effect of apraclonidine in long-term timolol users. Ophthalmology 1991;98:1543.
108. Yaldo MK, Shin DH, Parrow KA, et al: Additive effect of 1% apraclonidine hydrochloride to nonselective β-blockers. Ophthalmology 1991;98:1075.
109. Sonty SP, Sonty S, Viana MAG: The additive ocular hypotensive effect of topical 0.5% apraclonidine on glaucomatous eyes on topical beta blocker therapy. Invest Ophthalmol Vis Sci 1996;36:S738.
110. Koskela T, Brubaker RF: Apraclonidine and timolol: Combined effects in previously untreated normal subjects. Arch Ophthalmol 1991;109:804.
111. McCannel CA, Heinrich SR, Brubaker RF: Acetazolamide but not timolol lowers aqueous humor flow in sleeping humans. Invest Ophthalmol Vis Sci 1991;32(suppl):1256.
112. Bhattacharyya B, Krupin D, Bearelly S, et al: Ca-activated "Maxi" K-channel activity in rabbit ciliary epithelial cells is modulated by β-adrenergic agents. Invest Ophthalmol Vis Sci 1997;38:S819.
113. Maren TH: The rates of movement of Na^+, Cl^-, and HCO_3^- from plasma to posterior chamber: Effect of acetazolamide and relation to the treatment of glaucoma. Invest Ophthalmol 1976;15:356.
114. Cole DF: Electrochemical changes associated with the formation of the aqueous humor. Br J Ophthalmol 1961;45:202.
115. Lippa EA: Carbonic anhydrase inhibitors. *In* Ritch R, Shields MB, Krupin T (eds): The Glaucomas, 2nd ed, vol 3. St. Louis, Mosby–Year Book, 1996, p 1463.
116. Gross RL, Oram O: Update on carbonic anhydrase inhibitors. Ophthalmol Clin North Am 1997;10:327.
117. Bietti G, Virno M, Pecori-Giraldi J, et al: Acetazolamide, metabolic acidosis and intraocular pressure. Am J Ophthalmol 1975;80:360.
118. Camras CB, Bito LZ: Reduction of intraocular pressure in normal and glaucomatous primate *(Aotus trivirgatus)* eyes by topically applied prostaglandin $F_{2\alpha}$. Curr Eye Res 1981;1:205.
119. Camras CB, Bito LZ, Eakins KE: Reduction of intraocular pressure by prostaglandins applied topically to the eyes of conscious rabbits. Invest Ophthalmol Vis Sci 1977;16:1125.
120. Camras CB: Prostaglandins. *In* Ritch R, Shields MB, Krupin T (eds): The Glaucomas, 2nd ed, vol 3. St. Louis, Mosby–Year Book, 1996, p 1449.
121. Camras CB, Alm A, Watson P, et al: Latanoprost, a prostaglandin analog, for glaucoma therapy: Efficacy and safety after 1 year of treatment in 198 patients. Latanoprost Study Groups. Ophthalmology 1996;103:1916.
122. Villumsen J, Alm A: Prostaglandin $F_{2\alpha}$-isopropylester eye drops: Effects in normal human eyes. Br J Ophthalmol 1989;73:419.
123. Toris CB, Camras CB, Yablonski ME: Effects of PhXA41, a new prostaglandin $F_{2\alpha}$ analog, on aqueous humor dynamics in human eyes. Ophthalmology 1993;100:1297.
124. Nilsson SFE, Samuelsson M, Bill A, et al: Increased uveoscleral outflow as a possible mechanism of ocular hypotension caused by prostaglandin $F_{2\alpha}$-1-isopropylester in the cynomolgus monkey. Exp Eye Res 1989;48:707.
125. Poyer JF, Millar C, Kaufman PL: Prostaglandin $F_{2\alpha}$ effects on isolated rhesus monkey ciliary muscle. Invest Ophthalmol Vis Sci 1995;36:2461.
126. Fristrom B, Nilsson SEG: Interaction of PhXA41, a new prostaglandin analogue, with pilocarpine. Arch Ophthalmol 1993;111:662.
127. Chen J, Woodward DF: Prostanoid-induced relaxation of precontracted cat ciliary muscle is mediated by EP_2 and DP receptors. Invest Ophthalmol Vis Sci 1992;33:3195.
128. Lograno MD, Giovanazzi DS, Guarrera A, et al: Effects of prostaglandins and PAF on the contractility of the bovine ciliary muscle. Pharmacol Res 1992;25:195.
129. Yousufzai SY, Ye Z, Abdel-Latif AA: Prostaglandin $F_{2\alpha}$ and its analogs induce release of endogenous prostaglandins in iris and ciliary muscles isolated from cat and other mammalian species. Exp Eye Res 1996;63:305.
130. Lutjen-Drecoll E, Tamm E: Morphological study of the anterior segment of cynomolgus monkey eyes following treatment with prostaglandin $F_{2\alpha}$. Exp Eye Res 1988;47:761.
131. Lindsey JD, To HD, Weinreb RN: Induction of c-fos by prostaglandin $F_{2\alpha}$ in human ciliary smooth muscle cells. Invest Ophthalmol Vis Sci 1994;35:242.
132. Lindsey JD, Kashiwagi K, Boyle D, et al: Prostaglandins increase proMMP-1 and proMMP-3 secretion by human ciliary smooth muscle cells. Curr Eye Res 1996;15:869.
133. Weinreb RN, Lindsey JD, Kashiwagi K: Prostaglandin treatment reduces collagen types I and III in cultures of human ciliary smooth muscle cells. Invest Ophthalmol Vis Sci 1997;38:S813.
134. Diestelhorst M, Krieglstein GK: Der Einfluss von Mitomycin C auf die Kammerwassersekretion nach Trabekulektomie. Ophthalmologe 1995;92:542.
135. Nuyts RM, Felten PC, Pels E, et al: Histopathologic effects of mitomycin C after trabeculectomy in human glaucomatous eyes with persistent hypotony. Am J Ophthalmol 1994;118:225.
136. Mietz H, Addicks K, Diestelhorst M, Krieglstein GK: Intraocular toxicity to ciliary nerves after extraocular application of mitomycin C in rabbits. Int Ophthalmol 1995;19:89.
137. Murali S, Skubitz APN, Obritch WF, et al: Intraocular toxicity after extra-ocularly applied mitomycin C: Long-term histologic changes in rabbits. Invest Ophthalmol Vis Sci 1995;36:S876.
138. Hollo G, Suveges I: The effect of brief intrascleral or episcleral application of mitomycin C on the ciliary epithelium and pressure in the rabbit eye. Acta Ophthalmol (Copenh) 1994;72:739.
139. Mastrobattista JM, Luntz M: Ciliary body ablation: Where are we and how did we get here? Surv Ophthalmol 1996;41:193.
140. Weve H: Clinische lessen. Ned Tidjschr Geneeskd 1932;76:5335.
141. Troncoso M: Diathermic surgery of the ciliary body in glaucoma: Experimental and clinical observations. Am J Ophthalmol 1946;29:269.
142. Walton DS, Grant WM: Penetrating cyclodiathermy for filtration. Arch Ophthalmol 1970;83:47.
143. Waked N, Hamard H, Godde-Jolly D, et al: La cyclodiathermie: a-t-elle encore une valeur dans le traitement du glaucome? J Fr Ophthalmol 1990;13:159.
144. Bietti G: Surgical intervention on the ciliary body: New trends for the relief of glaucoma. JAMA 1950;142:889.
145. Quigley HA: Histologic and physiologic studies of cyclocryotherapy in primate and human eyes. Am J Ophthalmol 1976;82:722.
146. Ferry AP: Histopathologic observations on human eyes following cyclocryotherapy for glaucoma. Trans Am Acad Ophthalmol Otol 1977;83:90.
147. Green K, Hull Ds, Bowman K: Cyclocryotherapy and ocular blood flow. Glaucoma 1989;1:141.
148. Schubert HD, Federman JL: The role of inflammation in CW Nd:YAG contact transscleral photocoagulation and cryopexy. Invest Ophthalmol Vis Sci 1989;30:543.
149. Coleman DJ, Lizzi FL, Driller J, et al: Therapeutic ultrasound in the treatment of glaucoma. I: Experimental model. Ophthalmology 1985;92:339.
150. Coleman DJ, Lizzi FL, Driller J, et al: Therapeutic ultrasound in the treatment of glaucoma. II: Clinical applications. Ophthalmology 1985;92:347.
151. Samples JR: Laser cyclophotocoagulation for refractory glaucomas. Ophthalmol Clin North Am 1995;8:401.
152. Coleman AL, Jampel HD, Javitt JC, et al: Transscleral cyclophotocoagulation of human autopsy and monkey eyes. Ophthalmic Surg 1991;92:339.
153. Van der Zypen E, England C, Fankhauser F, et al: Blood flow status induced by cw-Nd:YAG laser light in melanin rich and melanin free tissue. Thromb Haemost 1991;65:87.
154. Marsh P, Wilson DJ, Samples JR, et al: A clinicopathologic correla-

tive study of noncontact transscleral Nd:YAG cyclophotocoagulation. Am J Ophthalmol 1993;115:597.
155. Gross RL, Smith JA, Font RL, et al: Transscleral Nd:YAG laser cycloablation in rabbits. Invest Ophthalmol Vis Sci 1986; 27(suppl):253.
156. Coleman AL, Jampel HD, Javitt JC, et al: Transscleral cyclophotocoagulation of human autopsy and monkey eyes. Ophthalmic Surg 1991;22:638.
157. Shields MB: Cyclodestructive surgery for glaucoma: Past, present and future. Trans Am Ophthalmol Soc 1985;83:282.

CHAPTER 4

Optic Nerve: Anatomy and Physiology

GEORGE A. CIOFFI

Increasingly, we are understanding that the group of diseases we refer to as *glaucoma* are optic neuropathies that have several characteristics in common. Given the central role of the optic nerve in this disease, it is vital that we understand the basic anatomy and physiology of this structure. Jack Cioffi has brought together this information to allow us to understand the anatomy and vascular supply of the retina, retinal nerve fiber layer, and optic nerve. Expanding into pathologic processes, he then discusses the factors that affect the optic nerve in glaucoma as well as other pathologic changes, such as peripapillary atrophy. In an attempt to get to the heart of the disease process, he puts current knowledge concerning optic nerve blood flow and neuroprotection in perspective. This chapter closely relates to Chapter 5, Optic Nerve Assessment, as well as Chapter 27, Optic Nerve Outcomes.

General Anatomy of the Optic Nerve[1–5]

The optic nerve serves as the neural connection between the visual sensory components of the eye and the brain. An understanding of the anatomy and physiology of the optic nerve is central to understanding glaucoma, because all forms of glaucoma are united by a characteristic dysfunction of the optic nerve. After processing by the inner and outer layers of the retina, neural signals are sent via the retinal ganglion cells and their axons to the lateral geniculate body of the midbrain. In addition, some ganglion cell axons connect with the superior colliculus, the hypothalamus, the pretectal nucleus, and other midbrain centers. As a tract of the central nervous system, the myelin of the optic nerve is produced by oligodendrocytes rather than Schwann cells.

The optic nerve extends from the superficial retinal ganglion cell layer within the eye to the optic chiasm. The optic disc, or optic nerve head, is the anteriormost aspect of the optic nerve and can be examined ophthalmoscopically. The optic disc is located approximately 3.5 mm nasal to the fovea. The optic disc is slightly oval, with an average vertical diameter of 1.7 mm and an average horizontal diameter of 1.5 mm. The optic nerve can then be separated into four anatomic regions:

- Intraocular, or anterior, optic nerve
- Retrobulbar, or intraorbital, optic nerve
- Intracannulicular optic nerve
- Intracranial optic nerve

The anterior optic nerve is the only portion of the optic nerve that is nonmyelinated. The anterior optic nerve is approximately 1 mm in length, extending from the retinal surface to posterior aspect of the globe.

In the adult, the retrobulbar or intraorbital optic nerve is approximately 30 mm long and extends from the posterior aspect of the globe to the optic canal. The distance between the posterior aspect of the globe and the optic canal is approximately 20 mm. Therefore, there is redundancy in the length of the intraorbital optic nerve, which results in an S-shaped configuration of the nerve. The orbital portion of the optic nerve becomes myelinated as it exits the globe and is also surrounded by the meningeal coverings of the central nervous system.

The intracannulicular optic nerve is the portion of the nerve that passes from the posterior orbit to the intracranial cavity, via the optic canal. The ophthalmic artery also passes through the optic canal. The intracannulicular portion of the optic nerve is typically 5 to 10 mm long.

The intracranial portion of the optic nerve is approximately 10 to 15 mm in length. At the posterior aspect of the nerve, the nerve fibers join with the optic chiasm, which subsequently extends to the optic tracks.

Retinal Ganglion Cell Layer and Retinal Nerve Fiber Layer[6–12]

The ganglion cell bodies are located anterior to the inner plexiform layer of the retina. Ganglion cells receive information via dendritic connections with the bipolar cells of the retina and interneural modifier cells, such as amacrine cells, after processing of the neural information within the retina. The ganglion cell layer is also known as the inner nuclear layer of the retina.

Multiple subclassifications of ganglion cells have been differentiated. Ganglion cells with larger cell bodies, more diffuse dendritic fields, and thicker axonal segments are principally located in the retinal periphery. These ganglion cells are known as *M cells* or *alpha cells*. The M cell is principally involved in transmitting information related to motion detection and rapid flicker as well as providing signals under scotopic illumination. A second group of retinal ganglion cells that have smaller dendritic fields, thinner axons, and are more common in the central foveal region of the retina (cone receptive fields) have also been described. These cells, known as *P cells* or *beta cells*, are more sensitive to color stimuli as well as to stimuli with high spatial frequencies associated with high levels of illumination.

There are approximately 1.2 million ganglion cells in the adult human retina, and approximately 100 photoreceptor cells for each retinal ganglion cell. The ganglion cell layer is thickest in the macular and parafoveal regions. In these regions, the ganglion cell bodies may be layered five to six deep, although the foveal region itself has no ganglion cells. Throughout most of the retina, ganglion cells are single-layered. The number of nerve fibers is indirectly correlated with age.

The retinal nerve fiber layer lies anterior to the ganglion cell layer and is composed primarily of the axons of the ganglion cells. Astrocytes and superficial retinal vessels also lie within this layer. The processes of Müller cells extend through the nerve fiber layer to form the internal limiting membrane. Axons extending from the ganglion cells closer to the optic nerve head lie more anterior within the nerve fiber layer than axons extending from peripheral ganglion cells.

Retinal ganglion cell axons or nerve fibers converge radially to form the optic nerve. The nerve fibers enter the optic nerve in a characteristic pattern (Fig. 4–1). Fibers entering the superior and inferior temporal aspects of the optic nerve originate from the peripheral retina, taking an arcuate course around the macula to enter the nerve. These fibers are the most susceptible to damage in early glaucomatous optic neuropathy. Fibers originating from the macular region, called the *papillomacular fibers*, occupy approximately one third of the temporal optic nerve. Arcuate fibers originate either superior or inferior to the median raphae and arch above and below the fovea. Papillomacular fibers take a more direct course from the macular and perimacular regions to the optic nerve.

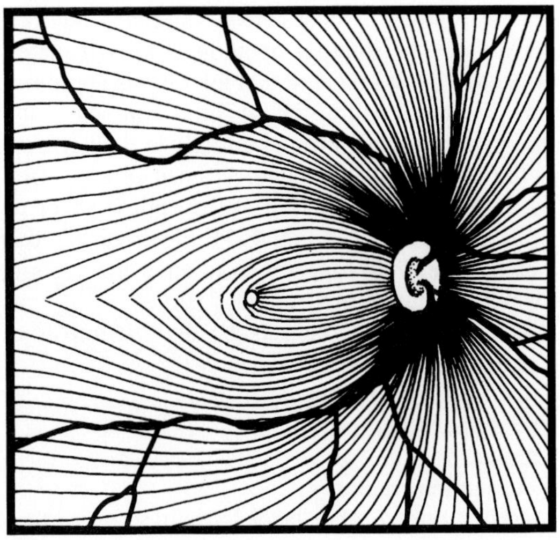

FIGURE 4–1. Nerve fiber layer organization. The retinal nerve fibers (ganglion cell axons) converge at the optic nerve. Arcuate fibers extend from the temporal retina above and below the macular region. (From Wright K (ed): Textbook of Ophthalmology. Baltimore, Williams & Wilkins, 1997.)

Other nerve fibers from the superior, inferior, and nasal retina converge directly to the optic nerve. The superotemporal and inferotemporal aspects of the optic nerve contain the greatest number of axons. The temporal and nasal regions are the thinnest regions of the optic disc. The neural glial cells (primarily astrocytes and Müller's cells) provide a structural framework that supports the axonal component of the nerve fiber layer. These glial structures partially separate groups of axons into nerve fiber bundles, and the distribution of these bundles can be detected ophthalmoscopically as they radiate from the optic nerve. This ophthalmoscopic observation is easiest in the superior and inferior temporal regions, corresponding to the regions of the thickest axonal distribution.

Anatomy of the Anterior Optic Nerve[1–4, 13–15]

The anterior optic nerve extends from the superficial retinal surface to the retrobulbar space, where the nerve exits the globe. The anterior optic nerve is composed of the axonal elements of the retinal ganglion cells, neural glial cells, blood vessels, and connective tissue. The normal adult human optic nerve contains approximately 1.2 million axons. At the superficial retinal level of the optic nerve, axons of the retinal nerve fiber layer constitute approximately 90% of the nerve tissue volume. As described previously, the ganglion cell bodies are located in the innermost nuclear layer of the retina.

At the optic nerve, the axons of the retinal nerve fiber layer turn to exit the eye. The retinal ganglion cell axons leave the eye via the posterior scleral canal or foramen. There are no photoreceptor cells overlying the optic disc.

The scleral foramen is most narrow internally and progressively widens. The internal opening is approximately 2.5 mm^2 in area, whereas the external aperture is approximately 3.5 mm^2. The nasal neural retinal rim is composed of axons from the nasal retina that travel directly to the nerve. Axons within the papillomacular bundle transit directly from the macula to the temporal margin of the optic disc, or temporal neural retinal rim (see Fig. 4–1). Fibers of the temporal retina arch around the foveal area to enter the superior and inferior poles of the temporal optic nerve.

The anterior optic nerve may be divided into four anatomic regions (Fig. 4–2):

- □ Superficial nerve fiber layer
- □ Prelaminar region
- □ Laminar region
- □ Retrolaminar region

The superficial nerve fiber layer is the portion of the optic nerve anterior to an imaginary plane extending across the optic nerve from the peripapillary Bruch's membrane. This layer is composed primarily of axons extending from the retinal nerve fiber layer and is similar in composition.

Immediately posterior to the superficial nerve fiber layer is the prelaminar region, which lies adjacent to the peripapillary choroid. The prelaminar region is distinguished by hypercellular glial septa (primarily astrocytes) with minimal connective tissue. The superficial nerve fiber layer and prelaminar region constitute the optic nerve head. The optic nerve head, or *optic disc*, is the anterior surface of the optic nerve, which is visible ophthalmoscopically. The optic disc is slightly oval, with a larger vertical diameter.

The laminar region is characterized by a gradual transition from glial columns to dense connective tissue plates, the *lamina cribrosa*. The lamina cribrosa is continuous with the peripapillary sclera but is fenestrated. Its primary function is to allow transit of the neural fibers and retinal vasculature. Each plate of laminar tissue has approximately 300 to 600 sieve-like perforations. The laminar plates are composed of fibroblasts, collagen, ground substance, glycosaminoglycans, and basement membrane. They are curved, with their concave surfaces in an anterior direction. Astrocytes are the predominant glial cells populating the laminar region.

Posterior to the lamina cribrosa is the retrolaminar region, which is marked by the beginning of the meningeal sheaths, myelinated axons, and delicate connective tissue septa. The optic nerve sheaths are composed of the innermost pia mater, the arachnoidea, and the outermost dura mater. The space between the optic nerve and sheaths communicates with the analogous cerebral space. The myelin is formed by the oligodendrocytes. The anterior aspect of the optic nerve dura mater fuses with the sclera. The meningeal sheaths enlarge the circumference of the optic nerve to approximately 3 mm as it exits the globe.

The neural glial cells of the anterior optic nerve are primarily astrocytes, whereas in the retrobulbar optic nerve, oligodendrocytes and microglia are more prevalent. An astrocytic network surrounds the fascicles of the nerve axons and is continuous from the superficial optic nerve to the laminar cribrosa and the retrobulbar optic nerve.

General Anatomy of the Orbital Vasculature[16–18]

The orbital contents receive their vascular supply from several arteries, including the ophthalmic artery, the menin-

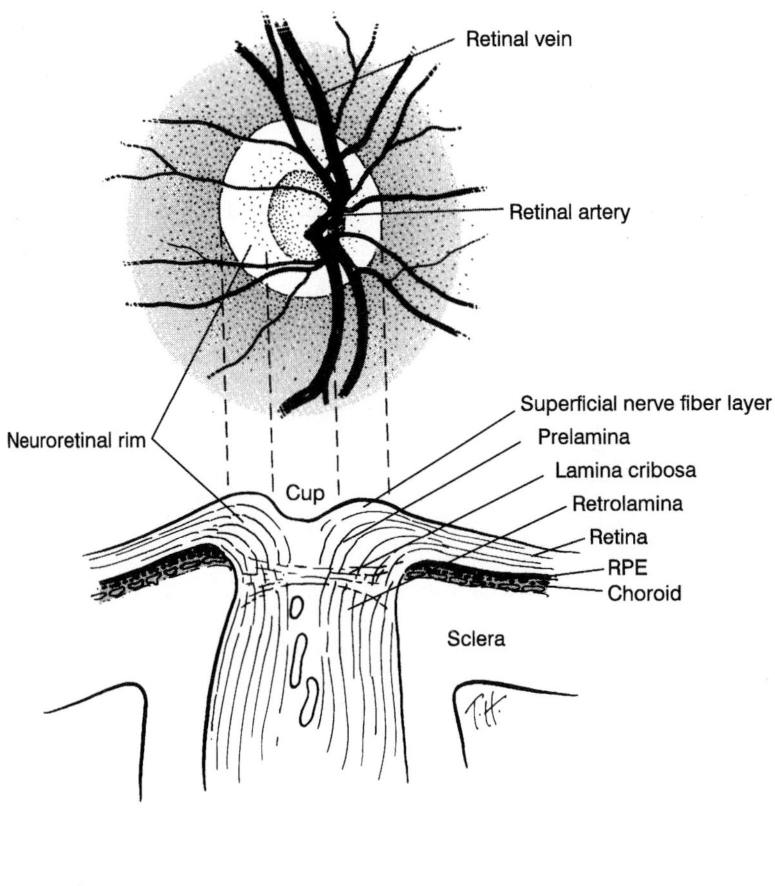

FIGURE 4–2. Normal optic nerve schematic (anterior optic nerve head and transverse view, right eye). (From Wright K (ed): Textbook of Ophthalmology. Baltimore, Williams & Wilkins, 1997.)

golacrimal artery (a branch from the middle meningeal artery), and the palpebral arteries, which branch from the facial artery. The middle meningeal artery and the facial artery belong to the external carotid arterial system.

The ophthalmic artery, which provides most of the blood supply to the eye, is the first branch of the internal carotid artery, arising as the internal carotid artery turns to pierce the dura and emerge from the cavernous sinus. The vascular supply to the intraorbital optic nerve, retina, and choroid arises predominantly from the ophthalmic arterial circulation via the posterior ciliary arteries, the central retinal artery, and the pial vascular network along the optic nerve. The ophthalmic artery exits the intracranial cavity through the optic canal and, in most individuals, lies inferolateral to the optic nerve. The ophthalmic artery has several intraorbital collateral vessels from the external carotid artery system. The most significant collaterals are the lacrimal and the ethmoidal anastomoses.

The ocular branches of the ophthalmic artery are the central retinal artery and one to five posterior ciliary arterial trunks. These trunks branch into the main posterior ciliary arteries (Fig. 4–3). Most individuals have two or three posterior ciliary trunks that supply the medial and lateral posterior ciliary arteries. Each main posterior ciliary artery further divides into several short posterior ciliary arteries just before or after entering the sclera. In addition, medial and lateral long posterior ciliary arteries arise from the ciliary trunks and travel anteriorly along the outside of the globe before penetrating the sclera at the horizontal meridian of the globe. The long posterior ciliary arteries supply the iris, the ciliary body, and the anterior region of the choroid.

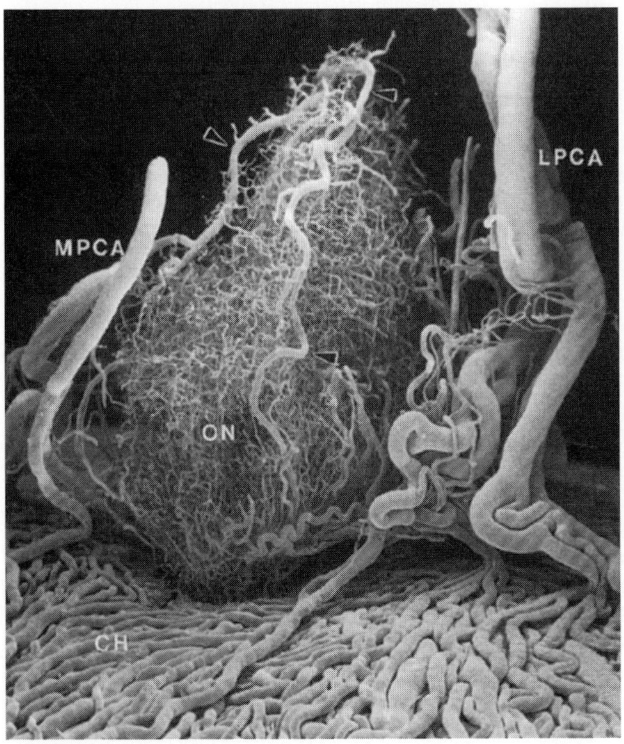

FIGURE 4–3. Posterior view of a vascular corrosion casting of a primate eye. The optic nerve enters the posterior aspect of the globe, with adjacent groups of posterior ciliary arteries. Pial arteries (*arrowheads*) course along the optic nerve. CH, choroid; LPCA, lateral posterior ciliary arteries; MPCA, medial posterior ciliary arteries; ON, optic nerve. (From Ritch R, Shields MB, Krupin T (eds): The Glaucomas. St. Louis, Mosby–Year Book, 1996.)

The short posterior ciliary arteries course anteriorly after branching from the main posterior ciliary arteries and pierce the sclera immediately adjacent to the optic nerve, predominantly in the nasal and temporal regions (Fig. 4–4). Occasionally, short posterior ciliary arteries may have extrascleral anastomoses. The short posterior ciliary arteries supply the posterior choroid as well as the majority of the anterior optic nerve. The size and shape of the area of the choroid and optic nerve supplied by each short posterior ciliary artery are variable among subjects and even between the eyes of a single person. Some short posterior ciliary arteries course, without branching, through the sclera directly into the choroid, and others divide within the sclera to provide branches to both the choroid and the anterior optic nerve.

Often, the medial and lateral short posterior ciliary arteries anastomose and form an elliptical circle around the optic nerve, the arterial circle of Zinn-Haller (Fig. 4–5). Branches derived from the circle of Zinn-Haller include the recurrent pial branches, choroidal branches, and branches penetrating the optic nerve. This arterial circle is usually intrascleral, but occasionally, an incomplete extrascleral arterial network is present. Human intravascular corrosion castings have demonstrated that the anastomoses between the lateral and medial short posterior ciliary arteries form a complete elliptical circle around the optic nerve in 77% of eyes, but that 43% of these eyes have narrowed segments along the interarterial anastomoses.

The venous drainage of the orbit generally does not follow the arterial supply. The orbital veins, in common with those of the head and neck, contain no valves. The largest of the orbital veins is the superior ophthalmic vein, which accommodates the majority of the orbital venous effluent. The venous drainage of the retina and the anterior optic nerve is almost exclusively via the central retinal vein and its tributaries, which subsequently empties into the superior ophthalmic vein. The choroid is drained through the vortex venous system that empties into the superior and inferior ophthalmic veins. It is often difficult to identify an inferior ophthalmic vein independent from the superior ophthalmic vein. Numerous anastomoses are generally present between the superior and inferior ophthalmic veins. Both vessels drain into the cavernous sinus. However, the inferior ophthalmic vein occasionally drains into the pterygoid plexus through the inferior orbital tissue.

Microvasculature of the Anterior Optic Nerve[3, 17–21]

The vasculature of the anterior optic nerve varies according to the region (Figs. 4–6 and 4–7). The superficial nerve fiber layer is supplied principally from the arterioles in the adjacent retina. Most of these vessels are capillaries originating in the peripapillary nerve fiber layer. These vessels, like all capillary beds within the optic nerve, are not fenestrated, and the tight junctions between their endothelial cells constitute the blood-ocular barrier. The tempo-

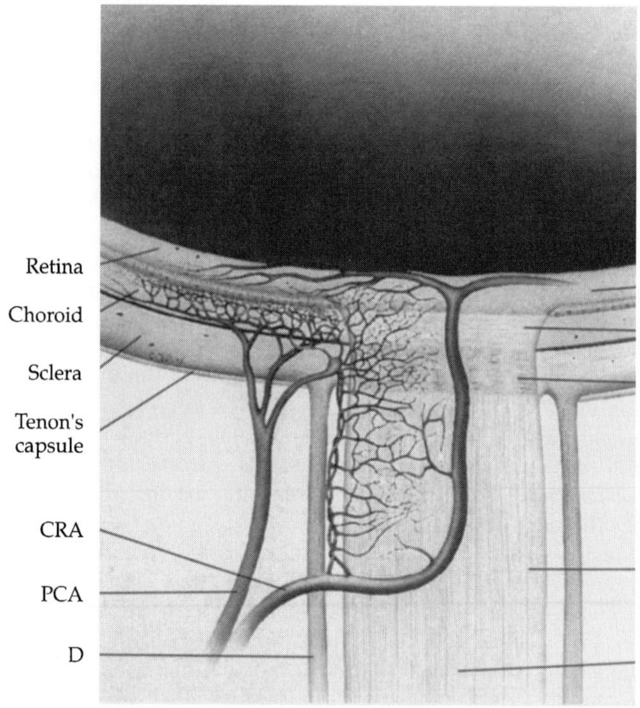

FIGURE 4–4. Arterial supply of the anterior optic nerve (ON). CRA, central retinal artery; D, dura mater; LC, laminar region; NFL, nerve fiber layer; PCA, posterior ciliary artery; PLC, prelaminar region; RLC, retrolaminar region. (From Ritch R, Shields MB, Krupin T (eds): The Glaucomas. St. Louis, Mosby–Year Book, 1996.)

ral nerve fiber layer may have an additional arterial contribution from the cilioretinal artery. No direct choroidal contribution is observed in the superficial nerve fiber layer region.

The prelaminar region receives its arterial supply via direct branches of the short posterior ciliary arteries and via vessels originating from the arterial circle of Zinn-Haller (Figs. 4–5 and 4–8). As detailed previously, the posterior ciliary arterial system provides input to both the choroid and the arterial circle of Zinn-Haller.

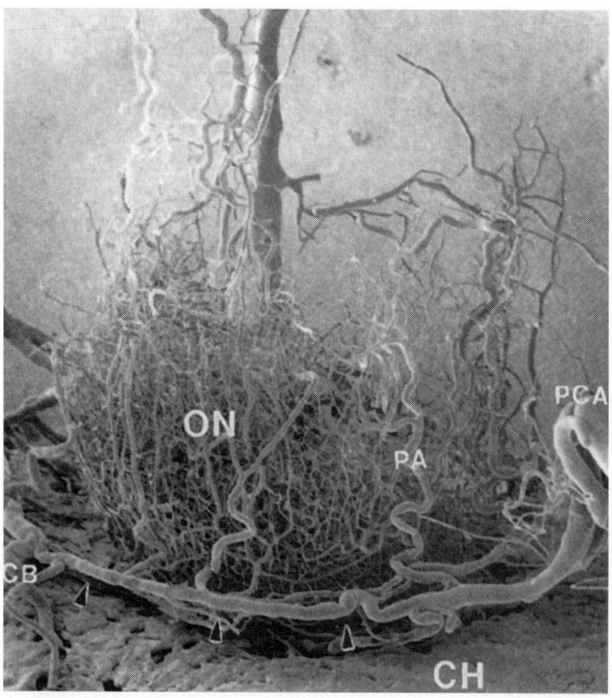

FIGURE 4–5. Posterior view of a vascular corrosion casting of a human eye. Note that the optic nerve (ON) is surrounded by a complete arterial circle of Zinn-Haller (*arrowheads*). CB, choroidal branches; CH, choroid; PA, pial arteries; PCA, posterior ciliary artery. (From Ritch R, Shields MB, Krupin T (eds): The Glaucomas. St. Louis, Mosby–Year Book, 1996.)

The origin of the blood supply to the prelaminar region of the anterior optic nerve has evoked controversy. Studies have suggested the presence of a choroidal arterial contribution to the prelaminar and laminar regions of the anterior optic nerve. Indeed, fluorescein angiography demonstrates the appearance of fluorescein in these deeper regions of the anterior optic nerve concomitant with the filling of the choroidal vasculature. This finding suggests that the anterior optic nerve and the choroid share a common arterial input. However, further investigations have demonstrated minimal anatomic vascular connections between the peripapillary choroid and anterior optic nerve. Branches from the short posterior ciliary arteries may actually course through the choroid and supply the prelaminar region. These vessels do not actually arise from the choroid but merely pass through it to directly supply the optic nerve. The direct arterial supply to the prelaminar region arising from the choroidal vasculature is minimal. Therefore, the simultaneous filling of the optic nerve vasculature and the peripapillary choroid on fluorescein angiography appears to be related to their common supply by the posterior ciliary arteries.

The arterial supply to the laminar region is similar to the supply of the prelaminar region (see Fig. 4–6). The short posterior ciliary arteries, either directly or via the arterial circle of Zinn-Haller, provide the principal arterial input to the laminar region of the optic nerve. As in the prelaminar region, the peripapillary choroid may contribute occasional small arterioles to the laminar region. The precapillary vessels perforate the outer aspect of the lamina cribrosa before branching into an intraseptal capillary network.

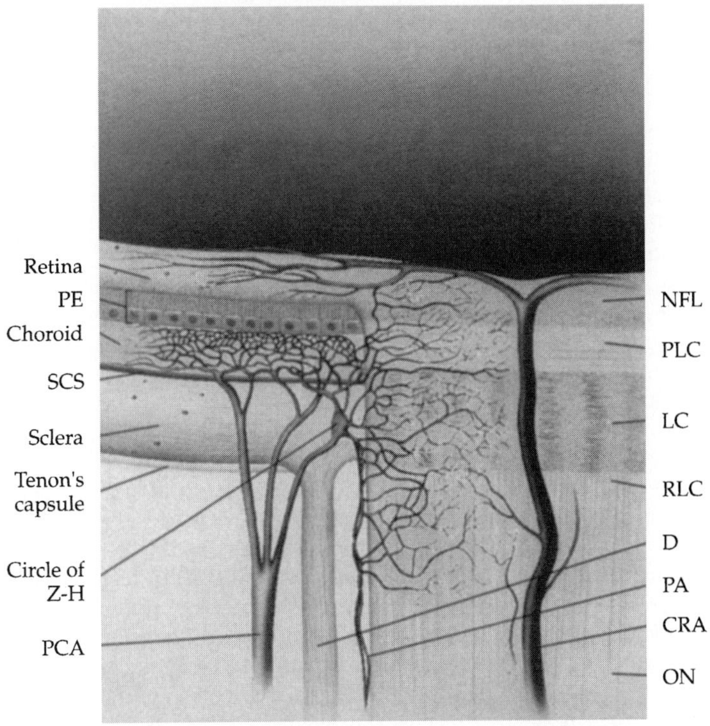

FIGURE 4–6. Arterial supply of the anterior optic nerve (ON) showing the contribution from the circle of Zinn-Haller (Z-H), the pial arteries (PA), and the central retinal artery (CRA). D, dura mater; LC, laminar region; NFL, nerve fiber layer; PCA, posterior ciliary artery; PE, pigment epithelium; PLC, prelaminar region; RLC, retrolaminar region; SCS, supraciliary space. (From Ritch R, Shields MB, Krupin T (eds): The Glaucomas. St. Louis, Mosby–Year Book, 1996.)

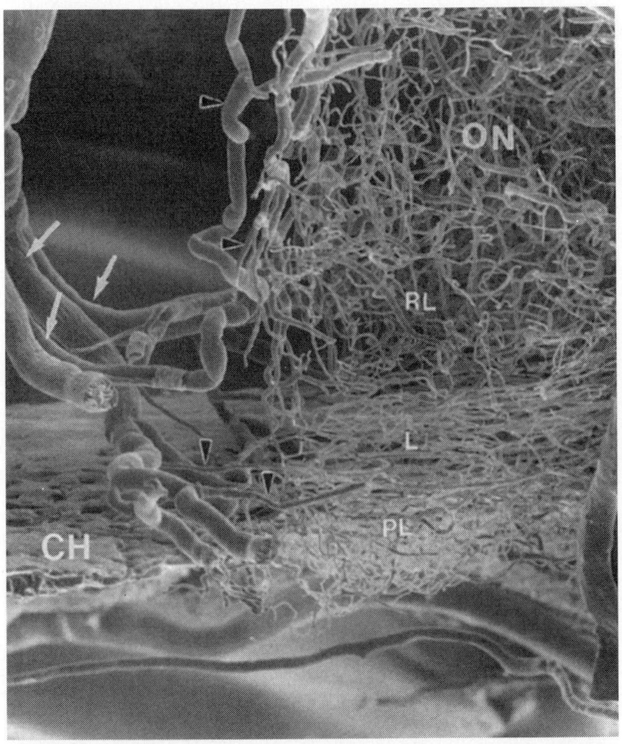

FIGURE 4–7. High magnification of a vascular corrosion casting of a human optic nerve (ON) demonstrating the direct supply of the posterior ciliary artery branches (*arrows*) to the anterior optic nerve. *Arrowheads* indicate pial arteries. CH, choroid, L, laminar region; PL, prelaminar region; RL, retrolaminar region. (From Ritch R, Shields MB, Krupin T (eds): The Glaucomas. St. Louis, Mosby–Year Book, 1996.)

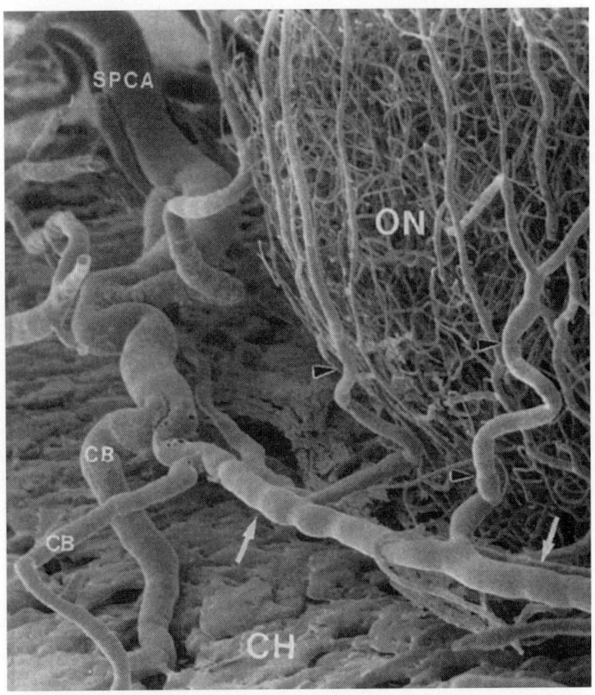

FIGURE 4–8. Vascular corrosion casting of a human optic nerve (ON) showing the circle of Zinn-Haller (*arrows*). Note the pial arteries (*arrowheads*) branching from the circle. CB, choroidal branches; CH, choroid; SPCA, short posterior ciliary arteries. (From Ritch R, Shields MB, Krupin T (eds): The Glaucomas. St. Louis, Mosby–Year Book, 1996.)

Most of the blood supply to the retrolaminar portion of the optic nerve occurs through numerous perforating vessels from the pia mater. These pial vessels obtain their supply either directly from the ophthalmic artery or indirectly from recurrent branches of the posterior ciliary arteries. The central retinal artery contributes occasional small branches within the retrolaminar optic nerve. The central retinal artery may also provide small branches to the retrobulbar optic nerve. Some investigators have described "central optic nerve artery equivalents," which are pial vessel–derived longitudinal arterioles in the retrolaminar nerve.

The rich capillary beds of the peripapillary retina, the anterior optic nerve, and the retrobulbar optic nerve are anatomically confluent and form a continuous vascular network along the anterior optic nerve. These capillary interconnections unite the microvasculature along the length of the anterior optic nerve. There is a subtle transition in the organization of the capillaries between the prelaminar and laminar regions. The capillaries of the prelaminar region are complex and randomly arranged, whereas the capillaries of the laminar region conform to the pattern of the connective tissue septa that compose the supportive architecture of the lamina cribrosa. The presence of this longitudinal anastomosis of capillaries might be viewed as a protective mechanism against regional ischemic insult, but the functional importance of these potential collaterals is not known. Flow resistance may be so high in these fine capillaries that it limits potential collateral flow.

The venous drainage of the anterior optic nerve is almost exclusively via the central retinal vein (Fig. 4–9). In the nerve fiber layer, blood is drained by small veins that converge and empty, ultimately, into the central retinal vein. In the prelaminar, laminar, and retrolaminar regions, venous drainage also occurs via the central retinal vein or centripetal tributaries to the central retinal vein. Occasionally, small venules connecting the optic nerve and the peripapillary choroid can be identified, mainly within the prelaminar region. In the peripheral aspects of the laminar and retrolaminar regions, some optic nerve venous drainage occurs via pial veins, but these pial veins ultimately drain into the central retinal vein as it exits the optic nerve.

Intrinsic and Extrinsic Factors in the Development of Glaucomatous Optic Neuropathy[22–29]

A multitude of factors, either intrinsic to or extrinsic to the optic nerve, alone or in combination, may adversely effect the health and function of the optic nerve. Potential extrinsic factors that may contribute to the development of glaucomatous optic neuropathy include elevated intraocular pressure and aberrations of the systemic cardiovascular status. Factors intrinsic to the optic nerve, which potentially contribute to axonal loss, include abnormalities of the composition of the support tissues of the optic nerve and anomalies of the microcirculatory physiology within the nerve. Some individuals may have optic nerves with particular anomalies of these intrinsic factors that lead to heightened susceptibility to glaucomatous optic neuropathy. Other individuals may possess optic nerves that develop glaucomatous damage primarily as the result of extrinsic insult. Thus, a spectrum of factors should be considered in each case of glaucoma.

Intraocular pressure plays a major role in the development of glaucomatous optic neuropathy for many patients. One hypothesis of the etiology of glaucoma proposes that neuronal damage results from mechanical pressure on the optic nerve. This hypothesis focuses primarily on the potential deleterious effects that elevated intraocular pressure has on the extracellular matrix and glial support structures of the anterior optic nerve. This hypothesis suggests that a direct, mechanical insult results from an increase in intraocular pressure above a tolerable threshold. The intraocular pressure causes backward bowing, stretching, and compres-

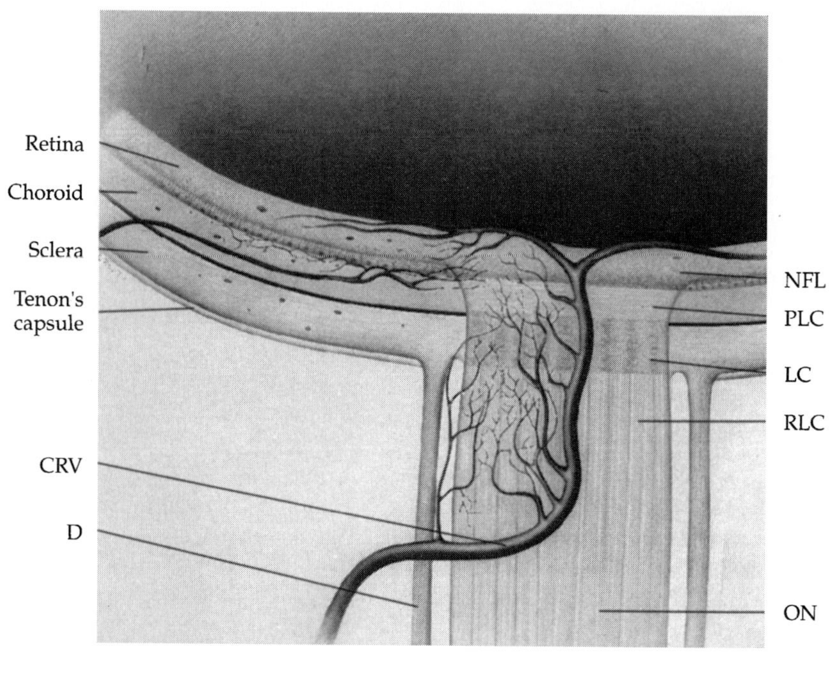

FIGURE 4–9. Venous drainage of anterior optic nerve (ON) and peripapillary choroid. The entire drainage is almost exclusively via the central retinal vein (CRV). LC, lamina cribrosa; NFL, nerve fiber layer; PLC, prelaminar region; RLC, retrolaminar region. (From Ritch R, Shields MB, Krupin T (eds): The Glaucomas. St. Louis, Mosby–Year Book, 1996.)

sion of the of the laminar plates within the lamina cribrosa (Fig. 4–10). Misalignment of the fenestrations within the lamina cribrosa and compression of the connective tissue plates results in the inhibition of axoplasmic flow within the axons of the ganglion cells. Interruption of axoplasmic flow or direct mechanical compression of the neural axons causes death of the nerve cells and results in glaucomatous optic neuropathy.

This extrinsic, pressure-induced hypothesis of glaucomatous optic neuropathy is supported by both laboratory models of glaucoma and clinical observations. Increased intraocular pressure in nonhuman primate models causes obstruction of axoplasmic flow in the laminar region. Histologic examination of such primate eyes demonstrates posterior bowing of the lamina cribrosa with compression of the connective tissue plates and distortion of the laminar fenestrae. Transverse sections through the lamina cribrosa have documented increases in the size of the laminar fenestrae in the superior and inferior poles of the optic nerve. These regional differences in the lamina cribrosa may account for asymmetric mechanical damage of the axons within the various regions. In early glaucomatous optic neuropathy, damage of the ganglion cell axons occurs primarily in the superior and inferior regions of the optic nerve. Histologic examination shows nonuniform distribution with higher numbers of large ganglion cell axons in the inferior and superior poles of the optic nerve. Large ganglion cell axons appear to be preferentially damaged early in glaucomatous optic neuropathy. This apparent greater susceptibility of the large cell axons may be due to the relative distribution of these axons within the regions of the optic nerve that are primarily distorted by mechanical forces. Other glial support tissues within the optic nerve also show changes in glaucomatous optic neuropathy. Extracellular matrix components, including elastin fibers of the lamina cribrosa, are altered in glaucomatous eyes and in experimental models of glaucoma. These changes may be the result of greater intraocular pressure with concomitant mechanical stress and may be associated with axonal death in glaucoma.

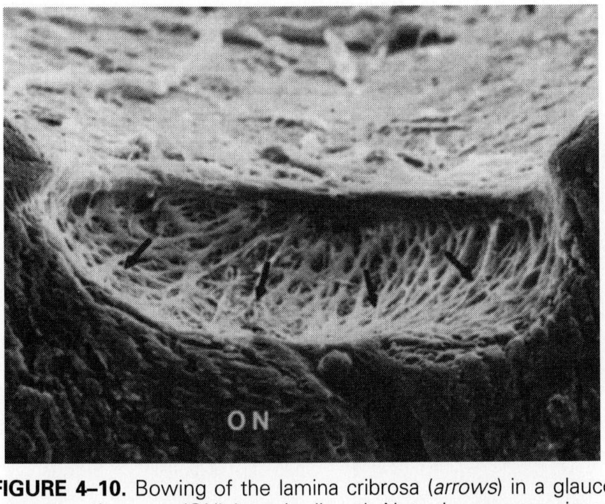

FIGURE 4–10. Bowing of the lamina cribrosa (*arrows*) in a glaucomatous optic nerve (ON) (trypsin digest). Note the compression of the laminar connective tissue plates. (Photograph courtesy of John Morrison.) (From Wright K (ed): Textbook of Ophthalmology. Baltimore, Williams & Wilkins, 1997.)

Accumulating epidemiologic and laboratory evidence, however, demonstrates that elevated intraocular pressure is not the sole cause of optic nerve injury in glaucoma. As many 20% to 30% of persons with glaucoma never exhibit statistically elevated intraocular pressures, and among patients treated for glaucoma, approximately 20% to 30% continue to lose vision despite maximal intraocular pressure–lowering therapy. Therefore, alternative hypotheses have been considered.

One commonly cited hypothesis proposes that intraneural ischemia leads to the development of glaucomatous optic neuropathy. This hypothesis proposes that vascular perfusion of the neural tissue within the optic nerve is deficient in eyes with glaucoma. Vascular perfusion depends on arterial blood pressure, venous outflow, tissue pressure surrounding the vasculature, autoregulation, and local and regional vasomodulators. Insufficiency or abnormality of any or all of these components may result in regional ischemia. In laboratory studies, axoplasmic flow of the ganglion cell axons is obstructed by interruption of the short posterior ciliary artery circulation to the optic nerve. This obstruction may lead to ganglion cell death similar to that found with mechanical compression. Autoregulatory mechanisms within regional vascular beds are believed to accommodate changes in arterial blood pressure in normal individuals. However, deficient autoregulation of the optic nerve vasculature would result in decreased optic nerve perfusion.

The vascular hypothesis for glaucoma suggests that elevated intraocular pressure results in increased tissue pressure within the optic nerve tissue surrounding the vasculature. This leads to vascular collapse and decreased neural perfusion, resulting in glaucomatous optic neuropathy. Greater tissue pressure from elevated intraocular pressure is only one possible cause of decreased vascular perfusion of the optic nerve. Individuals with glaucoma are more likely to have systemic vascular disorders, including diabetes mellitus, systemic hypertension, peripheral vascular disease, and vasospastic syndromes. These associations between extrinsic vascular factors and glaucoma support a vascular etiology in the development of glaucomatous optic neuropathy.

Glaucomatous optic neuropathy likely derives from many potential insults working independently or in concert. A combination of the various intrinsic and extrinsic factors may contribute to varying degrees in each person. Many possible scenarios may be considered. Increases in intraocular pressure with mechanical distortion of the optic nerve may result in elevated tissue pressure on the microvasculature of the optic nerve and reduced perfusion of the neuronal tissue. Mechanical distortion of the laminar cribrosa fenestrae could directly compromise ganglion cell axons, rendering them more susceptible to damage from an insufficient vascular supply. Further studies examining changes in the compliance and structure of the optic nerve resulting from increased intraocular pressure should improve our understanding of the mechanical component of the development of glaucomatous optic neuropathy. Greater understanding of autoregulatory mechanisms and of regional and systemic vasomodulation may also shed light on the possible contribution of the vascular system to glaucomatous optic neuropathy.

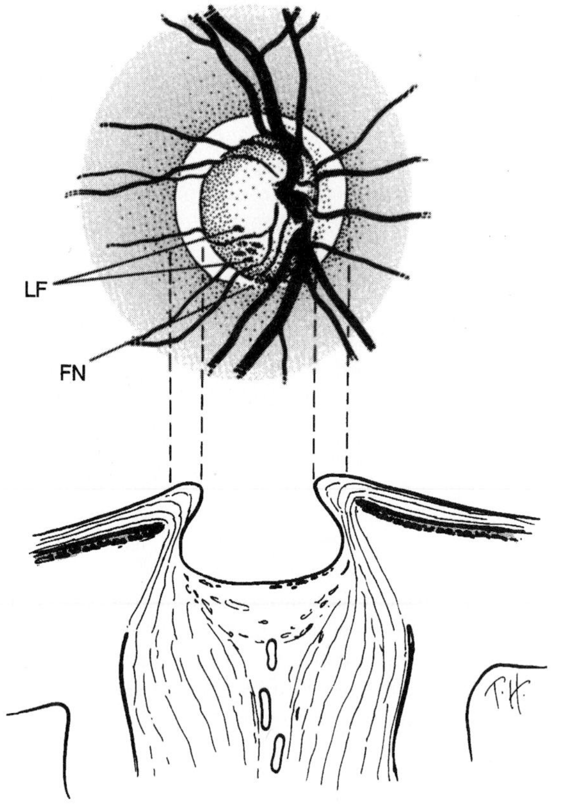

FIGURE 4–11. Glaucomatous optic nerve schematic (anterior optic nerve head and transverse view, right eye). Note the thinning and undermining of the inferior neuroretinal rim and focal notching (FN) with an enlarged cup and visible laminar pores, or laminar fenestrae (LF). (From Wright K (ed): Textbook of Ophthalmology. Baltimore, Williams & Wilkins, 1997.)

Glaucomatous Optic Neuropathy and Anatomic Variants[14, 30–38]

Glaucomatous optic neuropathy is the final common denominator of all forms of glaucoma. Characteristic changes in the clinical appearance of the optic nerve head are associated with the development of glaucomatous optic

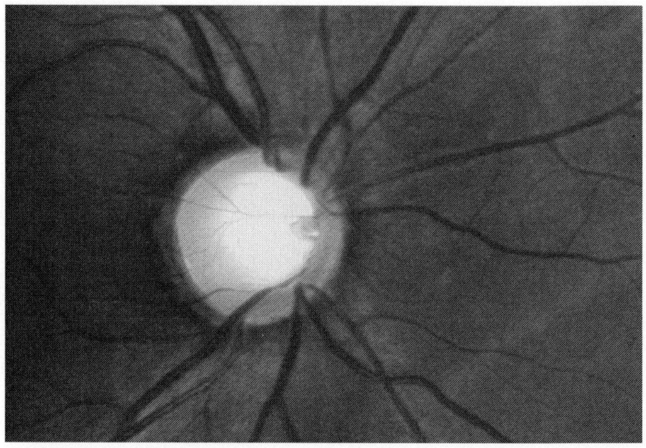

FIGURE 4–13. Photograph of an optic nerve with advanced glaucomatous cupping. Note the deep cup with laminar pores and nasalization of the central retinal vessels.

neuropathy and correlate with the histologic findings previously described. Initial changes of the glaucomatous optic nerve may include focal erosions of the neural retinal rim of the anterior optic nerve secondary to localized atrophy of the nerve fibers and overall enlargement of the cup-to-disc ratios with diffuse loss of the neural retinal rim secondary to diffuse axonal death (Figs. 4–11 to 4–13). Assessment of these clinical findings and other typical changes associated with the development of glaucomatous optic neuropathy are detailed elsewhere in this text (see Chapters 5 and 27).

Both localized and diffuse axonal atrophy may result in an increase in the depth of the cup, nasalization of the central retinal vessels, and baring of the underlying structure of the lamina cribrosa (see Fig. 4–13). With diffuse enlargement of the cup, asymmetry of the cup-to-disc ratios between the two eyes may develop (Fig. 4–14); significant asymmetry is uncommon in the normal population. As the neural retinal rim tissue atrophies and the central cup enlarges, the optic nerve often appears white. This appearance is secondary to the increased exposure of the underlying laminar tissue and should be distinguished from optic nerve pallor associated with an acute infarct of the nerve, as is seen in anterior ischemic optic neuropathy (Fig. 4–15).

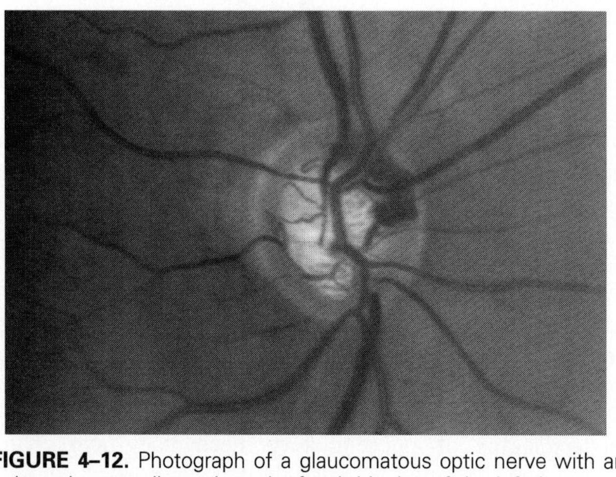

FIGURE 4–12. Photograph of a glaucomatous optic nerve with an enlarged cup-to-disc ratio and a focal thinning of the inferior neural retinal rim (notch) at the six o'clock position. Note the optic nerve hemorrhage.

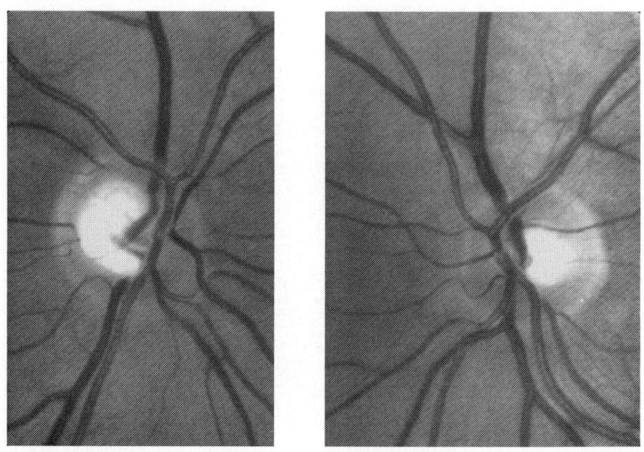

FIGURE 4–14. Bilateral optic nerve photographs demonstrating asymmetric cupping. Note the enlarged cup and thinning of the neural retinal rim in the right eye (*left*).

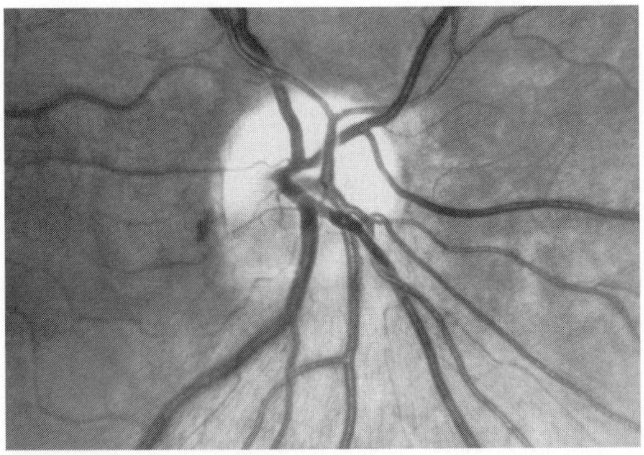

FIGURE 4–15. Photograph demonstrating marked pallor of the superior optic nerve from anterior ischemic optic neuropathy. Note that the cup is not enlarged and the central retinal vessels are not displaced.

Hemorrhages within the nerve fiber layer, of the anterior optic nerve, or in the peripapillary area are frequently associated with glaucomatous optic neuropathy (Fig. 4–16). These hemorrhages are believe to occur in as many as a third of patients with glaucoma at some point during the course of their disease and may be related to vascular abnormalities within the nerve. The appearance of nerve fiber layer hemorrhages may indicate inadequate therapeutic control and often precedes progression of glaucomatous nerve damage.

Peripapillary chorioretinal atrophy is also a common occurrence during the development of glaucomatous optic neuropathy, especially at the temporal aspect of the optic nerve (Fig. 4–17). Chorioretinal atrophy is often subdivided into two zones, alpha and beta. Beta-zone atrophy is immediately adjacent to the optic nerve and is characterized by visible sclera, occasional large choroidal vessels, and marked atrophy of the retinal pigment epithelium and choriocapillaris. Alpha-zone atrophy, which lies between the retina and the beta-zone, is characterized by irregular areas of both hyperpigmentation and hypopigmentation. The presence and extent of peripapillary atrophy should be noted during examination of the glaucomatous optic nerve. The casual observer often confuses a region of peripapillary atrophy and the limits of the optic nerve.

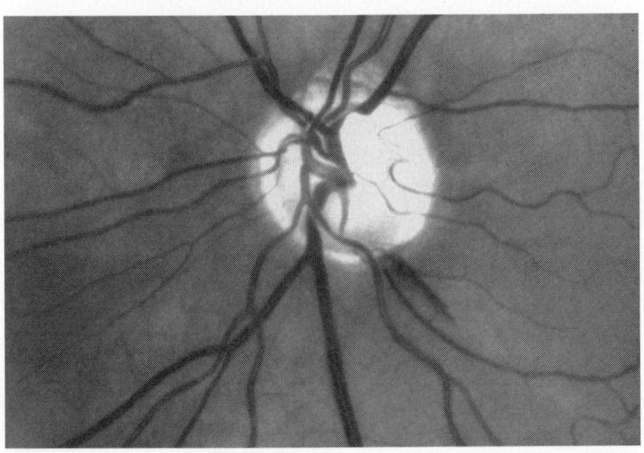

FIGURE 4–16. An optic nerve hemorrhage showing the characteristic feathery appearance of the blood within the nerve fiber layer.

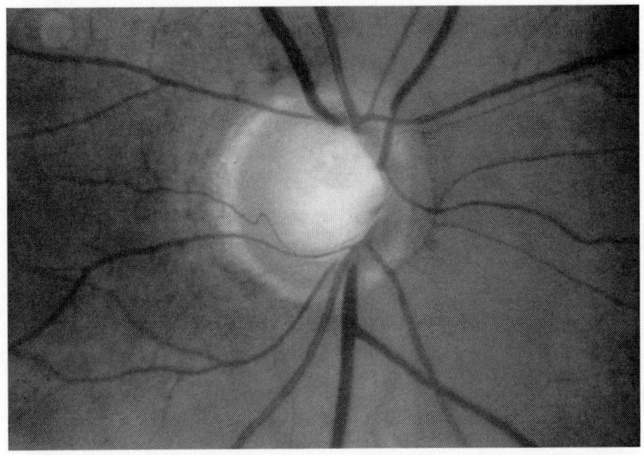

FIGURE 4–17. Photograph of a glaucomatous optic nerve with peripapillary chorioretinal atrophy. Beta-zone atrophy is immediately adjacent to the optic nerve (white crescent), and alpha-zone atrophy lies between the retina and the beta-zone (area of irregular pigmentation).

Three additional anatomic variants of the anterior optic nerve are common and may confuse the clinical interpretation of the glaucomatous optic nerve:

- □ Optic nerve pits, or pseudo-pits
- □ Optic nerve drusen
- □ Tilted insertion of the optic nerve

Optic nerve pits may be congenital or acquired (also known as optic nerve pseudo-pit). Congenital optic pits are rare but may be confused with glaucomatous enlargement of the cup. Congenital optic nerve pit, an anomaly most often seen in eyes with unusually large optic nerves, is a focal depression adjacent to the cup. Optic pits are usually located temporally and may be associated with serous retinal detachments. *Pseudo-pits* of the optic nerve are much more common and are the result of highly localized loss of anterior optic nerve tissue with focal thinning of the neural retinal rim (Fig. 4–18). It has been suggested that acquired optic nerve pits represent localized insufficiency of the

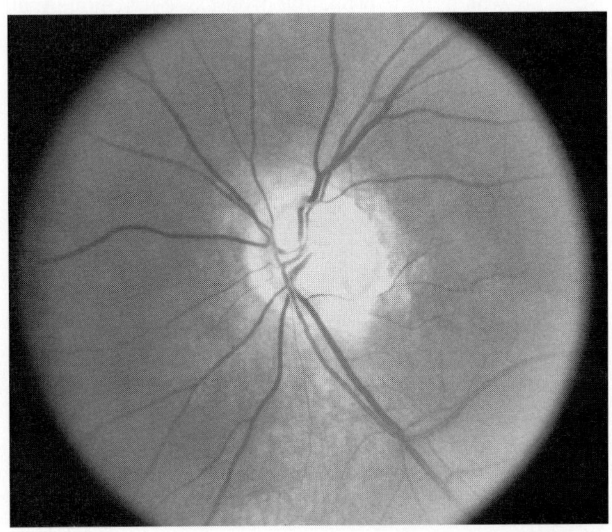

FIGURE 4–18. An optic nerve photograph demonstrating glaucomatous cupping with a localized notch and an acquired pseudo-pit with focal thinning of the neural retinal rim.

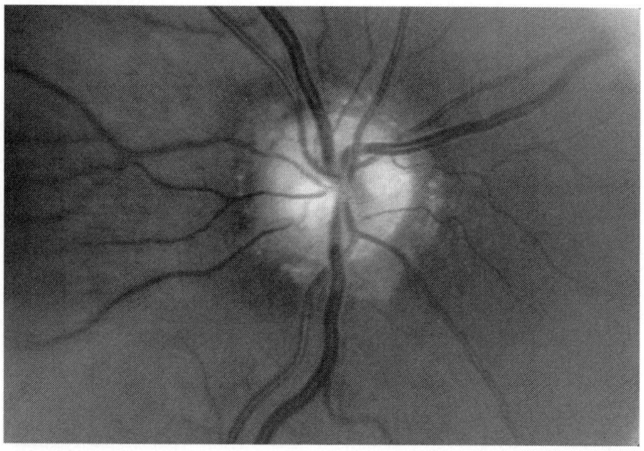

FIGURE 4–19. Photograph of an optic nerve with diffuse drusen appearing as raised irregularities of the optic nerve.

lamina cribrosa. *Optic nerve drusen* appears clinically as raised irregularities of the optic nerve and represents localized deposits of calcific cellular remnant (Fig. 4–19). It is often difficult to distinguish glaucomatous optic nerve changes in nerves with drusen. *Tilted insertion of the optic nerve* is often associated with a large area of visible sclera adjacent to the obliquely tilted optic nerve head and is more common in myopic eyes (Fig. 4–20). The sclera is visible through thinned neurosensory retina owing to absence of the retinal pigment epithelium and choroid. Assessment of the presence and extent of the optic nerve cupping is commonly difficult.

Optic Nerve Blood Flow and Glaucoma[39–46]

In 1885, Priestley Smith[39] wrote, "the excavation of the disc in glaucoma is not a purely mechanical result of exalted pressure; it is, in part at least, an atrophic condition which, though primarily due to pressure, includes vascular changes and impaired nutrition in the substance of the optic disc . . . which may probably progress even though all excess of pressure be removed." Currently, there is accumulating evidence that ischemia of the anterior optic nerve, retina, or choroid is involved in the development of glaucomatous optic neuropathy. There are many reasons to believe that microcirculatory changes are important in glaucoma. Many microvascular diseases, including diabetes mellitus, systemic hypertension or hypotension, and peripheral vascular disease, have been associated with glaucomatous optic neuropathy.

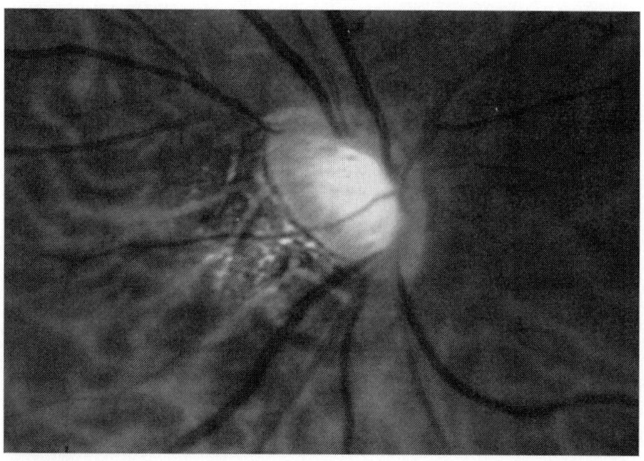

FIGURE 4–20. An optic nerve photograph of an eye with glaucoma. Note the tilted insertion of the optic nerve and a large area of visible sclera adjacent to the obliquely positioned optic nerve head.

Disorders associated with vasospasm, such as migraine headache and Raynaud's phenomenon, are seen in many patients with glaucoma, both with and without elevated intraocular pressure. Individuals also have been described with clinical vasospastic syndromes that exhibit glaucoma-like, but reversible, visual field defects in response to psychic or cold stress. Peripheral vasodilators, such as calcium channel antagonists, have been reported to slow the progression or even improve visual field damage in many of these vasospastic patients as well as in some patients with glaucoma and vasospasm.

Ischemia of the optic nerve associated with giant cell arteritis or resulting from a hemodynamic crisis can cause both optic nerve cupping and visual field loss indistinguishable from those found with primary open-angle glaucoma. Individuals with primary open-angle glaucoma also have been demonstrated to have abnormalities in microvascular autoregulation. Individually and collectively, these clinical observations support the role of microcirculatory changes in glaucoma, either as a primary abnormality or as a cofactor which enhances the susceptibility to pressure damage.

Both high and low blood pressure may contribute to the progression of glaucoma. Thirty years ago, it was observed that deterioration of visual field sensitivity was more rapid in individuals with glaucoma and systemic hypotension than in normotensive or hypertensive individuals. Subsequently, systemic hypotension, especially nocturnal hypotension, has been linked closely with glaucoma. Blood pressure normally decreases at night, during sleep, to levels 10% to 20% below the diurnal average. Individuals with glaucoma have lower nocturnal diastolic blood pressure and a greater mean decrease in nocturnal diastolic blood pressure. Among individuals with glaucoma who are taking systemic hypotensive medication, the nocturnal blood pressure dip is significantly larger for those with progressive visual field loss. This group with progressive visual field loss also shows a significantly lower mean minimum systolic nocturnal blood pressure than the group with stable disease. In patients with glaucoma and progressive visual field loss, significantly lower mean nocturnal blood pressure and significantly greater mean decrease in blood pressure at night have also been demonstrated.

In addition, high intraocular pressure and high systolic blood pressure appear concomitantly in many persons. Subjects with intraocular pressure greater than 20 mm Hg have significantly higher systolic blood pressure than age-matched controls. A relationship also has been established between the level of blood pressure and the presence of glaucoma. Persons with systolic blood pressure higher than 130 mm Hg or with diastolic perfusion pressure (diastolic blood pressure minus intraocular pressure) lower than 50 mm Hg are at higher risk for glaucoma. Although these data indicate an association between systemic blood pressure and glaucoma, the biologic basis for this association is not known. In the future, perhaps the relationship between blood pressure and ocular circulation will be elucidated by measurements of the hemodynamics within the eye.

Clinical assessment of blood flow of the eye, however, especially within the anterior optic nerve and in the retrobulbar circulation, requires the measurement of many different anatomic regions with a variety of techniques. Just within the anterior optic nerve, the capillary beds of the superficial nerve fiber layer and the prelaminar, laminar, and retrolaminar regions all potentially contribute to a circulatory aberrance that is involved in the development of glaucomatous optic neuropathy. Although there is no proven technology capable of providing hemodynamic information for all of these regions, pertinent ocular hemodynamic assessment is possible with a number of evolving techniques that employ laser and ultrasound-based technology.

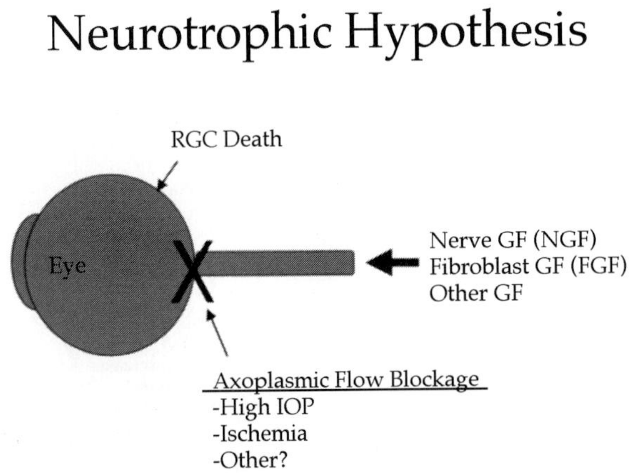

FIGURE 4–21. Diagram of the neurotrophic (growth factor) hypothesis of retinal ganglion cell (RPC) apoptosis. GF, growth factor; IOP, intraocular pressure.

Pathways of Neural Death and Neuroprotection[47–50]

Prior to the 1970s, it was thought that neural cell death following an ischemic insult, like many other cells, was primarily secondary to necrosis. Necrotic cell death is a cascade of events in which there is loss of the cellular membrane potential, calcium influx, and swelling of intracellular organelles resulting in fracture of the cellular membranes. This is followed by a localized inflammatory reaction to the cellular components via white blood cell response and is often accompanied by glial proliferation. However, histologic examinations of glaucomatous optic nerves have not demonstrated glial proliferation and scar tissue formation.

More recently, an alternative pathway of neural cell death, known as apoptosis, has been described. Apoptotic cell death involves a different cascade of events, with characteristic clumping of nuclear chromatin, DNA condensation, and fractionation of the nucleus. The breakdown of the nucleus results from the release of intracellular endonucleases and proteases. Nitric oxide and free radical production are also involved in intracellular destruction. Ultimately, the nerve cell shrinks but the cellular membranes remain intact. Finally, the involuted cell is engulfed by macrophages, without localized inflammation or glial proliferation. Apoptotic cell death has been demonstrated in the central nervous system, as a part of both developmental and degenerative neural cell reduction. It has been suggested that apoptosis is the body's mechanism to counterbalance overabundant cellular proliferation during development.

Preliminary findings suggest that apoptosis may be involved in ganglion cell death in both laboratory models of glaucoma and human glaucomatous eyes. Currently, a variety of hypotheses has been proposed concerning potential "triggers" that may initiate the apoptotic cascade in the retinal ganglion cell in glaucoma. Among these, the neurotrophic hypothesis, the excitotoxicity hypothesis, and the ischemic hypothesis have received the most attention.

The *neurotrophic hypothesis* states that the retinal ganglion cell bodies are deprived of trophic factors (growth factors) that are essential to the health and normal function of the ganglion cell. Cells depend on trophic support of these factors, which are produced by the target tissue of the particular nerve cell. In glaucoma, the lateral geniculate body is believed to produce several growth factors, which are transported to the ganglion cell body via the retrograde axoplasmic flow along the axon (Fig. 4–21). It is hypothesized that a blockade, likely occurring in the region of the lamina cribrosa, of transport of growth factors from the distal axon deprives the ganglion cell body. This blockade prevents the neurotrophic growth factors from reaching their site of action in the ganglion cell body, resulting in ganglion cell dysfunction and death.

An alternative hypothesis, the *excitotoxicity hypothesis*, involves an aberrant release or production of excitatory neurotransmitters, specifically glutamate (Fig. 4–22). The paradoxical effects of glutamate and certain excitatory amino acids was initially described in 1971. If released in abnormally high levels, glutamate is directly neurotoxic to postsynaptic or adjacent neurons. Glutamate potentiates calcium influx through *N*-methyl-D-aspartate (NMDA) channels and increases sodium influx, which also leads to

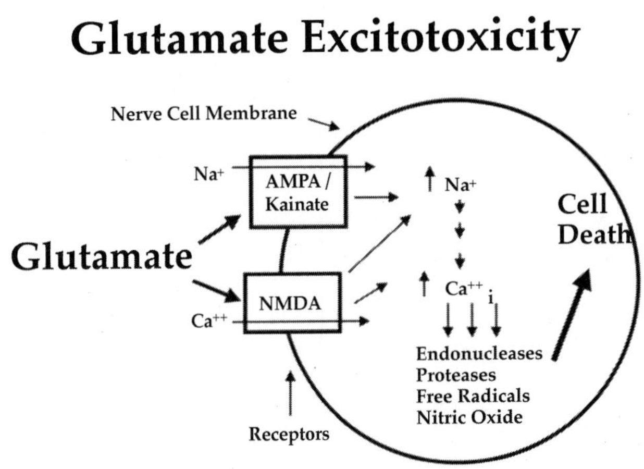

FIGURE 4–22. Diagram of the excitotoxicity hypothesis of retinal ganglion cell apoptosis. AMPA, α-amino-3-hydroxy-5-methyl-4-isoxazole propionic acid; NMDA, *N*-methyl-D-aspartate.

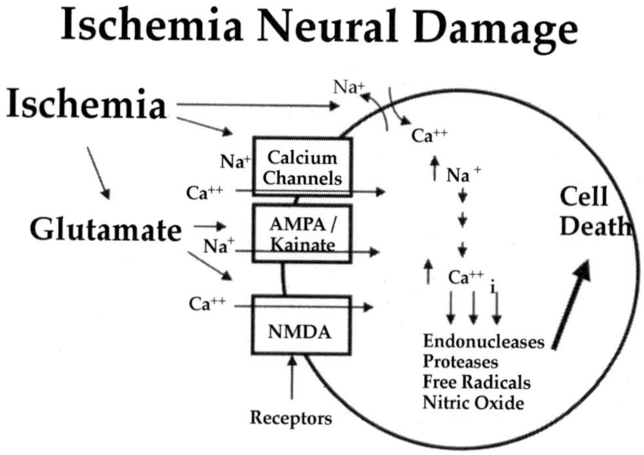

FIGURE 4–23. The ischemia hypothesis of retinal ganglion cell apoptosis. AMPA, α-amino-3-hydroxy-5-methyl-4-isoxazole propionic acid; NMDA, *N*-methyl-D-aspartate.

higher levels of intracellular calcium. Increased intracellular calcium stimulates a cascade of events resulting in production of free radicals and release of endonucleases, leading finally to cell death, as described previously for apoptosis. Excitotoxicity is believed to play a role in neural death following cerebral ischemia. Higher levels of glutamate have been found in vitreous samples of individuals with glaucoma compared with normal controls. Elevated vitreous glutamate has also been demonstrated in nonhuman primate eyes following extended periods of elevated intraocular pressure.

According to the *ischemic hypothesis,* ischemia of the ganglion cell, most likely in the anterior optic nerve, results in ganglion cell death, either directly or in conjunction with other factors (Fig. 4–23). Ischemia of the anterior optic nerve may be a potential cofactor in either the neurotrophic or excitotoxicity hypotheses. Blockade of growth factors within the optic nerve occurs secondary to both elevated intraocular pressure and anterior optic nerve ischemia. Ischemia also promotes release of glutamate from neural cells. In addition, ischemia directly increases intracellular calcium by potentiating calcium influx via cell membrane calcium channels. With each of these scenarios, ischemia would promote ganglion cell death.

Each of these hypotheses provides a potential yet unproven mechanism by which apoptotic ganglion cell death might be initiated in glaucoma.

On the basis of these hypotheses, many approaches have been developed to protect neurons (so-called neuroprotection) (Fig. 4–24). Neuroprotection may involve ameliorating risk factors, such as increased intraocular pressure or ischemia, or blocking cell-specific pathways, such as calcium channel activity or NMDA channels. Currently, a variety of neuroprotective agents is under investigation.

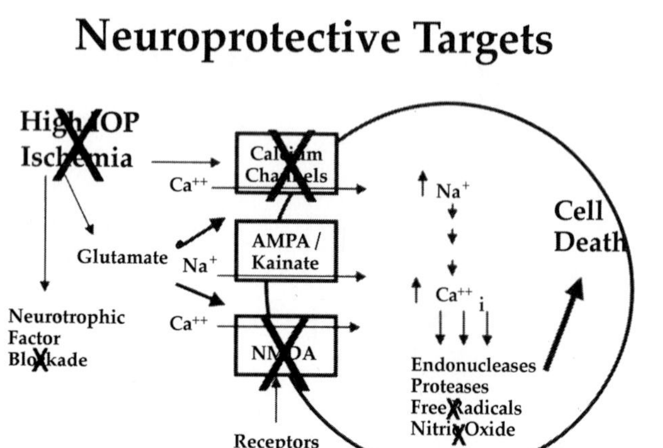

FIGURE 4–24. Potential targets for neuroprotection. The X marks demonstrate potential sites of action of neuroprotective agents. AMPA, α-amino-3-hydroxy-5-methyl-4-isoxazole propionic acid; IOP, intraocular pressure; NMDA, *N*-methyl-D-aspartate.

REFERENCES

1. Anderson DR: Ultrastructure of human and monkey lamina cribrosa and optic nerve head. Arch Ophthalmol 1969;82:800.
2. Anderson DR, Hoyt WF: Ultrastructure of intraorbital portion of human and monkey optic nerve. Arch Ophthalmol 1969;82:506.
3. Hayreh SS: Anatomy and physiology of the optic nerve head. Trans Am Acad Ophthalmol Otol 1974;78:240.
4. Minckler DS, Milam AA: Optic nerve axonal transport. *In* Tasman W, Jaeger EA (eds): Duane's Foundations of Clinical Ophthalmology, vol 1. Philadelphia, Lippincott-Raven, 1997, pp 1–24.
5. Witkovsky P: Functional anatomy of the retina. *In* Tasman W, Jaeger EA (eds): Duane's Foundations of Clinical Ophthalmology, vol 1. Philadelphia, Lippincott-Raven, 1997, pp 1–63.
6. Radius RL, Anderson DR: The histology of retina nerve fiber layer bundles and bundle defects. Arch Ophthalmol 1989;97:948.
7. Radius RL, Anderson DR: The course of axons through the retina and optic nerve head. Arch Ophthalmol 1979;97:115.
8. Gouras P, Charles S: Physiology of the retina. *In* Tasman W, Jaeger EA (eds): Duane's Clinical Ophthalmology. Philadelphia, JB Lippincott, 1993, pp 1–13.
9. Ogden TE: Topography of the Retina. *In* Ryan SJ (ed): Retina. St. Louis, Mosby–Year Book, 1994, pp 32–36.
10. Lennie P: Parallel visual pathways: A review. Vision Res 1980;20:561.
11. Van Essen DC, Anderson CH, Fellman DJ: Information processing in the primate visual system: An integrated systems perspective. Science 1992;255:419.
12. Balaszi AG, Rootman, J, Drance SM: The effect of age on the nerve fiber population of the human optic nerve. Am J Ophthalmol 1984;97:760.
13. Cioffi GA, Van Buskirk EM: Vasculature anatomy of the optic nerve. *In* Ritch R, Shields MR, Krupin T (eds): The Glaucomas, 2nd ed, vol 1. St. Louis, Mosby–Year Book, 1997, pp 177–188.
14. Jonas JB, Naumann GOH: The optic nerve: Its embryology, histology, and morphology. *In* Varma R, Spaeth GL (eds): The Optic Nerve in Glaucoma. Philadelphia, JB Lippincott, 1993, pp 3–26.
15. Cioffi GA, Van Buskirk MD: Anatomy of the optic nerve. *In* Wright KW (ed): Textbook of Glaucoma. Baltimore, Williams & Wilkins, 1997, pp 591–597.
16. Olver JM, Spalton DJ, McCartney ACE: Microvasculature study of the retrolaminar optic nerve in man: The possible significance in anterior ischaemic optic neuropathy. Eye 1990;4:7.
17. Onda E, Cioffi GA, Bacon DR, et al: Microvasculature of the human optic nerve. Am J Ophthalmol 1995;120:92.
18. Orgul S, Meyer P, Cioffi GA: Physiology of blood flow regulation and mechanisms involved in optic nerve perfusion. J Glaucoma 1995;4:427.
19. Hayreh SS: Blood supply of the optic nerve head and its role in optic atrophy, glaucoma, and oedema of the optic disc. Br J Ophthalmol 1969;53:721.
20. Liebermann MF, Maumenee AE, Green WR: Histologic studies of the vasculature of the anterior optic nerve. Am J Ophthalmol 1996;85:302.
21. Anderson DR: Vascular supply to the optic nerve of primates. Am J Ophthalmol 1970;70:341.
22. Cioffi GA, Van Buskirk EM: Introduction: What is glaucoma? *In*

Wright KW (ed): Textbook of Ophthalmology. Baltimore, Williams & Wilkins, 1997, pp 569–574.
23. Quigley HA, Hohman RM, Addicks EM, et al: Morphologic changes in the lamina cribrosa correlated with neural loss in open-angle glaucoma. Am J Ophthalmol 1983;95:673.
24. Quigley HA, Addicks EM: Chronic experimental glaucoma in primates. II: Effect of extended intraocular pressure elevation on optic nerve head and axonal transport. Invest Ophthalmol Vis Sci 1980;19:137.
25. Quigley HA, Addicks EM; Regional differences in the structure of the lamina cribrosa and their relation to glaucomatous optic nerve damage. Arch Ophthalmol 1982;99:137.
26. Drance SM: Some factors in the production of low tension glaucoma. Br J Ophthalmol 1972;56:229.
27. Hayreh SS: Pathogenesis of optic nerve damage and visual field defects in glaucoma. Doc Ophthalmol Proc Series 1980;22:89.
28. Hernandez MR, Luo XX, Igoe F, et al: Extracellular matrix of the human lamina cribrosa. Am J Ophthalmol 1987;104:567.
29. Cartwright MJ, Crajewski AL, Friedberg ML, et al: Immune-related disease and normal tension glaucoma: A case control study. Arch Ophthalmol 1992;110:500.
30. Cioffi GA, Van Buskirk EM: Clinical testing and examination techniques in glaucoma. *In* Wright KW (ed): Textbook of Ophthalmology. Baltimore, Williams & Wilkins, 1997, pp 575–590.
31. Quigley HA, Brown AE, Morrison JC, et al: The size and shape of the optic disc in normal human eyes. Arch Ophthalmol 1990;108:51.
32. Carpel EF, Engstrom PF: The normal cup-disk ratio. Am J Ophthalmol 1981;91:588.
33. Fishman RS: Optic disc asymmetry: A sign of ocular hypertension. Arch Ophthalmol 1970;84:590.
34. Kirsch RE, Anderson DR: Clinical recognition of glaucomatous cupping. Am J Ophthalmol 1973;75:442.
35. Read RM, Spaeth GL: The practical clinical appraisal of the optic disc in glaucoma: The natural history of cup progression and some specific disc-field correlations. Trans Am Acad Ophthalmol Otol 1974;78:255.
36. Drance SM, Fairclough M, Butler DM, et al: The importance of disc hemorrhage in the prognosis of chronic open angle glaucoma. Arch Ophthalmol 1977;95:226.
37. Dorrell D: The tilted disc. Br J Ophthalmol 1978;62:16.
38. Brown GC, Tasman WS: Congenital Anomalies of the Optic Disc. New York, Grune & Stratton, 1983.
39. Smith P: On a case of chronic glaucoma of unusually long duration. Ophthalmic Rev (Lond) 1885;4:261.
40. Weinreb RN, Cioffi GA, Harris A: Optic nerve blood flow. *In* Van Buskirk EM, Shields MB (eds): 100 Years of Progress in Glaucoma. Philadelphia, Lippincott-Raven, 1997, pp 59–78.
41. Harris A, Sergott RC, Spaeth GL, et al: Color doppler analysis of ocular vessel blood velocity in normal-tension glaucoma. Am J Ophthalmol 1994;118:642.
42. Hayreh SS, Zimmerman MB, Podhajsky P, et al: Nocturnal arterial hypotension and its role in optic nerve head and ocular ischemic disorders. Am J Ophthalmol 1994;117:603.
43. Leighton DA, Phillips CI: Systemic blood pressure in open-angle glaucoma, low tension glaucoma, and the normal eye. Br J Ophthalmol 1972;56:447.
44. Drance SM, Douglas GR, Wijsman K, et al: Response of blood flow to warm and cold in normal and low-tension glaucoma patients. Am J Ophthalmol 1988;105:35.
45. McLeaod SD, West SK, Quigley HA, et al: A longitudinal study of the relationship between intraocular and blood pressure. Invest Ophthalmol Vis Sci 1990;31:2361.
46. Gasser P, Flammer J: Influence of vasospasm on visual function. Doc Ophthalmol 1987;66:3.
47. Chalmers-Redman RME, Fraser AD, Ju WYH, et al: Mechanisms of nerve cell death: Apoptosis or necrosis after cerebral ischaemia. Int Rev Neurobiol 1997;40:1.
48. Small DL, Buchan AM: NMDA antagonists: Their role in neuroprotection. Int Rev Neurobiol 1997;40:137.
49. Quigley HA: Mechanisms of glaucomatous optic neuropathy. *In* Van Buskirk EM, Shields MB (eds): 100 Years of Progress in Glaucoma. Philadelphia, Lippincott-Raven, 1997, pp 79–98.
50. Dreyer EB, Zurakowski D, Schumer RA, et al: Elevated glutamate levels in the vitreous body of humans and monkeys with glaucoma. Arch Ophthalmol 1996;114:299.

CHAPTER 5

Optic Nerve Assessment

LISA S. GAMELL and JOEL S. SCHUMAN

Given the central role of the optic nerve in glaucoma, it is vital to translate the basic understanding of that role into the clinical ability to accurately assess the optic nerve during an examination. Lisa Gamell and Joel Schuman describe how to accomplish this very difficult task. Beginning with what instrument to use, proceeding with the key features to distinguish the normal from the glaucomatous optic nerve, and discussing how to look at the nerve fiber layer, they have given us the tools to be successful. Once we have seen the optic nerve and nerve fiber layer, how do we properly document findings? The next section of the chapter answers this question, presenting the available alternatives, including their strengths and weaknesses. The assessment of optic nerve function is also described, along with the basics of all forms of visual testing, electrophysiology, and psychophysical testing. Finally, the authors make some suggestions as to choices among the many options. With the information in this chapter, however, you will be able to reach your own conclusions. This chapter is closely related to Chapter 4, Optic Nerve: Anatomy and Physiology; Chapter 26, Visual Field; and Chapter 27, Optic Nerve Damage and Dysfunction in Glaucoma.

In patients in whom glaucoma is suspected, the clinician should make all attempts to carefully discern the state of the optic nerve head. This process requires a mastery of the various clinical tools available for subjective evaluation of the optic nerve, including its size, shape, contour, and nerve fiber layer. The clinician must also have a working knowledge of the many functional testing and imaging systems available today, such as visual field testing modalities, optic nerve head photography, and nerve fiber layer analysis. This chapter gives an overview of these examination techniques to give the reader the tools necessary to diagnose and, it is hoped, prevent or at least detect early glaucomatous damage.

Clinical Examination of the Optic Nerve Head

TECHNIQUES

The tools used for viewing the optic nerve head employ both monocular and binocular techniques. The direct ophthalmoscope is one of the oldest instruments available for evaluating the fundus and optic nerve head.[1] It is handheld and provides an upright, ×15 magnified, monocular view of the optic nerve. The clinician can use the direct ophthalmoscope to follow the course of vessels crossing the disc margin and thereby estimate changes in cup and rim contour.[2] The instrument is particularly useful in the absence of a slit lamp or for examining patients with undilated pupils.

Reflection of light off the iris is minimized when the smaller round light of the direct ophthalmoscope is used. In addition, the smaller light approximates the size of the normal disc, allowing recognition of a particularly large or small disc. The direct ophthalmoscope can also be useful in assessing the color of the disc. With a small light restricted to the illumination of the disc itself, there is no illumination of the surrounding red retina, the reflection of which can change the perception of disc rim color.

In order to best appreciate the depth and contour changes of the optic nerve, however, a stereoscopic view is neces-

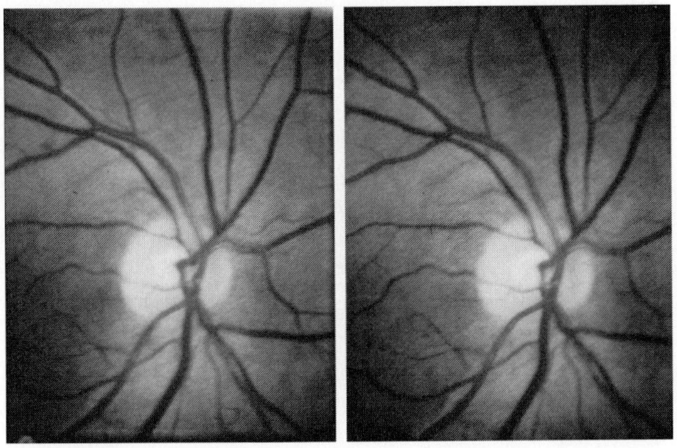

FIGURE 5–1. Healthy optic nerve head. Note the course of the vessels from the cup over the rim of the optic disc.

sary. Binocular indirect ophthalmoscopy at the slit lamp with the use of a hand-held, aspherical lens is the most useful technique.[2, 3] The 90D and 78D lenses are the most widely used. They give an inverted image of the optic nerve, with the 78D lens giving slightly higher magnification. Although this technique provides for an accurate three-dimensional assessment of the nerve, it requires an examiner who is skilled with such lenses and a compliant patient, and it is easiest with a dilated pupil. In circumstances when noncontact techniques are difficult to employ, a contact lens, such as the Goldmann three-mirror lens, may be used. It produces a stereoscopic, upright image and offers the advantage of stabilizing the patient's eye and holding open the lid during examination. Such contact lenses, however, require a coupling medium, such as hydroxymethylcellulose, which can be uncomfortable for the patient and may make subsequent fundus photography difficult.[4]

THE NORMAL OPTIC NERVE HEAD

In order to detect possible glaucomatous changes in the optic nerve, one must be familiar with its normal architecture. The optic nerve head is ovoid, with a horizontal diameter of 1.70 to 1.80 mm and a slightly larger vertical diameter of 1.85 to 1.95 mm.[4] It contains approximately 1.2 million axons, whose cell bodies form the ganglion cell layer of the retina.[5] As the axons exit the eye through the openings in the lamina cribrosa, they leave a central depression within the nerve known as the cup. The orange-pink tissue between the cup and the edge of the optic disc constitutes the neural or neuroretinal rim.[6] In a healthy optic nerve head, the course of the vessels can be fully traced from the cup over the rim of the optic disc (Fig. 5–1).

Glaucomatous Changes

ABNORMAL CUPPING

In patients with glaucoma, the optic cup enlarges and changes shape as a result of nerve fiber loss.[7] The enlargement is most notable in the vertical meridian of the disc, as most early axonal loss occurs at the superior and inferior poles.[8–10] It is this nonconcentric change in the cup that is typical of early glaucomatous damage. A loss of color often follows the loss of tissue, resulting in notably less pink rim tissue or a larger central yellow-white area, sometimes with the "cheesecloth" appearance of the lamina cribrosa in clear view (Fig. 5–2). Changes in color, however, are not accurate determinants of changes in cup size. In glaucoma, the area of cupping of the optic nerve should exceed the area of pallor. Glaucoma alters the natural contour of the rim tissue between the cup and the edge of the disc by causing a backward bowing of tissue.[2]

The normal shape of a physiologic cup is shown in frontal and cross-sectional view in Figure 5–3. One of the early signs of glaucomatous loss is a shelving or sloped appearance of the rim tissue (Fig. 5–4). It may seem that rim tissue is still present, but the delineation between rim and cup is less distinct. Another early change, termed *saucerization,* indicates a more subtle and more generalized depression of the entire disc (Fig. 5–5). Saucerization is a less common type of glaucomatous defect, but it is specific for glaucoma and can be an aid to early diagnosis.

Both shelving and saucerization defects tend to be early changes, and they are often not associated with visual field defects. When loss of neural tissue extends to the disc margin, visual field loss is noted (Fig. 5–6). Contour changes and configuration of the entire disc are important, but the superotemporal and inferotemporal portions of the disc are critical. The nerve fibers in this area represent the central and nasal portions of the visual field.[2]

ASYMMETRY

In a patient without glaucoma, it is rare to find a marked difference between the physiologic cups of the two eyes.[11–13] Asymmetry of the cups is an early sign of glaucoma until proven otherwise, and the index of suspicion rises if the intraocular pressure (IOP) is higher in the eye with the larger cup.[4]

Other factors that may contribute to seemingly asymmetric cups are (1) congenital anomalies, such as hypoplastic or tilted discs, (2) anisometropia, and (3) a physiologically large disc and scleral canal in one eye. Gross described a method of determining aberrations in disc size.[4, 14]

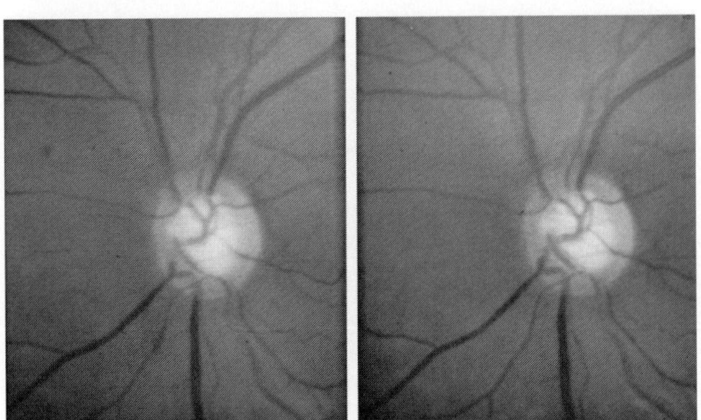

FIGURE 5–2. Optic nerve head of patient with primary open angle glaucoma.

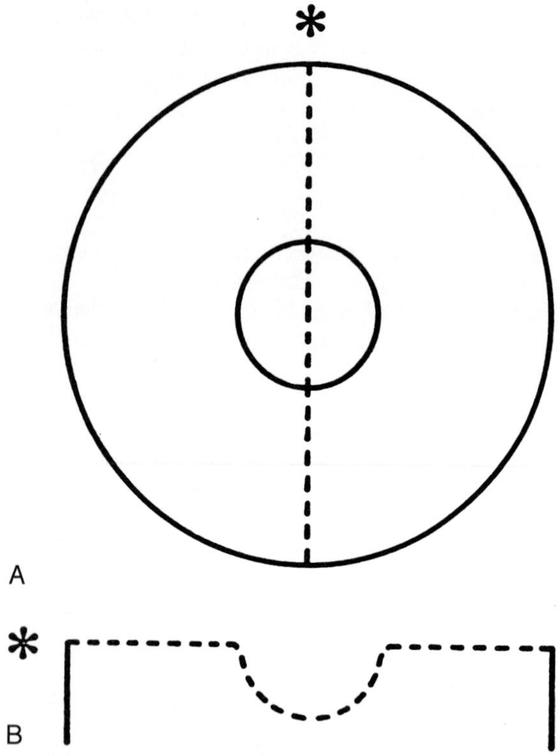

FIGURE 5–3. Frontal *(A)* and cross-sectional *(B)* views of a central physiologic cup. (From Epstein DL, Allingham RR, Schuman JS (eds): Chandler & Grant's Glaucoma, 4th ed. Baltimore, Williams & Wilkins, 1997, p 86.)

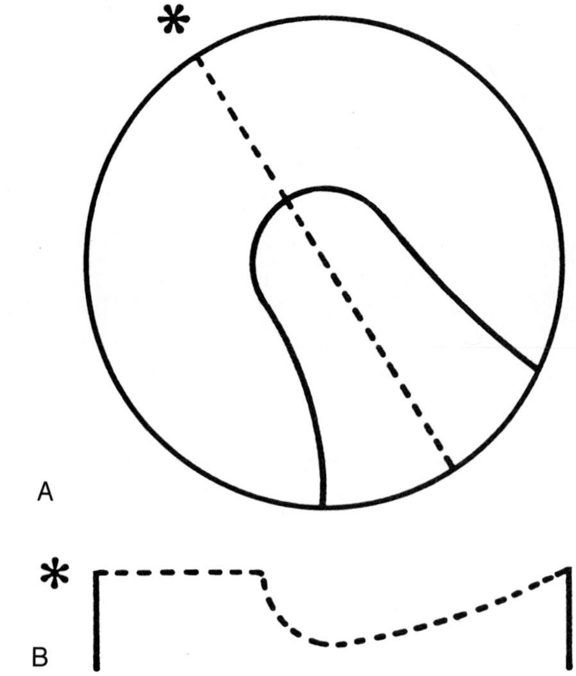

FIGURE 5–4. Frontal *(A)* and cross-sectional *(B)* views of a cup extending to the margin inferiorly and temporally (left eye). The cup is shelving, but it is not excavated and there is no visual field defect. (From Epstein DL, Allingham RR, Schuman JS (eds): Chandler & Grant's Glaucoma 4th ed. Baltimore, Williams & Wilkins, 1997, p 87.)

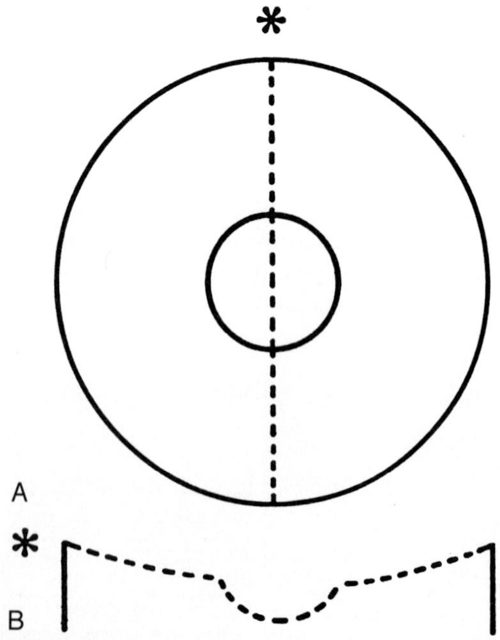

FIGURE 5–5. Frontal *(A)* and cross-sectional *(B)* views of a disc with saucerization. There is a backward bowing of the entire disc, but the physiologic cup is not enlarged. (From Epstein DL, Allingham RR, Schuman JS (eds): Chandler & Grant's Glaucoma, 4th ed. Baltimore, Williams & Wilkins: 1997, p 89.)

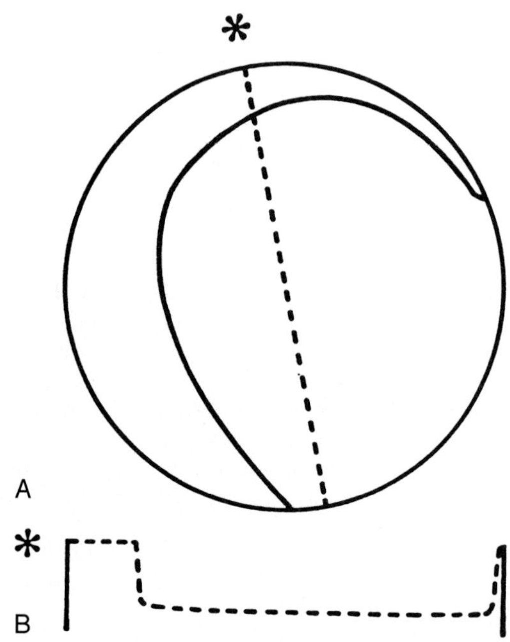

FIGURE 5–6. Frontal *(A)* and cross-sectional *(B)* views of a cup reaching the margin below and temporally (left eye). There is excavation both above and below as well as upper and lower visual fields defects. (From Epstein DL, Allingham RR, Schuman JS (eds): Chandler & Grant's Glaucoma, 4th ed. Baltimore, Williams & Wilkins, 1997, p 88.)

COLOR

As stated previously, in patients with glaucoma, cupping exceeds pallor, resulting in changes in rim contour that are more prominent than changes in color.[8, 15] In nonglaucomatous optic atrophy, there is often diffuse pallor but no change in the contour of the cup (Fig. 5–7). In some disorders, nonglaucomatous optic atrophy may be accompanied by cupping or pseudoglaucomatous cupping. These disorders include temporal arteritis, ischemic optic neuropathy, intracranial masses, toxic optic neuropathies (methanol), hereditary optic atrophy, syphilis, colobomas, and optic nerve pits.[16] Many of these disorders also produce glaucomatous-appearing visual field defects, which can be a confounding variable in diagnosis.[17] The key to differentiating these entities from true glaucoma lies within the intact neural rim; in glaucoma, the neural rim is pink, and in pseudoglaucoma, it is pale.

OTHER GLAUCOMATOUS SIGNS

With patients in whom glaucoma is suspected, there may be certain clinical clues to the progression toward actual disease. Flame-shaped disc hemorrhages, most commonly found inferotemporally, are a harbinger of future glaucomatous damage. Within 1 year after the presence of a disc hemorrhage, as many as 42% of patients in whom glaucoma was suspected had worsening of the nerve fiber layer reflectance, compared with 3.4% of those without disc hemorrhage.[18] Within 2 years, 22% of patients with disc hemorrhage had visual field progression, whereas only 7% of those without disc hemorrhage developed field loss.[18] The presence of a disc hemorrhage in a patient in whom glaucoma is suspected or diagnosed should therefore be regarded as a warning sign of possible disease progression.

One should bear in mind, however, that flame-type hemorrhages may also be found in association with other diseases, such as diabetic retinopathy, vascular occlusions, blood vessel abnormalities (optociliary shunt) and anterior ischemic optic neuropathy (AION). One needs, therefore, to use the history, clinical findings, symptoms, and visual field results to properly evaluate the patient with flame-shaped disc hemorrhages.

In the absence of disc hemorrhages or obvious excavation of the cup, the clinician must search for other clues to detect early signs of glaucoma. The orientation of the vessels on the disc can reveal subtle changes in the cup and rim contour. Nasalization of the vessels has been seen in association with glaucoma but may also be seen in physiologic cupping (Fig. 5–8).[4] *Undermining*, or the disappearance of vessels under the neural rim as they course over the rim of the cup, is also seen in glaucoma.[19] This appearance has also been called "bayoneting," for the sharp angle of the vessels has been likened to the edge of a bayonet. One should note that in a glaucomatous cupping, when the undermining vessels cross the disc, they pass over its scleral rim (Fig. 5–9). In physiologic cupping, the vessels pass around healthy disc tissue (Fig. 5–10). When rim tissue is lost and no longer present under a vessel, the vessel may appear suspended or floating. This phenomenon, known as *baring* of the circumlinear vessels, may be an indicator of loss of the neuroretinal rim tissue but is not specific for glaucoma (Fig. 5–11).[20] The main point here is that one should not use vessel configuration alone to diagnose glaucomatous change; one should use vessel findings as a means of detecting cup and rim contour changes, such as sloping and excavation, in order to diagnose optic nerve damage.

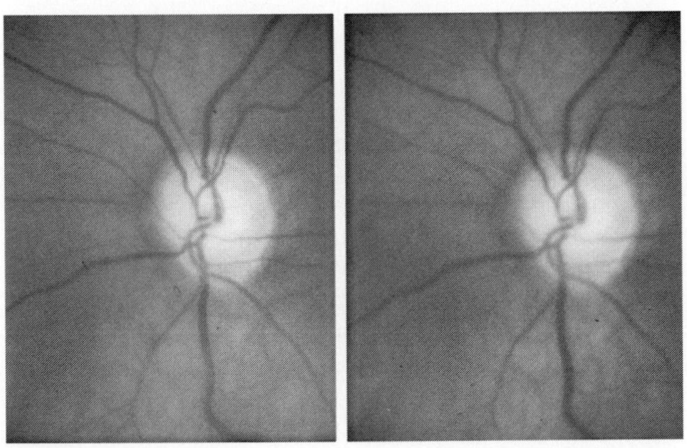

FIGURE 5–7. Nonglaucomatous optic atrophy. There is diffuse pallor exceeding the change in the contour of the cup.

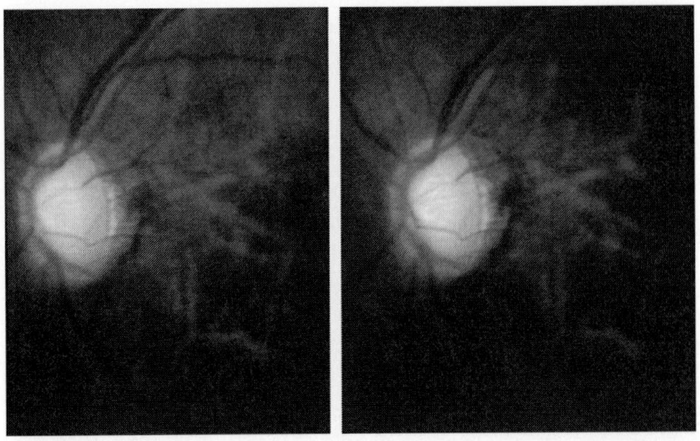

FIGURE 5–8. Optic nerve head with nasalization of the vessels. This can be seen in association with glaucoma or in physiologic cups.

However, rim contour can be difficult to delineate in the presence of peripapillary atrophy. This disorders manifests as an area of bare choroid or sclera surrounding the disc in a crescent or halo formation. When the atrophy is a large halo, as is often seen in high myopia, examining the caliber of the neural rim becomes a challenge (Fig. 5–12). These areas of atrophy sometimes have associated nerve fiber layer and visual field defects. Their relationship to glaucomatous optic nerve damage in particular remains unclear.[21] Some researchers suggest a relationship between peripapillary atrophy and glaucomatous damage and visual field changes.[22, 23] This nerve damage may be due in part to a compromised optic nerve or choroidal circulation in the areas of atrophy.[4] Similarly, the tilted appearance of many myopic discs can make early glaucomatous changes difficult to identify. These patients can have early field loss that extends into fixation.[24] This makes examination of the temporal portion of the disc especially important in myopic patients.[25] As a general rule, therefore, in patients with peripapillary atrophy or myopic-appearing discs, the clinician should have a lower threshold for obtaining visual

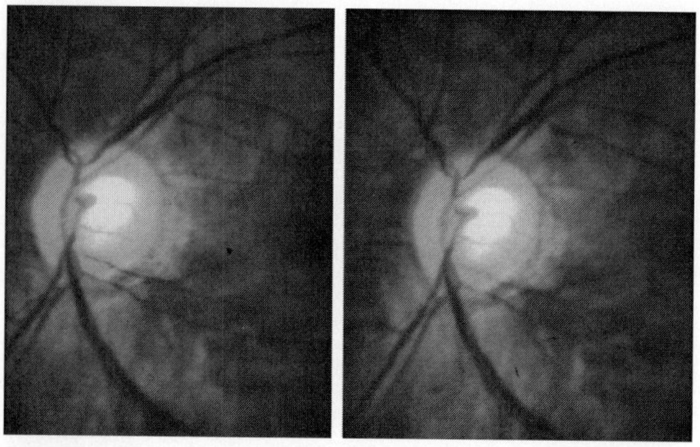

FIGURE 5–9. This glaucomatous cup shows undermining with blood vessels passing over the scleral rim.

field evaluations, treating elevated IOP, and suspecting a diagnosis of glaucoma.[2]

Clinical Examination of the Nerve Fiber Layer

NORMAL ANATOMY

The nerve fiber layer (NFL) of the retina contains the axons of the ganglion cells, neuroglia and astrocytes. The axons of the ganglion cells are anatomically separated along an imaginary horizontal demarcation line called the horizontal retinal raphe (Fig. 5–13). Ganglion cells from the superior retina travel toward the superior and superotemporal portions of the disc. Similarly, inferior ganglion cells enter the disc inferiorly and inferotemporally. The papillomacular bundle consists of ganglion cells between the fovea and the disc, and these fibers run directly to the temporal portion of the disc. Axons from the macular area temporal to the fovea arc around the papillomacular bundle fibers to enter the superior and inferior portions of the disc.[26, 27]

In addition to this horizontal segregation, the axons demonstrate a vertical stratification within the NFL based on anterior-to-posterior retinotopic location.[28] For example, the axons of peripheral retinal ganglion cells run deep within the NFL and enter the nerve toward the outer portion of the disc. The axons originating closer to the fovea course over these peripheral axons to lie more superficially within the NFL and enter the disc more centrally. The peripapillary axons lie most superficially and centrally within the optic nerve.[26]

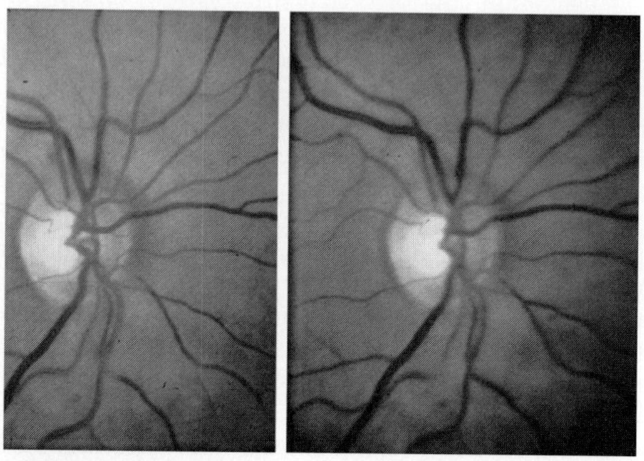

FIGURE 5–10. This physiologic cup shows blood vessels crossing over healthy disc tissue.

VIEWING THE NERVE FIBER LAYER

Clinically, the NFL covers the retina with a sheet of tubular fibers arranged in parallel. These nerve fibers are perpendicular to incoming rays of light. It is the organization of these nerve bundles that lends to their reflective pattern on examination. Viewing the NFL, however, is difficult and requires practice. It is most easily seen using red-free, or blue-green, wavelengths of light; the choroid and retinal pigment epithelium (RPE) absorb blue and green light, allowing for greater contrast between the nerve fibers and the remainder of the retina.[26] On the red-free background, axons can be seen as fine, silvery parallel lines in the posterior pole (Fig. 5–14). An absence of this typical pattern of reflectivity signifies loss of nerve fibers, the detection of which is crucial to monitoring glaucomatous damage.

Although the NFL can be seen with the red-free light and a direct ophthalmoscope, the best view is with stereoscopic biomicroscopy at the slit lamp.[29] A dilated pupil allows for easier visualization, and a 78D lens supplies adequate magnification to detect the delicate striations of the nerve bundles. A 90D lens can also be used if a broader field of view is preferred.

DETECTING NERVE FIBER LAYER LOSS

Understanding the normal reflective patterns of the NFL is a prerequisite for detecting its defects. The NFL is thickest at the superior and inferior poles of the disc, resulting in a higher reflectance in these areas (see Fig. 5–14). In these regions, one may also appreciate a texture similar to that of rice grains laid end to end.[26] Normally, there is lower reflectivity in the nasal area and papillomacular bundle because the NFL is thinner in these regions.[29] Another good clinical landmark is the medium-sized vessels, whose borders are usually obscured by an overlying layer of nerve fibers.

Damage to the ganglion cell axons can result in a pattern of diffuse NFL loss or focal NFL atrophy. When there is diffuse thinning of the NFL, the reflective pattern at the superior and inferior poles of the disc may acquire the same brightness as the papillomacular bundle and may lose its usual grainy texture. In addition, the borders of the medium-sized vessels, obscured in the healthy NFL, become more distinct.[29, 30] Diffuse dropout may be subtle, and often, comparing the diseased eye in question with the fellow eye may prove helpful.

Focal defects are usually wedge-shaped. They may be thin near the disc but they fan out in an arcuate pattern toward the periphery (Fig. 5–15). It is important to distinguish actual wedge defects from normally occurring slit defects. The key difference is that a normal slit defect is no larger in diameter than a retinal vein and does not

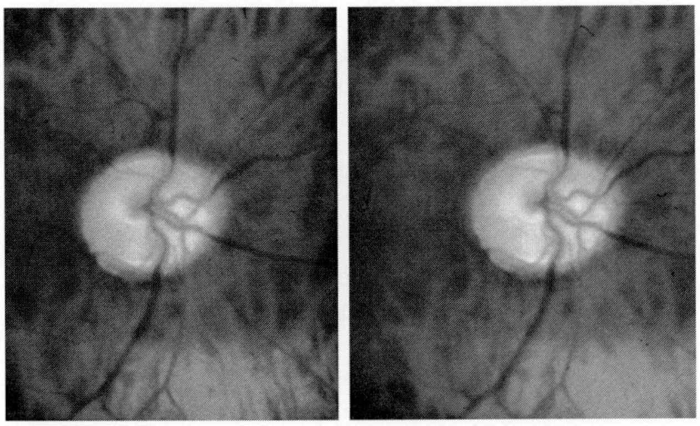

FIGURE 5–11. In this advanced glaucomatous cup, there is no neural rim tissue, and the vessels appear to be floating or suspended. This finding is known as "baring" of the circumlinear vessels.

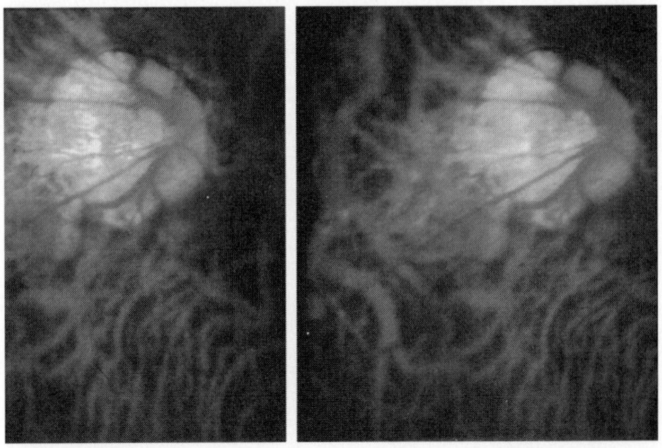

FIGURE 5–12. In this highly myopic patient with peripapillary atrophy, it can be a challenge to determine the amount of neural rim tissue.

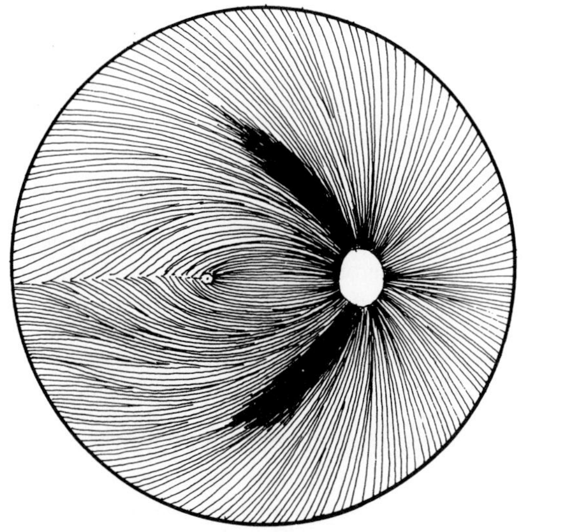

FIGURE 5–13. Representation of the typical arrangement of the human retinal nerve fiber layer (RNFL). Lower drawing represents the topography of the NFL where the more distal ganglion cell axons project to the more peripheral area of the optic disc rim. (Reprinted from Mattox C: Clinical examination of the nerve fiber layer. *In* Schuman JS (ed): Imaging in Glaucoma. Thorofare, NJ, Slack Inc, 1997, p 64.)

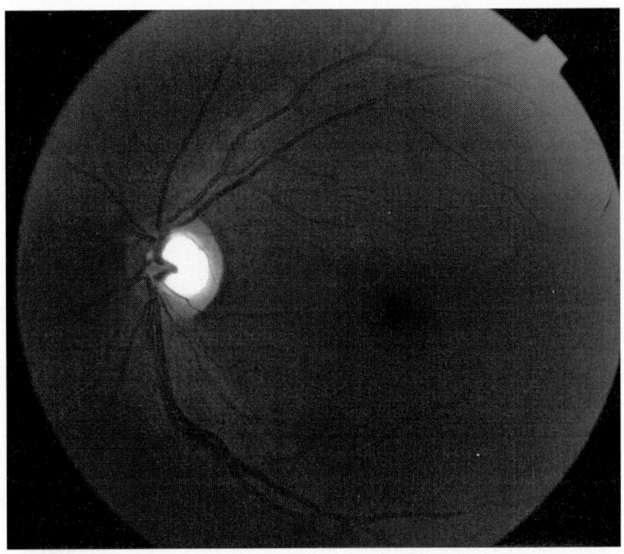

FIGURE 5–14. Red-free photograph of a healthy optic nerve head. Note very fine, silvery lines and the reflective pattern of the nerve fiber layer.

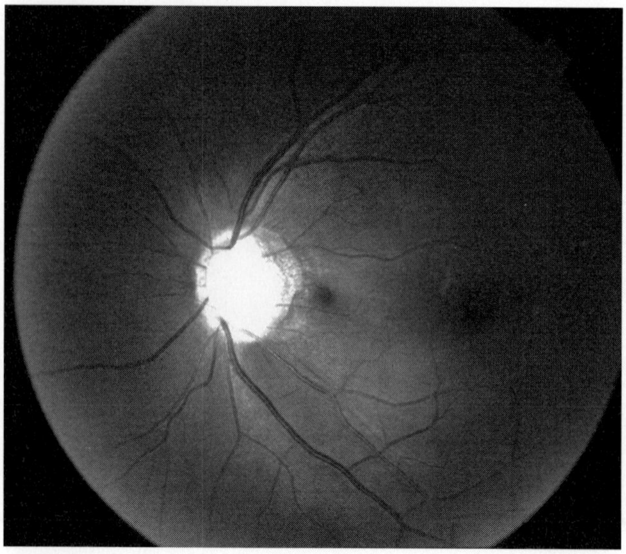

FIGURE 5–15. Red-free photograph of a glaucomatous optic nerve head. Note the loss of the reflectivity and a focal nerve fiber layer defect.

extend to the disc rim.[26] A wedge defect, in contrast, is larger than a retinal vessel and extends to the disc.

Once an NFL defect is detected, probably the best mode of documentation is NFL photography. This procedure, however, requires an experienced photographer. The various cameras used for this technique are described in Table 5–1. In the absence of photography, a consistent grading system becomes important for long-term follow-up and patient care. Intricate grading systems have been described to quantify NFL loss in patients.[31, 32] For clinical purposes, we prefer the use of descriptive terms, such as normal, thin, absent, focal, or diffuse, along with the location of the defects.[29] In addition, a small drawing of the optic nerve and NFL defect can be made for documentation.

WHY EXAMINE THE NERVE FIBER LAYER?

Although initially technically difficult, examining the NFL offers many advantages to the skilled clinician. Most evident is the ability to detect early loss of neural tissue, which is a hallmark of glaucomatous damage. Careful NFL examination, however, can also allow the practitioner to understand otherwise equivocal results of functional testing; for example, the first change on a visual field test or a change present on an unreliable field can be anatomically correlated with an area in the NFL. If a defect is present, the visual field changes are probably indicative of disease.

Methods of Optic Nerve Imaging and Analysis

We have discussed various techniques for subjectively and qualitatively examining the optic nerve head in order to detect possible glaucomatous damage. There is, however, great variation in interpretation of clinical optic nerve and NFL assessment. For this reason, we seek to develop objective, quantitative means to analyze the patient with glaucoma. Short of that, simple objective recording of the appearance of the eye is of value. By documenting information regarding the NFL, cup appearance, or neural rim caliber, we can establish an objective point of reference for evaluating disease progression. Some of the objective methods of documentation and quantitative analysis include stereoscopic optic nerve head photography, NFL photography, the Glaucoma Scope, confocal scanning laser ophthalmoscopy (CSLO), polarimetry, and optical coherence tomography (OCT).

PHOTOGRAPHY

Probably the longest-standing method of optic nerve imaging is photography. Stereoscopic disc photography is most valuable in following cases of glaucoma because it helps minimize interobserver and even intraobserver errors regarding optic nerve appearance and rim contour. The best technique for stereoscopic disc photography is simultaneous stereoscopic disc photography. Simultaneous devices allow the photographer to take a stereophotograph with a single exposure. There are two methods of achieving simultaneous photographs. One uses twin prisms mounted over the objective of a standard fundus camera. The Nidek 3Dx and Topcon TRC-SS2 employ this technique and are available for clinical use.[33] The other, the Donaldson fundus camera, has been considered the standard in simultaneous

TABLE 5–1. PHOTOGRAPHY TECHNIQUES FOR EVALUATION OF NERVE FIBER LAYER

	Airaksinen	Quigley	NEEC	NEEC
Camera	**Canon**	**Zeiss**	**Canon 6F60Z**	**Topcon 501A Digital System**
Field	60°	1.6× magnifier	60°	55°
Filter	Blue filter	Filter transmits <1% of light >580 nm, and 70% of light between 400 and 555 nm	Barrier filter out, exciter filter in	495 nm exciter filter only
Film settings	Kodak Pantomic-X	Kodak Technical Pan 480 to 720 watt-seconds	T-Max 400 Flash on 3 or 4	Digital Gain 6 dB, flash 25
Processing	7 minutes in Kodak HCl 10 mix 1:3	12 minutes at 70°F in D-11, 1:1 mix	8.5 minutes in D-19 process	Digital to prints or slides

NEEC = New England Eye Center, Boston, MA
From Mattox C: Clinical examination of the nerve fiber layer. *In* Schuman JS (ed): Imaging in Glaucoma. Thorofare, New Jersey, Slack Inc, 1997, p 65.

photography. It functions based upon the principles of binocular indirect ophthalmoscopy.[33] Unfortunately, the Donaldson camera is not commercially available, and repair of the existing units is extremely difficult. The Nidek 3Dx and Donaldson cameras have been shown to produce similar stereoscopic quality images.[34]

Another method of producing stereophotographs is to take consecutive exposures of the optic nerve head. This can be achieved by manually shifting the joystick to alter the viewing angle between frames.[33, 34] Alternatively, a device known as an Allen separator may be used. This is a motorized device that fits over the photographic tube of a standard Zeiss camera and contains a swiveling glass plate that directs light toward different portions of the pupil.[34]

GLAUCOMA SCOPE

Optic nerve photography and NFL photography allow the clinician to make qualitative assessments regarding the optic nerve and possible glaucomatous loss. The Glaucoma Scope (Ophthalmic Imaging Systems, Sacramento, CA) is a computerized system that allows for quantitative evaluation of the optic nerve topography. The computer projects a series of parallel lines onto the optic disc and can measure the peripapillary contour and the amount of change over time based upon the deflection of these lines. The lines are projected by a halogen lamp illumination system that projects 25 lines at an angle of 9 degrees to the optic nerve head.[35] This light wavelength is 750 nm, in the near-infrared light range, and a polarizing filter is employed to maximize reflection of the NFL. When using the images obtained by this mode of analysis, one must look at the quality scale rating. Usually, a rating of greater than 4 is adequate for analysis, 10 is very good, and greater than 15 is considered an excellent image.[36]

The technique works as follows: The examiner outlines the suspected disc margin with eight points and then maps the major disc vessels. The projected line data are then displayed, and an algorithm converts them into depth values based on a retinal reference point. The optic cup is defined as the area inside the disc margin that is 140 μm or more below the reference plane.[36] On the printout, up to 722 numeric depth values appear, with each value representing the average of 136 data points covering an area of 69 μm vertically by 138 μm horizontally. If there are no line data in an area, an "x" appears. Data are printed out as this numeric depth information and also as a change-from-baseline analysis report in which values that have changed by more than 75 μm are shown. One may also obtain three-dimensional false color topography map printouts, in which blue signifies shallow areas and red the deepest area. Other information provided comprises the cup-to-disc ratio, disc diameter, disc area, cup area, and the refraction of the eye.

There are some limitations to the Glaucoma Scope. The minimum pupil size necessary is about 4 mm, and pupillary dilation is preferable.[37] In addition, the quality of images may be influenced by hyperpigmentation of the fundus, pseudophakia, aphakia, corneal opacities, and cataracts.

Reproducibility

The Glaucoma Scope has a 90% specificity for identifying patients with glaucoma, which is not high enough for the clinician to rely upon this modality alone for screening.[36]

The best use for the Glaucoma Scope is in conjunction with careful clinical examination to detect changes in optic nerve head topography that may not be obvious to the naked eye. In addition, it may be helpful in detecting contour and depth changes in patients who (1) are noncompliant, (2) have ocular hypertension, or (3) have normal-tension glaucoma.

CONFOCAL SCANNING LASER OPHTHALMOSCOPY

Instruments such as the confocal scanning laser ophthalmoscope offer the advantage of providing real-time images of the fundus and nerve that can be evaluated at the time of the patient's visit. In contrast to the Glaucoma Scope, this system does not require pupillary dilation and clear media for good quality images. Two main systems have been clinically investigated: the Heidelberg Retina Tomograph (HRT, Heidelberg Engineering GmbH, Heidelberg, Germany) and the Topographic Scanning System (TopSS, Laser Diagnostic Technologies, Inc., San Diego, CA). The HRT uses a diode laser at a wavelength of 670 nm, and the TopSS uses a laser with a wavelength of 780 nm.[38] These imaging systems scan the surface of the optic nerve in three dimensions (x, y, and z) as a series of section images in 32 focal planes, producing an image consisting of 256 × 256 pixels. Total imaging and analysis time is approximately 1.6 seconds.

These scanning systems come with software programs that allow for ease of image acquisition, storage, retrieval, and data analysis. The systems record cup-to-disc ratio, cup volume, rim volume, disc area, cup area, rim area, cup depth, peripapillary retinal height, and NFL thickness. Topographic measurements can be obtained by placing a contour line around the disc margin. Topographic parameters are then calculated relative to a standard reference plane. With the HRT, this plane is 50 μm posterior to the surface of the papillomacular bundle. Parameters that may be determined include cup area, cup-to-disc area ratio, cup volume, rim area, rim volume, NFL thickness, and NFL cross-sectional area.[38]

Work is currently being conducted to determine the best way to analyze these data and help distinguish a normal optic nerve head from one with glaucoma. One technique is the ranked-segment distribution (RSD) curve.[39] This method measures topographic optic nerve parameters in 36 segments, each representing 10 degrees. The segments are ranked in descending order, and the fifth percentile value for rim area and NFL cross-sectional area from 39 age-matched nonglaucomatous eyes is used to establish normal limit values.[38] If a glaucomatous eye is evaluated, the fifth percentile data are used to construct an RSD curve, which is compared with an age-matched normal RSD curve. Three or more abnormal ranked segments indicates an abnormal RSD curve. More recent studies have investigated the use of other parameters to help detect potential glaucomatous damage and visual field loss.[40, 41]

One advantage of the CSLO units is that they do not rely heavily upon pupillary dilation or clear media to obtain quality images. In addition, real-time images allow for the assessment of optic nerve parameters during the patient's visit; there is no need for a skilled photographer and processing of film. Although variability of a single measurement can range from 25 to 40 μm, repetitive imaging may improve reproducibility.[42, 43]

Pupillary dilation is not necessary in most cases, but in patients with pupils less than 3 mm or with marked media opacities, dilation may allow good quality images to be obtained.[38] Another disadvantage is that this technology uses the papillomacular bundle as its reference plane, the thickness of which may be altered in glaucoma. In general, the HRT and other CSLO systems are currently good adjuncts to the clinical evaluation of patients with glaucoma. Future studies will determine the role of such instruments as aids in following disease progression or as screening devices.

OPTICAL COHERENCE TOMOGRAPHY

OCT allows noninvasive, noncontact, cross-sectional imaging of the optic nerve head and NFL.[35, 44–49] It is based on the principle of low-coherence reflectometry. It utilizes the coherence properties of light reflected back from a sample to determine time-of-light delay from the sample's reflective boundaries and back-scattering sites.[35] The longitudinal location of the reflection sites is found through the use of this delay information. By performing a series of these longitudinal scans at various lateral locations in the posterior pole, the OCT system can construct a two-dimensional, false-color printout. The resulting image is histologically comparable to the retinal layers and optic disc. OCT, therefore, is optically analogous to an ultrasound B-scan.[47] OCT, however, can achieve images at resolutions of up to 10 μm, higher than with computed tomography, magnetic resonance imaging, or ultrasound.

The commercial OCT unit is integral to a fundus camera (Humphrey Instruments, San Leandro, CA). Our prototype unit, on which we have analyzed more than 500 subjects, is coupled with a slit-lamp biomicroscope and computer-driven galvanometric scanners that permit manipulation of the beam. The beam passes through a 78D lens such that the beam is coincident with the slit-lamp image plane. This allows the eye to be visualized with a near-infrared charge coupled device (CCD) camera while scanning is in process (Fig. 5–16).[44] The image is usually attained in 2.5 seconds in the prototype and in less than 1 second in the commercial unit.

An image-processing computer program quantitates total retinal thickness and NFL thickness of the sections obtained by scanning the optic nerve head circumferentially. The NFL correlates with the highly reflective red layer at the vitreoretinal interface. The photoreceptor layer lies at the position of minimum reflectivity. The boundaries of the NFL and RPE are highlighted with a blue line, and the internal limiting membrane with a white line (Fig. 5–17). The NFL thickness is documented as an average of each quadrant of the optic nerve head, in the superior, inferior, temporal, and nasal quadrants, as well as by "clock hour" and for the entire 360 degrees.[44]

OCT has been found to show a high correlation not only with histopathologic findings[50] but also with clinical parameters such as visual fields and NFL appearance.[45, 51] Normally, the NFL is thickest in the superior and inferior quadrants, as the OCT printout shown in Figure 5–18 demonstrates. This produces a typical quadrifusiform pattern on OCT color printouts, representing the thinner NFL nasally and temporally alternating with the thicker areas superiorly and inferiorly. The NFL at 12 o'clock and 6 o'clock is slightly thinner, in general, than that on either side of each pole. In an eye with glaucoma, the NFL may be thinned in areas that correspond clinically with cupping and/or visual field loss (Fig. 5–19).

Although the development of a large-scale normative database is a focus of current research efforts, no definitive quantitative parameters exist for distinguishing glaucomatous from nonglaucomatous eyes. The most recent OCT findings, however, reveal that an NFL thickness greater than 125 to 130 μm in the superior and inferior quadrants is usually found in nonglaucomatous eyes. Eyes with glaucoma, however, often have an average NFL thickness less than 100 μm in these quadrants.[45, 46] These numbers are not absolute but are a general guideline to detecting glaucomatous changes; they are based on a circle diameter of 3.4 mm with our prototype device.[46]

NFL thinning that falls within the range for glaucomatous change as described previously also shows a significant correlation with defects found on visual field testing.[45] For example, defects in the inferior NFL corresponded to superior visual field changes. In contrast, cup-to-disc ratio is not significantly related to the presence of field defects. This finding is in agreement with earlier work that has shown the importance of NFL thickness with regard to glaucomatous status.[52–54]

Thus, OCT is a valuable imaging technique. The OCT device provides higher resolution images than optic nerve head analyzers and CSLO techniques. Unlike with other imaging modalities, no reference plane is required to determine the NFL thickness. OCT provides an absolute measurement of the retinal structure and thickness, from which the NFL thickness is calculated.[35] Reproducibility with OCT is also better than with other imaging devices, ranging from 10 to 20 μm for mean overall NFL thickness.[46] This more narrow range of variability can be critical in detecting potentially significant glaucomatous damage, because a reduction in NFL thickness of as much as 20% to 40% can be present before any defects are noted on visual field analysis.[53]

OCT, however, is new, and a normative database is currently being established. The technique is best used as an adjunct to clinical examination and functional testing, although studies are currently being conducted to determine its value as a screening tool for glaucoma. OCT may also prove particularly useful in patients who are unable to undergo functional testing or in whom visualization of the fundus is problematic.

SCANNING LASER POLARIMETRY

Scanning laser polarimetry is an imaging method that provides quantitative measurements of the peripapillary NFL. It relies on the birefringent nature of the NFL to assess

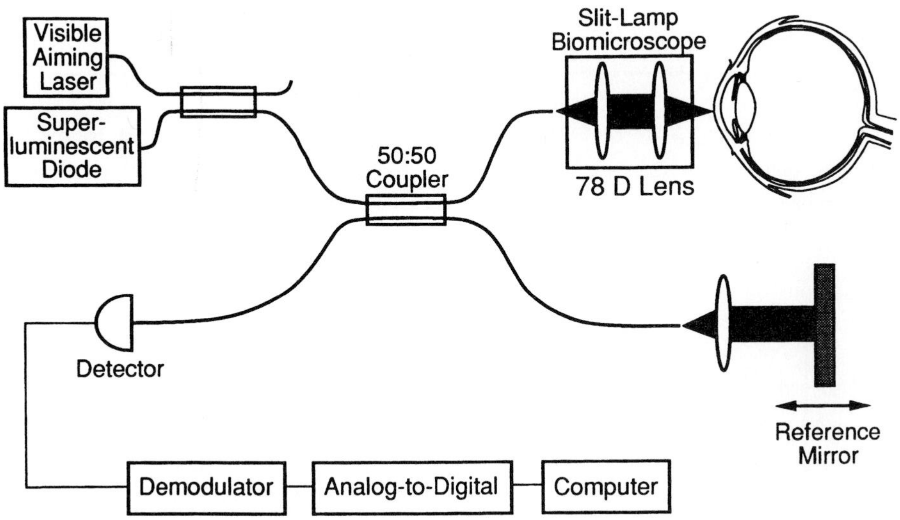

FIGURE 5–16. Schematic diagram of an optical coherence tomography scanner. (From Schuman JS, Hee MR, Puliafito CA, et al: Quantification of nerve fiber layer thickness in normal and glaucomatous eyes using optical coherence tomography: A pilot study. Arch Ophthalmol 1995; 113:586.)

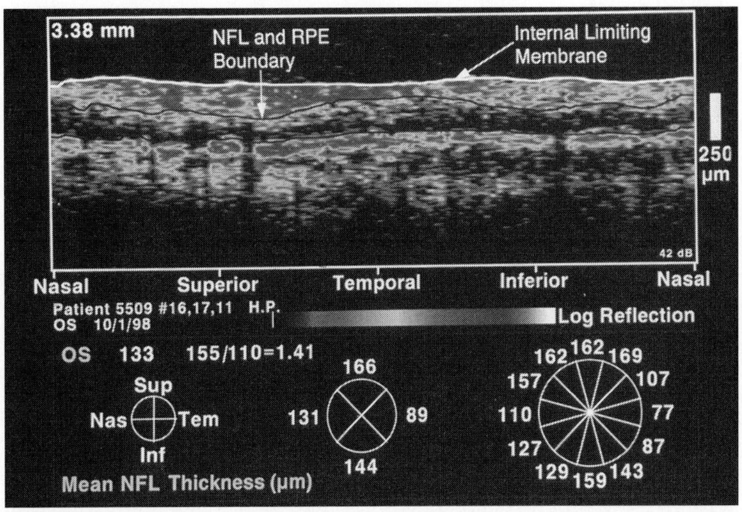

FIGURE 5–17. Optical coherence tomography scan showing the boundaries of the nerve fiber layer (NFL) and retinal pigment epithelium (RPE) (highlighted with a *blue line)*, and the internal limiting membrane *(white line)*. Inf, inferior; Nas, nasal; Sup, superior; Tem, temporal.

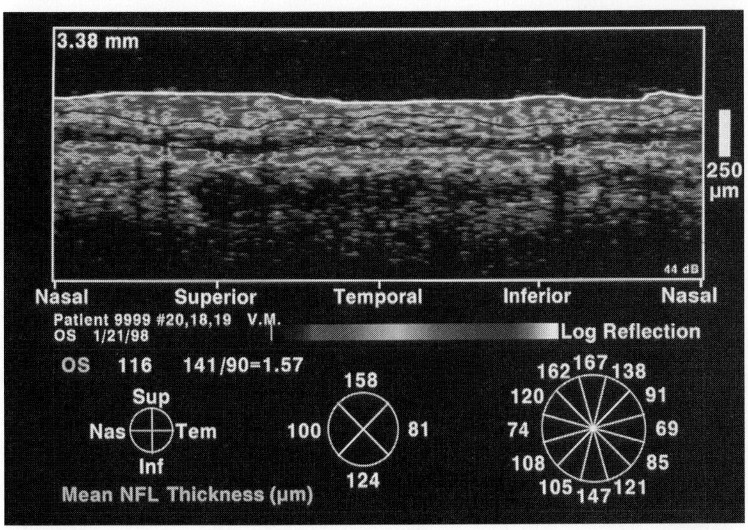

FIGURE 5–18. Double-hump pattern of an optical coherence tomography scan of a normal subject, showing thickest nerve fiber layer (NFL) in the superior and inferior quadrants. Inf, inferior; Nas, nasal; Os, left eye; Sup, superior; Tem, temporal.

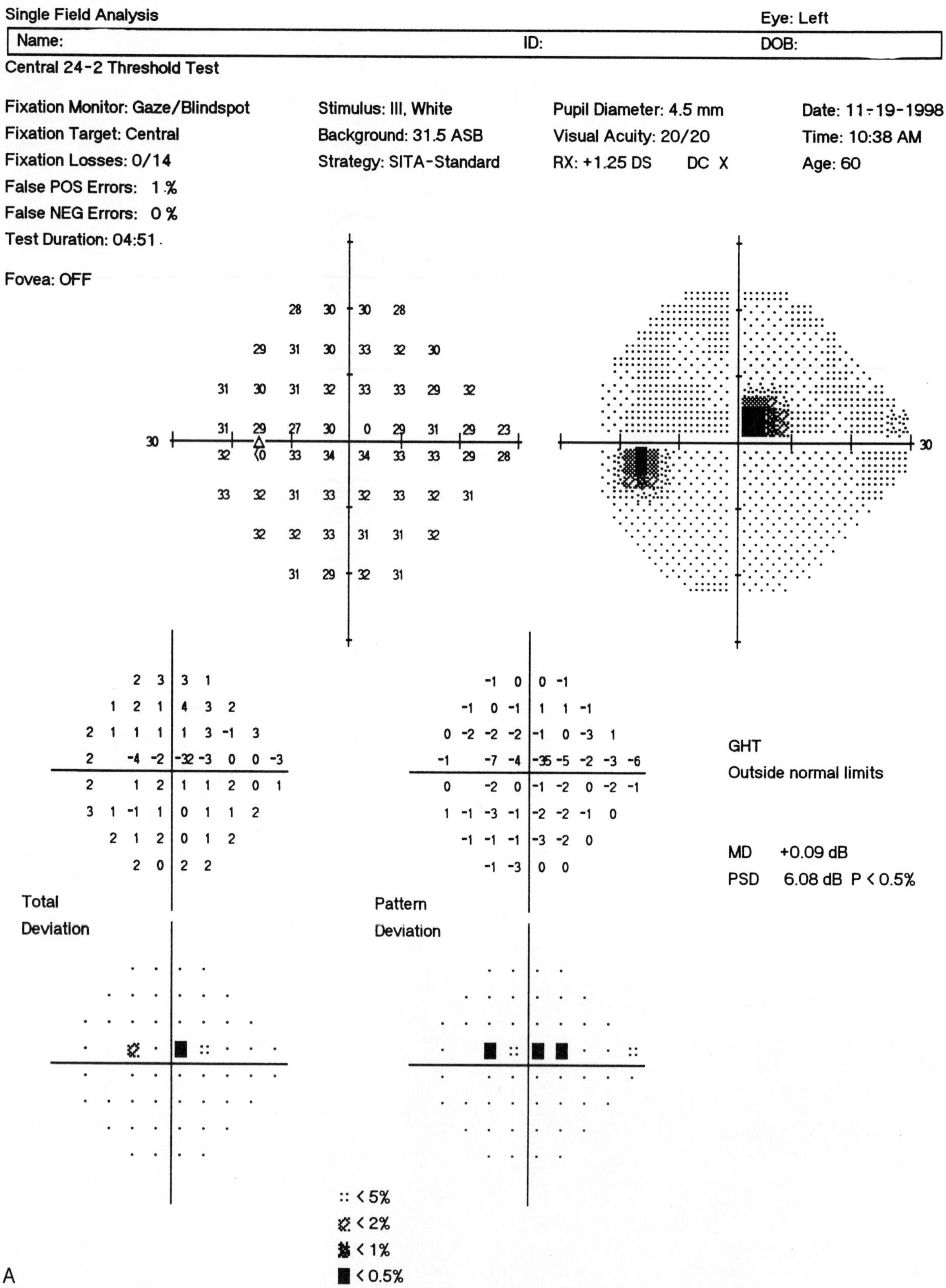

A

FIGURE 5–19. The defect in this visual field *(A)* corresponds well with the thinning of the nerve fiber layer (NFL) as seen in *(B)* the optical coherence tomograph of the same eye. Inf, inferior; Nas, nasal; OS, left eye; Sup, superior; Tem, temporal.

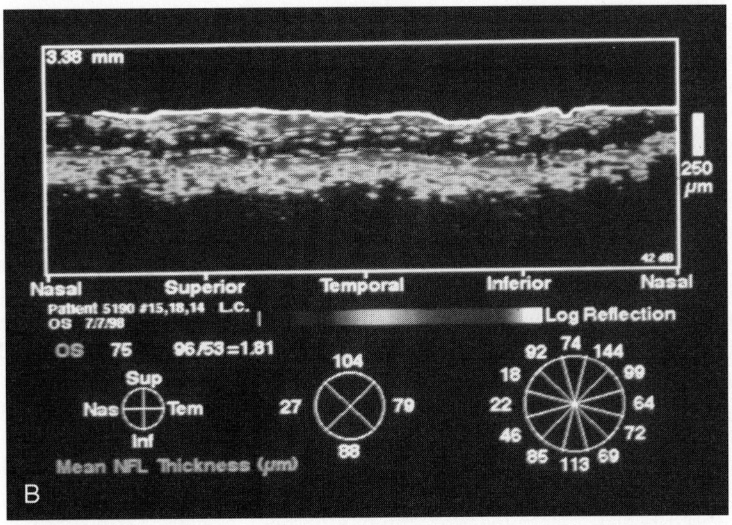

FIGURE 5–19 *Continued*

thickness.[53] As light travels back and forth along the NFL, it causes retardance, or a change of the polarization state of the illuminating laser beam. The thicker the NFL, the greater the retardance. NFL thickness is determined by Fourier ellipsometry, which measures the level of retardance. This technology utilizes a patented program to account for any polarization effects from areas anterior to the internal limiting membrane, such as the cornea and lens.[35]

The GDx (Nerve Fiber Analyzer-Laser Diagnostic Technologies, Inc., San Diego, CA) is a confocal scanning laser polarimeter that utilizes a polarization modulated laser beam at a wavelength of 780nm.[55] The beam is focused onto the retina, where it penetrates the NFL and is partially reflected from the retina's deeper layers. The light emitted back from the eye is separated from the illuminating beam by a nonpolarizing beam splitter and is analyzed by a polarization detection unit. This analyzed data is digitized and stored in a computer. Acquisition time for a scan consisting of 256 × 256 pixels is approximately 0.7 seconds.[55]

Once the data are obtained, a computer algorithm calculates the retardance at each pixel. It takes the system another 15 seconds to construct a retardance map from this information (Fig. 5–20). Retardation ratios have been shown to be significantly associated with global measures of field loss, mean deviation, and corrected pattern standard deviation.[56] Other studies have shown a resolution in vitro of up to 13 μm.[57]

One advantage of the GDx is that a reference plane is not needed to obtain images. In addition, the technique is not based on imaging principles, so there are no magnification errors.[55]

One important criticism of the GDx, however, is that it represents NFL thickness as retardation units. This is a relative measurement of the NFL, as opposed to measuring in microns, like the OCT unit. Studies in monkey eyes have revealed a correlation between histopathologic NFL measurements and retardation.[58] It is also unclear how cataract changes and corneal opacities influence retardance measurements. Also, the GDx can give erroneous values in areas of peripapillary atrophy and scarring, resulting in high retardance readings.[59] Further studies are needed to determine the quantitative parameters that will help detect early progression of glaucomatous damage.

Functional Testing in Glaucoma

In diagnosing glaucoma, the clinician considers factors such as IOP and the appearance of the optic nerve head and NFL, as discussed in earlier sections of the chapter. One must also, however, assess optic nerve function, because the ultimate concern is how changes in the optic nerve affect the patient's vision, visual field, and visual function. It is important to correlate clinical findings with results of functional testing in order to best determine the severity and progression of disease.

VISUAL FIELD TESTING

In the presence of cupping and/or NFL changes suspected to indicate glaucoma, a consistent change on visual field testing can often confirm the diagnosis of glaucoma. The normal visual field extends 60 degrees nasally and superi-

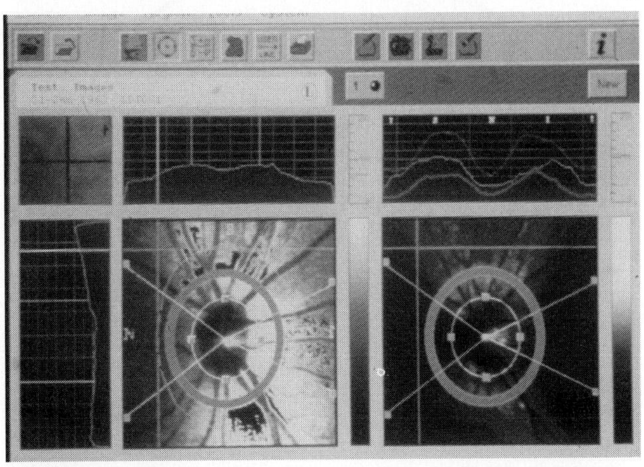

FIGURE 5–20. Scanning laser polarimetry showing a retardance map.

orly, 70 degrees inferiorly and 90 to 100 degrees temporally (Fig. 5–21). The blind spot, found 15 degrees temporal to central fixation, represents the area anatomically occupied by the optic nerve head.[60] The visual field has classically been described as an island of vision in a sea of blindness, which alludes to the rapid deterioration in retinal sensitivity radiating from the foveal peak to the periphery (Fig. 5–22).

Visual field defects can result in a change in the shape of the visual field. Many methods of perimetry are in use today to assess the visual field. They can be classified into two major groups: kinetic perimetry and static perimetry. Kinetic perimetry employs the moving of a test object of constant size and intensity from a non-seeing area toward a seeing area. This method relies upon a sloping hill of vision and is less accurate in detecting defects in the flatter areas of the visual field.

Static perimetry utilizes stationary objects of varying intensity. Threshold testing determines the stimulus intensity that is seen 50% of the time at a given location in the visual field. This is achieved by presenting stimuli of increasing or decreasing intensity at given points in the visual field.[60] Threshold testing provides the quantitative data necessary for early diagnosis and long-term follow-up of patients with glaucoma. Suprathreshold testing uses objects of a higher intensity than normally seen at any point within the visual field.[60, 61] This mode of testing can often be valuable for rapid screening. It cannot, however, detect early subtle defects. In general, static perimetry is the more popular mode of computerized perimetry used today, in part because the program algorithms needed for analysis are less complex and more reproducible than those for computerized kinetic perimetry.[61]

There are various ways to perform both static and kinetic perimetry. A confrontation visual field analysis can be performed quickly in order to assess any gross defects in the visual field. For more detailed visual field analysis, two methods of manual perimetry are particularly useful: Goldmann perimetry and the tangent screen. Both kinetic and static perimetry may be performed with these techniques. The tangent screen consists of a black, flat screen mounted on a wall with a fixation target in the center. With the patient seated 1 to 2 meters from the screen, the peripheral 30 degrees of the visual field can be assessed with the use of variously sized and colored objects. This method is not recommended for following small progressive defects so typical of glaucoma.[60]

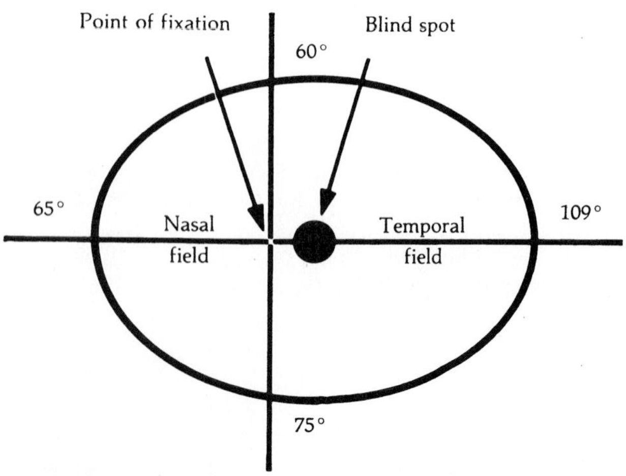

FIGURE 5–21. Limits of a normal visual field of the right eye: Nasally 65 degrees, superiorly 60 degrees, temporally 100 degrees, and inferiorly 75 degrees. The left visual field is a mirror image of the right. (From Ritch R, Shields MB, Krupin T (eds): The Glaucomas: Basic Sciences, 2nd ed, vol 1. St. Louis, Mosby–Year Book, 1996, p 492.)

The Goldmann perimeter uses an illuminated bowl onto which stimuli of various sizes and intensities can be projected. The patient's chin is placed on a rest, much like a slit lamp, and a lens holder allows for the appropriate refraction to be used during the test. While it is possible to obtain fairly accurate threshold testing with the Goldmann perimeter, it requires an experienced technician (Fig. 5–23). Computerized perimetry has replaced Goldmann perimetry for attaining reproducible, threshold measurements in an acceptable amount of time. The Goldmann perimeter, however, is still useful for patients who have trouble complying with the rapid response time needed for computerized techniques and for those with poor visual acuity.

Automated perimetry, as was mentioned earlier, most commonly employs static techniques for threshold and suprathreshold testing. The advantages of computerized perimetry, such as the Humphrey and Octopus systems, is that they are often performed quickly—approximately 30 minutes—and rely less heavily upon an experienced technician. A technician, however, is still an integral part of the testing to ensure that patients maintain proper head positioning, eye positioning, and attention to the test in progress. Like the Goldmann perimeter, the automated perimeters use light stimuli of varying intensity on an illuminated bowl with a central fixation target. The visual field printout provides a number of parameters to indicate test reliability, such as fixation losses, false-negative and false-positive errors, and short-term fluctuation. Inadequate pupil size, refractive errors, droopy upper lids, rim artifact from corrective lenses, and patient fatigue can also affect test quality.[60] (For a more complete discussion of acromatic automated visual field testing, the reader is referred to Chapter 26.)

As with more complicated systems of optic nerve and NFL analysis, visual field testing serves as an aid in the diagnosis and management of glaucoma. Nerve fiber loss is known to correlate with visual field changes in patients with glaucoma.[54] Glaucomatous defects classically respect the horizontal meridian, and patients with defects respecting the vertical meridian invariably need a neurologic evaluation. Generalized depression is considered the most common early defect in glaucoma, but it is fairly nonspecific. Defects characteristic of glaucoma usually fall within Bjerrum's area, which extends from the blind spot to the median raphe in an arcuate pathway 10 degrees from fixation.[61, 62] Within this region, one may see arcuate defects, paracentral scotomas, and nasal steps (Fig. 5–24). In more advanced cases of glaucoma, damage may progress to cause complete altitudinal defects or to involve the temporal area of the field.

Whereas diagnosing glaucoma at any stage of disease is critical to visual preservation, much of our emphasis today focuses on early detection and treatment. Blue-on-yellow or short-wavelength automated perimetry (SWAP) has been designed particularly for this purpose. It is based upon the

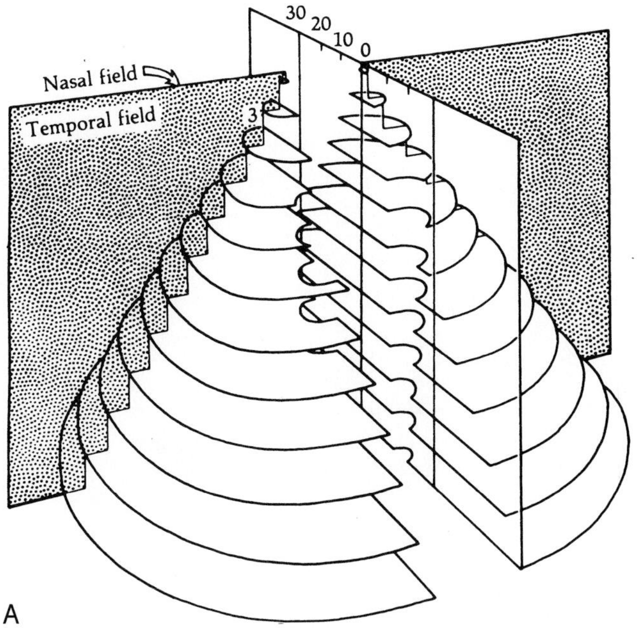

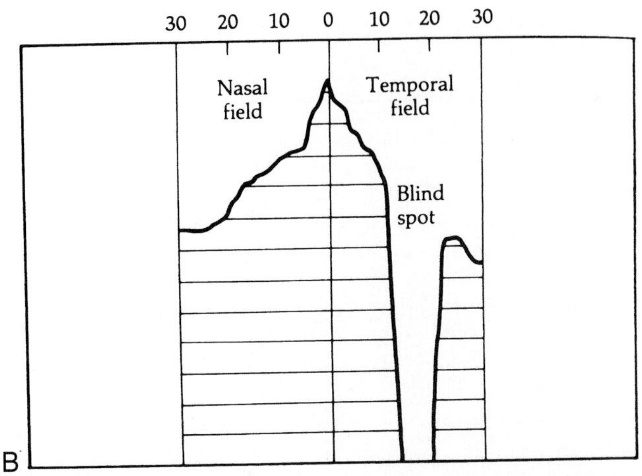

FIGURE 5–22. Traquair's hill of vision. *A*, Representation of the visual field as pieces of plywood cut in the shapes of isopters and stacked appropriately. Shaded plane separates the near temporal field from farther nasal field. Clear plane where plywood has been sectioned vertically and separated corresponds to *B*. *B*, A representation of the visual field as a profile, created by testing along a horizontal line through fixation (i. e., a 180-degree meridian by static perimetry). Thus the hill or island of vision may be visualized from above as kinetic isopters, or its profile may be visualized from any side as static meridians. (From Ritch R, Shields MB, Krupin T (eds): The Glaucomas: Basic Sciences, 2nd ed, vol 1. St. Louis, Mosby–Year Book, 1996, p 498.)

premise that loss of sensitivity to short-wavelength light is an early abnormality in eyes with glaucoma.[63] This mode of testing utilizes a size V blue stimulus on a yellow background. SWAP may be able to detect glaucomatous visual field changes sooner than standard white-on-white perimetry.[64–66] Studies have also shown that SWAP results correlate with topographic changes in the optic nerve head.[67] Interest in this mode of perimetry is currently high.

Other modes of visual field testing that show promise include the Swedish Interactive Thresholding Algorithm (SITA) and frequency-doubling perimetry. SITA allows for more efficient visual field testing by cutting test time almost in half. SITA-Standard runs in half the time of Standard Full Threshold algorithm. SITA-Fast, similarly, runs in half the time of the FastPac program—about 3 minutes per eye.[68] The SITA programs run on the newer Humphrey HFA-II perimeters (Humphrey Instruments, San Leandro, CA). More studies are needed to evaluate this program's screening ability. It is, however, useful in everyday management of patients with glaucoma who have difficulty with the longer Threshold programs. Studies have shown SITA to be associated with lower levels of fatigue and high concordance of visual field defects compared with Threshold 24-2 programs.[69, 70] It may be difficult, however, to compare SITA to Threshold testing, because SITA tends to improve the mean defect.[71]

Frequency-doubling perimetry (FDP) uses large flickering gratings as a stimulus. In healthy portions of the visual field, the patient sees an illusion of "double" the number of bars that exist in the grating.[68] In diseased portions of the visual field, this illusion is perceived only if the contrast is increased. One study showed a significant correlation of FDP threshold values with those of white-on-white and blue-on-yellow perimetry.[72] Threshold FDP also shows high sensitivity and specificity for detecting visual field defects in patients with glaucoma.[73] FDP screening tests, however, detected fewer defects than FDP threshold tests and conventional perimetry.[74]

ELECTROPHYSIOLOGY

Visual field testing can provide a fairly sensitive measure of optic nerve function, but it is a subjective test and therefore is influenced by the patient's attentiveness and mental agility. Research efforts are under way to develop modes of functional testing that are more objective and less dependent on patient participation. As an objective test of retinal function, the electroretinogram (ERG) has received much attention as a possible tool for visual function testing in glaucoma. The full-field ERG, however, mostly represents the outer retinal response, uses large stimuli, and is unable to detect the small areas of local damage that occur early in disease.[75] The pattern ERG, which uses smaller 2-mV responses, has been shown to be reduced in glaucoma.[76] Although the pattern ERG is believed to be an indicator of ganglion cell function, studies have shown that it has a low specificity for glaucomatous changes.[77]

The multifocal ERG is a promising new tool for this purpose. It uses a local flickering stimulus in a matrix composed of a hexagonal array of fields. The second-order kernel of the multifocal ERG can be divided into a retinal component and an optic nerve component, the latter of which may represent ganglion cell function.[78] In patients with glaucoma, the second-order component of the multifocal ERG is diminished, primarily because of the virtual

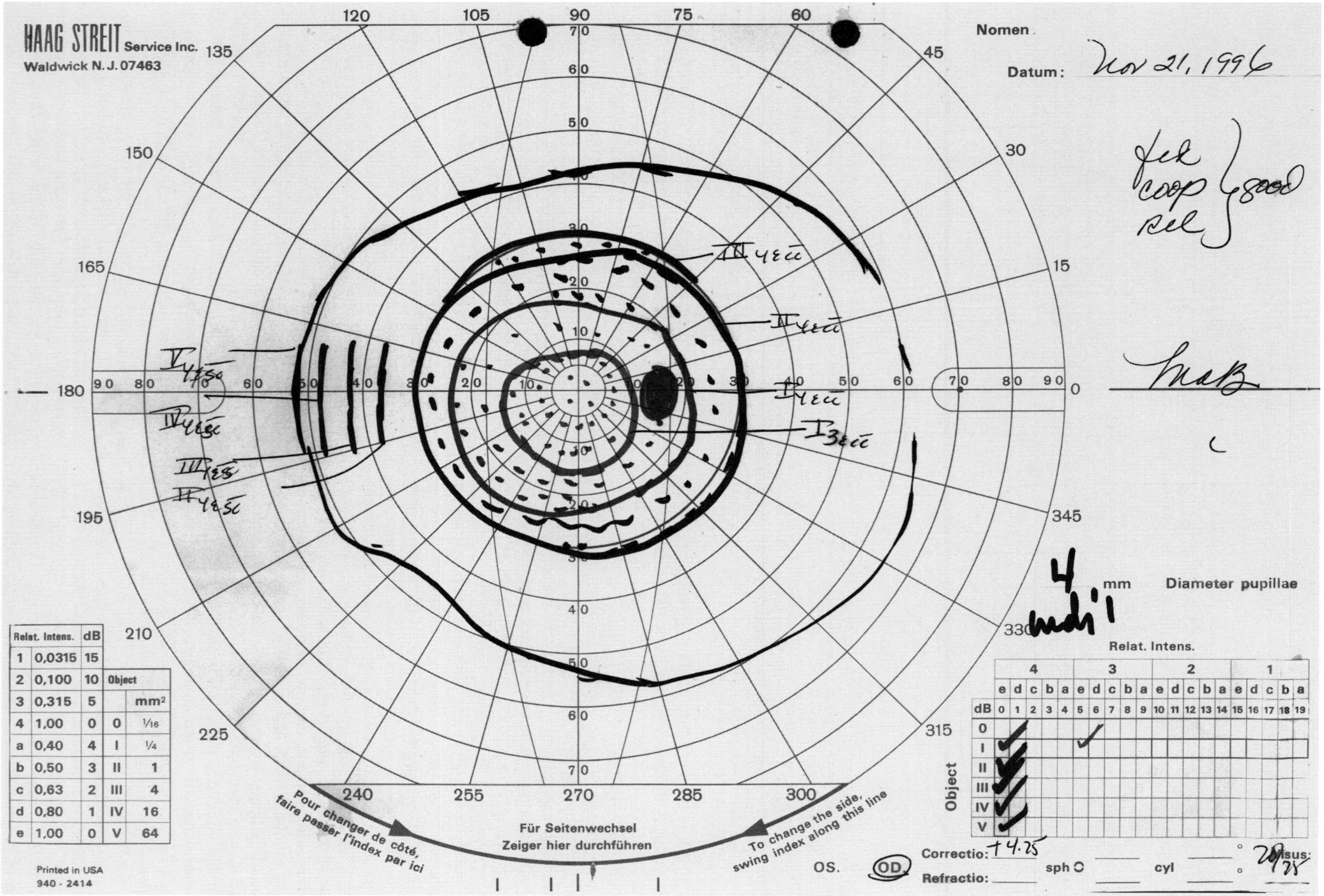

FIGURE 5–23. Goldmann visual field of normal eye.

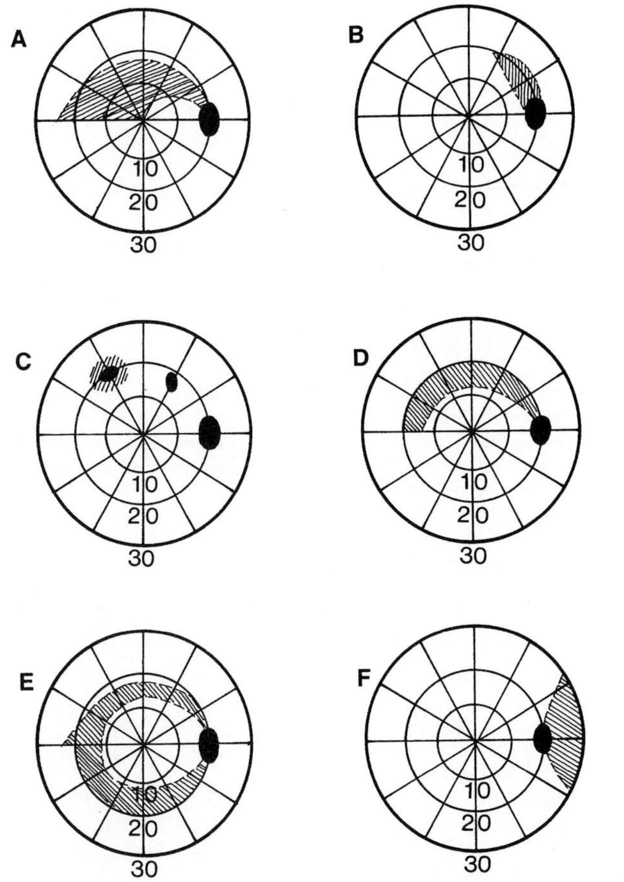

FIGURE 5–24. Arcuate visual field defects. *A*, Bjerrum's region: From the blind spot to the median raphe in an arcuate path that encompasses 10 to 20 degrees nasally from fixation. *B*, Seidel's scotoma. *C*, Paracentral scotoma. *D*, Arcuate or Bjerrum's scotoma. *E*, Double arcuate scotoma. *F*, Temporal wedge defects (not arcuate; are produced by damage to the nasal neuroretinal rim). (From Shields MB: Textbook of Glaucoma, 3rd ed. Baltimore, Williams & Wilkins, 1992, p 121.)

absence of the optic nerve head component. In particular, the second-order response components within the central 10 degrees show a loss of nasal to temporal asymmetry and a loss of latency delay at implicit time of 35 to 40 seconds.[79] In addition, depression of the optic nerve head component has been found in patients in whom glaucoma is suspected but who do not have visual field defects.[78] Although preliminary results with the multifocal ERG are certainly encouraging for providing a new objective, quantitative method of detecting ganglion cell dysfunction in glaucoma, this method of functional testing is still experimental. Studies are currently under way to determine the quantitative parameters that will help identify patients with early disease as well as detect early changes in patients with established disease.

Additional Psychophysical Testing

The wealth of modern technology now allows us to monitor glaucomatous changes closely, whether it be via sequential visual field testing, NFL photography, or optic nerve head analysis. Can we be sure, however, that these modalities allow us to detect glaucomatous damage early enough? Before defects are noted on perimetry, more than 40% of ganglion cells may be damaged in patients with glaucoma.[53] Similarly, eyes without field defects in patients with glaucoma may lose neural rim area at a rate of 1.7% per year.[80] Psychophysical testing is subjective and requires that the patient respond to a given stimulus. As a result, many factors can affect the utility of a psychophysical test, such as pupil size, refractive error, age, cataracts, attentiveness, and familiarity with testing techniques.[81] This section considers two modes of testing: color perception and contrast sensitivity.

COLOR PERCEPTION

The perception of color relies on a high degree of retinal integration, especially in the foveal area. When ganglion cells become damaged in glaucoma, this integrity is disturbed, and color vision is compromised.[82] Patients with glaucoma classically demonstrate diminished sensitivities in the blue short-wavelength cones.[81] There are many methods that may be used to detect this color dysfunction, such as the anomaloscope, the Farnsworth-Munsell 100-Hue Test, the Farnsworth D-15 Test, the Desaturated L'Anthony D-15 Test, and the Ishihara Plates. Although the anomaloscope is the most sensitive and specific of these methods, it is also the most difficult to interpret and is not used often in the clinical setting.[80] The Farnsworth-Munsell 100-Hue Test is a sensitive measure of color vision changes but requires 30 minutes of testing time. The Farnsworth D-15 and Desaturated L'Anthony D-15 tests are shorter and comparable to the 100-Hue test in detecting severity of color vision deficits.[83] In general, however, these tests have a low specificity for distinguishing normal eyes from eyes with suspicion or diagnosis of glaucoma.[81]

Color contrast sensitivity, on the other hand, isolates the blue cone system. If a blue stimulus is presented on a yellow background, the red and green cones adapt to the yellow light, leaving the blue cones to respond to the stimulus.[81] This premise has given rise to SWAP, described earlier in the chapter. This form of perimetry may detect glaucomatous damage earlier than conventional white-on-white perimetry and may therefore be useful in (1) following patients with suspicion of glaucoma and (2) monitoring changes in patients with existing visual field defects.[65–67]

Evaluation of the Glaucoma Patient

Table 5–2 summarizes the evaluation for possible techniques that can be used in the patient known to have glaucoma.

What Do We Actually Do?

When we evaluate a glaucoma patient, we consider the IOP, structure of the optic nerve head and NFL, and function of the optic nerve head. If a patient is suspected of having glaucoma but the patient has normal white-on-white perim-

TABLE 5–2. EVALUATION OF THE PATIENT WITH GLAUCOMA

Parameter Evaluated	Procedures/Instruments Used
Intraocular pressure	Tonometry
	Pneumatonometry
	Tonopen
	Schiøtz
	Non-contact tonometry
Optic nerve head and nerve fiber layer	Clinical examination
	Cupping:
	Is cup round or oval?
	Is rim intact?
	Focal notching
	Change over time
	Optic pits
	Disc size
	Nerve fiber layer:
	Small vessels obscured
	Good reflectance pattern
	Focal defects
	Change over time
	Imaging and analysis
	Optic nerve head:
	Photography
	Optic nerve head analyzers
	Confocal scanner laser ophthalmoscopy
	Nerve fiber layer:
	Polarimetry
	Optical coherence tomography
Visual function	Perimetry
	Static:
	Achromatic
	Blue-on-yellow (short wavelength)
	Swedish Interactive Thresholding Algorithm
	Frequency doubling technology (FDP)
	FastPac
	Kinetic:
	Goldmann
	Tangent screen
	Electrophysiology
	Multifocal electroretinography
	Experimental
	Movement detection perimetry
	Contrast sensitivity
	Color vision detection

etry, or if the patient has not undergone a visual field evaluation but has a good NFL or an intact neuroretinal rim, we perform a SWAP Humphrey Visual Field (HVF). We assess the NFL both clinically and by OCT, and we evaluate the optic nerve head clinically and by HRT. We are also investigating the role of ocular blood flow by Heidelberg Retina Flowmeter (HRF).

Our judgment of the patient's status is developed through a synthesis of all the information gathered regarding IOP and optic nerve head and NFL structure and function. We may judge a patient to have glaucoma who has a high IOP (e.g., >35 mm Hg) but with a normal-appearing optic nerve head and NFL, and with normal visual fields, even by SWAP. On the other hand, we may consider a patient to have glaucoma with a normal or low IOP, normal perimetry, but abnormally low NFL thickness or loss of neuroretinal rim. The technologic adjuncts become most valuable for individuals with IOPs in the middle to high ranges and normal visual fields. SWAP, OCT, or HRT may demonstrate an abnormality in such cases, leading to an increased suspicion of the diagnosis of glaucoma, or may reassure that the patient's eyes are structurally and functionally normal; these are patients we follow particularly closely.

ACKNOWLEDGMENTS

The authors are most grateful for the assistance of Helena Pakter, MD, in the preparation and review of this manuscript.

REFERENCES

1. Spaeth GL: Direct Ophthalmoscopy. *In* Varma R, Spaeth GL (eds): The Optic Nerve in Glaucoma. Philadelphia, JB Lippincott, 1993.
2. Epstein DL: Exam of the optic nerve. *In* Epstein DL, Allingham RR, Schuman JS (eds): Chandler & Grant's Glaucoma, 4th ed. Baltimore, Williams & Wilkins, 1997, p 102.
3. Friberg TR: Examination of the retina: Ophthalmoscopy & fundus biomicroscopy. *In* Albert DM, Jakobiec FA (eds): Principles and Practice of Ophthalmology, vol 2. Philadelphia, WB Saunders, 1994, p 686.
4. Airaksinen PJ, Tuuloren A, Werner EB: Clinical evaluation of the optic disc and retinal nerve fiber layer. *In* Ritch R, Shields MB, Krupin T (eds): The Glaucomas: Basic Sciences, 2nd ed, vol 1. St. Louis, Mosby–Year Book, 1996, p 617.
5. Mikelberg F, Drance S, Schilzer M, et al: The normal human optic nerve-axon diameter distribution. Ophthalmology 1989;96:1325.
6. Quigley HA: The size and shape of the optic disc in the human eye. Arch Ophthalmol 1990;108:51.
7. Quigley HA: Early detection of glaucoma damage. II: Changes in appearance of optic disk. Surv Ophthalmol 1985;30:111.
8. Kirsch RE, Anderson DR: Clinical recognition of glaucomatous cupping. Am J Ophthalmol 1973;75:442.
9. Spaeth GL: Development of glaucomatous changes of optic nerve. *In* Varma R, Spaeth GL (eds): The Optic Nerve in Glaucoma. Philadelphia, JB Lippincott, 1993.
10. Reed RM, Spaeth GL: The practical clinical appraisal of optic disc in glaucoma: Natural history of cup progression and. Trans Am Acad Ophthalmol Otorh 1974;78:225.
11. Armaly MF: Genetic determination of cup/disc ratio of the optic nerve. Arch Ophthalmol 1967; 8:35.
12. Jonas JB, Gusek GC, Naumann GO, et al: Optic disc, cup and neuroretinal rim size, configuration in the normal eye. Invest Opthalmol Vis Sci 1988; 29:1151.
13. Leibowitz HM, Krueger DE, Maunder LR, et al: The Framingham Eye Study monograph: An ophthalmological and epidemiological study of cataract, glaucoma, diabetic retinopathy, macular degeneration, and visual acuity in a general population of 2631 adults, 1973-1975. Surv Ophthalmol 1980;24(suppl):335–610.
14. Gross PG, inventor: Measuring Ophthalmoscope and Ophthalmoscopic Procedure, 10/1/91, U S patent 5 053 795. 1991.
15. Schwartz B: Cupping and pallor of the optic disc. Arch Ophthalmol 1973;89:272.
16. Brown GC: Differential diagnosis of the glaucomatous optic disc. *In* Varma R, Spaeth GL (eds): The Optic Nerve in Glaucoma. Philadelphia, JB Lippincott, 1993, p 99.
17. Wellington DP, Johnstone MA: Normal-tension glaucoma (low-tension glaucoma). *In* Albert DM, Jakobiec FA (eds): Principles and Practice of Ophthalmology, vol 3. Philadelphia, WB Saunders, 1994, p 1350.
18. Diehl DL, Quigley HA, Miller NR, et al: Prevalence and significance of optic disc hemorrhage in a longitudinal study of glaucoma. Arch Ophthalmol 1990;108:545.
19. Boeglin RT, Caprioli J: Contemporary clinical evaluation of optic nerve in glaucoma. Ophthalmol Clin North Am 1991;4:711.
20. Osher RH, Herschler J: The significance of baring of the circumlinear vessel: A prospective study. Arch Ophthalmol 1981;99:817.
21. Schuman JS: Peripapillary atrophy. *In* Epstein DL, Allingham RR, Schuman JS (eds): Chandler & Grant's Glaucoma, 4th ed. Baltimore, Williams & Wilkins, 1997, p 14.
22. Anderson DR: Correlation of the peripapillary anatomy with the disc damage and field abnormalities in glaucoma. *In* Greve EL, Hejil A

(eds): Fifth International Visual Field Symposium. The Netherlands: Dr. W Junk Publishers, 1983.
23. Anderson DR: Relationship of peripapillary haloes and crescents to glaucomatous cupping. *In* Krieglstein GK (ed): Glaucoma Update III. Berlin, Springer-Verlag, 1987.
24. Fong DS, Epstein DL, Allingham RR: Glaucoma and myopia: Are they related? Int Ophthalmol Clin 1990;30:215.
25. Epstein DL: Primary open angle glaucoma and myopia. *In* Epstein DL, Allingham RR, Schuman JS (eds): Chandler & Grant's Glaucoma, 4th ed. Baltimore, Williams & Wilkins, 1997, p 190.
26. Mattox C: Clinical examination of the nerve fiber layer. *In* Schuman JS (ed): Imaging in Glaucoma. Thorofare, NJ, Slack Inc, 1997, p 63.
27. Radius R, Anderson DR: The course of axons through the retina and optic nerve head. Arch Ophthalmol 1979;97:1154.
28. Radius R, Anderson DR: The histology of retinal nerve fiber layer bundles and bundle defects. Arch Ophthalmol 1979:97:948.
29. Schuman JS: Imaging of the optic nerve head and nerve fiber layer in glaucoma. *In* Epstein DL, Allingham RR, Schuman JS (eds): Chandler & Grant's Glaucoma, 4th ed. Baltimore, Williams & Wilkins, 1997, p 104.
30. Quigley H, Miller N, George T: Clinical evaluation of nerve fiber layer atrophy as an indicator of glaucomatous optic nerve damage. Arch Ophthalmol 1980;98:1564.
31. Airaksinen P, Drance S, Douglas G, et al: Diffuse and localized nerve fiber loss in glaucoma. Am J Ophthalmol 1984: 98:566.
32. Quigley H, Reacher M, Katz J, et al: Quantitative grading of nerve fiber layer photographs. Ophthalmology 1993;100:1800.
33. Greenfield DS, Zacharia P, Schuman JS: Comparison of Nidek 3Dx and Donaldson simultaneous stereoscopic disk photography. Am J Ophthalmol 1993;116:741.
34. Greenfield DS: Stereoscopic optic disc photography. *In* Schuman JS (ed): Imaging in Glaucoma. Thorofare, NJ, Slack Inc, 1997, p 3.
35. Schuman JS, Noecker RJ: Imaging of the optic nerve head and nerve fiber layer in glaucoma. Ophthalmol Clin North Am 1995;8:259.
36. Netland PA: The Glaucoma-Scope: Principle, techniques, and applications. *In* Schuman JS (ed): Imaging in Glaucoma. Thorofare, New Jersey, Slack Inc, 1997, p 17.
37. Hoskins HD, Hetherington J, Glenday M, et al: Repeatability of the Glaucoma-Scope measurements of optic nerve head topography. Glaucoma 1994;3:177.
38. Zangwill L, de Souza Lima M, Weinreb RN: Confocal scanning laser ophthalmoscopy to detect glaucomatous optic neuropathy. *In* Schuman JS (ed): Imaging in Glaucoma. Thorofare, New Jersey, Slack Inc, 1997, p 45.
39. Asawaphureekorn S, Zangwill L, Weinreb RN: The ranked-segment distribution curve for interpretation of optic nerve topography. J Glaucoma 1996;5:79.
40. Kamal DS, Garway-Heath DF, Hitchings RA, et al: Use of sequential Heidelberg Retina Tomograph (HRT) images to identify changes in the optic disc in ocular hypertensive patients at risk of developing glaucoma. Invest Opthalmol Vis Sci 1998;39(Suppl):1125.
41. Anton A, Williams J, Asawaphureekorn S, et al: Sensitivity and specificity of HRT rim parameters for detecting focal or diffuse optic disc damage in glaucoma. Invest Opthalmol Vis Sci 1998; 39(Suppl):1125.
42. Kruse Fe, Burk RO, Volcker HE, et al: Reproducibility of topographic measurements of the optic nerve head with laser tomographic scanning. Ophthalmology 1989;96:1320.
43. Weinreb RN, Lusky M, Bartsch DU, et al: Effect of repetitive imaging on topographic measurements of the optic nerve head. Arch Ophthalmol 1993; 111:636.
44. Schuman JS: Optical coherence tomography for imaging and quantitation of nerve fiber layer thickness. *In* Schuman JS (ed): Imaging in Glaucoma. Thorofare, NJ, Slack Inc, 1997.
45. Schuman JS, Hee MR, Arya AV, et al: Optical coherence tomography: A new tool for glaucoma diagnosis. Curr Sci 1995;6:89.
46. Schuman JS, Pedut-Kloizman T, Hertzmark E, et al: Reproducibility of nerve fiber layer thickness measurements using optical coherence tomography. Ophthalmology 1996;103:1889.
47. Izatt JA, Hee MR, Huang D, et al: Ophthalmic diagnostics using optical coherence tomography. *In* Ren Q, Pavel JM, (chairs/eds): Proceedings of Ophthalmic Technologies III, Los Angeles, January 16–18, 1992. (Progress in Biomedical Optics; Proceedings of SPIE, vol 1877.) Bellingham, WA: SPIE, 1993; 133.
48. Hee MR, Izatt JA, Swanson EA, et al: Optical coherence tomography of the human retina. Arch Ophthalmol 1995;113:325.
49. Schuman JS, Hee MR, Arya AV, et al: Optical coherence tomography: A new tool for glaucoma diagnosis. Curr Opin Ophthalmol 1995; 6:89.
50. Huang D, Swanson EA, Lin CP, et al: Optical coherence tomography. Science 1991;254:1178.
51. Pieroth L, Schuman JS, Hee MR, et al: Evaluation of focal defects in the nerve fiber layer using optical coherence tomography. Invest Ophthalmol Vis Sci 1996;37(Suppl):S1094.
52. Hoyt WF, Newman NM: The earliest observable defect in glaucoma? Lancet 1972;1:692.
53. Quigley HA, Addicks EM, Green RW: Optic nerve damage in glaucoma III: Quantitative correlation of nerve fiber loss and visual field defects in glaucoma, ischemic neuropathy, papilledema, and toxic neuropathy. Arch Ophthalmol 1982;100:135.
54. Sommer A, Katz J, Quigley HA, et al: Clinically detectable nerve fiber atrophy precedes the onset of glaucomatous field loss. Arch Ophthalmol 1991;109:77.
55. De Souza Lima M, Zangwill L, Weinreb RN: Scanning laser polarimetry to assess the nerve fiber layer. *In* Schuman JS (ed): Imaging in Glaucoma. Thorofare, NJ, Slack Inc, 1997, p 83.
56. Weinreb RN, Shakiba S, Sample PA, et al: Association between quantitative nerve fiber layer measurement and visual field loss in glaucoma. Am J Ophthalmol 1995;120:732.
57. Weinreb RN, Dreher AW, Coleman A, et al: Histopathologic validation of Fourier-ellipsometry measurements of retinal nerve fiber layer thickness. Arch Ophthalmol 1990;108:557.
58. Weinreb RN, Shakiba S, Zangwill L: Scanning laser polarimetry to measure the nerve fiber layer of normal and glaucomatous eyes. Am J Ophthalmol 1995;119:627.
59. Weinreb RN, Dreher AW, Coleman A, et al: Histopathologic validation of Fourier-ellipsometry measurements of retinal nerve fiber layer thickness. Arch Ophthalmol 1990;108:557.
60. Allingham RR: Visual fields and their relationship to the optic nerve. *In* Epstein DL, Allingham RR, Schuman JS (eds): Chandler & Grant's Glaucoma, 4th ed. Baltimore, Williams & Wilkins, 1997, p 120.
61. Caprioli J, Weitzman ML: Essentials of automated perimetry. *In* Walsh TJ (ed): Ophthalmology Monographs 3: Visual Fields, Examination and Interpretation, 2nd ed. San Francisco, American Academy of Ophthalmology, 1996, p 85.
62. Harrington DO: The Bjerrum scotoma. Am J Ophthalmol 1965;59:646.
63. Sample PA, Weinreb RN, Boynton RM: Acquired dyschromatopsia in glaucoma. Surv Ophthalmol 1986;31:54.
64. Johnson CA, Adams AJ, Casson EJ: Blue on yellow perimetry can predict the development of glaucomatous visual field loss. Arch Ophthalmol 1993;111:645.
65. Johnson CA, Adams AJ, Casson EJ, et al: Progression of early glaucomatous visual field loss as detected by blue-on-yellow and standard white-on-white perimetry. Arch Ophthalmol 1993:111:651.
66. Sample PA, Taylor JD, Martinez GA, et al: Short wavelength color visual fields in glaucoma suspects at risk. Am J Ophthalmol 1993;115:225.
67. Yamagishi N, Anton A, Sample A, et al: Mapping structural damage of the optic disk to visual field defect in glaucoma. Am J Ophthalmol 1997;123:667.
68. Anderson DR, Patella VM: Automated Static Perimetry, 2nd ed. St. Louis, Mosby–Year Book, 1999.
69. Fujimoto N, Kakinuma T, Adachi-Usami E: Fatigue and fluctuation in SITA and full-threshold perimetry of Humphrey Field Analyzer. Invest Ophthalmol Vis Sci 1998;39:s492.
70. Rueda JC, Parra JC, Platta, et al: SITA standard vs. full threshold 24-2 visual fields in glaucoma patients. Invest Ophthalmol Vis Sci 1998; 39:s492.
71. Nordmann JP, Mouton-Chopin D: Evaluation of the SITA accurate and SITA fast perimetric algorithms in normals and glaucoma patients. Invest Ophthalmol Vis Sci 1998;39:s493.
72. Inazumi K, Yamamoto T, Kondo Y, et al: A comparison of frequency doubling perimetry with W/W and B/Y perimetry in sensitivity threshold. Invest Ophthalmol Vis Sci 1998;39:s491.
73. Burnstein Y, Ellish NJ, Magbalon M, et al: A comparison of frequency doubling perimetry to Humphrey visual field analysis. Invest Ophthalmol Vis Sci 1998;39:s25.
74. Bass SJ, Sherman J, Feldman J: Correlation of screening vs threshold tests using frequency doubling perimetry (FDP). Invest Ophthalmol Vis Sci 1998;39:s25.

75. Sutter EE, Bearse MA Jr: Extraction of a ganglion cell component from the corneal response. *In* Vision Science and Its Applications, 1995 OSA Technical Digest Series, vol 1. Washington, DC, Optical Society of America, 1995, p 310.
76. Vaegan SL, Graham I, Goldberg, LB, et al: Flash and pattern electroretinogram changes with optic atrophy and glaucoma. Exp Eye Res 1995;60:697.
77. Nesher R, Trick GL: The pattern electroretinogram in retinal and optic nerve disease: A quantitative comparison of the pattern of visual dysfunction. Doc Ophthalmol 1991;77:225.
78. Sutter EE, Bearse MA Jr: The optic nerve head component of the human ERG. Vision Res 1999;39:419–436.
79. Pedut-Kloizman T, Sutter EE, Bearse MA, et al: Objective assessment of retinal function in normal and glaucomatous eyes using multifocal electroretinography. Invest Ophthalmol Vis Sci 1996;37(ARVO Suppl):S947.
80. Zeyen TG, Caprioli J: Progression of disc and field damage in early glaucoma. Arch Ophthalmol 1993;111:62.
81. Stamper RL, Lerner LE: Psychophysical techniques in glaucoma. *In* Ritch R, Shields MB, Krupin T (eds): The Glaucomas: Basic Sciences, 2nd ed, vol 1. St. Louis, Mosby–Year Book, 1996, p 617.
82. Stamper RL: Psychophysical changes in glaucoma. Surv Ophthalmol 1989;23(Suppl):309.
83. Bassi CJ, Galanis JC, Hoffman J: Comparison of the Farnsworth-Munsell 100-Hue, the Farnsworth D-15, and the L'Anthony D-15 desaturated color tests. Arch Ophthalmol 1993;111:639.

SECTION II

KEY PATIENT CHARACTERISTICS

CHAPTER 6

Genetics

DARRELL WUDUNN

There is an explosion of new information concerning the genetic basis for several types of glaucoma. In this chapter, Darrell WuDunn first educates us as to basic concepts of genetics, including patterns of inheritance and obtaining and interpreting the family history. Next, the implications for patients who have or are suspected of having glaucoma are presented. The majority of the chapter deals with the specific types of glaucoma with mendelian or nondistinct inheritance patterns. These include the genetic implications in common glaucomas, such as primary open-angle, and rarer types about which more genetic information is available. Because congenital and developmental glaucomas have a genetic basis, they are explored in much greater depth in this chapter. The distinctive manifestations of many of the other syndromes are discussed in more detail elsewhere, depending on the site of their distinctive sign. Finally, the physician's role in genetic counseling and monitoring is explored.

Over the past few years, advances in molecular genetics have greatly enhanced our understanding of several types of glaucoma. Genes relating to glaucoma have been mapped and even identified. Intense research is under way to characterize these genes and to identify other genes associated with glaucoma.

The aim of this chapter is to give a concise overview of genetics that relates to specific types of glaucoma or specific diseases associated with glaucoma. It is not meant to be a comprehensive review of the genetics of glaucoma but rather to emphasize the practical application of genetic concepts.

Recognizing Patterns of Inheritance

Many types of diseases causing, or associated with, glaucoma are inherited. A positive family history of glaucoma greatly increases the suspicion that a patient has, or is at high risk for, glaucoma. Certain glaucoma diseases follow recognizable patterns of inheritance, whereas others appear to be familial but lack a clear inheritance pattern. Recognizing a definite autosomal dominant or recessive pattern sometimes helps one make a diagnosis and has important implications for the patient's relatives and offspring.

The *autosomal dominant* pattern of inheritance (Fig. 6–1) is characterized by:

1. Vertical (generation-to-generation) transmission.
2. About equal numbers of male and females affected.
3. No skipping of generations.
4. 50% *recurrence risk* (the risk of the disease in subsequent offspring of parents with an affected child).

Offspring of unaffected parents do not have the disease. The risk that an affected parent will transmit an autosomal dominant disease to his or her offspring is one half. The presence of father–son transmission rules out certain other modes of transmission.

In *autosomal recessive* inheritance (Fig. 6–2), the disease:

1. Clusters in siblings and is not usually seen among parents or other ancestors.
2. Affects approximately equal numbers of affected males and females.
3. Sometimes demonstrates consanguinity, particularly in rare recessive diseases.

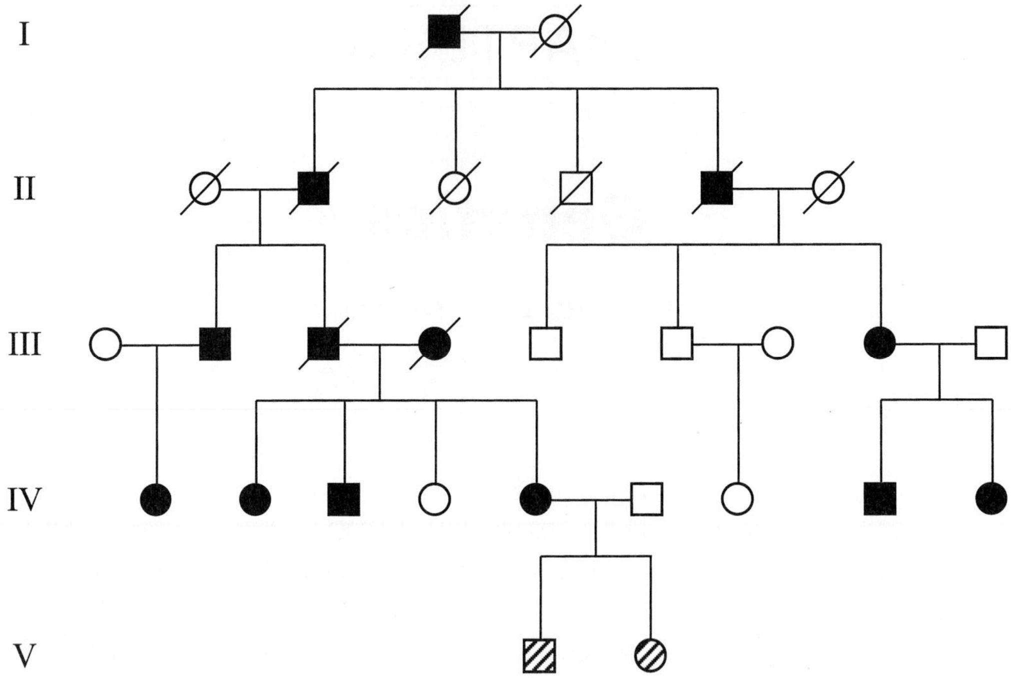

FIGURE 6–1. Pedigree of autosomal dominant juvenile glaucoma. Squares, males; circles, females; solid symbol, affected by the disorder; open symbol, unaffected; hashed symbol, affection status unknown; slash through a symbol, deceased.

4. Has a recurrence risk of 25% for each subsequent offspring if neither parent is affected.

However if an affected parent (homozygous) mates with an unaffected carrier (heterozygous), the recurrence risk is 50%.

In general, a dominant disease allele produces disease in a heterozygous individual, whereas a recessive disease allele does not. However, several confounding factors often make determining whether a disease is dominant or recessive difficult. The appearance of a disease in an individual with no family history of the disease may represent either an autosomal recessive disorder or a new mutation of an autosomal dominant disorder. The recurrence risk for the autosomal recessive disorder is 25%, whereas that for the dominant disorder is very low for subsequent siblings. The risk may be much higher for the offspring of the affected individual.

Reduced penetrance is another confounding factor in

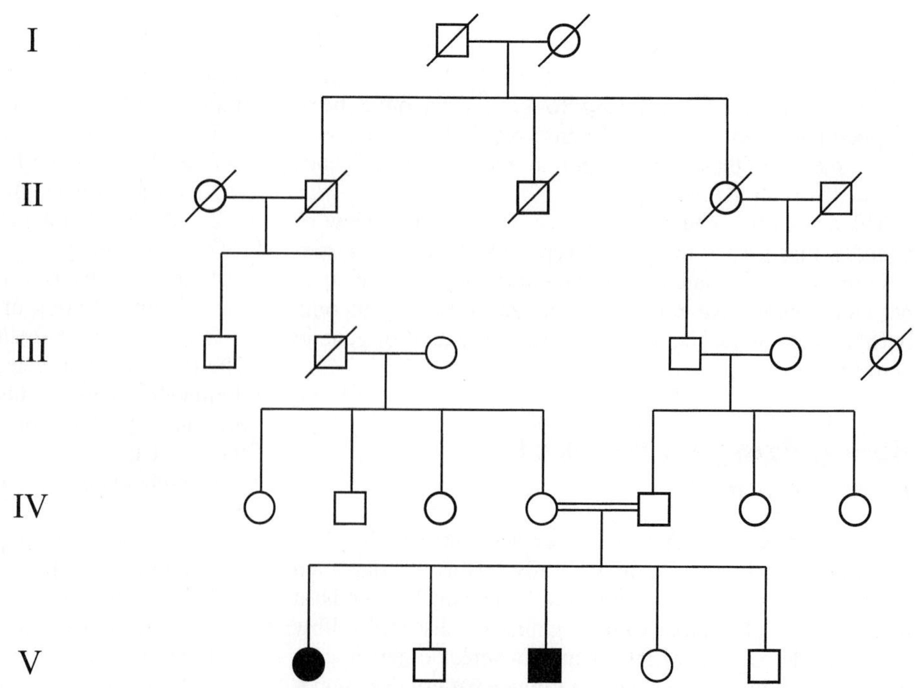

FIGURE 6–2. Pedigree of autosomal recessive congenital glaucoma. Squares, males; circles, females; solid symbol, affected by the disorder; open symbol, unaffected; slash through a symbol, deceased; double bars between symbols, consanguineous mating.

genetic diseases. An individual who has the genotype for a disease may not exhibit the disease phenotype even though he or she can pass the disease gene to the next generation. In addition, even in diseases with complete penetrance, the severity of the phenotype may vary (variable expression).

In *X-linked recessive* disorders:

1. Father–son transmission is absent.
2. Skipping of generations is present because genes are passed through female carriers.
3. Affected males greatly outnumber affected females.

The recurrence risk is somewhat more complicated than for the autosomal disorders. Most commonly, an affected father and a normal (noncarrier) mother produce all normal sons and all carrier daughters. If unaffected parents produce an affected son, the mother is most likely a carrier, and the recurrence risk is 50% for affected sons and 50% for carrier daughters.

Obtaining a Family History

In most clinical situations, a family history is obtained during the initial evaluation and consists of simply asking the patient whether he or she has any relatives with glaucoma. During this initial questioning, the patient often gives only a sketchy family history. The patient may state, for instance, that he or she is not aware of anyone else with glaucoma or knows only of one other affected relative. Frequently, the patient is unsure about relatives other than immediate family members.

For most patients with typical adult-onset glaucoma, these sketchy family histories are usually sufficient because the diagnosis is not in doubt. However, extensive family histories may be important in cases of congenital glaucoma, glaucoma associated with other ocular or systemic abnormalities, and other atypical types of glaucoma. Occasionally, a patient reports multiple affected relatives. This should alert the physician that a strongly positive family history is present and that the patient's glaucoma may be one of the inherited types of glaucoma described later in this chapter. When an inherited type of glaucoma is suspected, the physician can obtain a more extensive or precise family pedigree after the initial visit by instructing the patient to confer directly with relatives.

A population-based survey found that the odds ratio for a positive family history was two to three times higher for patients who knew they had glaucoma than for those who had just been diagnosed at the time of the survey.[1] This finding might suggest that when a patient is initially diagnosed with glaucoma, he or she may be unaware of relatives with glaucoma, but over time, he or she learns of other affected family members. Alternatively, relatives of patients with glaucoma may be more likely to undergo evaluation for glaucoma once they are aware that someone in the family is affected. Regardless, all patients diagnosed with glaucoma should be encouraged to learn whether other family members are affected and to report back to the ophthalmologist during subsequent visits.

An accurate family history may be difficult to achieve in cases of adult-onset glaucoma because of the delayed age of onset. At the time of initial diagnosis of glaucoma, the patient may be elderly with few living relatives from his or her parents' generation. The patient may know only of vision loss in members of the previous generation but not whether it was due to glaucoma or some other entity, such as cataract. Glaucoma may not have been diagnosed in the patient's generation until decades later. Furthermore, glaucoma may not be diagnosed in further generations until decades later. This delayed age of onset complicates the interpretation of inheritance patterns in families with glaucoma.

A "negative" family history of glaucoma does not necessarily exclude the diagnosis of an inherited type of glaucoma. The patient may not be aware of the presence of glaucoma in other family members. Some relatives may have glaucoma but are unaware that they are affected. As mentioned earlier, the initial appearance of the disease in a family may represent an autosomal recessive disorder or a new mutation of an autosomal dominant disorder.

Interpreting a Family History

Familial factors appear to be involved in many instances of glaucoma, even in the absence of a definable inheritance pattern. In a population-based study, 16% of individuals diagnosed with primary open-angle glaucoma had a positive family history among first-degree relatives, compared with 7% of controls.[1] For individuals with angle-closure glaucoma, the risk of a first-degree relative having angle-closure glaucoma may be as high as 6% to 12%.[2]

The presence of glaucoma among first-degree relatives appears to be a higher risk factor than the presence of glaucoma among more distant relatives. Data from the Baltimore Eye Survey[1] indicate that the relative risk of primary open-angle glaucoma is 3.7-fold higher for individuals who have a sibling with primary open-angle glaucoma than for individuals with no family history of the disease. The relative risk is lower for individuals who have a parent or child with primary open-angle glaucoma. The risk for having acute angle-closure glaucoma has been estimated to be about 2% to 5% for first-degree relatives and about 1% to 2.5% for second-degree relatives.[3]

The family history is most relevant in the evaluation of a patient in whom glaucoma is suspected. A positive family history should be considered a risk factor for glaucoma. The presence of glaucoma in a sibling is more significant than the presence of glaucoma in a more distant relative. Having multiple affected relatives also probably increases the relative risk and may also suggest an inherited form of glaucoma. The clinician may be more inclined to treat a patient with suspicion of glaucoma who has a positive family history. Similarly, the clinician may be more likely to recommend prophylactic laser iridotomy for narrow angles to a person with a relative who had an angle-closure attack. A positive family history, however, is just one of several important factors that may influence the decision to treat a patient in whom glaucoma is suspected. The ultimate decision to treat must be made on the basis of the overall clinical impression.

Although numerous studies have examined the incidence of glaucoma among relatives of affected individuals, few have examined the influence of familial factors on the natural progression of glaucoma. Hence, a positive family history may push the clinician to treat a patient with suspicion of glaucoma sooner, but it is unclear whether a patient with glaucoma who has a positive family history should be treated more aggressively than one who has a negative family history. However, a patient may prefer or may agree to more aggressive treatment if he or she knows a close relative with vision loss due to glaucoma.

Specific Types of Glaucoma with Mendelian Inheritance

Over the past few years, the rapidly advancing techniques of molecular genetics have enabled researchers to methodically search for and identify specific genes associated with glaucoma.[4, 5] A genetic factor associated with an observable disease or trait such as glaucoma may be localized to a specific chromosomal region by *genetic linkage analysis*. In this method, the researcher looks for a statistically significant association (linkage) between the disease phenotype and a polymorphic genetic marker. The likelihood of a successful genetic linkage analysis is greatly improved with large or multiple pedigrees that follow mendelian inheritance patterns. The energized efforts to find glaucoma genes has yielded a flurry of reports of pedigees that are affected by autosomal dominant or autosomal recessive forms of glaucoma (Table 6–1).

The types of glaucoma that are inherited in a distinct mendelian pattern are relatively rare. However, in small families with inheritable glaucoma, the autosomal dominant or autosomal recessive pattern of inheritance may be difficult to establish, especially if the family history is incomplete. Just one affected parent is consistent with an autosomal dominant form of glaucoma. A single distant cousin with glaucoma or a consanguineous mating is consistent with an autosomal recessive form of glaucoma. Furthermore, variable expression and incomplete penetrance may mask the inheritance pattern. Hence, the absence of a strong family history of glaucoma does not exclude the possibility of an inherited form of glaucoma.

TABLE 6–1. HERITABLE FORMS OF GLAUCOMA AND RELATED DISORDERS*

AUTOSOMAL DOMINANT PATTERN
Aniridia (PAX6)
Axenfeld-Rieger syndrome *(RIEG)*
Autosomal dominant juvenile-onset primary open-angle glaucoma *(TIGR/MYOC)*
Iridogoniodysgenesis anomaly
Iridogoniodysgenesis syndrome
Nail-patella syndrome
Pigment dispersion syndrome
Posterior polymorphous corneal dystrophy
Primary open-angle glaucoma—normal tension *(GCL1B)*
Primary open-angle glaucoma *(GLC1C)*
AUTOSOMAL RECESSIVE PATTERN
Congenital glaucoma *(CYP1B1)*
Congenital glaucoma *(GLC3B)*
Primary open-angle glaucoma
X-LINKED RECESSIVE PATTERN
Oculocerebrorenal syndrome of Lowe *(OCRL-1)*

* For certain conditions in which a gene has been mapped or identified, the assigned gene symbol is given in parentheses.

AUTOSOMAL DOMINANT JUVENILE-ONSET PRIMARY OPEN-ANGLE GLAUCOMA

This type of juvenile glaucoma is characterized by the onset of markedly elevated intraocular pressures during the second or third decade of life.[6–17] Pressures usually rise above 30 mm Hg, may even exceed 50 mm Hg, and do not respond well to medical therapy. Although the optic nerves may be fairly resistant considering the high pressures, some optic nerve damage usually occurs eventually without adequate treatment. The age at diagnosis may vary considerably (5 to over 50 years) even within a single pedigree.[12, 15] Most affected individuals have mild to moderate myopia. Gonioscopy may reveal normal-appearing open angles or angles with anterior iris insertion and an increased number of iris processes.[13]

Ultrasound biomicroscopy studies indicate reduced height of the trabecular meshwork in persons with juvenile glaucoma.[18] In addition, ultrastructural studies of the trabecular meshwork in eyes with juvenile glaucoma demonstrate large amounts of extracellular material arranged in fingerprint-like pattern, resembling basement membrane–like material and similar to that seen in steroid-induced glaucoma.[19, 20] However, the distinction between the autosomal dominant primary open-angle form and other types of juvenile glaucoma was not made in either of these studies.

Autosomal dominant juvenile-onset primary open-angle glaucoma follows an autosomal dominant pattern of inheritance. Penetrance of the disease is probably greater than 90%.[6, 9, 10, 12–14] Thus in affected families, almost every individual with markedly elevated intraocular pressure has an affected parent. Genetic linkage analysis studies indicate that in the majority of pedigrees with autosomal dominant juvenile glaucoma, a genetic mutation exists in the *GLC1A* gene located on chromosome 1 q23-25.[6–17] The *GLC1A* gene has been determined to be the *TIGR* (trabecular meshwork inducible glucocorticoid response) gene.[21] The *TIGR* gene product was initially identified in trabecular meshwork cell cultures after prolonged exposure to dexamethasone.[22–24] Studies indicate that the *TIGR* gene product is deposited into the extracellular matrix of the trabecular meshwork, and its accumulation may contribute to a decrease in aqueous outflow.[25] The *TIGR* gene is also known as the *MYOC* (myocilin) gene.

Genetic heterogeneity has been reported for autosomal dominant juvenile-onset primary open-angle glaucoma.[11, 13, 16] That is, families have been identified with this disorder that do not exhibit genetic linkage to the *TIGR* locus on chromosome 1q23-25. Hence, other gene(s) may be involved in this disorder. Another form of juvenile glaucoma, autosomal dominant iridogoniodysgenesis (see later), has also been studied, and two separate chromosomal loci have been mapped (4q25 and 6p25).

ADULT-ONSET PRIMARY OPEN-ANGLE GLAUCOMA

Adult-onset primary open-angle glaucoma probably represents a group of disorders characterized by slowly progressive glaucomatous optic nerve damage and visual field loss. Onset usually begins after the fourth decade of life. The optic neuropathy is thought to be pressure related, and treatment is designed to lower intraocular pressure. Most forms of adult-onset primary open-angle glaucoma are probably complex diseases with polygenic (multiple genes involved) or multifactorial (genes and environmental factors involved) inheritance.

Pedigrees of adult-onset primary open-angle glaucoma have been reported that follow mendelian inheritance patterns. Autosomal dominant, autosomal recessive, and X-linked patterns have been described.[26–34] For the most part, the clinical features of the inherited forms of adult-onset primary open-angle glaucoma do not differ significantly from those of the more typical primary open-angle glaucoma that lacks a clear inheritance pattern.

By analyzing large or numerous pedigrees, researchers have mapped chromosomal regions that contain putative genes for adult-onset primary open-angle glaucoma. In a genetic linkage study involving 17 pedigrees with the disorder, 6 of the pedigrees together demonstrated linkage to chromosome location 2 cen-q13 *(GLC1B)*.[31] The glaucoma in these families was notable for normal or only moderately elevated intraocular pressure (normal tension glaucoma), slow progression of disease, and onset between about 40 and 70 years (average, 47 years). Most cases were managed medically. No abnormal gonioscopy findings were noted.

Another study described a three-generation pedigree of autosomal dominant primary open-angle glaucoma. Genetic linkage analysis mapped the associated gene *(GLC1C)* to chromosome 3q21-24.[34] Affected individuals usually had intraocular pressures ranging from 20 to 25 mm Hg, increased vertical cup-to-disc ratios, and wide (grade IV) open angles on gonioscopy. Age of onset ranged from 38 years to more than 80 years, with most cases occurring in patients 45 to 65 years. Treatment varied from none to medications to laser or trabeculectomy.

Another potential genetic locus has been mapped to chromosome 9q34.[35] In two families affected with autosomal dominant nail-patella syndrome, open-angle glaucoma was diagnosed in more than half the individuals with the syndrome. Indeed, the glaucoma appeared to statistically cosegregate with the nail-patella syndrome. The gene for nail-patella syndrome was genetically linked to chromosome 9q34 in these two families, suggesting a possible locus for open-angle glaucoma in this region.

Mutations in the *TIGR* gene associated with autosomal dominant juvenile-onset glaucoma have been detected in about 3% of individuals with isolated primary open-angle glaucoma.[21] Moreover, glaucoma pedigrees linked to the *TIGR* gene locus include family members with adult-onset glaucoma in addition to members with juvenile-onset glaucoma.[12, 15] Other genetic loci for adult-onset primary open-angle glaucoma undoubtedly exist.

PIGMENT DISPERSION SYNDROME AND PIGMENTARY GLAUCOMA

Pigment dispersion syndrome is a fairly common disorder that may progress to pigmentary glaucoma. Key risk factors for the development of pigment dispersion syndrome are male gender, young age (20–45 years), myopia, and white race.[36]

Although pigment dispersion within the anterior segment can result from a number of ocular disorders, its association with certain other clinical findings suggests the diagnosis of pigment dispersion syndrome. A vertical accumulation of pigment on the lower midportion of the corneal endothelium (Krukenberg's spindle) results from convection currents within the anterior chamber.

The radial, spoke-like pattern of iris transillumination defects detected by retroillumination is another important characteristic sign of pigment dispersion syndrome. However, it is not always seen in affected individuals, especially in those with thick, brown irises. The radial slit defects, located in the iris periphery, may number from a few to almost one hundred and may involve the entire iris circumference. They correspond to the underlying anterior packets of lens zonules that presumably rub against the posterior iris.

Pigment accumulates in the chamber angle and may give the appearance on gonioscopy of a heavy, dark brown band over the posterior or entire trabecular meshwork. Gonioscopy may also reveal an unusually wide angle and concavity of the iris insertion. The peripheral iris may be fairly flaccid, so that the peripheral iris configuration varies during eye and eyelid movement.

Up to half of persons with pigment dispersion syndrome eventually demonstrate sustained elevation of intraocular pressure.[37] Pigmentary glaucoma, which may be very asymmetric between the fellow eyes, results from obstruction of the trabecular meshwork by accumulating pigment and subsequent insult to trabecular meshwork cells.[38] Management of pigmentary glaucoma is similar to that of primary open-angle glaucoma. Argon laser trabeculoplasty is associated with good initial success for pigmentary glaucoma; however, the effect does not appear to last as long as it does for primary open-angle glaucoma.

Pigment dispersion syndrome and pigmentary glaucoma do not typically demonstrate a mendelian inheritance pattern, but in many cases, autosomal dominant inheritance may be recognized.[39–44] Genetic linkage analysis of four white families affected with pigment dispersion syndrome mapped a responsible gene to chromosome 7q35-q36.[44] Half of the individuals affected with pigment dispersion syndrome had elevated intraocular pressure.

AXENFELD-RIEGER SYNDROME

Axenfeld-Rieger, or Rieger's, syndrome encompasses a clinical spectrum of ocular abnormalities associated with certain systemic anomalies. The ocular features in this autosomal dominant disorder, which are highly variable, include a prominent anteriorly displaced Schwalbe's line, iris processes that insert into Schwalbe's line, hypoplasia of the anterior iris stroma, corectopia, and pseudopolycoria. About half of affected individuals will develop high-tension glaucoma, usually by young adulthood. The systemic findings in Axenfeld-Rieger syndrome are also highly variable. The most common systemic anomalies are craniofacial, especially maxillary hypoplasia, dental hypoplasia, and failure of involution of periumbilical skin.

The ocular features of Axenfeld-Rieger syndrome are

bilateral and result from abnormal development of the anterior segment of the eye. The iris anomalies may be subtle but are often striking and are the principal reason the patient is brought to the ophthalmologist. Defects in the iris range from mild stromal thinning to marked atrophy with pseudopupil formation, corectopia, and ectropion uvea. These abnormalities are usually detected in infancy.

Gonioscopy reveals abnormal iris strands extending across the chamber angle and inserting into a prominent, anteriorly displaced ridge of Schwalbe's line. The iris strands vary from thin filaments to broad bands. The broad bands are typically in the same quadrant as the corectopia, with the iris holes in the opposite quadrant. In other areas the iris appears to insert anteriorly into the trabecular meshwork. The glaucoma associated with Axenfeld-Rieger syndrome may develop during infancy or at an elderly age, but usually occurs between childhood and early adulthood. It is often difficult to control medically, and eventually, surgical intervention is needed.

The systemic abnormalities of Axenfeld-Rieger syndrome also appear to be the result of abnormal morphogenesis. Although malar hypoplasia, dental hypoplasia, and prominent umbilicus are the most common findings, numerous other systemic defects have been reported.

Axenfeld-Rieger syndrome is inherited in an autosomal dominant manner. Isolated cases have been associated with chromosomal aberrations. A gene involved in this syndrome *(RIEG)* has been identified on chromosome 4q25.[45] Genetic linkage to 4q25 has been shown for several autosomal dominant pedigrees,[46, 47] and chromosomal defects involving 4q25 have been found for some isolated cases. The *RIEG* gene is a homeobox transcription factor gene that encodes for a protein called solurshin. The mouse homologue of *RIEG* is expressed in the eye mesenchyme, dental lamina, umbilical cord, and other tissues in mouse embryos, consistent with the abnormalities seen in Axenfeld-Rieger syndrome.

Not all cases of autosomal dominant Axenfeld-Rieger syndrome are due to mutations in the *RIEG* gene. In several affected pedigrees, genetic linkage to 4q25 has been statistically excluded.[47, 48] In one such pedigree, the ocular abnormalities ranged from iris hypoplasia, iris strands, and glaucoma to congenital buphthalmos.[47] Hypertelorism and maxillary hypoplasia were seen in affected individuals, but no dental or umbilical defects were present.

Another pedigree demonstrated genetic linkage to a second Axenfeld-Rieger syndrome gene locus at chromosome 13q14.[48] In this family, the ocular findings varied from mild (posterior embryotoxon and iris hypoplasia) to severe (iris adhesions, corectopia, severe glaucoma). Most of the affected individuals also had systemic findings, such as dental and hearing defects, mild craniofacial dysmorphism, hydrocephalus, cryptorchism, fetal kidney lobulations, congenital heart defects, and congenital hip abnormalities. None, however, had redundancy of the periumbilical skin. The clinical findings associated with the Axenfeld-Rieger syndrome linked to 4q25 and with that linked to 13q14 may be difficult to distinguish on the basis of only a few pedigrees. However, as more families are analyzed and the causative genes studied, differentiating features may become apparent.

A thorough family history for any patient in whom the disorder is suspected or has been diagnosed should include any relatives with the characteristic systemic features. Subtle ocular features such as posterior embryotoxon may escape diagnosis, so the presence of dental or umbilical anomalies in a relative should be considered an indication of Axenfeld-Rieger syndrome.

AUTOSOMAL DOMINANT IRIDOGONIODYSGENESIS

Autosomal dominant iridogoniodysgenesis anomaly is a rare disorder in which affected individuals have iris stromal hypoplasia and goniodysgenesis. It is thought to result from abnormal migration or differentiation of the neural crest cells involved in anterior segment formation. Most persons (67% to 74%) with this disorder go on to have juvenile glaucoma.[49–53]

Although the clinical features of iridogoniodysgenesis are variable, the iris hypoplasia in this disorder is usually quite marked. The condition is usually bilateral and symmetric. The iris color in affected individuals differs dramatically from that in unaffected relatives and is due to the exposure of the pigmented iris epithelium through the hypoplastic iris stroma. The iris collarette may be partial or absent, and the iris crypts may be thinned or absent. These defects help distinguish true iris stromal hypoplasia from the thin immature iris stroma of infants. The pupil is round and central but the normal pupillary sphincter stands out against the gray iris background. These congenital iris abnormalities do not change over time.

Gonioscopy may reveal overlying mesenchymal-like tissue or normal-appearing open angles. Occasionally, anomalous vascular loops lying along the circumference and fine iris processes extending to Schwalbe's line are seen in the angle.

Individuals with iridogoniodysgenesis are at high risk for juvenile-onset glaucoma. The glaucoma usually develops during the second or third decade, although wide variability in age of onset exists. Intraocular pressure elevation may be significant, although it usually does not reach the levels seen in autosomal dominant juvenile-onset glaucoma (discussed earlier). Medical therapy may be effective, but many cases eventually require surgical management.

Some individuals with autosomal dominant iridogoniodysgenesis have systemic abnormalities similar to those seen in Rieger's syndrome, including maxillary hypoplasia with dental abnormalities, abnormal umbilical skin, umbilical hernias, and hypospadias.[52, 54, 55] These patients may be considered to have autosomal dominant iridogoniodysgenesis syndrome, to differentiate them from patients lacking the systemic abnormalities (iridogoniodysgenesis anomaly). The iris stromal hypoplasias in iridogoniodysgenesis anomaly and iridogoniodysgenesis syndrome are very similar. However the overlying mesenchymal-like angle tissue often seen on gonioscopy of patients with the anomaly is apparently absent in patients with the syndrome.

Genetic linkage studies have yielded two chromosomal loci for autosomal dominant iridogoniodysgenesis. Two pedigrees with iridogoniodysgenesis anomaly (no nonocular manifestations) demonstrated linkage to chromosome 6p25.[53, 56] Other pedigrees with iridogoniodysgenesis showed linkage to the Rieger's syndrome locus at 4q25.[52, 55]

In these latter pedigrees, at least one affected family member also exhibited systemic abnormalities consistent with iridogoniodysgenesis syndrome. Hence, iridogoniodysgenesis syndrome and Rieger's syndrome may demonstrate allelic heterogeneity; that is, different mutations in the same gene *(RIEG)* may result in either iridogoniodysgenesis syndrome or Rieger's syndrome. It is important to note that even within a family with iridogoniodysgenesis syndrome, only a few of the affected individuals have the systemic features, so the distinction between the anomaly and the syndrome is not always easily made.

A patient diagnosed with iridogoniodysgenesis requires a systemic examination to rule out the abnormalities associated with iridogoniodysgenesis syndrome. As in cases of Rieger's syndrome, a thorough family history should be obtained in cases of iridogoniodysgenesis. In addition to information about ocular disorders, the physician should specifically ask about craniofacial, dental, and umbilical abnormalities, as well as hypospadias in males. Any family history of the nonocular features suggests the diagnosis of iridogoniodysgenesis syndrome. Subsequent offspring are thus at risk for the systemic abnormalities in conjunction with the ocular features. The absence of systemic features on physical examination or in the family history does not exclude the diagnosis of iridogoniodysgenesis syndrome in the particular family. In the future, genetic testing may allow unambiguous differentiation between iridogoniodysgenesis anomaly and iridogoniodysgenesis syndrome.

POSTERIOR POLYMORPHOUS CORNEAL DYSTROPHY

Posterior polymorphous dystrophy (PPMD) is an autosomal dominant disorder of the corneal endothelium. It encompasses a wide variety of corneal abnormalities ranging from mild vesicular opacities of the endothelium to more extensive geographic patterns of endothelial opacification associated with posterior corneal haze. The condition is usually bilateral, often progressive, and may be associated with normal or reduced vision. The endothelial cells in PPMD appear to have many features of epithelial cells, including desmosomes, microvilli, tonofilaments, and the ability to divide and form multiple layers.[57]

About 13% to 43% of persons with PPMD have glaucoma.[58, 59] Some patients have open angles, whereas other patients have closed angles secondary to the growth of abnormal endothelium over the trabecular meshwork. In patients with angle-closure glaucoma, fine or broad iridocorneal adhesions are found by gonioscopy. Occasionally, extensive iridocorneal adhesions are seen by slit-lamp biomicroscopy along with iris atrophy and corectopia.[60]

Autosomal dominant PPMD has been linked to chromosome 20q11 in a large pedigree.[59] Of the affected individuals in this pedigree, 38% had iris abnormalities and 43% had associated glaucoma.

ANIRIDIA

Aniridia is a hereditary condition that arises from a defect in the development of the eye. Although it is always associated with some degree of iris abnormality, aniridia is usually also associated with other anterior segment anomalies. The condition is caused by genetic defects in the *PAX6* gene located on chromosome 11p13. The *PAX6* gene is highly conserved in evolution and appears to play a critical role in the development of the eye.[61] Other ocular disorders, including Peters' anomaly and autosomal dominant keratitis, are also associated with mutations in the *PAX6* gene.

The most common hereditary form of this condition is isolated, autosomal dominant aniridia in which no systemic abnormalities are found. Less frequently, aniridia is associated with autosomal dominant WAGR syndrome.[62] This syndrome consists of Wilms' tumor, aniridia, genitourinary anomalies, and mental retardation and is associated with chromosomal defects (deletions, translocations, insertions) at 11p13. A rare autosomal recessive aniridia also occurs with cerebellar ataxia and mental retardation.[63] Although no defects within the *PAX6* gene have been reported, the PAX6 protein may be abnormal in this condition.

In a patient newly diagnosed with aniridia who has a family history of isolated, autosomal dominant aniridia, the likelihood of Wilms' tumor is extremely low. However, a patient with a sporadic case of aniridia (no family history) is at high risk for developing the kidney tumor.

Although the term aniridia denotes a lack of iris, individuals with aniridia always have at least some rudimentary iris structure. The clinical manifestations of aniridia are highly variable. Iris abnormalities range from small iris remnants to thin iris stroma with a normal pupil. The most typical features of aniridia are small rudimentary iris stump, photophobia, nystagmus, decreased vision, amblyopia, and strabismus. Other manifestations are corneal opacities, cataract formation, optic nerve hypoplasia, and macular hypoplasia. Most of these abnormalities are present at birth or develop during the first few years. Glaucoma frequently occurs in aniridia but usually not until the second decade. Progressive angle closure results from the developmental anomalies of the angle that may obstruct the trabecular meshwork. Angle-closure glaucoma is unlikely to occur in aniridic eyes with minimal iris abnormalities.

Proper genetic counseling is important for parents of a child newly diagnosed with aniridia. The family history inquiry should include any ocular or visual abnormality as well as systemic diseases, such as genitourinary anomalies, Wilms' tumor, and mental retardation. Even if the family history is reportedly negative, a thorough examination of both parents and close relatives should be undertaken, including iris fluorescein angiography to rule out mild subtle abnormalities in apparently normal irises. If the parents and other close relatives are not affected, the child has a sporadic case of aniridia and requires a full evaluation for evidence of the WAGR syndrome. Genetic studies of the patient's *PAX6* gene may be useful if available.

PRIMARY CONGENITAL GLAUCOMA (BUPHTHALMOS)

Primary (isolated) congenital glaucoma represents a group of disorders characterized by the onset of elevated intraocular pressures during infancy or early childhood in the absence of other ocular or systemic diseases or abnormalities. Although it is the most common type of glaucoma in infancy, primary congenital glaucoma is rare, occurring in about 1 in 10,000 to 1 in 30,000 live births in Western countries.[64] It is about four times more common in Middle Eastern countries.[65] The disorder usually affects both eyes and it is a leading cause of permanent blindness in children.

Congenital glaucoma is thought to result from maldevelopment of the trabecular meshwork.[66, 67] The iris and ciliary body appear immature, in that they have not receded posteriorly as they do in normally developed infant eyes. Hence, the iris insertion and anterior ciliary body overlap the posterior trabecular meshwork and obstruct aqueous outflow.

Most cases of congenital glaucoma occur sporadically. A small percentage of cases demonstrate autosomal recessive pattern of inheritance.[68–70] In these cases, multiple siblings may be affected or consanguinity may be present. The actual recurrence rate may be less than the expected 25% because of incomplete penetrance. In addition, males account for about two thirds of cases of primary congenital glaucoma. Hence, the inheritance pattern within some families may not be strictly autosomal recessive.

All of the signs and symptoms of primary congenital glaucoma are direct or indirect consequences of elevated intraocular pressure in the infant eye. Congenital glaucoma typically manifests as epiphora, photophobia, and blepharospasm. These symptoms result from the corneal irritation associated with corneal epithelial edema secondary to elevated pressure. Increased wall tension from the elevated intraocular pressure leads to enlargement of the eye (buphthalmos), especially at the corneoscleral junction, where the wall of the globe is thinnest.

Conjunctival injection and corneal haze from the pressure-induced edema may be mild initially. With stretching of the cornea, Descemet's membrane may rupture and allow rapid influx of aqueous into the corneal stroma and epithelium. The cornea then suddenly becomes more edematous and hazy, and the child experiences a sudden increase in tearing and photophobia.

Without adequate control of the intraocular pressure, the cornea and globe continue to enlarge, with more tears occurring in Descemet's membrane. Symptoms of tearing, photophobia, and blepharospasm may worsen, and corneal scarring, erosions, and ulcerations may develop. The globe may become more susceptible to hyphema, lens subluxation, or rupture due to blunt trauma.

Complete examination of an infant or young child (less than 5 years) with congenital glaucoma may be difficult and may require general anesthesia. In an otherwise healthy child, general anesthesia is relatively safe if administered by an anesthesiologist experienced in pediatric cases. Older children may cooperate adequately for an office examination with or without mild sedation. Chloral hydrate may slightly lower intraocular pressure.

During the initial and follow-up examinations in the office with the use of general anesthesia, certain critical signs should be noted. Because most general anesthetics lower intraocular pressure (ketamine may elevate the pressure slightly), intraocular pressure measurement (with hand-held applanation and/or TonoPen tonometer) should be made as soon as safely possible. Pressures greater than 21 mm Hg are probably abnormal, but as with other types of glaucoma, the intraocular pressure may not always be elevated. Similarly, a normal eye may occasionally have an elevated pressure. Hence, other signs must be taken into account in the evaluation of a child with or suspected of having congenital glaucoma.

An enlarging globe can be assessed by A-scan ultrasonography to measure axial length. Nomograms are available for reference. Retinoscopy may reveal a myopic shift as the eye lengthens. Horizontal corneal diameter should be determined with the use of calipers extending from the very edge of white sclera on each side. The normal horizontal corneal diameter is 10 to 10.5 mm in a newborn and grows to 11 to 12 mm by 1 year of age.

The cornea should also be assessed for clarity. The degree and location of edema, scarring, and tears in Descemet's membrane should be noted. Corneal opacities may affect visual acuity and contribute to amblyopia. The anterior segment is evaluated for other abnormalities that may suggest a diagnosis other than primary congenital glaucoma.

Gonioscopy may be performed with a mirrored lens viewed through the operating room microscope or with a Koeppe lens viewed through a hand-held binocular microscope. In the normal newborn eye, the iris typically inserts posterior to the scleral spur in a flat configuration with the ciliary body band visible anteriorly. During the first year, the angle recess forms as the iris turns slightly posteriorly before inserting into the ciliary body. The trabecular meshwork appears thick and translucent. In gonioscopy of the eye with congenital glaucoma, the iris appears to insert more anteriorly into the trabecular meshwork. The level of iris insertion may vary throughout the circumference of the angle.

Examination of an infant diagnosed with or suspected of having congenital glaucoma requires careful evaluation of the optic nerve. The operating microscope in conjunction with a fundus contact lens allows a magnified view of the nerve head. The optic nerves of infants and young children tend to have smaller cups than adult optic nerves. In young eyes, a cup-to-disc ratio of 0.1 or less is most common and a ratio of 0.3 should be treated with suspicion. In progressive congenital glaucoma, the optic cup tends to enlarge circumferentially; the enlargement may be reversible with control of the intraocular pressure, especially in children younger than 1 year.

A thorough family history is important in evaluating an infant in whom congenital glaucoma is suspected, as well as in genetic counseling of the parents. A history of an affected relative, especially a sibling, greatly increases the likelihood of an inherited disease. Consanguinity strongly suggests an autosomal recessive form of congenital glaucoma. The physician can inquire tactfully about consanguinity by asking whether the families of the two parents share a common ancestor.

At least two genetic loci for autosomal recessive primary congenital glaucoma have been identified.[71, 72] At least among Turkish and Saudi Arabian families with congenital glaucoma, the disease links most commonly to the GLC3A locus on chromosome 2p21.[71, 73] Frameshift, truncating mutations in cytochrome P4501B1 *(CYP1B1)* gene, located on chromosome 2p21, have been found in pedigrees affected with congenital glaucoma.[73] The cytochrome P4501B1 gene is expressed in the trabecular meshwork as well as in other tissues. It is a member of the cytochrome P450 enzyme family that is responsible for metabolizing a wide range of substrates. Cytochrome P4501B1 may play an important role in the development of the eye.

A second locus (GLC3B) for primary congenital glaucoma maps to chromosome 1p36.[72] Moreover, in several other families, the disease does not link to either the 2p21 or the 1p36 locus, indicating that at least one more locus for autosomal recessive congenital glaucoma must exist in the genome.[72] Any differences in the clinical features among the different genetic forms of autosomal recessive primary congenital glaucoma have not been described.

OCULOCEREBRORENAL SYNDROME OF LOWE

The oculocerebrorenal syndrome of Lowe is an X-linked recessive disorder characterized by ocular, renal, and musculoskeletal abnormalities as well as mental and growth retardation.[74] The most common ocular findings are cataracts and congenital glaucoma. Almost all patients with Lowe's syndrome have cataracts, which are usually dense nuclear or posterior cortical. In addition, the lens itself is small in both diameter and anteroposterior depth. Glaucoma occurs in the majority of cases. Although the precise mechanism of glaucoma is not known, the microphakia may contribute to abnormal development of the anterior chamber angle.

Patients with Lowe's syndrome are predominantly male, as expected for an X-linked recessive disease. Female carriers, however, may show progressive lenticular opacities. The gene for Lowe's syndrome *(OCRL-1)* has been identified on chromosome Xq25.[75–78] It appears to code for a protein similar to inositol polyphosphate-5-phosphatase, suggesting that the primary defect in Lowe's syndrome involves inositol metabolism.[77]

Glaucomas with Nondistinct Inheritance Pattern

For glaucoma not associated with a distinct inheritance pattern, a positive family history is still significant. In the evaluation and management of a patient in whom glaucoma is suspected, a positive family history may greatly influence the decision making. Such a patient may be followed more closely or started on therapy sooner than a patient without a positive family history. Family members of patients with glaucoma should be encouraged to undergo regular ophthalmologic evaluations, especially if other relatives are affected as well.

ADULT-ONSET PRIMARY OPEN-ANGLE GLAUCOMA

Although most cases of adult-onset primary open-angle glaucoma do not exhibit mendelian inheritance, a familial component appears to exist. The prevalence of glaucoma among first-degree relatives of patients with glaucoma may be as high as 16%, compared with a prevalence of about 2% in the general population older than 40 years. The risk of glaucoma in first-degree relatives may be up to five times that in the general population.

The genes causing the specific inherited forms of glaucoma described earlier may also be involved in other more common types of glaucoma. Mutations in the *TIGR* gene have been detected in at least 3% of patients with adult-onset primary open-angle glaucoma.[21] Increased *TIGR* gene expression in the meshwork occurs in approximately half of adult cases of primary open-angle glaucoma compared with age-matched control cases.[79] In addition, because prolonged steroid exposure stimulates *TIGR* gene expression, the *TIGR* gene may be involved in steroid-induced glaucoma as well. Moreover, many persons with primary open-angle glaucoma also experience increased intraocular pressure with long-term steroid use.

EXFOLIATION (PSEUDOEXFOLIATION) SYNDROME

Exfoliation (pseudoexfoliation) syndrome is a systemic disorder characterized by the presence of grayish white "exfoliation" material in or on various ocular tissues as well as various nonocular organs. The most recognizable sign is a distinct pattern of the material deposited on the anterior lens capsule. A clear zone separates a central white disc and an irregular peripheral white zone. The rubbing of the iris over the lens surface during normal pupil movement creates the clear zone. This iris-lens rubbing also causes dispersion of peripupillary pigment into the anterior chamber and peripupillary transillumination defects. Gonioscopy frequently reveals irregular pigment deposition on the trabecular meshwork, especially inferiorly.

Exfoliation syndrome is the most common identifiable cause of open-angle glaucoma.[80] Elevated intraocular pressure probably results from accumulation of pigment and exfoliation material in the trabecular meshwork, which leads to blockage of the outflow channels and damage to the trabecular cells.

Exfoliation syndrome may show familial occurrence, although a genetic basis for the disorder has not been established. Relatives of patients with the syndrome who are older than 40 years may be affected in up to 9.4% of cases, compared with 1% of relatives of nonaffected patients.[81] However, the high prevalence of exfoliation syndrome in certain geographic regions, especially in Scandinavia, suggests environmental factors and complicates interpretation. Furthermore, homozygous twins have been reported that are discordant for the presence of exfoliation syndrome.[81, 82]

ANGLE-CLOSURE GLAUCOMA

As mentioned earlier, close relatives of persons with angle-closure glaucoma are more likely to have angle-closure glaucoma than the normal population. First-degree relatives tend to have shallow anterior chambers and narrow angles,[83–85] which are predisposing conditions for angle closure. The risk of developing angle-closure glaucoma in first-degree relatives of affected patients may be especially high in certain ethnic groups, such as Eskimos.[86]

OCULAR FEATURES ASSOCIATED WITH GLAUCOMA

In addition to the familial inclination of glaucoma, the ocular characteristics associated with glaucoma may also

TABLE 6–2. INHERITED DISORDERS THAT MAY BE ASSOCIATED WITH GLAUCOMA

Ackerman's syndrome
Angiomatosis retinae (von Hippel–Lindau syndrome)
Anophthalmia-plus syndrome
Basal cell nevus syndrome
Bowen's syndrome
Cryptophthalmos
Cutis marmorata telangiectatica congenita
Cystinosis
Dandy-Walker–like malformation with atrioventricular septal defect
Dwarfism with stiff joints and ocular abnormalities
Dyssegmental dwarfism
Dyssegmental dysplasia and congenital glaucoma
Ehlers-Danlos syndrome type VI
Friedreich's ataxia and congenital glaucoma
Fuchs' endothelial dystrophy
GAPO (growth retardation, alopecia, pseudoanodontia, and optic atrophy) syndrome
Glaucoma with elevated episcleral venous pressure
GLEMSS (glaucoma, lens ectopia, microspherophakia, stiffness, shortness)
Histiocytic dermatoarthritis
Hyaloideoretinal degeneration of Wagner
Isolated ectopia lentis
Klippel-Trenaunay-Weber syndrome
Lowry-MacLean syndrome
Marfan's syndrome
Marshall's syndrome
Melnick-Needles syndrome
Microcornea, glaucoma, and absent frontal sinuses
Microphthalmos
Mucopolysaccharidosis type I (Hurler-Scheie syndrome)
Mucopolysaccharidosis type IV A (Morquio's syndrome)
Mucopolysaccharidosis type VI
Muscle-eye-brain disease
Nance-Horan syndrome
Neurofibromatosis type 1
Oculodentodigital dysplasia
Peters' anomaly
Polymorphous posterior corneal dystrophy
Prader-Willi syndrome
Primary familial amyloidosis
Renal tubular acidosis II
Rubenstein-Taybi syndrome
Spastic paresis, glaucoma, and mental retardation
Stickler's syndrome type 1
Sturge-Weber syndrome
Transthyretin
Tuberous sclerosis
Weill-Marchesani syndrome
Weissenbacher-Zweymuller syndrome
Zellweger's syndrome

have familial tendencies. Elevated intraocular pressure is much more likely in persons with a family history of primary open-angle glaucoma than in the general population.[87–89] Moreover, intraocular pressure shows significant correlation among close relatives.[90–94] Some studies suggest a familial association for the response of intraocular pressure to corticosteroids,[95–98] whereas other studies do not.[99–103] However, the variability in measuring and reproducing the steroid response complicates any genetic study. First-degree relatives may also show similarities in cup-to-disc ratio.[104–107]

Genetic Counseling

The physician should provide information about the risks of glaucoma in offspring and other close relatives. Family members should be encouraged to have early, regular monitoring for glaucoma. For disorders that exhibit mendelian inheritance, recurrence risks can be discussed. Parents must be aware that recurrence risks are true for each offspring and are not changed by the status of previous children. Furthermore, the 50% recurrence risk for an autosomal dominant disorder and the 25% recurrence risk for an autosomal recessive disorder are mitigated by reduced penetrance, variable expression, and perhaps environmental factors. For nonmendelian inherited glaucoma, genetic counseling may be useful in alerting relatives who may be at higher than normal risk than the general population.

In addition, many inherited systemic disorders are associated with glaucoma; this factor should be considered in all genetic counseling evaluations (Table 6–2).

Future Considerations

Advances in molecular genetics have already greatly enhanced our understanding of several types of glaucoma. In addition, results of genetic studies have prompted a new way of classifying glaucoma. For instance, iridogoniodysgenesis syndrome and Rieger's syndrome are both linked to the RIEG locus at 4q25, suggesting that the two syndromes are more closely related to each other than either is to its corresponding anomaly. Adult-onset primary open-angle glaucoma probably represents a collection of genetically distinct disorders that are grouped together on the basis of their clinical similarities. As more genes are discovered, the different types of glaucoma may be reclassified on their genetic basis rather than from their clinical features.

Identification of genetic mutations associated with glaucoma may also lead to genetic testing. This may allow determination of persons at risk for glaucoma, particularly relatives of affected individuals. Moreover, various mutations may be associated with different clinical aspects such as prognosis and responsiveness to certain therapies.

Characterization of specific genes will improve our understanding of the molecular basis of specific types of glaucoma. This will encourage development of specific therapies tailored to the underlying pathophysiology. Gene therapy may allow restoration of a defective gene. Alternatively, an agent that rescues or enhances the action of a defective gene product may reestablish the normal physiology. Furthermore, our understanding of glaucoma in general will be greatly enhanced by the identification and characterization of genes involved in specific inherited glaucoma diseases. Ultimately, molecular genetics will improve our ability to diagnose and manage our patients with glaucoma.

REFERENCES

1. Tielsch JM, Katz J, Sommer A, et al: Family history and risk of primary open angle glaucoma: The Baltimore Eye Survey. Arch Ophthalmol 1994;112:69.

2. Perkins ES: Family studies in glaucoma. Br J Ophthalmol 1974;58:529.
3. FranHois J: Multifactorial or polygenic inheritance in ophthalmology. *In* Henkind P (ed): Twenty-fourth International Congress of Ophthalmology. Philadelphia, JB Lippincott, 1985.
4. Damji KF, Allingham RR: Molecular genetics is revolutionizing our understanding of ophthalmic disease. Am J Ophthalmol 1997; 124:530.
5. Raymond V: Molecular genetics of the glaucomas: Mapping of the first five "GLC" loci. Am J Hum Genet 1997;60:272.
6. Johnson AT, Drack AV, Kwitch AE, et al: Clinical features and linkage analysis of a family with autosomal dominant juvenile glaucoma. Ophthalmology 1993;100:524.
7. Sheffield VC, Stone EM, Alward WLM, et al: Genetic linkage of familial open angle glaucoma to chromosome 1q21-q31. Nat Genet 1993;4:47.
8. Richards JE, Lichter PR, Boehnke M, et al: Mapping of a gene for autosomal dominant juvenile-onset open-angle glaucoma to chromosome 1q. Am J Hum Genet 1994;54:62.
9. Wiggs JL, Haines JL, Paglinauan C, et al: Genetic linkage of autosomal dominant juvenile glaucoma to 1q21-q31 in three affected pedigrees. Genomics 1994;21:299.
10. Meyer A, Valtot F, Bechetoille A, et al: Linkage between juvenile glaucoma and chromosome 1q in two French families [French]. C R Acad Sci III 1994;317:565.
11. Graff C, Urbak SF, Jerndal T, et al: Confirmation of linkage to 1q21-31 in a Danish autosomal dominant juvenile-onset glaucoma family and evidence of genetic heterogeneity. Hum Genet 1995;96:285.
12. Morissette J, Cote G, Anctil JL, et al: A common gene for juvenile and adult-onset primary open-angle glaucomas confined on chromosome 1q. Am J Hum Genet 1995;56:1431.
13. Wiggs JL, Del Bono EA, Schuman JS, et al: Clinical features of five pedigrees genetically linked to the juvenile glaucoma locus on chromosome 1q21-q31. Ophthalmology 1995;102:1782.
14. Johnson AT, Richards JE, Boehnke M, et al: Clinical phenotype of juvenile-onset primary open-angle glaucoma linked to chromosome 1q. Ophthalmology 1996;103:808.
15. Meyer A, Bechetoille A, Valtot F, et al: Age-dependent penetrance and mapping of the locus for juvenile and early-onset open-angle glaucoma on chromosome 1q (GLC1A) in a French family. Hum Genet 1996;98:567.
16. WuDunn D, Parrish RK II, Inana G: Genetic heterogeneity in Hispanic families with autosomal dominant juvenile glaucoma. Ophthalmic Genet 1996;17:87.
17. Lichter PR, Richards JE, Boehnke M, et al: Juvenile glaucoma linked to the GLC1A gene on chromosome 1q in a Panamanian family. Am J Ophthalmol 1997;123:413.
18. Stegman Z, Sokol J, Liebmann JM, et al: Reduced trabecular meshwork height in juvenile primary open-angle glaucoma. Arch Ophthalmol 1996;114:660.
19. Furuyoshi N, Furuyoshi M, Futa R, et al: Ultrastructural changes in the trabecular meshwork of juvenile glaucoma. Ophthalmologica 1997;211:140.
20. Johnson D, Gottanka J, Flugel C, et al: Ultrastructural changes in the trabecular meshwork of human eyes treated with corticosteroids. Arch Ophthalmol 1997;115:375.
21. Stone EM, Fingert JH, Alward WLM, et al: Identification of a gene that causes primary open angle glaucoma. Science 1997;275:668.
22. Nguyen TD, Huang W, Bloom E, et al: Glucocorticoid effects on HTM cells: Molecular biology approaches. *In* Lütjen-Drecoll E (ed): Basic Aspects of Glaucoma Research III. Stuttgart, Schattauer, 1993, p 331.
23. Polansky JR, Bloom E, Weinreb RN, et al: Hormonal responses in cultured human trabecular cells. Excerpta Med 1984;636:201.
24. Polansky JR, Kurtz R, Alvarado JA, et al: Eicosanoid production and glucocorticoid regulatory mechanisms in cultured human trabecular meshwork cells. Prog Clin Biol Res 1989;312:113.
25. Polansky JR, Fauss DJ, Chen P, et al: Cellular pharmacology and molecular biology of the trabecular meshwork inducible glucocorticoid response gene product. Ophthalmologica 1997;211:126.
26. Biró I: Notes upon the question of hereditary glaucoma. Ophthalmologica 1951;122:228.
27. Probert LA: A survey of hereditary glaucoma. Can Med Assoc J 1952;66:563.
28. Havener WH: Chronic simple glaucoma: Hereditary aspects. Am J Ophthalmol 1955;40:828.
29. FranHois J: Genetics and primary open-angle glaucoma. Am J Ophthalmol 1966;61:652.
30. Kitsos G, Cote G, Psilas K: An example of dominant heredity in the transmission of primary open-angle glaucoma in a northwestern region of Greece. J Fr Ophthalmol 1988;11:859.
31. Stoilova D, Child A, Trifan OC, et al: Localization of a locus (GLC1B) for adult-onset primary open-angle glaucoma to the 2cen-q13 region. Genomics 1996;36:142.
32. Avramopoulos D, Kitsos G, Economou-Petersen E, et al: Exclusion of one pedigree affected by adult onset primary open angle glaucoma from linkage to the juvenile glaucoma locus on chromosome 1q21-q31. J Med Genet 1996;33:1043.
33. Fossarello M, Zucca I, Galantuomo S, et al: Genetic mapping of autosomal dominant primary open-angle glaucoma (POAG) in Sardinia. Int Ophthalmol 1996–97;20:1.
34. Wirtz MK, Samples JR, Kramer PL, et al: Mapping a gene for adult-onset primary open-angle glaucoma to chromosome 3q. Am J Hum Genet 1997;60:296.
35. Lichter PR, Richards JE, Downs CA, et al: Cosegregation of open-angle glaucoma and the nail-patella syndrome. Am J Ophthalmol 1997;124:506.
36. Farrar SM, Shields MB: Current concepts in pigmentary glaucoma. Surv Ophthalmol 1993;37:233.
37. Richter CU, Richardson TM, Grant WM: Pigmentary dispersion syndrome and pigmentary glaucomas: A prospective study of the natural history. Arch Ophthalmol 1986;104:211.
38. Alvarado JA, Murphy CG: Outflow obstruction in pigmentary and primary open angle glaucoma. Arch Ophthalmol 1992;110:1769.
39. Becker B, Podos SM: Krukenberg's spindles and primary open-angle glaucoma. Arch Ophthalmol 1966;76:635.
40. Mandelkorn RM, Hoffman ME, Olander KW, et al: Inheritance and the pigmentary dispersion syndrome. Ann Ophthalmol 1983;15:577.
41. Kaiser-Kupfer MI, Kupfer C, McCain L: Asymmetric pigment dispersion syndrome. Trans Am Ophthalmol Soc 1983;81:310.
42. McDermott JA, Ritch R, Berger A, et al: Inheritance of pigmentary dispersion syndrome. Invest Ophthalmol Vis Sci Suppl 1987;28:153.
43. Paglinauan CM, Haines JL, del Bono EA, et al: Exclusion of chromosome 1q21-q31 from linkage to three pedigrees affected by the pigment-dispersion syndrome. Am J Hum Genet 1995;56:1240.
44. Andersen JS, Pralea AM, del Bono EA, et al: A gene responsible for the pigment dispersion syndrome maps to chromosome 7q35-q36. Arch Ophthalmol 1997;115:384.
45. Semina EV, Reiter R, Leysens NJ, et al: Cloning and characterization of a novel *bicoid*-related homeobox transcription factor gene, *RIEG*, involved in Rieger syndrome. Nat Genet 1996;14:392.
46. Murray JC, Bennett SR, Kwitek AE, et al: Linkage of Rieger syndrome to the region of the epidermal growth factor gene on chromosome 4. Nat Genet 1992;2:46.
47. Legius E, de Die-Smulders CEM, Verbraak F, et al: Genetic heterogeneity in Rieger eye malformation. J Med Genet 1994;31:340.
48. Phillips JC, del Bono EA, Haines JL, et al: A second locus for Rieger syndrome maps to chromosome 13q14. Am J Hum Genet 1996;59:613.
49. Weatherhill J, Hart C: Familial hypoplasia of the iris stroma associated with glaucoma. Br J Ophthalmol 1969;53:433.
50. Jerndal T: Goniodysgenesis and hereditary juvenile glaucoma: A clinical study of a Swedish pedigree. Acta Ophthalmol 1970; 107:100.
51. Pearce W, Wyatt H, Boyd T, et al: Autosomal dominant iridogoniodysgenesis: Genetic features. Can J Ophthalmol 1983;18:7.
52. Heon E, Sheth BP, Kalenak JW, et al: Linkage of autosomal dominant iris hypoplasia to the region of the Rieger syndrome locus (4q25). Hum Mol Genet 1995;4:1435.
53. Mears AJ, Mirzayans F, Gould DB, et al: Autosomal dominant iridogoniodysgenesis anomaly maps to 6q25. Am J Hum Genet 1996;59:1321.
54. Chisholm I, Chudley A: Autosomal dominant iridogoniodysgenesis with associated somatic anomalies: Four-generation family with Reiger's syndrome. Br J Ophthalmol 1983;67:529.
55. Walter MA, Mirzayans F, Mears AJ, et al: Autosomal-dominant iridogoniodysgenesis and Axenfeld-Rieger syndrome are genetically distinct. Ophthalmology 1996;103:1907.
56. Mirzayans F, Mears AJ, Guo SW, et al: Identification of the human

chromosomal region containing the iridogoniodysgenesis anomaly locus by genomic-mismatch scanning. Am J Hum Genet 1997; 61:111.
57. Rodrigues MM, Sun TT, Krachmer J, et al: Epithelialization of the corneal endothelium in posterior polymorphous dystrophy. Invest Ophthalmol Vis Sci 1980;19:832.
58. Rodrigues MM, Phelps CD, Krachmer JH, et al: Glaucoma due to endothelialization of the anterior chamber angle: A comparison of posterior polymorphous dystrophy of the cornea and Chandler's syndrome. Arch Ophthalmol 1980;98:688.
59. Heon E, Mathers WE, Alward WLM, et al: Linkage of posterior polymorphous corneal dystrophy to 20q11. Hum Mol Genet 1995;4:485.
60. Krachmer JH: Posterior polymorphous corneal dystrophy: A disease characterized by epithelial-like endothelial cells which influence management and prognosis. Trans Am Ophthalmol Soc 1985;83:413.
61. Churchill A, Booth A: Genetics of aniridia and anterior segment dysgenesis. Br J Ophthalmol 1996;80:669.
62. Pavilack MA, Walton DS: Genetics of aniridia: The aniridia–Wilms' tumor association. Int Ophthalmol Clin 1993;33:77.
63. Gillespie FD: Aniridia, cerebellar ataxia, and oligophrenia in siblings. Arch Ophthalmol 1965;73:338.
64. Francois J: Congenital glaucoma and its inheritance. Ophthalmologica 1972;181:61.
65. Jaffar MS: Care of the infantile glaucoma patient. *In* Reineck RD (ed): Ophthalmology Annual. New York, Raven Press, 1988, p 15.
66. Allen L, Burion HM, Braley AE: A new concept of development of anterior chamber angle: Its relationship to developmental glaucoma and other structural anomalies. Arch Ophthalmol 1955;53:783.
67. Barkan O: Pathogenesis of congenital glaucoma. Am J Ophthalmol 1955;40:1.
68. DeLuise V, Anderson D: Primary infantile glaucoma (congenital glaucoma). Surv Ophthalmol 1983;28:1.
69. Gencik A: Epidemiology and genetics of primary congenital glaucoma in Slovakia: Description of a form of primary congenital glaucoma in gypsies with autosomal recessive inheritance and complete penetrance. Dev Ophthalmol 1989;16:76.
70. Turacli ME, Aktan SG, Sayli BS, et al: Therapeutic and genetical aspects of congenital glaucomas. Int Ophthalmol 1992;16:359.
71. Sarfarazi M, Akarsu AN, Hossain A, et al: Assignment of a locus (GLC3A) for primary congenital glaucoma (buphthalmos) to 2p21 and evidence for genetic heterogeneity. Genomics 1995;30:171.
72. Akarsu AN, Turacli ME, Aktan SG, et al: A second locus (GLC3B) for primary congenital glaucoma (buphthalmos) maps to the 1p36 region. Hum Mol Genet 1996;5:1199.
73. Stoilov I, Akarsu AN, Sarfarazi M: Identification of three different truncating mutations in cytochrome P4501B1 (CYP1B1) as the principal cause of primary congenital glaucoma (buphthalmos) in families linked to the GLC3A locus on chromosome 2p21. Hum Mol Genet 1997;6:641.
74. Abassi V, Lowe CU, Calcagno PL: Oculo-cerebro-renal syndrome: A review. Am J Dis Child 1968;115:145.
75. Silver DN, Lewis RA, Nussbaum RL: Mapping the Lowe oculocerebrorenal syndrome to Xq24-q26 by use of restriction fragment length polymorphisms. J Clin Invest 1987;79:282.
76. Nelson DL, Ballabio A, Victoria MF, et al: Alu-primed polymerase chain reaction for regional assignment of 110 yeast artificial chromosome clones for the human X chromosome: Identification of clones associated with a disease locus. Proc Natl Acad Sci U S A 1991;88:6157.
77. Attree O, Olivos IM, Okabe I, et al: The Lowe's oculocerebrorenal syndrome gene encodes a protein highly homologous to inositol polyphosphate-5-phosphatase. Nature 1992;358:239.
78. Leahey AM, Charnas LR, Nussbaum RL: Nonsense mutations in the OCRL-1 gene in patients with the oculocerebrorenal syndrome of Lowe. Hum Mol Genet 1993;100:461.
79. Lütjen-Drecoll E, May CA, Polansky JR et al: Localization of the stress proteins αβ-crystallin and trabecular meshwork inducible glucocorticoid response protein in normal and glaucomatous trabecular meshwork. Invest Ophthalmol Vis Sci 1998;39:517.
80. Ritch R: Exfoliation syndrome: The most common identifiable cause of open-angle glaucoma. J Glaucoma 1994;3:176.
81. Aasved H: Study of relatives of persons with fibrillopathia epitheliocapsularis (pseudoexfoliation of the lens capsule). Acta Ophthalmol (Copenh) 1975;53:879.
82. Ringvold A, Blika S, Elsas T, et al: The Middle-Norway eye-screening study. I: Epidemiology of the pseudoexfoliation syndrome. Acta Ophthalmol (Copenh) 1988;66:652.
83. Lowe RF: Primary angle-closure glaucoma: Family histories and anterior chamber depths. Br J Ophthalmol 1964;48:191.
84. Spaeth GL: Gonioscopy: Uses old and new: The inheritance of occludable angles. Ophthalmology 1978;85:222.
85. Tornquist R: Chamber depth in primary acute glaucoma. Br J Ophthalmol 1956;40:421.
86. Alsbirk PH: Anterior chamber depth and primary angle-closure glaucoma: II: A genetic study. Acta Ophthalmol (Copenh) 1975;53:436.
87. Seddon JM, Schwartz B, Flowerdew G: Case-control of ocular hypertension. Arch Ophthalmol 1983;101:891.
88. Wilson MR, Hertzmark E, Walker AM, et al: A case-control study of risk factors in open angle glaucoma. Arch Ophthalmol 1987;105:1066.
89. Armaly MF: On the distribution of applanation pressure. I: Statistical features and the effect of age, sex, and family history of glaucoma. Arch Ophthalmol 1965;73:11.
90. Armaly MF: Genetic determination of ocular pressure in the normal eye. Arch Ophthalmol 1967;78:187.
91. Armaly MF, Monstavicius BF, Sayegh RE: Ocular pressure and outflow facility in siblings. Arch Ophthalmol 1968;80:354.
92. Becker B, Kolker AE, Roth FD: Glaucoma family study. Am J Ophthalmol 1960;50:557.
93. Davies TG: Tonographic survey of the close relatives of patients with chronic simple glaucoma. Br J Ophthalmol 1968;52:32.
94. Levene RZ, Workman PL, Broder SW, et al: Heritability of ocular pressure in normal and suspect ranges. Arch Ophthalmol 1970;84:730.
95. Armaly MF: The heritable nature of dexamethasone induced ocular hypertension. Arch Ophthalmol 1966;75:32.
96. Armaly MF: Inheritance of dexamethasone hypertension and glaucoma. Arch Ophthalmol 1967;77:747.
97. Becker B, Hahn KA: Topical corticosteroids and heredity in primary open angle glaucoma. Am J Ophthalmol 1964;57:543.
98. Becker B, Chevrette L: Topical corticosteroid testing in glaucoma siblings. Arch Ophthalmol 1966;76:484.
99. FranHois J, Heintz-de-Bree C, Tripathi RC: The cortisone test and the heredity of primary open angle glaucoma. Am J Ophthalmol 1966;62:844.
100. FranHois J: Corticosteroid glaucoma. Ann Ophthalmol 1977;9:1075.
101. Schwartz JT, Reuling FH, Feinleib M, et al: Twin study on ocular pressure after topical dexamethasone. I: Frequency distribution of pressure response. Am J Ophthalmol 1973;76:126.
102. Schwartz JT, Reuling FH, Feinleib M, et al: Twin study on ocular pressure following topically applied dexamethasone. II: Inheritance of variation in pressure response. Arch Ophthalmol 1973;90:281.
103. Schwartz JT, Reuling FH, Feinleib M, et al: Twin heritability study of the corticosteroid response. Trans Am Acad Ophthalmol Otol 1973;77:126.
104. Armaly MF: Genetic determination of cup/disc ratio of the optic nerve. Arch Ophthalmol 1967;78:35.
105. Bengtsson B: The inheritance and development of cup and disc diameters. Acta Ophthalmol (Copenh) 1976;54:27.
106. Schwartz TJ, Reuling FH, Feinleib M: Size of the physiologic cup of the optic nerve head: Heredity and environmental factors. Arch Ophthalmol 1975;93:776.
107. Teikari JM: Genetic influences in open-angle glaucoma. Int Ophthalmol Clin 1990;30:161.

CHAPTER 7

Race

BRUCE D. CAMERON and KEVIN C. GREENIDGE

Although often a sensitive and controversial subject, race is an important factor in the care of the patient with glaucoma. In this chapter, Bruce Cameron and Kevin Greenidge discuss the implications of the patient's race on glaucoma and its treatment. The racial origins of a patient are often indistinct, thus accounting for the variable findings. Nevertheless, the type of glaucoma a patient has, as well as its incidence, course, and treatment, appears to have at least a partial basis in race. The specific findings for the various racial groups are presented. These include patients seen routinely, such as those of European, African, and Asian descent. The authors also discuss specific races or groups for which less is known about the implications of glaucoma, such as Latin Americans, Native American Indians, and those of Indian descent. More intelligent decisions can be made about treatment when the implications of glaucoma in the patient's specific population are considered.

A *race* is defined as one of the group of populations constituting humanity, determined by gene frequencies differing from those of the other groups in the species.[1, 2] Races developed in response to genetic drift, mutation, natural selection, and geographic adaptation. As populations migrate and encounter other populations, the distinctions between races become less evident over time. It is often difficult, and usually unnecessary, to distinguish between members of different races.

In certain situations, however, it is helpful to be able to identify the racial origin of a person. In medicine, for example, the frequencies of certain disease processes vary according to race. The manner of disease presentation may differ from race to race, so methods of disease surveillance may need to be adjusted. The response of a disease to a particular treatment may vary from one race to another, so the physician may have to vary the approach to treatment. For all of these reasons, it is important to distinguish race in our patients, particularly for the diagnosis and management of glaucoma.

Historically, anthropologists have agreed on the existence of three relatively distinct groups of people differentiated mainly by physical traits, such as skin color, hair type, body morphology, and facial features. These three groups are Caucasoid or white, indigenous to Europe, northern Africa, western Asia, and India; Mongoloid, indigenous to eastern Asia; and Negroid or black, indigenous to western and southern Africa.[2]

Because disease frequencies vary not only by race but also by geographic location, the medical literature makes distinctions between groups of people on a geographic as well as racial basis. Persons of mixed racial origin present a challenge, in that they are not often easily assigned to a single racial category. The medical literature does not clearly address this dilemma. Epidemiologic literature addresses the issue but does not conclusively solve the problem. The difficulty of this problem is illustrated by the collection of data for the United States Census. Respondents to the Census often report their own race differently from how it is reported by official Census examiners, and methods of collecting racial data for the Census have changed over each of the past several decades.[3]

A wealth of information has been written about the various types of glaucoma as they pertain to different groups of people. Information is available on the prevalence, expression, course, and management of the glaucomas in each race and many geographic locales. Variations in presentation and course of the glaucomas occur from group to group, depending both on race and on the part of the world in which one looks. Because of the assimilation of people of different racial backgrounds over the years, it is extremely difficult to make distinctions on the basis of race alone. Therefore, one must make distinctions according to a combination of race and geographic location.

People of African Descent

TYPES OF GLAUCOMA

Open-Angle Glaucoma

Glaucoma is the leading cause of irreversible blindness in black Americans. Approximately 19% of all blindness in black Americans is due to glaucoma.[4] Primary open-angle glaucoma (POAG) occurs six times more frequently in black Americans than white Americans.[4] Compared with white Americans, black Americans with glaucoma are typically 10 years younger than whites on initial presentation,[4, 5] demonstrate disc and visual field damage earlier in the course of the disease, and experience a more rapid rate of disease progression.[5] Information in the literature about whether persons of African descent have higher intraocular pressures (IOPs) than other races is conflicting. The Barbados Eye Study found that mean IOP was significantly higher in black participants (18.7 mm Hg) than in white participants (16.5 mm Hg).[6] The Baltimore Eye Survey, on the other hand, found a significantly lower mean IOP in black Americans (21.48 mm Hg) with untreated POAG than in white Americans (24.15 mm Hg) with untreated POAG.[7] Other studies have found either no difference[5, 8] or an insignificant difference in IOP.[9, 10] The conflicting information on IOP leads some to speculate that people of African descent must have a greater susceptibility to damage from increased IOP or some other risk factor accounting for the aggressive nature of the disease in this population.

The prevalence of POAG is 1.23% in black Americans aged 40 to 49 years and increases to 11.26% in those older than 80 years.[11] Studies of patients presenting for eye care at academic centers in major cities in the United States find that although the racial distribution of these patients is equitable, 73% to 82% of patients with open-angle glaucoma are black.[9, 11, 12]

Age-adjusted prevalence of POAG is four to five times higher in black Americans than in white Americans.[11] The average age of these patients is 64 to 68 years, respectively. Only 27% to 56% of patients with ocular hypertension, however, are black.[8, 9] This finding may mean that most black Americans with increased IOP have glaucoma and not simply ocular hypertension. If this is the case, two things may be true: First, a finding of elevated IOP in a black American is a poor prognostic sign that forebodes glaucoma. Tolerance for simply observing such a patient should be minimal, and the threshold for initiating treatment for glaucoma should be low. Second, if a higher percentage of black American patients with elevated IOP have glaucoma than white Americans with elevated IOP, then black Americans may be more susceptible to glaucomatous optic nerve damage than white Americans. It has not been shown consistently that black Americans have higher IOP than whites.

Caribbean persons of African descent have an even higher prevalence of open-angle glaucoma than black Americans. In Barbados, for example, the prevalence of open-angle glaucoma is 6.7% in people older than 35 years. This number increases to 15% in the eighth decade and to 23% in the ninth decade.[6] Other studies of Caribbean populations reveal similar results.[13] The reasons for this higher prevalence of glaucoma in black West Indians are unknown.

Normal-Tension Glaucoma

Normal-tension glaucoma (NTG) is an entity that probably exists in individuals of African descent, although references to it in the medical literature are scarce. When caring for patients of African descent who are from the West Indies, one must remember that toxic optic neuropathy is in the differential diagnosis and may manifest as cupping of the optic nerve. The ingestion of "bush tea" in particular may cause a toxic optic neuropathy. In Curaçao, bush tea is made by boiling the leaves of the *Croton flavens* plant; an abstract from the seed of *Bixa orellana* is suspended in oil and is used in Jamaican folk medicine to treat diabetes mellitus. These types of "bush tea" have been implicated as causes of cirrhosis and esophageal cancer in the West Indies.[14–16] These toxins may also cause optic neuropathy. It is important, therefore, to specifically question patients from the West Indies about the past use of "bush tea" or other folk remedies for various ailments.

Angle-Closure Glaucoma

Angle-closure glaucoma is not as common as open-angle glaucoma in people of African descent. The literature on this subject, however, is relatively sparse.

In South Africa, the prevalence of angle-closure glaucoma is 0.002%.[17] Angle-closure glaucoma in black patients is usually chronic and may constitute as little as 13% of all cases of primary glaucoma in black Africans.[17, 18] Affected patients do not typically present with symptoms of acute angle-closure, such as pain, redness, and seeing colored halos around lights. Their disease is insidious and progresses quietly. It requires careful surveillance for prevention of irreversible loss of vision.

Because angle-closure glaucoma is so likely to exist without outward signs in people of African descent, routine gonioscopy is an essential component of the yearly eye examination in such patients. Routine gonioscopy is especially important in patients with hyperopia. In fact, the axiom that gonioscopy must be performed to rule out the possibility of chronic angle closure before a diagnosis of open-angle glaucoma is made is particularly true for patients of African descent.

Secondary Glaucomas

Secondary open-angle glaucoma does occur in black Americans, although reports in the literature are much less common than those of POAG.

One of the causes of secondary glaucoma in black Americans is the pigment dispersion syndrome (PDS). One relatively small screening of 83 black Americans found a

1.2% prevalence of PDS.[19] The manifestations of this syndrome in black patients may differ slightly from the classic description. The PDS in black Americans consists of heavy pigment deposition on the corneal endothelium and trabecular meshwork, along with increased IOP. Iris transillumination defects are rarely seen.[19] Black American patients with the PDS are often older than white patients with the syndrome, averaging 73 years. They are also less myopic than white patients with the syndrome, with an average refractive error of +2.15 diopters in one reported series of 20 black Americans with the syndrome.[20]

Fuchs' heterochromic iridocyclitis is another cause of secondary open-angle glaucoma in black Americans. Heterochromia, however, may be more difficult to distinguish in this group of patients because of their darker ocular pigmentation. Black Americans may be more prone than white patients to have secondary glaucoma in Fuchs' heterochromic iridocyclitis. In fact, up to 38% of black patients with this disease may have secondary glaucoma,[21] compared with approximately 11% of whites.

Pseudoexfoliation syndrome is another important cause of secondary open-angle glaucoma in black Africans. The prevalence of pseudoexfoliation syndrome in the black general ophthalmology population ranges from 0.16% of patients older than 20 years to 5% of patients older than 40 years.[22, 23] The prevalence of this syndrome in patients scheduled for cataract extraction is as high as 26%[23]; this finding is probably due to the higher average age of patients scheduled for cataract extraction. Pseudoexfoliation syndrome is present in 19% of patients with open-angle glaucoma[22].

There is one important difference between the characteristics of pseudoexfoliation syndrome in black patients and white patients. Black patients rarely demonstrate deposition of pseudoexfoliation material on the central lens capsule. Therefore, in order to make the diagnosis of pseudoexfoliation syndrome in a black patient, one must dilate the pupils in order to examine the anterior lens capsule for peripheral deposits of pseudoexfoliation material.

Pseudoexfoliation syndrome is also a cause of secondary glaucoma in black Americans, although it may occur less frequently in this population than in white Americans.[24] The syndrome occurs in approximately 0.4% of the black American population older than 50 years and in 2.7% of the white American population older than 50 years.

RISK FACTORS

Why is the prevalence of glaucoma so much higher in black patients than in white patients? It has not been shown consistently that the average IOP is higher in black people. Is the optic nerve of people of African descent more susceptible to glaucomatous damage? This question has led investigators to search for characteristics of the optic nerve that differ in these two groups of patients.

The average cup-to-disc ratio in the eyes of black subjects with no known optic nerve disease was found to be 0.35 by stereo disc photography[25] and 0.6 by scanning laser ophthalmoscopy.[26] The average cup-to-disc ratio in white patients was found to be 0.24 by stereo disc photography[25] and 0.4 by scanning laser ophthalmoscopy.[26] Although disc size and cup-to-disc ratio are larger in black American people, the actual neuroretinal rim area has been found to be the same in blacks and whites.[26] Despite these differences, it has not been proven that larger disc size or cup-to-disc ratio increases susceptibility to glaucomatous optic nerve damage.

Family history is thought to be an important factor in the assessment of glaucoma risk. The Baltimore Eye Survey found that black Americans who had a sibling with glaucoma had a four-fold greater risk of having glaucoma. For black Americans who had a parent with glaucoma, the risk of having glaucoma doubled.[27] White Americans, on the other hand, had only a two-fold higher risk of having glaucoma if they had a sibling with the disease and were not more likely to have glaucoma if one of their parents had the disease.

TREATMENT

The treatment of increased IOP in black Americans can be challenging. The darkly pigmented irides of black Americans may make their eyes resistant to treatment with topical medications. It has been shown, for example, that a higher concentration of timolol is required to control IOP in this group of patients.[28] Such patients may also need higher concentrations of pilocarpine to achieve the desired therapeutic effect.

Initial response to laser trabeculoplasty in black Americans is similar to that in white Americans. In one study, 85% of patients maintained a 15% reduction of IOP at 1 year, and 71% of patients had a persistent 15% decrease in IOP at 2 years.[29] However, another study of 38 eyes observed for more than 5 years after laser trabeculoplasty found that the median time to a post-treatment increase in IOP to more than 21 mm Hg was 12 months in blacks, compared with 60 months in whites.[30] The 5-year success rate, that is, the rate for maintaining IOP at less than 21 mm Hg, was 65% in white Americans but only 38% in black Americans.

The effect of filtering surgery is highly variable. Although the early response may be good, the long-term outcome of standard filtering surgery is almost uniformly dismal in patients of African descent. This outcome is due to proliferation of episcleral fibrous tissue.[31] The fibrous tissue proliferation is particularly problematic when standard surgical techniques and postoperative treatment regimens are used. Modification of surgical technique and postoperative treatment in patients of African descent may yield better results. Reports of successful reduction in IOP range from 78% to 92%[32, 33] to only 32% to 39%[34, 35] of eyes in which pressure was less than 22 mm Hg with or without medications in the first year following surgery. Success of partial-thickness filtering procedures continues to diminish over time. The 2-year success rate is less than 60% with or without medications.[36]

The IOP results for full-thickness filtering surgery are dramatically better than those for partial-thickness procedures. Full-thickness procedures provide an immediate, profound reduction in IOP. This pressure reduction is sustained in long-term follow-up and usually stabilizes in the range of 10 mm Hg.[37, 38] The sustained reduction of pressure is accompanied by greater risk of morbidity, however. The rate of complications following full-thickness procedures, including cataract formation, hypotony, serous choroidal detachment, and, possibly, retinal detachment, is higher than the rate of complications following trabeculectomy.

The use of adjunctive antifibrotic agents with partial-thickness filtering procedures markedly improves the success of filtering surgery in patients of African descent. Intraoperative application of 5-fluorouracil significantly improves IOP reduction compared with standard filtering surgery.[34] Intraoperative application of mitomycin has also been shown to provide a significantly lower IOP than standard trabeculectomy.[35, 39]

Adjunctive mitomycin C produces a lower mean IOP than adjunctive 5-fluorouracil in patients of African descent.[40] The IOP achieved after trabeculectomy with mitomycin C is almost as low as that after full-thickness filtering procedures, without many of the complications of the latter procedure. Adjunctive mitomycin C has also been shown to achieve a marked, sustained reduction in IOP at a mean of 20 months following trabeculectomy.[40]

One of the complications of adjunctive mitomycin C use is hypotony with associated maculopathy. This condition is often difficult, if not impossible, to treat effectively. Although hypotony does occur in patients of African descent, the incidence of hypotony maculopathy following trabeculectomy with mitomycin C in black Americans is approximately half that in white patients.[41, 42]

Because black Americans are less likely to experience a successful long-term reduction in IOP following standard trabeculectomy, the procedure of choice in these patients may be either full-thickness filtration or trabeculectomy with an adjunctive antifibrotic agent. This is especially true in patients with certain risk factors, such as young age, dark skin pigmentation, Caribbean ancestry, and keloid formation. The risk of complications from mitomycin C therapy is relatively low compared with that from full-thickness filtration, so trabeculectomy with mitomycin C may be the procedure of choice in patients with glaucoma that is not controlled by medicines or laser treatment. However, the use of mitomycin C results in increased complications than filtration surgery without the use of antifibrotics. Further study of the long-term outcome of trabeculectomy with mitomycin C, particularly with regard to preservation of visual function and quality of life, is needed.

Implantation of an aqueous drainage shunt may be necessary if the IOP fails to respond to trabeculectomy with mitomycin C. The use of aqueous drainage shunts in black Americans with refractory glaucoma yields results comparable to those in other races. Successful control of IOP (less than 21 mm Hg) with or without additional medications is achieved in 73% of patients with POAG, 83% of those with aphakic glaucoma, 80% of those with uveitic glaucoma, and 67% of those with neovascular glaucoma at an average of 2.5 years of follow-up.[43]

People of European Descent

TYPES OF GLAUCOMA

Open-Angle Glaucoma

Glaucoma is one of the second leading causes of irreversible blindness in whites, sharing the distinction with diabetic retinopathy.[4] Estimates of the prevalence of POAG in white Americans between the ages of 40 and 80 years range from 0.92% to 3.3%.[11, 44, 45] The prevalence of glaucoma increases to 2.16% to 7.2% in those older than 80 years.[11, 45]

Studies of patients presenting for eye care in urban academic centers in which the racial distribution was equal have shown that 7% to 18% of patients with open-angle glaucoma are white, and the average age of these patients is 69 to 72 years.[9, 11, 12] Of patients with ocular hypertension, 44% to 63% are white.[8, 9]

The estimated prevalence of glaucoma in whites outside the United States is similar to that within the United States. The overall prevalence of POAG in England is 0.71% in persons older than 40 years.[46] In Ireland and the Netherlands, the prevalence of POAG is 0.2% to 0.72% in middle-aged patients and increases to 3% in persons older than 80 years.[47, 48]

Normal-Tension Glaucoma

Although NTG has been described for years, it is only recently becoming recognized as a significant cause of glaucomatous optic neuropathy. As screening and diagnostic methods for glaucoma become more sensitive, more cases of NTG emerge. An essential part of routine screening for glaucoma and diagnosis of glaucoma in the past included an IOP greater than 21 mm Hg. As more visual field testing is performed in patients who have normal IOP but in whom glaucoma is suspected, more cases of NTG are diagnosed.

Population studies in which visual field testing is performed only on eyes with pressure above the normal range tend to underestimate the prevalence of NTG. In England, for example, the Bedford Glaucoma Survey estimated the prevalence of NTG to be 0.05% in persons older than 40 years.[46] Only 7% of all patients with open-angle glaucoma were found to have normal IOP.

Population studies in which visual field testing is performed on all patients regardless of IOP find the prevalence of NTG to be much higher. In Ireland, for example, 37% of cases of open-angle glaucoma are NTG, with a prevalence of 0.69%.[47] A similar prevalence of NTG is found in the Netherlands.[48] The Ferndale, Framingham, and Dalby studies found the proportion of cases of NTG to all cases of open-angle glaucoma to be 20%, 53%, and 62%, respectively.[49] The corresponding prevalence estimates of NTG in each study are 0.09%, 0.6%, and 0.5%, respectively. The Baltimore Eye Survey found that 16.7% of cases of open-angle glaucoma are NTG, with an estimated prevalence of 0.4%.[4]

Angle-Closure Glaucoma

Angle-closure glaucoma is much less common in whites than open-angle glaucoma. The prevalence of angle-closure glaucoma is 0.002% to 0.009%.[17, 47] The angle closure is acute in approximately two thirds of cases. Therefore, whites with this disease are more likely than persons of African descent to have symptoms of redness, pain, or blurred vision.

Secondary Glaucoma

Two of the most common causes of secondary glaucoma in whites are PDS and the pseudoexfoliation syndrome. The PDS seen in whites typically occurs in young, myopic males and consists of iris transillumination defects and pigment deposition on the corneal endothelium, trabecular meshwork, and other anterior segment structures. The prevalence of PDS in whites is 2.45%.[19]

The pseudoexfoliation syndrome usually occurs in older patients, and the prevalence increases with age. This syndrome in whites consists of iris transillumination defects at the pupil, deposition of characteristic pseudoexfoliation material on the iris and lens, and pigment deposition on the trabecular meshwork. Deposits on the lens often appear in a double-ring or "target" pattern because of iris-lens contact in the midperipheral region of the lens. This contact is thought to scrape the pseudoexfoliation material from the lens in this area. This material has also been demonstrated histologically in other ocular structures and in other organs.

There is a large geographic variation in the prevalence of the pseudoexfoliation syndrome in whites. Prevalence estimates vary from 0.09% to 18%.[22, 23, 47] In Great Britain, for example, pseudoexfoliation glaucoma accounts for approximately 5% of cases of open-angle glaucoma in whites and has a prevalence of 0.4%.[22, 47] White South Africans, however, have only a 0.09% prevalence of the syndrome.[23]

Scandinavia has a markedly higher prevalence of pseudoexfoliation syndrome than any other region of the world. The prevalence in Norway and Finland, for example, is approximately 18%. Eleven percent to 30% of Scandinavians with the syndrome have pseudoexfoliation glaucoma.[50, 51] Pseudoexfoliation glaucoma accounts for up to 75% of cases of open-angle glaucoma in Sweden.[52]

RISK FACTORS

Three factors have consistently been shown to be associated with increased risk of open angle glaucoma: increased IOP, increased cup-to-disc ratio, and family history of glaucoma. Whites have a two times higher risk for POAG if they have a sibling with glaucoma.[27] The average cup-to-disc ratio in healthy whites aged 27 to 37 years was found to be 0.24 by stereo disc photography[25] and 0.4 with a disc area of 1.73 mm^2 by scanning laser ophthalmoscopy.[26]

TREATMENT

Medical treatment of open-angle glaucoma in white patients is usually successful in lowering IOP, at least in the earlier stages of the disease. These cases usually respond well to beta-blockers, adrenergic agonists, carbonic anhydrase inhibitors, prostaglandin analogues, and miotics. Most of these classes of glaucoma medication have been advocated as first-line therapy, and various combinations of these agents have been proven effective in lowering IOP. In some cases, higher concentrations of medications may be required to achieve a significant pressure-lowering effect in eyes with darker pigmentation.[28]

The open-angle glaucomas in whites respond well to laser trabeculoplasty. Two types of glaucoma that respond particularly well are the secondary open-angle glaucomas of PDS and pseudoexfoliation syndrome. Initially, approximately 83% of cases respond with at least a 15% reduction in IOP.[28]

Long-term follow-up in the Glaucoma Laser Trial indicates that the initial response to laser trabeculoplasty decreases dramatically after 2 years. Two years postoperatively, control of IOP is maintained with laser therapy alone in only 44% of eyes.[53] The addition of up to two medications, however, raises this rate to 89%. Approximately 65% of eyes in white patients demonstrate a successful response to laser trabeculoplasty for at least 5 years.[30]

The eyes of white patients also respond well to filtering surgery. In uncomplicated POAG, the initial success rate of standard trabeculectomy is approximately 80%.[54] In eyes that are at risk for failure of filtering surgery, such as eyes with prior surgery, inflammation, or neovascularization, trabeculectomy with adjunctive antifibrotic agents, such as 5-fluorouracil or mitomycin C, often achieves a successful outcome. In these high-risk eyes, the short-term success rate for achieving pressure less than 21 mm Hg without medications is approximately 88% for trabeculectomy with adjunctive mitomycin C and 47% for trabeculectomy with 5-fluorouracil,[55] at an average of 10 months postoperatively. The 5-year follow-up results of the Fluorouracil Filtering Study indicate that the success rate for filtering surgery with adjunctive 5-fluorouracil is relatively stable over the long term at about 50%.[56] Long-term follow-up data for surgery with adjunctive mitomycin C indicate that the high success rate for this procedure is also stable over time. More than 80% of eyes so treated may have an IOP of 12 mm Hg or less with or without medications at an average of 32 months postoperatively.[57]

Native American Indians

No large population studies of glaucoma in Native American Indians have been published. However, smaller studies conducted in several tribes give a reasonable idea of the prevalence of the various types of glaucoma and, perhaps more importantly, the implications of glaucoma as a public health problem.

It is evident from these few studies that broad generalizations concerning glaucoma prevalence in all Native American Indian tribes are inaccurate. The risk of glaucoma seems to vary from one tribe to another. The Zuni tribe, for example, seems to have an extremely low prevalence of glaucoma of any type. In a small screening of 119 members of this tribe 40 years or older, no cases of glaucoma were found.[58] The prevalence of ocular hypertension in this small sample was 6.7%. This low glaucoma prevalence may be related to the fact that there was no age-related increase in IOP, even among the subjects older than 70 years. This finding is in distinct contrast to the increase in IOP with age found in people of European or African descent. The lack of an age-related increase in IOP, however, does not explain the fact that NTG is also not described in the Zuni population.

The prevalence of POAG in other Native American Indians, mostly members of the Navajo tribe, was found in one study to be 1.5%.[59] This estimate may be slightly high, because the subjects were patients drawn from a general ophthalmology clinic. Glaucoma may be the third leading cause of irreversible loss of vision in the Navajo tribe.

Pseudoexfoliation syndrome is a cause of secondary open-angle glaucoma in the Navajo tribe. In the study mentioned previously, the prevalence of pseudoexfoliation glaucoma was 0.45%. Another smaller study of 50 Navajo patients attending the general ophthalmology clinic found that 38% of patients had pseudoexfoliation syndrome and 6% had pseudoexfoliation glaucoma.[60]

Latin Americans

Latin Americans constitute a significant portion of the world population and thus deserve mention here. The racial background of this group is diverse, being derived mainly from European, indigenous American, and African roots. Unfortunately, literature on the prevalence of glaucoma in Latin Americans is virtually nonexistent. Therefore, the reader is referred to the sections of this chapter that deal with glaucoma in persons of European, Native American Indian, and African descent.

People of Indian Descent

Random samples of Indians seeking care for ocular complaints indicate that glaucoma is the primary cause of irreversible blindness in India.[61] The prevalence of glaucoma in Indians older than 30 years may be as high as 2.9%.[62] This figure is an estimate because (1) most of the 40,000 persons screened in the study cited were patients in eye camps and hospitals and (2) perimetry could not be performed in two thirds of subjects in the sample.

Pseudoexfoliation syndrome is very common in India. A random survey of ophthalmology patients older than 45 years found the prevalence of this syndrome to be 7.4%.[63] There is a marked increase in the prevalence of pseudoexfoliation syndrome with age, from 4.7% in the sixth decade to 13.4% in the eighth decade. The syndrome is more common in Indian males than females. Secondary glaucoma occurs in 9% of patients with pseudoexfoliation syndrome.

For patients whose glaucoma is inadequately controlled by medications or trabeculoplasty, filtering surgery becomes necessary. Indian patients may have a relatively high risk for failure of filtering surgery owing to their dark pigmentation. Therefore, the use of adjunctive antifibrotic agents during filtering surgery may be desirable.

The use of adjunctive mitomycin C has been studied in Indians with uncontrolled glaucoma. This agent has been found, at least in the short term, to be highly effective in assuring successful lowering of IOP in more than 90% of eyes.[64] Additional studies are needed to determine the long-term outcome of this surgical technique.

People of Middle Eastern Descent

Population-based surveys of blindness in Saudi Arabia estimate that glaucoma ranks from fourth to sixth as a leading cause of blindness in Arabs. Glaucoma accounts for 3.5% to 5.3% of all blindness in that country.[65, 66] Cataract, trachoma, and complications of ocular surgery are among the leading causes of blindness in Saudi Arabia.

In a study of bilateral blindness in Arabs living on the West Bank and in the Gaza Strip in Israel, glaucoma was found to be only the ninth most common cause of blindness.[67] More common causes of blindness are cataract, trachoma, and corneal scars.

People of Asian Descent

Early population studies show that glaucoma is second only to nonglaucomatous optic atrophy as a cause of blindness in China.[68] Because early glaucoma screening methods included an IOP above the "normal" range, cases of NTG would not be identified in those screenings. It is likely that some "nonglaucomatous" optic atrophy is actually due to NTG. Therefore, it is possible that glaucoma is actually a more common cause of blindness in China than currently reported.

TYPES OF GLAUCOMA

Open-Angle Glaucoma

The prevalence of open-angle glaucoma is quite variable in the Asian population. In Japan, for example, open-angle glaucoma is almost twice as common as angle-closure glaucoma. The prevalence of POAG in Japanese people older than 40 years is 0.58%.[69] This figure is slightly lower than that for whites. In Malaysians, open-angle glaucoma is three times as common as angle-closure glaucoma.[70]

Open-angle glaucoma in China, however, is much less common than angle-closure glaucoma. Open-angle glaucoma accounts for only 15% to 21% of all glaucoma in Chinese people.[68, 70] Estimates of the prevalence of POAG in China range from 0.07 to 0.11%.[71, 72]

Normal-Tension Glaucoma

NTG is the most common type of glaucoma in Japan. It is almost four times more common than high-pressure glaucoma and six times more common than angle-closure glaucoma. The prevalence of NTG is 2.04% in Japanese people older than 40 years and approximately 4% in those older than 70 years.[69]

Angle-Closure Glaucoma

Angle-closure glaucoma is the most common type of glaucoma in China. It is four times more common than open-angle glaucoma in Chinese people. The prevalence of this disorder in those older than 40 years is 1.17%.[73]

The prevalence of angle-closure glaucoma in Japan is 0.34% of people older than 40 years.[69, 74] The risk of angle closure increases with age, especially in Japanese women. The frequency of occludable angles increases from 0.48% in women aged 30 to 49 years to 3.44% in women older than 70 years. The frequency in men is 0.2% for those between 30 and 49 years of age and 1.03% for those older than 70 years.

Occludable angles are frequently found in the Vietnamese population. The overall frequency of occludable angles is 8.5%. This risk factor for angle-closure glaucoma increases from 16.5% in Vietnamese people younger than 40 years of age to 58% in those older than 70 years.[75]

Secondary Glaucomas

The prevalence of pseudoexfoliation syndrome in Japan is similar to that in non-Scandinavian whites. Pseudoexfoliation syndrome is found in approximately 1% of Japanese older than 40 years. Pseudoexfoliation glaucoma exists in 0.22% of Japanese older than 40 years.[69] Both conditions are more common in Japanese men than Japanese women. Pseudoexfoliation syndrome is extremely uncommon in China.

TREATMENT

Cases of open-angle glaucoma in Asians have been shown to respond to laser trabeculoplasty in a fashion similar to those in other races. Initially, 77% of cases are controlled with an IOP less than 20 mm Hg at an average of 11 months following trabeculoplasty.[76]

The response to standard filtering surgery in Asian patients is mediocre. The success rate of standard trabeculectomy for POAG and closed-angle glaucoma in China has been reported to be 49%.[77] Similar rates of success are reported for POAG in Japan.[78, 79] The rate of successful outcome in eyes with glaucoma that are refractory to treatment, such as aphakic, uveitic, or neovascular glaucoma, is even lower.

The use of antifibrotic agents dramatically improves the outcome of trabeculectomy in patients with primary and refractory glaucomas. For example, the use of postoperative subconjunctival 5-fluorouracil injections improves the 5-year success rate to approximately 93% for Japanese eyes with POAG and to 58% for eyes with refractory glaucoma.[78, 79]

Eskimos

Reports of glaucoma in Eskimos apply to Eskimos living in Canada, Greenland, and Alaska. The prevalence and characteristics of each type of glaucoma are similar for Eskimos living in all three of these areas.

TYPES OF GLAUCOMA

Open-Angle Glaucoma

Open-angle glaucoma is extremely unusual in Eskimos. The prevalence of open-angle glaucoma in Alaskan Eskimos is 0.01% to 0.06% in people older than 40 years.[80, 81]

Angle-Closure Glaucoma

Eskimos have a high prevalence of angle-closure glaucoma. This disease becomes more common with increasing age, and female Eskimos have at least twice the risk for angle closure compared with males.

The prevalence of angle-closure glaucoma in all Eskimos is 0.3% to 0.44%.[81–85] In Eskimos older than 40 years, the prevalence is 0.9% to 2.4% in males and 2.1% to 5.5% in females.[80, 83–85] For those older than 60 years, the prevalence of angle-closure glaucoma is 5.6% to 7% in males and 11.4% to 13.5% in females.[83, 85, 86] Eighty percent of cases of angle-closure glaucoma in Eskimos are acute.

The frequency of occludable angles in Eskimos older than 40 years is 2.3% for males and 3.4% for females. In those older than 70 years, the frequency of occludable angles increases to 13.6% for males and to 34.2% for females.[80]

Secondary Glaucoma

Pigment dispersion syndrome and pseudoexfoliation syndrome are not described in Eskimos.[51] Secondary angle-closure glaucoma, however, is usually reported as a consequence of uveitis.[81]

RISK FACTORS

Eskimos have the highest risk of angle-closure glaucoma in the world, possibly because on average, Eskimos have a slightly smaller anterior segment relative to the rest of the eye. Studies measuring the anterior chamber depth in Eskimos show that the average anterior chamber depth in those older than 60 years is 2.25 mm to 2.5 mm, whereas the average depth in whites older than 60 years is 2.7 mm.[84, 85, 87] The average corneal diameter in Eskimos is 11.1 mm in males and 10.98 mm in females, compared with 11.5 mm in whites.[84] The smaller anterior chamber depth and the smaller corneal diameter in Eskimos both contribute to a smaller anterior chamber volume, a feature thought to predispose an eye to risk of angle closure.

Australian Aborigines

Glaucoma is extremely uncommon in Australian Aborigines. The overall prevalence of glaucoma in this population has been reported to be less than 1%.[88, 89]

Pseudoexfoliation syndrome has been reported to occur in 1.3% of all Aborigines, and in 16.3% of those older than 60 years.[89] Secondary glaucoma has been found in 8% of those who had pseudoexfoliation syndrome. Therefore, the prevalence of this syndrome in Australian Aborigines approaches that in Scandinavian whites, although pseudoexfoliation glaucoma may not be as prevalent.

People of the South Pacific

No extensive population-based surveys of glaucoma have been conducted in the islands of the South Pacific, but there are several samples of groups on the various islands. In Samoa, for example, the prevalence of glaucoma is similar to that found in Asian populations. Estimates of glaucoma prevalence in Samoa range from 0.35% to 0.81%.[90] Estimates of the prevalence of the various types of glaucoma are not available, but most cases are probably acute angle-closure glaucoma.[91]

A preliminary study of the Maori people living on the North Island of New Zealand revealed no cases of glaucoma among the 333 persons aged 0 to 80 years who were examined.[92] The average IOP among the Maoris is 11 mm Hg. The ancestors of the Maori people are Mongoloid, and their roots are traced to Asia prior to the Han dynasty. Their Asian ancestry may make the Maoris more susceptible to normal tension or chronic angle-closure glaucoma than to POAG.

Using Racial Characteristics in Diagnosis and Treatment

It is evident that there is wide variation in the prevalence of the different glaucomas from race to race as well as within each race according to geographic location. Not only does the prevalence but also the expression, course, and management of the glaucomas vary according to race and location. These variations make the diagnosis and treatment of glaucoma somewhat difficult. Knowledge of these differences helps the physician deliver effective care to patients. Awareness of risk factors for the various types of glaucoma helps the physician identify and initiate appropriate treatment for affected individuals (Table 7–1).

PATIENTS OF AFRICAN DESCENT

In the care of persons of African descent, one must realize that glaucoma is the leading cause of irreversible blindness in this group. Individuals from the West Indies are at particularly high risk of glaucoma blindness.

The glaucoma that most commonly affects people of African descent is POAG. They present at a much younger age than people of other racial origins,[93] and their disease has a particularly aggressive course. Figure 7–1 illustrates the early onset of disease in persons of African descent compared with other races. Acute angle-closure glaucoma occurs rarely in persons of African descent. Chronic angle-closure glaucoma, although uncommon, manifests insidiously; therefore, gonioscopy is an indispensable part of the routine examination of patients of African descent.

PDS and pseudoexfoliation syndrome cause secondary open-angle glaucoma in people of African descent, but the presentations are different from those in whites. Persons of African descent rarely have iris transillumination defects in PDS, so the other manifestations of this entity are more important for diagnosis. These patients are also older and less myopic than the typical young, myopic white patient with PDS.

It is sometimes difficult to diagnose pseudoexfoliation syndrome in persons of African descent because deposition of pseudoexfoliation material usually does not occur on the central lens capsule. Therefore, such patients must undergo dilation for the diagnosis to be made.

Black patients with Fuchs' heterochromic iridocyclitis are at particularly high risk for secondary glaucoma, but the diagnosis of Fuchs' heterochromia is difficult to make in such patients because of the dark iris pigmentation.

The treatment of glaucoma in persons of African descent is challenging. Their glaucoma does not respond as well to medical treatment, and the response to surgical treatment is often short-lived. Laser trabeculoplasty is a good short-term solution in most black patients with open-angle glaucoma but provides long-term control in only a small minority. The outcome of standard trabeculectomy surgery is dismal because of a vigorous scarring tendency seen in the eyes of such patients. The use of adjunctive mitomycin C dramatically improves the outcome of trabeculectomy, making it a reasonable option for patients of African descent. Treatment of these patients must be prompt and aggressive in order to maintain visual function and quality of life.

WHITE PATIENTS

Although glaucoma is not as serious a problem among whites as among people of African descent, it is still an

TABLE 7–1. POPULATION GROUPS AT HIGH RISK FOR GLAUCOMA

	Type of Glaucoma			
Group	*Primary Open-Angle*	*Primary Angle Closure*	*Normal-Tension*	*Pseudoexfoliation*
African descent	Young age Treatment difficult	Low prevalence, but occurs insidiously Routine gonioscopy		
European descent	Elderly			Scandinavian Check for peripupillary iris transillumination and dilate to check lens surface for pseudoexfoliation material
Asian descent		Chronic in Chinese Acute in Vietnamese Routine gonioscopy	Japanese Careful examination of optic nerve Low threshold for VF testing	
Eskimo descent		Acute Routine gonioscopy beginning at young age		

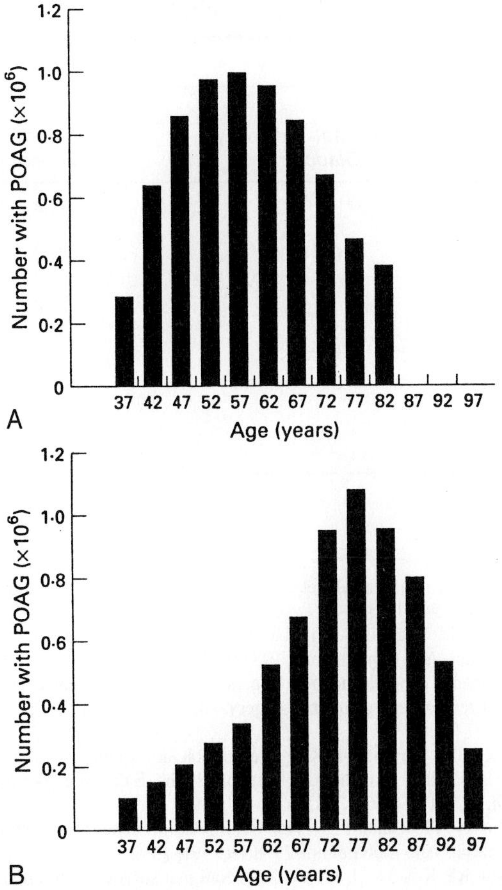

Figure 7–1. Comparison of primary open-angle glaucoma (POAG) distribution among African-derived *(A)* and European-derived *(B)* groups of people. All those older than 80 years in the African data are grouped in one age stratum, whereas for the European data, the proportion of those older than 80 years justified four additional 5-year groupings. (From Quigley HA: Number of people with glaucoma worldwide. Br J Ophthalmol 1996;80:389–393.)

important public health issue. Glaucoma is the second leading cause of irreversible blindness in whites, along with diabetic retinopathy. The most common type of glaucoma among persons of European descent is open-angle glaucoma. As screening techniques become less dependent on IOP measurement alone, evaluation of the optic disc and visual field are uncovering a greater number of cases of glaucomatous optic neuropathy with IOP values in the normal range, otherwise known as NTG. It is estimated that NTG may account for as many as one third to one half of all cases of open-angle glaucoma in white patients.

There is a marked geographic variation in the prevalence of pseudoexfoliation syndrome among whites. Scandinavians have a much higher prevalence than other whites, and pseudoexfoliation glaucoma is the most common type of glaucoma in that part of the world. Because Scandinavian whites have a high risk of secondary open-angle glaucoma from the pseudoexfoliation syndrome, routine examination of patients of this descent should include careful inspection of the anterior segment for pseudoexfoliation material and peripupillary iris transillumination defects. It is also important to dilate the pupil to look for pseudoexfoliation material on the anterior lens surface. Treatment of these patients with laser trabeculoplasty may be particularly successful.

Elderly white persons represent a high-risk group for glaucoma because of the increasing prevalence of POAG with age. Fortunately, the response to treatment in whites is relatively good. Prevention of visual disability in this group requires a high degree of suspicion and vigilance for the characteristic glaucomatous changes in the optic nerve and visual field.

NATIVE AMERICAN INDIAN PATIENTS

Most Native American Indians have a very low risk for glaucoma. One exception is the Navajo tribe, for whom the frequency of the pseudoexfoliation syndrome approaches that for Scandinavians. Pseudoexfoliation glaucoma, however, does not develop in as high a percentage of Navajo patients as in Scandinavian patients.

INDIAN PATIENTS

Glaucoma is the primary cause of irreversible blindness in India. Indians also have a high prevalence of pseudoexfoliation syndrome, almost as high as that found in Scandinavia. Secondary glaucoma from the syndrome, however, is less common in Indians than in Scandinavians.

ASIAN PATIENTS

Glaucoma is an important cause of blindness in persons of Asian descent. Angle-closure glaucoma is the most common type in Chinese and Vietnamese people, whereas open-angle glaucoma is the most common type in Japanese and Malaysian people. Pseudoexfoliation glaucoma occurs in people of Japanese descent with approximately the same frequency as in non-Scandinavian whites.

NTG has a particularly high prevalence in Japan. Japanese people may, in fact, have the highest risk for NTG in the world. Measurement of IOP alone is not sufficient to screen for NTG. Examination of Japanese patients must include (1) careful inspection of the optic nerve for characteristic glaucomatous changes and (2) visual field testing in patients with questionable disc changes. Prevention of progressive loss of vision is very difficult in patients with NTG, because it requires lowering of IOP to almost hypotonous levels. Achieving such a degree of pressure-lowering is difficult and may be accompanied by visual disability from hypotony maculopathy and other complications.

ESKIMO PATIENTS

The most common type of glaucoma in Eskimos is angle-closure glaucoma. Older Eskimos have an extremely high risk of angle closure as well as the highest rate of angle-closure glaucoma in the world. Onset of angle-closure glaucoma in the Eskimo is not difficult to detect because it usually manifests acutely as pain, redness, and blurred vision.

It is important, however, to detect patients at risk for acute angle closure before the onset of symptoms. Once symptoms appear, permanent loss of vision has already occurred. It is necessary, therefore, to perform routine goni-

TABLE 7–2. ESTIMATES OF GLAUCOMA PREVALENCE IN VARIOUS RACES

	Risk (%)			
Race or Descent	*Primary Open-Angle Glaucoma*	*Primary Angle-Closure Glaucoma*	*Normal-Tension Glaucoma*	*Pseudoexfoliation Glaucoma*
African descent	1.2–11.26*	0.002		0.04–0.5
West Indian	6.7–23*			
Caucasian	0.7–7.2*	0.002–0.009	0.09–0.69	0.009–5.4
Scandinavian				1.98–5.4
Indian				0.42–1.2
Asian				
Japanese	0.58	0.34	2.04–4	0.22
Chinese	0.07–0.11	1.17		
Eskimo	0.01–0.06	0.3–13.5*		
Australian Aborigine				0.1–1.3
Navajo Indian	1.5			

*Range indicates an increase in prevalence with age.

oscopy in all Eskimo patients. This part of the examination should be performed at as early an age as possible because, unlike open-angle glaucoma, acute angle closure is not necessarily a disease of the elderly.

SUMMARY

The physician who is aware of the prevalence and manifestations of the glaucomas in various racial and geographic groups may apply this knowledge during the examination of a particular patient at risk (Table 7–2). Doing so helps the physician maintain a suitable amount of suspicion for the diagnosis of glaucoma. Such knowledge also helps direct the management of glaucoma to the modality that is most effective for each patient.

Knowledge of the various high-risk groups affords one the opportunity to diagnose and treat affected patients early in the course of their disease (see Table 7–1). Proper vigilance in high-risk patients can prevent significant visual disability and preserve a satisfactory quality of life.

REFERENCES

1. The American Heritage Dictionary of the English Language, 3rd ed. New York, Houghton Mifflin, 1992.
2. The Concise Columbia Encyclopedia. New York, Columbia University Press, 1995.
3. McKenney NR, Bennet CE: Issues regarding data on race and ethnicity: The Census Bureau experience. Public Health Rep. 1994;109:16–25.
4. Sommer A, Tielsch JM, Katz J, et al: Racial differences in the cause-specific prevalence of blindness in East Baltimore. N Engl J Med 1991;325:1412–1417.
5. Wilson R, Richardson TM, Hertzmark E, et al: Race as a risk factor for progressive glauctomatous damage. Ann Ophthalmol 1985; 17:653–659.
6. Leske MC, Connell AMS, Schachat AP: The Barbados Eye Study: Prevalence of open angle glaucoma. Arch Ophthalmol 1994;112:821–829.
7. Sommer A, Tielsch JM, Katz J, et al: Relationship between intraocular pressure and primary open angle glaucoma among white and black Americans: The Baltimore Eye Survey. Arch Ophthalmol 1991;109:1090–1095.
8. Quigley HA, Enger C, Katz J, et al: Risk factors for the development of glaucomatous visual field loss in ocular hypertension. Arch Ophthalmol 1994;112:644–649.
9. Martin MJ, Sommer A, Gold E, et al: Race and primary open-angle glaucoma. Am J Ophthalmol 1985;99:383–387.
10. Coulehan JL, Helzlsouer KJ, Rogers KD: Racial differences in intraocular tension and glaucoma surgery. Am J Epidemiol 1980;111:759–768.
11. Tielsch JM, Sommer A, Katz J, et al: Racial variations in the prevalence of primary open-angle glaucoma: The Baltimore Eye Survey. JAMA 1991;266:369–374.
12. Wilensky JT, Gandhi N, Pan T: Racial influences in open-angle glaucoma. Ann Ophthalmol 1978;10:1398–1402.
13. Mason RP, Kosoko O, Wilson MR: National survey of the prevalence and risk factors of glaucoma in St. Lucia, West Indies. Part 1: Prevalence findings. Ophthalmology 1989;96:1363–1368.
14. Williams NA, Lee MG, Hanchard B: Hepatic cirrhosis in Jamaica. West Ind Med J 1997;46:60–62.
15. Hecken E: Cocarcinogens of the tumor-promoter type as potential risk factors of cancer in man: A first complete experimental analysis of an etiological model situation and some of its consequences. ARC Scientific Publications 1984;56:441–463.
16. Hecker E, Lutz D, Weber J: Multistage tumor development in the human esophagus: The first identification of cocarcinogens of the tumor-promoter type as principal carcinogenic risk factors in a local life style cancer. Prog Clin Biol Res 1983;132:219–238.
17. Salmon JF, Martell R: The role of ethnicity in primary angle-closure glaucoma. S Afr Med J 1994;84:623–626.
18. Luntz MH: Primary angle-closure glaucoma in urbanized South African caucasoid and negroid communities. Br J Ophthalmol 1973;57: 445–456.
19. Ritch R, Steinberger D, Leibman J: Prevalence of pigment dispersion syndrome in a population undergoing glaucoma screening. Am J Ophthalmol 1993;115:707–710.
20. Semple HC, Ball SF: Pigmentary glaucoma in the black population. Am J Ophthalmol 1990;109:518–522.
21. Tabbut BR, Tessler HH, Williams: Fuchs' heterochromic iridocyclitis in blacks. Arch Ophthalmol 1988;106:1688–1690.
22. Bartholomew RS: Incidence of pseudoexfoliation in South African Negroes and Scots. Trans Ophthalmol Soc U K 1979;99:299–301.
23. Luntz MH: Prevalence of pseudo-exfoliation syndrome in an urban South African clinic population. Am J Ophthalmol 1972;74:581–587.
24. Ball SF: Exfoliation syndrome prevalence in the glaucoma population of South Louisiana. Acta Ophthalmol 1988;66(Suppl):93–98.
25. Beck RW, Messner DK, Musch DC, et al: Is there a racial difference in physiologic cup size? Ophthalmology 1985;92:873–876.
26. Chi T, Ritch R, Stickler D, et al: Racial differences in optic nerve head parameters. Arch Ophthalmol 1989;107:836–839.
27. Tielsch JM, Katz J, Sommei A, et al: Family history and risk of primary open angle glaucoma. Arch Ophthalmol 1994;112:69–73.
28. Katz IM, Berger ET: Effects of iris pigmentation on response of ocular pressure to timolol. Surv Ophthalmol 1979;23:395–398.
29. Krupin T, Patkin R, Kurata FK, et al: Argon laser trabeculoplasty in

black and white patients with primary open-angle glaucoma. Ophthalmology 1986;93:811–816.
30. Schwarts AL, Love DC, Schwartz MA: Long-term follow-up of argon laser trabeculoplasty for uncontrolled open-angle glaucoma. Arch Ophthalmol 1985;103:1482–1484.
31. Welsh NH: Failure of filtration operations in the African. Br J Ophthalmol 1970;54:594–598.
32. Merrit JC: Filtering procedures in American blacks. Ophthalmic Surg 1980;11:91–93.
33. David R, Freedman J, Luntz M: Comparative study of Watson's and Cairns' trabeculectomies in a black population with open angle glaucoma. Br J Ophthalmol 1977;61:117–119.
34. Egbert PR, Williams AS, Singh K, et al: A prospective trial of intraoperative fluorouracil during trabeculectomy in a black population. Am J Ophthalmol 1993;116:612–616.
35. Mermoud A, Salmon JF, Murray ADN: Trabeculectomy with mitomycin C for refractory glaucoma in blacks. Am J Ophthalmol 1993;116:72–78.
36. Miller RD, Barber JC: Trabeculectomy in black patients. Ophthalmic Surg 1981;12:46–50.
37. Shingleton BJ, Distler JA, Baker BH: Filtration surgery in black patients: Early results in a West Indian population. Ophthalmic Surg 1987;81:195–199.
38. Wilson MR: Posterior lip sclerectomy vs trabeculectomy in West Indian blacks. Arch Ophthalmol 1989;107:1604–1608.
39. Kupin TH, Juzych MS, Shin DH, et al: Adjunctive mitomycin C in primary trabeculectomy in phakic eyes. Am J Ophthalmol 1995;119:30–39.
40. Singh K, Egbert PR, Byrd S, et al: Trabeculectomy with intraoperative 5-fluorouracil vs mitomycin C. Am J Ophthalmol 1997;123:48–53.
41. Smith MF, Doyle W, Nguyen QH: Results of intraoperative 5-fluorouracil or lower dose mitomycin-C administration on initial trabeculectomy surgery. J Glaucoma 1997;6:104–110.
42. Suner IJ, Greenfield DS, Miller MP, et al: Hypotony maculopathy after filtering surgery with mitomycin C: Incidence and treatment. Ophthalmology 1997;104:207–215.
43. Freedman J, Rubin B: Molteno implants as a treatment for refractory glaucoma in black patients. Arch Ophthalmol 1991;109:1417–1420.
44. Kahn HA, Leibowitz HM, Ganley JP, et al: The Framingham Eye Study. I: Outline and major prevalence findings. Am J Epidemiol 1977;106:17–32.
45. Klein BEK, Klein R, Sponsel WE, et al: Prevalence of glaucoma: The Beaver Dam Eye Study. Ophthalmology 1992;99:1499–1504.
46. Bankes JLK, Perkins ES, Tsolakis S, et al: Bedford Glaucoma Survey. Br Med J 1968;1:791–796.
47. Coffey M, Reidy A, Wormald R, et al: Prevalence of glaucoma in the west of Ireland. Br J Ophthalmol 1993;77:17–21.
48. Dielemans I, Vingerling JR, Wolfs RCW: The prevalence of primary open-angle glaucoma in a population-based study in the Netherlands. Ophthalmology 1994;101:1851–1855.
49. Leske MC: The epidemiology of open-angle glaucoma: A review. Am J Epidemiol 1983;118:166–187.
50. Ringvold A, Blika S, Elsas T: The Middle Norway eye-screening study. II: Prevalence of simple and capsular glaucoma. Acta Ophthalmol 1991;69:273–280.
51. Forsius H, Luukka H: Pseudoexfoliation of the anterior capsule of the lens in Lapps and Eskimos. Can J Ophthalmol 1973;8:274–277.
52. Lindblom B, Thorburn W: Observed incidence of glaucoma in Halsingland, Sweden. Acta Ophthalmol 1984;62:217.
53. The Glaucoma Laser Trial Research Group: The Glaucoma Laser Trial (GLT). 2: Results of argon laser trabeculoplasty versus topical medicines. Ophthalmology 1990;97:1403–1413.
54. Broadway D, Grierson I, Hitchings R: Racial differences in the results of glaucoma filtration surgery: Are racial differences in the conjunctival cell profile important? Br J Ophthalmol 1994;78:466–475.
55. Kitizawa Y, Kawase K, Matsushita H, et al: Trabeculectomy with mitomycin: A comparative study with fluorouracil. Arch Ophthalmol 1991;109:1693–1698.
56. The Fluorouracil Filtering Study Group: Five-year follow-up of the Fluorouracil Filtering Surgery Study. Am J Ophthalmol 1996; 121:349–366.
57. Katz GJ, Higginbotham EJ, Lichter PR, et al: Mitomycin C versus 5-fluorouracil in high-risk glaucoma filtering surgery: Extended follow-up. Ophthalmology 1995;102:1263–1269.
58. Kass MA, Zimmerman TJ, Alton E, et al: Intraocular pressure and glaucoma in the Zuni Indians. Arch Ophthalmol 1978;96:2212–2213.
59. Bettman JW: Eye disease among American Indians of the Southwest. I: Overall Analysis. Arch Ophthalmol 1972;88:263–268.
60. Faulkner HW: Pseudo-exfoliation of the lens among the Navajo Indians. Am J Ophthalmol 1971;72:206–207.
61. Sindal DK, Bhat RB, Shaligram CJ: Incidence of blindness around Miraj. Ind J Ophthalmol 1979;27:16–19.
62. Leydhecker W: A Glaucoma survey in South India. Doc Ophthalmol 1984;57:357–359.
63. Lamba PA, Giridhar A: Pseudoexfoliation syndrome: Prevalence based on random survey hospital data. Ind J Ophthalmol 1984;32: 169–173.
64. Ramakrishnan R, Michon J, Robin AL, et al: Safety and efficacy of mitomycin C trabeculectomy in southern India: A short-term pilot study. Ophthalmology 1993;100:1619–1623.
65. Al Faran MF, Al-Rajhi AA, Al-Othmar OM: Prevalence and causes of visual impairment and blindness in the south western region of Saudi Arabia. Int Ophthalmol 1993;17:161–165.
66. Tabbara KF, Ross-Degnan D: Blindness in Saudi Arabia. JAMA 1986;255:3378–3384.
67. Thomson IM, Chumbley LC: Eye disease in the West Bank and Gaza Strip. Br J Ophthalmol 1984;68:598–602.
68. Loh RCK: The problem of glaucoma in Singapore. Singapore Med J 1968;9:76–78.
69. Shiose Y, Kitazawa Y, Tsukahara S: Epidemiology of glaucoma in Japan—a nationwide glaucoma survey. Jpn J Ophthalmol 1991; 35:133–155.
70. Lim ASM: The pattern of ocular disease in Singapore. Trans Aust Col Ophthalmol 1971;3:122–125.
71. Gao Z: An epidemiologic study of glaucoma in Tongcheng County, Anhui Province. Chin J Ophthalmol 1995;31:149–151.
72. Hu CN: An epidemiologic study of glaucoma in Shunyi County, Beijing. Chin J Opthalmol 1989;25:115–119.
73. Zhao JL: An epidemiological survey of primary angle-closure glaucoma in Tibet. Chin J Ophthalmol 1990;26:47–50.
74. Okabe I, Tomita G, Sugiyama K: An epidemiological study on the prevalence of the narrow chamber angle in Japanese. Acta Soc Ophthalmol Jap 1991;95:279–287.
75. Nguyen N, Mora JS, Gaffney MM: A high prevalence of occludable angles in a Vietnamese population. Ophthalmology 1996;103:1426–1431.
76. Singh M, Kaur B: Argon laser trabeculoplasty in Asian eyes. Int Ophthalmol 1987;10:161–165.
77. Tan C, Chew PTK, Lum WL: Trabeculectomy: Success rates in a Singapore hospital. Singapore Med J 1996;37:505–507.
78. Nakano Y, Ariae M, Shirato S: Effect of postoperative subconjunctival 5-fluorouracil injections on the surgical outcome of trabeculectomy in the Japanese. Graefes Arch Clin Exp Ophthalmol 1989;227: 569–574.
79. Ariae M, Shoji N, Shirato S: Postoperative subconjunctival 5-fluorouracil injections and success probability of trabeculectomy in Japanese: Results of 5-year follow-up. Jpn J Ophthalmol 1992;36:158–168.
80. Arkell SM, Lightman DA, Sommer A: The prevalence of glaucoma among Eskimos of northwest Alaska. Arch Ophthalmol 1987;105: 482–485.
81. Cox JE: Angle-closure glaucoma among the Alaskan Eskimo. Glaucoma 1984;6:135–137.
82. Johnson GJ, Green JS, Paterson GD: Survey of ophthalmic conditions in a Labrador community. II: Ocular disease. Can J Ophthalmol 1984;19:224–233.
83. Drance SM: Angle closure glaucoma among Canadian Eskimos. Can J Ophthalmol 1973;8:252–254.
84. Alsbirk PH: Primary angle-closure glaucoma: Oculometry, epidemiology, and genetics in a high risk population. Acta Ophthalmol 1976;54(Suppl):5–31.
85. Clemmesen V, Alsbirk PH: Primary angle-closure glaucoma (ACG) in Greenland. Acta Ophthalmol 1971;49:47–58.
86. Van Rens GHMB, Arkell SM, Charlton W, et al: Primary angle-closure glaucoma among Alaskan Eskimos. Doc Ophthalmol 1988;70:265–276.
87. Alsbirk PH, Forsius H: Anterior chamber depth in Eskimos from Greenland, Canada (Igloolik) and Alaska (Wainwright): A preliminary report. Can J Ophthalmol 1973;8:265–269.

88. Mann I: Eye disease in the Eskimo and in the Australian Aboriginal: A brief comparison. Acta Ophthalmol 1972;50:543–548.
89. Taylor HR: Pseudoexfoliation of the lens in Australian Aborigines. Br J Ophthalmol 1977;61:473–475.
90. Holmes WJ: Glaucoma in the Central and South Pacific. Am J Ophthalmol 1961;51:253–261.
91. Elliott R: Ophthalmic disease in Western Samoa. Trans Ophthalmol Soc NZ 1959;12:87–97.
92. Mann I, Potter D: A Preliminary study of the Maoris of New Zealand. Am J Ophthalmol 1969;67:358–367.
93. Quigley HA: Number of people with glaucoma worldwide. Br J Ophthalmol 1996;80:389–393.

CHAPTER 8

Systemic Syndromes and Diseases and Glaucoma

JODY R. PILTZ-SEYMOUR and REBECCA WALKER

The past medical history is a vital component of any patient history. A thorough history aids in identifying other disease states that could have an impact on the diagnosis or treatment of glaucoma. This important chapter by Jody Piltz-Seymour and Rebecca Walker presents systemic abnormalities that impact the care of the patient with glaucoma. It begins with commonly seen problems in the glaucoma population, such as systemic hypertension, hypotension, vasospasm, cardiovascular disease, and diabetes mellitus. Identifying and properly treating these problems may well enhance the treatment of the glaucoma. Next, syndromes of which glaucoma may be a component are discussed, including the phakomatoses and anterior segment dysgenesis. Recognizing the associated findings is important not only for the treatment of the glaucoma but also to ensure identification of associated abnormalities. The causes of increased episcleral venous pressure are discussed because they all have a systemic etiology and often result in increased intraocular pressure. The discussion of the systemic causes of eye abnormalities, including dislocated crystalline lenses, ocular neovascularization, and ocular inflammation and infection will supplement the ocular diseases discussed in later chapters. Finally, less common systemic diseases and their relationship to glaucoma are addressed. This chapter provides the information needed to take the patient's past medical history and proceed with an improved ability for diagnosis and treatment.

Glaucoma can occur in people with a variety of systemic diseases. In some cases, there may be a direct relationship between the systemic disease and the development of glaucoma, as in the diabetic patient who has neovascular glaucoma. Often there is only a known association without a straightforward cause-and-effect relationship (Table 8–1). This fact should not be surprising given the complex nature of systemic diseases and the multifactorial nature of glaucoma. Most forms of glaucoma can be seen in conjunction with a myriad of systemic disorders. This chapter covers the basic relationships between several types of systemic conditions and glaucoma.

Systemic Abnormalities Associated with Primary Open-Angle Glaucoma

HYPERTENSION

Numerous studies have found an association between elevated systemic blood pressure and elevated intraocular pressure (IOP); however, the relationship between systemic hypertension and glaucoma is more controversial. Elevated diastolic and systolic blood pressures have been positively correlated to elevated IOP in a large number of studies.[1–4]

TABLE 8–1. SYSTEMIC DISEASES ASSOCIATED WITH OCULAR INFLAMMATION AND GLAUCOMA

UVEITIS (NONINFECTIOUS)
Arthridites (ankylosing spondylitis, juvenile rheumatoid arthritis)
Sarcoidosis
Vogt-Koyanagi-Harada syndrome
Behçet's disease
Crohn's disease
SCLERITIS OR EPISCLERITIS
Rheumatoid arthritis
Ankylosing spondylitis
Erythema nodosum
Tuberculosis
INFECTIOUS DISEASE
Viral infections
Syphilis
Toxoplasmosis
Parasitic diseases

Although the Rotterdam[5] and Framingham[6] studies found an association between systemic hypertension and elevated IOP, only the Rotterdam study found a relationship between systemic hypertension and primary open-angle glaucoma (POAG). Using a case-control study design, Wilson and associates[7] found that hypertension was strongly related to the risk of POAG. The Baltimore Eye Survey found a lower risk for glaucoma in young patients with hypertension, and a higher risk in subjects older than 80 years. These data from the Baltimore Eye Survey suggest that early hypertension may be associated with relative protection from optic nerve damage and that more prolonged hypertension increases the risk of glaucoma.[8]

In a prospective study of 647 patients followed by serial examinations of the optic nerve, nerve fiber layer, and visual field, Quigley and colleagues[9] found no significant association between initial field loss or nerve fiber layer status and hypertension. Similarly, investigators in the Barbados Eye Study concluded that high blood pressure alone was not a risk factor for open-angle glaucoma and was not a major contributor to the high prevalence of POAG in their study population.[10]

Although a correlation between systemic hypertension and increased IOP has been confirmed, the relationship between hypertension and glaucoma is complex and may change at different stages of the hypertensive-atherosclerotic process.

HYPOTENSION

Low systemic blood pressure has been reported to be a risk factor for glaucomatous damage.[11, 12] The Baltimore Eye Survey found a strong correlation between low diastolic perfusion pressure and POAG (Fig. 8–1). The prevalence of POAG remained stable until diastolic perfusion pressure decreased below 50 mm Hg, and there was a sixfold higher risk of POAG when the diastolic perfusion pressure was less than 30 mm Hg.[8]

It has been recognized since 1964 that both systolic and diastolic blood pressures decline during sleep.[13] The presumed mechanism for the nocturnal blood pressure "dip" is a reduction in sympathetic activity with decreased catecholamines, leading to reductions in heart rate, cardiac output, and peripheral resistance.[14] The development of ambulatory blood pressure monitoring devices now permits reliable and practical monitoring of blood pressure throughout the day and night.[15] Studies employing ambulatory monitoring devices have confirmed that most people have a 10% or greater dip in blood pressure typically between 2:00 AM and 4:00 AM, with a peak shortly after waking.[16, 17]

Investigators have demonstrated an association between nocturnal hypotension and progressive visual field deterioration.[14, 18] Graham and coworkers[14] reported that patients with glaucoma tend to have larger decreases in nocturnal blood pressure than normal control subjects, and that patients with worsening visual field defects tended to have greater nocturnal blood pressure dips than those with stable visual field defects (Fig. 8–2).[14]

It has been proposed that in glaucoma the normal autoregulatory mechanism may be compromised[19] and unable to respond appropriately to the reduction in perfusion caused by a fall in blood pressure. The effects of nocturnal hypotension may be particularly critical in patients with glaucoma and impaired autoregulation.[20]

Although there are subgroups of patients with glaucoma who have large nocturnal dips in blood pressure, there is substantial overlap with the general population. This fact led several investigators to conclude that nocturnal hypotension alone cannot be the sole mechanism in the development of glaucoma. Perhaps the risk posed by nocturnal hypotension may be more consequential when it occurs in conjunction with other factors that make the optic nerve more vulnerable to nocturnal dips in blood pressure. Such concurrent factors include the use of oral hypotensive therapy for systemic hypertension,[14] vasospastic diseases,[21] variability of blood pressure,[22] normal-tension glaucoma,[23] and focal ischemic glaucoma.[24]

VASOSPASM

Vasospasms are inappropriate constrictions of small vessels that may diminish blood flow and result in ischemia of

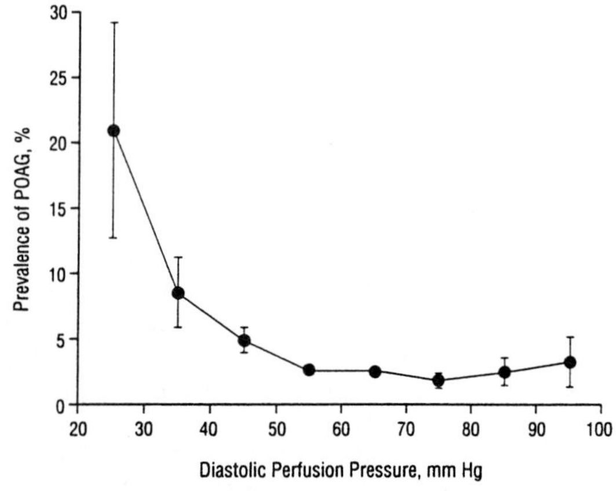

FIGURE 8–1. Prevalence (± standard error) of primary open-angle glaucoma (POAG) by diastolic perfusion pressure. (From Tielsch JM, Katz J, Sommer A, et al: Hypertension, perfusion pressure, and primary open-angle glaucoma: A population-based assessment. Arch Ophthalmol 113:216. Copyright 1995, American Medical Association.)

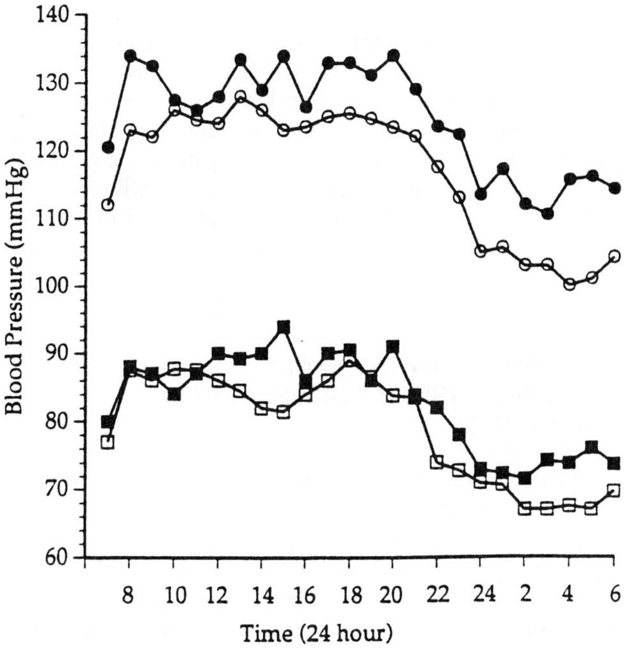

FIGURE 8–2. Mean hourly blood pressure for patients with progressive and stable visual field loss. The patients with progressive visual field loss have lower blood pressure levels, but the separation between the groups appears greatest at night. Circles, systolic blood pressure; squares, diastolic blood pressure; open symbols, patients with progressive visual field loss; solid symbols, patients with stable visual field loss. (From Graham SL, Drance SM, Wijman K, et al: Ambulatory blood pressure monitoring in glaucoma: The nocturnal dip. Ophthalmology 1995; 102:61.)

varying severity. Vasospastic diseases include Raynaud's disease, migraine, Prinzmetal's angina, and, possibly, Crohn's disease.[25] It is proposed that recurrent vasospasm in the eye may lead to axonal loss and manifest as normal-pressure glaucoma.

Evidence of vasospasm has been demonstrated in patients with normal-pressure glaucoma.[26–28] Drance and colleagues[29] used a laser Doppler flowmeter to measure fingertip blood flow; in subjects without migraine, a vasospastic response was detected in 65% of patients with normal-pressure glaucoma, compared with 26% of controls.[29] Systemic manifestations of vasospasm, such as Raynaud's phenomenon, cold extremities, and migraine, are more common in patients with normal-pressure glaucoma than in those with POAG and in controls.[30, 31] Patients with glaucoma, especially those with normal-pressure glaucoma, have an increased incidence of ischemic brain lesions as detected with magnetic resonance imaging (MRI).[32] There is also a higher incidence of silent myocardial ischemia, as detected by 24-hour Holter monitoring in patients with glaucoma.[20] Patients with vasospastic disease have demonstrated ocular vasospasm characterized by visual field defects induced by cold provocation, which in some cases is diminished by treatment with oral calcium channel blockers.[33, 34] Focal constriction of vessels at the edge of the optic disc occur more commonly in eyes with glaucoma than in eyes with ocular hypertension or controls (Fig. 8–3). Patients have been identified in whom these proximal arterial constrictions disappear, suggesting that these may represent focal vasospasms and not permanent constrictions.[35, 36]

Calcium channel antagonists have been proposed as therapy to diminish the impact of vasospasm in the development of glaucoma. Calcium channel antagonists, long used in coronary disease, have shown efficacy in improving the visual field[37–39] and contrast sensitivity[40] in patients with normal tension glaucoma, possibly by enhancing ocular circulation. Several calcium channel antagonists have been investigated, including nifedipine,[39] nimodipine,[37, 38, 40] and topical verapamil.[41] The long-term efficacy of these treatments has not been proven. Ophthalmologists must take care when prescribing calcium channel antagonists to avoid inducing systemic hypotension, which may pose additional risks for glaucomatous damage.

CARDIOVASCULAR DISEASE

Although many investigators have shown the statistical importance of cardiovascular disease status in patients with glaucoma,[42–44] it is not clear which features of cardiovascular disease raise the risk of glaucoma. The Beaver Dam Eye Study showed an association between elevated IOP, cholesterol level, and pulse,[44] and Winder[45] found higher levels of serum cholesterol in patients with normal-pressure glaucoma compared with POAG.[45] Other investigators have found that neither increased cholesterol levels nor increased triglyceride levels were risk factors for raised IOP.[46, 47]

Electrocardiograms (ECGs) have shown that patients with both normal-tension glaucoma and open-angle glaucoma have a higher prevalence of rhythm and conduction abnormalities than control subjects.[48] Normal-pressure glaucoma was found to be significantly associated with the occurrence of episodic, asymptomatic myocardial ischemia, which was characterized by ST-T segment depression on 24-hour ECG monitoring.[49]

Schulzer and colleagues[50] identified two distinct populations of patients with glaucoma. The smaller group, exhibited vasospasm in fingertip blood flow measurements and a significant correlation between visual field damage and highest recorded IOP. The larger group showed disturbed coagulation and biochemical measurements suggestive of vascular disease and did not demonstrate a correlation between visual field damage and IOP.[50] Although the asso-

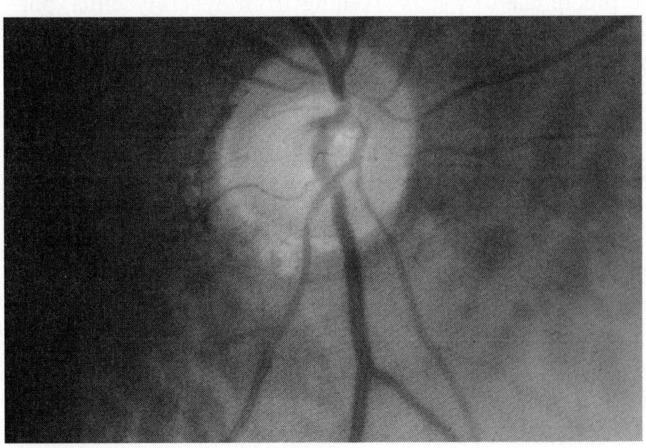

FIGURE 8–3. Focal constriction of the proximal aspect of the inferotemporal retinal artery.

ciation between cardiovascular disease and glaucoma remains vague at this time, it is known that regular aerobic exercise results in a decrease in IOP and may be an effective, nonpharmacologic intervention in patients with glaucoma.[51, 52]

DIABETES MELLITUS

Diabetes mellitus has significant ocular side effects, including retinopathy, cataract, and neovascular glaucoma.[53] The relationship among diabetes, elevated IOP, and POAG is less clear.

The majority of the literature, including population-based investigations, supports an association between elevated IOP and diabetes.[54–58] The connection between diabetes and POAG, however, continues to be debated. Much of the earlier literature suggested that POAG was more prevalent among patients with diabetes,[56, 59–62] although a number of studies showed no association.[63–65] Inherent problems in comparing these studies are the differing methods used to define both diabetes and POAG as well as the existence of selection bias. Several later population-based studies addressed some of these problems, using stricter criteria for the definition of both diabetes (glycosylated hemoglobin,[56] nonfasting glucose levels[58]) and POAG. Despite these improvements, no consistent conclusion has been reached.

The Beaver Dam Eye Study[66] showed a positive correlation between older-onset diabetes and POAG as determined by optic disc and visual field criteria. This conclusion was supported by the Rotterdam Study,[58] which found an association between diabetes and elevated IOP as well as a three-fold increase in the presence of glaucoma. In contrast, the Framingham Eye Study[67] did not find a significant association between diabetes and glaucoma. Similarly, the Baltimore Eye Survey did not find an association with POAG for either type I or type II diabetes.[57] A clear consensus remains to be reached.

Several observations suggest a possible relationship between diabetes mellitus and angle-closure glaucoma. Patients with angle-closure glaucoma have an abnormal response to oral glucose tolerance tests[65] and a high prevalence of non–insulin-dependent diabetes mellitus.[68] It has been suggested that acute angle-closure glaucoma may develop because of autonomic dysfunction[69] and a reduced anterior chamber depth.[70] Angle-closure attacks may also be precipitated by lens swelling from hyperglycemia, particularly in susceptible individuals.[71] Neovascular glaucoma can also develop as a consequence of diabetic retinopathy (see later).

Phakomatosis

(see Chapter 10)

The phakomatoses are a group of hereditary disorders characterized by the development of hamartias and hamartomas in the eye, central nervous system, viscera, and skin. *Hamartias* are nontumorous proliferations, and *hamartomas* are localized tumors; both arise from cells normally found at the location of the growth.

The prevalence of glaucoma varies among the phakomatoses, as do the mechanisms of development. Glaucoma develops commonly in encephalotrigeminal angiomatosis (Sturge-Weber syndrome), oculodermal melanosis (nevus of Ota) and Klippel-Trenaunay-Weber syndrome. There appears to be extensive overlap between these three syndromes, and it has been postulated that they present a spectrum of disease.[72] Glaucoma develops less commonly in patients with neurofibromatosis (von Recklinghausen's disease) and angiomatosis retinae (von Hippel–Lindau syndrome). It is unusual for glaucoma to develop with other phakomatoses.[73]

ENCEPHALOTRIGEMINAL ANGIOMATOSIS (STURGE-WEBER SYNDROME)

Encephalotrigeminal angiomatosis is characterized by vascular malformations of the face, eyes, and cerebral leptomeninges.[74] The cutaneous nevus flammeus (port wine stain) usually develops in the distribution of the ophthalmic (V_1) and maxillary (V_2) divisions of the trigeminal nerve and is usually unilateral. Ipsilateral facial hemihypertrophy, contralateral hemiplegia, and seizures may be seen.[75] Hemangiomas may involve multiple ocular sites, including the lid, conjunctiva, iris, ciliary body, and choroid.[76, 77] Glaucoma develops in the majority of cases when the nevus flammeus involves both the V_1 and V_2 distributions (Fig. 8–4).

The glaucoma in encephalotrigeminal angiomatosis generally occurs ipsilateral to the nevus flammeus and may develop from maldevelopment of the anterior chamber angle, elevated episcleral venous pressure,[78–80] or premature aging of the trabecular meshwork.[77, 81]

Filtering surgery may be complicated by choroidal effusions or choroidal hemorrhages.[82–86]

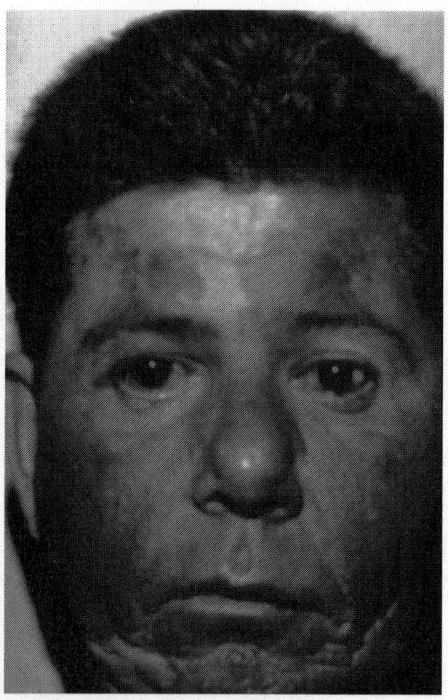

FIGURE 8–4. Nevus flammeus with bilateral involvement in the V_1, V_2, and V_3 distributions of the trigeminal nerve in a patient with encephalotrigeminal angiomatosis (Sturge-Weber syndrome).

KLIPPEL-TRENAUNAY-WEBER SYNDROME

Klippel-Trenaunay-Weber syndrome is characterized by cutaneous vascular malformations, venous and lymphatic malformations, arteriovenous shunts, and osseous and soft tissue hypertrophy.[87–89] Affected children present with cutaneous nevus flammeus and hemihypertrophy that usually involves a limb.[90] Neurologic abnormalities, such as seizures and mental retardation, may be present. Glaucoma occurs most commonly in patients with facial nevus flammeus (concomitant encephalotrigeminal angiomatosis).[91]

OCULODERMAL MELANOSIS (NEVUS OF OTA)

The hallmark of oculodermal melanosis is cutaneous pigmentation of the face in the ophthalmic (V_1) and maxillary (V_2) divisions of the trigeminal nerve; involvement of the mandibular division (V_3) occurs rarely.[92] Oculodermal melanosis is usually unilateral and is found more commonly in Asians. Thirty percent of patients have ocular hyperpigmentation of the episclera, sclera, trabecular meshwork, iris, and choroid.[93, 94] Glaucoma is seen in 10% of patients and may relate to abnormal angle development, impaired outflow due to melanocytic infiltration[95, 96] or uveitis[94] (Fig. 8–5).

NEUROFIBROMATOSIS

Neurofibromatosis (NF) is characterized by localized proliferations of peripheral nerve elements. There are multiple forms of neurofibromatosis. The clinical manifestations of NF1, von Recklinghausen's disease, are multiple neurofibromas of the skin, peripheral and central nervous system, and multiple café au lait spots.[97, 98] Other features are axillary, inguinal, or intertriginous freckling; sphenoid wing dysplasia or other osseous abnormalities; visceral neurofibromas; plexiform neuromas, regional hemihypertrophy; and fibroma mollusca.

Ocular features of NF1 include plexiform neuromas of the lids, optic nerve glioma, Lisch's nodules, ectropion uvea, retinal astrocytic hamartomas, and pulsating exophthalmos[73] (Fig. 8–6). Inheritance is typically autosomal dominant.

Glaucoma in NF1 is usually unilateral and rarely occurs in the absence of lid involvement.[99] Theories regarding the etiology of glaucoma in NF1 include developmental abnormalities of the anterior chamber angle structures and acquired mechanical obstructions to outflow, such as peripheral anterior synechiae formation from intraocular neurofibromas or neovascularization.[100–102]

The hallmarks of central neurofibromatosis (NF2) are bilateral acoustic meningiomas and posterior subcapsular cataracts. NF2 is generally not associated with glaucoma.[103, 104]

ANGIOMATOSIS RETINAE (RETINOCEREBELLAR ANGIOMATOSIS, VON HIPPEL–LINDAU SYNDROME)

The occurrence of angiomas of the retina and cerebellum characterize the von Hippel–Lindau syndrome.[105–107] This disorder has an autosomal dominant inheritance pattern with incomplete penetrance. The genetic abnormality has been localized to the short arm of chromosome 3.[108, 109] Untreated retinal lesions may cause exudative retinal detachments and neovascular glaucoma.[110] The cerebellar angiomas may result in headache, vertigo, and dystaxia. Angiomas may also develop in other viscera.

Anterior Segment Anomalies

The disorders highlighted in this section are also reviewed in Chapters 11 and 14. This discussion is limited specifically to nonocular findings.

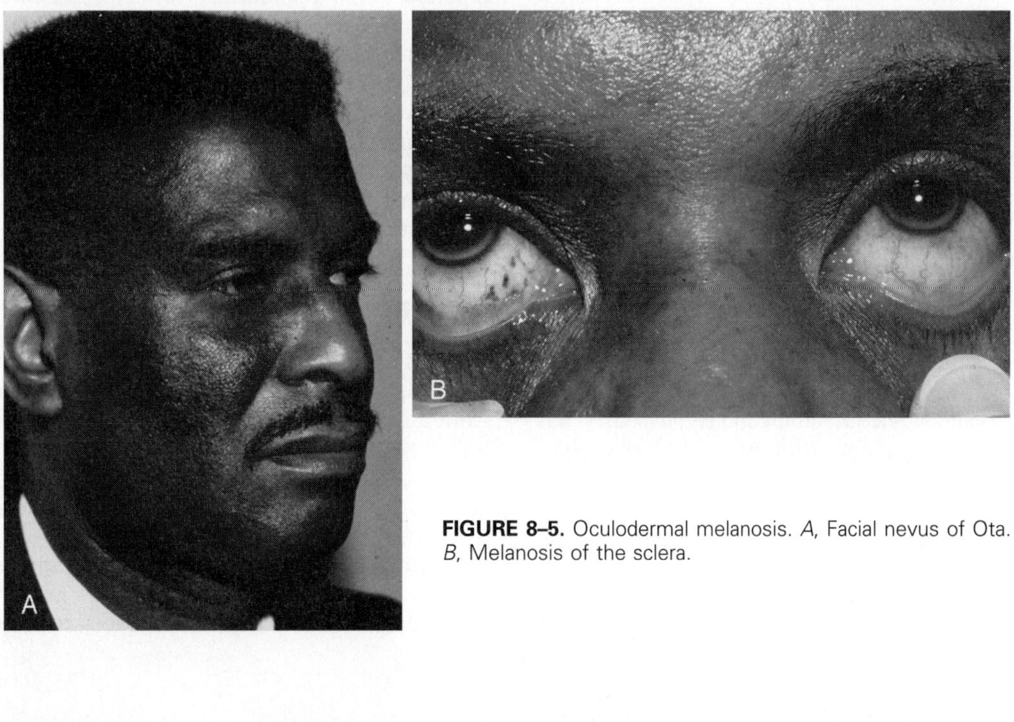

FIGURE 8–5. Oculodermal melanosis. *A*, Facial nevus of Ota. *B*, Melanosis of the sclera.

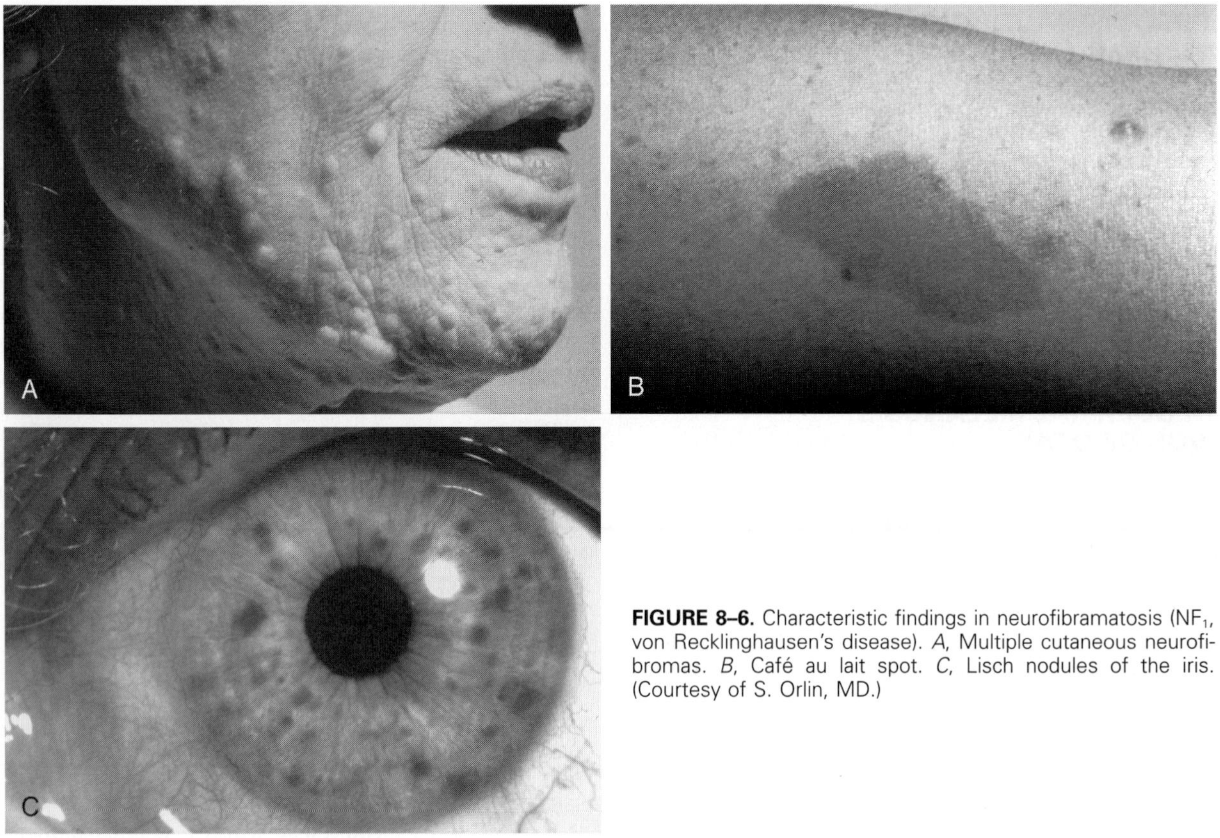

FIGURE 8–6. Characteristic findings in neurofibramatosis (NF_1, von Recklinghausen's disease). *A*, Multiple cutaneous neurofibromas. *B*, Café au lait spot. *C*, Lisch nodules of the iris. (Courtesy of S. Orlin, MD.)

AXENFELD-RIEGER SYNDROME

The Axenfeld-Rieger syndrome is a disorder of neural crest cell development with variable clinical presentations. The syndrome has an autosomal dominant pattern of inheritance, and the main locus has been mapped to the 4q25 chromosomal segment.[111, 112] A possible second locus has been mapped to chromosome 13q14.[113] Clinical features of the Axenfeld-Rieger syndrome include anterior segment anomalies, glaucoma, involvement of the facial bones and teeth, and failure of the periumbilical skin to involute (Fig. 8–7). Dental abnormalities include microdontia (small crown size), hypodontia (decreased number of teeth), and oligodontia (localized absence of teeth).[114] Anomalies of the facial bones manifest as maxillary hypoplasia with midface flattening, a receding upper lip, and a more protuberant lower lip.[115]

Pituitary anomalies are occasionally seen with the Axenfeld-Rieger syndrome. They include primary empty sella syndrome, congenital parasella arachnoid cysts, and growth hormone deficiency with short stature.[116, 117] Patients with this disorder may also have skeletal, neurologic, dermatologic, and cardiac defects. There have been reports associating Axenfeld-Rieger syndrome with mental deficiency, deafness, and oculocutaneous albinism. Hypospadias has also been reported in patients with Axenfeld-Rieger syndrome.[115]

PETERS' ANOMALY

Peters' anomaly is characterized by congenital bilateral central corneal leukomas with thinning of the posterior corneal stroma, defects in Descemet's membrane, and synechiae extending to the corneal opacity. Most cases of Peters' anomaly are sporadic, although there are isolated reports of possible autosomal recessive or autosomal dominant inheritance.[118] Various chromosomal abnormalities have been described with this disorder.[119–121]

Although Peters' anomaly usually occurs in isolation, it has been reported in association with a wide variety of nonocular anomalies. Defects have most commonly been reported in the genitourinary system, musculoskeletal system, heart, ears, and facial development. Mental deficiencies, cerebral palsy, myotonic dystrophy, cerebral maldevelopment, pulmonary disease, and dental anomalies have also been described.[122] It has been proposed that given the varied genetic patterns and systemic manifestations, Peters' anomaly may not actually be a unique single entity but rather may be a clinical pattern composed of multiple different disorders.

ANIRIDIA

Aniridia is a bilateral autosomal dominant condition associated with maldevelopment of the normal iris. It results from a dysgenesis of neuroectodermal tissue and has been linked to a mutation of the *PAX6* gene on the short arm of chromosome 11 (11p13).[111, 123] Two thirds of patients with aniridia have an affected parent, and one third represent new autosomal dominant mutations.[124]

Aniridia may manifest as isolated ocular involvement, such as poor vision, foveal and optic nerve hypoplasias, corneal pannus, microcornea, cataracts, nystagmus, and ec-

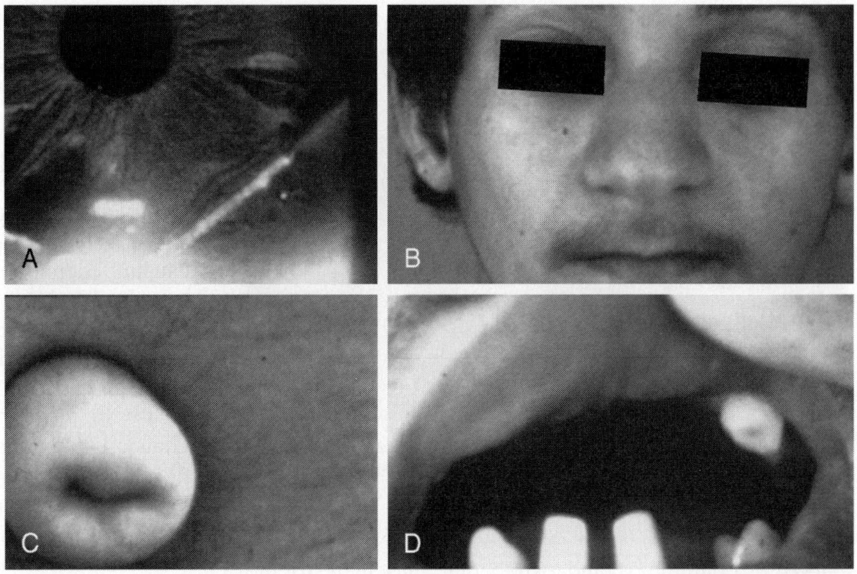

FIGURE 8–7. Typical findings in Axenfeld-Rieger syndrome. *A*, Polycoria. *B*, Midfacial flattening. *C*, Umbilical hernia, *D*, Dental anomalies. (Courtesy of David Kozart, MD.)

topia lentis. Large deletions in the region of 11p13 may result in the WAGR (Wilms' tumor, aniridia, genitourinary abnormalities, and mental retardation) syndrome.[111] Aniridia occurs infrequently in patients with Wilms' tumors (1:43 to 1:91 patients), Wilms' tumor occurs commonly in cases of sporadic aniridia (1:3 to 1:7).[125] A rare autosomal recessive form of aniridia is associated with mental retardation and cerebellar ataxia; it occurs in 2% of cases and does not seem to involve the *PAX6* gene.[126]

Glaucoma Associated with Elevated Episcleral Venous Pressure

(see Chapters 10 and 11)

Several systemic conditions can lead to elevated episcleral venous pressure (EVP) and dilated episcleral vessels. IOP is directly related to EVP, as approximated by the modified Goldmann equation:

$$IOP = F/C + EVP$$

where F is aqueous inflow and C is outflow facility. Any rise in EVP without a compensatory decrease in aqueous inflow or increase in outflow facility causes a corresponding rise in IOP.[127] Chronic elevation of IOP caused by increased EVP can lead to glaucomatous optic nerve damage similar to that found in open-angle glaucoma. Besides the direct effect on IOP, elevated EVP can also cause congestion and edema of the choroid, which may result in anterior displacement of the lens-iris diaphragm and secondary angle closure.[128] Alternatively, increased venous pressure can result in a decreased arterial supply, producing ocular ischemia and, ultimately, neovascular glaucoma.[129]

CAROTID ARTERY–CAVERNOUS SINUS FISTULA

Connections between the carotid artery and cavernous sinus of either the high-flow or low-flow type can occur spontaneously or as the result of trauma.

A high-flow fistula represents a direct communication of the intracavernous trunk of the internal carotid artery and the cavernous sinus; it typically occurs in young individuals following severe head trauma. These patients demonstrate pulsating exophthalmos, conjunctival chemosis, engorgement of the episcleral veins, decreased motility, and ocular ischemia. Visual loss and diplopia are present in about 50% of cases.[130, 131] Intraocular pressure is elevated in 60% to 70% of patients, most commonly because of elevated EVP as a result of these arteriovenous communications.[132, 133]

A low-flow fistula or dural fistula is a result of connections between smaller branches of the internal carotid artery or external carotid artery and the cavernous sinuses. These tend to occur spontaneously in middle-aged to elderly individuals. The fistula may be asymptomatic,[134] or a patient may present with minimal proptosis without pulsations, arterialized episcleral vessels, and no history of trauma.

The secondary glaucoma may be treated medically with drugs that decrease aqueous production. Because the majority of low-flow, dural fistulas resolve spontaneously, the IOP can usually be controlled until the fistula resolves. Occasionally, uncontrolled glaucoma or ischemic optic atrophy may occur, prompting the need for surgery. Depending on which vessel is feeding the shunt, treatment may involve either ligation of the carotid artery proximal to the ophthalmic artery or embolization with standard embolization methods or detachable balloon catheters.[135]

THYROID OPHTHALMOPATHY

Thyroid ophthalmopathy usually occurs in patients who are hyperthyroid but may occasionally occur in patients who are euthyroid or hypothyroid. Patients may have a diffuse goiter and dermatologic manifestations of the thyroid disease. It occurs more commonly in women than in men and typically develops in patients 30 to 50 years old.

The typical eye findings of Graves' thyroid ophthalmopathy include a characteristic stare and lid retraction. Exophthalmos is often mild. Approximately 10% of patients demonstrate an infiltrative ophthalmopathy with

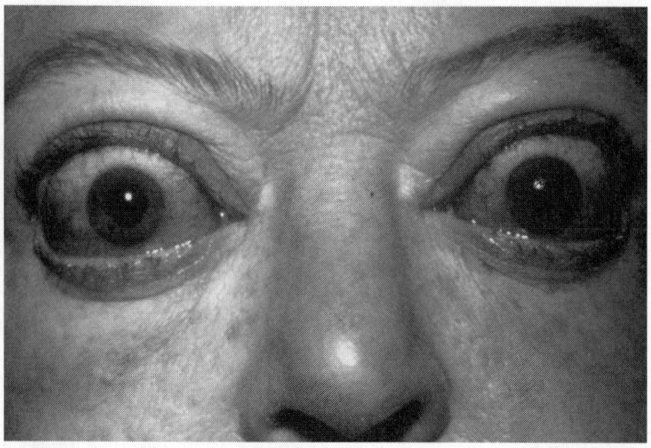

FIGURE 8–8. Bilateral exophthalmos with scleral show in thyroid ophthalmopathy. (Courtesy of S. Orlin, MD.)

marked exophthalmos and extraocular muscle restriction (Fig. 8–8); corneal exposure may lead to corneal ulceration and scarring.

Glaucoma may result from elevated EVP as a result of infiltration of the orbit and rectus muscles with inflammatory cells. It is speculated that the ophthalmic veins are compressed by swollen extraocular muscles, causing increased venous pressure and subsequently raised IOP.[136] A second mechanism involves contraction of thickened, infiltrated extraocular muscles on the globe that causes increased IOP, especially in particular gaze directions (Fig. 8–9). It may be difficult to distinguish whether vision loss is developing secondary to the infiltrative optic neuropathy or from the glaucoma (Fig. 8–10). A secondary angle-closure glaucoma may occur from the associated uveitis causing the formation of peripheral anterior synechiae.

Glaucoma resulting from orbital infiltration can generally be treated medically with topical medications or oral carbonic anhydrase inhibitors. In cases in which the optic nerve is compromised by direct compression, aggressive treatment with steroids, radiation, or surgical decompression may be necessary.

An association between hypothyroidism and POAG has been reported.[137] With use of the thyroid-stimulating hormone immunoradiometric assay, hypothyroidism was detected in 23% of POAG patients compared with 5% of control subjects. Half of the patients with glaucoma in this study were previously unaware that they were hypothyroid.

SUPERIOR VENA CAVA SYNDROME

Obstruction of the superior vena cava results in increased venous pressure in the head, neck, and upper extremities, causing edema and cyanosis of these areas. Increased IOP may lead to headache, visual distortion, and mental status changes. Ocular findings include edema of the lids, face, and conjunctiva, dilated conjunctival and episcleral vessels, papilledema, proptosis, and increased IOP. IOP may increase in the supine position and decrease with sitting. Glaucomatous cupping may not be present, depending on the duration of the underlying disorder[138] and the level of increased intracranial pressure.[139] Malignancy is the cause of 97% of all cases of superior vena cava syndrome.[140] Other causes are aortic aneurysm, enlarged hilar nodes, and thyroid disease. Treatment is aimed at the underlying disease process and conrol of the IOP.[141]

ORBITAL VARICES

The orbital venous plexus is formed by a shunt between the intracranial and extracranial venous systems. An orbital varix can result when there is posterior dilation of the intracranial vessels.[142] This disorder is typically found in a young person who gives a history of intermittent exophthalmos associated with bending over or Valsalva maneuvers.[143] The proptosis is a result of increased pressure within the jugular vein, causing the orbital varix to become distended. The episodes may be associated with symptoms of decreased vision, headache, nausea, and pain. Patients may have dilated veins in the eyelid and anterior orbit and may experience acute orbital hemorrhage.[144] Approximately 50% of patients may have other systemic venous abnormalities involving the scalp, palate, and forehead, and orbital varices may be associated with the Klippel-Trenaunay-Weber syndrome.[145] A 15% incidence of blindness due to repeated proptosis has been noted.[146] Fortunately, glaucoma is uncommon in this disorder because venous pressure is normal between attacks and the rise in EVP is typically

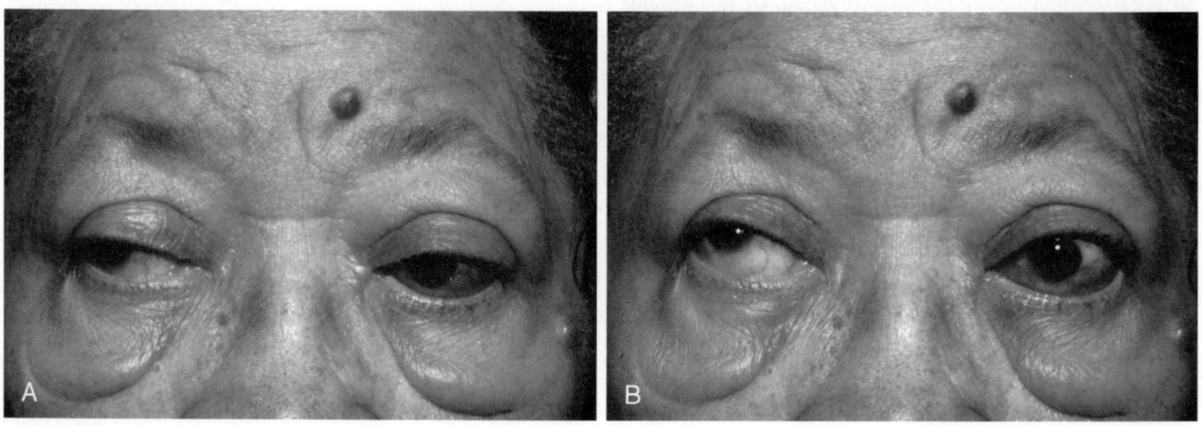

FIGURE 8–9. Restricted extraocular movements of the left eye of a patient with contracture of extraocular muscles from thyroid disease. *A*, In right gaze. *B*, In up gaze.

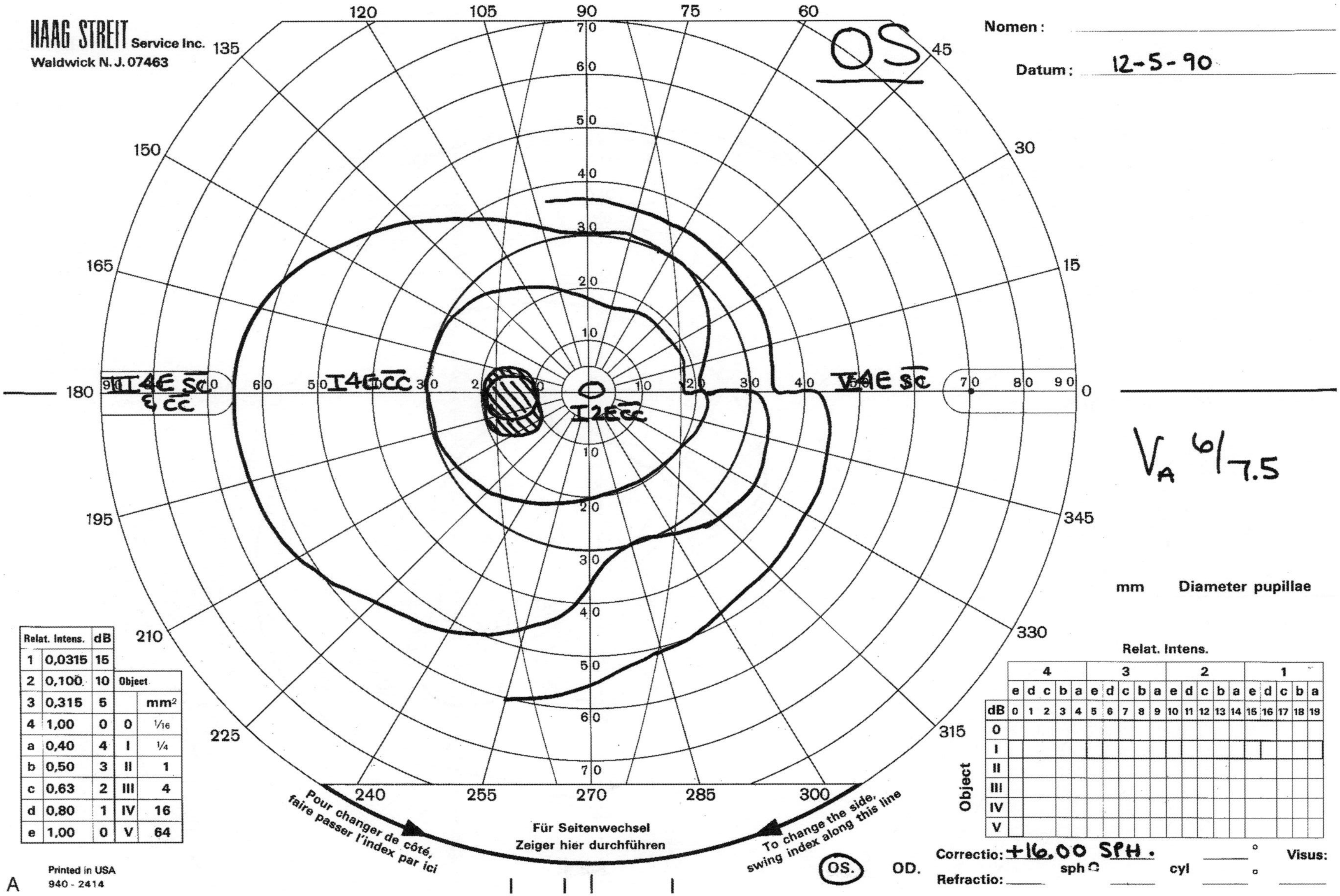

FIGURE 8–10. Reversibility of Goldmann visual field defects. *A* to *C*, Goldmann visual fields from a patient at different stages of disease and treatment. *A*, Before the development of the extraocular muscle contracture (December 5, 1990). *B*, In the active phases of infiltrative optic neuropathy and secondary glaucoma (April 20, 1992). *C*, After orbital decompression (October 25, 1993).

Illustration continued on following page

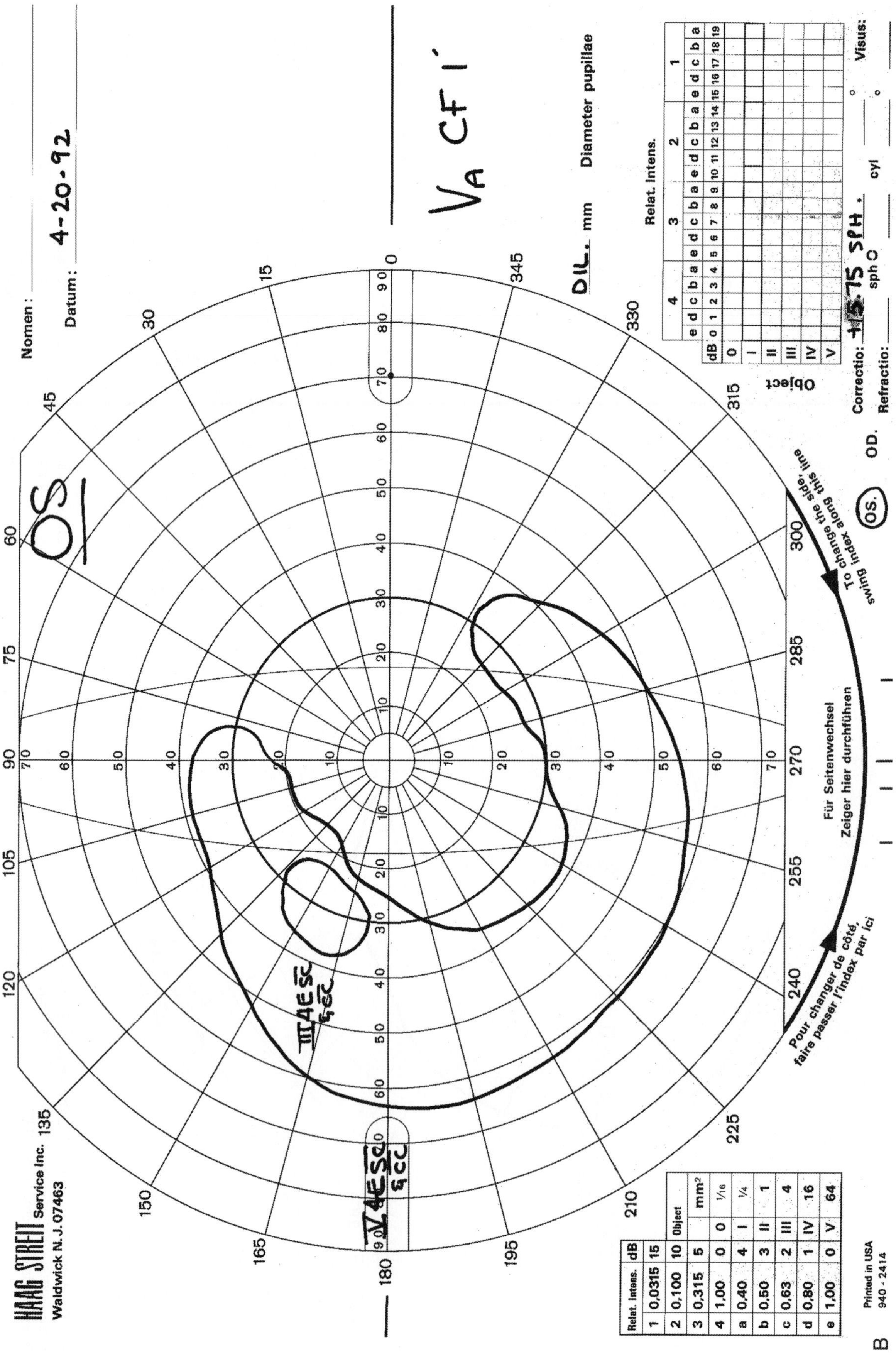

B

FIGURE 8–10. *Continued*

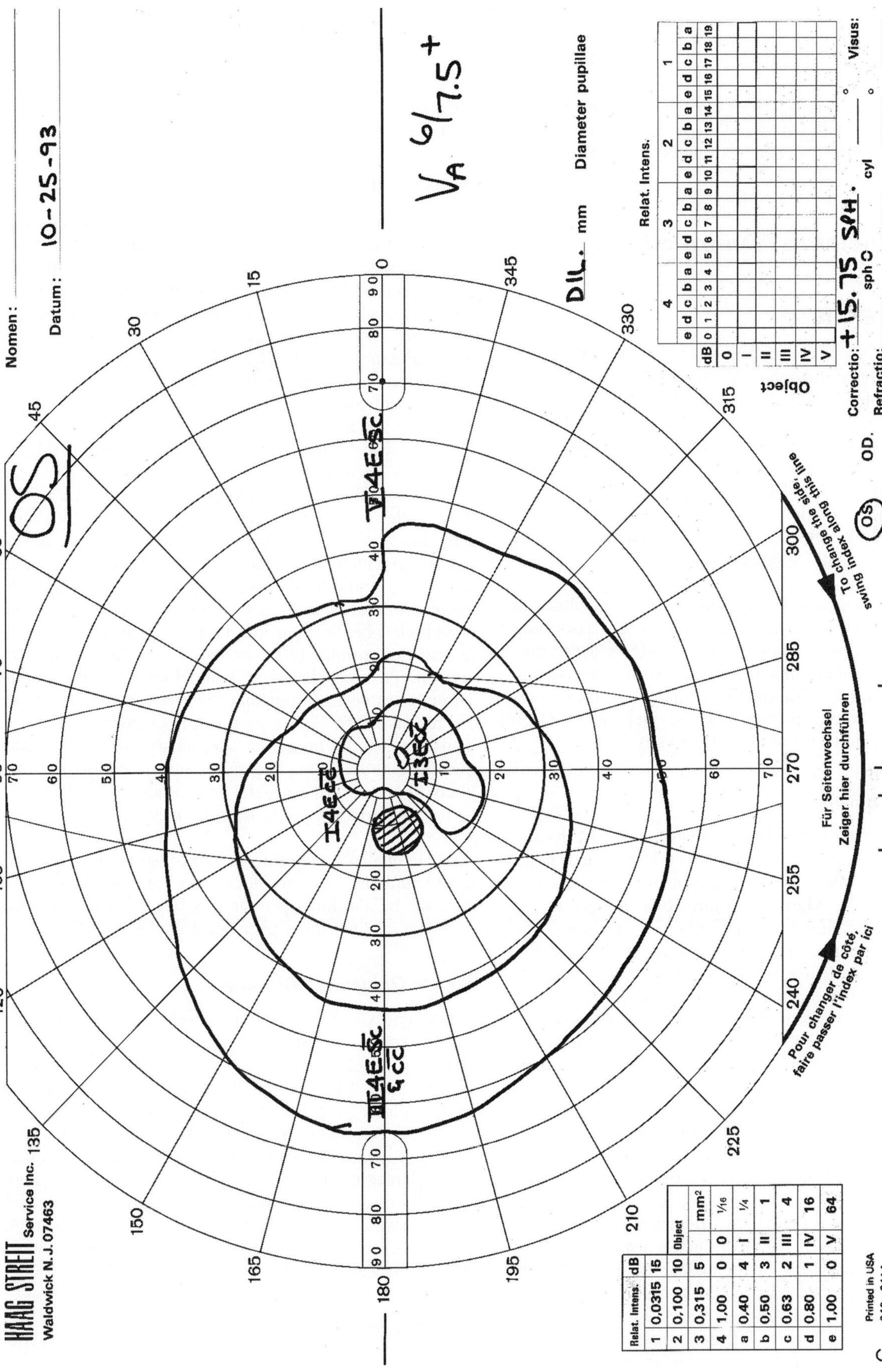

C

FIGURE 8–10. *Continued*

small and transient. Treatment is usually conservative, as the secondary glaucoma usually responds well to medical therapy.[147] Surgical intervention is generally performed for cosmetic purposes.[144]

Dilated episcleral vessels may also be caused by Sturge-Weber syndrome (discussed earlier) or retrobulbar tumors (meningiomas, pituitary adenomas, and metastases) or may be idiopathic.

Lens-Associated Abnormalities

(see Chapter 15)

ECTOPIA LENTIS

Ectopia lentis, or displacement of the lens with either partial or complete disruption of the zonules (dislocation), can cause angle-closure glaucoma. Patients with ectopia lentis often have symptoms of decreased vision, although with minimally subluxed lenses there may be no visual change. Glaucoma is present in approximately 8% of eyes with ectopia lentis,[148] and approximately one third of these cases are due to anterior movement of the lens resulting in pupillary-block angle closure. Glaucoma may also be associated with angle dysgenesis and prominent iris processes.[149, 150]

Ectopia lentis is most often due to trauma, although several hereditary systemic diseases may be associated with lens dislocation. They include Marfan's syndrome, homocystinuria, sulfite oxidase deficiency, hyperlysinemia, and Ehlers-Danlos syndrome. Recognition of these syndromes is important, as they may be fatal or result in significant morbidity if not treated correctly.

Marfan's Syndrome

Marfan's syndrome is the most common cause of a heritable lens dislocation, with a prevalence of about 4 to 6 cases per 100,000.[151] Inheritance is autosomal dominant with high penetrance.[152] Marfan's syndrome is a disorder of connective tissue, involving a variety of collagens and proteins that help maintain normal tissue architecture and function. The genetic abnormality responsible for Marfan's syndrome is located on the long arm of chromosome 15 (15q21.1) and involves a mutation of the fibrillin type 1 gene.[153, 154] Patients with the disorder have abnormal fibrillin in the skin and in cultures of fibroblasts[155]; fibrillin is also a component of lens zonules.

The typical marfanoid habitus is of disproportionately long limbs; abnormally long, slender fingers and toes (arachnodactyly); chest wall deformities (pectus excavatum); skull abnormalities; kyphoscoliosis; joint laxity; poor muscle development; and, most significant, cardiovascular anomalies (Fig. 8–11). There are often degenerative changes in the walls of the great vessels with aneurysmal dilation of the ascending aorta and aortic insufficiency. Early detection and screening of patients in whom Marfan's syndrome is suspected is critical, because life expectancy is reduced with this disease. The great majority of patients who die as a result of Marfan's syndrome do so from cardiac dysfunction, most commonly dissection of an aortic aneurysm.[156]

Glaucoma in a patient with Marfan's syndrome can be caused by anterior movement of the lens into the pupillary axis with subsequent pupillary block. In addition, many affected eyes exhibit angle dysgenesis with numerous iris processes, peripheral mounds of iris tissue, and vascular anomalies in the angle.[157]

Homocystinuria

Homocystinuria is an autosomal recessive disease with a prevalence of 1 case per 200,000. It is most often caused by a deficiency or abnormality of the enzyme cystathionine β-synthase, which catalyzes the conversion of homocysteine to cystathione. Two different forms of the enzyme deficiency have been defined on the basis of the response to pyridoxine (vitamin B_6), which is a precursor of the coenzyme for cystathionine β-synthase. In both types, the levels of methionine and homocysteine are elevated in the serum and excreted in excess amounts in the urine. The diagnosis can be made from the sodium nitoprusside test as well as electrophoresis.

Patients with homocystinuria have fair skin with a malar flush, pale, coarse hair, and poor peripheral circulation; 50% have mental retardation.[158] They may also have a marfanoid habitus with arachnodactyly, pectus deformities, joint laxity, and osteoporosis. Early death occurs in approximately 40% of patients and is most often related to thromboembolic phenomenon due to platelet dysfunction. This dysfunction results from increased platelet adhesiveness due to high blood levels of homocystine and methionine. Thromboses occur throughout the body, including the central retinal artery. They may result in cerebrovascular accidents, myocardial infarction, pulmonary emboli, and intermittent claudication. Thromboembolic events are most likely to occur during general anesthesia, and patients with homocystinuria are prone to pulmonary emboli after surgery.

Glaucoma in patients with homocystinuria is primarily due to pupillary block resulting from anterior dislocation of the lens. In addition, optic atrophy due to chronic vascular occlusion can resemble glaucomatous damage.[159]

Sulfite Oxidase Deficiency

Sulfite oxidase deficiency is inherited as an autosomal recessive trait. An enzyme found in mitochondria, sulfite oxidase is necessary for the breakdown of sulfur-containing amino acids. The enzyme deficiency leads to increased urinary concentrations of sulfur-containing compounds, which are excreted in the urine. The ectopia lentis seen in patients with the disorder is thought to result from excess sulfite damaging the disulfide bonds of fibrillin, a component of lens zonules.[160] Symptoms of sulfite oxidase deficiency develop in the first year of life, with muscular rigidity, severe mental retardation, seizures, and other neurologic abnormalities.[161]

Hyperlysinemia

Hyperlysinemia is a rare autosomal recessive disorder, with only seven reported cases.[162] It is due to a deficiency of lysine degradative enzyme. Systemic manifestations of the

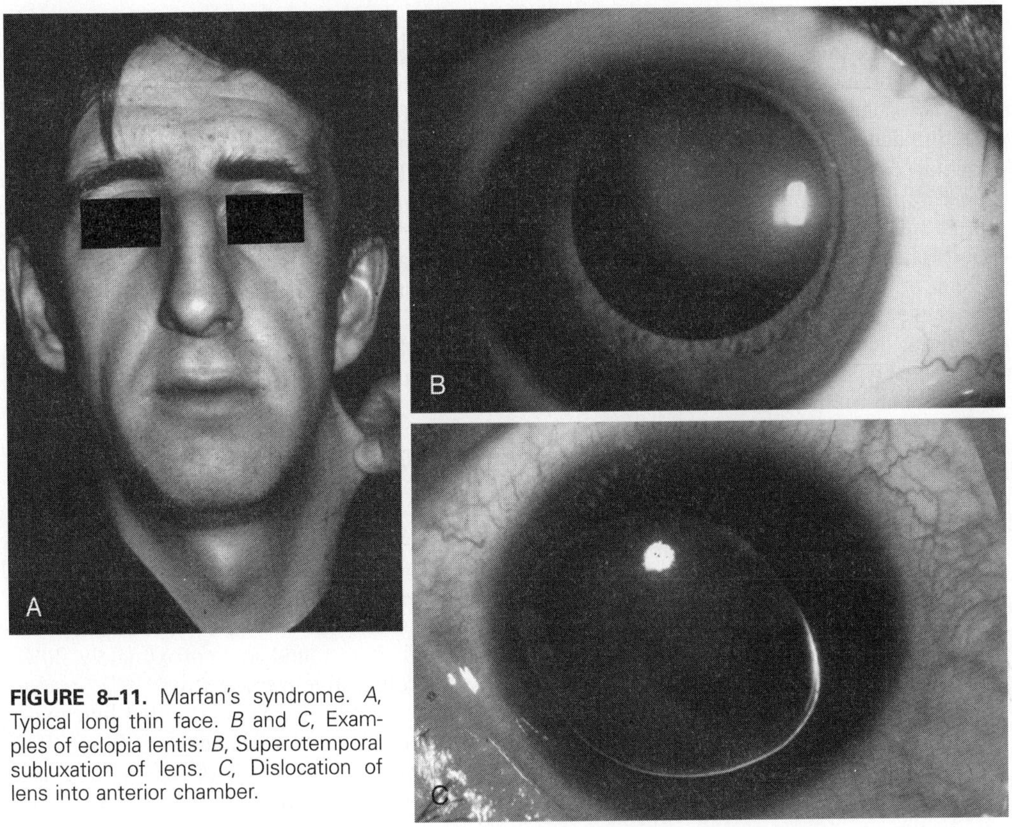

FIGURE 8–11. Marfan's syndrome. *A*, Typical long thin face. *B* and *C*, Examples of eclopia lentis: *B*, Superotemporal subluxation of lens. *C*, Dislocation of lens into anterior chamber.

disease include severe mental retardation, hypotonia, and convulsions,[163] as well as ectopia lentis.

Ehlers-Danlos Syndrome

Ehlos-Danlos syndrome is a group of connective tissue disorders characterized by fragile, hyperextensible skin, easy bruising, and joint laxity (Fig. 8–12). The various subtypes show abnormalities in collagen synthesis. Ectopia lentis is not as prominent in Ehlers-Danlos syndrome as in the entities previously discussed. Gonioscopy reveals angle abnormalities similar to those seen in Marfan's syndrome.[164] A notable consideration for the glaucoma surgeon is the extremely thin sclera found in patients with Ehlers-Danlos syndrome; the sclera may easily rupture after even minor trauma.[165]

MICROSPHEROPHAKIA

Microspherophakia can also be associated with ectopia lentis and glaucoma. The inheritance is typically autosomal recessive[166]; however, it may also be seen in an autosomal dominant pattern.[167] It has been associated with several syndromes including Marfan's syndrome,[148] homocystinuria, Alport's syndrome,[168] and Klinefelter's syndrome[169]; however, microspherophakia is most commonly associated with Weill-Marchesani syndrome.

The patient with Weill-Marchesani syndrome is short in

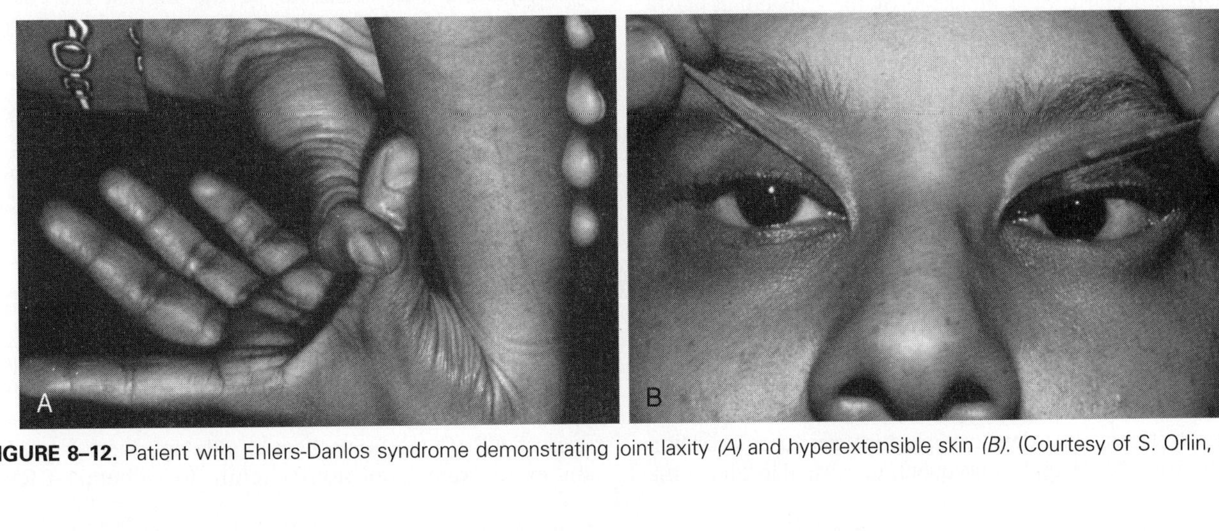

FIGURE 8–12. Patient with Ehlers-Danlos syndrome demonstrating joint laxity *(A)* and hyperextensible skin *(B)*. (Courtesy of S. Orlin, MD.)

stature with short, broad hands and feet, limited joint mobility, thick skin, and brachycephaly. The lens is small and spherophakic with a high degree of lenticular myopia. The presence of both microspherophakia and brachydactyly is necessary to make the diagnosis of this syndrome. In addition to the lenticular changes, the zonules may also be abnormal,[170] appearing loose and elongated.

Glaucoma may result from forward movement of the lens or dislocation of the lens into the anterior chamber. Anterior movement of the lens results in increased iris contact and may cause relative pupillary block and shallowing of the anterior chamber. Prolonged or recurrent attacks can result in peripheral anterior synechiae and blockage of the trabecular meshwork.

EXFOLIATION SYNDROME

Exfoliation syndrome (pseudoexfoliation) is a systemic disease characterized by the presence of a fibrillar material in the anterior segment of the eye. This syndrome is thought to be due to a disorder of extracellular matrix, but the exact biochemical nature of this material is unknown. Histologically, the material is found in and on the lens epithelium, iris stroma, and blood vessels as well as the subconjunctival tissue. Exfoliation material has also been detected along elastic fibers of the skin from various areas,[171] in the myocardium, lung, liver, gallbladder, kidney, and cerebral meninges.[172, 173]

No definite association has been found to link exfoliation syndrome with any systemic disease, although there have been reports of a greater frequency of HLA-Bw35 antigen in patients with exfoliation syndrome.[174] Several other investigators have found differences in ABO and Rh antigens among patients with exfoliative glaucoma, but there have been no relationships have been consistently confirmed.[175]

Exfoliation syndrome is associated with glaucoma in all populations, although the prevalence varies considerably.[176] In Scandinavian countries, exfoliation syndrome accounts for more than 50% of cases of open-angle glaucoma.[177] In the United States, the prevalence of exfoliation syndrome in glaucoma populations is approximately 12%,[178] with a lower prevalence in blacks than in whites.[179] This syndrome is also strongly correlated with age; typically, there is an almost 10-fold increase between patients younger than 60 years and patients older than 70 years.[180]

Exfoliation syndrome appears to result in open-angle glaucoma because of a blockage of the trabecular meshwork by the fibrillar material.[181] This corresponds to the finding of greater trabecular meshwork pigment in unilateral cases.[182] Exfoliation syndrome occasionally causes acute angle-closure glaucoma; however, the presence of narrow angles is common.[183, 184] It is hypothesized that angle closure, due to pupillary block may be caused by posterior synechiae, increased iris thickness, or anterior lens movement resulting from zonular weakness or dialysis.[185, 186]

Neovascular Glaucoma

(see Chapters 14 and 16)

Many systemic disorders can produce neovascularization of the iris (NVI) and subsequent neovascular glaucoma (NVG). Although a number of different entities are associated with NVG, they share the same basic pathophysiologic mechanism: ischemic retinopathy with retinal capillary nonperfusion. Histologically, NVI consists of a fibrovascular membrane overgrowing the iris and trabecular meshwork. This abnormal tissue eventually contracts to form synechial closure of the anterior chamber angle structures. Treatment is directed at decreasing angiogenesis factors by retinal ablation. Medical therapy is a temporizing measure; it is usually inadequate to control IOP once the outflow system is occluded. Filtering surgery is generally more successful after the neovascularization has regressed. Tube shunts or cyclodestructive procedures may be required.

DIABETES MELLITUS

Diabetes mellitus is a leading cause of blindness in the United States and the most common cause of NVG. Studies have shown that roughly one third to one half of cases of NVG are the result of diabetic retinopathy.[187] Fortunately, NVG occurs in only 2% of all patients with diabetes, although it is found in approximately 20% of those who have proliferative retinopathy.[188]

Diabetes mellitus is subdivided into two types. Type 1, or insulin-dependent diabetes mellitus (IDDM), accounts for approximately 20% of cases, and type 2, or non–insulin-dependent diabetes mellitus (NIDDM), for 80%.[189] The etiology of IDDM is likely the result of autoimmune destruction of the pancreatic islet cells, possibly triggered by viral infection. The etiology of NIDDM is unknown.

The long-term complications of diabetes mellitus are significant. They include retinopathy, nephropathy, myocardial infarction, stroke, peripheral vascular disease, cardiomyopathy, and skin lesions. The Diabetes Control and Complications Trial (DCCT)[191] has made important contributions to the understanding both of the role of hyperglycemia and diabetic complications and of the optimal therapy. This study, begun in the mid-1980s, randomly assigned patients to "standard" insulin therapy and intensive "experimental" therapy in which efforts were made to normalize blood glucose levels with frequent administration of insulin.[190] The DCCT clearly demonstrated that a regimen of intensive therapy aimed at maintaining blood glucose levels at near-normal levels markedly reduced the risks of retinopathy, nephropathy, and neuropathy.[191] Prolonged hyperglycemia was found to be the biggest risk factor for the development of long-term complications, including retinopathy.[192]

The current recommendation of the DCCT is that all patients with IDDM should attempt to maintain blood glucose levels as close to the "normal" range as possible.[191] Available treatment options now include external and implanted pumps; pancreatic islet cell transplants and artificial pancreases may be available in the future.[193, 194]

CENTRAL RETINAL VEIN OCCLUSION

Central retinal vein occlusion (CRVO) is the second most common cause of NVG. CRVO has been divided into two types, ischemic and nonischemic.[195] The majority (75%) of cases of CRVO are nonischemic, although there is a 16% conversion rate from nonischemic to ischemic CRVO within 4 months of the occlusion.[196] Although very few cases of nonischemic CRVO progress to NVG, 18% to 60% of cases of ischemic CRVO do so.[195, 197, 198] Traditionally, NVG has been noted 2 to 3 months after the CRVO ("100 day glaucoma") but it can occur at any point from 2 weeks to 2 years after the initial occlusion.[195, 197] CRVO has been associated with preexisting open-angle glaucoma and ocular hypertension.[195, 199, 200]

Many studies have found an association between CRVO and systemic diseases such as hypertension,[197, 201, 202] hyperlipidemia,[202, 203] abnormal glucose metabolism,[204] elevated ESR,[205] hyperviscosity syndromes,[206] and collagen vascular disorders including systemic lupus erythematosus.[207] Recent reports have linked CRVO to essential thrombocythemia, a rare myeloproliferative disorder with increased platelet counts.[208] CRVO and NVG may develop after ocular irradiation.

CAROTID ARTERY OCCLUSIVE DISEASE

Carotid artery occlusive disease (CAOD) is recognized as the third most common cause of NVG, accounting for approximately 13% of cases. Exact estimates may be inaccurate, however, because carotid disease is often a coexisting condition in patients who have NVG secondary to CRVO or diabetes mellitus.[209, 210]

Occlusions causing NVG can occur in the common carotid, internal carotid, and ophthalmic arteries.[211] In addition to NVG, CAOD may cause ocular ischemic syndrome.[212] Systemic manifestations of CAOD include transient ischemic attacks, strokes, and death.[213] Although auscultation of the carotid arteries may diagnose a carotid bruit, the absence of a bruit does not rule out the possibility of significant CAOD, and follow-up studies are necessary.[214] Noninvasive techniques, such as color-flow duplex scanning, are being used to screen for carotid obstruction.[215, 216] At present, contrast arteriography remains the "gold standard" for definitive diagnosis; MRI techniques are a useful adjunct.[217]

Treatment of CAOD has been evaluated by the North American Symptomatic Carotid Endarterectomy Trial[218] and the European Carotid Surgery Trial. These prospective, randomized studies have demonstrated reduction in risk of future stroke or death by surgical endarterectomy. Initial studies showed benefit in patients with high-grade stenosis (70–99% occlusion),[218] but later studies also demonstrated benefit for asymptomatic patients with stenoses of 60% or greater.[213] Medical management of CAOD consists of daily aspirin administration and aggressive medical treatment of associated risk factors.

OTHER VASCULAR DISEASES

NVG can be a sequela of systemic vascular disorders such as Takayasu's (pulseless) disease and temporal arteritis.[219] It has also been associated with Wyburn-Mason syndrome and congenital arteriovenous communication of the retina.[220] All of these entities can produce decreased retinal blood flow and retinal ischemia, leading to NVG.

CENTRAL RETINAL ARTERY OCCLUSION

Central retinal artery occlusion (CRAO) is also associated with NVG. The incidence of NVG ranges from 5% to 15%, although there is significant overlap with CAOD.[195, 221] The interval between the occurrence of CRAO and the development of NVG ranges from 1 week to 5 months.[195] As with all other causes of NVG, the common denominator is retinal ischemia. There is debate as to whether the ischemia is due to CRAO or to long-standing carotid occlusive disease.[195, 221, 222]

SICKLE CELL HEMOGLOBINOPATHIES

Sickle cell hemoglobinopathies result from an amino acid substitution that causes hemoglobin A (HbA) to form hemoglobin S (HbS). These erythrocytes may become sickled in hypoxic conditions. Approximately 10% of blacks have HbS. These mutations can manifest as sickle cell trait (AS hemoglobin) or sickle cell anemia (SS disease). SS disease has the most severe systemic manifestations, with painful hemolytic crises. Patients with sickle cell trait have milder symptoms.

Ocular findings include nonproliferative and proliferative retinopathy, retinal detachment, CRAO, and CRVO.[223] Although NVI and NVG can result from ocular ischemia, only a few cases of NVG have been reported.[224, 225] Ghost cell or hemolytic glaucoma may develop following vitreous hemorrhage due to sickle cell retinopathy. Patients with either sickle cell disease or sickle cell trait may experience profound elevation of intraocular pressure with hyphemas[226, 227] and may be more prone to CRAO and optic atrophy due to increased IOP.[228]

Inflammatory Conditions

(see Chapter 12)

Many systemic diseases are associated with ocular inflammatory conditions, such as uveitis, episcleritis, and scleritis, which can lead to open-angle or closed-angle forms of glaucoma. In the acute phases of iridocyclitis, IOP is generally low as a result of decreased aqueous humor production or increased uveoscleral outflow. Secondary open-angle or closed-angle glaucoma may subsequently develop. Secondary open-angle glaucoma may result from trabecular obstruction (by white blood cells, particulate debris, or an increased viscosity of the aqueous humor), trabecular inflammation (trabeculitis), or elevated EVP (particularly in scleritis). Secondary closed-angle glaucoma can result from the formation of peripheral anterior synechiae, posterior synechiae leading to pupillary block, or ciliochoroidal effusions causing anterior rotation of the ciliary body. The treatment of these inflammatory conditions with corticosteroids can also produce elevated IOP and glaucoma. Cycloplegia can also raise IOP by antagonizing either resting parasympathetic tone or topical miotic therapy.

ARTHRITIDES

Ankylosing spondylitis occurs predominantly in males between the ages of 15 and 40 years.[229] It typically involves

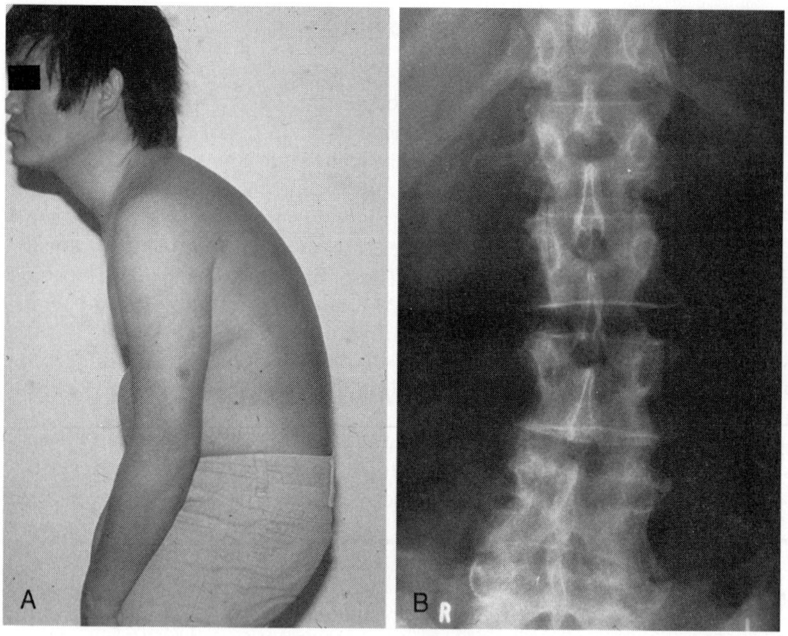

FIGURE 8–13. Vertebral involvement in a patient with ankylosing spondylitis. *A*, Clinical photograph. *B*, Radiograph. (Courtesy of S. Orlin, MD.)

the sacroiliac joints, lumbosacral spine, and cervical vertebrae (Fig. 8–13). Ninety-six percent of patients with ankylosing spondylitis are HLA-B27 antigen–positive.[230] Between 15% and 25% of patients with the disorder experience acute, nongranulomatous anterior uveitis,[230] and some patients have secondary open-angle or closed-angle glaucoma (Fig. 8–14).

Juvenile rheumatoid arthritis (JRA) may cause chronic uveitis and multiple ocular complications. This disorder is divided into three subgroups: acute systemic JRA (Still's disease), polyarticular JRA, and pauciarticular JRA. The pauciarticular subtype, which accounts for approximately 60% of all cases of JRA, typically affects girls around 2 years of age. JRA most commonly involves the knees, ankles, and elbows. Uveitis is most frequent in patients with the pauciarticular subtype, with an incidence of 78% to 91%.[231] Patients at highest risk for uveitis are those with positive antinuclear antibody (ANA) titers and negative rheumatoid factors. In patients with pauciarticular, ANA-positive JRA, secondary glaucoma occurs in 19% to 30%.[232–234] Treatment requires long-term systemic corticosteroids, which can also contribute to the development of glaucoma.

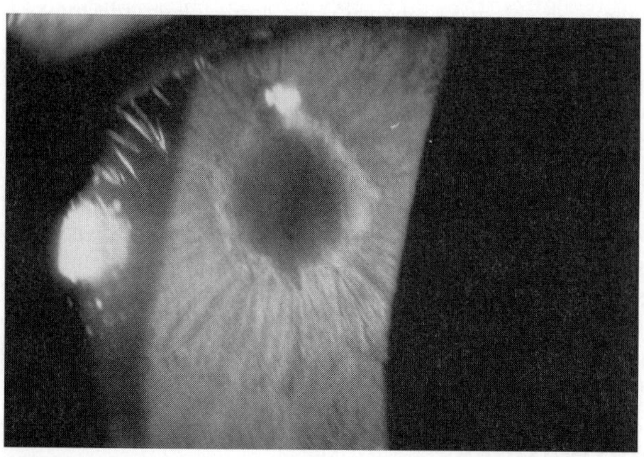

FIGURE 8–14. Slit-lamp photographs from a patient with ankylosing spondylitis showing 360 degrees of posterior synechiae resulting in iris bombé.

SARCOIDOSIS

Sarcoidosis is a multisystem disorder that typically affects blacks between 20 and 40 years of age. The disease may involve the lungs, liver, spleen, musculoskeletal system, central nervous system, and skin (Fig. 8–15).[235] Ocular involvement consists of anterior and posterior uveitis, chorioretinitis, retinal periphlebitis, optic neuritis, and orbital disease. Diagnosis is based on a chest radiograph, which shows abnormal findings in greater than 90% of patients with ocular sarcoidosis.[236] Other findings are positive Kveim skin test result,[237] elevation of serum lysozyme,[238] and elevation of serum angiotensin-converting enzyme.[239] A tissue biopsy reveals typical noncaseating granulomas. A "blind" conjunctival biopsy may yield a diagnosis in 10% to 30% of patients in whom the disorder is suspected; if the patient has conjunctival nodules, the diagnostic yield is approximately 75%.[240, 241] Systemic corticosteroids are usually effective in treating systemic sarcoidosis, although occasionally, stronger immunosuppressive agents are required.[242]

VOGT-KOYANAGI-HARADA SYNDROME

Vogt-Koyanagi-Harada (VKH) syndrome, or uveomeningitic syndrome, is a systemic disease that involves multiple organ systems, including the eyes, ears, skin, and meninges.[243] This disorder affects dark-skinned or Asian individuals between 30 and 50 years of age. Ocular findings include granulomatous anterior uveitis, posterior uveitis with exudative retinal detachment, vitritis, and papilledema. Systemic findings consist of hearing loss, vitiligo, poliosis, and alopecia. Patients may have prodromal symptoms such as headache, stiff neck, and vertigo.

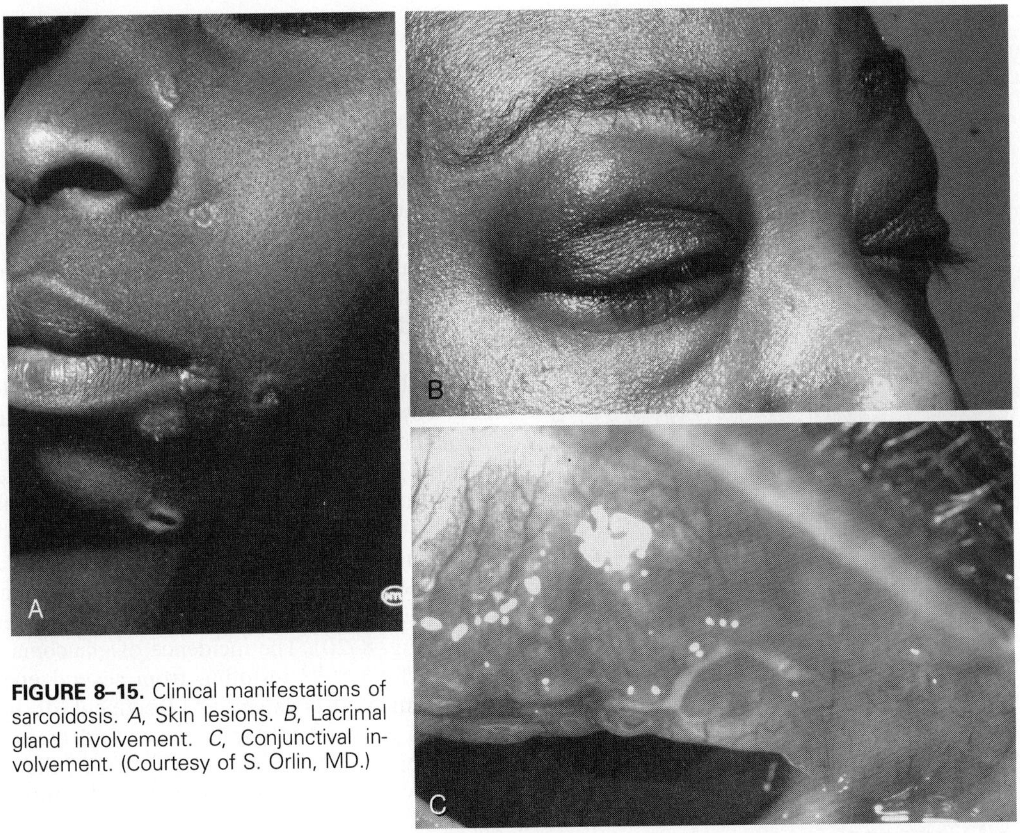

FIGURE 8–15. Clinical manifestations of sarcoidosis. *A*, Skin lesions. *B*, Lacrimal gland involvement. *C*, Conjunctival involvement. (Courtesy of S. Orlin, MD.)

VKH syndrome is associated with shallowing of the anterior chamber and elevated IOP.[244] The incidence of glaucoma is 20% to 38%.[245, 246] In one study of patients with associated glaucoma, approximately 56% were found to have open angles, and 44% had closed angles secondary to pupillary block.[245]

BEHÇET'S DISEASE

Behçet's disease is a multisystem disorder characterized by aphthous stomatitis, genital ulceration, and intraocular inflammation (Fig. 8–16).[247] Other systemic findings are arthritis, erythema nodosum, intestinal ulcers, thrombophlebitis, and central nervous system disorders. The systemic manifestations of this disease are due to occlusive vasculitis. Behçet's disease is more common in individuals from the Far East and Mediterranean areas. This disorder is associated with HLA-Bw51 and HLA-B5 antigens.

The principal ocular finding is bilateral, nongranulomatous anterior uveitis with hypopyon. Occlusive events involving the retina and optic nerve can lead to retinal necrosis and optic atrophy. Glaucoma has been reported in 17% of patients with anterior uveitis. Neovascular glaucoma has also been associated with this disease.[247–249] Treatment of Behçet's disease requires immunosuppressive therapy, typically cyclosporine alone or in combination with prednisone.[250]

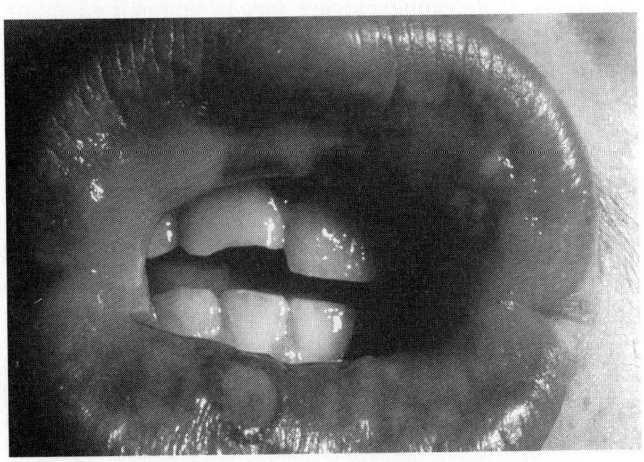

FIGURE 8–16. Aphthous ulcers in patient with Behçet's disease. (Courtesy of D. Kozart, MD.)

CROHN'S DISEASE

Crohn's disease is an inflammatory bowel disease involving the lower intestinal tract. Other systemic findings are peripheral arthritis (resembling rheumatoid arthritis) and erythema nodosum. Acute, nongranulomatous anterior uveitis occurs in 2% to 3% of patients with Crohn's disease.[251] Additional ocular manifestations are episcleritis, keratitis, scleritis, optic neuritis, and retinal vasculitis.[252, 253] Patients with uveitis and inflammatory bowel disease tend to be HLA-B27 antigen–positive and are more likely to have arthritis.[251] Treatment depends on the extent and site of involvement. Options are medical treatment (corticosteroid therapy with or without azathioprine), enteral nutrition, and surgical resection.[254, 255]

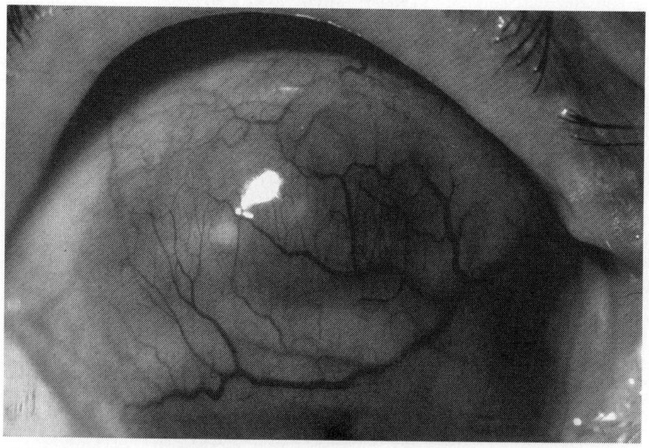

FIGURE 8–17. Scleral thinning superiorly after scleritis in a patient with rheumatoid arthritis. (Courtesy of S. Orlin, MD.)

SCLERITIS OR EPISCLERITIS

Glaucoma can occur in patients with either scleritis or episcleritis associated with a variety of systemic diseases. The most common cause is rheumatoid arthritis (Figs. 8–17 and 8–18). Scleritis may also develop in patients with ankylosing spondylitis, erythema nodosum, and tuberculosis.[256]

Infectious Diseases

Numerous infectious diseases, including viral, bacterial, and protozoan diseases, can result in glaucoma. Elevated IOP may result from blockage of the trabecular meshwork by cellular debris or trabecular inflammation. Secondary angle closure may be caused by peripheral anterior synechiae formation, pupillary block, or anterior rotation of the ciliary body.

HERPES VIRUSES

Herpes simplex virus (HSV), both type 1 (oral) and, less commonly, type 2 (genital), can cause ocular infection. Although the majority of affected adults demonstrate antibodies to the type 1 virus, the virus remains inactive, and few patients have ocular infection. Recurrent ocular herpes simplex can cause conjunctivitis, keratitis, and uveitis (Fig. 8–19). Elevated IOP is seen in approximately 28% of patients with herpes simplex keratouveitis[257]; the incidence is much higher in cases of keratouveitis associated with anterior segment ischemia.[258] IOP usually returns to normal as the inflammation resolves, although roughly 10% of patients have persistent elevations in IOP and require filtration surgery.[257] Treatment of systemic HSV requires systemic antiviral agents administered either orally or intravenously, depending on the patient's immune status.[259]

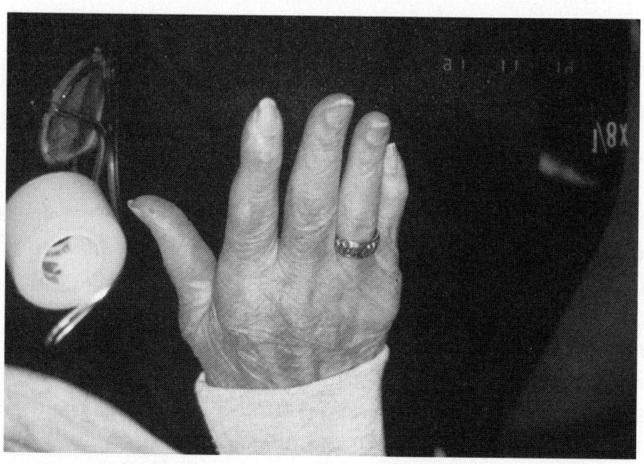

FIGURE 8–18. Joint changes and ulnar deviation of the hand in rheumatoid arthritis. (Courtesy of N. Volpe, MD.)

Herpes zoster is caused by the varicella-zoster virus, which also causes varicella (chicken pox). Herpes zoster produces a vesicular rash on an erythematous base in a dermatomal distribution. Lancinating pain may precede the rash by 24 to 48 hours. Although herpes zoster is usually a self-limited disease, invasion of the ophthalmic branch (V_1) of the trigeminal nerve produces herpes zoster ophthalmicus. The ocular disease is usually mild, but more severe complications, such as corneal scarring, glaucoma, optic neuritis, retinitis,[260] and postherpetic neuralgia, can occur (Fig. 8–20). The incidence of glaucoma ranges from 16% to 50%,[261–263] resulting from several open-angle and closed-angle mechanisms.[264] Treatment of herpes zoster infection with oral antiviral agents can decrease the severity of the episodes.[265] Varicella rarely affects the eye, although there have been reports of associated keratitis, uveitis, and glaucoma.[260]

HUMAN IMMUNODEFICIENCY VIRUS

The human immunodeficiency virus (HIV) causes acquired immune deficiency syndrome (AIDS). A wide range of systemic infections and neoplasms result from this serious disorder of cellular immunity.[266] Ocular manifestations include Kaposi's sarcoma, molluscum contagiosum, cotton-wool spots, uveitis, retinitis, retinal detachment, papilledema, and cranial nerve palsies (Fig. 8–21).[267] Interestingly, IOP appears to be lower than normal in patients affected with HIV, a finding that may be associated with a decreased CD+ T lymphocyte count.[268] Elevated IOP may be found in association with anterior uveitis and as a result of secondary angle-closure glaucoma due to ciliochoroidal effusions and anterior rotation of the ciliary body.[269]

Bilateral acute angle closure has been reported in patients with AIDS. It may respond to cycloplegia, aqueous suppressants, peripheral iridoplasty,[270] iridotomy, or drainage of choroidal effusions.[269]

MUMPS

Mumps is a contagious systemic infection resulting in painful enlargement of the salivary glands (usually the parotid glands). In older males, it can produce orchitis. Reports of meningitis and pancreatitis have also been described. Ocular findings include dacryoadenitis, keratitis, iritis, scleritis, and optic neuritis. Glaucoma can occur in association with iritis.[271] Some investigators describe episodes of open-angle glaucoma without signs of episcleritis or iritis.[272]

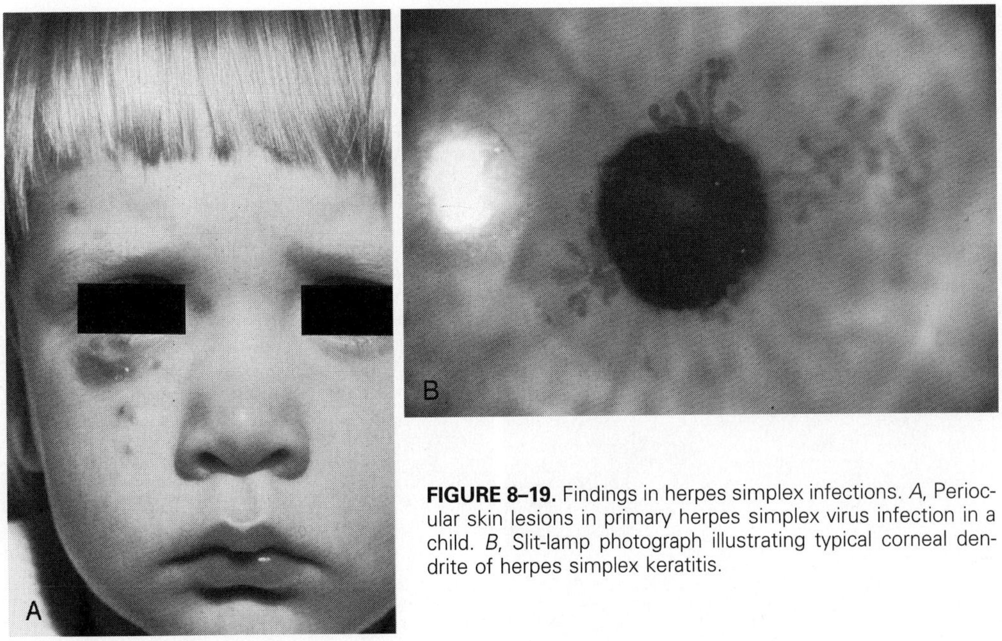

FIGURE 8–19. Findings in herpes simplex infections. *A,* Periocular skin lesions in primary herpes simplex virus infection in a child. *B,* Slit-lamp photograph illustrating typical corneal dendrite of herpes simplex keratitis.

RUBELLA

Congenital rubella can produce a wide range of congenital defects, including heart disease, deafness, microcephaly, and mental retardation. The severity of these manifestations is greater the earlier in the pregnancy that transmission of the virus to the fetus occurs, particularly during the early first trimester. Ocular disorders due to congenital rubella include cataracts, pigmentary retinopathy, micro-ophthalmous, corneal clouding, and glaucoma. Although cataract occurs commonly, glaucoma may develop in the more severe cases.[273]

SYPHILIS

Syphilis can occur in a congenital or acquired form. Congenital syphilis can produce a variety of findings, including rash, dental abnormalities, osteochondritis, deafness, meningitis, anemia, hepatosplenomegaly, nephritis, and pneumonia. Ocular manifestations are interstitial keratitis, uveitis, "salt-and-pepper" retinopathy, optic neuritis, and cataracts.

Acquired syphilis has several stages. Patients with primary syphilis demonstrate skin lesions or chancres. Secondary syphilis may result in lymphadenopathy, meningitis, and optic nerve involvement. Eye findings include uveitis and chorioretinitis. Tertiary syphilis results in severe central nervous system involvement and cardiovascular disease.

Diagnosis is based on positive serologic test results. The rapid plasma reagin (RPR) test is used to screen for active disease; the result reverts to negative when a patient has been treated adequately. The serum fluorescent treponemal antibody absorption (FTA-ABS) test is the definitive test,

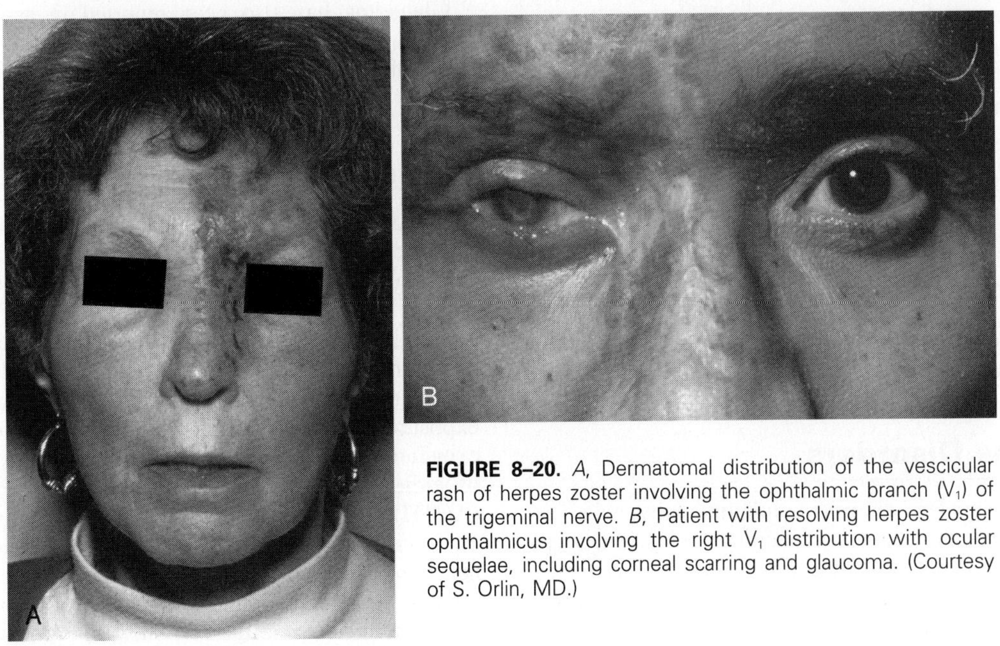

FIGURE 8–20. *A,* Dermatomal distribution of the vescicular rash of herpes zoster involving the ophthalmic branch (V_1) of the trigeminal nerve. *B,* Patient with resolving herpes zoster ophthalmicus involving the right V_1 distribution with ocular sequelae, including corneal scarring and glaucoma. (Courtesy of S. Orlin, MD.)

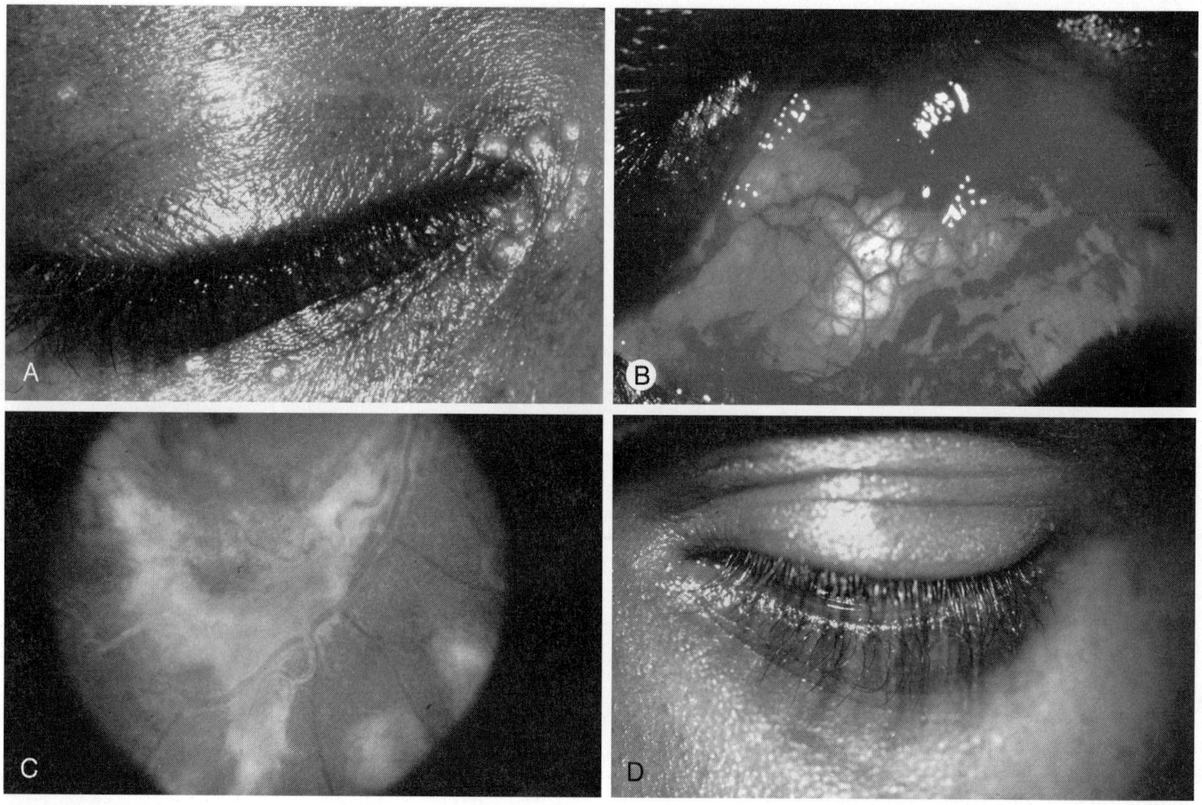

FIGURE 8–21. Clinical findings in acquired immunodeficiency syndrome (AIDS). *A*, Molluscum contagiosum lesions around the eyelid. *B*, Kaposi's sarcoma of the conjunctiva. *C*, Cytomegalovirus retinitis. *D*, Trichomegaly. (Courtesy of A. Ho, MD.)

because the result remains positive even after therapy.[274] Glaucoma can occur acutely, concomitant with active uveitis, or can occur years after the original inflammation has become qurescent.[275] Treatment of systemic syphilis involves intravenous or intramuscular penicillin.

TOXOPLASMOSIS

Toxoplasmosis is caused by *Toxoplasma gondii*, a protozoon. In immunocompetent patients, infection results in a flu-like illness. In immunocompromised hosts, however severe encephalitis, pneumonitis, or myocarditis can occur.[276–278] Congenital toxoplasmosis produces hydrocephaly, cerebral calcifications, seizures, hepatosplenomegaly, and retinochoroiditis. Open-angle glaucoma is a potential complication of acute retinochoroiditis, occurring in 13% of patients.[279]

PARASITIC DISEASES

Parasitic infection, such as onchocerciasis (river blindness) or gnathostomiasis, can produce uveitis and glaucoma.[280, 281]

Endocrine Disorders

Diabetes mellitus and thyroid ophthalmopathy were discussed earlier in the chapter. Glaucoma occurs in association with several endocrine disorders; however, it is unclear whether any endocrine abnormality directly causes chronic open-angle glaucoma.[282]

PITUITARY ABNORMALITIES

Eosinophilic pituitary adenomas causing acromegaly have been associated with impaired IOP regulation in glaucoma.[283, 284] The incidence of elevated intraocular pressure in acromegaly, however, may be artifactually high. Central corneal thickness is increased in patients with acromegaly, possibly producing an artifactual increase in applanation tonometry readings.[285, 286]

Glaucoma has also been reported in association with chromophobe adenomas[287, 288] and basophil adenomas of the pituitary. Normal-tension glaucoma has been associated with primary empty sella syndrome.[289]

CUSHING'S SYNDROME

Elevation of intraocular pressure related to decreased outflow facility has been described in patients with Cushing's syndrome.[290–292] Glaucomatous optic nerve and visual field damage has been described in selected cases.[291]

Cushing's syndrome is characterized by truncal obesity, abdominal striae, hypertension, hirsutism, edema, glucosuria, and osteoporosis. The disorder results from long-term exposure to excess glucocorticoid, which is due to either exogenous administration or endogenous overproduction of either glucocorticoid or adrenocorticotropic hormone (ACTH). Endogenous causes of excess glucocorticoid secretion include adrenal hyperplasia, cortisol-secreting adrenal tumors, and excess ACTH synthesis from pituitary tumors, pituitary hypothalamic dysfunction, or ACTH-producing nonendocrine tumors, such as bronchogenic carcinoma, thymoma, pancreatic carcinoma, and bronchial adenoma.

Renal Failure

Patients with chronic renal failure who are undergoing hemodialysis exhibit fluctuations in IOP during hemodialysis treatments. Initially, IOP decreases, but after the first 2 hours, most patients show a gradual rise in IOP. The average increase in IOP in patients experiencing a rise in pressure is 7 mm Hg; however, the magnitude of these elevations is variable.[293–295] This increase in IOP may relate to a decrease in serum osmolality causing osmotic movement of water into the globe,[296] or it may be related to central nervous system mechanisms.[294] Although these transient IOP elevations are generally not associated with the development of glaucoma, people with impaired outflow facility can experience more significant spikes in IOP.[297]

Patients who have undergone renal transplantation may demonstrate elevated IOP in association with systemic administration of corticosteroids.[298–300]

Primary Familial Amyloidosis

Patients with primary familial amyloidosis may have bilateral open-angle glaucoma. In patients with amyloidosis, weakness and peripheral neuropathy may develop, as well as other manifestations resulting from amyloid deposition in the cardiovascular, renal, gastrointestinal, and endocrine systems. Amyloid accumulates with the characteristic appearance in the vitreous, causing sufficient opacification to impair visual acuity. Other signs of ocular involvement are lid abnormalities, extraocular muscle weakness, proptosis, pupillary abnormalities, retinal perivasculitis, and internal ophthalmoplegia. Amyloidosis usually exhibits an autosomal dominant inheritance pattern.[301, 302] Up to one fourth of affected patients have glaucoma, and the risk of glaucoma increases with longer duration of the disease.

REFERENCES

1. Klein BE, Klein R: Intraocular pressure and cardiovascular risk variables. Arch Ophthalmol 1981;99:837.
2. Leske MC, Podgor MJ: Intraocular pressure, cardiovascular risk variables, and visual field defects. Am J Epidemiol 1983;118:280.
3. Shiose Y: The aging effect on intraocular pressure in an apparently normal population. Arch Ophthalmol 1984;102:883.
4. Shiose Y, Kawase Y: A new approach to stratified normal intraocular pressure in a general population. Am J Ophthalmol 1986;191:714.
5. Dielemans I, Vingerling JR, Algra D, et al.: Primary open-angle glaucoma, intraocular pressure and systemic blood pressure in the general elderly population. The Rotterdam Study. Ophthalmology 1995;102:54.
6. Kahn HA, Leibowitz HM, Galey JP, et al: The Framingham Eye Study. II: Association of ophthalmic pathology with single variables previously measured in the Framingham Heart Study. Am J Epidemiol 1977;106:33.
7. Wilson MR, Hertzmark E, Walker AM, et al.: A case-control study of risk factors in open angle glaucoma. Arch Ophthalmol 1987;105:1066.
8. Tielsch JM, Katz J, Sommer A, et al: Hypertension, perfusion pressure, and primary open -angle glaucoma: A population-based assessment. Arch Ophthalmol 1995;113:216.
9. Quigley HA, Enger C, Katz J, et al: Risk factors for the development of glaucomatous visual field loss in ocular hypertension. Arch Ophthalmol 1994;112:644.
10. Leske MC, Connell AMS, Wu SY, et al: Risk factor for open-angle glaucoma: The Barbados Eye Study. Arch Ophthalmol 1995; 113:918.
11. Drance SM: Some factors in the production of low tension glaucoma. Br J Ophthalmol 1972;56:229.
12. Drance SM, Sweeney VP, Morgan RW, et al: Studies of factors involved in the production of low tension glaucoma. Arch Ophthalmol 1973;89:457.
13. Richardson DW, Honour AJ, Fenton GW, et al: Variation in arterial pressure throughout the day and night. Clin Sci 1964;26:445.
14. Graham SL, Drance SM, Wijsman K, et al: Ambulatory blood pressure monitoring in glaucoma: The nocturnal dip. Ophthalmology 1995;102:61.
15. National High Blood Pressure Education Program Coordinating Committee: National High Blood Pressure Education Program Working Group report on ambulatory blood pressure monitoring. Arch Intern Med 1990;150:2270.
16. Verdecchia P, Porcellati C: The day-night changes in ambulatory blood pressure: Another risk indicator in hypertension? G Ital Cardiol 1992;22:879.
17. Pickering TG: The clinical significance of diurnal blood pressure variations: Dippers and non-dippers. Circulation 1990;81:700.
18. Hayreh SS, Zimmerman MB, Podhajsky P, et al: Nocturnal arterial hypotension and its role in optic nerve head and ocular ischemic disorders. Am J Ophthalmol 1994;117:603.
19. Grunwald JE, Riva CE, Stone RA, et al: Retinal autoregulation in open-angle glaucoma. Ophthalmology 1984;91:1690.
20. Kaiser HJ, Flammer J: Systemic hypotension: A risk factor for glaucomatous damage? Ophthalmologica 1991;203:105.
21. Orgul S, Kaiser HJ, Flammer J, et al: Systemic blood pressure and capillary blood-cell velocity in glaucoma patients: A preliminary study. Eur J Ophthalmol 1995;5:88.
22. Bresson-Dumont H, Bechetoille A: Role of arterial blood pressure in the development of glaucomatous lesions. J Fr Ophthalmol 1996;19:435.
23. Bresson-Dumont H, Bechetoille A: Arterial hypotension in glaucoma of normal or moderately high pressure. J Fr Ophthalmol 1995;18:128.
24. Bechetoille A, Bresson-Dumont H: Diurnal and nocturnal blood pressure drops in patients with focal ischemic glaucoma. Graefes Arch Clin Exp Ophthalmol 1994;232:675.
25. Gasser P: Clinical syndromes with vasoconstrictor response. Wein Klin Worchenschr 1991;103:217.
26. Flammer J: Psychophysical mechanisms and treatment of vasospastic disorders in normal-tension glaucoma. Bull Soc Belge Ophtalmol 1992;244:129.
27. Flammer J, Prunte C: Ocular vasospasm. 1: Functional circulatory disorders in the visual system, a working hypothesis. Klin Monatsbl Augenheilkd 1991;198:411.
28. O'Brien C, Butt Z: Blood flow velocity in the peripheral circulation of glaucoma patients. Ophthalmologica 1999;213:150–153.
29. Drance SM, Douglas GR, Wijsman K, et al: Response of blood flow to warm and cold in normal and low tension glaucoma patients. Am J Ophthalmol 1988;105:35.
30. Gasser P, Flammer J: Blood-cell velocity in the nailfold capillaries of patients with normal-tension and high-tension glaucoma. Am J Ophthalmol 1991;111:585.
31. Phelps CD, Corbett JJ: Migraine and low-tension glaucoma: A case control study. Invest Ophthalmol Vis Sci 1985;26:1105.
32. Stroman GA, Stewart WC, Golnik KC, et al: Magnetic resonance imaging in patients with low-tension glaucoma. Arch Ophthalmol 1995;113:168.
33. Gasser P, Flammer J: Influence of vasospasm on visual function. Doc Ophthalmol 1987;66:3.
34. Bouvier P, Berrod JP, Garniche J, et al: Ocular vasospasm in cold provocation test and primary vascular acrosyndrome. J Fr Ophtalmol 1995;18:151.
35. Rader J, Feuer WJ, Anderson DR: Peripapillary vasoconstriction in the glaucomas and the anterior ischemic optic neuropathies. Am J Ophthalmol 1994;117:72.
36. Rankin SJA, Drance SM: Peripapillary focal retinal arteriolar narrowing in open angle glaucoma. J Glaucoma 1996;5:22.
37. Piltz JR, Bose S, Lanchione D: The effect of nimodipine, a centrally

active calcium antagonist, on visual function and macular blood flow in patients with normal-tension glaucoma and controls. J Glaucoma 1998;7:336.
38. Kitazawa Y, Shirai H, Go FJ: The effect of calcium antagonist on visual field in low-tension glaucoma. Graefes Arch Clin Ophthalmol 1989;227:408.
39. Gaspar AZ, Flammer J, Hendrickson P: Influence of nifedipine on the visual fields of patients with optic-nerve-head diseases. Eur J Ophthalmol 1994;4:24.
40. Bose S, Piltz JR, Breton ME: Nimodipine, a centrally active calcium antagonist, exerts a beneficial effect on contrast sensitivity in patients with normal-tension glaucoma and in control subjects. Ophthalmology 1995;102(8):1236.
41. Netland PA, Grosskreutz CL, Feke GT, et al: Color Doppler ultrasound analysis of ocular circulation after topical calcium channel blocker. Am J Ophthalmol 1995;119:694.
42. Goldberg I, Hollows FC, Kass MA, et al: Systemic factors in patients with low-tension glaucoma. Br J Ophthalmol 1981;65:56.
43. Mermoud A: Glaucoma and risk factors: Comparative study of cardiovascular risk factors in primary open-angle glaucoma, normal-pressure glaucoma and simple ocular hypertension. Rev Med Suisse Romande 1996;116:51.
44. Klein BE, Klein R, Linton KL: Intraocular pressure in an American community: The Beaver Dam Eye Study. Invest Ophthalmol Vis Sci 1992;33:2224.
45. Winder AF: Circulating lipoprotein and blood glucose levels in association with low-tension and chronic simple glaucoma. Br J Ophthalmol 1977;61:641.
46. Stewart WC, Sine C, Sutherland S, et al: Total cholesterol and high-density lipoprotein levels as risk factors for increased intraocular pressure. Am J Ophthalmol 1996;122:575.
47. Chisholm IA, Stead S: Plasma lipid patterns in patients with suspected glaucoma. Can J Ophthalmol 1988;23:164.
48. Demailly P, Cambien F, Plouin PF, et al: Do patients with low tension glaucoma have particular cardiovascular characteristics? Ophthalmologica 1984;188:65.
49. Waldmann E, Gasser P, Dubler B, et al: Silent myocardial ischemia in glaucoma and cataract patients. Graefes Arch Clin Exp Ophthalmol 1996;234:595.
50. Schulzer M, Drance SM, Carter CJ, et al: Biostatistical evidence for two distinct chronic open angle glaucoma populations. Br J Ophthalmol 1990;74:196.
51. Passo MS, Goldberg L, Elliot DL, et al: Exercise training reduces intraocular pressure among subjects suspected of having glaucoma. Arch Ophthalmol 1991;109:1096.
52. Qureshi IA: The effects of mild, moderate, and severe exercise on intraocular pressure in glaucoma patients. Jpn J Physiol 1995;45:561.
53. Benson WE, Brown GC, Tasman W: Diabetes and Its Ocular Complications. Philadelphia; WB Saunders, 1988.
54. Christiansson J: Intraocular pressure in diabetes mellitus. Acta Ophthalmol 1961;39:155.
55. Leske MC, Podgor MJ: Intraocular pressure, cardiovascular risk variables and visual field defects. Am J Epidemiol 1983;118:280.
56. Klein BE, Klein R, Moss SE: Intraocular pressure in diabetic persons. Ophthalmol 1984;91:1356.
57. Tielsch JM, Katz J, Quigley HA, et al: Diabetes, intraocular pressure, and primary open-angle glaucoma in the Baltimore Eye Survey. Ophthalmology 1995;102:48.
58. Dielemans I, de Jong PT, Stolk R, et al: Primary open-angle glaucoma, intraocular pressure, and diabetes mellitus in the general elderly population: The Rotterdam Study. Ophthalmology 1996;103:1271.
59. Armaly MF, Baloglou PJ: Diabetes mellitus and the eye. II. Intraocular pressure and aqueous outflow facility. Arch Ophthalmol 1967;77:493.
60. Becker V: Diabetes mellitus and primary open-angle glaucoma: The XXVII Edward Jackson Memorial Lecture. Am J Ophthalmol 1971;71:1.
61. Kass MA, Sears ML: Hormonal regulation of intraocular pressure. Surv Ophthalmol 1977;22:153.
62. Nielsen NV: The prevalence of glaucoma and ocular hypertension in type 1 and 2 diabetes mellitus. Acta Ophthalmol (Copenh) 1983;61:662.
63. Kahn HA, Milton RC: Alternative definitions of open-angle glaucoma: Effect on prevalence and associations in the Framingham Eye Study. Arch Ophthalmol 1980;98:2172.
64. Armaly MF, Frueger DE, Maunder L, et al: Biostatistical analysis of the Collaborative Glaucoma Study. I. Summary report of the risk factors for glaucomatous visual-field defects. Arch Ophthalmol 1980;98:2163.
65. Mapstone R, Clark CV: Prevalence of diabetes in glaucoma. Br Med J 1985;291:93.
66. Klein BE, Klein R, Jensen SC: Open-angle glaucoma and older-onset diabetes: The Beaver Dam Eye Study. Ophthalmology 1994;101(7):1173.
67. Kahn HA, Leibowitz HM, Ganley JP, et al: The Framingham Eye Study 2: Association of ophthalmic pathology with single variables previously measured in the Framingham Heart Study. Am J Epidemiol 1977;106:33.
68. Clark CV, Mapstone R: The prevalence of diabetes mellitus in the family history of patients with primary glaucoma. Doc Ophthalmol 1986;62:161.
69. Mapstone R, Clark CV: The prevalence of autonomic neuropathy in glaucoma. Trans Ophthalmol Soc UK 1985;104:265.
70. Moore MV, Jeffcoate WJ, Haworth S: Autonomic neuropathy and the pathogenesis of glaucoma in diabetes mellitus. Diabet Med 1989;6:717.
71. Sorokanich S, Wand W, Nix HR: Angle-closure glaucoma and acute hyperglycemia. Arch Ophthalmol 1986;104:1434.
72. Teekhasaenee C, Ritch R: Glaucoma in phakomatosis pigmentovascularis. Ophthalmology 1997;104:150.
73. Weiss J, Ritch R: Glaucoma in the phakomatoses. *In* Ritch R, Shields MB, Krupin T (eds): The Glaucomas. St. Louis, CV Mosby, 1996, pp 899–924.
74. Sturge WA: A case of partial epilepsy due to a lesion of one of the vasomotor centers of the brain. Trans Clin Soc London 1879;12:162.
75. Beck RW, Hanno R: The phakomatoses. Int Ophthalmol Clin 1985;25:97.
76. Sullivan TJ, Clarke MP, Morin JD: The ocular manifestations of the Sturge-Weber syndrome. J Pediatr Ophthalmol Strabismus 1992;29:349.
77. Cibis GW, Tripathi RC, Tripathi BJ: Glaucoma in Sturge-Weber syndrome. Ophthalmology 1984;91:1061.
78. Weiss DI: Dual origin of glaucoma in encephalotrigeminal angiomatosis. Trans Ophthalmol Soc UK 1973;93:477.
79. Jorgenson JS, Guthoff R: Sturge-Weber syndrome: Glaucoma with elevated episcleral venous pressure. Klin Monatsbl Augenheilkd 1987;191:275.
80. Phelps CD: The pathogenesis of glaucoma in Sturge-Weber syndrome. Ophthalmology 1978;85:276.
81. Kranemann CF, Pavlin CJ, Trope GE: Ultrasound biomicroscopy in Sturge-Weber–associated glaucoma. Am J Ophthalmol 1998; 125:119.
82. Christensen GR, Records RE: Glaucoma and expulsive hemorrhage mechanisms in the Sturge-Weber syndrome. Ophthalmology 1979;86:1360.
83. Bellows AR, Chylack LT Jr, Epstein DL, et al: Choroidal effusion during glaucoma surgery in patients with prominent episcleral vessels. Arch Ophthalmol 1979;97:493.
84. Ritch R, Simmons RT, Krupin T, et al: Serous retinal detachment after glaucoma filtration surgery in Sturge-Weber syndrome. J Glaucoma 1992;1:58.
85. Turut P, Madelain T, Milazzo S: Uveal effusion following trabeculectomy in a case of Sturge-Weber-Krabbe syndrome. Bull Soc Ophtalmol Fr 1985;85:33.
86. Iwach AG, Hoskins HD Jr, Hetherington J Jr, et al: Analysis of surgical and medical management of glaucoma in Sturge-Weber syndrome. Ophthalmology 1990;97:904.
87. Klippel M, Trenaunay P: Du naevus variqueux ostéohypertrophique. Arch Gén Méd 1900;77:641.
88. Weber FP: Angioma formation in connection with hypertrophy of limbs and hemihypertrophy. Br J Dermatol 1907;190:231.
89. Weber FP: On the association of extensive hemangiomatosis nevus of the skin with cerebral (meningeal) hemangioma. Proc R Soc Med 1928;22:431.
90. Kontras SB: The Klippel-Trenaunay syndrome. Birth Defects 1974;10:177.
91. Reynolds JD, Johnson BL, Gloster S, et al: Glaucoma and Klippel-Trenaunay-Weber syndrome. Am J Ophthalmol 1988;106:494.

92. Teekhasaenee C, Ritch R, Rutnin U, et al: Ocular findings in oculodermal melanocytosis. Arch Ophthalmol 1990;108:1114.
93. Gonder JR, Nichol J, Augsburger JJ, et al: Ocular and oculodermal melanocytosis. Can J Ophthalmol 1985; 20:176.
94. Teekhasaenee C, Ritch R, Rutnin U, et al: Glaucoma in oculodermal melanocytosis. Ophthalmology 1990;97:562.
95. Goncalves V, Sandler T, O'Donnell FE: Open-angle glaucoma in melanosis oculi: Response to laser trabeculoplasty. Ann Ophthalmol 1988;17:33.
96. Shaffer RN, Weiss DI: Congenital and Pediatric Glaucomas. St. Louis, CV Mosby, 1970.
97. Von Recklinghausen F: Über die multiplen Fibrome der Haut und ihre Beziehung zu den multiplen Neuromen. Berlin, Hirschwald, 1882.
98. NIH Concensus Development Conference: Statement on neurofibromatosis. Arch Neurol 1988;45:575.
99. Lieb WA, Wirth WA, Geeraets WJ: Hydrophthalmos and neurofibromatosis. Confin Neurol 1958;19:230.
100. Gaas JDM: The phakomatoses. *In* Smith JL, (ed): Neuro-ophthalmology, vol 2. St. Louis, CV Mosby, 1965.
101. Grant WM, Walton DS: Distinctive gonioscopic findings in glaucoma due to neurofibromatosis. Arch Ophthalmol 1968;79:127.
102. Friedman MW, Ritchey CL: Unilateral congenital glaucoma, neurofibromatosis, and pseudoarthrosis. Arch Ophthalmol 1963;70:294.
103. Kaye LD, Rothner AD, Beauchamp GR, et al: Ocular findings associated with neurofibromatosis type II. Ophthalmology 1992; 99:1424.
104. Pearson-Webb JA, Kaiser-Kupfer MI, Eldridge R: Eye findings in bilateral acoustic (central) neurofibromatosis: Association with presenile lens opacities and cataracts but absence of Lische nodules. N Engl J Med 1986;315:1553.
105. Von Hippel E: Über eine sehr seltene Erkrankung der Netzhaut. Graefes Arch Clin Exp Ophthalmol 1904;59:83.
106. Lindau A: Studien uber Kleinhirncysten. Acta Pathol Microbiol Scand 1926;1(suppl):1.
107. Maher ER, Yates JR, Harries R, et al: Clinical features and natural history of von Hippel–Lindau disease. Q J Med 1990;77:1151.
108. Hosoe S, Brauch H, Yatif F, et al: Localization of the von Hippel–Lindau disease gene to a small region of chromosome 3. Genomics 1990;8:634.
109. Maher ER, Iselius L, Yates JR, et al: Von Hippel–Lindau diseases: A genetic study. J Med Genet 1991;28:443.
110. Watzke RC, Weingeist TA, Constantine JB: Diagnosis and management of von Hippel–Lindau disease. *In* Peyman GA, Apple DJ, Saunders DR, (eds): Intraocular Tumors. New York, Appleton-Century-Crofts, 1977.
111. Alward WLM, Johnson AT, Nishimura DY, et al: Molecular genetics of glaucoma: Current status. J Glaucoma 1996;5:276.
112. Serville FAB: Pericentric inversion and partial monosomy 4q associated with congenital anomalies. Hum Genet 1977;39:239.
113. Phillips JC, del Bono EA, Haines JL, et al: A second focus for Rieger syndrome maps to chromosome 13q14. Am J Hum Genet 1996;59:613.
114. Wesley RK, Baker JD, Golnick AL: Rieger's syndrome (oligodontia and primary mesodermal dysgenesis of the iris): Clinical features and report of an isolated case. J Pediatr Ophthalmol Strabismus 1978;15:67.
115. Shields MB: Axenfeld-Rieger syndrome. *In* Ritch R, Shields MB, Krupin T (eds): The Glaucomas. St. Louis, CV Mosby, 1996, pp 875–885.
116. Kleinman RE, Ketarian EL, Raptopoulos V, et al: Primary empty sella and Rieger's anomaly of the anterior chamber of the eye. N Engl J Med 1981;304:90.
117. Sadeghi-Nejad A, Senior B: Autosomal dominant transmission of isolated growth hormone deficiency in iris-dental dysplasia (Rieger's syndrome). J Pediatr 1974;85:644.
118. Kivlin JD, Fineman RM, Crandall AS, et al: Peters' anomaly as a consequence of genetic and nongenetic syndromes. Arch Ophthalmol 1986;104:61.
119. Azuma I: Peters' anomaly associated with glaucoma and chromosomal abnormality. Folia Ophthalmol Jpn 1984;35:1869.
120. Bateman JB, Maumenee IH, Sparkes RS: Peters' anomaly associated with partial deletion of the long arm of chromosome 2. Am J Ophthalmol 1984;97:11.
121. Cibis GW, Waeltermann J, Harris D: Peters' anomaly in association with ring 21 chromosomal abnormality. Am J Ophthalmol 1985; 100:733.
122. Trabousi EI, Maumenee IH: Peters' anomaly and associated congenital malformations. Arch Ophthalmol 1992;110:1739.
123. Franke U, George DL, Brown MG, et al: Gene dose effect: Intraband mapping of the LDH A locus using cells from four individuals with different interstitial deletions of 11p. Cytogenet Cell Genet 1977;19:197.
124. Churchill A, Booth A: Genetics of aniridia and anterior segment dysgenesis. Br J Ophthalmol 1996;80:669.
125. Nelson LB, Spaeth GL, Nowinski TS, et al: Aniridia: A review. Surv Ophthalmol 1984;28:621.
126. Gillespie, FD: Aniridia, cerebellar ataxia, and oligophrenia in siblings. Arch Ophthalmol 1965;73:338.
127. Goldmann H: Der Druck im schlemmschen canal bei normalen und glaucoma simplex. Experientia 1950;6:110.
128. Harris GJ, Rice PR: Angle closure in carotid cavernous fistula. Ophthalmology 1979;86:1521.
129. Weiss DI, Shaffer RN: Neovascular glaucoma complicating carotid-cavernous fistula. Arch Ophthalmol 1963;69:304.
130. Henderson JW, Schneider RC: The findings in carotid-cavernous fistula in a series of 17 cases. Am J Ophthalmol 1959;48:585.
131. Kupersmith MJ, Berenstein A, Flamm E, et al: Neuroophthalmology abnormalities and intravascular therapy of traumatic carotid cavernous fistulas. Ophthalmology 1986;93:906.
132. Weekers R, Delmarcelle Y: Pathogenesis of intraocular hypertension in cases of arteriovenous aneurysm. Arch Ophthalmol 1952;48:338.
133. Sanders M, Hoyt W: Hypoxic ocular sequelae of carotid cavernous fistulae: Study of the causes of visual failure before and after neurosurgical treatment in a series of 125 cases. Br J Ophthalmol 1969;53:82.
134. Miller N: Walsh and Hoyt's Clinical Neuro-Ophthalmology, 4th ed. Baltimore, Williams & Wilkins, 1988.
135. Haneken AM, Miller NR, Debrun GM, et al: Treatment of carotid-cavernous fistulas using a detachable balloon catheter through the superior ophthalmic vein. Arch Ophthalmol 1989;107:87.
136. Jorgensen JS, Guthoff R: Die rolle des episkleralen venedrucks bei der entstehung von sedundarglaukomen. Kllin Monatsbl Augenheilkd 1988;193:471.
137. Smith KD, Arthurs BP, Saheb N: An association between hypothyroidism and primary open-angle glaucoma. Ophthalmology 1993;100:1580.
138. Alfano JE, Alfano PA: Glaucoma and the superior vena caval obstruction syndrome. Am J Ophthalmol 1956;42:685.
139. Yablonski ME, Podos SM: Glaucoma secondary to elevated episcleral venous pressure. *In* Sheilds MD, Ritch R, (eds): The Secondary Glaucomas. St. Louis, CV Mosby, 1982.
140. Lokich JJ, Goodman R: Superior vena cava syndrome. JAMA 1975;231:58.
141. Bedrossian EH: Increased intraocular pressure secondary to mediastinal syndrome. Arch Ophthalmol 1952;47:641.
142. Flanagan JC: Vascular problems of the orbit: Symposium: Tumors of the lids and orbit. Ophthalmology 1979;86:896.
143. Lloyd GAS, Wright JE, Morgan G: Venous malformations in the orbit. Br J Ophthalmol 1971;55:505.
144. Wright JE: Orbital vascular anomalies. Trans Am Acad Ophthalmol Otolaryngol 1974;78:OP606.
145. Rathbun JE, Hoyt WF, Beard C: Surgical management of orbitofrontal varix in Klippel-Trenaunay-Weber syndrome. Am J Ophthalmol 1970;70:109.
146. Duke-Elder S, MacFaul PA: System of Ophthalmology: XIII. The Ocular Adnexa. St. Louis, CV Mosby, 1974.
147. Kollarits C, Gaasterland D, DiChiro G, et al: Management of a patient with orbital varices, visual loss, and ipsilateral glaucoma. Ophthalmol Surg 1977;8:54.
148. Cross HE, Jensen AL: Ocular manifestations in the Marfan syndrome and homocystinuria. Am J Ophthalmol 1973;75:405.
149. Wachtel JF: The ocular pathology of Marfan's syndrome. Arch Ophthalmol 1966;76:512.
150. Burian HM, Allen L: Histologic study of the chamber angle of patients with Marfan's syndrome. Arch Ophthalmol 1961;65:323.
151. Pyeritz RE, McKusick VA: The Marfan syndrome: Diagnosis and management. N Engl J Med 1979;300:772.
152. Maumenee IH: The eye in the Marfan syndrome. Trans Am Ophthalmol Soc 1981;79:684.

153. Dietz HC, Cutting GR, Pyeritz RE, et al: Marfan syndrome caused by recurrent de novo missense mutation in the fibrillin gene. Nature 1991;352:337.
154. Francke U, Furthmayr H: Marfan's syndrome and other disorders of fibrillin. N Engl J Med 1994;330:1384.
155. Hollister DW, Godfrey M, Sakai LY, et al: Immunohistologic abnormalities of the microfibrillar-fiber system in the Marfan syndrome. N Engl J Med 1990;323:152.
156. Murdoch JL, Walker BA, Halpern BL, et al: Life expectancy and causes of death in the Marfan syndrome. N Engl J Med 1972;286:804.
157. von Noorden GG, Schutz RO: A gonioscopic study of the chamber angle in Marfan's syndrome. Arch Ophthalmol 1960;64:929.
158. Nelson LB, Maumenee IH: Ectopia lentis. Surv Ophthalmol 1982;27:143.
159. Spaeth GW: Glaucomatous changes in homocystinuria. *Discussion of* Jay B: Glaucoma associated with spontaneous displacement of the lens. Br J Ophthalmol 1972;56:258.
160. Mudd SH, Levy HL, Skovby F: Disorders of transsulfuration. *In* Scriver CR, et al (eds): The Metabolic Basis of Inherited Disease, 6th ed, vol I. New York, McGraw-Hill, 1989, p 1463.
161. Irreverre F, Mudd SH, Heizer WD, et al: Sulfite oxidase deficiency: Studies of a patient with mental retardation, dislocated ocular lenses, and abnormal urinary excretion of S-sulfo-L-cysteine sulfite and thiosulfate. Biochem Med 1967;1:187.
162. Smith TH, Holland ME, Woody MC: Ocular manifestations of familial hyperlysinemia. Trans Am Acad Ophthalmol Otolaryngol 1971;75:355.
163. Dancis J, Hutzler J, Cox RP, et al: Familial hyperlysinemia with lysine-ketoglutarate reductase insufficiency. J Clin Invest 1969; 48:1447.
164. Durham DG: Cutis hyperelastica (Ehlers-Danlos syndrome) with blue scleras, microcornea, and glaucoma. Arch Ophthalmol 1953;49:220.
165. Beighton P: Serious ophthalmological complications in the Ehlers-Danlos syndrome. Br J Ophthalmol 1970;54:263.
166. Johnson VP, Grayson M, Christian JC: Dominant microspherophakia. Arch Ophthalmol 1971;85:534.
167. Probert LA: Spherophakia with brachydactyly. Am J Ophthalmol 1953;36:1571.
168. Sohar E: Renal disease, inner ear deafness and ocular changes: A new heredofamilial syndrome. Arch Intern Med 1956;97:627.
169. Bessiere E, Riviere J, Leuret JP: An association of Klinefelter's disease and congenital anomalies (captodactyly, microphakia). Bull Soc Ophthalmol Belge 1970;54:263.
170. Jensen AD, Cross HE, Paton D: Ocular complications in the Weill-Marchesani syndrome. Am J Ophthalmol 1974;77:261.
171. Streeten BW: Pseudoexfoliative fibrillopathy in the skin of patients with ocular pseudoexfoliation. Am J Ophthalmmol 1990;110:490.
172. Schlotzer-Schrehardt UM: Pseudoexfoliation syndrome: Ocular manifestation of a systemic disorder? Arch Ophthalmol 1992; 110:1752.
173. Streeten BW, Li ZY, Wallace RN, et al: Pseudoexfoliative fibrillopathy in visceral organs of a patient with pseudoexfoliation syndrome. Arch Ophthalmol 1992;110:1757.
174. Olivus E, Polland W: Histocompatibility (HLA) antigens in capsular glaucoma and simplex glaucoma. Acta Ophthalmol (Copenh) 1980;58:406.
175. Ringvold A, Blika S, Elsas T: The middle-Norway eye-screening study. III: The prevalence of capsular glaucoma is influenced by blood-group antigens. Acta Ophthalmol (Copenh) 1993;71:207.
176. Ritch R: Exfoliation syndrome: The most common identifiable cause of open-angle glaucoma. J Glaucoma 1994;3:176.
177. Taylor HR: Pseudoexfoliation, an environmental disease? Trans Ophthalmol Soc UK 1979;99:302.
178. Roth M, Epstein DL: Exfoliation syndrome. Am J Ophthalmol 1980;89:477.
179. Cashwell LF, Shields MB: Exfoliation syndrome: Prevalence in a southeastern United States population. Arch Ophthalmol 1988; 106:335.
180. Hiller R, Sperduto RD, Kreuger DE: Pseudoexfoliation, intraocular pressure, and senile lens changes in a population-based survey. Arch Ophthalmol 1982;100:1080.
181. Layden WE, Shaffer RN: Exfoliation syndrome. Am J Ophthalmol 1974;78:835.
182. Puska P: The amount of lens exfoliation and chamber-angle pigmentation in exfoliation syndrome with or without glaucoma. Acta Ophthalmol Scand 1995;73:226.
183. Bartholomew RS: Pseudoexfoliation and angle-closure glaucoma. Glaucoma 1981; 3:213.
184. Wishart PK, Spaeth GL, Poryzees EM: Anterior chamber angle in the exfoliation syndrome. Br J Ophthalmol 1985;69:103.
185. Ritch R: Exfoliation syndrome: Clinical findings and occurrence in patients with occludable angles. Trans Am Ophthalmol Soc 1994;92:845.
186. Futa R, Furuyoshi N: Phacodenesis in capsular glaucoma: A clinical and electron microscope study. Jpn J Ophthalmol 1989;33:311.
187. Brown GC, Magargal LE, Schachat A, et al: Neovascular glaucoma. Etiologic considerations. Ophthalmology 1984;91:315.
188. Nielsen NV: The prevalence of glaucoma and ocular hypertension in type 1 and 2 diabetes mellitus on the island of Falster, Denmark. Acta Ophthalmol (Copenh) 1983;61:662.
189. Gerich JE: Insulin-dependent diabetes mellitus: Pathophysiology. Mayo Clin Proc 1986;61:787.
190. Saudek CD: Non-ophthalmologic findings of the Diabetes Control and Complications Trial. Surv Ophthalmol 1995;40:157.
191. Diabetes Control and Complications Trial: The relationship of glycemic exposure (HbA1c) to the risk of development and progression of retinopathy in the Diabetes Control and Complications Trial. Diabetes 1995;44:68.
192. Diabetes Control and Complications Trial: Progression of retinopathy with intensive versus conventional treatment in the Diabetes Control and Complications Trial Research Group. Ophthalmology 1995;102:647.
193. Saudek CD, Selam JL, Pitt HA, et al: A preliminary trial of the programmable implantable medication system for insulin delivery. N Engl J Med 1989;321:574.
194. Saudek CD: Future developments in insulin delivery systems. Diabetes Care 1993;16(Suppl 3):122.
195. Hayreh SS: Classification of central retinal vein occlusion. Ophthalmology 1983;90:458.
196. Central Vein Occlusion Study Group: Baseline and early natural history report. Arch Ophthalmol 1993;111:1087.
197. Magargal LE, Donoso LA, Sanborn GE: Retinal ischemia and risk of neovascularization following central retinal vein obstruction. Ophthalmology 1982;89:1241.
198. Laatikainen L, Kohner EM, Khoury D, et al: Panretinal photocoagulation in central retinal vein occlusion: A randomised controlled clinical study. Br J Ophthalmol 1977;61:741.
199. David R, Zangivill L, Badasna M, et al: Epidemiology of retinal vein occlusion and its association with glaucoma and increased intraocular pressure. Ophthalmologica 1988;197:69.
200. Frucht J, Shapero A, Merin S: Intraocular pressure in retinal vein occlusion. Br J Ophthalmol 1984;68:26.
201. Cole MD, Dodson PM, Hendeles S: Medical conditions underlying retinal vein occlusion in patients with glaucoma or ocular hypertension. Br J Ophthalmol 1989;73:693.
202. McGrath MA, Wecksler F, Hunyor AB, et al: Systemic factors contributory to retinal vein occlusion. Arch Intern Med 1978; 138:216.
203. Dodson PM, Galton DJ, Hamilton AM: Retinal vein occlusion and the prevalence of lipoprotein abnormalities. Br J Ophthalmol 1982;66:161.
204. Elman MJ, Bhatt AK, Quonlan PM, et al: The risk for systemic vascular diseases and mortality in patients with central retinal vein occlusion. Ophthalmology 1990;97:1543.
205. Appiah AP, Trempe CL: Differences in the contributory factors among hemicentral, central, and branch retinal vein occlusions. Ophthalmology 1989;96:365.
206. Arend O, Remky A, Jung F, et al: Role of rheologic factors in patients with acute central retinal vein occlusion. Ophthalmology 1996;103:80.
207. Prince HM, Thurlow PJ, Buchanan RC, et al: Acquired protein S deficiency in a patient with systemic lupus erythematosus causing central retinal vein thrombosis. J Clin Pathol 1995;48:387.
208. Yoshizumi MO, Townsend-Pico W: Essential thrombocythemia and central retinal vein occlusion with neovascular glaucoma. Am J Ophthalmol 1996;121:728.
209. Brown GC, Shah HG, Magasgal LE, et al: Central retinal vein obstruction and carotid artery disease. Ophthalmology 1984; 91:1627.

210. Lazzaro EC: Retinal-vein occlusions: Carotid artery evaluation indicated. Ann Ophthalmol 1986;18:116.
211. Wagner WH, Weaver FA, Brinkley JR, et al: Chronic ocular ischemia and neovascular glaucoma: A result of extracranial carotid artery disease. J Vasc Surg 1988;8:551.
212. Bennett LW: Ocular ischemic syndrome as initial manifestation of bilateral carotid occlusive disease. J Am Optom Assoc 1997;68:250.
213. Executive Committee for the Asymptomatic Carotid Atherosclerosis Study: Endarterectomy for asymptomatic carotid artery stenosis. JAMA 1995;273:1421.
214. Riles TS, Liberman A, Kopelman I, et al: Symptoms, stenosis, and bruit: Interrelationships in carotid artery disease. Arch Surg 1981;116:218.
215. Ho AC, Fieb WE, Flaharty PM, et al: Color Doppler imaging of the ocular ischemic syndrome. Ophthalmology 1992;99:1453.
216. Hood DB, Mattos MA, Mansour A: Prospective evaluation of new duplex criteria to identify 70% internal carotid artery stenosis. J Vasc Surg 1996;23:254.
217. Hu WY, TerBruggee KG: The role of angiography in the evaluation of vascular and neoplastic disease in the external carotid artery circulation. Neuroimaging Clin N Am 1996;6:625.
218. North American Symptomatic Carotid Endarterectomy Trial Collaborators: Beneficial effect of carotid endarterectomy in symptomatic patients with high-grade carotid stenosis. N Engl J Med 1991;325:445.
219. Boberg-Ans J, Vesti Nielsen N: Neovascular glaucoma as the primary ocular complication in temporal arteritis. Glaucoma 1986; 8:138.
220. DeJong PTVMP: Neovascular glaucoma and the occurrence of twin vessels in congenital arteriovenous communications of the retina. Doc Ophthalmol 1988;68:205.
221. Duker JS, Sivalingam A, Brown GC: A prospective study of acute central retinal artery obstruction: The incidence of secondary ocular neovascularization. Arch Ophthalmol 1991;109:339.
222. Duker JS, Brown GC: Iris neovascularization associated with obstruction of the central retinal artery. Ophthalmology 1988;95:1244.
223. Cohen SB, Fletcher ME, Goldberg MF, et al: Diagnosis and management of ocular complications of sickle hemoglobinopathies: Part V. Ophthalmic Surg 1986;17:369.
224. Bergren RL, Brown GC: Neovascular glaucoma secondary to sickle-cell retinopathy. Am J Ophthalmol 1992;113:718.
225. Goldberg MF, Tso MO: Rubeosis iridis and glaucoma associated with sickle cell retinopathy: A light and electron microscopic study. Ophthalmology 1978;85:1028.
226. Friedman AH, Halpern BL, Freedberg DN, et al: Transient open-angle glaucoma associated with sickle cell trait: Report on four cases. Br J Ophthalmol 1979;63:832.
227. Shapiro AL, Baum JL: Acute open-angle glaucoma in a patient with sickle cell trait. Am J Ophthalmol 1964;58:292.
228. Goldberg MF: The diagnosis and treatment of secondary glaucoma after hyphema in sickle cell patients. Am J Ophthalmol 1979;87:43.
229. Nussenblatt RB, Palestine AG: Ankylosing spondylitis. *In* Uveitis: Fundamentals and Clinical practice, St Louis, Mosby, 1989.
230. Brewerton DA, Hart FD, Nicholls A, et al: Ankylosing spondylitis and HLA-B27. Lancet 1973;1:904.
231. Olmo S, Char DH, Kimura SJ, et al: HLA antigens and antinuclear antibody titers in juvenile chronic iridocyclitis. Br J Ophthalmol 1977;61:59.
232. Kanski JJ: Anterior uveitis in juvenile rheumatoid arthritis. Arch Ophthalmol 1977;95:1974.
233. Wolf MD, Lichter PR, Ragsdale CG: Prognostic factors in the uveitis of juvenile rheumatoid arthritis. Ophthalmology 1987; 94:1242.
234. Tugal-Tutkun I, Havrlikova K, Power WJ, et al: Changing patterns in uveitis of childhood. Ophthalmology 1966;103:375.
235. Mitchell DN, Scadding JG, Heard BE, et al: Sarcoidosis: Histopathological definition and clinical diagnosis. J Clin Pathol 1977;30:395.
236. Obenauf CD, Shaw HE, Sydnor CF, et al: Sarcoidosis and its ophthalmic manifestations. Am J Ophthalmol 1978;86:648.
237. Hurley TH, Sullivan JR, Hurley JV: Reaction of Kveim test material in sarcoidosis and other diseases. Lancet 1975;1:494.
238. Weinberg RS, Tessler HH: Serum lysozyme in sarcoid uveitis. Am J Ophthalmol 1976;82:105.
239. Weinreb RN, Kimura SJ: Uveitis associated with sarcoidosis and angiotensin-converting enzyme. Trans Am Ophthalmol Soc 1979; 77:280.
240. Bornstein JS, Frank MI, Radner DB: Conjunctival biopsy in the diagnosis of sarcoidosis. N Engl J Med 1962;267:60.
241. Merritt J, Lipper SI, Peiffer RL, et al: Conjunctival biopsy in sarcoidosis. J Natl Med Assoc 1980;72:347.
242. Akova YA, Foster CS: Cataract surgery in patients with sarcoidosis-associated uveitis. Ophthalmology 1994;101:473.
243. Nussenblatt RB, Palestein AG: Vogt-Koyanagi-Harada syndrome (uveomeningitic syndrome). *In* Schachat AP, Muphy RB, Patz A (eds): Retina, vol 2. St. Louis, Mosby, 1989.
244. Kimura R, Sakai M, Okabe H: Transient shallow anterior chamber as initial symptom in Harada's syndrome. Arch Ophthalmol 1981;99:1604.
245. Forster DJ, Rao NA, Hell RA, et al: Incidence and management of glaucoma in Vogt-Koyanagi-Harada syndrome. Ophthalmology 1993;100:613.
246. Sugiura S: Vogt-Koyanagi-Harada disease. Jpn J Ophthalmol 1978;22:9.
247. Michelson JB, Chisari FV: Behçet's disease. Surv Ophthalmol 1982;26:190.
248. Mishima S, Masuda K, Izawa Y, et al: The Eighth Frederick H Verhoeff Lecture: Behçet's disease in Japan: Ophthalmologic aspects. Trans Am Ophthalmol Soc 1979;77:225.
249. Winter FC, Yukin RE: The ocular pathology of Behçet's disease. Am J Ophthalmol 1966;62:257.
250. Wakefield D, McCluskey P: Cyclosporine: A therapy in inflammatory eye disease. J Ocul Pharmacol 1991;7:221.
251. Salmon J, Wright JP, Murray AD: Ocular inflammation in Crohn's disease. Ophthalmology 1991;98:480.
252. Hopkins DJ, Horan E, Burton IL, et al: Ocular disorders in a series of 332 patients with Crohn's disease. Br J Ophthalmol 1974;58:732.
253. Petrell EA, McKinley M, Troncale FJ: Ocular manifestations of inflammatory bowel disease. Ann Ophthalmol 1982;14:356.
254. Walmsley RS, Gillen CD, Allen RN: Prognosis and management of Crohn's disease in the over-55 age group. Postgrad Med J 1907;73:225.
255. Griffiths AM, Ohlsson A, Sherman PM, et al: Meta-analysis of enteral nutrition as a primary treatment of active Crohn's disease. Gastroenterology 1995;108:1056.
256. Watson PG, Hayreh SS: Scleritis and episcleritis. Br J Ophthalmol 1976;60:163.
257. Falcon MG, Williams HP: Herpes simplex keratouveitis and glaucoma. Trans Ophthalmol Soc UK 1978;98:101.
258. Johns KJ, O'Day DM, Webb RA, et al: Anterior segment ischemia in chronic herpes simplex keratouveitis. Curr Eye Res 1991;10:117.
259. Erlich KS: Management of herpex simplex and varicella-zoster virus infections. West J Med 1997;166:211.
260. Ostler HG, Thygeson P: The ocular manifestations of herpes zoster, varicella, infectious mononucleosis, and cytomegalovirus disease. Surv Ophthalmol 1976;21:148.
261. Panek WC, Holland GN, Lee DA, et al: Glaucoma in patients with uveitis. Br J Ophthalmol 1990;74:223.
262. Womack LW, Liesegang TJ: Complications of herpes zoster ophthalmicus. Arch Ophthalmol 1983;101:42.
263. Nigam P, Kumar A, Kapaar KK, et al: Clinical profile of herpes zoster ophthalmicus. J Indian Med Assoc 1991;89:117.
264. Alhalel A: Bilateral simultaneous acute angle closure glaucoma in a herpes zoster. Br J Ophthalmol 1991;75:510.
265. Cobo LM, Faulks GN, Liesegang T, et al: Oral acyclovir in the therapy of acute herpes zoster ophthalmicus. An interim report. Ophthalmology 1985;92:1574.
266. Palestine AG, Rodrigues MM, Macher AM, et al: Ophthalmic involvement in acquired immunodeficiency syndrome. Ophthalmology 1984;91:1092.
267. Holland GN, Pepose JS, Pettit TH, et al: Acquired immune deficiency syndrome: Ocular manifestations. Ophthalmology 1983; 90:859.
268. Arvalo JF, Munguia D, Faber D, et al: Correlation between intraocular pressure and CD4+ T-lymphocyte counts in patients with human immunodeficiency virus with and without cytomegalovirus retinitis. Am J Ophthalmol 1996;1221:91.
269. Ullman S, Wilson RP, Schwartz L: Bilateral angle-closure glaucoma in association with the acquired immune deficiency syndrome. Am J Ophthalmol 1986;101:469.
270. Koster HR, Liebmann JM, Ritch R, et al: Acute angle-closure glaucoma in a patient with acquired immunodeficiency syndrome

successfully treated with argon laser peripheral iridoplasty. Ophthalmic Surg 1990;21:501.
271. Riffenburgh RS: Iritis and glaucoma associated with mumps. Arch Ophthalmol 1954;51:702.
272. Polland W, Thorburn W: Transient glaucoma as a manifestation of mumps. Acta Ophthalmol (Copenh) 1976;54:779.
273. Wolff SMK: The ocular manifestations of congenital rubella. Trans Am Ophthalmol Soc 1972;70:577.
274. Tuffanelli DL, Wuepper KD, Bradford LL, et al: Fluorescent treponemal antibody absorption tests: Studies of false positive reactions to test for syphilis, N Engl J Med 1967;276:258.
275. Tsukahara S: Secondary glaucoma due to inactive congenital syphilitic interstitial keratitis. Ophthalmologica 1977;174:188.
276. Elkins BS, Holland GN, Opremcak EM, et al: Ocular toxoplasmosis misdiagnosed as cytomegalovirus retinopathy in immunocompromised patients. Ophthalmology 1994;101:499.
277. Moorthy RS, Smith RE, Rao NA: Progressive ocular toxoplasmosis in patients with acquired immunodeficiency syndrome. Am J Ophthalmol 1993;115:742.
278. Ruskin J, Remington JS: Toxoplasmosis in the compromised host. Ann Intern Med 1976;84:193.
279. Friedmann CT, Knox DL: Variations in recurrent active toxoplasmic retinochoroiditis. Arch Ophthalmol 1969;81:481.
280. Whitworth JA, Gilbert CE, Mabey DM, et al: Visual loss in an onchocerciasis endemic community in Sierra Leone. Br J Ophthalmol 1993;77:30.
281. Kittiponghansa S, et al: Intracameral gnathostomiasis: A cause of anterior uveitis and secondary glaucoma. Br J Ophthalmol 1987; 71:618.
282. Kass MA, Sears ML: Hormonal regulation of intraocular pressure. Surv Ophthalmol 1977;22:153.
283. Kushner LF: Disorders of regulation of intraocular pressure in acromegaly and in pregnant women with acromegaloid syndrome. Vestn Oftalmol 1966;79:89.
284. Howard GM, English FT: Occurrence of glaucoma in acromegalics. Arch Ophthalmol 1965;73:765.
285. Bramson T, Klauber A, Bjerre P: Central corneal thickness and intraocular tension in patients with acromegaly. Acta Ophthalmol (Copenh) 1980;58:971.
286. Ehlers N, Bramsen T, Sperling S: Applanation tonometry and central corneal thickness. Acta Ophthalmol (Copenh) 1975;53:34.
287. Van Bijsterveld OP, Richards RD: Pituitary tumors and intraocular pressure. Am J Ophthalmol 1964;57:267.
288. Schmelzer H: Hypophyse and glaukomgenese. Klin Monatsbl Augenheilkd 1956;129:114.
289. Yamabayashi S, Yamamoto T, Sasaki T, et al: A case of 'low tension glaucoma' with primary empty sella. Br J Ophthalmol 1988;72:852.
290. Krasnovid TA: A new hypothesis on the mechanism of diurnal variations in intraocular tension. Oftalmol Zh 1966;21:185.
291. Haas JS, Nootens RH: Glaucoma secondary to benign adrenal adenoma. Am J Ophthalmol 1974;78:497.
292. Kass MA, Sears ML: Hormonal regulation of intraocular pressure. Surv Ophthalmol 1977;22:153.
293. Burn RA: Intraocular pressure during hemodialysis. Br J Ophthalmol 1973;57:511.
294. Ramsell JT, Ellis PP, Patterson CA, et al: Intraocular pressure changes during hemodialysis. Am J Ophthalmol 1971;72:926.
295. Sitprija V, Holmes JH, Ellis PP, et al: Intraocular pressure changes during artificial kidney therapy. Arch Ophthalmol 1964;72:626.
296. Lentzch S, Colombi A: Intraocular pressure (IOP) in patients on long-term hemodialysis treatment. Kidney Int 1975;7:365.
297. Jaeger PH, et al: Prevention of glaucoma during hemodialysis by mannitol and acetazolamide. N Engl J Med 1980;303:702.
298. Blomdahl S, Calissendorff B, Magnusson G: Ocular complications in recipients of kidney transplants. Scand J Urol Nephrol 1977; 42(suppl):195.
299. Hovland KR, Ellis PP: Ocular changes in renal transplant patients. Am J Ophthalmol 1967;63:283.
300. Wilson DM, Martin JHS: Raised intraocular tension in renal transplant recipients. Med J Aust 1973;1:482.
301. Chandler PA, Grant WM: Amyloidosis and open-angle glaucoma. *In* Glaucoma, 2nd ed. Philadelphia, Lea & Febiger, 1979.
302. Paton D, Kuke JR: Primary familial amyloidosis (ocular manifestations with histopathologic observations). Am J Ophthalmol 1966; 61:736.

CHAPTER 9

Normal-Pressure Glaucoma*

MARTIN B. WAX

There are many locations within this book to place the chapter that discusses normal-pressure glaucoma. This particular position was chosen to emphasize the possible impact of systemic factors on the care of all patients with glaucoma and how each patient's history must play a key role in identification. Although it increasingly appears that these systemic attributes may have particular significance in the normal-pressure glaucomas, they can be important in other forms of glaucoma as well. The better we understand these factors, the better we will understand and be able to treat glaucoma. In this chapter, Marty Wax presents the definition, natural history, diagnosis, variants, and patient evaluation for normal-pressure glaucoma. He also discusses the key ocular and systemic signs and symptoms that prompt a higher level of suspicion of the diagnosis. Finally, he considers the unique implications of treatment for the patient with normal-pressure glaucoma.

Definition

WHAT'S IN A NAME?

Open-angle glaucoma (OAG), the second leading cause of irreversible blindness in the United States,[1] comprises two major syndromes: primary OAG (POAG) and normal-pressure glaucoma (NPG). POAG is a disease generally characterized by a clinical triad consisting of (1) elevated intraocular pressure (IOP), (2) the appearance of optic atrophy, presumably resulting from elevated IOP, and (3) a progressive loss of peripheral visual sensitivity in the early stages of the disease, which may ultimately progress to impair central visual acuity.[2] POAG affects approximately 0.5% of the American population,[3] occurring in 1.3% of white Americans and 4.7% of black Americans older than 40 years (1.6 million people).[4] Studies have indicated, however, that a surprisingly high percentage of patients with OAG have findings identical to those in patients with POAG but with a singular exception, namely, that the IOP has never been demonstrated to be elevated. This form of glaucoma is often called "low-tension glaucoma," but also goes by the names "normal-tension glaucoma" and "normal-pressure glaucoma."

Numerous arguments and custom may be used to justify either of these two latter terms, but it is prudent to state the obvious: (1) there is nothing "low" about the range of IOPs in these patients, and (2) the use of the word "tension" is idiosyncratic to the field of ophthalmology, because it is a term used to describe tonometric readings. I and my colleagues prefer the word "pressure" because it is more readily understood by our medical colleagues and patients alike. Furthermore, since there is no widely acknowledged effective therapy for this disorder, "tension" is, unfortunately, most descriptive of the interactions that commonly occur between the physician and the patient with this disorder, and it is often anything but low! In this chapter, therefore, "normal-pressure glaucoma" is used for this syndrome.

NATURAL HISTORY

Several large population-based studies have documented the high prevalence of NPG.[5] Although a few of these

*This study was supported in part by EY06841, the American Health Assistance Foundation, Washington, DC, and the Glaucoma Research Foundation, San Francisco, CA, and by an unrestricted grant to Washington University from Research to Prevent Blindness, Inc, New York, NY.

studies suggest that as many as 50% of patients with OAG may indeed have NPG, more conservative estimations prevail in numerous population studies. It is reasonable, therefore, to consider that approximately 25% of cases with OAG occur in the presence of normal IOP.[6]

Little is known about the natural history of NPG. Most experts, however, believe that although the hallmark of this syndrome is progression of visual field loss (as it is for POAG), there are often long periods, often years, in which the visual fields are stable. Unfortunately, in some patients, episodes of rapid deterioration can and do occur within a relatively short time, typically several months to a year. One long-term, population-based study found that 62% of patients with NPG showed progression of visual field loss over 5 years.[7] This rate was significantly worse than that in the 42% of patients with POAG who were tested and followed similarly during the same period. NPG is therefore often a disease marked by continued progression of visual field loss, but not all patients experience such progression even during long periods of follow-up. In many patients, episodic deterioration is interrupted by long intervals of stable visual function.

Several findings make NPG particularly difficult for the ophthalmologist to treat. Most apparent, however, is that IOP, the target of conventional glaucoma therapy, is no longer an attractive parameter to lower, because it is already within the normal range in these cases. Several investigators have speculated, however, that further lowering of IOP may still be beneficial, presumably by facilitating vascular perfusion in the region of the lamina cribrosa, because blood flow will occur against less resistance if the IOP is lowered. There is limited but controversial data from a national prospective study that suggests the rate of visual field loss in patients with NPG is reduced when the IOP is further lowered by 30% from baseline values.[8]

Ongoing studies in Britain have suggested that visual field deterioration may indeed be minimized or limited in patients in whom IOP is lowered effectively by filtration surgery.[9, 10] Furthermore, in eyes with asymmetric IOPs lower than 21 mm Hg and visual field loss in one eye, the eye with the field loss almost invariably has the higher IOP.[11, 12] Such studies, coupled with our inability to offer better alternatives, serve as the basis for our rationale that effective lowering of IOP, by medication, laser, or surgery, may be a useful therapeutic intervention for many patients with NPG.

Making the Diagnosis

A DIAGNOSIS OF EXCLUSION

The diagnosis of NPG is a diagnosis of exclusion. NPG is defined by the clinical constellation of (1) open iridocorneal angles, (2) normal IOP, (3) optic nerve damage, and (4) visual field loss that is progressive and may ultimately impair central vision.

The first issue that must be evaluated as an inclusion criterion is what precisely is meant by normal IOP. Although it is well known that IOP obeys a non-gaussian distribution in humans,[13] several studies specify IOP values as acceptable threshold levels for the diagnosis of NPG. These values generally range between 20 and 24 mm Hg, and although they may have some utility for clinical studies, they should be viewed with less importance in an office setting. These threshold values certainly are *not* criteria for defining glaucoma. The key question the practitioner must ask is, "Do I think my patient has a component of pressure-related glaucomatous neuropathy or not?" When a patient's IOPs are elevated to more than 3 standard deviations above the population mean (e.g., >25 mm Hg), it is often easier to guess the right answer. When pressures are between 15 and 20 mm Hg, however, the answer to this question is not nearly so easy to ascertain.

Another well-accepted inclusion criterion for NPG is progressive changes in either visual fields or optic nerve cupping. In many patients, changes in both visual fields and cupping occur. However, deterioration of either constitutes legitimate glaucomatous progression.

Most importantly, the definition of NPG implies the absence of alternative causes of optic neuropathy, such as meningeal disease, infections (e.g., syphilis), inflammation, ischemic disease, and compressive lesions that may account for anterior nerve fiber bundle loss. Other causes of optic neuropathy, of course, are those in which episodic or transient elevation of IOP has been documented previously, such as occurs in steroid responsiveness, or as a sequela of some forms of trauma or intraocular disease.

Simple ophthalmoscopic examination is often helpful in ruling out ocular conditions that may mimic glaucomatous nerve fiber layer damage, such as congenital anomalies of the optic disc, choroidopathies (e.g., toxoplasmosis lesions), and retinal lesions (e.g., retinoschisis). Most often such conditions are easily recognized. Furthermore, they generally constitute nonprogressive lesions and are therefore not easily confused with genuine glaucoma.

VARIANTS

Now that we have satisfactorily ruled out numerous possible causes of intrinsic glaucomatous neuropathy, as well as other conditions that may resemble glaucomatous damage, we are left with a clinical entity whose name, normal-pressure glaucoma, unfortunately tells us little about its underlying pathophysiology. Because the hallmark of medical therapy is that it is directed at preventing or ameliorating specific pathologic processes, it should be no surprise that we have little to offer to patients with this disorder. Fortunately, however, the clinician can often gain useful insight into the factors underlying glaucomatous damage in individual patients. It is becoming increasingly clear that NPG is likely composed of numerous clinical variants affecting subsets of patients in whom there appear distinct similarities and thus clues as to the etiology of neuronal cell death. The most common variants of NPG may be characterized by the following features:

- No known cause identified (idiopathic)
- History of migraine headaches and/or peripheral vasospasm
- Evidence of aberrant systemic, serum, or retinal autoimmunity (i.e., specific antiretinal antibodies)
- Presence of nocturnal systemic hypotension
- Occurrence of hypovolemic shock (e.g., blood loss that usually requires transfusions)

□ Hyposecretion coexisting with impaired outflow (so-called burnt-out glaucoma)
□ Falsely low IOP recordings due to excessive corneal thinness[13]

Although distinctions in these heterogeneous patients with NPG may often be made clinically, the advent of modern genetic techniques makes it likely that a hereditary factor will be identified for one or more of the subsets of patients with these variants. The chromosomal loci (2cen-q13) of genes responsible for at least one form of NPG that typically manifests in the fifth decade has already been identified.[14]

The finding that there are identifiable subsets of patients within the population with NPG is not surprising, in light of contemporary views of the pathogenesis of glaucoma. In addition to high IOP, evidence is rapidly accumulating that prompts us to consider that damage to the optic nerve may be initiated or sustained by any number of the factors listed previously, in addition to others, such as excitotoxicity, neurotrophin insufficiency, and peroxynitrite damage as well as yet undefined factors. These different injurious influences then act through common final pathways that eventually disturb ion transport and activate the cellular proteases that accompany neuronal programmed cell death.

LABORATORY EVALUATION

Certainly, in order to rule out certain systemic considerations to help confirm the diagnosis of NPG, it is reasonable to perform several laboratory and radiologic tests. In general, two schools of thought have always tempered the clinical judgment of ophthalmologists regarding testing of patients in whom NPG is suspected. Some practitioners order almost no tests whatsoever, and others arrange for every test imaginable. We would advocate that, in general, it is reasonable to perform limited testing to detect certain obvious disorders that are treatable, or require further medical evaluation to assess potential treatment, in all patients with NPG. The following tests should be viewed as the minimal essential testing to be performed, with the rationale for choosing them:

1. *Complete blood count with differential and platelet counts:* There is no easier test with which to identify obvious blood dyscrasias or common anemias, which may impair the delivery of oxygen to the high-energy requirement tissues of the retina and optic nerve.
2. *Antinuclear antibody (ANA) panel:* A useful screen for collagen vascular disease and other autoimmune abnormalities. A hospital generally offers ANA panels of varying complexity, and we would advocate that the most complete panel offered, which typically tests for antibodies to extractable nuclear antigens such as Ro/SSA, La, and Sm antibodies, are the most useful. Confirmation of the presence of any of these autoantibodies may signify the identification of the autoimmune subset of patients with NPG.[15]
3. *Venereal Disease Research Laboratory (VDRL) test and fluorescent treponemal antigen (FTA).* One of the great imitators of glaucomatous optic neuropathy is indeed luetic disease. In our experience, 2 of every 100 patients with optic atrophy who have been referred for NPG have tertiary syphilis that requires treatment.
4. *Serum immunofixation for paraproteins:* In our experience, in a tertiary care setting, approximately 10% to 15% of patients with NPG have a monoclonal gammopathy (i.e., paraproteinemia), a clonal expansion of B cells that produces excessive serum immunoglobulin.[16] The majority of monoclonal gammopathies in an older adult population generally represent benign conditions (monoclonal gammopathy of undetermined significance). Approximately one third of the gammopathies, however, turn out to be caused by lymphoproliferative disorders, such as multiple myeloma and other neoplastic conditions. It is recommended, therefore, that the ophthalmologist test for this condition and refer that patient in whom a paraproteinemia is found to a hematologist for further evaluation, which may include a bone marrow aspirate. Although paraproteinemias can often be determined by obtaining full serum protein electrophoresis profiles, a much easier and cheaper test is available in most laboratories in which immunofixation testing is performed in order to detect a serum monoclonal protein.

Additional laboratory tests that may be useful in selected patients are:

1. *SMA 12/60 (Sequential Multiple Analyzer [12 tests in 60 minutes]):* It is not unreasonable to obtain electrolyte determinations and studies of liver and renal function in patients in whom there is a high index of suspicion of such disease. We have found, however, that routine testing for these values has been rather unproductive in virtually all patients with NPG.
2. *Complement studies:* Testing for C3 and C4 complement components has been unproductive in our experience as an assessment of potential collagen vascular disease.
3. *Vitamin B12 and folate measurements:* These two tests have likewise been unrevealing in our patients. Although they are often obtained when there is a high degree of suspicion of an intrinsic neuropathy affecting central vision, we have not found them to be of value in assessing patients with NPG.
4. *Cryoglobulin measurements:* These may be useful in patients in whom there is Raynaud's phenomenon or evidence of marked peripheral vasospasm, but are otherwise not very helpful.

RADIOLOGIC EVALUATION

There is considerable debate about the utility of obtaining a computed tomography (CT) scan or magnetic resonance imaging (MRI) in patients with NPG. Obviously, these evaluations are more useful in patients in whom there is a loss of central vision with preservation of peripheral vision or in whom chiasmal lesions are suspected. On the other hand, one might argue that it is not unreasonable to "leave no stone unturned," especially in the evaluation of a patient in whom central vision is threatened (e.g., a progressive paracentral scotoma very near fixation).

We have never found that a positive MRI or CT scan result uncovers a lesion accounting for glaucomatous optic neuropathy, although anecdotal reports exist of such findings.[17, 18] However, we would consider it wise to obtain radiologic studies of the brain or orbit to help eliminate any suspected source of optic nerve damage resembling glaucoma. This is perhaps especially true if a physician is practicing in a "hostile" medicolegal environment like the United States.

Finally, another useful clinical measurement that may be relevant in some cases is the assessment of corneal thickness. Certainly, patients who have had corneal refractive surgery, and high myopia, should have pachymetry performed, because applanation tonometry underestimates IOP by 3 mm Hg for a 50-μm decrease in corneal thickness.[19]

Signs and Symptoms

OCULAR CLUES

Intraocular Pressure

It is well known that IOP fluctuates throughout the day. In most humans, the highest IOP occurs in the midmorning. The patient who is evaluated at a single visit, however, may have IOP values within the normal range during the visit, because he or she does not necessarily manifest elevated IOP at that time. For this reason, we often prefer to obtain IOP measurements not only during multiple office visits but also at various times of the day in order to gain a truer sense of an individual's IOP range. Furthermore, we find that serial recording of diurnal pressure measurements is often useful to obtain an accurate representation of the average IOP readings in the eye.

Although the procedure sounds quite simple, it is not easy in practice to obtain detailed recordings over a 24-hour period. Most practitioners have the capability of recording pressure measurements throughout the day when their office is open, say from 8 AM to 5 PM. In general, when we determine diurnal measurements for this period, we are usually satisfied that we have obtained a sampling that can detect an episodic increase during the day. Our own diurnal measurements, however, are made throughout the night as well, leaving out the period from midnight to 6 AM. Of course, patients who have an aberrant light/dark cycle, such as those who work in the evening, should undergo IOP testing preferably during the 12 to 16 hours after their arousal from sleep.

Optic Nerve Atrophy

Documenting progressive optic nerve atrophy is generally straightforward. Admittedly, many sophisticated instruments have the ability to define numerous optic nerve parameters in a moderately objective way. Some of the nerve fiber layer or optic nerve analyzers on the market give fairly reproducible and reliable estimates of specific measurements, such as cup-to-disc diameter, neuroretinal rim area, and nerve fiber layer height. It is important to keep in mind, however, that no computer has yet been able to answer the obvious question we would like to ask about the key parameters of interest: What, exactly, constitutes a significant change of any given parameter measured at various time points? More important, can a practitioner without access to research-grade instruments make such assessments at all?

Fortunately, there is evidence that a good set of stereo disc photographs interpreted by an astute observer constitutes perhaps the most reliable way to assess meaningful changes in the optic nerve head.[20] By far the most important change that should be assessed is a loss of neural tissue. This parameter is assessed according to the presence of cupping, which of course represents atrophy of both neural and glial tissue. We would advocate that three-dimensional viewing is extremely advantageous in this assessment. Certain clues, such as the displacement of vessels or the increased visualization of laminar pores, may assist the viewer who has access only to two-dimensional analysis. In short, one does not need high-technology instrumentation to assess optic nerve progression; rather, all that is needed is a good brain.

It should be noted that patients with NPG often present at a later stage of disease than their counterparts with POAG. Therefore, it is not unusual for the ophthalmologist to encounter patients in whom cupping is quite advanced and, in many cases, almost complete. In such patients, the progression of optic nerve cupping is not nearly as productive as the clinical assessment of progressive visual field loss for the characterization of the clinical course of glaucoma.

Another parameter that has received increased attention is the appearance of parapapillary (also called "peripapillary") atrophy. This atrophy of the retinal pigment epithelium adjacent to the optic nerve head has been found to be active and dynamic and accompanies the glaucomatous process.[21] By itself, an increase in parapapillary atrophy is not considered a diagnostic indicator of optic nerve progression. However, the clinician's index of suspicion for progressive nerve damage should certainly be elevated if progressive changes in parapapillary atrophy occur with time.

Optic Disc Hemorrhages

The presence or recurrence of one or more splinter hemorrhages on the optic disc surface has long been considered an important prognostic sign of the development or progression of glaucomatous damage.[22, 23] The greater incidence of these hemorrhages in patients with NPG than in those with POAG[24] is particularly troubling. It suggests that such hemorrhages are not merely the result of structural changes that accompany glaucomatous optic neuropathy but, in the patient with NPG, are an ominous sign of neurovascular infarction and, hence, eventual progressive optic nerve deterioration. Some observers believe that the appearance of such hemorrhages is not always followed by further field loss. In fact, such hemorrhages have been observed in patients without glaucoma.

However, when present, field loss does indeed occur in the nerve fiber bundles in which such disc hemorrhages have been present. Such hemorrhages usually occur at the upper and lower poles of the optic nerve head, especially inferotemporally. They are often found in association with disc "notching" of the neuroretinal rim, which also is strong evidence that the presence of hemorrhages is of pathogenic importance. We are inclined to view the appearance of optic disc hemorrhages most pessimistically. When such hemorrhages occur, they often prompt our serious reconsideration of current therapy (or lack thereof). Succinctly put, the appearance of hemorrhages in a patient with NPG tell us that whatever we are doing to minimize future vision loss is not working.

Visual Field Loss

No assessment of glaucoma can be made without confirmation that there has been a progressive decrease in light sensitivity of the peripheral or paracentral visual field or both. Because visual field analysis is performed with the use of several different instruments among practitioners, no generalized statement can be made regarding the precise definition of what constitutes visual field progression.

With the use of the Humphrey field analyzer (Humphrey Instruments, San Leandro, CA), our criterion for visual field abnormalities on the computerized parametric test is either (1) a corrected pattern standard deviation with a p value <0.05 or (2) a glaucoma hemifield test value outside normal limits that was obtained with at least two reliable and reproducible visual field examinations. Visual field damage is considered to have progressed if there was a change in 5 or more points, with at least 3 being contiguous compared with their baseline values based on the glaucoma change probability analysis (STATPAC). With the use of Goldmann manual perimetry, kinetic visual field defects typically consist of reproducible nasal steps at least 10 degrees in width or paracentral scotomas more than 5 degrees in width, in addition to classic Seidel and Bjerrum scotomas. The criteria for progression of visual field loss commonly consist of a reproducible and meaningful increase in either the depth or the extent of the scotoma.

Although it has been the subject of considerable controversy, most observers would agree that characteristic changes of the visual field often seen in patients with NPG include visual field defects that are steeper, deeper, and closer to fixation than those seen in patients with POAG. If paracentral defects are present, it is often helpful to utilize the 10-2 program of the Humphrey instrument; and if visual acuity is poor, the use of a size V stimulus as opposed to a III stimulus is often preferred.[25] In many patients, we alternate the 30-2 and 10-2 programs on sequential visits.

SYSTEMIC CLUES

Vasospasm

Patients with vasospasm constitute one of the earliest and best-characterized subsets of patients with NPG.[26] The literature is replete with studies that measure the vascular diameter of fingernail bed capillaries in response to temperature changes in order to assess peripheral vasospasm in these patients.[27] Should the clinician feel inadequate who does not have access to such technology? The answer of course is a resounding "No!" The eminent Dr. Stephen Drance has taught us that the easiest way to assess the presence of vasospasm is simply to shake a patient's hands. Naturally, some patients may have cold hands if they are nervous, as they may be for a visit to the doctor, but the clinician's perception of cold hands should prompt directed questions to ascertain whether or not the patient is vasospastic. Are their feet cold? Does the patient sleep with socks on, particularly in the summertime? There is a high yield of positive responses to these questions in patients who have cold hands as detected with a simple handshake.

An additional piece of history that is often given by vasospastic individuals with NPG is that of migraine headaches.[28] In attempting to elicit this history, it is important to keep in mind that the presentation of migraine headaches spans the gamut from classic migraine to acephalgic migraine, in which the headaches are not nearly as prominent as the visual disturbances associated with spasm of either retinal or cerebral vessels.

The subset of patients with NPG who are vasospastic are not only one of the largest subsets but also constitute a group for whom some rational, however unproven, therapy may be considered. The use of calcium channel antagonists has been popularized for the treatment of this subset of patients with NPG. We consider the evidence that this family of compounds is efficacious in this disorder to be anecdotal and not utterly convincing.[29, 30] In addition, many studies have shown that these compounds do not favorably alter visual field loss progression in either normal-pressure or high-pressure glaucoma.[31, 32]

Complicating this issue even further are a number of interesting reports suggesting that patients who use these drugs as long-term therapy may experience a higher risk of cancer.[33] Before offering patients calcium channel blockers, the practitioner should consider this: If the practitioner does not experience enough "tension" already in dealing with patients with this disease, one can only imagine what happens when informing patients of these studies. We nevertheless do advocate the use of calcium channel antagonists in selected patients, particularly those with frank and overt manifestations of peripheral vasospasm or migraine headaches, in which visual field worsening has occurred despite other therapeutic efforts such as maximum reduction of IOP.

Calcium channel antagonists vary in their selectivity of cardiac as opposed to vascular receptors. Although ideally one would expect that the most vasoselective calcium channel antagonist is the one that should be used, the reality is that initiating therapy with these compounds often has untoward side effects, such as headache and lethargy. Therefore, we generally initiate therapy with nonselective agents such as verapamil (Calan SR) prior to escalating the therapy with more selective compounds such as nifedipine (Procardia). (Nimodipine, the most vasoselective compound, is prohibitively expensive and therefore not a practical choice.)

The use of calcium channel antagonists is a two-edged sword in more than one way. Effective concentrations may ameliorate vasospasm to a significant extent. However, excessive doses of this compound may decrease cardiac inotropy and chronotropy, thereby diminishing cardiac output and thus resulting in reduced ocular perfusion, which is counterproductive. Patients should be explicitly told to monitor the pulse rate and blood pressure when using this family of compounds.

Systemic Hypotension

System hypotension is one of the most treatable of conditions affecting a subset of patients with NPG. Many factors affect blood flow to the optic nerve, including systemic blood pressure, vascular resistance, and IOP. A meaningful way to integrate the relationship between IOP and blood pressure is to refer to "perfusion pressure," which is the systemic diastolic blood pressure minus IOP. Studies suggest that the risk of glaucomatous damage increases markedly when diastolic perfusion pressure decreases below 50 mm Hg.[34] Several studies have demonstrated that patients with both the high-pressure and low-pressure forms of glaucoma (in fact, all individuals) may experience nocturnal hypotension, in which the blood pressure drops precipitously during the evening hours of sleep.[35, 36] This drop, of course, decreases perfusion pressure and likely increases the risk of optic neuropathy. In our experience, this syndrome occurs most typically in thin, older patients, particularly women.

We have been impressed that self-monitoring of blood pressure with automated sphygmomanometry devices readily available at the local pharmacy can reveal profound decreases in diastolic pressures (e.g., <50 mm Hg) in some patients. In such cases, we take a commonsense approach and prescribe the use of a salt tablet after dinner as a dietary supplement. Salt tablets, generally available in any health food store, usually consist of 450 mg sodium chloride and 50 mg potassium chloride. We are often successful in preventing nocturnal hypotension in patients with this feature by having them increase salt and fluid intake prior to retiring. Of course, the long-term effect on the optic neuropathy is unknown. However, we believe it is reasonable to advocate such an approach to facilitate ocular circulation and minimize the potential harm of lowered systemic blood pressure.

Is There a Role for Aberrant Autoimmunity?

Many patients in whom we suspect an autoimmune component to the optic neuropathy can be identified easily from the history. Questions relating to the presence of musculoskeletal and joint involvement, skin rashes, and sicca complex are all useful in order to identify these potential cases. We should recognize, however, that the presence of such symptoms is generally nonspecific. In fact, we all know that sicca syndrome, or dry eyes, is quite common in elderly persons, not just patients with glaucoma. The most useful means of detecting potential autoimmune involvement in glaucomatous optic neuropathy is eliciting a history in patients in whom there is another autoimmune disease. We have identified several patients who belong to this subset of NPG from clues that they have other autoimmune diseases, such as Paget's disease, Addison's disease, multiple myeloma, chronic inflammatory peripheral neuropathy, and hypothyroidism. In fact, the epidemiologic association of patients with autoimmune disorders obtained from their histories was the first clue that identified the subset of patients in whom autoimmunity may mediate the optic neuropathy that occurs in this disease.[37]

Of course, it is beyond the scope of the ophthalmologist to treat these other disorders. Also discouraging is that the treatment of autoimmune diseases is in its infancy. The use of global suppressants such as steroids is often successful in ameliorating certain symptoms of several diseases, but the price is often high. Furthermore, there is no evidence to suggest that the relief of symptoms by the use of steroids or other immunosuppressants will have any favorable bearing on the glaucomatous process, if indeed a similar autoimmune mechanism underlies both diseases. Nevertheless, it is the responsibility of the ophthalmologist to be alerted by the presence of accompanying autoimmune diseases, and to work closely with a patient's internist throughout the course of the patient's care. Certainly, any use of steroids in these patients must be monitored closely in order to detect a steroid-related rise in IOP, which, if it occurs, can certainly compromise an already glaucomatous nerve.

Treatment

WHEN AND WHY TO TREAT CONSERVATIVELY

Although it may seem like anathema to the practicing glaucoma specialist, we nevertheless believe that not all patients with progressive visual field loss require treatment. Let us take for example a 92-year-old woman who has had documented NPG for 30 years. During that time, she has had excellent visual acuity in both eyes, with perhaps a paracentral scotoma in one eye and an arcuate defect in the other eye that has been noted to undergo episodic worsening over the 30 years. We do not believe it would be unreasonable to consider that minimal, if any, impairment in functional vision would occur in this patient's expected lifespan if the NPG was left untreated.

Thus, the ophthalmologist's decision to treat should be tempered by several considerations, such as the age of the patient, the level of visual function, and the level of visual needs. On the other hand, there are patients in whom we would advocate aggressive treatment, although it must be emphasized that the efficacy of any treatment is unclear. Certainly, the younger the patient, the more inclined we are to consider treatment, because of the likely longer remaining life span during which such a patient may experience further visual deterioration.

The decision to treat based on the usual hallmarks of progression, namely, changes in the visual field or the optic nerve, garners the most attention. However, we believe that in many patients, the occurrence of repetitive optic nerve hemorrhages are the harbinger of future field loss, and their appearance often prompts us to treat aggressively. This is particularly true in younger patients.

Assuming one has made the decision that treatment should be initiated to minimize future damage, the basic tenets for treatment vary little for NPG from those for other glaucomas. The risks and benefits of any individual therapy, whether it be medical, laser, or surgical, must be ascertained on an individual basis. Patients with multiple allergies to topical drops would make the further use of that modality inadvisable. Similarly, patients who are tremulous or uncooperative may not be able to successfully undergo argon laser trabeculoplasty. Finally, older patients who have undergone either multiple ocular surgical procedures or multiple filtering procedures that were unsuccessful may not be the best candidates for further filtering surgery owing to the risk of intraoperative complications such as expulsive hemorrhage.

In general, we do not advocate surgery for patients in whom the IOP is controlled to values in the low teens. We are much more likely to recommend pressure lowering by whatever means necessary for patients whose IOP exceeds 15 mm Hg. The reason for this recommendation is twofold and rather obvious. First, it is difficult to guarantee successful filtering surgery that yields pressure in single digits or the low teens. The desired potential benefit following filtering is limited in an eye whose initial pressures are not that different from those likely to be obtained postoperatively. Second, although it appears that there is a continuum of visual field loss with IOP in glaucoma (with low pressures generally being associated with the least loss), it is again by no means clear that a pressure of 9 mm Hg is necessarily better than a pressure of 12 mm Hg in a disease in which the contributing role of any level of IOP is poorly understood. We would also add that we have no quarrel with those who feel differently and for whom the reduction of IOP to the single digits is an important goal in all patients.

For filtering surgery, we generally prefer a guarded trabeculectomy procedure employing releasable sutures to obtain low pressures early in the postoperative course and avoid the common complications of full-thickness procedures, such as choroidal effusions and flat chambers. We routinely employ antimetabolites in virtually all filtering surgeries, although the dose and duration vary according to individual patient characteristics. We use low doses of mitomycin C (0.2 mg/mL for 2 minutes) in individuals with thin sclerae, such as those with myopia and particularly in young myopic males. This group is one in whom the occurrence of hypotonous maculopathy has been well documented following antimetabolite therapy. We rarely employ intraoperative mitomycin in patients with very thin or atrophic conjunctivae or in those in whom there is a virtually absent Tenon's layer.

FUTURE OUTLOOK

The best opportunities for treatment will obviously be based on evidence that a specific pathologic mechanism mediates neuronal cell death in any or all of the variants of NPG. At present, there is little evidence that any presumed mechanism of glaucomatous neuropathy is specific to NPG as opposed to POAG. Although it is likely that the neuropathy in many patients with NPG and high-pressure glaucoma may have a common mechanism, such mechanisms must be identified before optimum strategies for treatment can be chosen. Unfortunately, it is entirely too early to know whether neuroprotectants, immunosuppressive agents, or gene therapy will be available to us in the immediate future. At present, common sense tempering sound medical judgment offers the best opportunity to decrease the morbidity of the diminished optic nerve function that may accompany this most perplexing optic neuropathy.

ACKNOWLEDGMENTS

The author wishes to thank Michael A. Kass, MD, and William Hart, MD, PhD, for their critical review of this manuscript.

REFERENCES

1. Tielsch JM, Sommer A, Witt K, et al: Blindness and visual impairment in an American urban population. Arch Ophthalmol 1990;108:286–290.
2. Quigley HA: Open angle glaucoma. N Engl J Med 1993;328:1097–1106.
3. Hart WM Jr: The epidemiology of primary open-angle glaucoma and ocular hypertension. *In* Ritch R, Shields MB, Krupin T (eds): The Glaucomas, vol 2. St. Louis, CV Mosby, 1989, pp 789–795.
4. Tielsch JM, Sommer A, Katz J, et al: Racial variations in the prevalence of primary open-angle glaucoma. JAMA 1991;266:369–374.
5. Sommer A: Intraocular pressure and glaucoma. Am J Ophthalmol 1989;107:186–188.
6. Sommer A: Doyne Lecture: Glaucoma: Facts and fancies. Eye 1996;10:295–301.
7. Gliklich RE, Steinman WC, Spaeth G: Visual field change in low tension glaucoma over a five-year follow-up. Ophthalmology 1989;96:316–320.
8. Comparison of glaucomatous progression between untreated patients with normal-tension glaucoma and patients with therapeutically reduced intraocular pressures. Collaborative Normal-Tension Glaucoma Study Group. Am J Ophthalmol 1998;126:487–497.
9. Hitchings RA, Wu J, Poinoosawmy D, McNaught A: Surgery for normal-tension glaucoma. Br J Ophthalmol 1995;79:402–406.
10. Bhandari A, Crabb DP, Poinoosawmy D, et al: Effect of surgery on visual field progression in normal-tension glaucoma. Ophthalmology 1997;104:1131–1137.
11. Crichton A, Drance SM, Douglas GR, Schulzer M: Unequal intraocular pressure and its relation to asymmetric visual field defects in low-tension glaucoma. Ophthalmology 1989;96:1312–1314.
12. Cartwright MJ, Anderson DR: Correlation between asymmetric damage with asymmetric intraocular pressure in normal-tension glaucoma (normal-tension glaucoma). Arch Ophthalmol 1988;106:898–900.
13. Hollows FC, Graham PA: Intra-ocular pressure, glaucoma and glaucoma suspects in a defined population. Br J Ophthalmol 1966;50:570–586.
14. Stoilova D, Child A, Trifan OC, et al: Localization of a locus (GLC1B) for adult-onset primary open angle glaucoma to the 2cen-q13 region. Genomics 1996;36:142–150.
15. Wax MB, Tezel G, Saito I, et al: Anti-Ro/SS-A positivity and heat shock protein antibodies in patients with normal pressure glaucoma. Am J Ophthalmol 1998;125:145–157.
16. Wax MB, Barrett DA, Pestronk A: Increased incidence of paraproteinemia and autoantibodies in patients with normal pressure glaucoma. Am J Ophthalmol 1994;117:561–568.
17. Gutman I, Melamed S, Ashkenazi I, Blumenthal M: Optic nerve compression by carotid arteries in low tension glaucoma. Graefes Arch Clin Exp Ophthalmol 1993;231:711–717.
18. Kalenak JW, Kosmorsky GS, Hassenbusch SJ: Compression of the unilateral optic nerve mimicking unilateral normal-pressure glaucoma. J Clin Neuroophthalmol 1992;12:230–235.
19. Mardelli PG, Piebenga LW, Whitacre MM, Siegmund KD: The effect of excimer laser photorefractive keratectomy on intraocular pressure measurements using the Goldmann applanation tonometer. Ophthalmology 1997;104:945–948.
20. Caprioli J, Prum B, Zeyen T: Comparison of methods to evaluate the optic nerve head and nerve fiber layer for glaucomatous change. Am J Ophthalmol 1996;121:659–667.
21. Tezel G, Kass MA, Kolker AE, Wax MB: Comparative optic disc analysis in normal pressure glaucoma, primary open angle glaucoma and ocular hypertension. Ophthalmology 1996;103:2105–2113.
22. Drance SM, Begg IS: Sector haemorrhage—a probable acute ischemic disc change in chronic simple glaucoma. Can J Ophthalmol 1970;5:137–141.
23. Kitazawa Y, Shirato S, Yamamoto T: Optic disc hemorrhage in low-tension glaucoma. Ophthalmology 1986;93:853–857.
24. Levene RZ: Low tension glaucoma: A critical review and new material. Surv Ophthalmol 1980;24:621–624.
25. Zalta AH: Use of a central 10 degrees field and size V stimulus to evaluate and monitor small central islands of vision in end stage glaucoma. Br J Ophthalmol 1991;75:151–154.
26. Gasser P, Flammer J, Guthauser U, et al: Bedeutung des vasospastischen syndroms in der augenheilkunde. Klin Monatsbl Augenheilkd 1986;183:503–509.

27. Drance SM, Douglas GR, Wijsman K, et al: Response of blood flow to warm and cold in normal and low-tension glaucoma patients. Am J Ophthalmol 1988;105:35–39.
28. Phelps CD, Corbett JJ: Migraine and low-tension glaucoma: A case-controlled study. Invest Ophthalmol Vis Sci 1985;26:1105–1108.
29. Kitazawa Y, Shiirai H, Go FJ: The effect of Ca2(+)-antagonist on visual field in low-tension glaucoma. Graefes Arch Clin Exp Ophthalmol 1989;227:408–412.
30. Netland PA, Chaturvedi N, Dreyer EB: Calcium channel blockers in the management of low-tension glaucoma. Am J Ophthalmol 1993;115:608–613.
31. Lumme P, Tuulonen A, Airaksinen PJ, et al: Neuroretinal rim area in low tension glaucoma: Effect of nifedipine and acetazolamide compared to no treatment. Acta Ophthalmol 1991;69:293–298.
32. Liu S, Araujo SV, Spaeth GL, et al: Lack of effect of calcium channel blockers on open angle glaucoma. J Glaucoma 1996;5:187–190.
33. Pahor M, Guralnik JM, Ferrucci L, et al: Calcium-channel blockade and incidence of cancer in aged populations. Lancet 1996;348:493–497.
34. Tielsch JM, Katz J, Sommer A, et al: Hypertension, perfusion pressure and primary open angle glaucoma: A population based assessment. Arch Ophthalmol 1995;113:216–221.
35. Kaiser LJ, Flammer J, Graf T, Stümfig D: Systemic blood pressure in glaucoma patients. Graefes Arch Clin Exp Ophthalmol 1993;231:677–680.
36. Hayreh SS, Zimmerman MB, Podhajsky P, Alward WLM: Nocturnal arterial hypotension and its role in optic nerve head and ocular ischemic disorders. Am J Ophthalmol 1994;117:603–624.
37. Cartwright MJ, Grajewski AL, Friedberg ML, et al: Immune-related disease and normal-tension glaucoma. Arch Ophthalmol 1992;110:500–502.

SECTION III

KEY DIAGNOSTIC SIGNS

CHAPTER 10

Glaucomas Associated with External Eye Signs

ANTHONY ECONOMOU and STEVEN T. SIMMONS

When one examines a patient suspected of having glaucoma, the external examination is typically the starting point. This chapter, by Anthony Economou and Steve Simmons, presents a systematic approach for identifying the key signs that may be of help. You may wish to refer to Chapter 6, Genetics, and Chapter 8, Systemic Syndromes and Diseases and Glaucoma, for additional information on these topics. Chapter 20, Eyelids, Lacrimal Apparatus, Orbit, Motility, deals with findings of the external examination that may result from glaucoma treatment.

The glaucomas discussed in this chapter represent those that occur with external signs. They represent a unique category of conditions that may be diagnosed initially from their external presentations. The underlying mechanisms for the development of the glaucoma are divided into four catagories: episcleral venous pressure (EVP), masses, pigmentary mechanism, and developmental abnormalities.

Entities Associated with an Increase in Episcleral Venous Pressure

STURGE-WEBER SYNDROME

Encephalotrigeminal angiomatosis (Sturge-Weber syndrome) manifests with striking external signs. A facial cutaneous angioma (nevus flammeus, port wine stain) and facial hypertrophy secondary to cutaneous angiomas may be present (Fig. 10–1). The complete Sturge-Weber syndrome encompasses (1) a facial hemangioma,[1] (2) ipsilateral meningeal racemose hemangioma, (3) ipsilateral choroidal hemangioma, and (4) congenital glaucoma.[2] The presence of at least two of these factors is necessary to establish the diagnosis of this syndrome. The cutaneous angioma, glaucoma, and associated intraocular abnormalities are nearly always unilateral and ipsilateral.[1, 3, 4]

The most likely cause of the elevated intraocular pressure (IOP) seems to be a combination of developmental abnormalities and elevated EVP (Fig. 10–2). The developmental abnormalities consist of prominent iris processes adherent to the trabecular meshwork and an amorphous granular material that can be seen throughout the trabecular meshwork and juxtacanalicular region. The endothelial lining of Schlemm's canal is attenuated, giving the appearance of advanced aging of the aqueous outflow system. Phelps[1] proposed that the elevated EVP may be secondary to the episcleral hemangioma with its numerous arteriovenous shunts.

The glaucoma occurs in about 30% of patients with Sturge-Weber syndrome.[5–7] The facial angioma is present at birth and is unilateral in 90% of the cases involving the first and second divisions of the trigeminal nerve.[8] The lesion involves the dermis and is composed of dilated, telangiectatic, cutaneous capillaries lined by a single layer of endothelial cells. It has been suggested that the lesion is secondary to localized autonomic nerve loss that results in an inability to regulate blood flow through the dermal vasculature.[9] The lesion usually becomes more pronounced with age because of an increased depth of color, which blanches with external pressure.

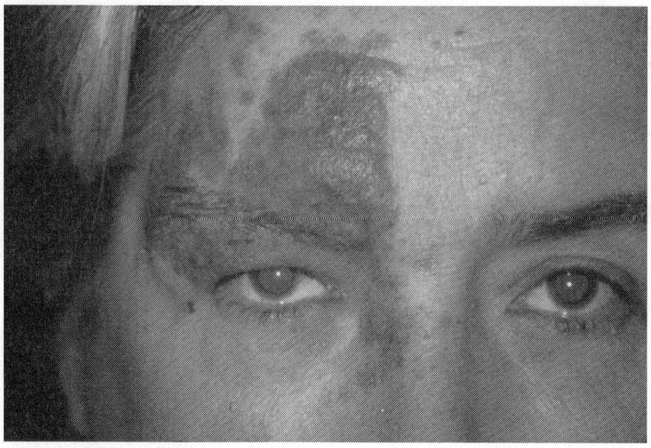

FIGURE 10–1. The cutaneous angioma of Sturge-Weber syndrome. The lesion involves the dermis and is composed of dilated, telangiectatic cutaneous capillaries.

Management of the glaucoma secondary to Sturge-Weber syndrome may include goniotomy and trabeculotomy in children less than 5 years of age for whom medical therapy has failed. Trabeculectomy should be performed in adults, with tight sutures applied to the scleral flap. This maneuver decreases the risk of a flat chamber secondary to a serous choroid effusion, which commonly occurs in this condition.

KLIPPEL-TRENAUNAY-WEBER SYNDROME

Klippel and Trenaunay[10] in 1900 and Weber[11] in 1907 described another ocular syndrome. It comprises (1) a cutaneous hemangioma that extends over one limb, (2) varicosities in the affected limb, and (3) hypertrophy of the underlying bone and soft tissue. The syndrome may be inherited in a dominant pattern.[12] Ocular findings of Klippel-Trenaunay-Weber syndrome include cutaneous angioma of the face, heterochromia iridis, orbital and retinal varices, choroidal angiomas, disc anomalies, and an enlargement of the globe (buphthalmos) with or without glaucoma.[13, 14] The ocular findings are more common when the cutaneous angioma involves the face. The elevated EVP may be secondary to varicosities, arteriovenous fistulas, and telangiectasias.

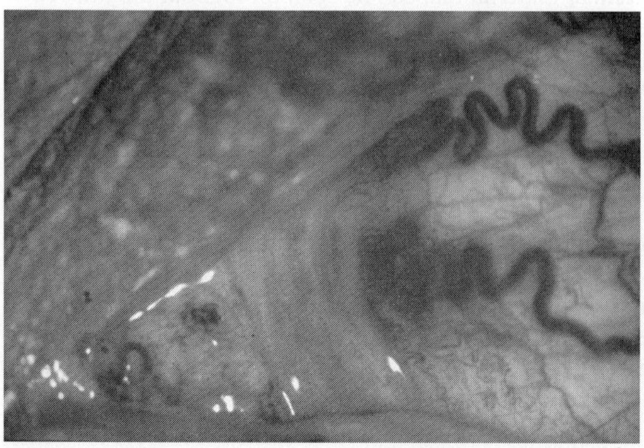

FIGURE 10–2. Prominent episcleral vessels in a patient with Sturge-Weber syndrome. Increased episcleral venous pressure is believed to be the underlying cause of the increased intraocular pressure in this syndrome.

ORBITAL VARIX

Orbital varix also manifests with external eye signs. The key external diagnostic signs seen with this disorder are (1) intermittent unilateral proptosis, (2) dilated veins in the eyelid, anterior orbit, or both, and (3) an enlarged orbit with phleboliths seen on imaging (Fig. 10–3).[15–17] The glaucoma seen with orbital varices is rare but may occur if the varix is large and causes an increase in episcleral pressure. Orbital varices are dilations of existing orbital veins usually found in young people at birth or in early childhood.[18] They do not have an arterial component. The proptosis may worsen with Valsalva maneuver, sneezing, or bending over.[19] Between the episodes of increased IOP, the involved eye may be enophthalmic. Because the venous pressure is normal between attacks, the brief episodes of elevated IOP rarely lead to glaucomatous damage.[20]

CAROTID-CAVERNOUS AND ARTERIOVENOUS FISTULAS

Key external diagnostic signs with carotid-cavernous and arteriovenous (AV) fistulas are (1) orbital bruits, (2) restricted ocular motility, (3) proptosis, and (4) pulsating exophthalmos (Fig. 10–4). Another external sign is the caput medusa of the conjunctival vessels secondary to blood reversal through the conjunctival vessels. Widening of the superior orbital fissure with erosion of the adjacent sella and sphenoidal sinus wall can be seen radiographically.[21–23]

Fistula formations are abnormal communications between previously normal arteries and veins without an intervening capillary bed. These abnormal communications may be secondary to trauma or spontaneous degeneration. The most common trauma associated with AV fistulas is basal skull fractures.[24] The internal carotid artery is the most common source of arterial blood, and the cavernous sinus is the most common venous structure. Outflow facility may become impaired secondary to increased episcleral

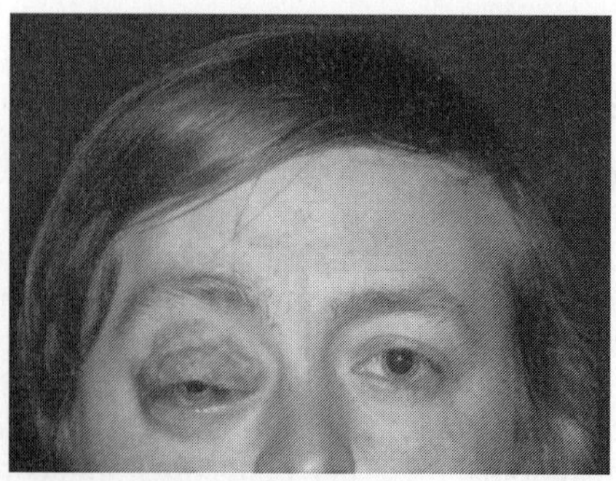

FIGURE 10–3. Unilateral proptosis with dilated veins of the eyelid and anterior orbit in a patient with an orbital varix.

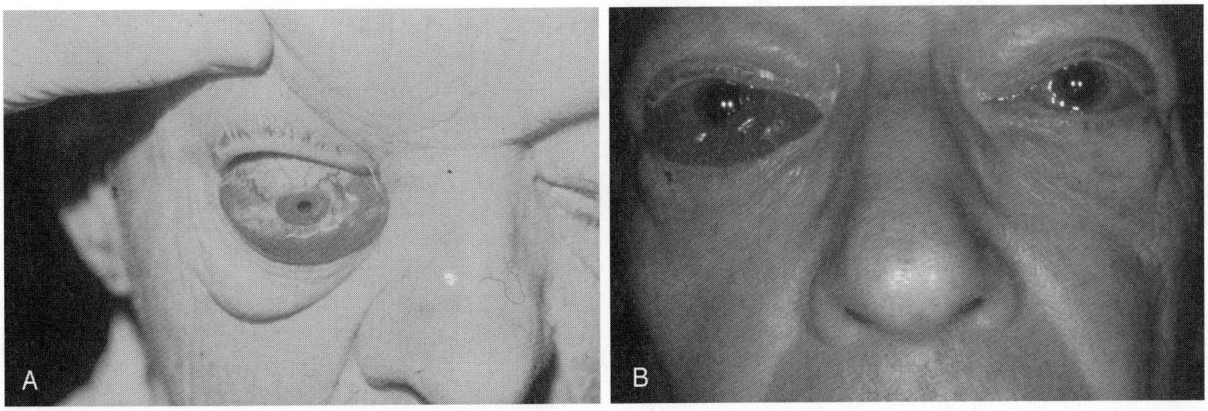

FIGURE 10–4. Proptosis and pulsatile exophthalmos with excessive inferior chemosis seen with a carotid cavernous sinus fistula *(A)* and with an arteriovenous fistula *(B)*.

pressure, leading to glaucoma in 60% to 70% of patients with AV fistulas (Fig. 10–5).[25, 26] In addition to increased EVP, carotid-cavernous fistulas may be associated with neovascular glaucoma. Capillary nonperfusion leads to retinal ischemia with liberation of angiogenic factors by the hypoxic retinal tissue.

SUPERIOR VENA CAVA SYNDROME

Superior vena cava syndrome occurs secondary to obstruction of venous blood return to the heart along the great vessels, which causes elevated EVP. External presenting signs of superior vena cava syndrome are (1) edema of the lid, face, and conjunctiva and (2) proptosis.[27] Ninety-seven percent of cases are secondary to an underlying malignancy.[28] Other etiologies for superior vena cava syndrome are aortic aneurysms, hilar node enlargement, and thyroid disease. The glaucoma is sometimes found bilaterally and worsens when the patient is in the supine position.[29]

THYROID OPHTHALMOPATHY

Another condition that can manifest with an increase in EVP is thyroid ophthalmopathy. The disorder is characterized by inflammation and enlargement of the extraocular muscles and orbital tissues. The key external diagnostic signs are exophthalmos and a typical stare with lid lag and lid retraction in downgaze. Early in the disease, the lid retraction (Dalrymple's sign) is due to sympathomimetic response; in its later course, the retraction results from the fibrosis of lid tissues. The retrobulbar infiltrative process and extraocular muscle enlargement can compromise the orbital venous system, leading to an increased EVP and glaucoma (Fig. 10–6).

In addition, a high IOP can occur secondary to contraction of fibrosed, infiltrated extraocular muscles in certain directions of gaze.[30] Fibrosis affects the inferior rectus muscle most frequently, and a significant increase in IOP can occur in up gaze.[31] Because of changes in IOP related to gaze, the IOP should be measured in different directions of gaze. Other causes of increased IOP are a generalized, chronic exposure leading to chronic inflammation and secondary angle closure, and increased mucopolysaccharide deposition in the angle.[32]

In patients with infiltrative ophthalmopathy and normal outflow facilities, pressure elevations only in isolated fields of gaze do not require therapy. For those with sustained elevations in all fields of gaze, treatment is analogous to that for chronic open-angle glaucoma. The most effective

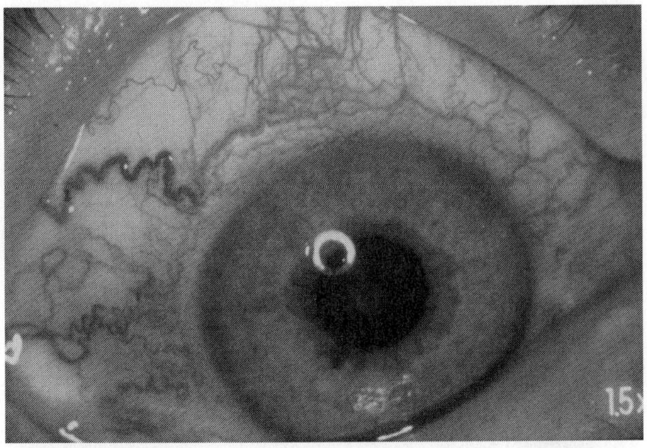

FIGURE 10–5. Prominent conjunctival vessels seen with an arteriovenous (AV) fistula. Increased episcleral venous pressure leads to secondary glaucoma in more than 60% of the patients with AV fistula.

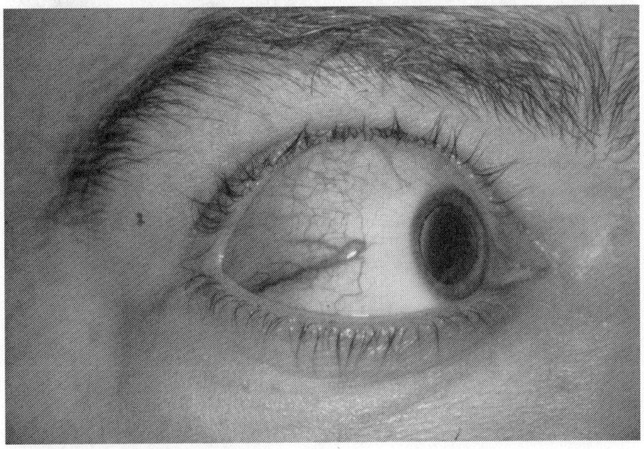

FIGURE 10–6. Dilated venous tree overlying lateral rectus in thyroid ophthalmopathy, in which increased episcleral venous pressure can lead to secondary glaucoma.

treatments for infiltrative ophthalmopathy include high-dose corticosteroids, radiotherapy, and surgical decompression.

Entities Associated with Masses

TUBEROUS SCLEROSIS

Tuberous sclerosis (Bourneville's syndrome) is a rare condition transmitted as an autosomal dominant trait and present in approximately 1 in 15,000 births.[33] External signs constitute the hallmarks of tuberous sclerosis, which is one of the rare phakomatoses. A red-brown papular rash, *adenoma sebaceum*, located on the malar regions of the face and chin is present in 83% of the cases.[34] Histologically these lesions are angiofibromas. The other classic external sign is the *ash leaf sign*, which occurs in up to 90% of patients.[35] It is a hypopigmented lesion best seen under an ultraviolet Wood's lamp. Along with the cutaneous involvement, 90% of patients with tuberous sclerosis have seizures, and approximately 50% of patients may have mental retardation.[36] The most common ocular finding in tuberous sclerosis is an astrocytic retinal hamartoma, or mulberry lesion, seen in more than 50% of cases (Fig. 10–7).[37] The glaucomas associated with tuberous sclerosis may occur from vitreous hemorrhage, rubeosis irides, and retinal detachment.[38]

JUVENILE XANTHOGRANULOMA

Another syndrome in this category is juvenile xanthogranuloma, which is commonly seen in young children. The typical external skin signs are yellow or orange papules located on the skin of the head and neck. The diagnosis is made after biopsy of the skin lesions, which displays layers of histiocytes and the Touton giant cell that is pathognomonic for juvenile xanthogranuloma (Fig. 10–8).

A salmon-colored or lightly pigmented lesion can sometimes be seen on the iris that can lead to a spontaneous hyphema. Juvenile xanthogranuloma is the most common cause of spontaneous hyphema in children. Ocular examination reveals hyphema, iris tumor, and elevated IOP. Glaucoma occurs secondary to obstruction of aqueous outflow by histiocytes and red blood cells following the spontaneous hyphema. Treatment includes systemic corticosteroids and medical treatment for the glaucoma.[39]

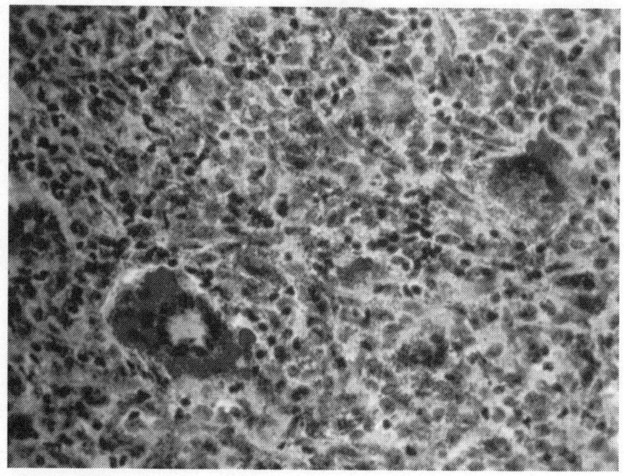

FIGURE 10–8. Skin biopsy specimen demonstrates the pathognomonic Touton's giant cell of juvenile xanthogranuloma.

NEUROFIBROMATOSIS

The key external diagnostic signs in neurofibromatosis are plexiform neuromas of the upper lid secondary to distended nerves and thickened perineural sheaths (Fig. 10–9).[40] These plexiform neurofibromas can also be present in the orbit, causing displacement of the globe with proptosis. In addition to the neurofibromas, one can see a pulsating exophthalmos unassociated with bruits, which results from orbital wall defects or meningoceles and tumor erosion with orbital extension leading to pulsation and muscle palsies. The plexiform neuromas have a characteristic feeling of a "bag of worms" and usually affect the upper lid unilaterally, creating the characteristic S-shaped deformity (Fig. 10–10).

Another striking skin finding associated with neurofibromatosis type 1 (NF1, von Recklinghausen's disease) is the presence of multiple neurofibromas, which appear as

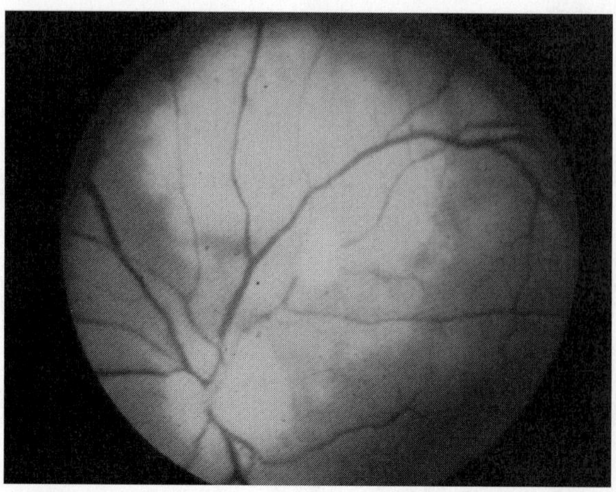

FIGURE 10–7. Astrocytic retinal hamartoma (mulberry lesion) seen in tuberous sclerosis. Other findings are the "adenoma sebaceum" on the malar region of the face and the "ash-leaf sign."

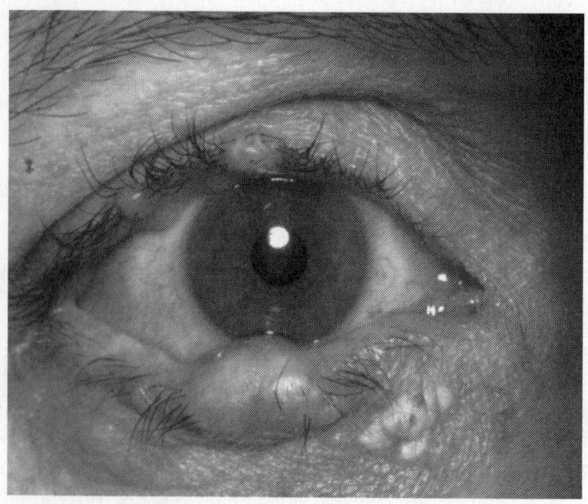

FIGURE 10–9. Plexiform neuromas of the upper and lower lids in neurofibromatosis.

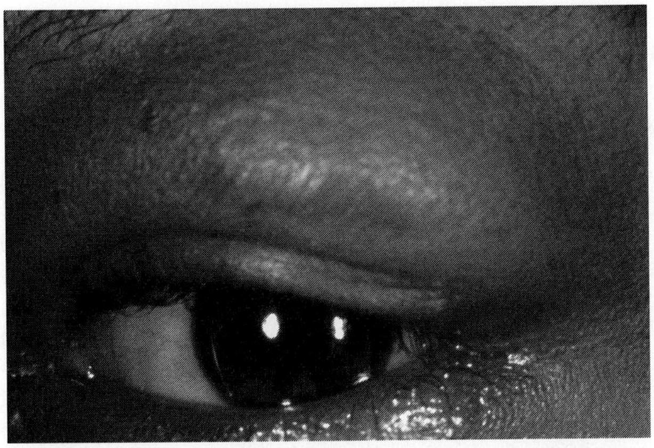

FIGURE 10–10. S-shaped deformity of the upper eyelid caused by a plexiform neuroma in neurofibromatosis.

isolated pedunculated nodules (fibroma molluscum) to large subcutaneous skin masses. Histopathologically, they appear to be enlarged cutaneous nerves in association with Schwann's cells, fibroblasts, and connective tissue components.[40] Of the two distinct variants of neurofibromatosis, cutaneous manifestations exist with the NF1 variant only. Glaucoma is present in about 50% of eyes with plexiform neuromas. The most likely cause of the increased IOP seems to be a combination of developmental abnormalities and tissue hypertrophy of the iris (Fig. 10–11) and of the angle.[41, 42] The proposed mechanisms of the glaucoma are numerous. Treatment depends on the severity of the glaucoma, the patient's age at onset, and the mechanism of the glaucoma. Congenital glaucomas should be managed surgically, whereas treatment for juvenile-onset and adult-onset glaucomas utilizes conventional medical and surgical therapies.

Entity Associated with Pigmentary Mechanism

Key external diagnostic signs of oculodermal melanocytosis (nevus of Ota) are (1) pigmentation of the deep dermal layers and (2) associated hyperpigmentation of structures of the ipsilateral globe.[43] This condition is commonly found in patients of dark-skinned races, particularly Asians. The dermal pigmentation manifests as a blue nevus of the periocular skin (Fig. 10–12). The nevus contains fusiform dendritic melanocytes that are usually unilateral and follow the distribution of the first and second divisions of the trigeminal nerve.[44]

The glaucomas noted with oculodermal melanocytosis vary in classification with the underlying assumption that the eye with the elevated IOP characteristically has the intraocular nevus involving the trabecular meshwork.[45] It has thus been postulated that the elevated IOP occurs in patients with a pre-existing compromised angle, and the melanocytic involvement overwhelms the outflow component of the trabecular meshwork. However, two separate studies contraindicate the association of melanocytic involvement of the angle and increased IOP. These studies showed no correlation in 227 patients between melanocytic involvement of the trabecular meshwork and elevated IOP.[46, 47]

Entities Associated with Developmental Abnormalities

CONGENITAL GLAUCOMAS

The diagnostic signs of *primary congenital glaucoma* are photophobia, blepharospasm, and epiphora secondary to corneal edema and tears in Descemet's membrane (Haab's striae). These signs arise from elevated IOP, which is often recognized between 3 and 9 months of age. Buphthalmos is often a presenting sign. When present, particularly in unilateral cases, buphthalmos may be a helpful key to diagnosis (Fig. 10–13).

Primary congenital glaucoma is the most common congenital glaucoma, occurring in about 1 in 30,000 live births.[48] Its inheritance pattern is multifactorial, with 10% of cases believed to be autosomal recessive.[49] This is in contrast to *juvenile open-angle glaucoma*, which is autoso-

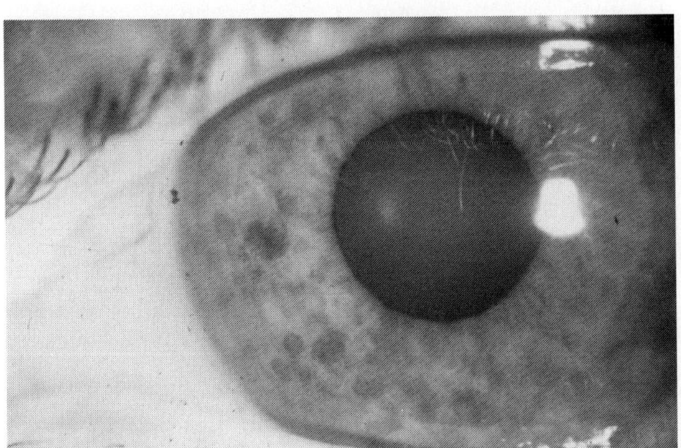

FIGURE 10–11. Numerous melanocytic hamartomas (Lisch nodules) occupying the iris in a patient with neurofibromatosis.

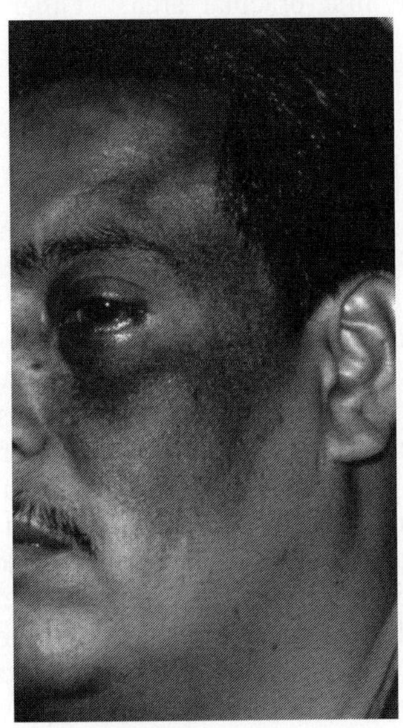

FIGURE 10–12. Typical facial appearance in oculodermal melanocytosis.

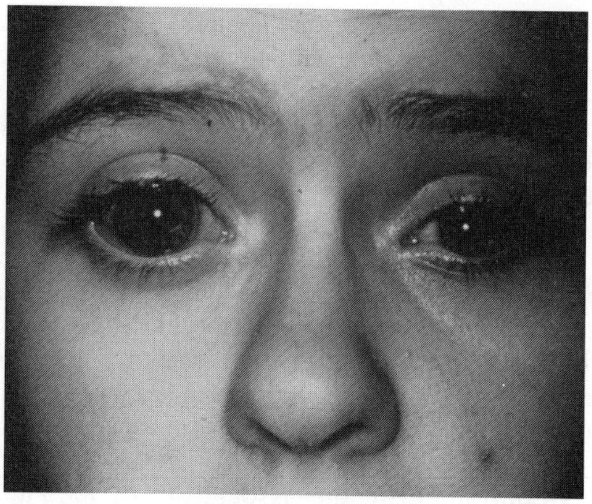

FIGURE 10–13. Unilateral buphthalmos from unilateral congenital glaucoma.

mal dominant, occurs in children older than 3 years, and does not cause buphthalmos.[50] There are two schools of thought for the inherited defect in the congenital glaucomas. Some investigators believe the elevated IOP may be secondary to arrested development of the angle.[51] Others have proposed that a Barkan's membrane may cover the trabecular meshwork, obstructing aqueous outflow.[52]

STICKLER'S SYNDROME

Open-angle glaucoma commonly occurs with Stickler's syndrome,[53] a connective tissue disease that is autosomal dominant with variable penetrance. Ocular examination may show axial myopia and the presence of cataracts in 50% of patients. Various fundus changes can be seen, including chorioretinal pigment changes, retinal detachments, and retinal breaks.[54] The glaucoma is secondary to anomalies of the anterior chamber angle. The external orofacial signs are (1) midfacial flattening and (2) the Pierre Robin malformation complex, which consists of micrognathia, cleft palate, and glossoptosis from maldevelopment of the first brachial arch.[55] Other abnormalities sometimes present are hearing loss, arthritis, and hyperextensive joints.[54]

NANOPHTHALMOS

Nanophthalmos is a rare, usually bilateral, inherited defect that is sporadic in its inheritance.[56, 57] External signs are (1) deeply set eyes in small bony orbits, (2) narrow palpebral fissures, and (3) an increased hyperopic correction. Angle closure secondary to a short axial length characterizes the glaucoma found. It usually manifests in patients between 40 and 60 years of age.[58] The short axial length with a normal to large lens predisposes to angle crowding, relative pupillary block, and subsequent glaucoma.[58, 59] Peripheral iridectomies should be performed to avoid angle closure if gonioscopy confirms impending angle closure. If chronic angle-closure glaucoma exists, medical therapy should be initiated. Special care should be taken to avoid postoperative hypotony in an attempt to prevent choroidal effusions, shallowing of the anterior chamber, and aqueous misdirection more commonly seen in these patients. Goniosynechiolysis may be a surgical option if the angle closure is relatively recent.

AXENFELD-RIEGER SYNDROME

Axenfeld-Rieger syndrome represents a rare spectrum of developmental disorders. This syndrome includes changes in ocular and extraocular structures derived from neural crest tissue.[60] The term "anterior cleavage syndrome"[61] has been used in the past but has been shown to be incorrect. All clinical variations of this syndrome have now been classified as Axenfeld-Rieger syndrome. The condition involves the anterior segment bilaterally and is associated with secondary glaucoma due to arrested development in about 50% of cases.

Axenfeld-Rieger syndrome is a rare autosomal dominant inherited disorder. Shields and coworkers[62] postulate that developmental arrest, occurring late in gestation, causes retention of primordial endothelium over parts of the iris and anterior chamber angle. Contraction of this primordial monolayer causes iris stromal thinning, corectopia, and hole formation. With contraction, the anterior uvea is hindered from migrating posteriorly, resulting in a high insertion of the iris into the anterior chamber angle.[60] Developmental defects associated with Axenfeld-Rieger syndrome are most commonly associated with teeth and facial bones. Microdontia (peg-like incisors), hypodontia (decreased number of evenly spaced teeth) and anodontia (focal absence of teeth) are most commonly noted (Fig. 10–14).[61, 63] The facial abnormalities include maxillary hypoplasia and a protruding lower lip. Telecanthus and hypertelorism have also been described in association with Axenfeld-Rieger syndrome.[64] Medical therapy is recommended prior to initiation of standard filtration surgery.

TRISOMY 21

Of the numerous congenital disorders associated with external signs and glaucoma, the most prevalent is trisomy 21 (Down syndrome). The incidence is 1 in 800 births and increases with advancing maternal age. Trisomy 21 is the most common of the autosomal trisomy syndromes.[65] External ocular abnormalities are common; they include mongoloid slant of the palpebral fissures, epicanthus of the

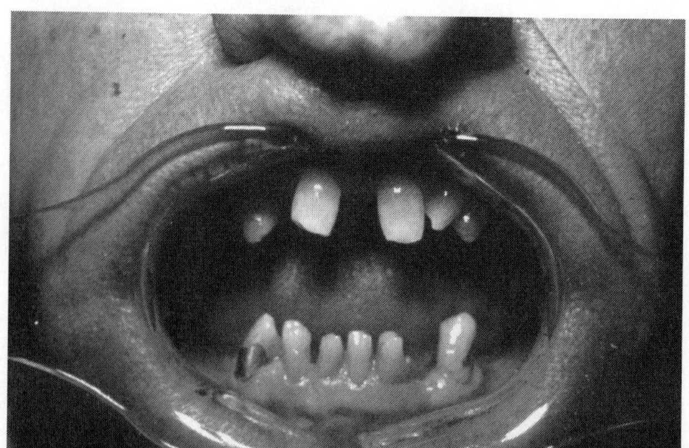

FIGURE 10–14. Dental abnormalities in Axenfeld-Rieger syndrome, including microdontia, hypodontia, and anodontia.

TABLE 10–1. DEVELOPMENTAL CONDITIONS ASSOCIATED WITH EXTERNAL SIGNS AND GLAUCOMA

Turner's syndrome
Ring chromosome 6 syndrome
Prader-Willi syndrome
Dental-ocular-cutaneous syndrome
Familial histiocytic dermatoarthritis
Hallermann-Streiff syndrome
Hereditary angioedema
Krause's syndrome
Multiple basal cell nevi syndrome
Nieden's syndrome
Oculocutaneous albinism
Oculodentodigital dysplasia
Osteogenesis imperfecta
Pierre Robin syndrome
Rubinstein-Taybi syndrome
Zellweger's syndrome

nasal portion of the upper lids, esotropia, nystagmus, myopia, and blepharitis.[66] The internal ocular findings noted are Brushfield's spots on the anterior surface of the iris, iris stromal atrophy, cataract, and keratoconus.[67] The most common systemic features are mental retardation, short stature, cardiac abnormalities, hypotonia, and characteristic facial features. Congenital glaucoma in patients with trisomy 21 is rare. Mesodermal dysgenesis has been observed, but no direct correlation of trisomy 21 and glaucoma has been proven, and the occurrence of glaucoma may be by chance.[68, 69]

TRISOMY 18

The second most common chromosomal trisomy is trisomy 18 syndrome (Edward's syndrome). Systemic findings include low-set ears, rocker-bottom feet, short sternum, and ventricular septal defects. The ocular abnormalities include ptosis, narrow palpebral fissures, blepharophimosis, hypertelorism and hypotelorism, corneal and lens opacities, uveal colobomas, blue sclera, microphthalmos, myopia, abnormal retinal pigmentation, shallow orbits, eyelash and eyebrow abnormalities, nystagmus, and strabismus. The glaucoma is related to trabeculodysgenesis and incomplete maturation of the anterior chamber.[70]

OTHER CONGENITAL DISORDERS

There are numerous other congenital disorders with external signs and glaucoma. The mechanisms of the glaucoma can include both open-angle and closed-angle forms of glaucoma and may occur at various times throughout life. Each condition listed in Table 10-1 has known cases in which glaucoma is present with one or both of the mechanisms.

REFERENCES

1. Phelps CD: The pathogenesis of glaucoma in Sturge-Weber syndrome. Ophthalmology 1978;85:276.
2. Elrich LM: Bilateral glaucoma associated with unilateral nevus flammeus. Arch Ophthalmol 1941;25:1002.
3. Dunphy EB: Glaucoma accompanying nevus flammeus. Am J Ophthalmol 1935; 18:709.
4. Weiss DI: Dual origin of glaucoma in encephalotrigeminal hemangiomatosis. Trans Ophthalmol Soc U K 1971;93:477.
5. Tripathi RC, Tripathi BJ, Cibis GW: Sturge-Weber syndrome. *In* Gold DH, Weingeist TA (eds): The Eye in Systemic Disease. Philadelphia, JB Lippincott, 1987.
6. Font RL, Ferry AP: The phakomatoses. Int Ophthalmol Clin 1972; 12:1.
7. Cibis GW, Tripathi RC, Tripathi B: Glaucoma in Sturge-Weber syndromes. Ophthalmology 1984;91:1061.
8. Duke-Elder S, Jay B: System of Ophthalmology: Diseases of Lens and Vitreous: Glaucoma and Hypotony, vol 11. St. Louis, CV Mosby, 1969, pp 637–640.
9. Rosen S, Smoller BR: Port-wine stains: A new hypothesis. J Am Acad Dermatol 1987;17:164.
10. Klippel M, Trenaunay P: Du naevus variques ostéohypertrophique. Arch Gen Med 1900;77:641.
11. Weber FP: Angioma formation in connection with hypertrophy of limbs and hemihypertrophy. Br J Dermatol 1907;190:231.
12. Waardenburg PJ, Franceschetti A, Klein D: Genetics and Ophthalmology, vol 2. Oxford, Blackwell, 1973.
13. Miller N: Walsh and Hoyt's Clinical Neuro-Ophthalmology, 4th ed. Baltimore, Williams & Wilkins, 1988.
14. Kontras SB: The Klippel-Trenaunay syndrome. Birth Defects 1974;10:177.
15. Bullock JD, Goldberg SH, Connelly PJ: Orbital varix thrombosis. Ophthalmology 1990;97:251.
16. Lloyd GAS: Phleboliths in the orbit. Clin Radiol 1965;16:339.
17. Wright JE: Orbital vascular anomalies. Trans Am Acad Ophthalmol Otolaryngol 1974;78:606.
18. Song GX, Tian WF, Qiang DF, Liu JI: Surgical treatment of orbital varices. Chin Med J 1979;92:723.
19. Winter J, Centeno RS, Bentson JR: Maneuver to aid diagnosis of orbital varix by computerized tomography. AJNR 1982;3:30.
20. Brauston BB, Norton EWD: Intermittent exophthalmos. Am J Ophthalmol 1963;55:701.
21. Elliot AJ: Ocular manifestations of carotid-cavernous fistulas. Postgrad Med 1954;15:191.
22. Henderson JW, Schneider RC: The ocular findings in carotid-cavernous fistula in a series of 17 cases. Am J Ophthalmol 1959;48:585.
23. Newton TH, Cronquist S: Involvement of dural arteries in intracranial arteriovenous malformation. Radiology 1969;93:1071.
24. Flanagan JC: Vascular problems of the orbit. Ophthalmology 1979;86:896.
25. Kupersmith MJ, Berenstein A, Flamm E, et al: Neuroophthalmologic abnormalities and intravascular therapy of traumatic carotid cavernous fistulas. Ophthalmology 1986;93:906.
26. Sugar HS, Meyer SJ: Pulsating exophthalmos. Arch Ophthalmol 1940;23:1288.
27. Urschel HC Jr: Superior vena cava canal obstruction. Dis Chest 1966;49:155.
28. Lokich JJ, Goodman R: Superior vena cava syndrome. JAMA 1975;231:58.
29. Yablonski ME, Podos SM: Glaucoma secondary to elevated episcleral venous pressure. *In* Shields MB, Ritch R (eds): The Secondary Glaucomas. St. Louis, CV Mosby, 1982.
30. Duke-Elder S (ed): System of Ophthalmology, vol 13. St. Louis, CV Mosby, 1974.
31. Spierer A, Eisenstein Z: The role of increased intraocular pressure on upgaze in the assessment of Grave's ophthalmopathy. Ophthalmology 1991;98:1491.
32. Manor RS, Kurz O, Lewitus Z: Intraocular pressure in endocrinological patients with exophthalmos. Ophthalmologica 1974;168:241.
33. Hunt A, Lindenbaum RH: Tuberous sclerosis: A new estimate of prevalence within the Oxford region. J Med Genet 1984;21:272.
34. Lagos JC, Gomez MR: Tuberous sclerosis: Reappraisal of clinical entity. Mayo Clin Proc 1967;42:26.
35. Gomez MR (ed): Tuberous Sclerosis. New York, Raven Press, 1979.
36. Williams R, Taylor D: Tuberous sclerosis. Surv Ophthalmol 1985; 30:143.
37. Robertson DM: Ophthalmic manifestations of tuberous sclerosis. Ann N Y Acad Sci 1991;615:17.
38. Robertson DM: Ophthalmic findings. *In* Gomez M (ed): Tuberous Sclerosis. New York, Raven Press, 1979.

39. Shields J, Shields C, Shields MB: Glaucoma associated with intraocular tumors. *In* Ritch R, Shields MB, Krupin T (eds): The Glaucomas. St. Louis, CV Mosby, 1996, p 1138.
40. Font RL, Ferry AP: The phakomatoses. Int Ophthalmol Clin 1972;12:1.
41. Poloti F, Sachs R, Barishak R: Neurofibromatosis and congenital glaucoma: A case report. Ophthalmologica 1978;176:155.
42. Wheeler JM: Plexiform neurofibromatosis involving the choroid, ciliary body, and other structures. Am J Ophthalmol 1937;20:368.
43. Hidano A, Kajima H, Ikeda S, et al: Natural history of nevus of Ota. Arch Dermatol 1967;95:187.
44. Teekhasaenee C, Ritch R, Rutnin U, et al: Ocular findings in oculodermal melanocytosis. Arch Ophthalmol 1990;108:1114.
45. Weiss DL, Krohn DL: Benign melanocytic glaucoma complicating oculodermal melanocytosis. Am Ophthalmol 1971;3:958.
46. Gonder JR, Nichols J, Augsburger JJ, et al: Ocular and oculodermal melanocytosis. Can J Ophthalmol 1985;20:176.
47. Teekhasaenee C, Ritch R, Rutnin U, et al: Glaucoma in oculodermal melanocytosis. Ophthalmology 1990;97:562.
48. Duke-Elder S (ed): System of Ophthalmology, vol 3, part 2: Congenital Deformities. St. Louis, CV Mosby, 1969.
49. Shaffer RN: Genetics in the congenital glaucomas. Trans Am Acad Ophthalmol Otolaryngol 1965;69:253–259.
50. Vidie B, Lerchner H: Long-term biometric results in glaucoma in children. Fortschr Ophthalmol 1990;87:25.
51. Broughton WL, Fine BS, Zimmerman LE: A histologic study of congenital glaucoma associated with a chromosomal defect. Ophthalmology 1980;87:96.
52. Maumenee AE: The pathogenesis of congenital glaucoma. Am J Ophthalmol 1959;47:827.
53. Phelps CD: Glaucoma associated with retinal disorders. *In* Ritch R, Shields MB (eds): The Secondary Glaucomas. St. Louis, CV Mosby, 1982, p 159.
54. Blair NP, Albert DM, Liberfarb RM, Hirose T: Hereditary progressive arthro-ophthalmopathy of Stickler. Am J Ophthalmol 1979;88:876.
55. Schreiner RL, McAlister WH, Marshall RE, et al: Stickler syndrome in a pedigree of Pierre Robin syndrome. Am J Dis Child 1973;126:86.
56. O'Grady RB: Nanophthalmos. Am J Ophthalmol 1971;71:1251.
57. Duggan JW, Hassard DTR: Familial microphthalmos classification and definition of terms. Trans Can Ophthalmol Soc 1961;24:210.
58. Kimbrough RL, Trempe CL, Brockhurst RJ, et al: Angle closure glaucoma in nanophthalmos. Am J Ophthalmol 1979;88:572.
59. Calhoun FP Jr: The management of glaucoma in nanophthalmos. Trans Am Ophthalmol Soc 1975;73:97.
60. Shields MB: Axenfeld-Rieger syndrome: A theory of mechanism and distinctions from iridocorneal endothelial syndrome. Trans Am Ophthalmol Soc 1983;81:736.
61. Reese AB, Ellsworth RM: The anterior chamber cleavage syndrome. Arch Ophthalmol 1966;75:307.
62. Shields MB: Axenfeld-Rieger syndrome. *In* Ritch T, Shields MB, Krupin T (eds): The Glaucomas. St. Louis, CV Mosby, 1996.
63. Burian HM, Braley AE, Allen L: External and gonioscopic visibility of ring of Schwalbe and trabeculum, an interpretation of the posterior corneal embryotoxon and the so-called congenital hyaline membranes on the posterior corneal surface. Trans Am Ophthalmol Soc 1955;51:389.
64. Wesley RK, Baker JD, Golnick AL: Rieger's syndrome, oligodontia and primary mesodermal dysgenesis of the iris: Clinical features and report of an isolated case. J Pediatr Ophthalmol Strabismus 1978;15:67.
65. Thompson JB, Thompson MW (eds): Genetics in Medicine. Philadelphia, WB Saunders, 1980.
66. Cantor LB: Glaucoma associated with congenital disorders. *In* Ritch T, Shields MB, Krupin T (eds): The Glaucomas. St. Louis, CV Mosby, 1996.
67. Williams RDB: Brushfield spots and Wofflin nodules in the iris: An appraisal in handicapped children. Dev Med Child Neurol 1982;23:646.
68. Catalano R: Down syndrome. Surv Ophthalmol 1990;34:385.
69. Howard RO: Classification of chromosomal eye syndrome. Int Ophthalmol 1981;4:77.

CHAPTER 11

Conjunctiva and Cornea

MARY ANN LLOYD and DALE K. HEUER

We are in our element when examining the eye with a magnified binocular view. This examination begins with the biomicroscopic observation of the ocular surface structures, including the conjunctiva, episclera, sclera, and cornea. In this chapter, Mary Ann Lloyd and Dale Heuer offer a discussion of the critical areas that are often affected by glaucoma. Inflammatory diseases of the episclera and sclera may result in glaucoma. Increased episcleral venous pressure, also discussed in Chapters 8 and 10, is considered. Scleral abnormalities, including pigmentation and thinning, may also be related to glaucoma. Changes in conjunctiva may represent key signs in the identification of ocular inflammation, ocular ischemia, drug toxicity, and vascular anomalies. Similarly, the cornea provides insight into potential diagnoses. Identifying corneal edema or toxic, infectious, or interstitial keratitis gives valuable insight into the underlying process. Examination of the corneal endothelium is particularly important because of its close relationship with the trabecular meshwork. Developmental and acquired abnormalities of the cornea, particularly the endothelium, may often be diagnostic alone. The authors include a very useful section on two common clinical problems, postkeratoplasty and steroid-induced glaucomas. Finally, they address the potential for glaucoma in the patient with excessively large or small corneal structures.

Glaucoma may be associated with a number of clinical syndromes and diseases affecting the anterior structures of the eye. Careful history and clinical examination allow the observer to make the correct diagnosis and treatment plan when elevated intraocular pressure (IOP) is found in conjunction with findings in the episclera, sclera, conjunctiva, and cornea. Although such findings may be caused by elevated IOP or its treatment, they may also be directly or indirectly related to the pathogenesis of the elevation in IOP.

Episclera and Sclera

INFLAMMATION

Episcleritis

Inflammation of the episclera and sclera can be associated with glaucoma.[1] Episcleritis is a common, benign condition affecting women more often than men and occurring most often in the fourth decade of life. The etiology remains obscure, although the initial episode often follows a viral infection and may act like a type I hypersensitivity reaction.

The presenting symptoms vary from minor to more severe conjunctival and episcleral hyperemia and chemosis lasting from a few to several weeks, but discomfort is generally mild to absent. Episcleritis may also manifest as nodule formation within episcleral tissue.[2] Eyelid edema, miosis, and myopia may also result. Up to 60% of patients with the disorder have recurrent attacks. Episcleritis can be distinguished from scleritis on the basis of two features seen only in episcleritis:

- Blanching of surface vessels in response to topical vasoconstrictors
- Minimal discomfort present

Treatment of episcleritis is indicated only if symptoms warrant. Topical steroidal and nonsteroidal medications may give symptomatic relief but do not reduce the duration of disease.[3, 4] Systemic nonsteroidal agents may be useful if attacks are frequent or severe.

Although uncommon, acute open-angle glaucoma can be associated with episcleritis. It most often occurs in patients with severely infiltrated, edematous episclera and lids. Such patients present with pain and decreased vision.[5] The IOP is high, and corneal edema and miosis are present. The angle is open without blood reflux into Schlemm's canal. The predominant cause is probably trabecular meshwork edema rather than elevated episcleral venous pressure (EVP). The IOP usually normalizes with administration of aqueous suppressants, cycloplegia, and topical steroids.

Acute angle-closure glaucoma has also been reported in episcleritis. It responds to standard therapy.[1] Steroid-induced glaucoma may occur with long-term topical steroids and infrequently with systemic steroid therapy. Filtering surgery may be useful if open-angle or closed-angle glaucoma persists.

Scleritis

Scleritis is a significantly more painful and potentially devastating inflammation than episcleritis.[1, 2] The discomfort may extend from the globe to the orbit and is a result of edema or destruction of the sclera. Inflammation can manifest as diffuse anterior scleritis with edema of the deep scleral tissue and episcleral hyperemia up to the equator of the globe that fails to blanch in response to topical vasoconstrictors. In scleritis, vascular plexuses detour from their uniform arrangements to form large bypass channels, unlike in episcleritis. Anterior scleritis may also manifest in more focal nodules or less commonly as necrotizing scleritis, which is always associated with marked pain and congestion and may result in loss of the eye if not aggressively treated. The conjunctiva and sclera may be avascular over the foci of the lesions, which can break down and result in tissue necrosis. Anterior scleritis is treated with systemic steroidal or nonsteroidal anti-inflammatory agents; in necrotizing scleritis, high-dose systemic steroids or immunosuppressive agents are usually necessary to stop progression of the disease.

Posterior scleritis involves inflammation posterior to the equator of the globe. It is often more difficult to diagnose than anterior scleritis. In one study, 45% of eyes enucleated for scleritis were undiagnosed at the time of enucleation.[6] The location of the inflammation determines the signs and symptoms, which range from pars planitis to exudative retinal detachment, papilledema, and proptosis.[7] Ultrasound and computed tomography (CT) scanning can aid in the diagnosis. Treatment with systemic nonsteroidal agents can be attempted, although systemic steroids are usually necessary.

Glaucoma is sometimes associated with scleritis. In one study, IOP elevation was found in 12% of patients with scleritis, 3% of whom underwent surgery for its control.[1] However, another histologic study revealed that 49% of the eyes enucleated for scleral disease had glaucoma, the majority of cases being a combination of anterior and posterior disease.[8] Different mechanisms may be responsible for the development of glaucoma in patients with scleritis. Patients may present with variable IOP elevations and open angles, with or without intraocular inflammation. Uveitis is often seen on histologic examination but less commonly on clinical examination, and severe uveitis is usually limited to eyes with marked inflammation around the globe or extending posteriorly.

Glaucoma in patients with scleritis may be a consequence of a combination of trabecular damage, impairment of the episcleral outflow channels, anterior segment ischemia, and involvement of the uveal tract by granulomas. It may be more common in diffuse anterior scleritis involving the limbus or in circumferential necrotizing scleritis, which may directly involve the meshwork.[1, 8] Glaucoma associated with scleritis can also represent steroid response, more often if topical treatment has been used. In addition, glaucoma may much less commonly be a result either of secondary angle closure with formation of peripheral anterior synechiae (PAS) or of pupillary block; both mechanisms are seen in cases of severe or chronic uveitis. Angle-closure glaucoma may also result from anterior choroidal effusions secondary to inflammation around the ciliary body. In these cases, the entire anterior chamber shallows and on gonioscopic examination appears to be occluded unilaterally (Fig. 11–1).[9, 10]

Management of glaucoma in scleritis is primarily aimed at reduction of inflammation with topical and systemic anti-inflammatory agents, although aqueous suppressants may be needed until inflammation subsides. Peripheral iridectomy be necessary in those rare cases of pupillary block glaucoma. Cycloplegic agents may be helpful in cases of angle closure due to choroidal effusion, and miotic agents should certainly be avoided in such cases. Trabeculectomy is occasionally warranted if IOP elevation is intractable.[11] In general, glaucoma associated with episcleritis or scleritis may have varied underlying mechanisms that are often preventable and usually treatable with attention to diagnosis and management of glaucoma and inflammation.

EPISCLERAL CONGESTION (INCREASED EPISCLERAL VENOUS PRESSURE)

Conditions causing elevated EVP can lead to glaucoma. The predominant route for aqueous drainage is through the trabecular meshwork and Schlemm's canal, which is connected to episcleral and conjunctival veins by intrascleral aqueous vessels. The episcleral vessels connect to the cavernous sinus by way of the anterior ciliary and superior

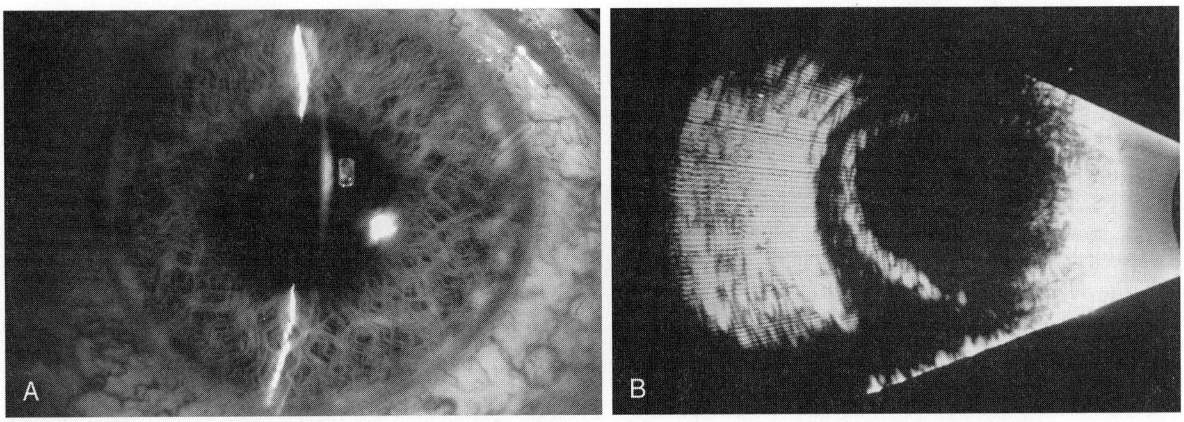

FIGURE 11–1. Posterior scleritis with shallow anterior chamber (*A*) associated with 360-degree ciliochoroidal detachment, as demonstrated by B-scan echography (*B*). (Courtesy of Kirk Wilhelmus, MD.)

ophthalmic veins, and the conjunctival veins drain into the superior ophthalmic vein or the facial veins via the angular and palpebral veins. Conditions that increase pressure in the venous system can therefore impair drainage of aqueous and lead to elevated IOP. In addition, increased venous pressure may lower the perfusion pressure to the optic nerve, making it more susceptible to damage.[12, 13]

Patients with increased EVP have tortuous and dilated episcleral veins (caput medusa) , and the condition may be unilateral or bilateral, depending on the location of the cause of the increased pressure. The angle is open and appears normal except for the presence of blood in Schlemm's canal in some cases; neovascularization due to ischemia is less commonly seen.[14] Venous stasis in the posterior segment may lead to uveal congestion, causing forward displacement of the lens diaphragm and angle-closure glaucoma.[15]

Carotid Artery–Cavernous Sinus Fistula

EVP can be elevated by arteriovenous anomalies. As the term implies, carotid artery–cavernous sinus fistula involves anastomosis between the carotid artery and cavernous sinus. It can be traumatic or spontaneous. Owing to intracranial connections between the two cavernous sinuses, bilateral symptoms may result from a unilateral fistula. Because arterial pressure may be reduced by the shunt, ischemic ocular necrosis may result.[14] Presenting signs and symptoms include conjunctival and orbital vascular engorgement from reversal of blood flow into the orbital veins (Fig. 11–2), a bruit or subjective sensation of a pulsating sound, pulsating exophthalmos, and pain. Diplopia may result from orbital compression, traumatic paresis, or ischemia, and vision may be impaired by corneal exposure, ischemia, or glaucoma. Choroidal detachment, disc edema, and retinal hemorrhage are less common.[16] The diagnosis is made by carotid arteriography, although in long-standing cases, radiographs may reveal widening of the superior orbital fissure and erosion of the sella and sphenoid sinus.

IOP is elevated in 60% to 70% of patients with carotid artery–cavernous sinus fistula,[17] although glaucomatous optic neuropathy is less common.[12] Such a fistula can cause increased EVP as well as increased pressure in the central retinal and vortex veins. The angle usually appears open in glaucoma associated with elevated EVP, although reduced ocular perfusion can result in ischemia and neovascularization of the disc and retina as well as the iris and angle, causing neovascular glaucoma.[18] Angle-closure glaucoma can occasionally be seen as a result of forward movement of the lens from choroidal engorgement or detachment.

Treatment of glaucoma due to carotid artery–cavernous sinus fistula is aimed at treating the underlying structural problem. Usually, IOP can be controlled with aqueous suppressants. The decision to perform intracranial surgery is sometimes difficult and should be based on the severity of the findings, because in many cases, the fistula spontaneously improves or resolves, and surgery can be associated with complications.[18] Transvascular surgical procedures have reduced the potential for complications and are now the standard approach for carotid artery–cavernous sinus fistula that is unresponsive to conservative management.[17]

Orbital Varices

Other structural lesions causing increased IOP associated with unilaterally elevated EVP are orbital varices. They are most commonly found in young patients who have had intermittent episodes of unilateral proptosis since birth or early childhood. Proptosis can be evoked or exacerbated

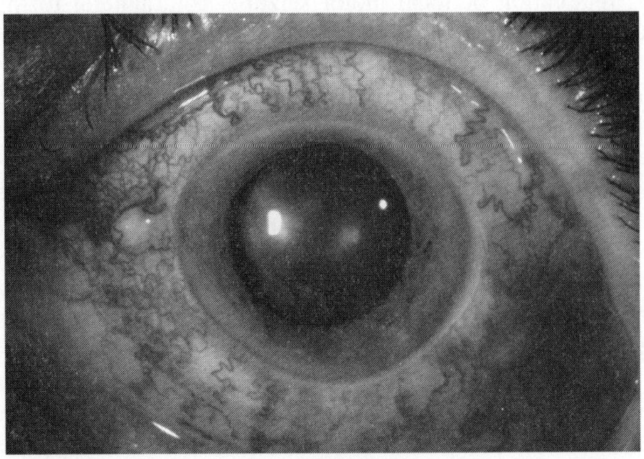

FIGURE 11–2. Conjunctival vascular engorgement due to carotid artery–cavernous sinus fistula. (Courtesy of Andrew Lee, MD.)

with any action that increases venous pressure in the head and neck, such as a Valsalva maneuver or bending over.[19, 20] Enophthalmos may be seen in between episodes on the affected side. Other presenting symptoms are dilated veins in the eyelid and anterior orbit, spontaneous orbital hemorrhage, and thrombophlebitis. Roughly half of patients with orbital varices have other systemic venous anomalies involving the scalp, palate, and forehead. Less commonly, orbital varices may be associated with the Klippel-Trenaunay-Weber syndrome.

Multiloculated cysts may be seen in the conjunctiva of a patient with orbital varices; such findings should not be mistaken for orbital lymphangioma. The diagnosis may be confirmed by orbital radiographs showing orbital phleboliths and an enlarged orbit; ultrasound and CT may reveal a soft tissue mass. B-scan echography may demonstrate retro-ocular fluid-filled spaces with Valsalva maneuver, and venography usually shows an abnormal venous pattern.[12]

Glaucoma may result if an orbital varix causes a chronic or extreme elevation of EVP. Because this situation is rare, glaucoma is uncommon, and vision is only rarely affected unless the varix directly compresses the optic nerve.[19] Medication usually controls the glaucoma due to optic varices, and surgery is rarely performed except for cosmetic reasons.

Encephalotrigeminal Angiomatosis (Sturge-Weber Syndrome)

Patients who present at birth with unilateral or bilateral hemangiomas of the lids in the presence or absence of intracranial and ocular hemangiomas should be suspected of having encephalotrigeminal angiomatosis or Sturge-Weber syndrome. The facial cutaneous angioma (nevus flammeus or port-wine stain) is often seen in the distribution of the first and second divisions of the trigeminal nerve. The angioma is variable in size and consists of a loose arrangement of dilated capillaries in the dermis and subcutaneous tissue. It is bilateral in 10% to 30% of cases, and facial hypertrophy in the affected region is common. A meningeal racemose hemangioma usually occurs ipsilateral to the dermal angioma and may be associated with progressive calcification of the meningeal arteries and atrophy of the cerebral cortex, sometimes associated with mental retardation or focal motor seizures contralateral to the facial angioma that begin in the first few years of life. Various combinations of structural involvement may occur, and other visceral organs may be involved with angiomas, although Sturge-Weber syndrome classically involves the leptomeninges, eyes, and face.[21]

Ocular involvement of the hemangiomas may affect the lid, episclera, conjunctiva, iris, and ciliary body (Fig. 11–3). Although there are exceptions, when the angioma involves the upper lid, usually there is ipsilateral intraocular involvement, but the eye is generally spared if the lid is spared (Anderson's rule).[22] Iris hyperchromia, tortuous retinal vessels, and scleral melanosis may occur in a smaller number of patients. Choroidal hemangiomas, which occur in 40% of cases, are usually flat and diffuse and involve the posterior pole. They may appear as a diffuse flush, described as "tomato catsup fundus,"[23] or as an orange-yellow mass; histopathologic examination reveals them to be cavernous hemangiomas.[21]

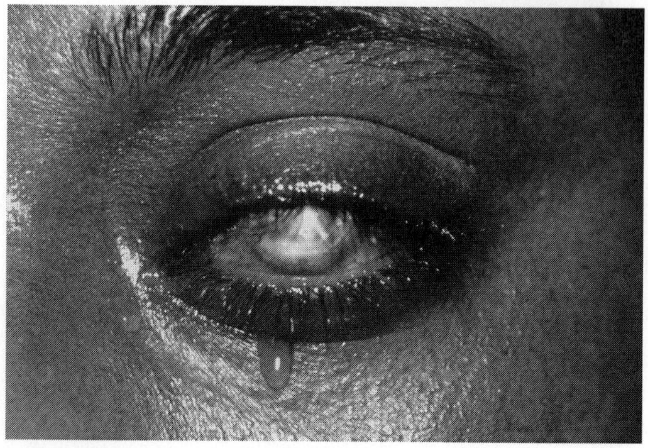

FIGURE 11–3. Sturge-Weber syndrome with lid and conjunctival hemangiomas. This patient had secondary glaucoma and corneal opacification.

Approximately one third of patients with Sturge-Weber syndrome have increased IOP, usually when the angioma involves the lid, tarsus, and conjunctiva. IOP elevation is more common when choroidal hemangioma is present. Although glaucoma is more often unilateral, bilateral angiomas may be associated with bilateral IOP elevation. Glaucoma may occur any time from infancy to adulthood. Theories abound as to the cause of glaucoma in this syndrome. The most plausible involve developmental abnormalities of the angle structures, with anterior insertion of the iris root and thick uveoscleral meshwork. Choroidal hemangiomas may result in fluid transudation or hemorrhage and a hypersecretory glaucoma or may lead to forward displacement of the lens, causing angle-closure glaucoma.[12, 24, 25] IOP elevation may be the result of vascular malformations that increase production, decrease outflow, or change the components of aqueous.[21] Increased EVP has been measured in a majority of patients in some studies; theoretically, it may result from arteriovenous shunts.[24] The most plausible mechanism for elevated IOP may be a combination of developmental angle anomalies and increased EVP, the role of each varying among individuals.

Treatment of glaucoma associated with Sturge-Weber syndrome is often difficult, because medical therapy is commonly ineffective. Goniotomy or trabeculotomy is occasionally successful in cases of congenital glaucoma. Trabeculectomy or tube shunt surgery is more often successful, although filtering surgery is associated with increased incidence of uveal effusion and choroidal detachment,[24, 26, 27] the risks of which may be lessened by posterior sclerotomy.

Other Arteriovenous Anomalies

Other arteriovenous anomalies that may lead to elevated EVP are orbital-meningeal shunts, including dural venous fistulas; carotid jugular venous shunts; and intraocular vascular shunts.[12] In patients with low-flow systems, such as dural venous shunts, the signs and symptoms of elevated EVP are generally more subtle than in those with higher flow fistulas.

Superior Vena Cava Syndrome

Another cause of elevated venous pressure is obstruction of the venous system, such as in the superior vena cava syndrome. The presenting signs are edema and cyanosis of the head, neck, and upper extremities. Chest wall veins may become dilated from development of collateral circulation.[28] Symptoms include headache, blurred vision, and altered consciousness from increased intracranial pressure. Ocular findings include prominent conjunctival, episcleral, and retinal veins; lid and disc edema; and elevations of EVP and IOP, particularly in the supine position. Glaucomatous cupping of the optic nerve is usually absent, possibly because of an opposing effect of increased intracranial pressure.[12]

The cause of superior vena cava syndrome had most commonly been mediastinitis secondary to pulmonary infections such as syphilis and tuberculosis, but currently malignancy is the cause in 97% of cases.[29] Other causes are aortic aneurysm, enlarged hilar nodes, and thyroid disease. Management of superior vena cava syndrome is aimed at treating the cause.

Thyroid Ophthalmopathy

Another possible cause of elevated EVP is thyroid ophthalmopathy, in which lymphocytes, mast cells, and plasma cells infiltrate the orbit. Congestion of the orbit may impair the orbital venous system and raise EVP. Less commonly, EVP may be elevated as a result of thrombosis of the orbital veins. Increased EVP may result in elevation of IOP. Patients with symptoms of elevated EVP due to thyroid ophthalmopathy often present with exophthalmos, limitation of extraocular muscle function, and keratopathy related to corneal exposure. Contraction of extraocular muscles may also raise IOP, most often on down gaze. Orbital infiltration may be treated with systemic steroids, irradiation, or surgical decompression of the orbit.

Other Causes of Elevated Episcleral Venous Pressure

Other mechanisms of venous obstruction that may lead to elevated EVP are retrobulbar tumors, congestive heart failure, thrombosis of the cavernous sinus or orbital vein, vasculitis involving episcleral or orbital veins, and jugular vein obstruction.[12]

Although in most patients, increased EVP has a local or systemic cause, both sporadic and familial idiopathic cases have been reported.[13, 26, 27, 30] Idiopathic elevation of EVP may occur in all age groups, and the right eye is more often or more severely affected.[31] The angle appears open, and blood may or may not be visible in Schlemm's canal. Medical therapy is the initial treatment, and surgery can be performed in cases unresponsive to medication.

INCREASED PIGMENTATION

Oculodermal melanocytosis, or nevus of Ota, usually manifests as a unilateral hyperpigmentation of the dermis in the distribution of the first and second divisions of the trigeminal nerve, more often in patients of Asian descent. Hyperpigmentation of the globe usually occurs and may involve the sclera, conjunctiva, cornea, iridocorneal angle, iris, and fundus. Angioid streaks are sometimes present, and the condition is associated with a greater incidence of uveal and orbital melanoma.[21]

Both primary open-angle and angle-closure glaucomas have been identified.[32–35] Although secondary glaucomas have been reported in association with melanocytic infiltration of the angle, increased numbers of iris processes, malignant melanoma of the iris, and nevus flammeus with retinal angiomatosis,[36–29] a larger study of patients with oculodermal melanocytosis reported no correlation between melanocytic infiltration of the trabecular meshwork and elevated IOP.[40] One study found that when oculodermal melanocytosis and nevus flammeus occur together (phakomatosis pigmentovascularis) and each extensively involves the globe, there is a strong predisposition for congenital glaucoma, but the associated vascular anomalies play a larger role in the predisposition to glaucoma than the melanocytosis.[41] Treatment of glaucoma associated with oculodermal melanocytosis is similar to that of primary open-angle glaucoma.

SCLERAL THINNING

Patients presenting with blue sclerae, brittle bones, deafness at birth, and glaucoma may have osteogenesis imperfecta (van der Hoeve's syndrome, Lobstein's syndrome, brittle bone disease, or osteopsathyrosis idiopathica).[42, 43] This disorder occurs in 1 of 50,000 births without race or gender predilection and is inherited in an autosomal dominant pattern in most cases. Although the cause is unknown, osteogenesis imperfecta is thought to be a diffuse collagen disorder. It has two clinical forms:[44]

1. Osteogenesis imperfecta congenita, which manifests early in life and has more severe symptoms, often leading to early death
2. Osteogenesis imperfecta tarda, which is less severe and may be associated with deafness, brittle bones, soft skull, caput medusae, short stature, dental defects, hypotonia, hyperflexibility, and small facies.

A characteristic ocular finding in osteogenesis imperfecta is a blue appearance to the sclerae, resulting from decreased thickness and increased translucency of the sclerae. Shallow orbits, hypertelorism, megalocornea, keratoconus, cataracts, and optic atrophy may also be seen. Open-angle glaucoma may be diagnosed in the first or second decade. Surgery can be used to manage the glaucoma if it is unresponsive to medical therapy, although surgical treatment can be complicated by the abnormally thin sclerae, which may also predispose to postoperative scleral collapse, flat anterior chamber, or suprachoroidal hemorrhage.[42]

Conjunctiva

INFLAMMATION

Uveitis

Conjunctival inflammation can be associated with a number of conditions in which elevated IOP may be present. Uveitis is one of the more common conditions that can be associated with inflamed conjunctiva and glaucoma. Typically, patients present with varying degrees of conjunctival injection (often perilimbal), miosis, anterior chamber and sometimes posterior segment inflammatory reaction (cell, flare, and keratic precipitates), IOP elevation, pain, blurred vision, and photophobia (Fig. 11–4).

Although a number of conditions may be associated with uveitis, it is often idiopathic. A careful history and examination guide the examiner to the correct diagnosis, and ancillary testing may prove helpful in establishing any associated conditions. Specific inflammatory conditions that may be associated with glaucoma include infections such as syphilis, tuberculosis, rubella, herpesvirus infection, Lyme disease, and, less commonly, mumps. Associated systemic inflammatory conditions include ankylosing spondylitis and Reiter's syndrome (conjunctivitis, urethritis, arthritis, mucocutaneous lesions), both of which are associated with the HLA-B27 genotype, adult or juvenile rheumatoid arthritis, systemic lupus erythematosus, sarcoidosis, and Behçet's disease. Conditions associated with uveitis and glaucoma that typically do not cause conjunctival inflammation or pain include Fuchs' heterochromic cyclitis, glaucomatocyclitic crisis (Posner-Schlossman syndrome), and, sometimes, juvenile arthritis.

Initial IOP elevation associated with uveitis usually occurs via an open-angle mechanism and is likely due to obstruction of the outflow channels caused either by swelling or dysfunction of the trabecular sheets or endothelial cells or by the accumulation of inflammatory cells and debris in the trabecular meshwork. Prostaglandins may also contribute to a breakdown of the blood-aqueous barrier that contributes to elevation of IOP.[45] Chronic or severe uveitis can lead to pupillary block glaucoma from posterior synechiae formation or to secondary angle closure from PAS formation. Treatment is directed at establishing and treating any underlying disease entity and managing the intraocular inflammation with topical and sometimes systemic steroid therapy, cycloplegia, and glaucoma medication. The IOP usually normalizes as the inflammation subsides, although it can remain elevated if the uveitis is chronic. Steroid-induced glaucoma is also common; however, it is frequently incorrectly suspected when IOP rises, because the rise often occurs when reduced outflow related to inflammatory trabecular meshwork damage is unmasked by the increased in aqueous humor production that occurs in response to the decrease in inflammation.

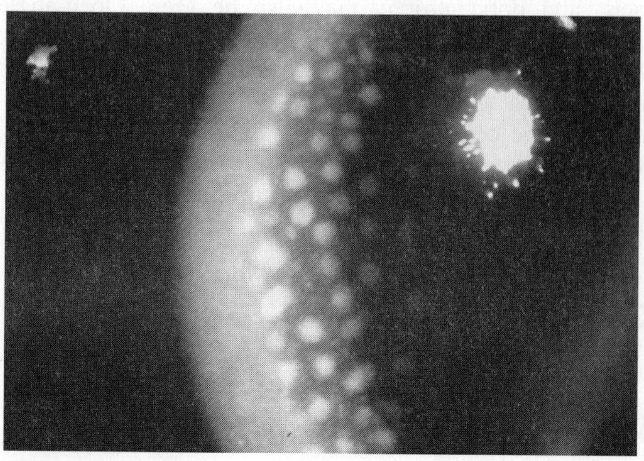

FIGURE 11–4. Granulomatous uveitis with mutton-fat keratic precipitates.

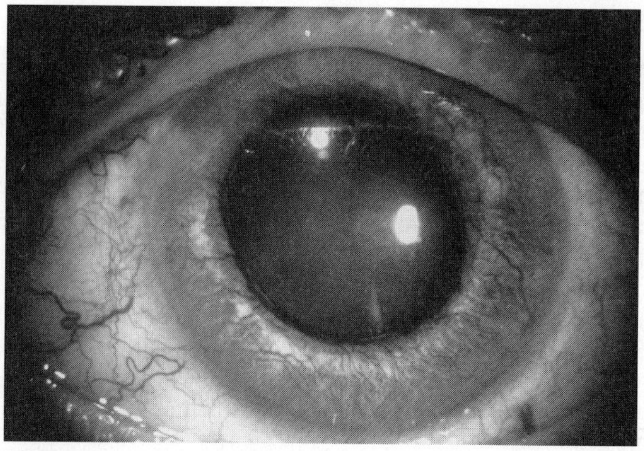

FIGURE 11–5. Rubeosis iridis.

Ocular Ischemia

Conjunctival inflammation associated with glaucoma can also be a sign of ocular ischemia. Patients presenting with congested conjunctiva, steamy cornea, new iris vessels, ocular pain, decreased visual acuity, and markedly elevated IOP should be suspected of having neovascular glaucoma (Fig. 11–5). Hyphema may be present. The angle may be open with vessels crossing the scleral spur into the trabecular meshwork, or closed to varying degrees by fibrovascular membrane proliferation and PAS formation.

Local ocular ischemia from central retinal artery or vein occlusion can result in rubeosis iridis. Ocular ischemia may also result from arteriovenous malformations or carotid artery–cavernous sinus fistula, as previously discussed. In addition, ocular ischemia and rubeosis iridis may result from systemic vascular diseases, such as carotid occlusive disease, Takayasu's disease (aortic arch syndrome), and temporal arteritis, which have in common decreased blood flow to the ophthalmic and central retinal arteries with secondary retinal and ocular ischemia. The IOP may be normal or low despite extensive rubeosis and synechial angle closure because decreased perfusion of the ciliary body in carotid occlusive disease reduces aqueous production.[46, 47]

Other causes of glaucoma associated with rubeosis iridis are diabetes mellitus, chronic retinal detachment, previous vitrectomy or retinal detachment repair, intraocular tumors, sickle cell retinopathy, Stickler's syndrome, and other conditions associated with chronic diffuse retinal or anterior segment ischemia. The glaucoma is managed through treatment of the underlying condition, along with panretinal photocoagulation, medical treatment, and, often, surgical intervention.

Drug-Induced Conjunctivitis

Conjunctival erythema noted in patients who are taking medications for glaucoma may be drug-related. Patients who have been receiving such medication for variable lengths of time may present with mild to marked conjunctival injection often associated with punctate corneal epithelial defects. Adrenergic agonists such as epinephrine and, to a lesser extent, the pro-drug dipivefrin[48] are commonly associated with congestion of conjunctival vessels due to vasodilation following the initial vasoconstriction. The incidence of allergy due to apraclonidine 1% and 0.5% may be as high as 48% and 36%, respectively, after at least 3 months of use.[49, 50] Brimonidine is also associated with conjunctival injection, but to a lesser degree. The topical carbonic anhydrase inhibitor dorzolamide is also associated with a 10% to 15% incidence of conjunctival hyperemia and keratitis.[51] Similar reactions can also be seen in up to 30% of cases with the prostaglandin analogue latanoprost. Any topical glaucoma medication, however, can cause conjunctival inflammation or allergy, the preservatives in the solutions often being the cause.

VASCULAR ANOMALIES

Vascular anomalies in the conjunctival vessels can serve as warning signs of potential underlying glaucoma. Conjunctival telangiectasis noted early in life may be part of a condition known as Klippel-Trenaunay syndrome, a neurocutaneous disorder consisting of a cutaneous capillary vascular malformation or nevus flammeus associated with venous and lymphatic malformations and soft tissue or skeletal hypertrophy or both.[41, 52] Weber[53] described a similar syndrome in which arteriovenous shunts were prominent, and the two conditions are often linked into one, known as the Klippel-Trenaunay-Weber syndrome. The condition may be inherited in an irregular dominant pattern, and formes frustes may occur. Patients may have seizures, mental retardation, and cerebral hemangiomas. Ocular findings in addition to conjunctival telangiectasis include enophthalmos, iris heterochromia or coloboma, oculosympathetic palsy, retinal varicosities, choroidal angiomas, strabismus, orbital varices, disc anomalies, buphthalmos (with or without glaucoma), and glaucoma. Ocular findings may occur without the facial hemangioma. Glaucoma is relatively uncommon in this condition and is usually associated with a facial nevus.[21, 54]

A far less common congenital disorder associated with conjunctival hemangiomas and sometimes glaucoma is diffuse congenital hemangiomatosis.[21, 55] In this condition, multiple small cutaneous hemangiomas occur with visceral hemangiomas, and death results in the first few months of life as a result of cardiac failure due to a large hepatic hemangioma. Ocular findings in 50% of patients in a series of 16 cases included hemangiomas of the iris, conjunctiva, and lid, abnormal chorioretinal vasculature, and microphthalmos. Cortical blindness as well as third and sixth nerve palsies occurred secondary to central nervous system hemangiomas. Glaucoma was reported in 12.5% of the cases in this study.[55]

NODULES

Conjunctival nodules or diffuse infiltration of the episclera by nerve fibers or small tumors can occasionally be seen in neurofibromatosis. This condition, which is detailed in other chapters, is a neuroectodermal dysplasia characterized by tumor-like formations derived from the proliferation of peripheral nerve elements. Neurofibromatosis may involve the eyelids, orbit, uvea, optic nerve, retina, cornea, tarsal conjunctiva, and bulbar conjunctiva. Glaucoma is relatively rare in this condition but can occur at birth or at any time thereafter. It is usually unilateral and associated with involvement of the upper lid.[21] Glaucoma occurs in half of patients with plexiform neuroma.[56]

Cornea

EDEMA

Corneal edema may be related to intrinsic diseases of the cornea, such as congenital hereditary endothelial dystrophy, Fuchs' dystrophy, inflammation, infection, trauma, and surgery. It may also be a sign of an underlying increase in IOP due to many conditions other than primary glaucoma. Therefore, evaluation of IOP is imperative in patients presenting with corneal edema. Acute IOP elevation most commonly leads to epithelial or microcystic edema, whereas chronic elevation sometimes results in endothelial dysfunction and. in some cases. stromal edema. The globe is more distensible in children younger than 3 years, and raised IOP may result in disruptions of Descemet's membrane (Haab's striae) and corneal enlargement associated with buphthalmos.

EPITHELIAL DISORDERS

Drug-Induced Keratitis

Medications used to treat glaucoma and other ocular diseases not infrequently cause ocular surface changes, most often in the epithelium but sometimes in the stroma as well.[57, 58] Preservatives such as benzalkonium chloride, found in most glaucoma medications, are frequently the cause of drug-induced surface changes, although other substances can also play a role. Pilocarpine occasionally causes conjunctival hyperemia or allergic keratoconjunctivitis, and pilocarpine gel has been implicated in punctate epitheliopathy in up to 40% of patients and in mild diffuse subepithelial haze in up to 20% of patients using the medication for more than 8 weeks. Symblepharon and conjunctival scarring have been associated with the use of echothiophate iodide (Phospholine Iodide).

Epinephrine compounds can induce punctate epitheliopathy, conjunctival hyperemia and allergy, and adrenochrome pigmentation of the conjunctiva and cornea, especially in the presence of vascularized scarring or pre-existing corneal edema. The pro-drug of epinephrine, dipivefrin, does not cause adrenochrome deposits but occasionally may produce conjunctival scarring.

Beta-blockers such as timolol may produce acute and chronic punctate epitheliopathy as well as delayed epithelial healing (sometimes resulting in persistent epithelial defects) and may worsen keratitis sicca. The α_2-agonists apraclonidine and, less commonly, brimonidine may be associated with allergy and punctate keratitis, as may the topical carbonic anhydrase inhibitor dorzolamide and the prostaglandin analogue latanoprost.

Chemical-Induced Keratitis

The history is usually revealing when a patient presents with corneal findings consistent with chemical exposure. The amount of ocular damage correlates with the ease of ocular penetration, chemical concentration, and duration of exposure. Alkaline chemicals usually incite more significant damage than acid burns because of the destruction of the lipid barriers of the anterior segment. Ischemia of the anterior circulation results after even brief strong alkali exposure, manifesting as whitened sclera and conjunctiva; the cornea often takes on a hazy, edematous, beaten-silver appearance. Acids cause coagulation of tissue proteins and a more superficial, corrosive injury, unless exposure is prolonged, in which case the clinical appearance is like that of the more severe alkali burn.

Accurate measurement of IOP may be difficult early after chemical injury to the cornea because of a number of factors, such as periorbital edema and a thickened and irregular corneal surface. Applanation or Schiøtz tonometry readings may underestimate IOP in the presence of corneal edema; Tono-Pen (Mentor O & O, Norwell, MA) or pneumatonometer readings may be more accurate. IOP may be elevated early because of scleral shrinkage secondary to the chemical injury, and released prostaglandins may also be a factor. Increased IOP associated with corneal chemical injury is usually treated with aqueous suppressants. The ciliary body may be damaged in severe injuries, resulting in hypotony.[59]

As tissue reparation and re-epithelialization occur, IOP elevation may continue because of trabecular meshwork damage, peripheral anterior and posterior synechiae formation from inflammation (particularly in the presence of hypopyon), and even pupillary block.[60] Corticosteroids may be contraindicated early in the course if there is corneal epithelial or stromal damage.

IOP elevation may persist after tissue reparation is complete, and measurement may be difficult because of corneal edema, scarring, or surface irregularities. Optic nerve and visual field evaluations may also be limited due to corneal opacification. Glaucoma surgery may be indicated if medical therapy fails to control the IOP, but conjunctival scarring may make the filtration procedure more difficult and less successful. Cyclodestruction must be performed with caution because of possible underlying ciliary body necrosis and the risk of hypotony with overtreatment.

Infectious Keratitis

Another entity that causes epithelial and stromal opacification and can be associated with elevated IOP is infectious keratitis. The rise in IOP is most often a result of obstruction of the trabecular meshwork by inflammatory debris, but prostaglandin release and corneal and limbal edema may also contribute in some cases. Filamentous organisms causing fungal keratitis can gain entry into the anterior chamber through an intact Descemet's membrane and raise the IOP by directly blocking the meshwork or through pupillary block secondary to posterior synechiae.[58] In cases of bacterial and fungal keratitis, the IOP usually normalizes as the inflammation resolves.

Chronic IOP elevation more commonly occurs with infections with herpesviruses, such as herpes simplex and herpes zoster. Up to 90% of adults have antibodies to type 1 herpes simplex virus. Ocular herpetic disease may develop despite the presence of circulating antibodies, however, and manifests as conjunctivitis, keratitis (epithelial or stromal), uveitis (in the presence or absence of keratitis), or trophic (postherpetic) keratitis.[45] The initial presentation is that of a dendritiform corneal epithelial defect (Fig. 11–6); later, stromal edema and opacification and anterior uveitis may occur. Glaucoma most often results in patients with stromal disease, either disciform or stromal keratouveitis, less commonly in patients with disciform keratitis, stromal keratitis, scleral keratitis, and metaherpetic ulcer, and not usually in patients with active corneal ulcers. Elevated IOP is often intermittent early in the course of the disease and later may become persistent. The IOP elevation is related to trabecular blockage or trabeculitis.[61, 62] Treatment of epithelial disease is usually with antiviral agents such as trifluridine or acyclovir. Corticosteroids are used to reduce ocular inflammation, but they can reactivate epithelial disease and carry the potential for steroid-induced glaucoma. Approximately 12% of patients have chronic glaucoma after the uveitis has resolved, requiring medical or, in some cases, surgical intervention.[62]

Herpes zoster ophthalmicus is caused by reactivation of the virus in the gasserian ganglion and the ophthalmic branch of the trigeminal nerve. It manifests as a painful erythematous vesicular rash along the affected nerve distribution. Lesions involving the skin over the tip of the nose, which is supplied by the nasociliary branch of the fifth nerve, often are followed by keratitis and uveitis, with mutton-fat keratic precipitates, posterior synechiae, and sector iris atrophy, along with reduced corneal sensation (Fig. 11–7). Secondary glaucoma is less commonly associated with herpes zoster keratouveitis than with herpes simplex infection but still occurs in up to 25% of affected eyes.[45] IOP may be elevated by meshwork blockage with inflammatory debris or liberated iris pigment, or by pupillary block if there is posterior synechiae formation. Treatment consists of topical steroids to suppress inflammation along with glaucoma medications and filtering surgery, if necessary, although steroid-induced glaucoma may result from their use.

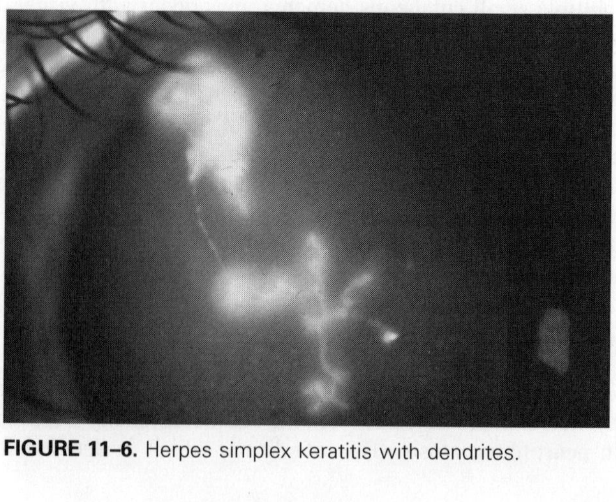

FIGURE 11–6. Herpes simplex keratitis with dendrites.

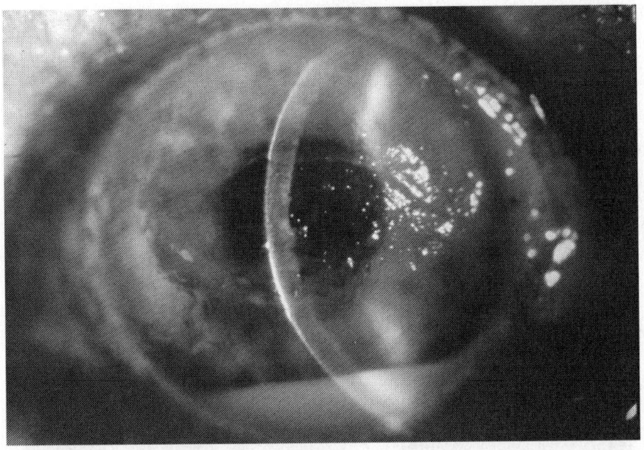

FIGURE 11–7. Herpes zoster keratouveitis with central epithelial defect and sterile hypopyon.

STROMAL DISORDERS (INTERSTITIAL KERATITIS)

One of the most characteristic presentations of glaucoma associated with stromal opacification is that of congenital syphilitic interstitial keratitis. Although it most often occurs in isolation, interstitial keratitis can be seen together with peg teeth and labyrinthine deafness, the combination known as Hutchinson's triad.

Interstitial keratitis occurs in approximately 15% of cases of congenital syphilis, appearing in patients between 6 and 12 years of age and becoming bilateral in 90% of patients. First presenting in the active stages with pain and photosensitivity, it is followed by corneal edema, infiltrates, and vascularization of the deep corneal layers associated with anterior uveitis. A pink or "salmon patch" appearance may result if vascularization is pronounced. The vascularization may remain active for weeks to months. As the inflammation resolves, the channels at the level of Descemet's membrane persist as ghost vessels associated with stromal scarring and endothelial alterations such as collagenous membrane deposition that may also involve the iris and angle (Fig. 11–8). The diagnosis should be confirmed through serologic testing, because interstitial keratitis may also be associated with tuberculosis, leprosy, mumps, lymphogranuloma venereum, trypanosomiasis, onchocerciasis, and Cogan's syndrome.[45, 58]

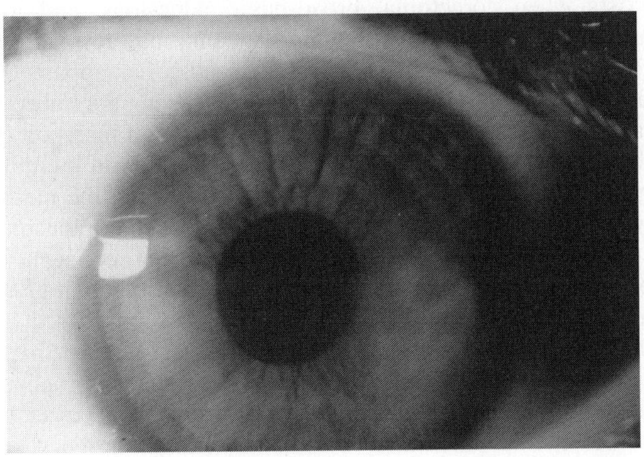

FIGURE 11–8. Interstitial keratitis.

Glaucoma secondary to interstitial keratitis does not correlate with the amount of corneal disease and can occur early or later in life. It may occur acutely with the uveitis, which can be associated with any phase, or later in the course with postinflammatory scarring, steroid use, or intraocular surgery such as penetrating keratoplasty. Open-angle and angle-closure glaucomas occur with equal frequency in patients with interstitial keratitis and may affect one or both eyes.[63, 64] Open-angle glaucoma has an insidious onset and a course similar to that of primary glaucoma, whereas angle-closure glaucoma may occur acutely or chronically. Structural changes associated with interstitial keratitis that may lead to reduction in aqueous outflow include focal and broad PAS formation, pigment deposition in the meshwork, and distortion of trabecular architecture. Interstitial keratitis in infancy may result in eyes with small anterior chambers and vertically oval corneas, inflammatory PAS formation, and intraepithelial iris and ciliary body cysts, all of which can predispose to angle closure.[65] Antiglaucoma medications and, possibly, steroids and surgery are used to treat open-angle glaucoma. Iridectomy, however, is successful in controlling angle-closure glaucoma in 60% to 70% of patients without medications and in up to 90% of patients with medications; the remaining patients undergo filtering surgery.[66, 67]

ENDOTHELIAL DISORDERS

Iridocorneal Endothelial Syndrome

Several disorders manifesting as corneal endothelial findings may be associated with glaucoma. Iridocorneal endothelial (ICE) syndrome, which often occurs unilaterally in early to middle adulthood (more often in women and rarely familially), affects the cornea, angle, and iris. It may be associated with blurred vision, pain, and corneal edema. The corneal endothelium may have a characteristic fine, hammered-silver appearance on slit-lamp examination, and specular microscopy shows variable cellular pleomorphism and polymegathism with intracellular dark areas as well as loss of the clear hexagonal margins.[68] These abnormal cells line multilayered collagenous tissue posterior to Descemet's membrane. Fellow, uninvolved eyes may also show focal areas of endothelial abnormalities. The abnormal endothelial membrane may proliferate to include the anterior chamber angle and iris; the contraction of this membrane may lead to structural changes in the iris, PAS formation, and glaucoma (due to PAS or the membrane itself covering the angle).[69] Abnormal endothelial permeability may also result in corneal edema at normal or mildly elevated IOPs. While various theories have been suggested, the cause of ICE syndrome is unknown.

Iridocorneal endothelial syndrome encompasses three clinical presentations, depending on the nature of the iris findings, all with involvement of the corneal endothelium[70]:

1. Progressive iris atrophy characterized by iris atrophy with hole formation and differing degrees of corectopia and ectropion uveae (Fig. 11–9).[71]
2. Chandler's syndrome in which corneal endothelial findings may be associated with little, if any, iris atrophy and corectopia (Fig. 11–10).[72, 73]
3. Cogan-Reese syndrome present with variable

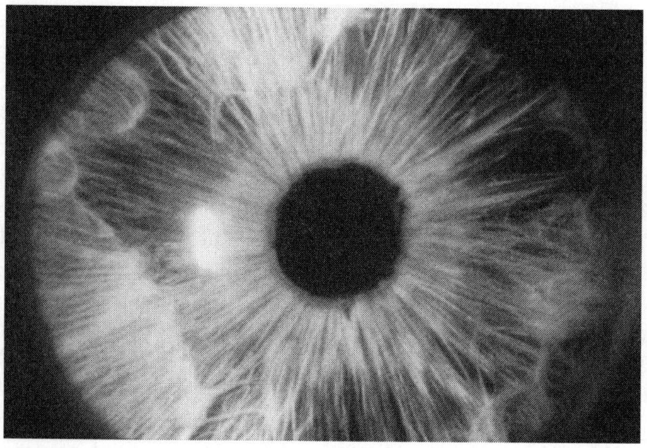

FIGURE 11–9. Progressive iris atrophy.

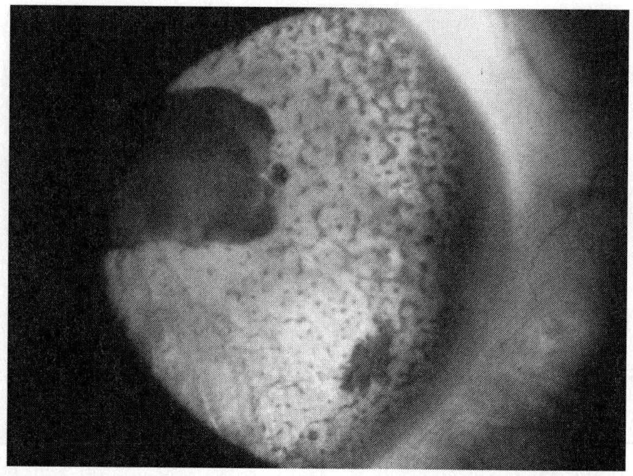

FIGURE 11–11. Cogan-Reese syndrome with pigmented iris lesions.

amounts of iris atrophy and pedunculated, pigmented lesions on the iris surface (iris stromal tissue) (Fig. 11–11).[74, 75]

The iris nevus syndrome causes more diffuse, flat iris lesions with a histologic structure of nevi and may be either a fourth variation of ICE syndrome or a separate condition.[76]

Common to all variations of ICE syndrome are PAS, most often extending up to or beyond Schwalbe's line. Histologically, a single sheet of endothelial cells and a Descemet-like membrane extending from peripheral cornea are seen. The angle may remain open or may be variably closed by the synechiae, which are usually progressive. Glaucoma is common and does not correlate with the amount of synechial closure, as it may be caused by membrane itself.

Treatment of glaucoma and the accompanying corneal edema in ICE syndrome may first be attempted with antiglaucoma medications, hypertonic saline solutions, and soft contact lenses, although filtering surgery may be necessary to control IOP, because laser trabeculoplasty is ineffective. Endothelialization of the filtering site may cause surgical failure; aqueous shunting procedures may be the most effective way to avoid this complication. Penetrating keratoplasty may be performed to improve visual function in patients in whom corneal edema persists despite normalization of IOP.[77]

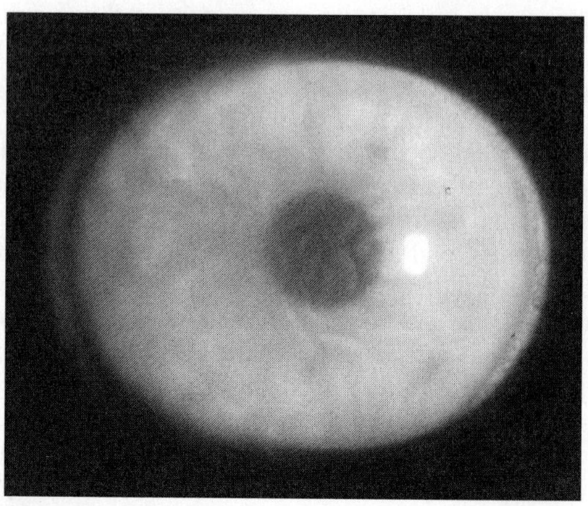

FIGURE 11–10. Chandler's syndrome with corneal edema. The iris is normal.

Posterior Polymorphous Dystrophy

Posterior polymorphous dystrophy (PPMD) is usually a congenital, autosomal dominant, bilateral, familial disorder of the corneal endothelium that remains asymptomatic until adulthood. It may represent a range of clinical and histologic variations. Although edema may occur, the cornea may be clear and the visual acuity unaffected. Geographic, vesicular, or band-like opacities are noted on the posterior layers of the cornea (Fig. 11–12). A relatively small number of patients have broad PAS that may also cause corectopia, ectropion uvea, and iris atrophy similar to those seen in the ICE syndrome. The cause of PPMD may be proliferation and contraction of the corneal endothelium across the anterior chamber. Histologic examination shows endothelial cells to have epithelial characteristics and Descemet's membrane to be thickened and multilayered, with an abnormal posterior collagenous layer.[77–80]

Secondary glaucoma occurs in about 13% of patients with PPMD, manifesting as adult open-angle or angle-closure or juvenile forms. In adult open-angle and juvenile glaucomas, the angle appears normal except for a high insertion of the iris, whereas in angle-closure glaucoma, variably sized PAS are present. Glaucoma nearly always exists when corectopia, broad-based adhesions, and iris atrophy are present.[78] Although glaucoma may result from PAS, it may also occur (1) in the presence of an apparently open angle as a result of a membrane overlying the trabecular meshwork or (2) in association with a high insertion of the iris into the meshwork (similar to that seen in infantile glaucoma, in which a membrane does not cover the meshwork). In high insertion of the iris, the intertrabecular spaces are compressed and obliterated, and collagen is present in the trabeculae, with phagocytosed pigment granules in the endothelial cells. Abnormal tension caused by the high insertion of the iris may lead to collapse of the meshwork and resistance to outflow. One theory proposes that this angle configuration results from a spectrum of developmental anomalies associated with tissues derived from neural crest cells.[58, 77, 81–83]

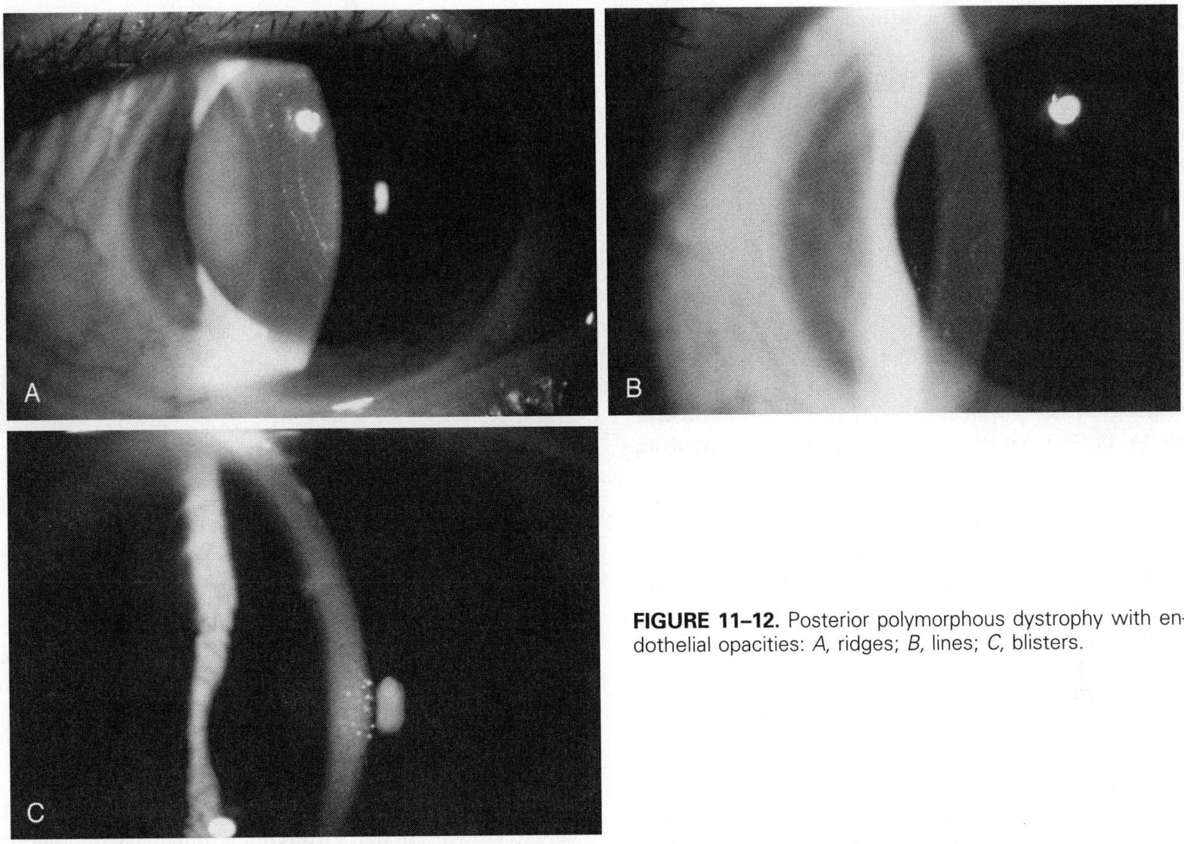

FIGURE 11–12. Posterior polymorphous dystrophy with endothelial opacities: *A*, ridges; *B*, lines; *C*, blisters.

Management of corneal edema is with hypertonic saline and with antiglaucoma medications if the IOP is elevated. Penetrating keratoplasty may be necessary to restore vision if corneal decompensation is significant.[78] Treatment of glaucoma is similar to that of ICE syndrome: medications are tried first, followed by filtering or aqueous shunting procedures if IOP control is inadequate.

Fuchs' Endothelial Dystrophy

Although corneal guttata are a very common finding, particularly in elderly patients, associated corneal edema is less often seen. The combination of cornea guttata and corneal edema without an identifiable cause is known as Fuchs' endothelial dystrophy. This condition is usually a bilateral primary disease of the corneal endothelium that occurs more frequently in women, in some cases with familial tendency, and in at least some cases with autosomal dominant inheritance. Slit-lamp examination reveals corneal guttata that are variably pigmented and in later stages may be associated with stromal and epithelial edema, most often in patients between 40 and 70 years of age. The endothelium may resemble hammered silver, as in ICE syndrome, but specular microscopy distinguishes these conditions; a characteristic pattern of enlarged endothelial cells with dark areas that overlap cell borders is noted in Fuchs' dystrophy.[84] The major pathologic finding is an alteration in the corneal endothelium that results in deposition of collagen on the posterior surface of Descemet's membrane, histologically appearing as warts or excrescences (guttata). Additional basement membrane may also cover such focal accumulations, or the posterior collagen layers may be uniformly thickened.[85]

Although open-angle glaucoma has been reported in patients with Fuchs' dystrophy, further studies have suggested that the two diseases are probably not directly related but may occur concomitantly. However, angle-closure glaucoma may occur in Fuchs' dystrophy because of gradual corneal thickening from edema and eventual narrowing of the angle in patients with shallow anterior chambers. Management of open-angle glaucoma associated with Fuchs' dystrophy is the same as for primary open-angle glaucoma. Miotic therapy is generally not effective in patients with impending angle closure. Iridectomy or filtering operations are usually necessary. Reduction of IOP may lessen corneal edema; however, penetrating keratoplasty may be indicated to restore vision in cases of marked corneal decompensation with associated functional visual impairment.[77]

Pigment Dispersion Syndrome

Pigmented guttata seen on the corneal endothelium must be distinguished from endothelial pigment dusting seen in association with pigment dispersion syndrome (PDS). Pigmentary glaucoma is a bilateral, autosomal dominant disorder that is usually associated with myopia. It is more common in men and in relatively younger patients (35 to 45 years at onset in men and 40 to 50 years in women, with the IOP elevation occurring as early as the teen years).

In contrast to pigmented guttata of Fuchs' dystrophy, which are usually scattered evenly on the endothelium, the

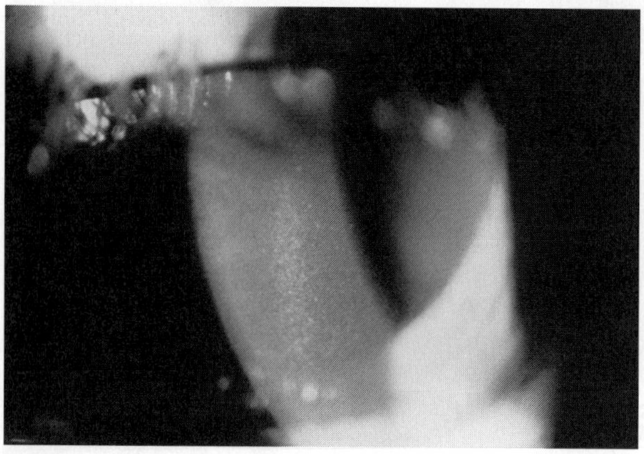

FIGURE 11–13. Pigment dispersion syndrome with Krukenberg's spindle.

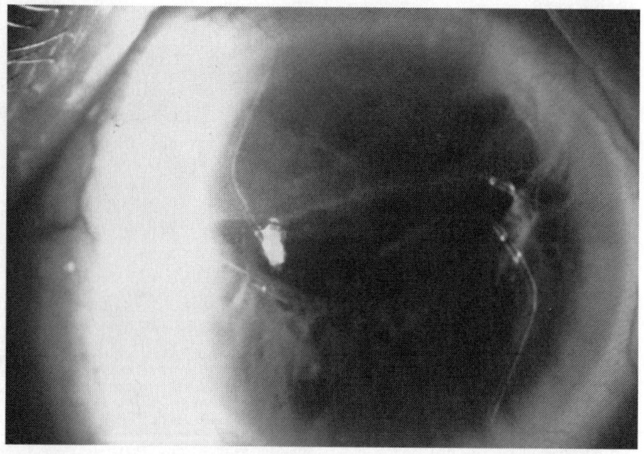

FIGURE 11–14. Epithelial downgrowth, seen as a membrane extending over the superior portion of the endothelium, 2 years after cataract removal and intraocular lens implantation. (Courtesy of Kirk Wilhelmus, MD.)

pigment deposits in PDS usually have the configuration of a central, vertical, brown band (Krukenberg's spindle), although they can also be more diffusely distributed (Fig. 11–13). The shape is attributable to the vertical meeting of aqueous convection currents. On retroillumination of the iris during slit-lamp examination, a variable number of radial, slit-like, midperipheral transillumination defects can be seen; they are the sources of the pigment. Pigment may also be seen on the anterior iris surface, anterior or posterior lens capsule, and the zonules. The anterior chamber is deep, and gonioscopy reveals a homogeneously dense band of pigment in the trabecular meshwork and a ring of pigment along or anterior to Schwalbe's line (Sampaolesi's line). The midperipheral iris may have a flat or, more often, concave configuration.[86–91] PDS is often completely asymptomatic, but affected patients sometimes present with complaints of blurred vision or halos due to transient rises in IOP from pigment liberation, particularly during exercise or after pupillary dilation.

The mechanism for glaucoma development in PDS is unknown but may be related to trabecular dysfunction due to accumulation of melanin pigment in the meshwork or in the cells lining the meshwork, or a mesodermal angle anomaly. There may be a deficiency of the mesodermal support tissues in the iris that leads to the concave iris structure and chafing against the zonules, causing pigment liberation from the pigmented epithelium of the iris that corresponds to the midperipheral iris transillumination defects. A reverse pupillary block mechanism leading to pigment dispersion and glaucoma has also been proposed.[86, 92–94]

Although the prevalence of PDS in the general population and the frequency with which glaucoma develops is unknown, one long-term retrospective study found glaucoma to occur in 36% of male and 33% of female patients with PDS after a mean follow-up interval of 17 years.[95] An association exists between active pigment dispersion and progression of glaucoma. Thus, in patients with pigmentary glaucoma, increasing numbers of iris transillumination defects or increasing amounts of cornea, lens capsule, or angle pigment deposition may be risk factors for increasing IOP.[96] Although pigmentary glaucoma may have a mild course or may become less severe as a patient ages, it is often a progressive disease requiring medical or surgical treatment (with laser trabeculoplasty or filtering procedures). The role of laser iridectomy, if any, to relieve the potential reverse pupillary block has yet to be determined.

Epithelial Ingrowth

Epithelial ingrowth and fibrous ingrowth (see later) are also included in the differential diagnosis of endothelial findings associated with glaucoma. These conditions generally occur in patients who have had previous intraocular surgery (often difficult or complicated) or penetrating eye trauma.

In epithelial downgrowth, patients present with aching discomfort and sometimes with blurred vision and photophobia. Ciliary injection is seen, often along with wound gape or leaking bleb or fistula, on Seidel's testing. Band keratopathy may be present, and a posterior corneal membrane is seen, demarcated by a gray line representing the leading edge of the multicellular epithelial sheet that is often scalloped with focally thickened areas (Figs. 11–14 and 11–15). Vascularization of the corneal stroma, which is thought to provide nutrients to the epithelium, may also be present. Descemet's striae, related to hypotony,

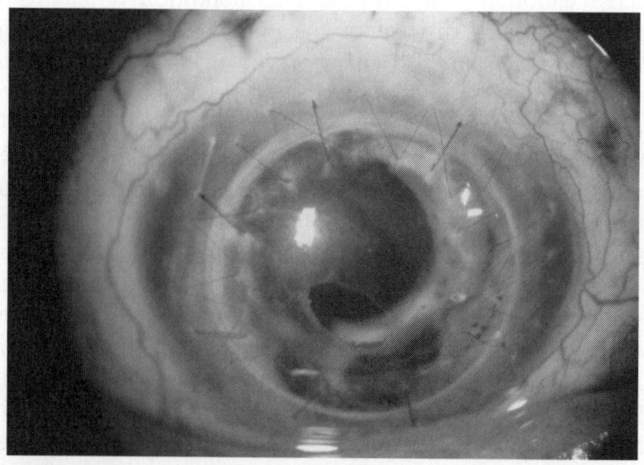

FIGURE 11–15. Epithelial ingrowth after penetrating keratoplasty. The posterior corneal membrane extends over much of the graft.

inflammation, and corneal edema, as well as anterior chamber flare and cells are evident. The anterior chamber cells may include larger cells, which are presumably desquamated corneal epithelium from the ingrowth.

Gonioscopic examination often reveals iris, lens cortex or capsule, or vitreous incarcerated in the internal aspect of the traumatic or surgical wound. Epithelium may be seen along suture tracts or along the internal opening of a bleb or fistula. It may occur as a sheet obscuring details of the trabecular meshwork, and PAS may be present. Epithelium also grows over the iris and ciliary body, obscuring details or causing pupillary distortion. The time from surgery to presentation can vary from days to years.[97–101]

Histopathologic examination reveals one to eight layers of nonkeratinized, stratified squamous epithelium extending over the posterior cornea and lining the iris and surface of the angle or "false angle" made by PAS continuous with the iris surface. The underlying meshwork may appear sclerotic and necrotic, and a chronic inflammatory cell infiltrate may be seen in the episclera, iris, and ciliary body. Endothelium may be missing or may have been replaced by epithelial metaplasia in areas where the membrane is present.

Although the pathogenesis of epithelial ingrowth has yet to be fully determined, it is presumed that complicated surgery or penetrating trauma results in incarceration of tissue that acts as a wick and facilitates wound gape, creating access for epithelial ingrowth. Hypotony, inflammation, and iris incarceration may work together to provide conditions ideal for ingrowth as well as a nutrient source.[102–105]

Hypotony is usually seen early in the course of epithelial ingrowth, but glaucoma is often observed in the later stages, particularly if the original fistula closes. Hypotony, inflammation, and anterior chamber shallowing may result in broad PAS, as well as the epithelial membrane extending over the meshwork and leading to additional PAS with contraction. Pupillary block glaucoma may result from membrane seclusion of the pupil. Hemorrhagic and ghost cell glaucoma may also be consequences of recurrent bleeding from neovascularization.

Medical treatment is directed at controlling the IOP and inflammation. Surgical treatment is usually complicated and often ineffective, directed at delineating the extent of the membrane (such as with argon laser) and removing as much of it as possible. The wound is débrided of incarcerated tissue, and cryotherapy is applied in a transcorneal and trans-scleral fashion to devitalize the remaining epithelium on the posterior surface of the cornea, in the angle, and on the ciliary body.[105–108] Aqueous shunting procedures are an alternative palliative approach for eyes with advanced epithelial ingrowth in which the intraocular extent of the epithelium is such that excisional or cryosurgical techniques are not appropriate.[109]

Fibrous Ingrowth

Fibrous ingrowth occurs under the same circumstances as epithelial downgrowth, that is, complicated surgery, vitreous loss, incarceration of tissues in the wound, inadequate wound closure, postoperative hypotony, chronic postoperative inflammation, and trauma. This disorder consists of proliferation of subconjunctival connective tissue continuous with the ocular surface and extending over the anterior chamber structures. Fibrous ingrowth can be seen as a retrocorneal membrane, most often after penetrating keratoplasty. The graft-host junction may develop a plaque-like thickening as early as 2 weeks postoperatively, later becoming an opacified, even vascularized crescent that is more easily seen behind the donor button. Proceeding from a defect in Descemet's membrane, this fibrous proliferation can extend into the anterior chamber and appear as a fenestrated membrane, or it can diffusely cover the posterior surface of the donor button. Fibrous ingrowth has also been reported after cataract surgery, trauma, goniotomy, and filtering surgery.[110–112]

The clinical presentations of fibrous ingrowth may differ; inflammation and pain are variably present. It may resemble epithelial ingrowth with a translucent membrane appearance but more often is adjacent to the wound and extends onto the posterior corneal surface, appearing as a thicker felt-like or woven gray-white opacity with a frayed edge. Corneal edema is usually seen in the area of ingrowth, which may extend to involve the angle, iris, and vitreous.[97]

The origin of the fibrocellular material (sometimes vascular) may be uncertain (stromal, episcleral, or endothelial). Histologic examination shows wound gape is filled with this fibrocellular material. There may be vascularization and chronic inflammation of the corneal stroma, and endothelium is often missing adjacent to the wound; Descemet's membrane may also be stripped or may be thickened, irregular, and covered by fibroblastic endothelium. Fibrous tissue or PAS may cover the trabecular meshwork, which often shows inflammatory or pigment cells and later has a sclerotic or atrophic appearance. Corectopia, ectropion uveae, pupillary membranes, and even retinal detachment have been reported secondary to massive fibrous ingrowth.

Fibrous ingrowth occurring in association with corneal incisions appears different from that occurring in association with limbal incisions; the fibroblastic cells apparently originate from metaplastic endothelium or from stromal keratocytes in the former. The retrocorneal membrane consists of Descemet's membrane (which has been ruptured at the surgical wound), as opposed to a multilaminar, PAS-positive layer of variable thickness and cellularity. Endothelium may be absent or may appear metaplastic, pigmented, or attenuated.[113–114]

The factors predisposing to epithelial ingrowth appear also to contribute to fibrous ingrowth, along with recurrent hemorrhaging into the eye from an inflamed and vascularized wound, which provides a fibrin scaffold for fibrous growth. Potential sources of fibrous ingrowth include subepithelial connective tissue, corneal stromal fibroblasts, metaplastic corneal endothelium, migratory cells from the anterior chamber angle, and metaplastic uveal monocytes.[97, 110, 115, 116] Fibrous ingrowth is often more slowly progressive than epithelial ingrowth. Treatment is also directed at controlling inflammation; in some cases, the eyes remain quiescent and the fibrous scar matures without causing progressive damage to anterior segment structures. Surgical removal is difficult and is aimed at relieving the consequences of the ingrowth, such as glaucoma.[109, 116]

DEVELOPMENTAL DISORDERS

Several developmental disorders in which the cornea is affected may be associated with glaucoma. These are mentioned briefly here and are covered in greater detail in other chapters.

Presenting symptoms of *congenital glaucoma* are epiphora, photophobia, and blepharospasm secondary to irritation from corneal epithelial edema that is caused by elevated IOP. Corneal and scleral tissue elasticity allows the eyes to become enlarged or buphthalmic with IOP elevation. Corneal diameter and axial length measurements can be used to confirm the diagnosis and to follow disease progression. The angle appears poorly developed, with an anterior insertion of the iris directly into the trabecular meshwork. The cornea may be variably hazy. As corneal tissues stretch, ruptures of Descemet's membrane permit aqueous to permeate corneal stoma and epithelium, sometimes causing sudden increases in corneal edema and haze as well as symptoms (Fig. 11–16). The breaks in Descemet's membrane (Haab's striae) appear as elliptical, glassy, parallel ridges on the posterior cornea in a variety of locations and orientations. If the IOP remains uncontrolled, progression of these corneal findings may lead to scarring, erosions, and ulcerations.

Peters' anomaly is a congenital disorder in which patients present with central corneal opacities; it is usually a bilateral, sporadic condition and is associated with glaucoma in half the cases. Slit-lamp examination shows a central defect in Descemet's membrane involving the corneal endothelium and associated with thinning and opacification of the adjacent stroma. Adhesions from the central iris to the posterior corneal defect are frequently seen; keratolenticular contact or cataract may also be present (Fig. 11–17).[117]

Congenital corneal staphyloma is an unusual developmental anomaly in which the cornea is ectatic and opacified. It is typically unilateral, and the anterior segment is markedly abnormal, with the ectatic, vascularized cornea protruding through the palpebral fissure. Other ocular abnormalities seen in congenital corneal staphyloma are microphthalmos, keratoglobus, cornea plana, and congenital leukoma. Congenital corneal staphyloma is often associated with severe glaucoma, which is secondary to an obliterated anterior chamber with iris adherent to the posterior cornea. This condition may be similar to Peters' anomaly, in that its pathogenesis is likely due to a failure of normal migration of neural crest cells.[42]

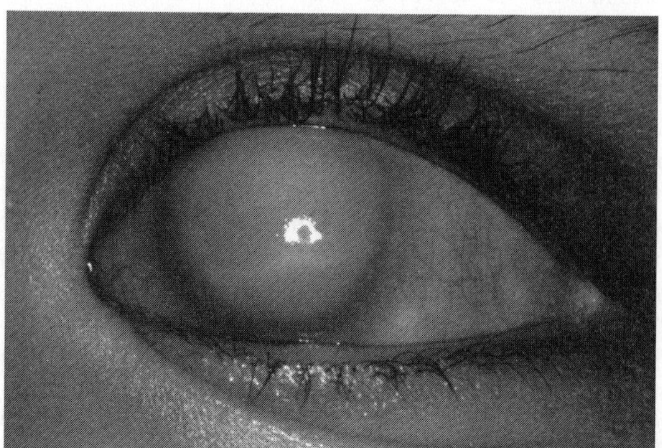

FIGURE 11–16. Congenital glaucoma with buphthalmos, corneal edema, and horizontal Haab's striae.

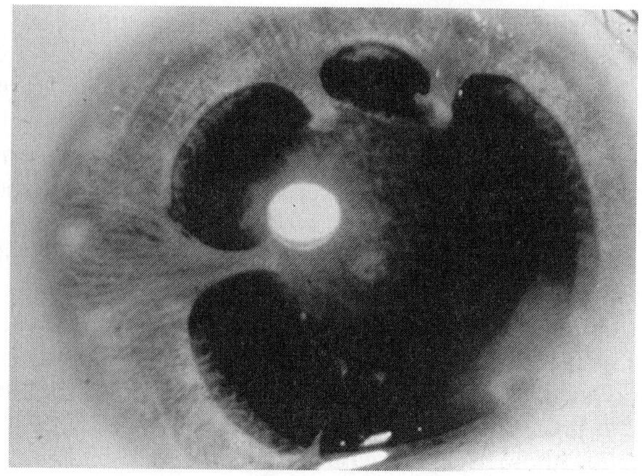

FIGURE 11–17. Peters' anomaly with central iridocorneal adhesions.

Glaucoma is sometimes associated with *sclerocornea*, a developmental disorder in which the cornea is vascularized and opacified and blends with the sclera, the cornea being more opaque peripherally than centrally. It can be unilateral or bilateral and is usually sporadic, not associated with systemic findings. *Cornea plana* is a rare congenital disorder that can be associated with sclerocornea or microcornea. It probably results from an arrest of the corneal tissue in the fourth month of gestation when the corneal curvature changes relative to that of the sclera. It is characterized by diffuse corneal stromal opacities and shallow appearance to the anterior chamber secondary to the flat cornea. The limbus may be poorly defined and the refractive power of the cornea lessened. Other findings are iris colobomas, cataract, ectopia lentis, retinal and macular aplasia, amblyopia, and glaucoma from progressive angle closure due to crowding of the angle.[42]

Aniridia is another bilateral developmental disorder with which glaucoma is often associated. The iris is a rudimentary stump of variable width. Glaucoma occurs in 50% to 75% of aniridic patients and may be present at birth in association with congenital angle anomalies. The angle often remains open early in life, but between the ages of 5 and 15 years, it can become occluded by the iris rudiment, leading to secondary angle-closure glaucoma. Aniridia is usually inherited in an autosomal dominant fashion, but sporadic cases also occur (sometimes associated with Wilms' tumor). Other ocular findings are congenital lens opacities, corneal pannus that advances centrally with age, and foveal hypoplasia.

In *Axenfeld-Rieger (A-R) syndrome*, a bilateral developmental eye disorder inherited in an autosomal dominant manner, systemic developmental defects are often seen (dental anomalies, maxillary hypoplasia, hypertelorism, telecanthus, a broad, flat nose, and genitourinary anomalies). Glaucoma occurs in about half the patients with this disorder, most commonly becoming manifest in childhood or young adulthood but sometimes during infancy. The characteristic corneal finding is an anteriorly displaced Schwalbe's line, appearing as a prominent white line on

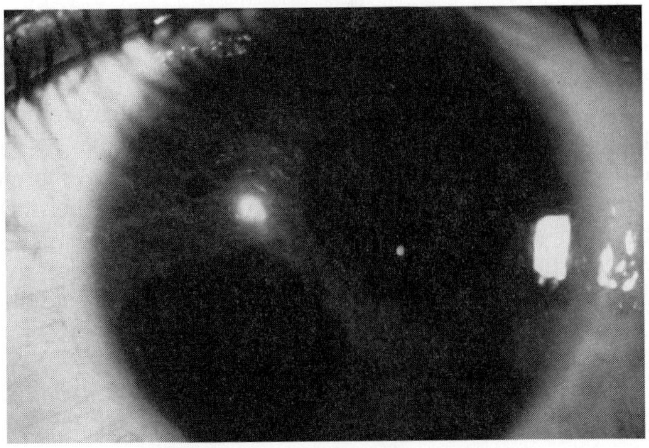

FIGURE 11–18. Rieger's syndrome with polycoria.

the posterior cornea adjacent to the limbus (posterior embryotoxon). Tissue strands from the peripheral iris to Schwalbe's line and a high insertion of the iris into the posterior trabecular meshwork are noted on gonioscopy. Centrally, the iris structure may range from normal to mild stromal thinning to significant atrophy with hole formation, corectopia, and ectropion uveae (Fig. 11–18).[118]

GLAUCOMA ASSOCIATED WITH PENETRATING KERATOPLASTY

The reported incidence of IOP elevation after penetrating keratoplasty is variable but substantial. IOP elevation can occur transiently soon after penetrating keratoplasty or as a chronic condition.

Early IOP elevation usually occurs in the presence of a clear graft, is often quite high (up to 50 mm Hg), and may respond poorly to medical therapy. The IOP elevation can be due to retained viscoelastic agents, inflammation, pupillary block, aqueous misdirection, or mechanical distortion or collapse of the trabecular meshwork. IOP elevation may occur more commonly with same-sized donor grafts in which tight suturing is done, and less commonly when slightly oversized grafts are used. Pupillary block glaucoma is more common in patients with a history of inflammatory conditions such as uveitis and herpetic keratitis and in patients with Fuchs' dystrophy. Although the IOP is usually quite elevated, the diagnosis of angle closure may be difficult to confirm because the peripheral cornea is often distorted, edematous, and opacified, making gonioscopic evaluation challenging.[119–126]

Although acute IOP elevation often resolves after the first postoperative week, chronic IOP elevation is not uncommon after penetrating keratoplasty. One study has determined that preoperative glaucoma and aphakia are risk factors for its development but that other variables, such as method of cataract removal, intraocular lens implant type, and performance of vitrectomy, are not.[126] Chronic glaucoma may be caused by the open-angle or angle-closure mechanisms listed previously, as well as by angle closure due to progressive PAS formation secondary to inflammation. Patients may also be at risk of steroid-induced glaucoma as a result of long-term use of topical steroids to treat inflammation or graft rejection.

Treatment of postkeratoplasty glaucoma depends on the underlying mechanism. Reduction of inflammation, treatment of pupillary block, and suppression of aqueous production are initial measures. Filtering surgery with antimetabolites, aqueous shunting procedures, or cyclodestruction may be undertaken if adequate IOP control is not achieved by the initial measures, although such procedures may potentially increase the risk of graft failure in some cases.

STEROID-INDUCED GLAUCOMA

Patients receiving long-term steroid therapy for corneal inflammatory disorders or after penetrating keratoplasty may experience steroid-induced glaucoma. In patients who are steroid-responsive, a chronic elevation in IOP may develop after a few weeks of treatment with topical, periocular, or, less commonly, systemic steroids.

Histologic studies of eyes with steroid-induced glaucoma show increased density of the cribriform meshwork and thinning of the endothelial lining of Schlemm's canal, but whether these are primary or secondary changes is unclear. Many theories have been suggested to explain the reduction in outflow facility seen in steroid-induced glaucoma, but its pathophysiology remains unclear. Evidence suggests that some individuals may be genetically predisposed to the disorder; however, a relatively small number of individuals in the general population are steroid "responders." Nonetheless, patients who have primary open-angle glaucoma (or first-degree relatives with the disorder), diabetes, or high myopia may be at higher risk for steroid-induced glaucoma.[127–130]

IOP levels may become quite high in steroid-induced glaucoma, with elevations occurring a week to several years after steroid therapy is begun. A careful history of past or present corticosteroid use is critical in leading to the diagnosis of steroid-induced glaucoma. Young children with steroid-induced glaucoma may present with signs and symptoms similar to those of primary infantile glaucoma, but older children and adults are usually asymptomatic. Occasionally, however, if IOP in an older child or adult is sufficiently high or has been elevated for a prolonged period, the patient may present with corneal edema, diminished vision, or both because of advanced glaucomatous optic neuropathy. The diagnosis of steroid-induced glaucoma may be complicated by the presence of other ocular conditions, such as uveitis, that may also be associated with glaucoma.

Management consists of stopping the steroid therapy, if possible, and changing to another medication less likely to raise IOP, if necessary. If the disease is discovered early, discontinuation of steroid therapy usually normalizes the pressure. However, later in the course of steroid therapy, the IOP may remain elevated even after steroid therapy is stopped. Antiglaucoma medications may be necessary in such cases or for the patient in whom an underlying condition requires continued steroid therapy. Patients with steroid-induced glaucoma that is inadequately controlled with medical management may eventually require filtering surgery, which if successful usually controls pressure despite continued steroid use.[131, 132]

MEGALOCORNEA

Megalocornea may be an indication of glaucoma. In its pure form, it is a nonprogressive developmental anomaly of the cornea without associated glaucoma; the horizontal corneal diameter at birth must be at least 12 mm for this diagnosis to be made.[133] Megalocornea is most commonly inherited through an X-linked recessive pattern, but autosomal dominant and autosomal recessive patterns have been documented.[134, 135] Abnormal tissue in the anterior chamber angle has been noted in some patients with normal IOPs. Because megalocornea and congenital glaucoma have been reported together in a number of pedigrees and because glaucoma may occur later in life in patients with X-linked recessive megalocornea, IOP should be evaluated when corneal enlargement is noted, even in the absence of corneal edema. The relationship between megalocornea and congenital glaucoma is not fully understood.[136]

Two forms of megalocornea have been described. The cornea and anterior segment appear normal in the presence of multiple iris processes and pigmented trabecular meshwork in incomplete megalocornea. In complicated megalocornea (anterior megalophthalmos), posterior embryotoxon, Krukenberg's spindles, pigmentation of the trabecular meshwork, iris tissue bridging the angle, lax zonular fibers, iridodonesis, and cataract or dislocated lens occur in addition to enlarged corneal diameter. Glaucoma may occur primarily in patients who have megalocornea in association with A-R syndrome.[42]

MICROCORNEA AND MICROPHTHALMOS

Glaucoma may be associated with small corneal diameter. Microcornea is a rare congenital condition in which the corneal diameter is less than 10 mm. The eye may be otherwise normal or other conditions may coexist, such as anterior chamber dysgenesis with anterior iris insertion and glaucoma or anterior microphthalmos with crowded anterior chamber and angle-closure glaucoma. Glaucoma may also coexist, as may congenital cataracts and Peters' anomaly, uveal coloboma, high myopia, posterior staphyloma, and microphthalmia. A syndrome consisting of microcornea and congenital cataracts, nystagmus, abnormal iris, and congenital glaucoma has been reported. Microcornea may rarely be associated with other systemic disorders, such as Ehlers-Danlos syndrome.[42, 137]

Microphthalmos, a condition in which the entire globe is unusually small, may manifest in different forms, may be inherited in different patterns, and may be associated with elevated IOP. Nanophthalmos is a familial syndrome characterized by hypermetropia, short axial length, small corneal diameters, thickened sclera, narrow angles, and glaucoma.[138] Microphthalmos may be associated with orbital cyst caused by failure of the choroidal fissure to close during development. Retinal tissue grows through the fissure into the orbital space and, along with connective tissue, forms a cyst.[139] Microphthalmos may also be associated with a number of congenital systemic syndromes, congenital infectious syndromes (rubella, toxoplasmosis, cytomegalic inclusion disease), and congenital ocular disorders (sclerocornea, congenital cataracts, iris and uveal colobomata, cornea plana, microcornea, persistent hyperplastic primary vitreous, and Rieger's anomaly),[42] as previously discussed.

The glaucoma in conditions associated with microphthalmos is due to crowding of the anterior chamber by the normal-sized lens within the small globe. Of the chronic angle-closure type, glaucoma occurs most often between the third and fifth decades. Medical and laser treatments may not effectively control IOP because of the progressive angle-closure, and filtering surgery may be complicated by choroidal effusions and other problems.[138, 140, 141]

SUMMARY

Glaucoma may be associated with many findings in the episclera, sclera, conjunctiva, and cornea. Developmental, hereditary, infectious, inflammatory, and drug-induced and surgery-induced conditions may engender characteristic findings involving these structures. Accurate assessment facilitates the correct diagnosis and treatment planning for control of IOP and other complications.

REFERENCES

1. Watson PG: Glaucoma secondary to keratitis, episcleritis, and scleritis. *In* Ritch R, Shields MB, Krupin T (eds): The Glaucomas, vol II. St. Louis, CV Mosby, 1989, pp 1187–1204.
2. Watson PG, Hazleman BL: The Sclera and Systemic Disorders. London, WB Saunders, 1976.
3. Lloyd-Jones D, Tokarewicz A, Watson PG: Clinical evaluation of clobetasone butyrate eye drops in episcleritis. Br J Ophthalmol 1981;65:641.
4. Watson PG, McKay DA, Clemett RS, Wilkinson P: Treatment of episcleritis: A double blind trial comparing beta-methasone 0.1%, oxyphenbutazone 10%, and placebo eye ointments. Br J Ophthalmol 1973;57:866.
5. Harbin T, Pollack J: Glaucoma in episcleritis. Arch Ophthalmol 1975;93:948.
6. Fraunfelder FT, Watson PG: Evaluation of eyes enucleated for scleritis. Br J Ophthalmol 1976;60:227.
7. Cleary PE, Watson PG, McGill JI, Hamilton AM: Visual loss due to posterior segment disease in scleritis. Trans Ophthalmol Soc UK 1975;95:297.
8. Wilhemu K, Grierson I, Watson PG: Histolopathologic and clinical associations of scleritis and glaucoma. Am J Ophthalmol 1981;91:697.
9. Gass JDM: Retinal detachment and narrow angle glaucoma secondary to pseudotumour of the uveal tract. Am J Ophthalmol 1967;64:612.
10. Watson PG, Grierson I: The place of trabeculectomy in the treatment of glaucoma. Ophthalmology 1981;88:175.
11. Brockhurst RJ, Schepens CL, Okamura ID: Uveitis II: Peripheral uveitis: Clinical description, complications and differential diagnosis. Am J Ophthalmol 1960;49:1257.
12. Weinreb RN, Jeng S, Goldstick BJ: Glaucoma secondary to elevated episcleral venous pressure. *In* Ritch R, Shields MB, Krupin T (eds): The Glaucomas, vol II. St. Louis, CV Mosby, 1989, pp 1127–1140.
13. Radius RL, Maumenee AE: Dilated episcleral vessels and open angle glaucoma. Am J Ophthalmol 1968;86:31.
14. Spencer WH, Thompson HS, Hoyt WF: Ischemic ocular necrosis from carotid-cavernous fistula. Br J Ophthalmol 1973;57:145.
15. Harris GJ, Rice PR: Angle closure in carotid cavernous fistula. Ophthalmology 1979;86:1521.
16. Harbison JW, Guerry D, Wiesinger H: Dural arteriovenous fistula and spontaneous choroidal detachment: New cause of an old disease. Br J Ophthalmol 1978;62:483.
17. Kupersmith MJ, Berenstein A, Flamm E, Ransohoff J: Neurooph-

thalmologic abnormalities and intravascular therapy of traumatic carotid cavernous fistulas. Ophthalmology 1986;93:906.
18. Weiss DI, Shaffer RN: Neovascular glaucoma complicating carotid-cavernous fistula. Arch Ophthalmol 1963;69:60.
19. Kollarits CR, Gaasterland D, DiChiro G, et al: Management of a patient with orbital varices, visual loss and ipsilateral glaucoma. Ophthalmic Surg 1977;8:54.
20. Lloyd GAS, Wright JE, Morgan G: Venous malformations in the orbit. Br J Ophthalmol 1971;55:505.
21. Weiss JS, Ritch R: Glaucoma in the phakomatoses. *In* Ritch R, Shields MB, Krupin T (eds): The Glaucomas, vol II. St. Louis, CV Mosby, 1989, pp 905–929.
22. Anderson JR: Hydrophthalmia or Congenital Glaucoma. London, Cambridge University Press, 1939.
23. Susac JO, Smith JL, Scelfo RJ: The "tomato-catsup" fundus in Sturge-Weber syndrome. Arch Ophthalmol 1974;92:69.
24. Phelps CD: The pathogenesis of glaucoma in Sturge-Weber syndrome. Trans Am Acad Ophthalmol Otolaryngol 1978;85:276.
25. Weiss DL: Dual origin of glaucoma in encephalotrigeminal hemangiomatosis. Trans Ophthalmol Soc UK 1971;93:477.
26. Bellows RA, Chylack LT, Epstein DL, Hutchinson T: Choroidal effusion during glaucoma surgery in patients with prominent episcleral vessels. Arch Ophthalmol 1979;97:493.
27. Bigger JF: Glaucoma with elevated episcleral venous pressure. South Med J 1975;68:1444.
28. Urschel HC, Paulson DL: Superior vena cava canal obstruction. Dis Chest 1966;49:155.
29. Lokich JJ, Goodman R: Superior vena cava syndrome. JAMA 1975;231:58.
30. Minas TF, Podos SM: Familial glaucoma associated with elevated episcleral venous pressure. Arch Ophthalmol 1968;80:202.
31. Talusan ED, Schwartz B: Episcleral venous pressure: Difference between normal, ocular hypertensive and primary open angle glaucoma. Arch Ophthalmol 1983;99:824.
32. Fishman FRA, Anderson R: Nevus of Ota. Am J Ophthalmol 1962;54:453.
33. Foulks GN, Shields MB: Glaucoma in oculodermal melanocytosis. Ann Ophthalmol 1977;9:1299.
34. Teekhasaenee C, Ritch R, Rutnin U, Leelawongs N: Ocular findings in oculodermal melanocytosis. Arch Ophthalmol 1990;108:1114.
35. Teekhasaenee C, Ritch R, Rutnin U, Leelawongs N: Glaucoma in oculodermal melanocytosis. Ophthalmology 1990;97:562.
36. Shaffer RN, Weiss DI: Congenital and Pediatric Glaucomas. St. Louis, CV Mosby, 1970.
37. Dev D, Jain IS, Nayo K: Naevus of Ota associated with glaucoma. Orient Arch Ophthalmol 1969;7:251.
38. Font RL, Reynolds AN, Zimmerman LE: Diffuse malignant melanoma of the iris in the nevus of Ota. Arch Ophthalmol 1967;77:513.
39. Reinke RT, Haber K, Josselson A: Ota nevus, multiple hemangioma and Takayasu arteritis. Arch Dermatol 1974;110:447.
40. Gonder JR, Nichol J, Augsburger JJ, Shields JA: Ocular and oculodermal melanocytosis. Can J Ophthalmol 1985;20:176.
41. Teekhasaenee C, Ritch R: Glaucoma in phakomatosis pigmentovascularis. Ophthalmology 1997;104:150.
42. Cantor LB: Glaucoma associated with congenital disorders. *In* Ritch R, Shields MB, Krupin T (eds): The Glaucomas, vol II. St. Louis, CV Mosby, 1989, pp 931–960.
43. Dessoff J: Blue sclerotics, fragile bones and deafness. Arch Ophthalmol 1934;12:60.
44. Goodman M, Gorlin RJ: The Face in Genetic Disorders. St. Louis, CV Mosby, 1970.
45. Krupin T, Feitl ME: Glaucoma associated with uveitis. *In* Ritch R, Shields MB, Krupin T (eds): The Glaucomas, vol II. St. Louis, CV Mosby, 1989, pp 1205–1223.
46. Huckman MS, Haas J: Reversed flow through the ophthalmic artery as a cause of rubeosis iridis. Am J Ophthalmol 1972;74:1094.
47. Swan KC, Raff J: Changes in the eye and orbit following carotid ligation. Trans Am Ophthalmol Soc 1951;49:435.
48. Yablonski ME, Shin DH, Kolker AE, et al: Dipivefrin in use in patients with intolerance to topically applied epinephrine. Arch Ophthalmol 1977;95:2157.
49. Butler P, Mannschreck M, Lin S, et al: Clinical experience with the long-term use of 1% apraclonidine: Incidence of allergic reactions. Arch Ophthalmol 1995;113:293.
50. Nagasubramanian S, Hitchings RA, Demailly P, et al: Comparison of apraclonidine and timolol in chronic open-angle glaucoma: A three month study. Ophthalmology 1993;100:1318.
51. Strahlman E, Tipping R, Vogel R, et al: A double-masked, randomized 1-year study comparing dorzolamide (Trusopt), timolol, and betaxolol. Arch Ophthalmol 1995;113:1009.
52. Klippel M, Trenaunay P: Naevus variqueux ostéo-hypertrophique. J Arch Gen Méd Pract 1900;14:65.
53. Weber FP: Angioma-formation in connection with hypertrophy of limbs and hemihypertrophy. Br J Dermatol 1907;190:231.
54. Reynolds JD, Johnson BL, Bloster S, Biglan AW: Glaucoma and Klippel-Trenaunay-Weber syndrome. Am J Ophthalmol 1988; 106:494.
55. Haik BG, Clancy P, Ellsworth RM, et al: Ocular manifestations in diffuse neonatal hemangiomatosis. J Pediatr Ophthalmol 1983;20:101.
56. Lieb WA, Wirth WA, Geeraets WJ: Hydrophthalmos and neurofibromatosis. Confin Neurol 1958;19:230.
57. Shihab ZM: Antiglaucoma therapy. *In* Lamberts DW, Potter DE (eds): Clinical Ophthalmic Pharmacology. Boston, Little Brown, 1987.
58. Miller KN, Carlson AN, Foulks GN, Shields MB: Associated glaucoma and corneal disorders. *In* Shults WT (ed): Focal Points 1989: Clinical Modules for Ophthalmologists, vol VII, module 4. San Francisco, American Academy of Ophthalmology, 1989.
59. Herschler J, Cobo M: Trauma and elevated intraocular pressure. *In* Ritch R, Shields MB, Krupin T (eds): The Glaucomas, vol II. St. Louis, CV Mosby, 1989, pp 1233–1235.
60. Brown SI, Tragakis MP, Pearce DB: Treatment of the alkali-burned cornea. Am J Ophthalmol 1972;74:316.
61. Hogan MJ, Kimura ST, Thygeson P: Pathology of herpes simplex kerato-iritis. Am J Ophthalmol 1964; 7:551.
62. Falcon MG, Williams HP: Herpes simplex kerato-uveitis and glaucoma. Trans Ophthalmol Soc UK 1978;98:101.
63. Knox DL: Glaucoma following syphilitic interstitial keratitis. Arch Ophthalmol 1961;64:44.
64. Sugar HS: Late glaucoma associated with inactive syphilitic interstitial keratitis. Am J Ophthalmol 1962;53:602.
65. Lichter PR, Shaffer RN: Interstitial keratitis and glaucoma. Am J Ophthalmol 1969;68:24.
66. Grant WM: Late glaucoma after interstitial keratitis. Am J Ophthalmol 1975;79:87.
67. Tsukahara S: Secondary glaucoma due to inactive congenital syphilitic interstitial keratitis. Ophthalmologica 1977;174:188.
68. Eagle RC Jr, Font RL, Yanoff M, Fine BS: The iris naevus (Cogan-Reese) syndrome: Light and electron microscopic observations. Br J Ophthalmol 1980; 4:446.
69. Eagle RC, Font RL, Yanoff M, Fine BS: Proliferative endotheliopathy with iris abnormalities: The iridocorneal endothelial syndrome. Arch Ophthalmol 1979;97:2104.
70. Shields MB: Progressive essential iris atrophy, Chandler's syndrome, and the iris nevus (Cogan-Reese) syndrome: A spectrum of disease. Surv Ophthalmol 1979;24:3.
71. Campbell DG, Shields MB, Smith TR: The corneal endothelium and the spectrum of essential iris atrophy. Am J Ophthalmol 1978;86:317.
72. Chandler PA: Atrophy of the stroma of the iris: Endothelial dystrophy, corneal edema, and glaucoma. Am J Ophthalmol 1956;41:607.
73. Quigley HA, Forster RF: Histopathology of cornea and iris in Chandler's syndrome. Arch Ophthalmol 1978;96:1878.
74. Cogan DG, Reese AB: A syndrome of iris nodules, ectopic Descemet's membrane, and unilateral glaucoma. Doc Ophthalmol 1969;26:424.
75. Radius RL, Herschler J: Histopathology in the iris-nevus (Cogan-Reese) syndrome. Am J Ophthalmol 1980;89:780.
76. Sugar HS: The iris nevus and Cogan-Reese syndromes: Separate entities? Ann Ophthalmol 1981;13:405.
77. Shields MB, Bourgeois JE: Glaucomas associated with primary disorders of the corneal endothelium. *In* Ritch R, Shields MB, Krupin T (eds): The Glaucomas, vol II. St. Louis, CV Mosby, 1989, pp 963–980.
78. Krachmer JH: Posterior polymorphous corneal dystrophy: A disease characterized by epithelial-like endothelial cells which influence management and prognosis. Trans Am Ophthalmol Soc 1985;83:413.
79. Grayson M: The nature of hereditary deep polymorphous dystrophy of the cornea: Its association with iris and anterior chamber dysgenesis. Trans Am Ophthalmol Soc 1974;72:516.

80. Tripathi RC, Casey TA, Wise G: Hereditary posterior polymorphous dystrophy: An ultrastructural and clinical report. Trans Am Ophthalmol Soc UK 1974;94:211.
81. Bourgeois J, Shields MB, Thresher R: Open-angle glaucoma associated with posterior polymorphous dystrophy. Ophthalmology 1984;91:420.
82. Kupfer C, Kaiser-Kupfer MI, Datilies M, McCain L: The contralateral eye in the iridocorneal endothelial (ICE) syndrome. Ophthalmology 1983;90:1343.
83. Tripathi BJ, Tripathi RC: Embryology of the anterior segment of the human eye. *In* Ritch R, Shields MB, Krupin T (eds): The Glaucomas, vol I. St. Louis, CV Mosby, 1989, pp 3–40.
84. Laing RA, Leibowitz HM, Oak SS, et al: Endothelial mosaic in Fuchs' dystrophy: A qualitative evaluation with the specular microscope. Arch Ophthalmol 1981;99:80.
85. Magovern M, Beauchamp GR, McTigue JW, et al: Inheritance of Fuchs' combined dystrophy. Ophthalmology 1979;86:1897.
86. Richardson TM: Pigmentary glaucoma. *In* Ritch R, Shields MB, Krupin T (eds): The Glaucomas, vol II. St. Louis, CV Mosby, 1989, pp 981–995.
87. Epstein DL: Pigment dispersion and pigmentary glaucoma. *In* Chandler PA, Grant WM (eds): Glaucoma, vol II. Philadelphia, Lea & Febiger, 1979.
88. Gillies WE: Pigmentary glaucoma: A clinical review of anterior segment pigment dispersal syndrome. Aust N Z J Ophthalmol 1985;13:325.
89. Lichter PR, Shaffer RM: Diagnostic and prognostic signs in pigmentary glaucoma. Trans Am Acad Ophthalmol Otolaryngol 1970;74:984.
90. Scheie HG, Cameron JD: Pigment dispersion syndrome: A clinical study. Br J Ophthalmol 1981;65:264.
91. Sugar HS: Pigmentary glaucoma: A 25-year review. Am J Ophthalmol 1966;62:499.
92. Fine BS, Yanoff M, Scheie HG: Pigmentary "glaucoma": A histologic study. Trans Am Acad Ophthalmol Otolaryngol 1974;78:314.
93. Campbell DG: Pigmentary dispersion and glaucoma: A new theory. Arch Ophthalmol 1979;97:1667.
94. Karickhoff JR: Pigmentary dispersion syndrome and pigmentary glaucoma: A new mechanism concept, a new treatment, and a new technique. Ophthalmic Surg 1992;23:269.
95. Migliazzo CV, Shaffer RN, Nykin R, Magee S: Long-term analysis of pigmentary dispersion syndrome and pigmentary glaucoma. Ophthalmology 1986;93:1528.
96. Richter CU, Richardson TM, Grant WM: Pigmentary dispersion syndrome and pigmentary glaucoma: A prospective study of the natural history. Arch Ophthalmol 1986;104:211.
97. Smith P, Stark WJ, Maumenee AE, Green WR: Epithelial, fibrous, and endothelial proliferation. *In* Ritch R, Shields MB, Krupin T (eds): The Glaucomas, vol II. St. Louis, CV Mosby, 1989, pp 1299–1335.
98. Allen JC: Epithelial and stromal ingrowths. Am J Ophthalmol 1968;65:179.
99. Bettman JW Jr: Pathology of complications of intraocular surgery. Am J Ophthalmol 1969;68:1037.
100. Jaffe NS: Epithelial invasion of the anterior chamber. *In* Jaffe NS: Cataract Surgery and Its Complications. St. Louis, CV Mosby, 1981.
101. Bernardino VB, Kim JC, Smith TR: Epithelialization of the anterior chamber after cataract extraction. Arch Ophthalmol 1969;82:742.
102. Sidrys LA, Demong T: Epithelial downgrowth after penetrating keratoplasty. Can J Ophthalmol 1982;17:29.
103. Burris TE, Rowsey JJ, Nordquist RE: Model of epithelial downgrowth. II: Scanning and transmission electron microscopy of corneal epithelialization. Cornea 1984;3:141.
104. Burris TE, Nordquist RE, Rowsey JJ: Model of epithelial downgrowth. III: Scanning and transmission electron microscopy of iris epithelialization. Cornea 1985;4:249.
105. Zavala EY, Binder PS: The pathologic findings of epithelial ingrowth. Arch Ophthalmol 1980;98:2007.
106. Maumenee AE, Paton D, Morse PH, Butner R: Review of 40 histologically proven cases of epithelial downgrowth following cataract extraction and suggested surgical management. Am J Ophthalmol 1970;69:598.
107. Stark WJ, Michels RG, Maumenee AE, Cupples H: Surgical management of epithelial ingrowth. Am J Ophthalmol 1978;85:772.
108. Stark WJ: Management of epithelial ingrowth and cysts. Dev Ophthalmol 1981;5:64.
109. Fish LA, Heuer DK, Baerveldt G, et al: Molteno implantation for secondary glaucomas associated with advanced epithelial ingrowth. Ophthalmology 1990;97:557.
110. Sherrard ES, Rycroft PV: Retrocorneal membranes. I: Their origin and structure. Br J Ophthalmol 1967;51:379.
111. Sherrard ES, Rycroft PV: Retrocorneal membranes. II: Factors influencing their growth. Br J Ophthalmol 1967;51:387.
112. Werb A: The postgraft membrane. Int Ophthalmol Clin 1962;2:771.
113. Hales RH, Spencer WH: Unsuccessful penetrating keratoplasties: Correlation of clinical and histologic findings. Arch Ophthalmol 1963;70:805.
114. Rycroft PV: Corneal graft membranes. Trans Ophthalmol Soc UK 1965;85:317.
115. Swan KC: Fibroblastic ingrowth following cataract extraction. Arch Ophthalmol 1973;89:445.
116. Bloomfield SE, Jakobiec FA, Iwamoto F: Fibrous ingrowth with retrocorneal membrane. Ophthalmology 1981;88:459.
117. Townsend WM, Font RL, Zimmerman LE: Congenital corneal leukomas. 2: Histopathologic findings in 19 eyes with central defect in Descemet's membrane. Am J Ophthalmol 1974;77:192.
118. Shields MB, Buckley E, Klintworth GK, et al: Axenfeld-Rieger syndrome: A spectrum of developmental disorders. Surv Ophthalmol 1985;29:387.
119. Olson RJ, Lee JS, Zimmerman TJ: Glaucoma associated with penetrating keratoplasty. *In* Ritch R, Shields MB, and Krupin T (eds): The Glaucomas, vol II. St. Louis, CV Mosby, 1989, pp 1337–1347.
120. Bourne WM, Davison JA, O'Fallon WM: The effects of oversize donor buttons on postoperative intraocular pressure and corneal curvature in aphakic penetrating keratoplasty. Ophthalmology 1982;89:242.
121. Thoft RA, Gordon JM, Dohlman CH: Glaucoma following keratoplasty. Trans Am Acad Ophthalmol Otolaryngol 1974;78:352.
122. Irvine AR, Kaufman HE: Intraocular pressure following penetrating keratoplasty. Am J Ophthalmol 1969;68:835.
123. Goldberg DB, Schanzlin DJ, Brown SI: Incidence of increased intraocular pressure after keratoplasty. Am J Ophthalmol 1981;92:372.
124. Karesh JW, Nirankari VS: Factors associated with glaucoma after penetrating keratoplasty. Am J Ophthalmol 1983;96:160.
125. Olson RJ, Kaufman HE: Prognostic factors of intraocular pressure after aphakic keratoplasty. Am J Ophthalmol 1978;86:510.
126. Foulks GN: Glaucoma associated with penetrating keratoplasty. Ophthalmology 1987;94:871.
127. Kass MA, Johnson T: Corticosteroid-induced glaucoma. *In* Ritch R, Shields MB, Krupin T (eds): The Glaucomas, vol II. St. Louis, CV Mosby, 1989, pp 1161–1168.
128. Armaly MF: Inheritance of dexamethasone hypertension and glaucoma. Arch Ophthalmol 1967;77:747.
129. Becker B, Hahn KA: Topical corticosteroids and heredity in primary open-angle glaucoma. Am J Ophthalmol 1964;57:543.
130. Schwartz B: Corticosteroids and the eye. Int Ophthalmol Clin 1966;6:753.
131. Kronfeld PC: The effects of topical steroid administration on intraocular pressure and aqueous outflow after fistulizing operations. Trans Am Ophthalmol Soc 1964;62:375
132. Kolker AE: *Discussion of* Wilensky JT, Synder D, Gieser D: Steroid-induced ocular hypertension in patients with filtering blebs. Ophthalmology 1980;87:243.
133. Schweitzer NMJ: Megalocornea. Ophthalmologica 1962;144:304.
134. Mets MB, Maumenee IH: The eye and the chromosome. Surv Ophthalmol 1983;28:20.
135. Rogers GL, Polomeno RC: Autosomal-dominant inheritance of megalocornea associated with Down's syndrome. Am J Ophthalmol 1974;78:526.
136. Malbran E, Dodds R: Megalocornea and its relation to congenital glaucoma. Am J Ophthalmol 1960;49:908.
137. Green JS, Johnson GJ: Congenital cataract with microcornea and Peters' anomaly as expressions of one autosomal dominant gene. Ophthalmic Paediatr Genet 1986;7:187.
138. Singh OS, Simmons RJ, Brockhurst RJ, Trempe CL: Nanophthalmos, a perspective on identification and therapy. Ophthalmology 1982; 89:1006.
139. Ladenheim J, Metrick S: Congenital microphthalmos with cyst formation. Am J Ophthalmol 1956;41:1059.
140. Kimbrough RL, Trempe CS, Brockhurst RJ, Simmons RJ: Angle-closure glaucoma in nanophthalmos. Am J Ophthalmol 1979;88:572.
141. Calhoun FP: The management of glaucoma in nanophthamos. Trans Am Ophthalmol Soc 1975;73:97.

CHAPTER 12

Anterior and Posterior Chambers

SHERIF M. EL-HARAZI and ROBERT M. FELDMAN

The examination of the anterior and posterior chambers is one of the most important parts of the examination of the patient with glaucoma. Combined with gonioscopy (discussed in Chapter 13), it provides invaluable information to assist in diagnosis. Deviations from normal are relatively easily identified, because under normal circumstances, the anterior and posterior chambers are essentially optically empty fluid spaces. Therefore, any change noted by critical observation is an abnormality. In this chapter, Sherif El-Harazi and Robert Feldman discuss the changes that can be observed. Intraocular inflammation, as discussed in Chapters 11, 14, and 16, can be diagnosed from cells and flare in the anterior chamber. This chapter subdivides the inflammatory response on the basis of severity to facilitate correct identification of the underlying etiology. Another important and often obvious sign in the anterior chamber is blood, either hyphema, red cell components, or clot. Debris of various types may also be identified, including parasites, lens particles, pigment, exfoliative material, viscoelastic substances, tumor cells, and silicone oil. There is great variety in what may be observed in the anterior chamber, but when identified, any abnormality often represents a key finding for diagnosis.

Examination of the anterior chamber is vital in determining the etiology and the proper management of glaucoma. There are only a few ways to classify changes in the aqueous humor: flare, cells, and foreign bodies, debris, clotted blood, or fibrin clots. However, closer examination may divulge something useful in determining etiology.

Intraocular Inflammation

(See Chapter 16)

Intraocular inflammation disrupts the blood-aqueous barrier, leading to leakage of high-molecular-weight proteins into the anterior chamber.[1-3] Through the Tyndall effect, these proteins can be seen on slit-lamp examination and are interpreted as flare. Flare is graded from 0+ to 4+, 0+ being no flare and 4+ being a plasmoid aqueous (Fig 12–1; Table 12–1).[4] Disruption of the blood-aqueous barrier also leads to leakage of white or red cells from the iris and ciliary vessels into the anterior chamber. These, too, can be seen on slit-lamp examination and are graded on a scale of 1+ to 4+ (Table 12–2).[4] Cells, however, come in a variety of sizes and shapes, and the cell type may assist in diagnosis. White blood cells are easily seen against the dark pupil if a slit beam is shone at an angle across the pupil. The beam should not normally be visible in aqueous. However, with anterior chamber inflammation, flare can be homogeneously visualized, with focal cells evident. When cells are present, their number, size and color should be noted.

Mechanisms of glaucoma associated with a breakdown of the blood-aqueous barrier include (1) blockage of the trabecular meshwork with inflammatory debris and (2) in-

TABLE 12–1. GRADING OF ANTERIOR CHAMBER FLARE

Flare	Description
0	Complete absence
1+	Faint flare (barely detectable)
2+	Moderate flare (iris and lens details clear)
3+	Marked flare (iris and lens details hazy)
4+	Intense flare (fixed coagulated aqueous humor with considerable fibrin)

From Hogan MH, Kimura SJ, Thygeson P: Signs and symptoms of uveitis. I: Anterior uveitis. Am J Ophthalmol 1959;47:155.

TABLE 12–2. GRADING OF ANTERIOR CHAMBER CELLS

Cells per Field	Grade
0	No cells
1–2	Rare cells
3–7	Occasional cells
7–10	1+
10–15	1–2+
15–20	2+
20–50	3+
50+	4+

From Hogan MH, Kimura SJ, Thygeson P: Signs and symptoms of uveitis. I: Anterior uveitis. Am J Ophthalmol 1959;47:155.

filtration of the trabecular meshwork by lymphocytes, polymorphonuclear cells, or fibrin, resulting in decreased aqueous outflow, increased viscosity of aqueous humor, and hypersecretion associated with prostaglandin-mediated vascular hyperpermeability.[5–10] Formation of peripheral anterior synechia (PAS) may lead to secondary angle-closure glaucoma. PAS results from adhesion of the peripheral iris to the angle structures as inflammatory debris consolidates in the angle, usually initially in the inferior angle.[11] Other possible mechanisms of angle closure are pupillary block from an occluded or secluded pupil and fibrovascular contraction and scarring after rubeosis iridis.[12] Inflammation of the ciliary body may also lead to choroidal effusions, which can cause angle closure due to anterior rotation and swelling of the ciliary body. Initially, with active inflammation, the intraocular pressure (IOP) is often low because of decreased aqueous production as a result of breakdown of the blood-aqueous barrier, diminishing the osmotic gradient necessary for aqueous production. When inflammation resolves, the blood-aqueous barrier and osmotic gradient are re-established and normal aqueous production resumes, at which time pressure may rapidly become elevated as a result of normal aqueous production and diminished aqueous outflow.

Evaluation can be simplified by a determination of the amount of inflammation and the cell type involved. Although any etiology that produces severe inflammation may begin with mild inflammation, several causes of inflammation lead only to mild flare and the presence of cells.

GLAUCOMAS ASSOCIATED WITH MILD INFLAMMATION

Glaucomatocyclitic Crisis (Posner-Schlossman Syndrome)

Glaucomatocyclitic crisis is typically diagnosed in adults between the ages of 20 and 50 years and rarely initially manifests in patients older than 60 years. Patients present with a recurrent acute elevation of IOP, which results in blurred vision and mild to moderate ocular discomfort. It is generally unilateral, but bilateral cases do occur.[13–17] The condition is self-limited, but optic nerve damage from elevated IOP can be permanent.

On examination, the eye is quiet, and the conjunctiva is generally not injected. The cornea rarely may be edematous owing to the acutely elevated IOP. Edema is generally microcystic, although corneal stromal edema may be present. The IOP elevation is generally in the range of 40 to 60 mm Hg during attacks. The extent of elevation is out of proportion to the amount of inflammation in the anterior chamber. There is minimal flare, and rare cells are present in the anterior chamber. A few keratic precipitates (Fig. 12–2) may be found; they are usually round, flat, and nonpigmented and may persist after the attack.[18, 19] Gonioscopically, the angles are open. Visual field loss may occur after repeated episodes.

The cause of the disorder is unclear but can be considered a recurrent trabeculitis that is suspected to be caused

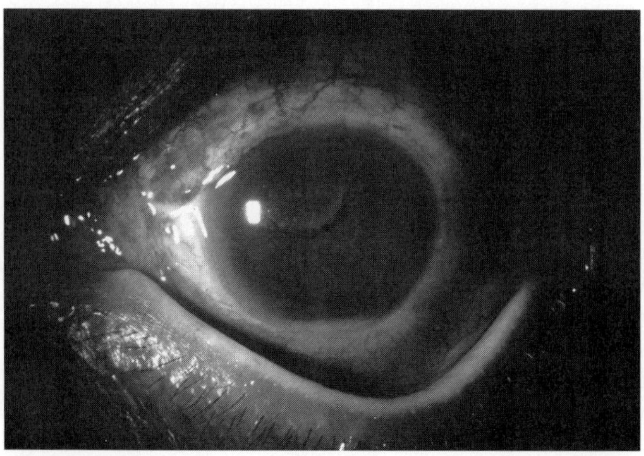

FIGURE 12–1. Slit-lamp photograph showing 4+ flare; note the fixed coagulated fibrin at the pupillary margin and the anterior chamber hypopyon.

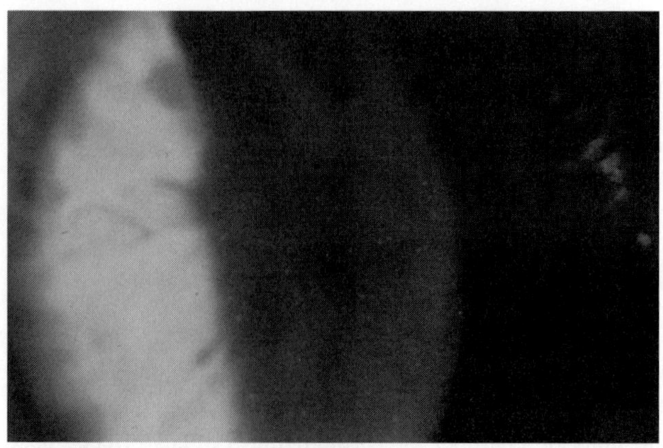

FIGURE 12–2. Slit-lamp photograph showing keratic precipitates on the corneal endothelium.

by herpesviruses.[20, 21] There is a significant reduction in trabecular outflow facility during the attacks.

The increased IOP responds quickly to treatment with topical corticosteroids. Suppression of aqueous production is also recommended for a few days. Prophylactic treatment between attacks is usually unnecessary. However, if frequent attacks occur, prophylaxis may be necessary; nonsteroidal anti-inflammatory drugs (NSAIDs) or topical corticosteroids may be used.[22, 23] Treatment of presumed elevations of IOP may also be appropriate prior to definitive IOP determination in patients with frequent attacks or those with previously markedly elevated IOP.

Fuchs' Heterochromic Iridocyclitis

Fuchs' heterochromic iridocyclitis is characterized by a triad of heterochromia, anterior segment inflammation, and cataract. Men and women are approximately equally affected, and the disease is usually diagnosed in the third or fourth decade of life.[24] It is usually unilateral, although bilateral presentations have been reported in up to 13% of cases.[24, 25] Patients may be asymptomatic or may present with mild blurred vision or floaters. Visual deterioration is generally due to formation of posterior subcapsular cataract. The affected eye has a slightly lighter colored iris (hypochromic); however, this phenomenon is difficult to demonstrate in dark irides, and iris color should be evaluated in natural lighting (sunlight, not fluorescent lighting).[26] In light-colored eyes, the loss of iris stroma may lead the affected eye to appear darker.[24]

Inflammation is usually mild, and characteristic keratic precipitates are found: round, small, or stellate, with fine interconnecting filaments. Gonioscopically, fine radial blood vessels may be seen crossing the scleral spur and trabecular meshwork. Amsler and Verrey[27] reported these fragile vessels to bleed in the angle opposite to the site of entry of paracentesis.

Glaucoma is found in 5% to 60% of cases.[28–32] Mechanisms proposed to account for the glaucoma include angle neovascularization and trabecular sclerosis.[33, 34]

The specific cause of Fuchs' heterochromic iridocyclitis is still unknown. An association between the disease and *Toxoplasma gondii* has been assumed on the basis of the presence of chorioretinal scars clinically consistent with toxoplasmosis.[35, 36] Other theories include immunologic origin,[33] a primary vascular disease,[37] and intrauterine insult.[38]

Treatment is usually not required unless glaucoma develops. Topical corticosteroids are ineffective and may cause progression of cataracts. The glaucoma is often refractory to medical treatment. Trabeculectomy can be effective in these cases.

Reiter's Syndrome

Reiter's syndrome consists of a triad of conjunctivitis or mild anterior uveitis, urethritis, and polyarthritis. Mucocutaneous lesions are common.[39] Men are more frequently affected than women, and most patients are positive for the HLA-B27 antigen.[40, 41] Ophthalmic manifestations include mucopurulent conjunctivitis, nongranulomatous iridocyclitis, keratitis, and episcleritis. Glaucoma is very rare in Reiter's syndrome and might be due to uveitis.[42]

Vogt-Koyanagi-Harada Syndrome

Vogt-Koyanagi-Harada (VKH) syndrome is a multisystem disorder of unknown etiology. The disease most commonly affects Asians or American Indians between the ages of 30 and 50 years. Ophthalmic manifestations are chronic iridocyclitis, multifocal choroiditis, and the hallmark of multifocal exudative retinal detachment.[43] Systemic manifestations include alopecia, poliosis, vitiligo, meningismus, and central auditory system dysfunction.

Glaucoma can be associated with VKH syndrome. The reported incidence varies from 20% to 38%. Patients present with transient shallowing of the anterior chamber and increased IOP. The mechanism of glaucoma is most commonly anterior rotation of the ciliary body with choroidal effusions causing an angle-closure glaucoma.[44–46] Treatment of the glaucoma is cycloplegia, which returns the ciliary body to a more normal position. Systemic corticosteroids are the treatment of choice for the inflammation and exudative retinal detachment.[44]

Sympathetic Ophthalmia

Sympathetic ophthalmia is a bilateral, granulomatous panuveitis occurring weeks, months, or years after penetrating ocular trauma or intraocular surgery to one eye.[47, 48] Anterior uveitis is common in both the traumatized eye (exciting eye) and the fellow eye (sympathizing eye). Clinical signs and symptoms are usually detected in the traumatized eye. Following an interval of months to years, anterior chamber inflammation is detected in the sympathizing eye.[49, 50]

The incidence of sympathetic ophthalmia is unknown. During the American Civil War, sympathetic ophthalmia developed in 16% of all cases of ocular injury. However, in 1972, the incidence was reported to be 0.19% following penetrating injuries and 0.007% following intraocular surgery.

The etiology of the disease is believed to be an immunologic response to soluble proteins associated with retinal photoreceptors or other retinal or choroidal antigens.[47, 49, 51, 52]

Glaucoma can occur in association with sympathetic ophthalmia; however, its incidence is unknown. Both open-angle and closed-angle mechanisms have been reported.[47, 53] Glaucoma associated with sympathetic ophthalmia is difficult to manage and requires frequent adjustment of corticosteroid and antiglaucoma medications. Surgery should be reserved for cases refractory to medical treatment.

Juvenile Rheumatoid Arthritis

Juvenile rheumatoid arthritis (JRA) is an idiopathic inflammatory arthritis of at least 3 months' duration in a child younger than 16 years. Unlike in adult rheumatoid arthritis, the rheumatoid factor test is negative, and the disease is associated with a high incidence of uveitis. Females are more commonly affected, in a ratio of 3:1. According to the American Rheumatism Association, the disease is divided into three types.

ACUTE SYSTEMIC JRA. Acute systemic JRA (Still's disease) accounts for about 20% of patients presenting with JRA. Still's disease is a multisystem disease characterized by high recurrent fever, lymphadenopathy, maculopapular rash on the trunk and limbs, and leukocytosis. Pericarditis, polyarthritis, and splenomegaly may also be seen. The disease is more prominent in young boys. Uveitis and uveitic glaucoma are very rarely observed.

POLYARTICULAR JRA. Polyarticular JRA accounts for 20% of cases of JRA. Females are more commonly affected, with an incidence rate of about 80%. The disease usually affects more than five joints, especially the knees, hands, and wrists. Uveitis is observed in about 10% of patients.[54] The main morbidity in this type is due to destructive arthritis.

PAUCIARTICULAR JRA. Pauciarticular JRA accounts for about 37% to 60% of cases of JRA. The disease affects younger patients, and females are more commonly affected. The disease affects fewer joints, and the arthritis is rarely destructive. Uveitis is observed in more than 75% of cases.[54, 55]

Glaucoma is common in patients with JRA, and its incidence varies with the chronicity of the intraocular inflammation. Several mechanisms contribute to the development of glaucoma. Most commonly, angle-closure glaucoma occurs from anterior and posterior synechiae, although open-angle glaucoma from trabecular obstruction by inflammatory debris and steroid-induced glaucoma also are observed.[56, 57]

Medical therapy is difficult, and steroid-induced glaucoma must always be considered. Miotics should be avoided because of disruption to the blood-aqueous barrier. Pupillary block glaucoma can be treated with iridotomy. The results of filtration surgery in children with JRA and glaucoma are very poor, although the use of adjuvant antifibrotic agents appears to be helpful. Finally, drainage implant devices may be effective in cases refractory to the previous measures. Pars plana insertion of tube shunts is especially useful when the anterior chamber is severely distorted from synechia.

Herpes Simplex Keratouveitis

This disease is characterized by recurrent attacks of uveitis, conjunctivitis, and keratitis. It accounts for approximately 5% of all cases of uveitis occurring in adults.[58] This keratouveitis is sometimes associated with IOP elevation, lasting 3 to 10 weeks.[59] The mechanism of IOP elevation is generally inflammation of trabecular cells and blockage of the trabecular meshwork with inflammatory debris.[60, 61] However, in severe cases of keratouveitis, angle-closure glaucoma might occur.

The management of glaucoma is primarily medical. Beta-blockers, alpha-agonists, and carbonic anhydrase inhibitors (CAIs) are usually effective in controlling the IOP. As the inflammation subsides, the glaucoma usually resolves. Corticosteroid therapy often results in an initial rapid decrease in IOP, but with continued treatment, corticosteroid-induced glaucoma may occur from frequent intense topical therapy.

Herpes Zoster Keratouveitis

Herpes zoster keratouveitis results from primary invasion of the ophthalmic division of the trigeminal nerve by the zoster virus or from reactivation of latent infection in the gasserian ganglion. Keratitis and uveitis are the main ocular presentations. Glaucoma is associated with this disorder, being found in up to half of cases.[62, 63] The mechanisms of IOP elevation and treatment are similar to those in herpes simplex keratouveitis.

Cytomegalic Inclusion Retinitis

Cytomegalic inclusion retinitis was initially reported in two adult recipients of renal transplants. Open-angle glaucoma developed in both patients and was associated with anterior uveitis.[64] Although cytomegalovirus (CMV) retinitis is now more frequent in the setting of human immunodeficiency virus (HIV) infection, glaucoma is exceedingly rare.

GLAUCOMAS ASSOCIATED WITH SEVERE INFLAMMATION

Behçet's Disease

Behçet's disease is a systemic disorder associated with increased prevalence of HLA-Bw51 and HLA-B5 antigens. The disease typically occurs in the Far East and the eastern Mediterranean region and is rare in the United States. It is characterized by oral ulceration, genital ulceration, and recurrent intraocular inflammation.[65] Other lesions are arteritis, gastrointestinal ulcers, thrombophlebitis, and cardiovascular and central nervous system (CNS) lesions.

Ocular involvement is usually bilateral, and about 70% of patients present with recurrent, nongranulomatous anterior uveitis. The basic lesion in Behçet's disease is obliterative vasculitis, which is thought to be due to neutrophil and platelet hyperfunction. Glaucoma in Behçet's disease is secondary to anterior uveitis, although neovascular glaucoma has been reported.[66, 67]

High-dose corticosteroids are usually effective in controlling the inflammation, but steroid resistance eventually develops. Cyclosporine (immunosuppressant) has been used successfully in the treatment of ocular manifestations of this disease.[68–70] Combined prednisone and cyclosporine have been shown to be effective and may be less toxic than cyclosporine monotherapy. The high IOP in Behçet's disease should initially be treated medically.

Syphilis

Syphilis is a sexually transmitted disease caused by the spirochete *Treponema pallidum*. The disease has congenital and acquired forms, and both forms have ocular involvement. The reported incidence of uveitis in patients infected with syphilis varies from 4% to 14%. However, because the incidence of syphilis is rising at present, the incidence of uveitis can be expected to increase. The ocular disease may be unilateral or bilateral, and both anterior and posterior uveitis occur. As there are no pathognomonic features of syphilitic uveitis, it must be suspected in any case of intraocular inflammation that is resistant to conventional treatment. Patients infected with syphilis are also at increased risk to be infected with other sexually transmitted diseases, including HIV. Infections related to acquired immune deficiency syndrome (AIDS), such as CMV, might coexist with syphilis and contribute to the uveitis.

Both open-angle and closed-angle glaucomas complicate syphilitic ocular involvement.[71, 72] The incidence of glaucoma varies between 15% and 20% in patients infected with syphilis. The glaucoma can occur during the active phase of inflammation or later in life.[73] In addition to treatment of the underlying infection, glaucoma associated with syphilitic uveitis is difficult to control; there is a poor response to antiglaucoma medications, and most patients require surgery.[74] Closed-angle glaucoma can be controlled with iridectomy with or without antiglaucoma medications.[74]

Leprosy (Hansen's Disease)

Leprosy is a systemic infection caused by *Mycobacterium leprae*. The disease occurs in two forms, lepromatous and tuberculoid. Ocular involvement, including uveitis, is common. The incidence of uveitis varies from 16% to 22% in the lepromatous form and from 5% to 7% in the tuberculoid form of leprosy.[75, 76]

Glaucoma has been associated with about 4% of cases of leprosy.[77] Both open-angle and closed-angle mechanisms are associated with the disease.

Sarcoidosis

Sarcoidosis is a systemic granulomatous disease of unknown etiology.[78, 79] The pathologic hallmark of the disease is a noncaseating granuloma. This disorder is more common in blacks, and women are more commonly affected than men. Adults between the ages of 20 and 40 years are generally affected. Ocular manifestations occur in about 30% of patients and may involve any part of the eye. However, uveitis is the most common ocular manifestation of sarcoidosis.[80, 81] Inflammation is initially unilateral, but with progression of the disease, bilateral involvement is frequent.

Glaucoma has been associated with ocular sarcoidosis.[78, 79] Several mechanisms contribute to the development of glaucoma in sarcoidosis, including infiltration of the trabecular meshwork with inflammatory cells, PAS, and obstruction of the trabecular meshwork with particulate matter.[82] Closed-angle glaucoma also develops from pupillary block due to secluded pupil from posterior synechiae.

Sarcoid-induced glaucoma initially is treated medically; however, miotics and prostaglandin analogues should be avoided if possible. Trabeculectomy with antimetabolites or tube shunt surgery may eventually become necessary in cases refractory to medical treatment. Laser iridotomy is the treatment of choice for pupillary block glaucoma, but it is ineffective in the presence of complete synechial angle closure.

Ankylosing Spondylitis

Ankylosing spondylitis is an idiopathic chronic inflammatory arthritis involving the cervical spine, lumbosacral spine, or sacroiliac joint.[83] There is a strong association with presence of the HLA-B27 antigen. Ninety-six percent of patients with ankylosing spondylitis have positive reactions to HLA-B27 testing.[84] Males are more commonly affected, in a ratio of 3:1.

Ocular manifestations are common, and the disease is usually associated with nongranulomatous, recurrent iritis, which may precede the onset of systemic symptoms. Open-angle glaucoma and steroid-induced glaucoma may occur. PAS or posterior synechiae frequently lead to the development of angle-closure glaucoma.

BLOOD (HYPHEMA) IN THE ANTERIOR CHAMBER

Hyphema is the accumulation of blood in the anterior chamber after penetrating and nonpenetrating ocular injuries (Fig 12–3) (see also Chapter 24). Clinically, hyphema is graded according to the amount of blood in the anterior chamber. The amount of blood varies from occasional red blood to total clotted hyphema filling the entire anterior chamber, becoming a "black-ball" or "eight-ball" hyphema. However, the majority of hyphemas fill less than one third of the anterior chamber.

Elevated Intraocular Pressure

One of the most dreaded complications of hyphema is elevated IOP. The risk of hyphema-related glaucoma correlates with the size of the hyphema, and its incidence varies from 27% for hyphemas filling half of the anterior chamber to 100% for "eight-ball" hyphemas.

Several mechanisms contribute to the elevated IOP, mainly obstruction of the trabecular meshwork by red blood cells and fibrin, angle recession, and pupillary block with "eight-ball" hyphemas.

If the hyphema is traumatic in origin, angle recession should be considered. In the eight-ball type, the clot is in the shape of a collar button filling the entire anterior and posterior chambers and resulting in pupillary block.

Rebleeding or secondary hemorrhage into the anterior chamber often leads to glaucoma. The incidence of rebleeding is almost 25%, with most cases occurring within 4 to 7 days. It is frequently associated with glaucoma and may result in corneal blood staining.

The management of glaucoma associated with hyphema is initially with antiglaucoma medications, mainly aqueous suppressants. However, oral CAIs should be avoided in

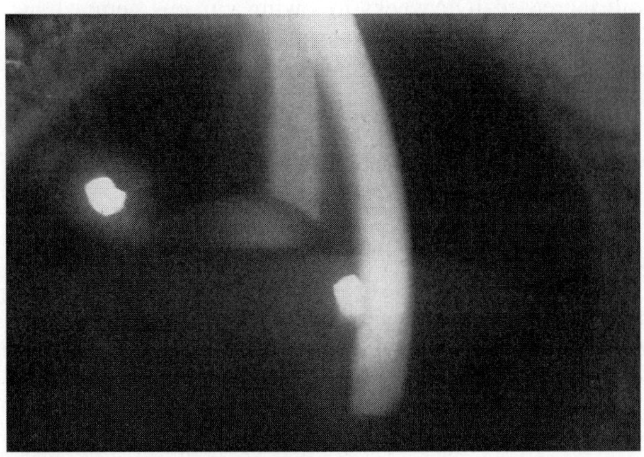

FIGURE 12–3. Slit-lamp photograph showing blood accumulation in the anterior chamber (hyphema).

cases of bleeding associated with sickle cell hemoglobinopathies, because lowering the pH may exacerbate the sickling. Trabeculectomy is indicated in cases refractory to medical treatment. Anterior chamber washout and removal of clots should be avoided, as they may cause additional bleeding.

Sickle Cell Hemoglobinopathies

The sickle cell hemoglobinopathies arise from a single gene mutation in the normal adult hemoglobin A, substituting the amino acid valine for glutamic acid to form hemoglobin S. Under hypoxic conditions, this abnormal hemoglobin sickles, deforming red blood cells and occluding small blood vessels. The disease is most common in blacks but can be found in other races. The most common forms of the disease are sickle cell anemia (SS disease) and sickle cell trait (AS hemoglobin).

Intraocular hemorrhages, including vitreous hemorrhage and hyphema, are common in patients with sickle cell hemoglobinopathies and this possibility should be evaluated in any black patient who presents with hyphema.

Several mechanisms contribute to the elevated IOP, including obstruction of Schlemm's canal with blood, neovascular glaucoma, ghost cell glaucoma, and uveitic glaucoma.[85, 86] Sickle cells are less pliable than normal red blood cells. Their egress through the trabecular meshwork is limited and is associated with additional blockage of the meshwork. The optic nerve may be more susceptible to IOP elevation in patients with sickle cell hemoglobinopathies than in the normal population.

Ghost Cell Glaucoma

Ocular trauma, retinal diseases, and vitreous surgery are often accompanied by vitreous hemorrhage. The fresh red blood cells in the vitreous are normally biconvex and nonrigid and can easily pass through the trabecular meshwork. Within 2 weeks, morphologic changes occur, slowly transforming them into rigid, spherical, khaki-colored, empty cells (ghost cells).[87] These cells subsequently migrate forward toward the anterior chamber through openings in the anterior hyaloid face. The IOP elevation results from mechanical obstruction of the trabecular meshwork by these rigid cells. Clinically, patients usually present with increased IOP weeks following vitreous hemorrhage. Sometimes a heavy accumulation of ghost cells in the anterior chamber leads to the formation of a pseudohypopyon.

Medical treatment with antiglaucoma medications might be sufficient to control the high IOP.[87] Vitrectomy is often indicated to clear the ghost cells.[88]

Hemolytic Glaucoma

Hemolytic glaucoma is another sequela of intraocular hemorrhage. On slit-lamp examination, reddish brown cells can be seen floating in the anterior chamber.[89] Hemoglobin-filled macrophages can obstruct the trabecular meshwork, leading to the elevation of the IOP. The elevated IOP often responds to antiglaucoma medications. Anterior chamber washout[89] or trabeculectomy may be indicated.

Hemosiderotic Glaucoma

Hemosiderotic glaucoma is a rare condition associated with long-standing intraocular hemorrhage. Siderosis of the trabecular meshwork due to iron liberated from hemoglobin may cause trabecular endothelial cell dysfunction, leading to obstruction of the trabecular meshwork.[90]

UVEITIS-GLAUCOMA-HYPHEMA SYNDROME

Uveitis-glaucoma-hyphema (UGH) syndrome was first described by Ellingson[91] in 1977. He attributed the condition to the poorly finished footplates of injection-molded anterior chamber lenses. However, the disorder still occurs with newer lenses, and posterior chamber intraocular lenses (IOLs) have been implicated as well.[92] The classic triad is anterior uveitis, hyphema, and elevated IOP.[93] Reported mechanisms include localized contact between the implant and the iris, which leads to chafing, and erosion of angle structures by improperly sized implants. The disease should be suspected in any patient with pseudophakia who demonstrates this triad of symptoms. However, it is possible to have just uveitis with hyphema, uveitis with glaucoma, or glaucoma with hyphema.

PARASITES

Onchocerciasis (River Blindness)

Onchocerciasis is a parasitic infection caused by the nematode *Onchocerca volvulus*.[94] The disease is rare in the United States but endemic in Central America and central Africa. The adult worm produces microfilariae, which when dead incites a severe inflammatory response. Both anterior uveitis and posterior uveitis have been associated with the disease.[95] On slit-lamp examination, scar tissue surrounding dead microfilaria can be seen in the anterior chamber. Uveitic glaucoma has been reported. The management consists of removal of the organism. Filtration surgery may be required to control the elevated IOP.

Gnathostomiasis

Gnathostomiasis is a parasitic infection caused by the nematode *Gnathostoma spinigerum*.[96] The disease is rare in the United States but has been frequently reported in Asia, especially in Thailand. It infects humans through ingestion of raw or inadequately cooked meat or fish. The intraocular parasite may be found in either the anterior or posterior segment.[97] Intracameral third-stage larvae may cause anterior uveitis and glaucoma. The management of the disease consists of removal of the parasite.

Pentastomiasis

Pentastomiasis is a rare parasitic infection caused by the larva *Linguatula serrata* or *Armillifer armillatus*. Humans are usually infected through consumption of contaminated water or vegetables and sometimes from intimate contact with an infected dog or cat. Intracameral pentastomiasis has been reported to cause anterior uveitis and unilateral glaucoma.[98]

Leishmaniasis

Leishmaniasis is caused by a protozoan from the genus *Leishmania*. Two forms have been identified, visceral leishmaniasis (kala-azar) and cutaneous leishmaniasis. Humans are infected through the bite of the sand fly. Post–kala-azar uveitis has been reported; it causes marked elevation of IOP requiring medical intervention.[99]

Toxocariasis

Toxocariasis is caused by the nematode *Toxocara canis*. Two forms have been identified, visceral larva migrans and ocular toxocariasis. The disease normally resides in the small intestine of dogs, and humans are infected through the ingestion of eggs present in contaminated soil or by direct contact with puppies.

Ocular toxocariasis is characterized by leukocoria, retinitis, and uveitis. Glaucoma might be associated with posterior synechiae and iris bombé.[100]

Debris

RETAINED LENS CORTEX (LENS PARTICLE GLAUCOMA)

Lens particle glaucoma is associated with disruption of lens capsule leading to the liberation of cortical material and, sometimes, parts of the lens capsule into the anterior chamber (Fig 12–4).[101] The disruption usually occurs after cataract extraction, penetrating injuries, or Nd:YAG laser capsulotomy. On slit-lamp examination, fluffy material can be seen floating in the anterior chamber. Flare and cells can also be seen, and in severe cases, a hypopyon may be observed. Patients usually present with elevated IOP correlated with the amount of lens material in the anterior chamber. The glaucoma is due to blockage of the trabecular meshwork with lens particles; however, the associated inflammation may often contribute to the elevated IOP.[102] The severity of uveitis and glaucoma is usually related to the amount of lens remnants in the anterior chamber.

The elevated IOP often responds to aqueous suppressants. Steroids should be used to control inflammation, and in severe cases, surgical removal of the lens material might be indicated.

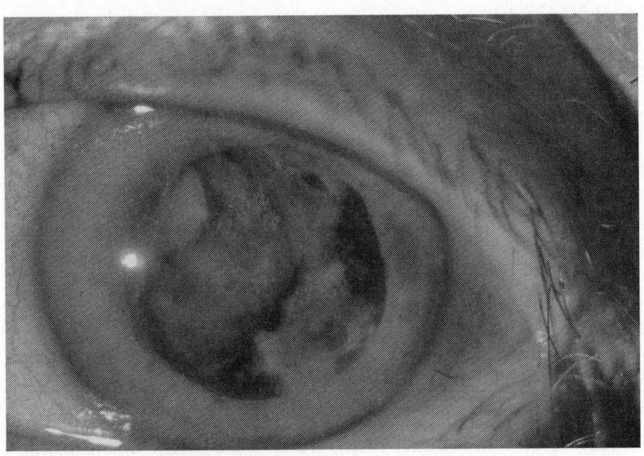

FIGURE 12–4. Slit-lamp photograph showing retained cortical material in the anterior chamber.

PIGMENT

Pigment dispersion syndrome and pseudoexfoliation syndrome are the two most common causes of increased pigmentation of the trabecular meshwork. Free-floating pigment may be seen in the anterior chamber. Iris trauma following surgery or laser can also lead to release of pigment into the anterior chamber.

Pigment Dispersion Syndrome

Pigment dispersion syndrome may or may not be associated with glaucoma. However, it is estimated that about one third of cases progress to pigmentary glaucoma over 15 years. Pigmentary glaucoma constitutes about 1% to 1.5% of the glaucomas in the western world.[103, 104] Risk factors associated with progression to pigmentary glaucoma include male gender, myopia, young age, and white race. Although the disease is most common in whites, it does occur in all races.[105, 106]

Pigmentary glaucoma is characterized by wide fluctuations in IOP, and the amount of pigment in the trabecular meshwork correlates with extent of IOP elevation. The accumulation of pigment in the angle obstructs aqueous outflow, causing chronic elevation of IOP. Exercise and pupillary dilation have been described to increase shedding of the pigment, resulting in IOP spikes.

The symptoms are usually those of primary open-angle glaucoma (POAG); however, the IOP in pigmentary glaucoma may fluctuate widely in some patients. The IOP elevation may be associated with halos or blurred vision. The treatment is usually medical, with ocular hypotensive agents. Laser surgery is another alternative. Good initial results can be achieved using argon laser trabeculoplasty (ALT) because of the heavy pigmentation, but the success rate decreases over time. Laser peripheral iridostomy (PI) can also be used; it causes flattening of the iris, which leads to a decrease in iridozonular contact and pigment shedding. Trabeculectomy is the surgical procedure of choice if the pressure is still uncontrolled; however, antimetabolites should be used with caution, especially in young patients, to avoid hypotonous maculopathy.

Pseudoexfoliation or Exfoliation Syndrome

It is estimated that more than 50% of patients with pseudoexfoliation or exfoliation syndrome eventually experience glaucoma. The disease is mainly seen in patients in their late 60s and early 70s, with no gender predilection. It is mainly bilateral but usually asymmetric. No hereditary pattern has been established. There is a high prevalence in Scandinavian countries, but pseudoexfoliation syndrome occurs in every part of the world.[107–109] The prevalence of the disease is underestimated mainly because of a low index of suspicion for it and because the pupils of an affected patient are difficult to dilate. The differential diagnosis is mainly composed of capsular delimitation, primary amyloidoses, and pigment dispersion.

Gonioscopically, the angle is open, and there is hyperpig-

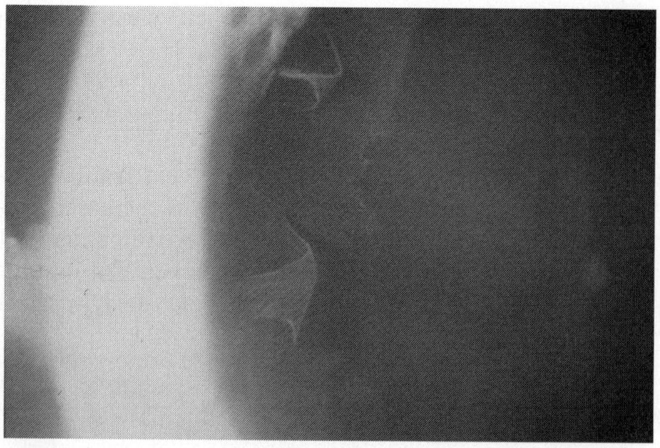

FIGURE 12–5. Slit-lamp photograph showing pseudoexfoliation material on the anterior lens capsule.

mentation of the trabecular meshwork that is more prominent inferiorly. The pigment has uneven and patchy distribution on the surface of the trabecular meshwork, and in unilateral cases, pigment is denser in the more severely affected eye.[110–112] Pigment also deposits on or anterior to Schwalbe's line (Sampaolesi's line), a finding considered pathognomonic of the disease.[113] Pseudoexfoliation material has a dandruff-like appearance, and is seen mainly in the inferior angle. After dilation, pseudoexfoliative material may be seen floating freely in aqueous humor (Fig 12–5). The glaucoma in pseudoexfoliation syndrome is of the open-angle type; however, sporadic cases of closed-angle glaucoma have been reported.[113–115] The mechanism of glaucoma is most likely due to obstruction of the trabecular meshwork by pigment and pseudoexfoliation material.

HYPOPYON

Mild anterior chamber inflammation is a common finding in acute angle-closure glaucoma. Hypopyon has been reported with acute angle-closure glaucoma (Fig 12–6). The etiology of the hypopyon is related to the necrosis of the iris. Another report related this intense inflammatory response to postischemic vascular leakage of leukocytes into the anterior chamber after resolution of the acute glaucoma attack. The hypopyon usually resolves spontaneously after the IOP is controlled.

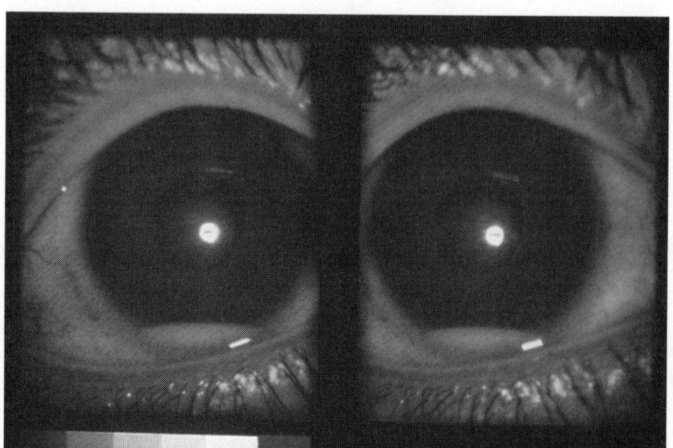

FIGURE 12–6. Slit-lamp photographs showing anterior chamber hypopyon.

VISCOELASTIC SUBSTANCES

Viscoelastic substances are widely used to re-form the anterior chamber and to protect the corneal endothelium during intraocular surgery. These substances should be removed from the anterior chamber at the end of surgery to prevent angle obstruction and IOP elevation. However, a significant rise of IOP may still occur despite the removal of the substances at the end of surgery. The remaining viscoelastic substance can be detected in the anterior chamber by a search for cells, which appear to be stagnant, trapped within the viscoelastic material.

The postoperative IOP spikes have been shown to occur with use of all the viscoelastics on the market. An extreme example of elevation of IOP occurred only with Orcolon. This viscoelastic caused a severe elevation of IOP, which led to its removal from the market by the U.S. Food and Drug Administration.

TUMOR CELLS AND TUMOR PSEUDOHYPOPYON

Anterior chamber involvement by intraocular malignancies is relatively rare. Tumor cells can migrate into the aqueous and manifest as free-floating opacities. In advanced cases, tumor cells deposit in the inferior angle, with the subsequent formation of a pseudohypopyon. These atypical presentations might lead to a false diagnosis of ocular inflammation.[116] The most accurate diagnostic technique is cytologic examination after anterior chamber paracentesis.[117] Intraocular neoplasms that can simulate an anterior uveitis include multiple myeloma, retinoblastoma, anterior uveal melanoma, metastatic carcinoma, and leukemia. The mechanism of glaucoma is either obstruction of the aqueous outflow by tumor cells or tumor-laden macrophages or the cells' direct infiltration of the trabecular meshwork.

Retinoblastoma

Retinoblastoma is the most common primary intraocular malignancy of childhood.[118] Barrett and colleagues reported 30 cases of retinoblastoma with anterior chamber involvement.[116] Of 30 patients, 17 presented with pseudohypopyon, and 4 patients with free anterior chamber cells and clusters. In a study by Shields and associates,[119] IOP elevation developed in 17% of eyes diagnosed with retinoblastoma. The mechanisms of IOP elevation are iris neovascularization, angle closure secondary to anterior displacement of the iris-lens diaphragm, and tumor seeding of the trabecular meshwork.[119] The presence of anterior chamber extension is a poor prognostic sign.

Metastatic Melanomas

Metastatic melanoma to the eye might manifest as ocular inflammation, dark hypopyon, or secondary glaucoma.[120, 121] Albert and coworkers[122] reported a case of disseminated cutaneous melanoma with a secondary mass in the ciliary body. A black hypopyon formed in the anterior chamber, and diagnostic paracentesis confirmed the presence of tumor cells and pigment-laden macrophages. Char and colleagues[120] presented another case of disseminated cutaneous melanomatosis with a black hypopyon in the anterior chamber. Secondary glaucoma occurred in both cases. Wormald and Harper[121] reported a patient with metastatic malignant melanoma who presented with bilateral black hypopyons and secondary glaucoma.

Metastatic Carcinomas

Anterior segment metastasis is a known cause of ocular inflammation, and the metastasis may antedate the detection of the primary site of the tumor.[123] In one series, iridocyclitis was the presenting sign in 40% of anterior segment metastases, and was the diagnosis in 19%.[124] Metastatic carcinoma to the eye is considered the most common form of intraocular malignancy.[125] Anterior segment metastases account for approximately 10% of ocular metastases.[124] The most common primary sites for ocular metastases are the breast and the lung. Glaucoma has been reported as a complication of iris and ciliary body metastases. One of the mechanisms of IOP elevation is outflow obstruction by free tumor cells or tumor-laden macrophages. Tumor cells might seed into the aqueous, producing a pseudohypopyon composed of layered tumor cells.

Leukemias

The presence of tumor cells in the anterior chamber is one of the presenting signs of leukemic infiltrates to the eye. In one study, 28% of children with leukemia presented with flare and cells in the anterior chamber.[126] The leukemic infiltrate to the eye leads to the development of glaucoma, which might be associated with hyphema or hypopyon.[127, 128] The management of these cases is directed toward the treatment of malignancy; however, one report documented an improvement in IOP after washing of necrotic tumor cells from the anterior chamber.[129]

Multiple Myeloma

Intraocular multiple myeloma has been reported.[130–132] The disease affects the eye by either direct extension or hematogenous spread. Nongranulomatous anterior uveitis with glaucoma has been reported in association with the disease.[133] In one report of associated glaucoma, microscopic examination of the anterior chamber aspirate disclosed multiple inflammatory cells, but no tumor cells were detected.[134] In another report, tumor cells were documented in the anterior chamber.[133]

Anterior Uveal Melanomas

An association between uveal melanoma and increased IOP has been documented in some reports.[135–137] Several mechanisms may contribute to the development of glaucoma, including obstruction of the trabecular meshwork from seeding of tumor cells in the anterior chamber angle and direct invasion of this area by the melanoma.[138, 139] Another mechanism, melanomalytic glaucoma, had been described in which melanin-laden macrophages are found in the anterior chamber angle of eyes with necrotic melanomas.[140] Both melanin-laden macrophages and free-floating tumor cells may be seen in aqueous.

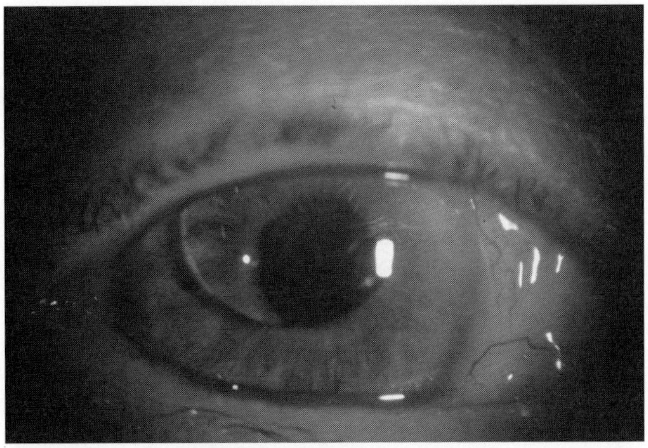

FIGURE 12–7. Slit-lamp photograph showing silicone oil droplet in the anterior chamber.

SILICONE OIL–INDUCED GLAUCOMA

Silicone oil is used in retinal surgery to provide long-term tamponade for the retina (see Chapters 16 and 24). Silicone bubbles are resistant to emulsification in aqueous owing to viscosity or interface tension and may be seen as droplets in the anterior chamber (Fig 12–7). IOP elevation is a common problem following silicone oil use.[141] Several mechanisms might contribute to the increased IOP. Pupillary block after oil injection has been reported.[142, 143] Emulsified oil in aqueous might block the trabecular meshwork, with subsequent increase in IOP.

Silicone oil–induced glaucoma can be managed medically; however, medical treatment eventually fails.[144, 145] Surgical procedures, including tube shunts, are alternative measures to control the high pressure.

REFERENCES

1. Krause U, Raunio V: The proteins of the pathologic human aqueous humor. Ophthalmologica 1970;160:280.
2. Dernochamps JP: The proteins of the aqueous humor. Doc Ophthalmol 1982;53:193.
3. Dernochamps JP, Michiels J: Molecular sieve properties of the blood-aqueous barrier in uveitis. Exp Eye Res 1977;25:25.
4. Hogan MH, Kimura SJ, Thygeson P: Signs and symptoms of uveitis. I: Anterior uveitis. Am J Ophthalmol 1959;47:155.
5. Belfort R, Nussenblatt RB: Surgical approaches to uveitis. Int Ophthalmol Clin 1990;30:314.
6. Roth M, Simmons RJ: Glaucoma associated with precipitates in the trabecular meshwork. Ophthalmology 1979;86:1613.
7. Krupin T, Feitl ME, Karalekas D: Glaucoma associated with uveitis. In Rich R, Shields MB, Krupin T (eds): The Glaucomas. St. Louis, Mosby–Year Book, 1996.
8. Toris CB, Pederson JE: Aqueous humor dynamics in experimental iridocyclitis. Invest Ophthalmol Vis Sci 1987;28:477.
9. Kass MA, Podos SM, Moses RA, Becker B: Prostaglandin E_1 and aqueous humor dynamics. Invest Ophthalmol 1972;11:1022.
10. Podos SM, Becker B, Kass MA: Prostaglandin synthesis, inhibition, and intraocular pressure. Invest Ophthalmol 1973;12:426.

11. Wallace AM: Uveitic glaucoma. In Tasman W, Jaeger EA (eds): Duane's Clinical Ophthalmology. Philadelphia, JB Lippincott, 1992.
12. Ritch R: Pathophysiology of glaucoma in uveitis. Trans Ophthalmol Soc UK 1981;101:321.
13. Brooke AM, Grant G, Young T, et al. Cyclitic glaucoma. Aust N Z J Ophthalmol 1989;17:157.
14. Higgitt AC: Secondary glaucoma. Trans Ophthalmol Soc UK 1956;76:73.
15. Knox DL: Glaucomatocyclitic crises and systemic disease. Trans Am Ophthalmol Soc 1988;86:473.
16. Levatin P: Glaucomatocyclitic crises occurring in both eyes. Am J Ophthalmol 1956;41:1056.
17. Posner A: Present status of the syndrome of glaucomatocyclitic crises. EENT Monthly 1958;37:402.
18. Posner A, Schlossman A: Syndrome of recurrent attacks of glaucoma with cyclitic symptoms. Arch Ophthalmol 1948;39:517.
19. Bloch-Michel E, Dussaix E, Cerqueti P, Patarin D: Possible role of cytomegalovirus in the etiology of Posner-Schlossman syndrome. Int Ophthalmol 1987;11:95.
20. Dernouchamps JP: The Posner-Schlossman Syndrome. Bull Soc Belg Ophthalmol 1989;230:13.
21. Masuda K, Izawa Y, Mishima S: Prostaglandins and glaucomatocyclitic crisis. Jpn J Ophthalmol 1975;19:368.
22. Posner A, Sclossman A: Further observations on the syndrome of glaucomatocyclitic crises. Trans Am Acad Ophthalmol Otolaryngol 1953;57:531.
23. Theodor FH: Observations on glaucomatocyclitic crisis: Posner Sclossman syndrome. Br J Ophthalmol 1952;36:207.
24. Franceschetti A: Heterochromic cyclitis: Fuchs' syndrome. Am J Ophthalmol 1955;39:50.
25. Ciarnella Cantani A, Leonardi E: Bilateral Fuchs' syndrome of heterochromic cyclitis. Clin Ocul Pathol Ocul 1982;3:91.
26. Kimura SJ: Fuchs' syndrome of heterochromic cyclitis in browneyed patients. Trans Am Ophthalmol Soc 1987;76:76.
27. Amsler M, Verrey F: Heterochromie de Fuchs et fragilité vasculaire. Ophthalmologica 1946;111:177.
28. Huber A: Das Glaukom bei komplizieretер heterochromic Fuchs. Ophthalmologica 1961;142:66.
29. Tabbut BR, Tessler HH, Williams D: Fuchs' heterochromic iridocyclitis in blacks. Arch Ophthalmol 1988;106:1688.
30. Liesegang TJ: Clinical features and prognosis in Fuchs' uveitis syndrome. Arch Ophthalmol 1982;100:1622.
31. Jones NP: Fuchs' heterochromic uveitis: A reappraisal of the clinical spectrum. Eye 1991;5:649.
32. Huber A: Glaucoma as a complication in heterochromia of Fuchs. Ophthalmologica 1961;142:66.
33. O'Connor GR: Heterochromic iridocyclitis. Trans Ophthalmol Soc UK 1985;104:219.
34. Lerman S, Levy C: Heterochromic iritis and secondary neovascular glaucoma. Am J Ophthalmol 1964;57:479.
35. Schwab IR: The epidemiologic association of Fuchs' heterochromic iridocyclitis and ocular toxoplasmosis. Am J Ophthalmol 1991; 111:356.
36. DeAbreu MT, Belfort R, Hirata PS: Fuchs' heterochromic iridocyclitis and ocular toxoplasmosis. Am J Ophthalmol 1982;93:739.
37. Saari M, Vuorre I, Nieminen H: Fuchs's heterochromic cyclitis: A simultaneous bilateral fluorescein angiographic study of the iris. Br J Ophthalmol 1978;62:715.
38. Fuchs E: Ueber komplikationen der heterochromie. Z Augenheilkd 1906;15:191.
39. Reiter H: Ueber eine bisher unerkannte Spirachateninfektion. Dtsch Med Wochenschr 1916;42:1535.
40. Sharp JT: Reiter's syndrome (reactive arthritis). *In* McCarthy DJ (ed): Arthritis and Allied Conditions. Philadelphia, Lea & Febiger, 1985, p 841.
41. Lee DA, Barker SM, Su WPD, et al: The clinical diagnosis of Reiter's syndrome: Ophthalmic and nonophthalmic aspects. Ophthalmology 1986;93:350.
42. Amett FG: Incomplete Reiter's syndrome: Discriminating features and HLA-W27 in diagnosis. Ann Intern Med 1976;84:8.
43. Shields MB: Glaucoma associated with ocular inflammation. *In* Shields MB (ed): Textbook of Glaucoma. Baltimore, Williams & Wilkins, 1997, p 317.
44. Shirato S, Hayashi K, Masuda K: Acute angle closure glaucoma as an initial sign of Harada's disease: Report of two cases. Jpn J Ophthalmol 1980;24:260.
45. Kimura R, Kasai M, Shoji K, Kanno C: Swollen ciliary processes as an initial symptom in Vogt-Koyanagi-Harada syndrome. Am J Ophthalmol 1983;95:402.
46. Kimura R, Kasai M, Okabe H: Transient shallow anterior chamber as initial symptom in Harada's syndrome. Arch Ophthalmol 1981;99:1604.
47. Lubin JR, Albert DM, Weinstein M: Sixty-five years of sympathetic ophthalmia: A clinicopathologic review of 105 cases. Ophthalmology 1980;87:109.
48. Thies O: Gedanken über den Ausbruch der sympathischen ophthalmia. Klin Monatsbl Augenheilkd 1947;112:185.
49. Marak GE Jr: Recent advances in sympathetic ophthalmia. Surv Ophthalmol 1979;24:141.
50. Morse PH, Duke JR: Sympathetic ophthalmia: Report of a case, proven pathologically, 8 years after original injury. Am J Ophthalmol 1969;68:508.
51. Duke-Edler S, Perkins EA: Diseases of the uveal tract. *In* Duke-Edler S (ed): System of Ophthalmology, vol IX. St. Louis, CV Mosby, 1966.
52. Lindy BSL, Stuart J: Sympathetic ophthalmia in Canada. Can J Ophthalmol 1972;7:157.
53. Samuels B: Glaucoma and sympathetic ophthalmia. Arch Ophthalmol 1937;17:1031.
54. Schaller J, Kupfer C, Wedgewood RJ: Iridocyclitis in juvenile rheumatoid arthritis. Pediatrics 1969;44:92.
55. Ohno S, Char DH, Kimura SJ, O'Connor GR: HLA antigens and antinuclear antibody titres in juvenile chronic iridocyclitis. Br J Ophthalmol 1977;61:59.
56. Kanski JJ: Uveitis in juvenile chronic arthritis: Incidence, clinical features, and prognosis. Eye 1988;2:641.
57. Merriam JC, Chylack LT, Albert DM: Early-onset pauciarticular juvenile rheumatoid arthritis: A histopathologic study. Arch Ophthalmol 1983;101:1085.
58. Panek WC: Glaucoma in patients with uveitis. Br J Ophthalmol 1990;74:223.
59. Oh JO: Effect of cyclophosphamide on primary herpes simplex kerato-uveitis and glaucoma. Invest Ophthalmol Vis Sci 1987; 17:769.
60. Falcon MG, Williams HP: Herpes simplex keratouveitis and glaucoma. Trans Ophthalmol Soc UK 1978;98:101.
61. Townsend WM, Kaufman HE: Pathogenesis of glaucoma and endothelial changes in herpetic keratouveitis in rabbits. Am J Ophthalmol 1971;71:904.
62. Nigam P, et al: Clinical profile of herpes zoster ophthalmicus. J Indian Med Assoc 1991;89:117.
63. Reijo A, Antti V, Jukka M: Endothelial cell loss in herpes zoster keratouveitis. Br J Ophthalmol 1983;67:751.
64. Merit JC, Callender CO: Adult cytomegalic inclusion retinitis. Ann Ophthalmol 1978;10:1059.
65. Michelson JB, Chisari FV: Behçet disease. Surv Ophthalmol 1982;26:190.
66. Wakefield D, McCluskey P: Behçet syndrome: Ocular features in an Australian population. Aust NZ J Ophthalmol 1990;18:129.
67. Winter FC, Yukin RE: The ocular pathology of Behçet disease. Am J Ophthalmol 1966;62:257.
68. Benezra D, Cohen E: Treatment and visual prognosis in Behçet disease. Br J Ophthalmol 1986;70:589.
69. Masuda K, Nakajima A, Urayama A, et al: Double-masked trial of cyclosporine versus colchicine and long-term open study of cyclosporine in Behçet disease. Lancet 1989;1:1093.
70. Nussenblatt RB, Palastine AG, Chan CC: Cyclosporine A therapy in the treatment of intraocular inflammatory disease resistant to systemic corticosteroids and cytotoxic agents. Am J Ophthalmol 1983;96:275.
71. Knox DL: Glaucoma following syphilitic interstitial keratitis. Arch Ophthalmol 1961;64:44.
72. Sugar HS: Late glaucoma associated with inactive syphilitic interstitial keratitis. Am J Ophthalmol 1962;63:602.
73. Tsukahara S: Secondary glaucoma due to inactive congenital syphilitic keratitis. Ophthalmologica 1977;174:188.
74. Grant DM: Late glaucoma after interstitial keratitis. Am J Ophthalmol 1975;79:87.
75. Brandt F, Malla OK, Anten JGF: Influence of untreated chronic plastic iridocyclitis on intraocular pressure in lepromatous patients. Br J Ophthalmol 1981;65:240.

76. Michelson JB, Roth AM, Waring GO III: Lepromatous iridocyclitis diagnosed by anterior chamber paracentesis. Am J Ophthalmol 1979;88:674.
77. Spaide R, Nattis R, Lipka A, D'Amico R: Ocular involvement in leprosy in the United States. Am J Ophthalmol 1985;100:411.
78. Jobs DA, Johns CJ: Ocular involvement in chronic sarcoidosis. Am J Ophthalmol 1986;102:297.
79. Obenauf CD, Shaw HE, Sydnor CF, Klintworth GK: Sarcoidosis and its ophthalmic manifestations. Am J Ophthalmol 1978;86:6648.
80. James DC, Anderson R, Langley D, Ainslie D: Ocular sarcoidosis. Br J Ophthalmol 1964;48:461.
81. James DJ, Neville E, Langley DA: Ocular sarcoidosis. Trans Ophthalmol Soc UK 1976;96:133.
82. Jobs DA: The rheumatic diseases. *In* Schachat AP, Murphy RB, Patz A (eds): Retina, vol 2. St. Louis, Mosby–Year Book, 1989.
83. Russel AS, Lentle BC, Percy JS, Jackson FI: Scintigraphy of sacroiliac joints in acute anterior uveitis: A study of thirty patients. Ann Intern Med 1976;85:606.
84. Brewerton DA, et al: Ankylosing spondylitis and HLA-B27. Lancet 1973;1:904.
85. Goldberg MF: The diagnosis and treatment of secondary glaucoma after hyphema in sickle cell patients. Am J Ophthalmol 1979;87:43.
86. Goldberg MF: Sickled erythrocytes, hyphema, and secondary glaucoma: The diagnosis and treatment of sickled erythrocytes in human hyphemas. Ophthalmic Surg 1979;10:17.
87. Campbell DG, Simmons RJ, Grant WM: Ghost cells as a cause of glaucoma. Am J Ophthalmol 1976;81:441.
88. Singh H, Grand MG: Treatment of blood-induced glaucoma by trans plana vitrectomy. Retina 1981;1:255.
89. Phelps CD, Watzke RC: Hemolytic glaucoma. Am J Ophthalmol 1975;80:690.
90. Vannas S: Hemosiderosis in eyes with secondary glaucoma after delayed intraocular hemorrhages. Acta Ophthalmol 1960;38:254.
91. Ellingson FT: Complications with the Choyce Mark anterior chamber lens implant (uveitis-glaucoma-hyphema). Am Intra-Ocular Implant Soc J 1977;3:199.
92. Pazandak B, Johnson S, Kratz R, Faulkner GD: Recurrent intraocular hemorrhage associated with posterior chamber lens implantation. Am Intra-Ocular Implant Soc J 1983;9:327.
93. Bergo RO: Fox shield treatment of the UGH syndrome. J Cataract Refract Surg 1986;12:419.
94. Whitworth JA, Gilbert CE, Mabey DM, et al: Visual loss in onchocerciasis endemic community in Sierra Leone. Br J Ophthalmol 1993;77:30.
95. Olsen KP, Gass JDM: Diffuse unilateral subacute neuroretinitis. *In* Schachat AP, Murphy RB, Patz A (eds): Retina, vol 2. St. Louis, Mosby–Year Book, 1989.
96. Owen R: Anatomical description of two species of Entozoa from the stomach of a tiger. Proc Zool Soc Lond 1836;47:123.
97. Kittiponghansa S, Prabriputaloong A, Pariyanonda S, Ritch R: Intracameral gnathostomiasis: A cause of anterior uveitis and secondary glaucoma. Br J Ophthalmol 1987;71:618.
98. Lang Y, Garzozi H, Epstein Z, et al: Intraocular pentastomiasis causing unilateral glaucoma. Br J Ophthalmol 1987;71:391.
99. Dechant W, Rees PH, Kager PA, et al: Post kala-azar uveitis. Br J Ophthalmol 1980;64:680.
100. Shields JA: Ocular toxocariasis: A review. Surv Ophthalmol 1984; 28:361.
101. Epstein DL: Diagnosis and management of lens-induced glaucoma. Ophthalmology 1982;89:227.
102. Epstein DL, Jedziniak JA, Grant WM: Obstruction of aqueous outflow by lens particles and by heavy-molecular-weight soluble lens proteins. Invest Ophthalmol Vis Sci 1978;17:272.
103. Mapstone R: Pigment release. Br J Ophthalmol 1981;65:258.
104. Scheie HG, Fleischauer HW: Idiopathic atrophy of the epithelial layers of the iris and ciliary body. Arch Ophthalmol 1958;59:216.
105. Scheie HG, Cameron JD: Pigment dispersion syndrome: A clinical study. Br J Ophthalmol 1981;65:264.
106. Weber PA, Dingle JB: Pigmentary glaucoma in a black albino. Ann Ophthalmol 1983;15:454.
107. Aasved H: The geographical distribution of fibrillopathia epitheliocapsularis. Acta Ophthalmol (Copenh) 1969;47:792.
108. Tarkkanen A: Pseudoexfoliation of the lens capsule. Acta Ophthalmol (Copenh) 1962;71:1.
109. Taylor HR: Pseudoexfoliation, an environmental disease. Trans Ophthalmol Soc UK 1979;99:302.
110. Meyer E, Haim T, Zonis S, et al: Pseudoexfoliation: Epidemiology, clinical, and scanning electron microscopic study. Ophthalmologica 1984;188:141.
111. Prince AM, Streeten BW, Ritch R, et al: Preclinical diagnosis of pseudoexfoliation syndrome. Arch Ophthalmol 1987;105:1076.
112. Wishart PK, Spaeth GL, Poryzees EM: Anterior chamber angle in the exfoliation syndrome. Br J Ophthalmol 1985;69:103.
113. Amalric P, Sampaolesi R, Bessou P: Early diagnosis and heredity of pseudocapsular exfoliation. Bull Soc Ophthalmol Fr 1960;5–6:341.
114. Bartholomew RS: Anterior chamber depth in eyes with pseudoexfoliation. Br J Ophthalmol 1980;64:322.
115. Dark AJ, Streeten BW, Conward CC: Pseudoexfoliative syndrome of the lens: A study in electron microscopy and histochemistry. Br J Ophthalmol 1977;61:462.
116. Haik BG, Dunleavy SA, Cooke C, et al: Retinoblastoma with anterior chamber extension. Ophthalmology 1987;94:367.
117. Jakobiec FA, Chattock A: The role of cytology and needle biopsies in the diagnosis of ophthalmic tumors and simulating conditions. *In* Jakobiec FA (ed): Ocular and Adnexal Tumors. Birmingham, AL, Aesculapius Publishing, 1978, p 341.
118. Reese AB: Tumors of the Eye, 3rd ed. New York, Harper & Row, 1976, p 89.
119. Shields CL, Shields JA, Shields B, Augsburger JJ: Prevalence and mechanisms of secondary intraocular pressure elevation in eyes with intraocular tumors. Ophthalmology 1987;94:839.
120. Char DH, Schwartz A, Miller TR, Abele JS: Ocular metastases from systemic melanoma. Am J Ophthalmol 1980;90:702.
121. Wormald RPL, Harper JI: Bilateral black hypopyon in a patient with self-healing cutaneous malignant melanoma. Br J Ophthalmol 1983;67:231.
122. Albert DM, Lahav M, Troczynski E, Bahr R: Black hypopyon: Report of two cases. Graefes Arc Klin Ophthalmol 1975;193:81.
123. Rotkis WM, Kulander BG, Chandler JW, Kaiser FS: Diagnosis of anterior chamber metastasis by serologic marker found during anterior chamber paracentesis. Am J Ophthalmol 1986;102:179.
124. Ferry AP, Font RL: Carcinoma metastatic to the eye and orbit: A clinicopathologic study of 26 patients with carcinoma metastatic to the anterior segment of the eye. Arch Ophthalmol 1975;93:472.
125. Scholz R, Green WR, Baranano EC, et al: Metastatic carcinoma to the iris: Diagnosis by aqueous paracentesis and response to irradiation and chemotherapy. Ophthalmology 1983;90:1524.
126. Nelson CC, Hertzberg BS, Klintworth GK. A histopathologic study of 716 unselected eyes in patients with cancer at the time of death. Am J Ophthalmol 1983;95:788.
127. Rosenthal AR: Ocular manifestations of leukemia: A review. Ophthalmology 1983;90:899.
128. Zakka KA, Yee RD, Shorr N, et al: Leukemic iris infiltration. Am J Ophthalmol 1980;89:204.
129. Ayliffe W, Foster CS, Marcoux P, et al: Relapsing acute myeloid leukemia manifesting as hypopyon uveitis. Am J Ophthalmol 1995;119:361.
130. Clark E: Ophthalmic complications of multiple myelomatosis. Br J Ophthalmol 1955;39:233.
131. Ashton N: Ocular changes in multiple myelomatosis. Arch Ophthalmol 1965;73:487.
132. Bronstein M: Ocular involvement in multiple myeloma. Arch Ophthalmol 1956;55:188.
133. Shakin EP, Augsburger JJ, Eagle, Jr RC, et al: Multiple myeloma involving the iris. Arch Ophthalmol 1988;106:524.
134. Baker T, Spencer W: Ocular findings in multiple myeloma. Arch Ophthalmol 1974;91:110.
135. Terry TL, Johns JP: Uveal sarcoma-malignant melanoma: A statistical study of ninety four cases. Am J Ophthalmol 1935;18:903.
136. Foos RY, Hull SN, Straatsma BR: Early diagnosis of ciliary body melanomas. Arch Ophthalmol 1969;81:336.
137. Yanoff M: Glaucoma mechanisms in ocular malignant melanomas. Am J Ophthalmol 1970;70:898.
138. Hopkins RE, Carriker FR: Malignant melanoma of the ciliary body. Am J Ophthalmol 1958;45:835.
139. Ashton N: Primary tumors of the iris. Br J Ophthalmol 1964;48:650.
140. Yanoff M, Scheie HG: Melanomalytic glaucoma: Report of a case. Arch Ophthalmol 1970;84:471.
141. Unosson K, Stenkula S, Tornqvist P, Weijdegard L: Liquid silicone in the treatment of retinal detachment. Acta Ophthalmol 1985; 63:656.

142. Ando F: Intraocular hypertension resulting from pupillary block by silicone oil. Am J Ophthalmol 1985;99:87.
143. Barr CC, Lai MY, Lean JS, et al: Postoperative intraocular pressure abnormalities in the silicone oil study.: Silicone oil study report 4. Ophthalmology 1993;100:1029.
144. Haunt J, Ullern M, Chermet M, Van Effenterre G: Complications of intraocular injections of silicone combined with vitrectomy. Ophthalmologica 1980;180:29.
145. Okun E: Intravitreal surgery utilizing liquid silicone: A long-term follow-up. Trans Pac Coast Oto-Ophthalmol Soc 1968;49:141.

CHAPTER 13

Gonioscopy

SHERIF M. EL-HARAZI and ROBERT M. FELDMAN

A discussion of gonioscopy could be placed in several different locations in this text, because it represents a key concept in the glaucoma care process. It is included in the section on diagnosis because gonioscopy is a vital component in the diagnosis of essentially every form of glaucoma. Additionally, prior to the making of decisions concerning therapy, the status of the angle must be known. In this chapter, Sherif El-Harazi and Robert Feldman systematically examine the key findings observed gonioscopically. They differentiate these distinctive signs by their location on the trabecular meshwork and by what the observed abnormality is—pigment, blood, blood vessels, debris, or membranes. They also discuss structural abnormalities that may be observed gonioscopically, including tears, disinsertion, and synechiae. Referring to this information should greatly enhance your ability to decipher gonioscopic findings on examination.

No anatomical area plays as pivotal a role in the diagnosis and management of glaucoma as the iridocorneal angle. Specific diseases can be diagnosed from the clinical finding of a single structure in this area, the entire angle, or its anatomical configuration. Furthermore, in the evaluation of treatment success or failure, gonioscopy often plays a key role.

The normal adult iridocorneal angle consists of five anatomical landmarks, from anterior to posterior: Schwalbe's line, anterior (nonpigmented) trabecular meshwork, posterior (pigmented) trabecular meshwork, scleral spur, and ciliary body band (Fig. 13–1).

Observation of the iris as part of gonioscopy is important because the iris itself may contribute to disease of the angle in the ability to occlude structures directly from scars across the angle (synechiae), and iris processes may project anteriorly to the trabecular meshwork.

Total internal reflectivity of the cornea precludes direct observation of angle structures without special viewing techniques. To overcome this optical barrier, either direct or indirect methods are used (Fig. 13–2). Gonioscopy using a Koeppe's lens allows direct visualization of the angle by changing the corneal refractive surface through the use of a viewing lens. The light rays can then overcome internal reflectivity, allowing direct viewing. This technique is used primarily in the operating room as the patient is supine. The operating microscope is tilted to allow visualization for diagnostic or therapeutic intervention (i.e., goniotomy). The image is erect and panoramic.

Most commonly in the clinical setting, indirect visualization is used and is accomplished using a mirrored lens to change the angle of the light rays, allowing them to pass through the cornea. This results in an inverted image. Indirect systems are of two types. Both require topical anesthesia. The first uses a viscous coupling agent between the cornea and the viewing lens, such as the Goldmann or Ritch type. The advantage is a very stable viewing system. The major disadvantages are (1) the time required to establish the image and (2) the leaving of viscous agent on the ocular surface after removal of the lens and its interference with subsequent visualization. This technique is preferred during treatment of the angle, such as with argon laser trabeculoplasty, which requires the stable view and excellent visualization that this technique provides.

Increasingly, indirect viewing without a viscous agent is being used because of its advantages. This technique uses the Zeiss (glass) or Posner (plastic) four-mirror gonioprism with handles or the Sussman lens. The most important

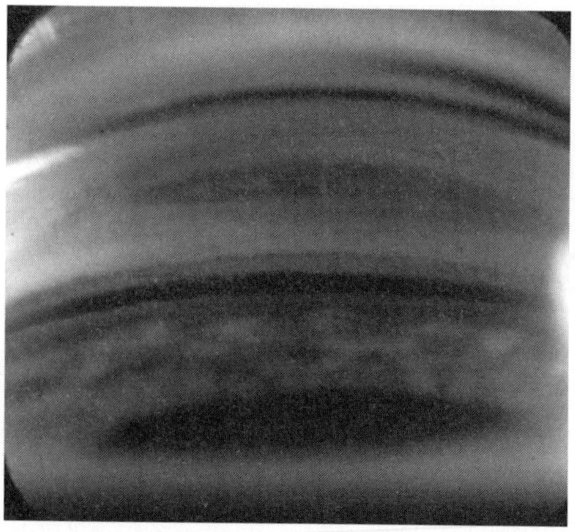

FIGURE 13–1. Identification of angle structures (from top to bottom, anterior to posterior): cornea, Schwalbe's line, anterior nonpigmented trabecular meshwork, posterior pigmented trabecular meshwork, scleral spur, ciliary body band, iris. This is an eye with pigment dispersion. Note the heavy amount of pigmentation in the posterior trabecular meshwork.

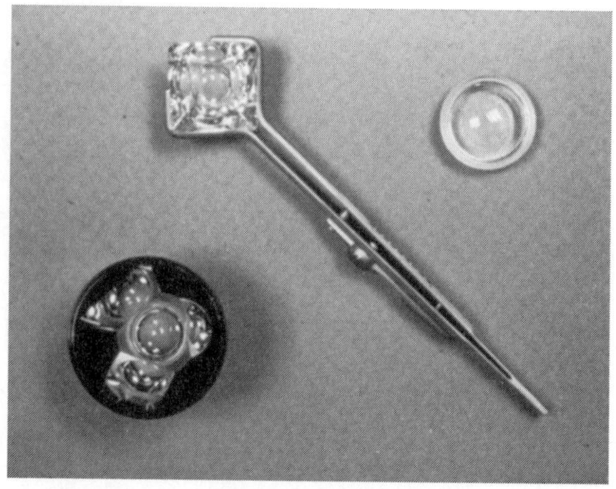

FIGURE 13–2. Lenses commonly used for gonioscopy. Left to right: Goldmann three-mirror, Zeiss four-mirror, Koeppe.

advantage is the ability to perform dynamic or compression gonioscopy. After initial visualization of the angle structures, gentle pressure is applied with the lens directly posteriorly on the corneal surface. The pressure forces aqueous into the peripheral recesses of the angle, expanding its depth. This maneuver allows differentiation of appositional from synechial angle closure (Fig. 13–3). The technique is much faster than the others with no distortion of subsequent visualization after it is completed. The primary disadvantage is that the lens is not as stable on the corneal surface, and greater experience is needed to successfully master the technique.

TECHNIQUE OF INDIRECT GONIOSCOPY

After topical anesthesia is instilled (and *after* intraocular pressure is measured), the patient should be comfortably seated at the slit lamp. The lens should be grasped and the patient instructed to look up with the eyes only. This upper lid elevation widens the lid fissure. The examiner should then bring the lens gently into contact with the globe while retracting the lower eyelid with the other fingers of the hand holding the lens. The patient is then told to look straight ahead. During performance of gonioscopy, it is important for the examiner's hand to be stabilized. The examiner can place the fingers that are not holding the lens on the patient's cheek or on the slit lamp structure. There should be elbow support also, if necessary.

Signs of Glaucoma According to Structure

The clinical signs of glaucoma in most cases can be evaluated on a structure-by-structure basis. They are listed here according to the five anatomical landmarks of the iridocorneal angle previously mentioned.

CHANGES ANTERIOR TO SCHWALBE'S LINE

Sampaolesis's Line

Sampaolesis's line typically is a black pigment line found on or anterior to Schwalbe's line in pseudoexfoliation syn-

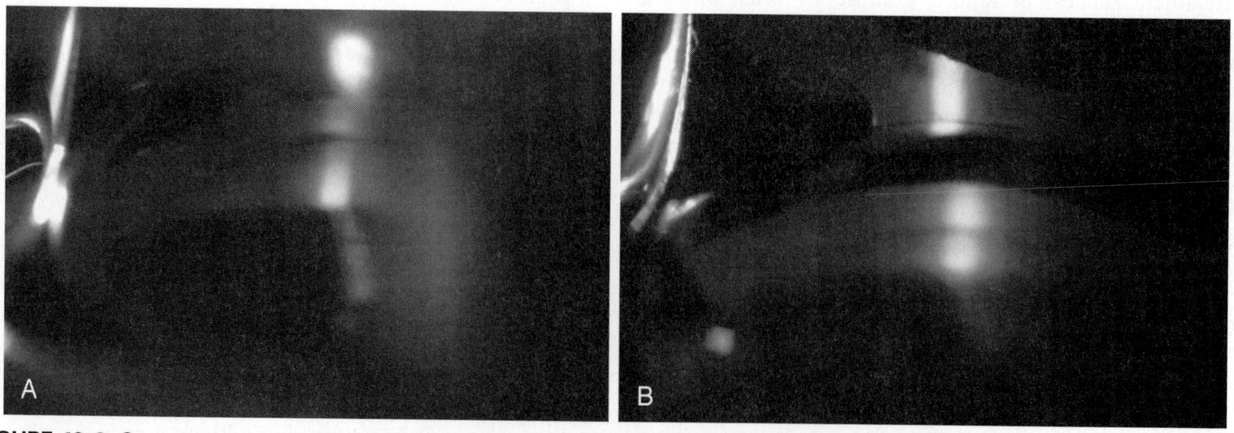

FIGURE 13–3. Compression gonioscopy. *A*, Typical view trough Zeiss gonioprism. Note that no angle structures are visible with marked peripheral iris bow. It is not possible to determine whether the iris is permanently adherent to meshwork (synechial) or not (appositional). *B*, With compression gonioscopy, the peripheral chamber deepens and the iris is separated from the meshwork, confirming appositional closure.

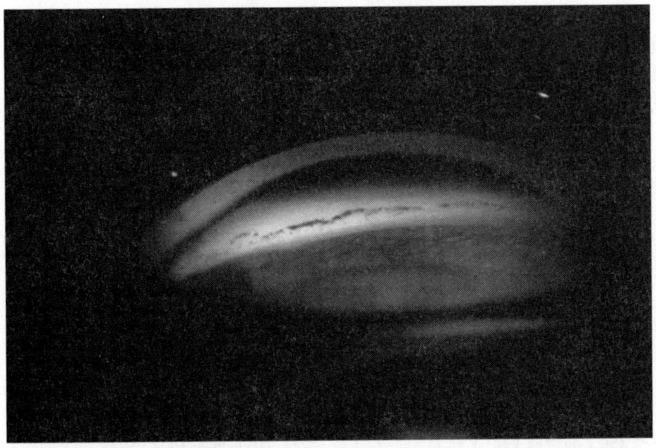

FIGURE 13–4. Sampaolesis's line is seen as the black pigment on or anterior to Schwalbe's line.

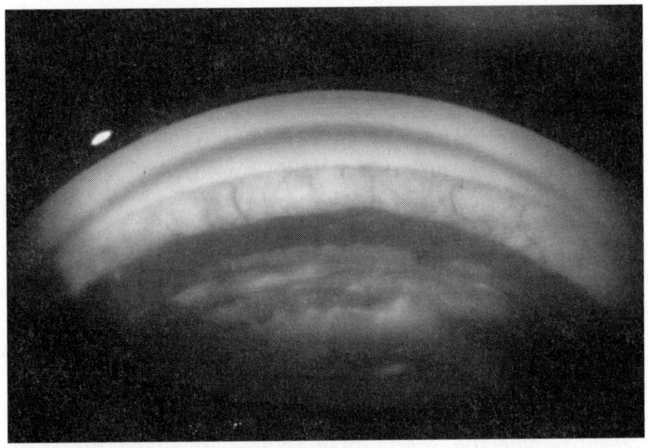

FIGURE 13–5. Neovascular glaucoma. Mature vessels on iris surface result in synechial angle closure.

drome (Fig. 13–4).[1] The line may be segmental (inferior) or may extend 360 degrees. Similar nonspecific pigment lines may often be seen inferiorly but tend to be brown in color.

Pigment Smudging

Irregular pigment that appears wiped on the angle structures is called pigment smudging. It indicates previous appositional closure. When this sign is observed in an occludable angle, consideration should be given to intermittent (or subacute) angle closure.

ANTERIOR TRABECULAR MESHWORK

Anterior trabecular meshwork extends from Schwalbe's line posteriorly to the pigmented portion of the trabecular meshwork. It normally is very light gray or brown but may contain greater amounts of pigmentation.

Pigmentation

Increased pigmentation of the anterior trabecular meshwork may be seen in the same disorders that cause pigmentation of the posterior trabecular meshwork and anterior to Schwalbe's line, such as pseudoexfoliation syndrome and pigment dispersion syndrome. See later discussion of the posterior trabecular meshwork.

Vessels

NEOVASCULAR GLAUCOMA

In neovascular glaucoma, irregular vessels may be seen crossing the angle. The fine vessels arborize before terminating.[2] They are generally first seen at the pupillary margin but may become visible in the angle first.[3, 4] The vessels exist in a fibrovascular membrane, which prevents aqueous from entering the trabecular meshwork. Later in the disease, the membrane contracts, causing angle closure (Fig. 13–5).[5, 6] Treatment of the retina prior to the angle closure may portend a better outcome.[7–10] Some researchers advocate goniophotocoagulation as a means of therapy at the stage of open-angle neovascularization.[11, 12] The success of this procedure is variable and may well primarily depend on the effect of retinal photocoagulation, which remains the primary therapy.

FUCHS' HETEROCHROMIC IRIDOCYCLITIS

Radial vessels may be seen crossing the scleral spur onto the trabecular meshwork in Fuchs' heterochromic iridocyclitis (Fig. 13–6).[13] These vessels are responsible for the hemorrhages that may occur during anterior segment surgery.[14]

FIBROUS INGROWTH

Fibrous ingrowth results from the ingrowth of fibroblasts from the external eye internally through a wound. Vasculature may follow as growth factors are produced by the membrane. Most often, fibrous ingrowth occurs through a poorly closed wound that furnishes a path for entrance.[15] The ingrowth is clearly visible, in contrast to the clear membrane of epithelial downgrowth. The membrane may cover the angle, eventually closing it entirely. Observation of growth over time is essential in differentiating this progressive disorder from synechia.[16]

Blood in Anterior Trabecular Meshwork (Schlemm's Canal)

Blood in Schlemm's canal indicates increased episcleral venous pressure (EVP) or ocular hypotony.[17] It can occur

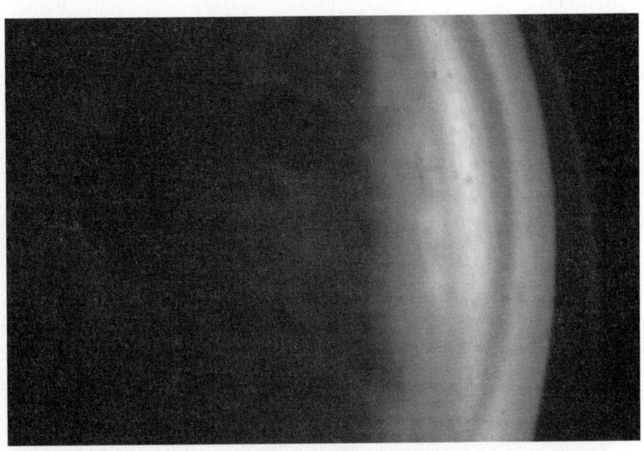

FIGURE 13–6. Fuchs' heterochromic iridocyclitis. Note the fine branching vessels in the angle crossing the scleral spur.

only when the EVP is greater than the IOP and is uncommon. It may not be clearly visible in highly pigmented trabecular meshwork but may be seen as a light red tinge.

Causes of elevated episcleral venous pressure are:

- □ Carotid cavernous sinus fistula (high-flow)[18–20]
- □ Dural cavernous sinus fistula (low-flow)[20]
- □ Familial
- □ Idiopathic[22, 23]
- □ Sturge-Weber syndrome[24, 25]
- □ Superior vena cava syndrome[26–28]
- □ Thyroid ophthalmopathy[29]

Occasionally, blood may be seen in Schlemm's canal in a normal patient after extended periods of Valsalva maneuver. More commonly for the novice gonioscopist, lens pressure over the sclera may induce localized blood in Schlemm's canal.

Exfoliation Material

Exfoliation material may appear as fluffy white deposits on the darkened trabecular meshwork. It is generally found in more than one angle structure.[30]

Epithelial Membrane

For discussion of this finding, see Angle as a Whole.

Sclerostomy

A sclerostomy formed at the time of trabeculectomy is often clearly visible in the anterior trabecular meshwork and generally extend anteriorly through Schwalbe's line. With proper visualization, internal patency can be confirmed (Fig. 13–7*A*). In the setting of elevated IOP and a flat bleb, one must consider the possibility of internal obstruction of the sclerotomy site. Gonioscopy can also allow identification of intraocular contents that may be responsible, such as lens particles, vitreous, iris, Descemet's flap, or an intraocular lens haptic (Fig. 13–7*B*).

Viscocanalostomy or Deep Sclerectomy

The Descemet's window remaining after nonpenetrating techniques such as viscocanalostomy or deep sclerectomy can be seen to reflect light. A gray shadow is seen behind it, confirming the presence of a intrascleral cavern or lake. In deep sclerectomy with implant, the implant may be visible through Descemet's window.

Sutures

Although corneoscleral sutures are usually seen as an aside, it is sometimes important to identify their presence. They can be associated with wound neovascularization, particularly if the suture material is full-thickness through the cornea.

POSTERIOR TRABECULAR MESHWORK

The posterior trabecular meshwork may be lightly to darkly pigmented, and its pigmentation is independent of eye color. The pigmentation increases with age. The pigment of the posterior trabecular meshwork may become intracellular while surface pigment remains extracellular. The meshwork pigmentation is believed to come from pigmented iris epithelium. Normally, the pigmentation is regular and is greater inferiorly than superiorly.

Irregular Pigmentation

Irregular pigmentation is seen in pseudoexfoliation syndrome and early pigment dispersion syndrome.[31] With time, the increase in pigmentation may become so dark that it appears homogeneous.

SIDEROSIS

Siderosis is rusty pigmentation secondary to a metallic intraocular foreign body (iron or steel).[32] It may cause dysfunction of trabecular cells, leading to elevated IOPs.

Inflammatory Deposits

Inflammatory deposits may be seen with any granulomatous uveitis or severe nongranulomatous uveitis. They appear as trabecular precipitates and may be similar to mutton-fat keratic precipitates.[33, 34] This finding is discussed further in Chapters 11 and 12 on the anterior chamber.

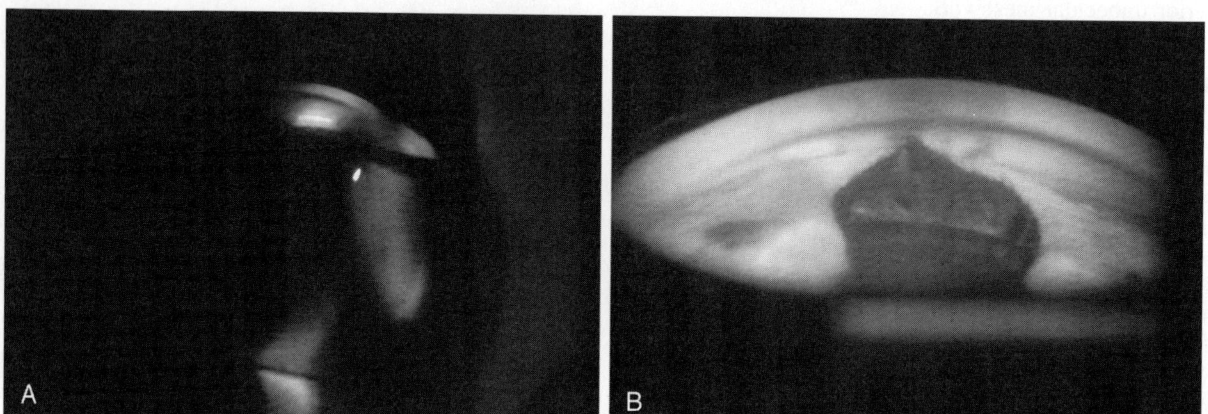

FIGURE 13–7. Internal view of sclerostomy portion of glaucoma filtration surgery. *A*, Patent. *B*, Occluded with iris.

Exfoliation Material

Exfoliation material is commonly seen deposited against the dark pigmentation of the trabecular meshwork and is diagnostic of the pseudoexfoliation syndrome.

SCLERAL SPUR

The scleral spur may be difficult to visualize, but once identified, it is the key to identifying all other angle structures. Its visibility without indentation gonioscopy ensures a nonoccludable angle.[30]

CILIARY BODY BAND

Widened Band

A widened ciliary body band may be seen in angle-recession glaucoma.[35–37] The recessed area often has a grayer appearance than the surrounding normal ciliary body band because of surface fibrosis (Fig. 13–8). This finding is generally the result of blunt trauma. Usually, it represents a tear between the longitudinal and circular muscles of the ciliary body. The name is somewhat misleading because the trabecular meshwork itself is not directly damaged, but dysfunction occurs because of the massive concussive trauma.

The glaucoma usually does not develop immediately. There are two peaks of occurrence: at weeks and at years after the angle recession occurred. Even without trauma, the other eye is at high risk for primary open-angle glaucoma.[37] A widened ciliary body band may also occur with processes that pull the iris posteriorly or may indicate invasion by tumor, typically, melanoma of the ciliary body.

Band Disinserted from Scleral Spur

CYCLODIALYSIS CLEFT

A cyclodialysis cleft appears as an empty space between the ciliary body band and the scleral spur and represents disinsertion of the ciliary muscle from the spur (Fig. 13–9).[38] Cyclodialysis clefts generally cause hypotony. When a thin slit of light is projected into a cleft, sclera is visible deep within the cleft. Clefts can be difficult to see in a soft eye but are more easily visible with a Goldmann-type lens that uses a viscous coupling fluid. A cleft as small as 50 μm may be responsible for hypotony.[39, 40] Detection of a cleft in a soft eye may be aided by filling (or overfilling) the anterior chamber with a viscoelastic prior to gonioscopy.[39–42]

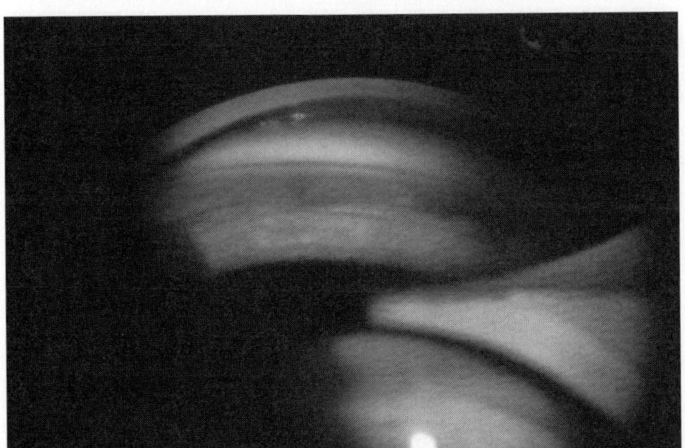

FIGURE 13–8. Angle recession. Widened ciliary body band with gray fibrotic membrane covers the exposed ciliary body.

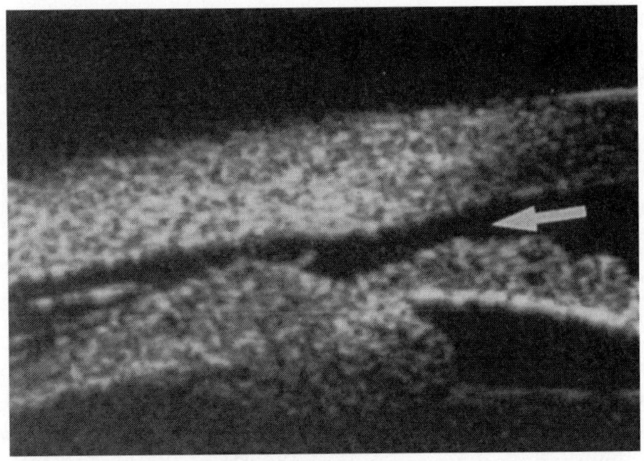

FIGURE 13–9. Cyclodialysis cleft. Ultrasound biomicroscopic identification of a direct connection between the anterior chamber and the supraciliary space.

Iris Root Disinsertion

Iridodialysis, or separation of the iris root from its insertion into the ciliary body band (or scleral spur), may be associated with trabecular damage and glaucoma. Angle recession may also be associated. If small, this finding can be mistaken for a surgical peripheral iridotomy. Larger iridodialyses may result in corectopia.

Angle Closure

Angle closure can be appositional or synechial. The distinction must be made with the use of indentation gonioscopy (see Fig. 13–3).

Indentation gonioscopy is a technique of opening an appositionally closed angle for viewing or breaking an acute attack of primary angle-closure glaucoma. It can be performed only with a lens that has a coupling surface smaller than the cornea. Lenses that can be used include the Zeiss 4-mirror, Posner, Sussman, and similar gonioprisms. Applying pressure to the central area of the cornea forces fluid peripherally, opening the angle for viewing. This maneuver may also be effective in breaking an acute angle-closure attack. Under conditions in which the appositional closure is reversed and the angle is visible, aqueous has access to the trabecular meshwork and outflow is reestablished. It is important to limit the duration of the compression to a few seconds due to the associated rise in IOP from an already elevated level.

APPOSITIONAL ANGLE CLOSURE

Generally, appositional angle closure occurs early in chronic intermittent angle closure or during an acute attack of primary acute angle-closure glaucoma. The angle structures are generally not visible until pressure is placed on the goniopprism. If the angle opens upon indentation with the gonioscope, it is said to be appositionally closed; if the angle cannot be opened, it is scarred closed either by direct adhesion of iris to the angle (or anterior to it) or by membrane contraction (see Fig. 13–3). This is one of the most important concepts in understanding glaucoma.

PRIMARY ACUTE ANGLE CLOSURE

Acute angle closure is characterized by a red painful eye, cloudy cornea, and shallow anterior chamber (but centrally formed) with an occluded angle. Other forms of angle closure may be differentiated according to the mechanism through which they occur, for example, as pushing mechanisms or pulling mechanisms.

Primary acute angle closure generally has two components: pupillary block and pre-existing narrow angles possibly secondary to an increase in lens size with age.[43, 44] Other causes of acute angle closure are ciliary swelling with anterior rotation, aqueous misdirection syndrome,[45–47] neovascular glaucoma,[5, 6] phakomorphic glaucoma,[48] and plateau iris syndrome.[49–51] These conditions do not improve with peripheral iridectomy despite angle closure. It is important to remember that only pupillary block is responsive to iridectomy. Once an attack is broken medically or surgically, it is vital to confirm the status of the angle by gonioscopy and visualization of angle structures. If allowed to persist, nonsynechial angle closure may become synechial in nature.

Risk factors for primary acute angle closure include increasing age, large crystalline lens, and hyperopia.[52, 53]

It is also important to perform gonioscopy after the institution of miotic therapy to avoid an unrecognized narrowing of the angle due to increased pupillary block.

PERSISTENCE OF AN OCCLUDED ANGLE DESPITE PATENT IRIDECTOMY

Nonpatency

To confirm patency, the anterior lens capsule must be visible through the iridectomy. The iridectomy also must be at least 50 μm in size to both allow adequate flow and prevent later closure.[54–56]

Vitreous

The vitreous face or vitreous strands may occlude an iridectomy that appears patent.

Obstruction by Intraocular Lens

Both anterior and posterior chamber lenses have been found to occlude iridectomies. Additionally, capsular flaps or remnants of the crystalline lens can also occlude an iridectomy.

Ciliary Swelling with Anterior Rotation

Ciliary swelling and rotation may be associated with an anterior annular choroidal effusion, which is being recognized more commonly as a cause of acute angle closure since the advent of the ultrasound biomicroscope. This finding has been associated with scleral buckling procedures that occlude venous outflow.

Malignant Glaucoma (Aqueous Misdirection Syndrome)

Malignant glaucoma is rapid acute elevation of IOP in the presence of a flat or very shallow anterior chamber, following filtration surgery or a wound leak (more commonly in eyes with hyperopia). The IOP may only be 8 or 10 mm Hg.[47, 57] Gonioscopically, it can be identified as an anterior chamber that is uniformly shallow both centrally and peripherally (Fig. 13–10).

Phakomorphic Glaucoma

In the setting of a large lens relative to the size of the eye (it may be of normal size but in a small eye), the lens may push the peripheral iris anteriorly into the angle. A superimposed papillary block mechanism may accelerate the IOP rise. If the angle remains narrow after resolution of the pupillary block, this diagnosis should be considered.

Subluxed Lens

In cases of mild luxation of the crystalline lens, gonioscopy can be useful in allowing a comparison of the distance between the pupillary border and the lens surface in several areas. Typically, this distance is increased and is not uniform. In more severe cases, gonioscopy allows direct visualization of the presence or absence of zonular support (Fig. 13–11).

Plateau Iris Syndrome

The angle structures may not be visible despite a centrally deep chamber and absence of pupillary block. The flat iris goes directly toward the angle, but the insertion is very steep within the angle recess.[58, 59] Dilation would increase the thickness of the last iris roll, causing appositional closure. Treatment is iridoplasty or pilocarpine. Lens extraction can also be effective.

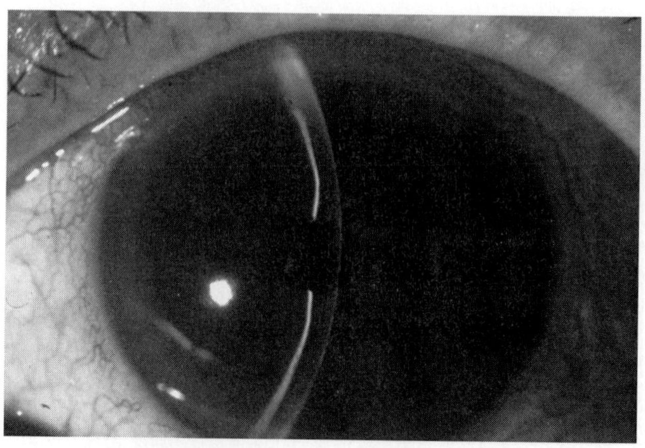

FIGURE 13–10. Aqueous misdirection. Note the uniform very shallow anterior chamber depth.

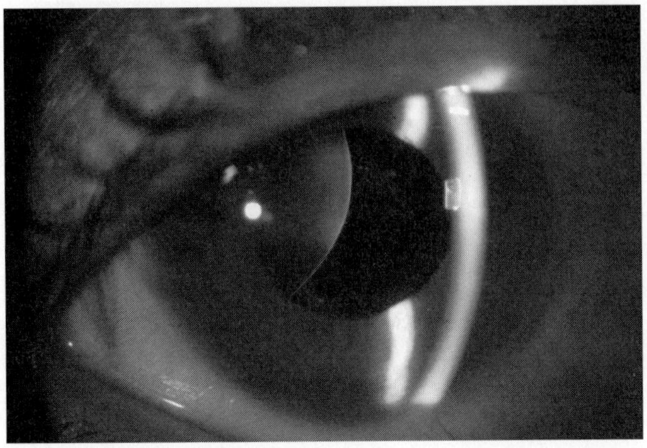

FIGURE 13–11. Dislocated lens (severe) with zonular dehiscence.

Iris Bow

Occasionally, the angle is not visible but is still open. This finding can be caused by a large iris bow. The bow can usually be overcome by having the patient look toward the gonioprism mirror being viewed. Iris bow should not be confused with the more localized iris bulges caused by tumors, epithelial cysts, or iris bombé.

Iridoschisis

Iridoschisis is a rarely seen split in the layers of the iris that causes angle closure. See the discussion of the iris in Chapter 14.

Iris Cysts

Cysts of the iris pigment epithelium may be seen as localized areas of anteriorly protruding iris (Fig. 13–12). Rarely are they large enough to cause appositional angle closure. Laser of the cyst is often effective treatment, although this can lead to an elevation in IOP due to release of debris.

Tumors

The angle structures may be partially or fully covered with tumor infiltrates. The most common tumors are ring

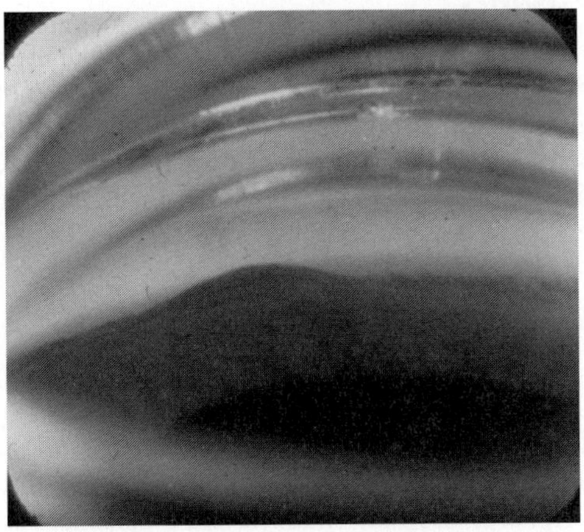

FIGURE 13–12. Iris pigment epithelial cyst.

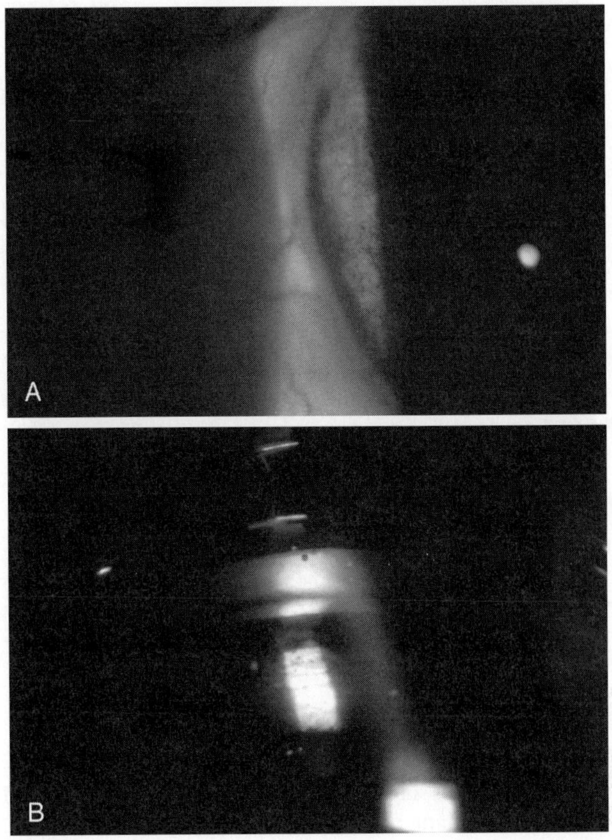

FIGURE 13–13. Angle ring melanoma. *A*, Slit-lamp appearance. *B*, Gonioscopic appearance.

melanomas (Fig. 13–13); metastases, frequently from breast carcinoma; and leukemic infiltrates.[60, 61] Leukemic infiltrates may appear as a pseudohypopyon in the angle.[62–64]

ANGLE INFILTRATES

Angle infiltrates are commonly caused by:

- Leukemia
- Lymphoma
- Adenocarcinomas
- Trabeculitis

The angle usually appears normal but may be histologically inflamed. The trabecular beams may be thickened and edematous.[2] Occasionally, an infiltrate may be seen gonioscopically. Members of the herpes simplex virus family might cause trabeculitis and may be the cause of Posner-Schlossman syndrome.[65]

Angle as a Whole

RADIAL VESSELS

Radial iris vessels may be found in the normal angle; however, they will not project anterior to the scleral spur. Fine single radial vessels may be found in Fuchs' heterochromic iridocyclitis.

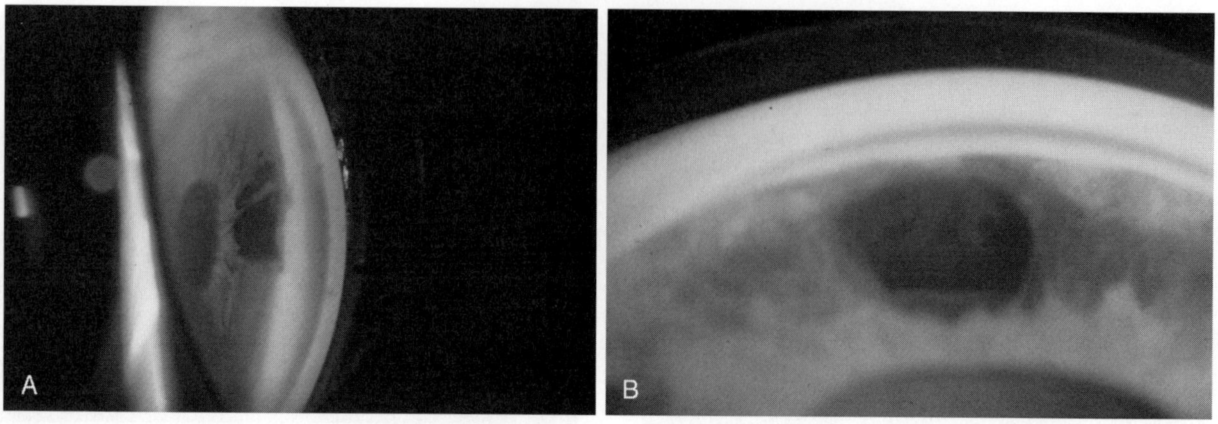

FIGURE 13–14. *A* and *B*, Iridocorneal endothelial (ICE) syndrome. Note the synechiae formation with iris atrophy leading to hole formation.

MEMBRANES

The angle may appear open or closed but may still be covered by a membrane. The most common membranes are neovascular, but a number of other entities may cause membranes. The entities can often be differentiated according to the appearance of the membrane.

Fibrovascular Membranes

Fibrovascular membranes may be seen in neovascular glaucoma and fibrous ingrowth, both of which are discussed earlier in this chapter.

Clear (or Opaque) Membranes

EPITHELIAL DOWNGROWTH

Synechiae may be present in part or all of the angle. A sheet of multilayered epithelial cells grows from a wound over the corneal endothelium, and overlying edema usually occurs. The leading edge of the membrane may be visible on the cornea as a gray endothelial line that rapidly progresses. It also grows onto the iris, eventually covering it. Loss of normal iris architecture may be the only clue. Presence of the membrane can be confirmed by applications of the argon laser at low power with a large spot size that turn the membrane white.[66] The earliest sign of epithelial downgrowth is often a persistent steroid-nonresponsive "uveitis."

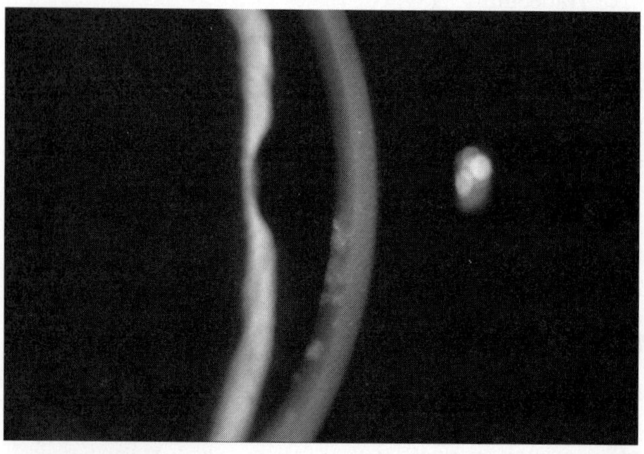

FIGURE 13–15. Posterior polymorphous dystrophy showing deep corneal deposits.

IRIDOCORNEAL ENDOTHELIAL (ICE) SYNDROMES

In the ICE syndromes, abnormal corneal endothelium grows over the angle and iris, causing peripheral anterior synechiae and synechial angle closure (Fig. 13–14).[67–69] Diagnosis is made from specular microscopy of the corneal endothelium. The disease is almost always unilateral; it is more prevalent in women in the fourth and fifth decades of life (see Chapters 11 and 14).

POSTERIOR POLYMORPHOUS DYSTROPHY

Posterior polymorphous dystrophy is characterized by corneal endothelial vesicles with surrounding haze (Fig. 13–15).[70] It is an autosomal dominant disease that has been associated with glaucoma. The glaucoma arises from a clear membrane that causes synechial angle closure.

Developmental Abnormalities

Examination of the angle is mandatory in a newborn, infant, or child with suspected glaucoma. In the very young, it is almost always necessary to perform gonioscopy as part of an examination under anesthesia. At this time, gonioscopy plays a key role in differentiating primary developmental diseases from diseases with specific identifiable abnormalities.

CONGENITAL OR DEVELOPMENTAL GLAUCOMA

In primary congenital glaucoma, the trabecular meshwork takes on a "ground-glass" appearance with a muting of the angle structures (Fig. 13–16). This appearance has been described as Barkan's membrane, which also may explain the efficacy of goniotomy. However, this membrane has not been confirmed pathologically.

AXENFELD-RIEGER SYNDROME

Axenfeld-Rieger syndrome represents a continuum of disease that is developmental in nature. Gonioscopically, posterior embryotoxon can be seen, as well as the large, broad-based synechiae that insert on or anterior to Schwalbe's line. Peripheral iris abnormalities may also be visualized (Fig. 13–17).

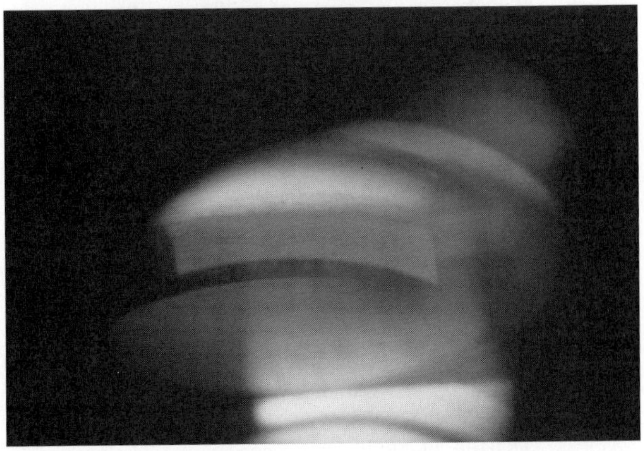

FIGURE 13–16. Developmental glaucoma with typical "ground-glass" appearance of the trabecular meshwork.

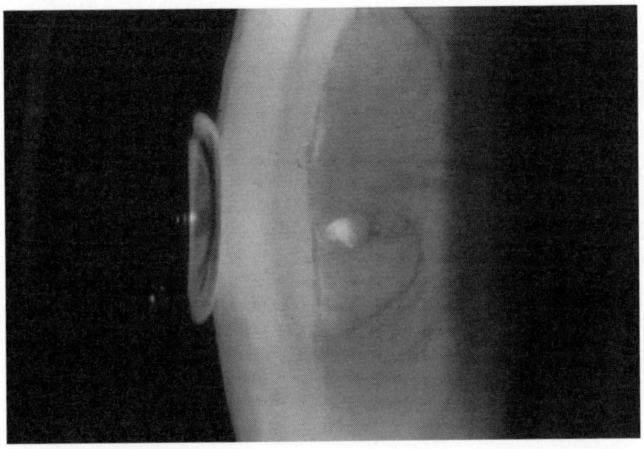

FIGURE 13–17. Axenfeld-Rieger syndrome. Gonioscopic appearance with prominent peripheral anterior synechiae inserting anterior to Schwalbe's line.

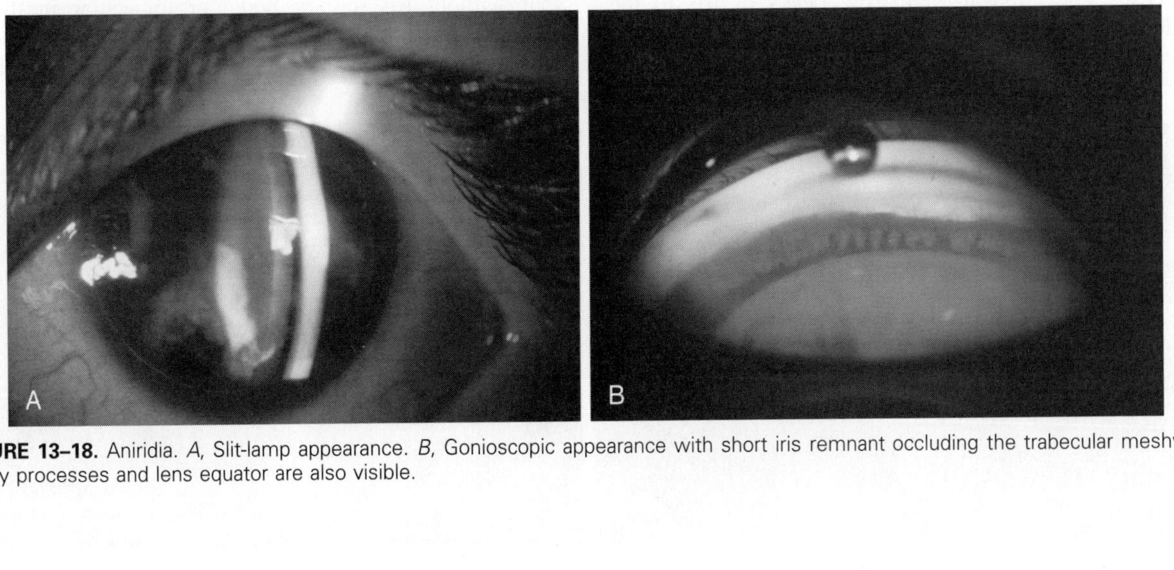

FIGURE 13–18. Aniridia. *A*, Slit-lamp appearance. *B*, Gonioscopic appearance with short iris remnant occluding the trabecular meshwork. Ciliary processes and lens equator are also visible.

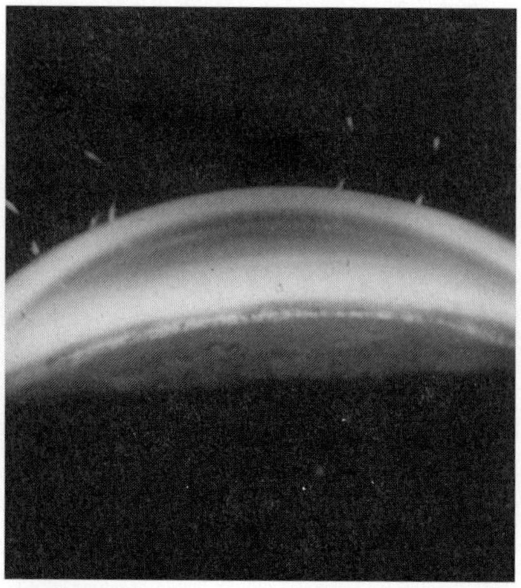

FIGURE 13–19. Iris processes.

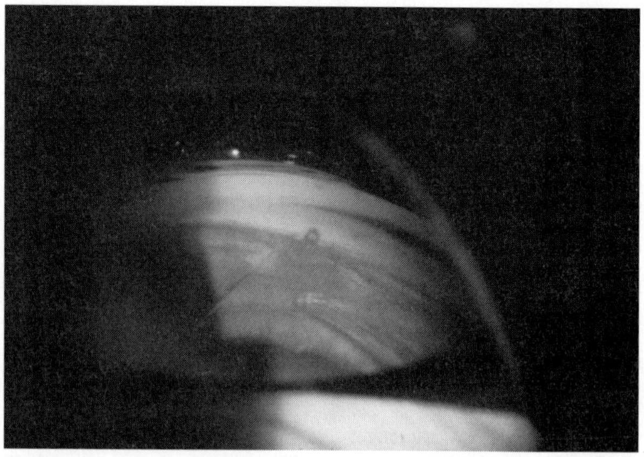

FIGURE 13–21. Gonioscopy of anterior chamber intraocular lens (IOL) with proper IOL haptic location.

ANIRIDIA

The term *aniridia*, implying complete absence of the iris, is a misnomer; in fact, a small amount of iris tissue can be identified gonioscopically. The diagnosis can usually be made at slit-lamp examination (Fig. 13–18*A*). It is also possible to determine the amount of trabecular meshwork occluded by the iris remnant. Because of the absence of iris, it is possible to directly visualize the ciliary processes as well as the lens equator (Fig. 13–18*B*).

IRIS PROCESSES

Iris processes are not actually abnormalities, but rather a normal anatomic variant. They represent remnants of iris that bridge across the trabecular meshwork. Beneath them, the meshwork is developed normally. The only importance of iris processes is that they must be differentiated from synechiae that are acquired and pathologic (Fig. 13–19).

Acquired Findings

MULTIPLE LOCALIZED SYNECHIAE

One type of synechiae deserves special attention—"teepees." They appear as narrow peaks of iris to the location of the trabeculoplasty spots. These are a result of argon laser trabeculoplasty being performed posteriorly within the trabecular meshwork. They do not require treatment and appear to have no effect on the success of the trabeculoplasty but should not be confused with other causes of synechiae.

UVEITIC PERIPHERAL ANTERIOR SYNECHIAE

Permanent adhesions between iris and angle structures, peripheral anterior synechiae, have many causes, including primary angle closure and structural abnormalities discussed previously. However, one of the most common causes is intraocular inflammation. These adhesions tend to form first inferiorly and are generally broad-based and of variable height on the meshwork (Fig. 13–20). The extent of angle occluded and the remaining function of the open angle determine the presence of glaucoma.

INTRAOCULAR LENS

Particularly in the presence of an anterior chamber intraocular lens, it is important to examine the eye gonioscopically to determine the position of the lens haptics in the angle. It is most desirable to have the haptic on the scleral spur without iris, ciliary body, or trabecular meshwork contact (Fig. 13–21). Complications can occur if the haptic is buried in tissue or in apposition to corneal endothelium.

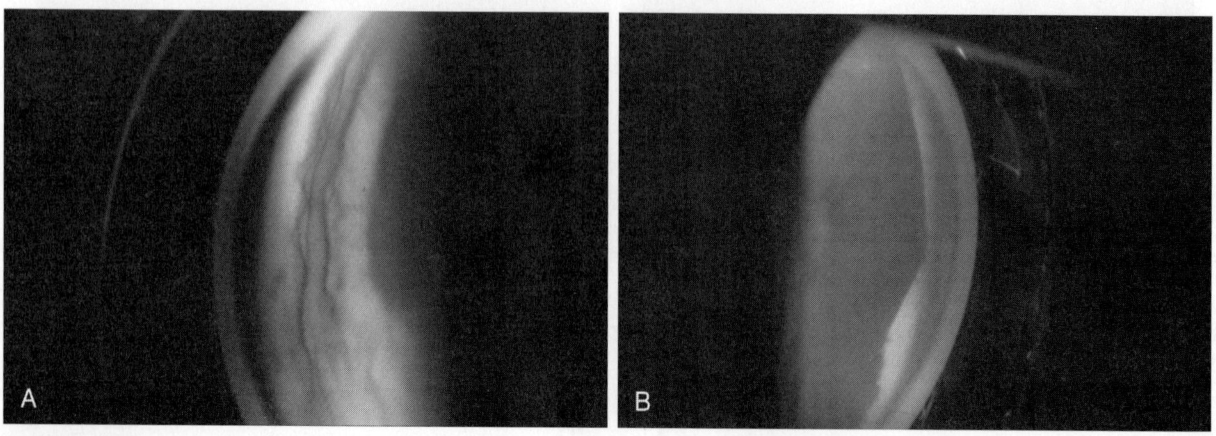

FIGURE 13–20. Peripheral anterior synechiae in uveitis.

SUMMARY

Gonioscopy plays a vital role in the care of all glaucoma patients with glaucoma. Practice is required to master the art of angle observation. Once mastered, gonioscopy makes diagnosis much more accurate and appropriate.

REFERENCES

1. Wishart PK, Spaeth GL, Poryzees EM: Anterior chamber angle in the exfoliation syndrome. Br J Ophthalmol 1985;69:103.
2. Chandler PA, Grant WM: Lectures on Glaucoma. Philadelphia, Lea & Febiger, 1965.
3. Anderson DM, Morin JD, Hunter WS: Rubeosis iridis. Can J Ophthalmol 1971;6:183.
4. Schulze RR: Rubeosis iridis. Am J Ophthalmol 1967;63:487.
5. Nomura T: Pathology of anterior chamber angle in diabetic neovascular glaucoma: Extension of corneal endothelium onto iris surface. Jpn J Ophthalmol 1983;27:193.
6. John T, Sassani JW, Eagle RC Jr: The myofibroplastic component of rubeosis iridis. Ophthalmology 1983;90:721.
7. Callahan MA, Hilton GF: Photocoagulation and rubeosis iridis. Am J Ophthalmol 1974;78:873.
8. Krill AE, Archer D, Newell FW: Photocoagulation in complications secondary to branch vein occlusion. Arch Ophthalmol 1971;85:48.
9. Little HL, Rosenthal AR, Dellaporta A, et al: The effect of pan-retinal photo-coagulation on rubeosis iridis. Am J Ophthalmol 1976;81:804.
10. Jacobson DR, Murphy RP, Rosenthal AR: The treatment of angle neovascularization with panretinal photocoagulation. Ophthalmology 1979;86:1270.
11. Simmons RJ, Dueker DK, Kimbrough RL, Aiello LM: Gonio-photocoagulation for neovascular glaucoma. Trans Am Acad Ophthalmol Otolaryngol 1977;83:80.
12. Simmons RJ, Deppermann SR, Dueker DK: The role of goniophotocoagulation in neovascularization of the anterior chamber angle. Ophthalmology 1980;87:79.
13. Huber A: Das Glaukom bei komplizierter heterochromic Fuchs. Ophthalmologica 1961;142:66.
14. Amsler M, Verrey F: Heétérochromie de Fuchs et fragilité vasculaire. Ophthalmologica 1946;3:117.
15. Swan KC: Fibroplastic ingrowth following cataract extraction. Arch Ophthalmol 1973;89:445.
16. Friedman AH, Henkind P: Corneal stromal overgrowth after cataract extraction. Br J Ophthalmol 1970;54:528.
17. Kolker AE, Hetherington J: Becker and Shaffer's Diagnosis and Treatment of Glaucoma, 5th ed. St. Louis, CV Mosby, 1984.
18. De Keiyer RJW: Spontaneous carotid-cavernous fistulas: The importance of the typical limbal vascular loops for the diagnosis, the recognition of glaucoma and the uses of conservative therapy in this condition. Doc Ophthalmol 1979;46:403.
19. Elliot AJ: Ocular manifestations of carotid-cavernous fistulas. Postgrad Med 1954;15:191.
20. Keltner JL, Satterfield D, Dublin AB, Lee BCP: Dural and carotid cavernous sinus fistulas: Diagnosis, management and complications. Ophthalmology 1987;94:1585.
21. Minas TF, Podos SM: Familial glaucoma associated with elevated episcleral venous pressure. Arch Ophthalmol 1968;80:202.
22. Talusan ED, Fishbein SL, Schwartz B: Increased pressure of dilated episcleral veins with open-angle glaucoma without exophthalmos. Ophthalmology 1983;90:257.
23. Jorgensen JS, Guthoff R: Pathogenesis of glaucoma in patients with idiopathic dilated episcleral vessels. Klin Monatsbl Augenheilkd 1987;190:428.
24. Dunphy EB: Glaucoma accompanying nevus flammeus. Am J Ophthalmol 1935;18:709.
25. Phelps CD: The pathogenesis of glaucoma in Sturge-Weber syndrome. Trans Am Acad Ophthalmol Otolaryngol 1978;85:276.
26. Alfano LE: Glaucoma following ligation of the superior vena cava. Am J Ophthalmol 1965;60:412.
27. Alfano JE, Alfano PA: Glaucoma and the superior vena caval syndrome. Am J Ophthalmol 1956;42:685.
28. Bedrosian EH: Increased intraocular pressure secondary to mediastinal syndrome. Arch Ophthalmol 1952;47:641.
29. Lorgensen JS, Guthoff R: Die Rolle des episkleralen Venendrucks bei der Entstehung von Sekundarglaukomen. Klin Monatsbl Augenheilkd 1988;193:471.
30. Mizuno K, Muroi S: Cycloscopy pseudoexfoliation. Am J Ophthalmol 1979;87:513.
31. Lichter PR, Sfaffer RN: Iris processes and glaucoma. Am J Ophthalmol 1970;70:905.
32. Sneed SR, Weingeist TA: Management of siderosis bulbi due to a retained iron-containing intraocular foreign body. Ophthalmology 1990;97:375.
33. Belfort R, Nussenblatt RB: Surgical approaches to uveitis. Int Ophthalmol Clin 1990;30:314.
34. Toris CB, Pederson JE: Aqueous humor dynamics in experimental iridocyclitis. Invest Ophthalmol Vis Sci 1987;28:477.
35. Alper MG: Contusion angle deformity and glaucoma: Gonioscopic observations and clinical course. Arch Ophthalmol 1963;69:445.
36. Blanton FM: Anterior chamber angle recession and secondary glaucoma. Arch Ophthalmol 1964;72:39.
37. Salmon JF, Mermoud A, Ivey A, et al: The detection of post-traumatic angle recession by gonioscopy in a population-based survey. Ophthalmology 1994;101:1844.
38. Gentile RC, Pavlin CJ, Liebmann JM, et al: Diagnosis of traumatic cyclodialysis by ultrasound biomicroscopy. Ophthalmic Surg Lasers 1996;27:97.
39. Ormerod LD, Baerveldt G, Murad AS, Riekhof FT: Management of the hypotonous cyclodialysis cleft. Ophthalmology 1991;98:1384.
40. Chandler PA, Maumenee AE: A major cause of hypotony. Am J Ophthalmol 1961;52:609.
41. Partamian LG: Treatment of cyclodialysis cleft with argon laser photocoagulation in a patient with a shallow anterior chamber. Am J Ophthalmol 1985;99:5.
42. Alparr JJ: Sodium hyaluronate (Healon) in glaucoma filtering procedures. Ophthalmic Surg 1986;17:724.
43. Chandler PA: Narrow-angle glaucoma. Arch Ophthalmol 1952; 47:695.
44. Chandler PA, Trotter RR: Angle-closure glaucoma: Subacute types. Arch Ophthalmol 1955;53:305.
45. Dueker GR: Ciliary-block glaucoma—differential diagnosis and management. J Glaucoma 1994;3:167.
46. Duy TP, Wollensak J: Ciliary block (malignant) glaucoma following posterior chamber lens implantation. Ophthalmic Surg 1987;18:741.
47. Simmons RJ: Malignant glaucoma. Br J Ophthalmol 1972;56:273.
48. Abramson DH, Franzen LA, Coleman DJ: Pilocarpine in the presbyope: Demonstration of an effect on the anterior chamber and lens thickness. Am J Ophthalmol 1973;89:100.
49. Tornquist R: Angle-closure glaucoma in an eye with a plateau type of iris. Acta Ophthalmol (Copenh) 1958;36:413.
50. Ritch R: Plateau iris is caused by abnormally positioned ciliary processes. J Glaucoma 1992;1:23.
51. Wand M, Pavlin CJ, Foster FS: Plateau iris syndrome: Ultrasound biomicroscopy and histological study. Ophthalmic Surg 1993;24:129.
52. Fontana ST, Brubacker RF: Volume and depth of the anterior chamber in the normal aging human eye. Arch Ophthalmol 1980;98:1803.
53. Markowitz SN, Morin JD: Angle-closure glaucoma: Relation between lens thickness, anterior chamber depth and age. Can J Ophthalmol 1984;19:300.
54. Abraham RK: Procedure for outpatient argon laser iridectomies for angle closure glaucoma. Int Ophthalmol Clin 1976;16:1.
55. Harrad RA, Stannard KP, Shilling JS: Argon laser iridotomy. Br J Ophthalmol 1985;69:368.
56. Fleck BW: How large must an iridotomy be? Br J Ophthalmol 1990; 74:583.
57. Chandler PA, Simmons RJ, Grant WM: Malignant glaucoma: Medical and surgical treatment. Am J Ophthalmol 1968;66:495.
58. Tornquist R: Angle-closure glaucoma in an eye with a plateau type of iris. Acta Ophthalmol 1958;36:413.
59. Wand M, Grant WM, Simmons RJ, Hutchinson BT: Plateau iris syndrome. Trans Am Acad Ophthalmol Otol 1977;83:122.
60. Bloch RS, Gartner RS: The incidence of ocular metastatic carcinoma. Arch Ophthalmol 1971;85:673.
61. Ferry AP, Font RL: Carcinoma metastatic to the eye and orbit: A clinicopathologic study of 227 cases. Arch Ophthalmol 1974;92:276.
62. Zakka KA, Yee RD, Shorr N, et al: Leukemic iris infiltration. Am J Ophthalmol 1980;89:204.
63. Kincaid MC, Green WR: Ocular and orbital involvement in leukemia. Surv Ophthalmol 1983;27:211.

64. Rosenthal AR: Ocular manifestations of leukemia: A review. Ophthalmology 1983;90:899.
65. Bloch-Michael E, Dussaix E, Cerqueti P, Patarin D: Possible role of cytomegalovirus in the etiology of the Posner-Schlossman Syndrome. Int Ophthalmol 1987;11:95.
66. Maumenee AE: Treatment of epithelial down-growth and intraocular fistula following cataract extraction. Trans Am Ophthalmol Soc 1964;62:153.
67. Eagle RC Jr, Font RL, Yanoff M, Fine BS: Proliferative endotheliopathy with iris abnormalities: The iridocorneal endothelial syndrome. Arch Ophthalmol 1979;97:2104.
68. Eagle RC Jr, Shields JA: Iridocorneal endothelial syndrome with contralateral guttate endothelial dystrophy: A light and electron microscopic study. Ophthalmology 1987;94:862.
69. Campbell DG, Shields MB, Smith TR: The corneal endothelium and the spectrum of essential iris atrophy: A clinicopathologic study. Arch Ophthalmol 1978;86:317.
70. Laganowski HC, Sherrard ES, Kerr Muir MG, Buckley RJ: Distinguishing features of the iridocorneal endothelial syndrome and posterior polymorphous dystrophy: Value of endothelial specular microscopy. Br J Ophthalmol 1991;75:212.

CHAPTER 14

Iris and Pupil

REBECCA K. MORGAN and GREGORY L. SKUTA

This chapter by Rebecca Morgan and Greg Skuta reviews the key diagnostic signs of the iris. This structure offers a huge diversity of disease manifestations and often plays a pivotal role in the arrival at the correct diagnosis. Often, the iris is one of the areas where abnormality is first recognized. The chapter logically describes the changes that are associated with glaucoma. It begins with entities in which the entire iris tissue is decreased and proceeds through those conditions associated with loss of specific components, such as transillumination defects. The pupil is intimately related to the iris structure. Abnormalities related to mydriatic, miotic, and corectopic pupils are discussed. More subtle signs of iris abnormality, such as abnormal structure, configuration, and position, are included. Finally, the common pathologic findings of synechiae, cysts, pigmentation changes, and iris vessels are presented.

Variations in iris and pupillary findings are numerous. The observant clinician should note these unusual findings, because they can be helpful in determining the mechanism of increased intraocular pressure (IOP) and glaucoma. This portion of the ocular examination may alert the clinician to search for other specific ocular findings or history that may help identify an underlying cause of secondary glaucoma. In still other cases, notation of iris or pupillary abnormalities may indicate a need to search for nonocular abnormalities, and may prompt the eye care specialist to refer the ophthalmic patient for a systemic evaluation to rule out an associated treatable syndrome.

Abnormal Amount of Iris Tissue

ABSENCE OF OR DECREASE IN IRIS TISSUE (Table 14–1)

One of the most striking iris abnormalities associated with secondary glaucoma is that of aniridia. In this developmental condition, only a rudimentary stump of iris, often not visible without gonioscopic examination, is typically present (Fig. 14–1). Variable expressivity is possible, however, and a patient may also present with (1) a small iris remnant visible on slit-lamp examination, (2) typical or atypical iris colobomas, or (3) iris stromal thinning with absence of the collarette and either a central or eccentrically located pupil.[1–3] Persistent iris strands may also be a finding in aniridia.[1]

Genetically, aniridia is most commonly an isolated, autosomal dominant form without systemic manifestations. A sporadic form associated with Wilms' tumor and genitourinary abnormalities also occurs and may be associated with the deletion of the short arm of chromosome 11. Still other cases may be autosomal recessive and may be associated with mental retardation and cerebellar ataxia. Other ocular manifestations of aniridia are photophobia, nystagmus, decreased vision, amblyopia, strabismus, corneal opacities, cataracts, foveal hypoplasia, and glaucoma.

Glaucoma in aniridia is due to obstruction of trabecular

TABLE 14–1. CAUSES OF ABSENCE OF OR DECREASE IN IRIS TISSUE AND ASSOCIATED GLAUCOMA

Aniridia
Axenfeld-Rieger syndrome
Peters' anomaly
Prior ocular trauma
Prior intraocular surgery

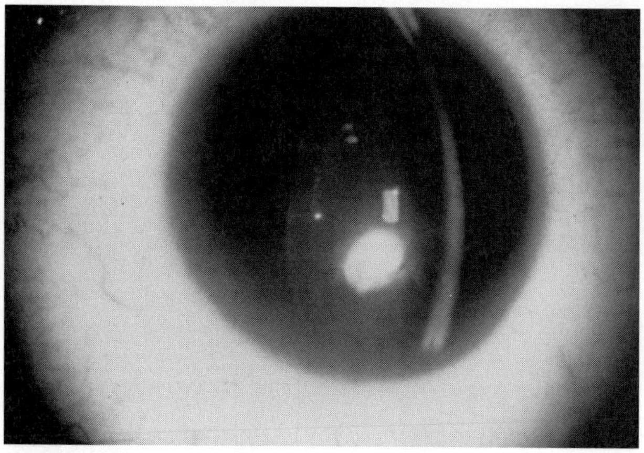

FIGURE 14–1. Slit-lamp view of an eye with aniridia, with no visible iris.

meshwork outflow from progressive angle anomalies and angle closure from rudimentary iris tissue. Patients with minimal iris abnormalities, such as a missing collarette or small coloboma, generally do not experience these complications.[4, 5] Although the iris findings in aniridia are present at birth, poor aqueous outflow and increased IOP generally do not develop until preadolescence or early adulthood. Once glaucoma develops, treatment becomes difficult. Medical glaucoma therapy is usually successful only initially, and invasive surgery is often fraught with complications.

Other developmental disorders associated with a decreased amount of iris tissue and associated glaucoma are the Axenfeld-Rieger syndrome and Peters' anomaly (each discussed later in this chapter), either of which may be confused with aniridia because of phenotypic similarities to the less pronounced form of aniridia. Glaucoma in the presence of minimal or no evident iris tissue may also have nondevelopmental causes. Ocular injuries in which iris tissue is lost from the injury itself or in which a resultant prolapsed iris is surgically removed may lead to a secondary traumatic glaucoma. A total or large peripheral iridectomy may be purposely or inadvertently performed at the time of anterior segment surgery, with subsequent development of glaucoma from the effects of the primary surgical procedure.

TABLE 14–2. CAUSES OF IRIS TRANSILLUMINATION DEFECTS DUE TO STROMAL OR PIGMENT EPITHELIAL THINNING OR TO HYPOPLASIA AND ASSOCIATED GLAUCOMA

Midperipheral iris defects—pigment dispersion syndrome
Peripupillary iris defects—exfoliation syndrome
Far peripheral iris defects
Congenital glaucoma
Marfan's syndrome
Axenfeld-Rieger syndrome (not typical)
After laser peripheral iridoplasty or gonioplasty
Other focal, multifocal, or diffuse defects
Current or previous ocular inflammation
Prior ocular surgical procedures
Prior ocular trauma
Previous unsuccessful laser peripheral iridotomy
Previous episode of acute angle closure
Any iridocorneal endothelial syndrome
Posterior polymorphous dystrophy
Axenfeld-Rieger syndrome
Iridoschisis

IRIS TRANSILLUMINATION DEFECTS

Stromal or Pigment Epithelial Thinning or Hypoplasia

Iris transillumination defects, best demonstrated with retroillumination of the slit-lamp beam through the pupil, may be seen in a number of patterns and in a variety of glaucomas (Table 14–2).

PIGMENT DISPERSION SYNDROME

A classic example of a specific transillumination pattern associated with a well-defined entity is that seen with the pigment dispersion syndrome (PDS). No other ocular conditions have pigment defects resembling those of this entity. The defects are generally slit-like, radial, and in the midperipheral and outer half of the iris (Fig. 14–2). They may also be dot-like or round. The defects may be in a distribution of a few to all "clock hours" of the iris, with increasing numbers or even coalescence with the passage of time. Posterior bowing of the iris, often more evident on gonioscopy than on slit-lamp examination, may be present.

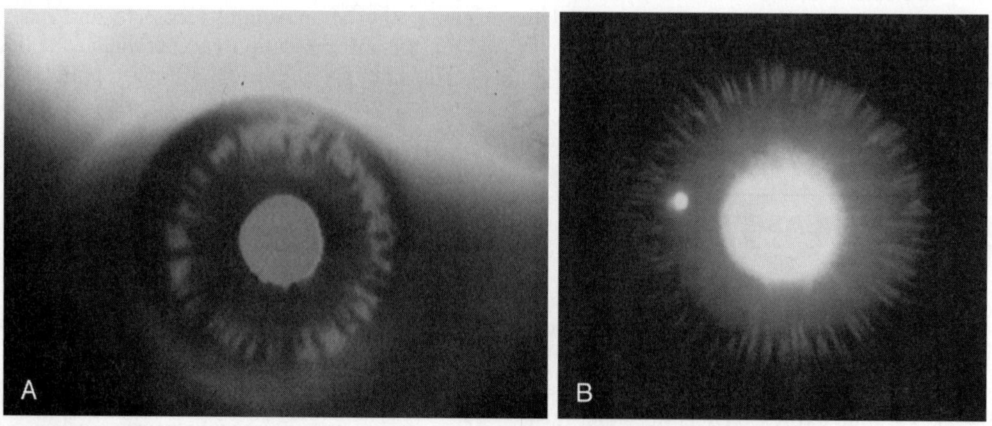

FIGURE 14–2. *A* and *B*, Slit-lamp views of the eyes of two patients with pigment dispersion, showing radial, slit-like midperipheral iris transillumination defects.

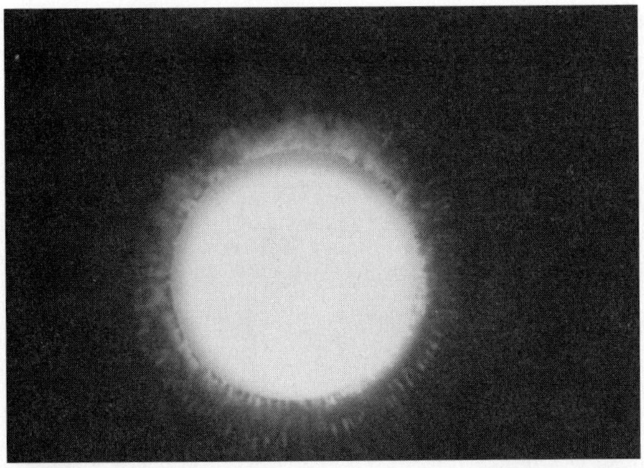

FIGURE 14–3. Slit-lamp view of the eye of a patient with exfoliation syndrome, showing moth-eaten peripupillary iris transillumination defects.

Other typical ocular findings are often seen; they are described in other chapters (see Chapters 11, 12, and 13).

PDS may progress to pigmentary glaucoma, which constitutes about 1% of glaucomas in the western hemisphere.[6, 7] Although PDS itself has no gender predilection, pigmentary glaucoma typically affects males and tends to occur in myopic, young, white adults.[8, 9] The pigment dispersion and midperipheral iris defects seen in this disorder are believed to be due to chafing of the iris pigment epithelial layer against the lens zonules with repeated change in pupillary size. Increased IOP and glaucoma in PDS occur when pigment swept into the trabecular meshwork causes dysfunction of aqueous outflow, but the exact mechanism of this damage is unknown.[10–12] Pigmentary glaucoma is usually treated with standard glaucoma medical therapy, laser trabeculoplasty, and incisional filtration. Some have recommended placement of a peripheral iridotomy to relieve a presumed reverse pupillary block in pigment dispersion, thereby allowing flattening of the concave iris and relief of the pigment-epithelial contact and chafing against the lens zonules.[13–15]

EXFOLIATION SYNDROME

Another ocular syndrome in which a particular pigment epithelium defect is generally present is the exfoliation syndrome. In contrast to the midstromal slit-like defects of PDS, the defects in this disorder are found at the pupillary border. Patchy or total loss of the pupillary ruff typically gives the sphincter a moth-eaten transillumination pattern (Fig. 14–3).[16–18] These defects may occur in eyes without the exfoliation syndrome but are much more commonly associated with the disorder (6.1% vs. 74% in one report).[16] A similar moth-eaten appearance of the pupillary border may also be seen in Fuchs' heterochromic iridocyclitis, but other findings of this syndrome, such as iritis and heterochromia (described in a later section), readily distinguish this disorder from the exfoliation syndrome. The exfoliation findings may be significantly more pronounced in one eye, with the ruff in the fellow eye sometimes totally intact (Fig. 14–4). More peripheral findings, described as diffuse, "starry-sky" transillumination defects, may also be present.[19]

The exfoliation syndrome usually affects older patients, commonly those in their 60s and 70s, and has no definite sex predilection. It is now known to be a systemic syndrome, likely a disorder of extracellular matrix; deposits of exfoliative material are found in a number of ocular and nonocular tissues. The source of the exfoliative deposits in the eye, which may appear as whitish material adhering to the pupillary border (Fig. 14–5) and elsewhere (see Chapter 15 for a more detailed description), is believed to be the epithelia of the lens, iris, and ciliary body.[20–24]

Although only unilateral slit-lamp findings may be evident with apparent unilateral glaucoma, the exfoliation syndrome is more likely always bilateral but sometimes very asymmetric in its presentation.[22, 25] The reported incidence of associated glaucoma varies widely, from near zero to 93%.[16, 26–29] The mechanism of increased IOP is most likely blockage of the trabecular meshwork by exfoliation material and dispersed pigment in an open angle. Potentially occludable narrow angles and peripheral anterior synechiae (PAS) are also reported to occur in up to 32% of affected eyes.[17, 30–32] Although typically more resistant to medical therapy than primary open-angle glaucoma (POAG), exfoliative glaucoma is similarly managed with medications, laser trabeculoplasty, and filtering surgery; peripheral iridotomies are recommended for those eyes with occludable angles.

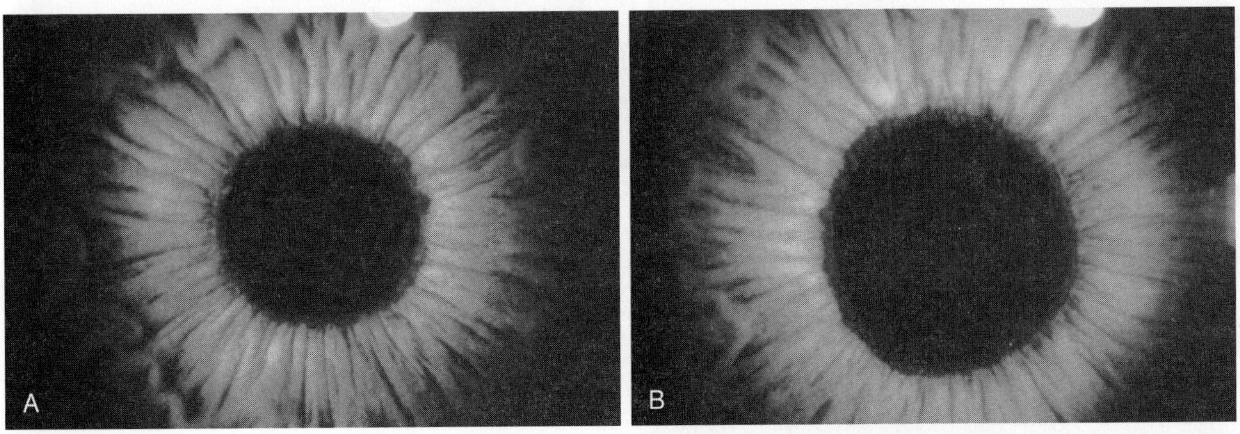

FIGURE 14–4. Slit-lamp views of the eyes of a patient with unilateral exfoliation syndrome. *A,* Note the loss of the pupillary ruff. *B,* The pupillary ruff in the other eye is normal.

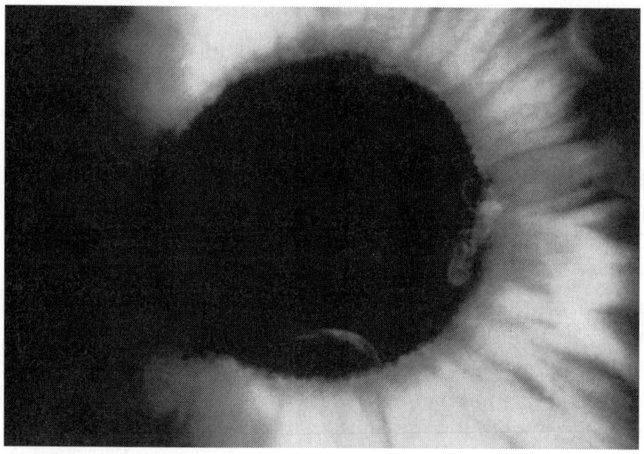

FIGURE 14–5. Slit-lamp view of exfoliation material adherent to the pupillary border.

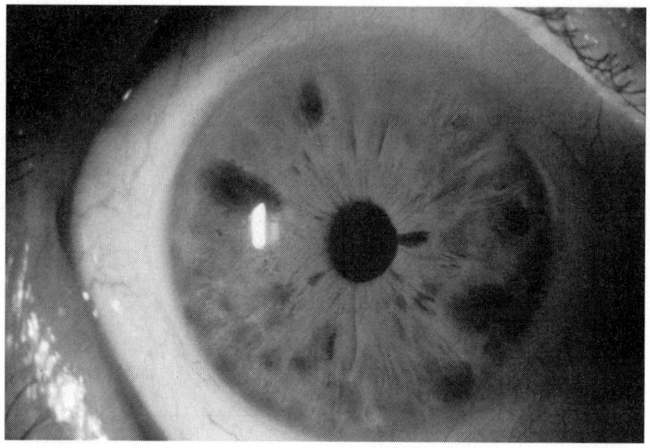

FIGURE 14–6. Slit-lamp view of peripheral thinning of the iris due to previous laser iridoplasty.

CONDITIONS WITH FAR PERIPHERAL IRIS DEFECTS

In addition to peripupillary and midperipheral iris pigment defects, patterns of transillumination in the far peripheral iris may be seen. Although not typical findings, these may occur in congenital glaucoma, a condition in which the elastic nature of the eye in very young children allows enlargement of the globe in the presence of increased IOP. The peripheral iris, thin even in normal infants, is thinned further with stretching of the irides. Marfan's syndrome, an autosomal dominant systemic disorder discussed more fully in Chapter 8, may be associated with a number of ocular abnormalities, including ectopia lentis, high myopia, retinal detachment, and glaucoma, and may also have findings of peripheral transillumination defects with iris stromal and dilator muscle hypoplasia. Rarely, peripheral spoke-like transillumination defects may be seen in the Axenfeld-Rieger syndrome. Previous laser gonioplasty or peripheral iridoplasty, both of which involve placement of large slow laser burns near the angle to stretch open a narrow outlet, may also result in enough iris thinning to produce peripheral transillumination defects (Fig. 14–6).

CONDITIONS WITH FOCAL, MULTIFOCAL, OR DIFFUSE TRANSILLUMINATION DEFECTS

Less distinct patterns of transillumination defects occur with diffuse, focal, or multifocal areas of iris atrophy from a variety of causes. Intraocular inflammation, intraocular surgical procedures, and ocular trauma may be responsible for such defects and may lead to secondary glaucoma as well. Herpes zoster keratouveitis, for example, is a classic entity in which both sector iris atrophy and inflammatory glaucoma may be observed (Fig. 14–7). Focal thinning at

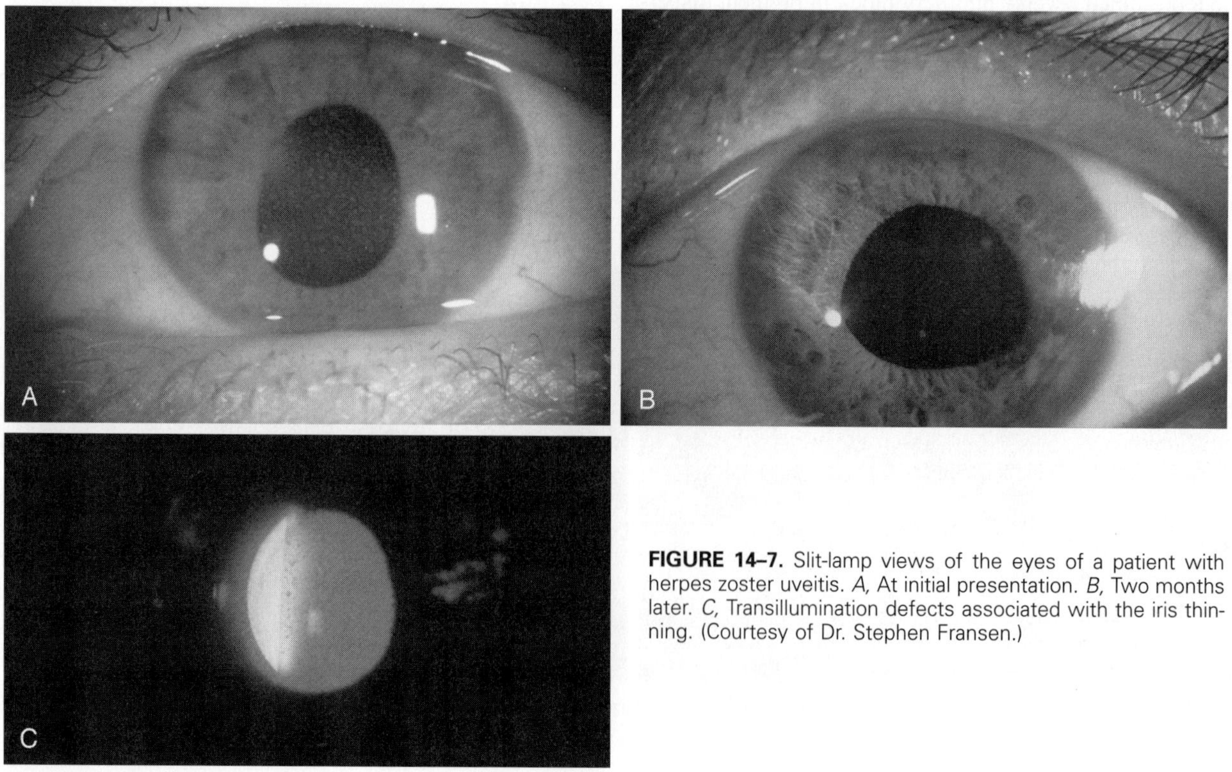

FIGURE 14–7. Slit-lamp views of the eyes of a patient with herpes zoster uveitis. *A,* At initial presentation. *B,* Two months later. *C,* Transillumination defects associated with the iris thinning. (Courtesy of Dr. Stephen Fransen.)

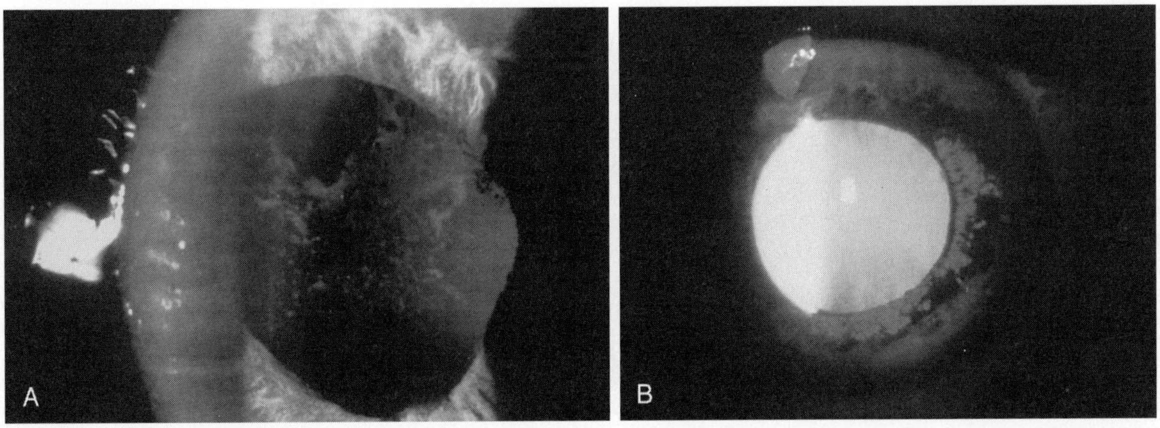

FIGURE 14–8. *A,* Slit-lamp view of segmental iris atrophy in a patient who suffered an episode of acute angle-closure glaucoma. *B,* Iris transillumination defects from iris thinning in another patient after acute angle-closure glaucoma; also note transillumination of the superior peripheral iridotomy, performed to break the attack.

one or more peripheral sites in one or both eyes of a patient may result from previous unsuccessful attempts at laser peripheral iridotomy. An episode of acute angle closure itself may lead to segmental iris atrophy (Fig. 14–8). Either or both of these findings in an eye with glaucoma suggest an angle-closure mechanism as the cause of increased IOP.

A more specific group of disorders known as the *iridocorneal endothelial (ICE) syndromes* can also be associated with various patterns of iris transillumination defects. This group of syndromes, almost always unilateral in its clinical presentation, consists of a spectrum of entities known as progressive or essential iris atrophy, Chandler's syndrome, and Cogan-Reese syndrome. Each of these disorders is typically found in early to middle adulthood and is more likely to affect women than men. ICE syndromes are characterized by an abnormality of the corneal endothelium and cause a number of iris changes as well as corneal and anterior chamber angle findings discussed elsewhere in this book (see Chapter 11).

Various degrees of iris atrophy and other iris findings, including full-thickness defects and pigmented nodules (both discussed later in this chapter), help distinguish the three entities of ICE syndrome. The most profound transillumination defects are found in progressive iris atrophy (Fig. 14–9). The iris atrophy, along with hole formation and corectopia, indeed occurs in a progressive fashion and is located opposite the displaced pupil (Fig. 14–10).[33] In Chandler's syndrome, corneal findings are more prominent; iris atrophy and transillumination defects may not be detectable and, when present, are mild and are not generally associated with hole formation (Fig. 14–11). Any extent of transillumination defects and iris atrophy may be seen with the Cogan-Reese syndrome, which is distinguished from the other two entities by pigmented nodular iris lesions (Fig. 14–12).[34–36]

The corneal endothelial abnormality found in the ICE syndromes has been hypothesized to cause the formation of the cellular membrane found on histologic examination in the chamber angle and on the surface of the iris in this disorder.[33] The contraction of this membrane stretches the iris and is believed to be the cause of the atrophy with hole formation. Associated glaucoma is likely due to outflow obstruction of the trabecular meshwork by the cellular membrane or resultant PAS. Secondary glaucoma is found in about half of patients with ICE syndromes, and tends to be more severe in progressive iris atrophy and the Cogan-Reese syndrome.[37] Treatment consists of medical therapy with aqueous suppressants and surgical filtration.

A familial corneal endothelial disorder known as *posterior polymorphous dystrophy,* detailed in Chapter 11, may occasionally manifest as an associated glaucoma and rarely as iris atrophy exhibiting transillumination defects.[38–40] This disorder is similar to the ICE syndromes in that it is characterized by production of a dystrophic membrane responsible for a spectrum of anterior segment findings, including posterior corneal abnormalities and iridocorneal adhesions. In contrast to the ICE variants, however, posterior polymorphous dystrophy is familial and always bilateral.

Another condition that causes varied iris transillumination defects on slit-lamp examination is the developmental disorder known as *Axenfeld-Rieger syndrome.* As in the ICE syndromes, affected patients may have mild iris stromal thinning or marked iris atrophy with hole formation and corectopia (Fig. 14–13), as well as chamber angle abnormalities. When iris thinning is present, it is typically located in the quadrant opposite the displaced pupil, as in the ICE syndromes. However, Axenfeld-Rieger syndrome

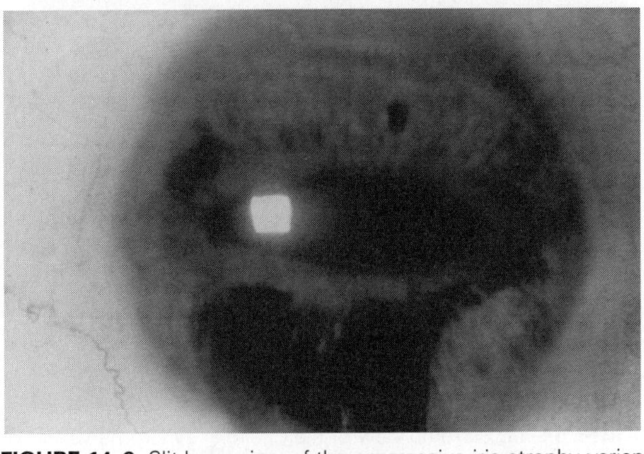

FIGURE 14–9. Slit-lamp view of the progressive iris atrophy variant of iridocorneal endothelial syndrome.

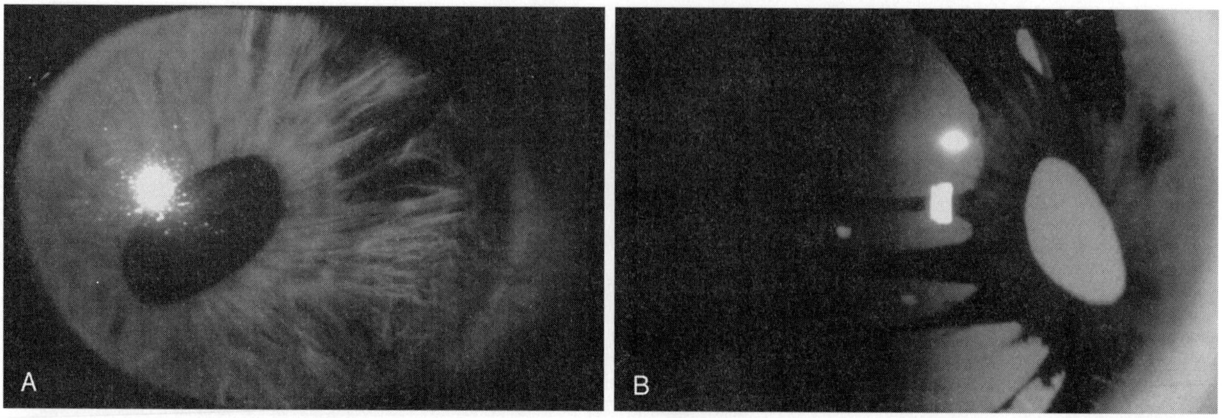

FIGURE 14–10. Photographs of progressive iris atrophy, showing an ectopic pupil *(A)* and transillumination defects *(B)*.

is distinguished from the ICE syndrome by (1) usual diagnosis in infancy or childhood, (2) bilaterality, (3) autosomal dominant inheritance, and (4) lack of corneal endothelial abnormalities. Typically, the iris changes do not progress in Axenfeld-Rieger syndrome, but changes in central iris appearance, including increased thinning, may occur, usually in the first year of life.[41–43] As mentioned previously, peripheral spoke-like pigment defects have been observed in this disorder, but they are not typical.

Axenfeld-Rieger syndrome may be associated with a number of chromosomal aberrations, with most evidence pointing to a locus in 4q25. It involves a spectrum of clinical presentations,[43–47] from peripheral anterior segment defects only to additional iris changes with associated systemic abnormalities. The extraocular defects primarily involve the teeth and facial bones, but a variety of other developmental defects are also possible (see Chapter 6). Both the ocular and nonocular structures involved are primarily of neural crest cell origin, and it is theorized that a developmental arrest of anterior segment ocular structures derived from these cells results in the ocular anomalies.[43, 48]

Glaucoma, which develops in approximately 50% of patients with Axenfeld-Rieger syndrome, is believed to be secondary to compression or incomplete development of the trabecular meshwork and Schlemm's canal. It does not always correlate with the extent of iris and chamber angle abnormalities. Increased IOP may occur in infancy but more typically is seen in childhood or early adulthood. All patients with this syndrome should be monitored for development of glaucoma. If present in infancy, it may be managed with trabeculotomy or goniotomy, but in older patients, treatment with aqueous suppressants first, followed by filtering surgery, is recommended.

An uncommon condition known as *iridoschisis* has transillumination defects due to dissolution of the iris stroma like those seen in the ICE and Axenfeld-Rieger syndromes. Iridoschisis, however, occurs at a much later age (the sixth to seventh decade). It is progressive and is characterized by bilateral separation of the iris stromal layers with shedding of the anterior iris leaf, usually in the inferior quadrants (Fig. 14–14). Full-thickness holes and systemic abnormalities are not present.[49] Glaucoma may be associated with this disorder in about 50% of cases. The mechanism is believed to be due in some cases to angle closure with pupillary block and in others to obstruction of the trabecular meshwork by released iris pigment or iris shreds.[50] Management of the glaucoma includes placement of an iridotomy for pupillary block and otherwise standard medical and surgical therapy for open-angle glaucoma.

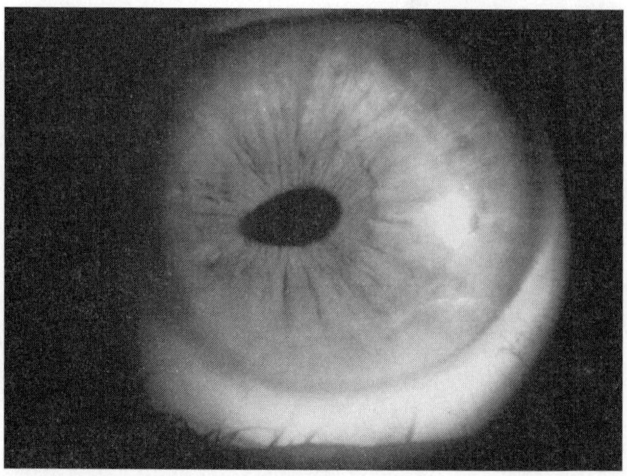

FIGURE 14–11. Slit-lamp view of the Chandler syndrome variant of the iridocorneal endothelial syndrome. Note the rather mild iris and pupillary findings.

Full-Thickness Iris Defects

Full-thickness iris defects may be seen in a number of situations in which glaucoma is also present (Table 14–3). A patent laser iridotomy or surgical iridectomy can usually be identified with direct slit-lamp examination, but a small or very peripheral defect may best be detected with a transillumination technique. If present, an iridotomy or iridectomy may be helpful in signifying previous acute or chronic angle closure as a contributing cause of a patient's

TABLE 14–3. CAUSES OF FULL-THICKNESS IRIS DEFECTS AND ASSOCIATED GLAUCOMA

Previous laser peripheral iridotomy or surgical iridectomy
Iridocorneal endothelial syndrome
Axenfeld-Rieger syndrome
Iridodialysis
Iris coloboma

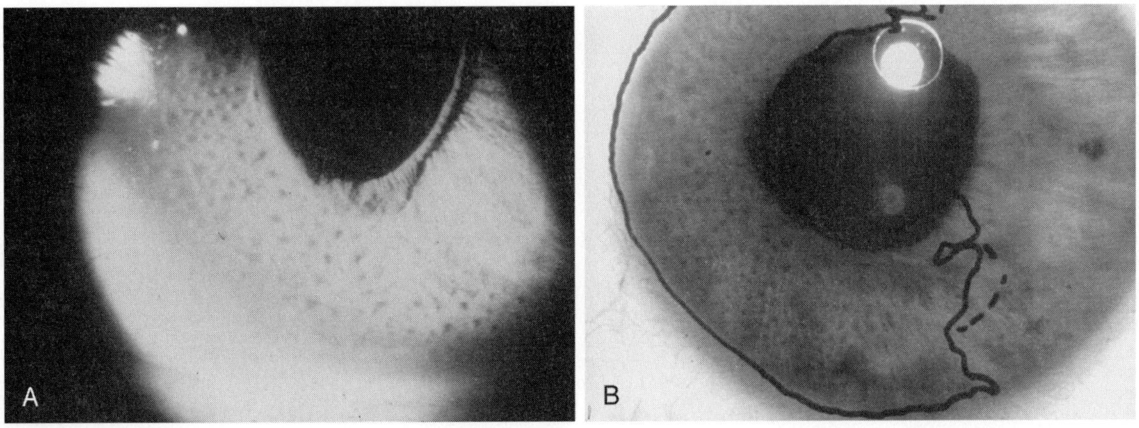

FIGURE 14–12. *A* and *B*, Slit-lamp views of the eyes of two patients with the Cogan-Reese syndrome variant of ICE syndrome. Note the pigmented iris nodules.

glaucoma, particularly if gonioscopic examination is not possible (see Fig. 14–8*B*). An obvious full-thickness iris opening may help rule out pupillary block as a cause of increased IOP in the patient with a shallow anterior chamber and may guide the clinician to appropriate management of other mechanisms of angle closure, such as aqueous misdirection and other causes of anterior rotation of the iris-lens diaphragm.

As noted in the section on transillumination defects associated with thinning of the iris, patients with ICE syndromes or Axenfeld-Rieger syndrome may have full-thickness defects as well. Among the ICE variants, progressive iris atrophy is distinguished by hole formation within the iris. Stretch holes occur in an area in which the iris becomes progressively thinned, opposite the direction of a characteristically displaced pupil (see Fig. 14–10).[51] Other full-thickness defects in this variant are referred to as *melting holes*, which develop independent of iris thinning or corectopia and may be due to iris ischemia.[51] In their purest forms, the Cogan-Reese and Chandler's syndrome variants of the ICE syndrome typically do not cause iris hole formation. Some patients with Axenfeld-Rieger syndrome may have full-thickness iris holes (see Fig. 14–13*B* and *C*), which are almost always nonprogressive and are located in the quadrant of stromal thinning away from an eccentric pupil.

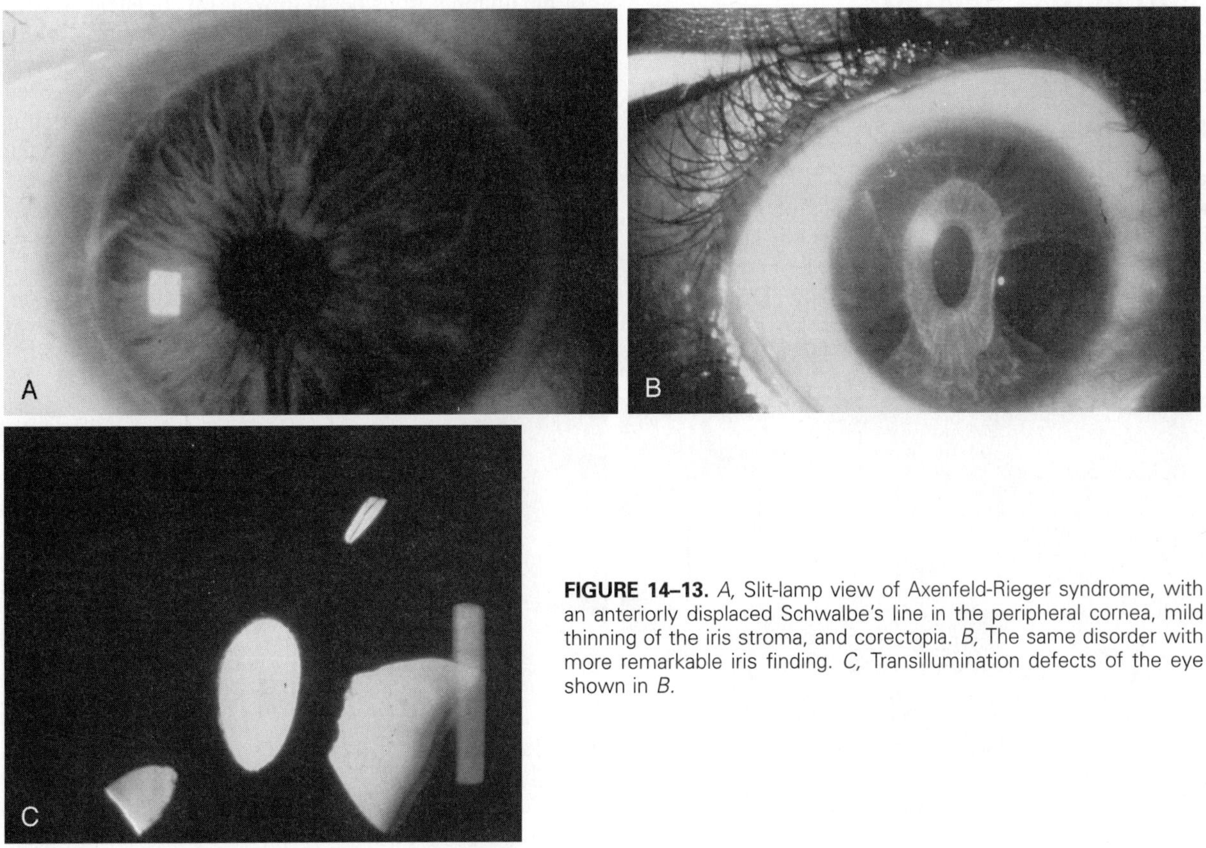

FIGURE 14–13. *A*, Slit-lamp view of Axenfeld-Rieger syndrome, with an anteriorly displaced Schwalbe's line in the peripheral cornea, mild thinning of the iris stroma, and corectopia. *B*, The same disorder with more remarkable iris finding. *C*, Transillumination defects of the eye shown in *B*.

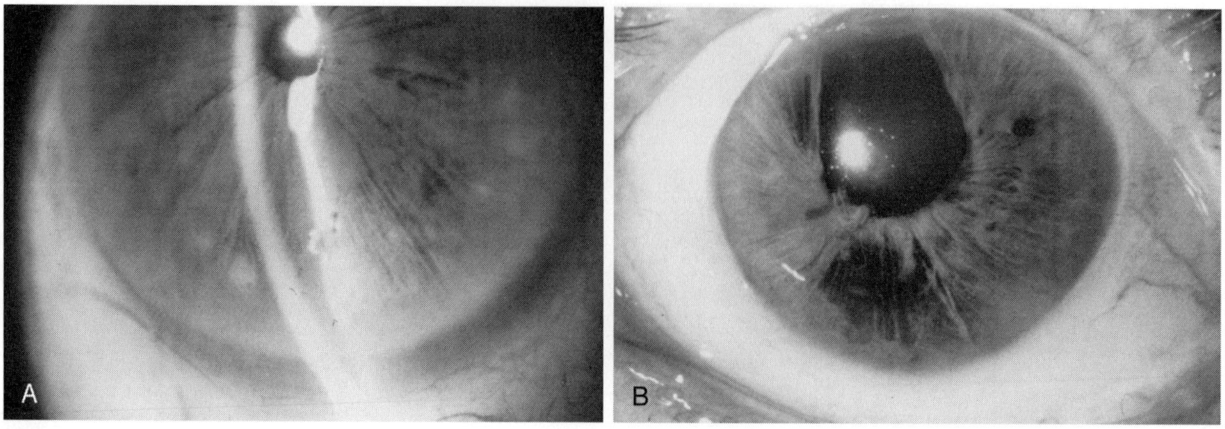

FIGURE 14–14. *A* and *B,* Slit-lamp views of eyes with iridoschisis, showing separation of anterior layers of the iris stroma in the inferior quadrants.

A peripheral full-thickness iris defect that is not due to hole formation or actual loss of iris tissue may be the result of iridodialysis. This defect occurs with detachment of the iris root from the ciliary body, typically after a blunt ocular injury (Fig. 14–15). The iridodialysis itself provides no mechanism for increased IOP, but its presence provides a clue to trauma as a cause of glaucoma. Traumatic glaucoma may be due to a number of mechanisms, including hemorrhage, inflammation, and direct trabecular meshwork injury. Iridodialysis may also occur at the time of anterior segment surgery, other effects of which later lead to the development of a secondary glaucoma.

Abnormalities Related to the Pupil

(Table 14–4)

LARGE PUPIL

A large pupil is most commonly due to mydriasis, but some of the less pronounced expressions of aniridia may exhibit enough peripheral iris remnants at slit-lamp examination to mimic a dilated pupil; this disorder and its associated glaucoma were discussed previously. Occasionally, contraction of the fibrovascular membrane covering the iris in the late stages of neovascular glaucoma may retract the iris peripherally to enlarge the pupil, sometimes to the extent that the eye appears aniridic. Traumatic mydriasis may occur, with a coincident glaucoma due to other effects of the injury. Glaucoma secondary to previous intraocular surgery may be present in the patient with a pupil enlarged by stretching or sphincterotomy maneuvers performed at the time of the procedure to allow easier removal of a cataractous lens or better visualization of the fundus.

A patient who presents with increased IOP and a large pupil from recent pharmacologic dilation should be suspected of having an angle-closure episode. The mechanism for this disorder is usually pupillary block, occurring in a patient with an occludable angle, generally after the affects of the dilating drops begin to wear off. In an acute episode, other ocular findings, such as unilateral conjunctival hyperemia, corneal edema, and iris bombé, as well as classic symptoms, such as halos, pain, tearing, and decreased vision, are usually present and make the diagnosis straightforward. Such an episode, whether iatrogenic or spontaneous, usually prompts the patient to seek medical care. Occasionally, poor access to health facilities, a mistaken diagnosis, or more vague symptoms result in a delay between the acute episode and examination. The pupil may later remain fixed in a mid-dilated position owing to iris sphincter ischemia from the sudden pressure elevation,

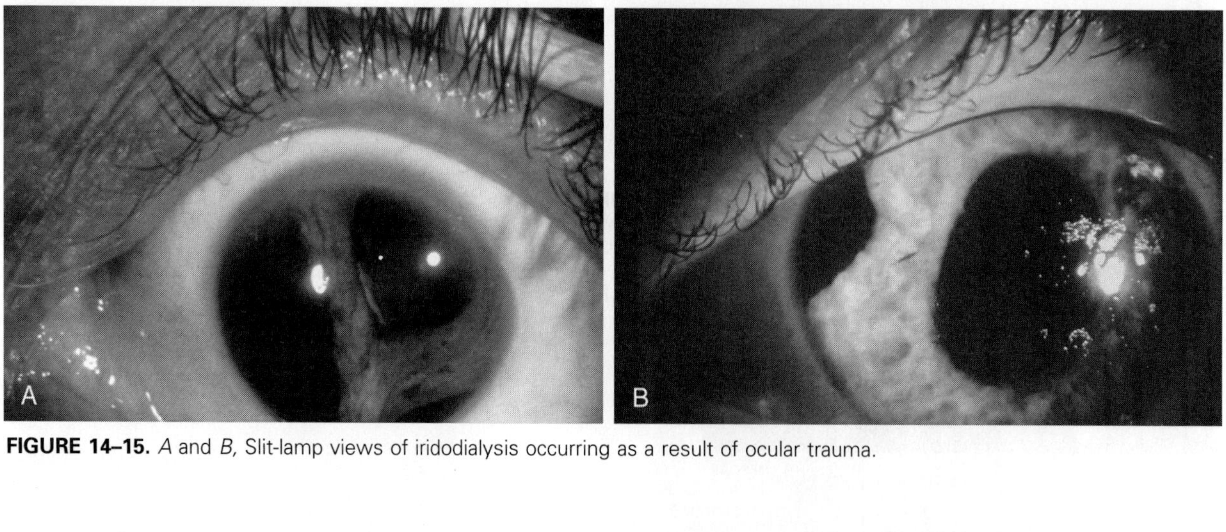

FIGURE 14–15. *A* and *B,* Slit-lamp views of iridodialysis occurring as a result of ocular trauma.

TABLE 14–4. CAUSES OF ENLARGED OR CONSTRICTED PUPIL AND ASSOCIATED GLAUCOMA

- Enlarged pupil with associated glaucoma
  - Aniridia
  - Later stages of neovascular glaucoma
  - Pharmacologic dilation
    - With associated acute angle closure
    - With increased intraocular pressure in the presence of an open angle
    - With increased intraocular pressure due to increased pigment release in pigment dispersion syndrome or exfoliation syndrome
  - Previous episode of acute angle closure
- Constricted pupil and increased intraocular pressure
  - Installation of miotic drops
    - Exacerbation of angle closure
    - Increased intraocular pressure due to interference with uveoscleral outflow

with a coincident residual glaucoma from the angle closure (Fig. 14–16). In either situation, the pupil is classically vertically elongated but may exhibit other unusual shapes. As described earlier, segmental iris atrophy may also be evident at some point after the acute episode (see Fig. 14–8). These iris findings all suggest an acute episode of angle closure, a possibility that can be further confirmed with gonioscopic examination (see Chapter 13).

Significantly increased IOPs may also occur more immediately after diagnostic dilation in the presence of open angles.[52] This situation may be seen in POAG, especially in patients taking pilocarpine, in whom it is presumably due to interference with the IOP-lowering effect of the miotic. Pupillary dilation may also elevate pressures through an increased dispersion of pigment into the trabecular meshwork of eyes with PDS or exfoliation syndrome. A rarer cause of increased IOPs after pharmacologic pupillary dilation is an angle-closure mechanism due to actual crowding of the angle with peripheral rolls of iris in the plateau iris syndrome,[53] described more fully in Chapter 13. Gonioscopic examination is helpful in differentiating these entities from angle closure due to pupillary block. The presence or absence of iris bombé (described later) may also be helpful in the differential diagnosis for IOP elevation in this setting.

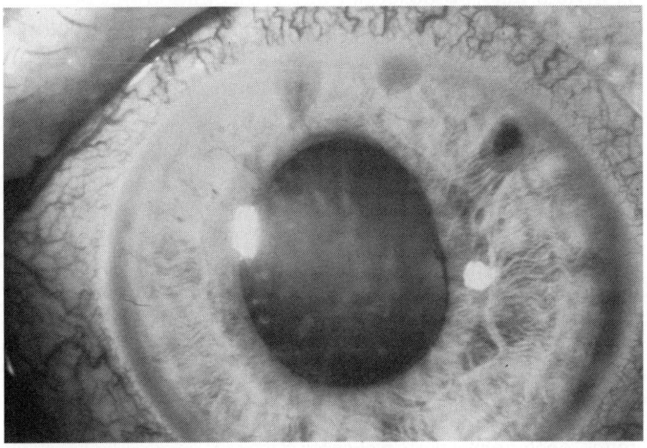

FIGURE 14–16. A mid-dilated, vertically elongated pupil resulting from an acute attack of angle-closure glaucoma attack.

SMALL PUPIL

A constricted pupil is usually associated with the instillation of miotics utilized (1) to increase aqueous outflow in the management of open-angle glaucoma, (2) to break an attack of primary acute angle closure by pulling peripheral iris out of the chamber angle, or (3) less commonly, as prophylaxis against angle closure in plateau iris syndrome. Miotics also induce ciliary muscle contraction with a resultant axial thickening and forward shift of the crystalline lens. This phenomenon results in anterior chamber shallowing and, along with increased iris lens contact due to the miotic effect itself, may promote angle closure in a patient with a potentially occludable angle.[54–56]

Miosis may also be responsible for secondary angle closure with exacerbation of anterior chamber shallowing in patients with posterior pushing forms of closure, in which a posterior space-occupying lesion (e.g., choroidal effusion) is present. Pilocarpine, the miotic in most widespread use for management of glaucoma, also decreases uveoscleral outflow.[57] If started on miotic therapy, a patient with little or no conventional trabecular meshwork outflow may present with an increased IOP and a constricted pupil because of a paradoxical pressure rise due to loss of the unconventional drainage.[58]

ABNORMAL PUPIL POSITION OR SHAPE (Table 14–5)

As mentioned earlier, corectopia, or eccentrically positioned pupil, may occur in ICE syndromes or Axenfeld-Rieger syndrome. Progressive iris atrophy may be associated with varying degrees of corectopia (see Fig. 14–10), and in Chandler's syndrome, the pupillary displacement is usually mild (see Fig. 14–11). The pupil is pulled toward the quadrant in which prominent PAS, a characteristic gonioscopic finding in these disorders, occur. Similarly, corectopia is in a direction toward bands of iridocorneal adhesions that bridge the chamber angle in Axenfeld-Rieger syndrome (Fig. 14–17). Glaucoma and other iris findings associated with these disorders have already been discussed. The pupil in a patient with Marfan's syndrome or a patient with posterior polymorphous corneal dystrophy,

TABLE 14–5. CAUSES OF ABNORMAL PUPIL POSITION OR SHAPE AND ASSOCIATED GLAUCOMA

- Ectopic pupil
  - Iridocorneal endothelial syndrome
  - Posterior polymorphous dystrophy
  - Axenfeld-Rieger syndrome
  - Marfan's syndrome
- Abnormal pupil shape
  - Previous trauma or surgical procedure (irregular)
  - Incarceration of iris in wound or filtering ostomy (peaked pupil)
  - Posterior synechiae (irregular)
  - Acute angle closure (vertically or horizontally)

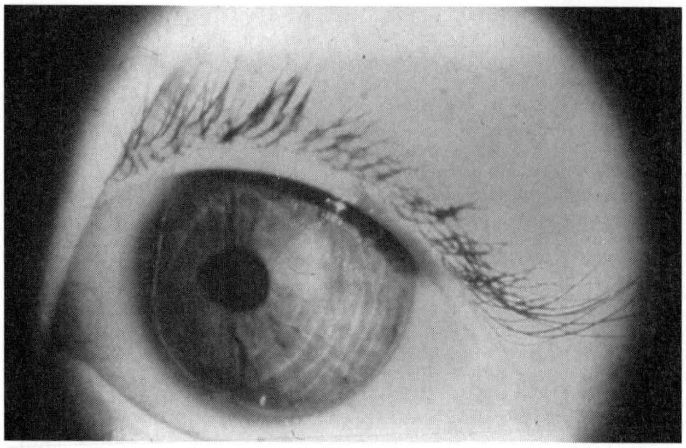

FIGURE 14–17. Slit-lamp view of corectopia in a patient with Axenfeld-Rieger syndrome. The pupil is displaced nasally toward a prominent Schwalbe's line.

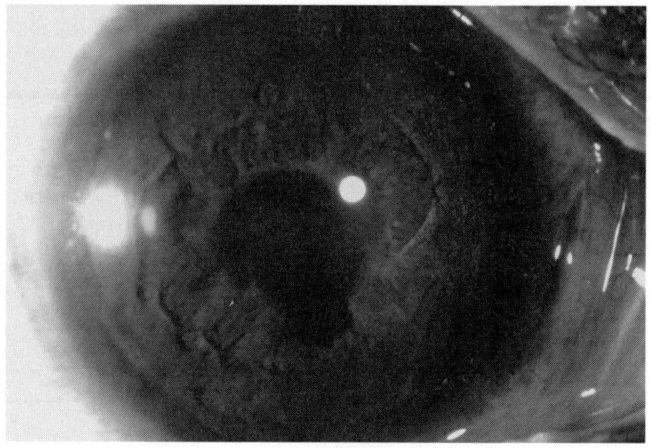

FIGURE 14–19. Slit-lamp view of pupillary distortion due to posterior synechiae resulting from sarcoid uveitis.

each of which may have iris findings as previously described, may also be ectopic.

Various irregularities in the shape of the pupil may occur as a result of prior IOP elevations or abnormalities due to trauma or inflammation. A peaked pupil may indicate prolapse or incarceration of iris in a limbal wound or incision. Increased IOP in spite of recent filtration surgery may indicate occlusion of the ostomy by iris. In the presence of hypotony, this presentation should lead one to suspect incarcerated iris as a cause of a wound gape with facilitation of a wound leak or inadvertant filtration bleb. Moreover, a wound gape may predispose an eye to epithelial downgrowth (Fig. 14–18) or fibrous ingrowth (both described more fully later), each of which may cause updrawing or distortion of the pupil. Small nicks at the pupillary border occur with sphincter tears from trauma or from sphincterotomies performed to enlarge the pupil for cataract or vitreoretinal procedures. Posterior synechiae due to inflammation may result in a distorted pupil (Fig. 14–19). A mid-dilated, vertically elongated pupil due to ischemia of the iris sphincter typically occurs after the acute pressure elevation of an acute episode of angle closure (see Fig. 14–16); the clinician should suspect this diagnosis when observing this finding. Less commonly, the sphincter ischemia may result in a horizontally elongated or simply irregularly shaped pupil.

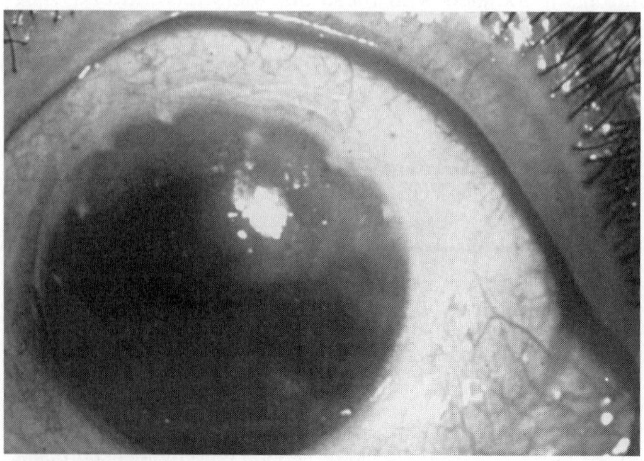

FIGURE 14–18. Slit-lamp view of an eye with epithelial downgrowth. Note the updrawn pupil and membrane on the posterior corneal surface superiorly.

ABNORMALLY REACTING PUPIL
(Table 14–6)

A nonreactive or poorly reactive pupil may be noted with pharmacologic dilation or constriction. Causes of increased IOP in these situations were discussed previously. Iris ischemia from an acute pressure rise, also mentioned earlier, may result in a nonreactive pupil in the mid-dilated position. Posterior synechiae from inflammation or manipulation of the iris during anterior segment procedures can also cause a fixed pupil. In neovascular glaucoma, a fibrotic, nonresponsive iris may prevent motion of the pupil. Finally, an afferent pupillary defect is possible with optic nerve compromise due to glaucoma; the severity of the defect correlates with the extent of the damage.

Abnormal Iris Architecture

(Table 14–7)

OBSCURATION OF DETAILS OR LOSS OF CRYPTS

Iris details may be obscured in an uncommon but devastating ocular condition known as *epithelial downgrowth* or ingrowth. This complication occurs when a sheet-like epithelial membrane grows into the eye through a surgical or traumatic penetrating wound. The membrane proliferates

TABLE 14–6. CAUSES OF A POORLY REACTING OR NONREACTIVE PUPIL AND ASSOCIATED GLAUCOMA

Pharmacologic dilation (see Table 14–4) or constriction (see Table 14–5) of the pupil
Iris ischemia from acute angle closure
Posterior synechiae
Prior surgical manipulation of the iris
Fibrotic iris in neovascular glaucoma
Afferent pupil defect due to glaucomatous optic nerve damage

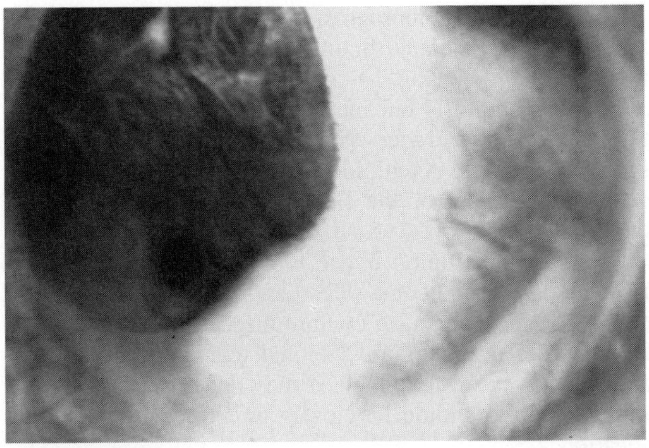

FIGURE 14–20. Slit-lamp view of an eye with fibrous ingrowth, showing a thick gray membrane on the surface of the iris and corneal endothelium.

over the posterior corneal surface (see Chapter 11), across the chamber angle, and over the iris (see Fig. 14–18). Although it is difficult to see the actual membrane covering the iris, this abnormality typically causes flattening of the stroma, and occasionally, the edge of the membrane indents the iris surface. The epithelial tissue may also cause ectropion uveae and may distort the pupil or completely cover the pupillary opening. Identification and delineation of the extent of the iris membrane may be achieved with application of photocoagulation. Argon laser burns placed on areas of involved iris produce characteristic fluffy white lesions.[59]

Presenting features of epithelial downgrowth are (1) retrocorneal membrane, (2) corneal edema, (3) detection of wound leak by Seidel's test, and (4) glaucoma (43% in one series).[60] Resultant glaucoma may be secondary to inflammation, formation of PAS, occlusion of the trabecular meshwork by exfoliated epithelial cells or the membrane itself, necrosis of the covered trabecular meshwork, pupillary block from an occluded pupil, or other causes.[61–64] Management of the eye with epithelial downgrowth may be attempted with surgical excision of the membrane and other techniques, but the ultimate prognosis is often poor.

Sometimes difficult to distinguish from epithelial downgrowth, *fibrous ingrowth* may also occur after anterior segment surgical procedures or trauma and may flatten or obscure the iris surface architecture. Fibrous proliferation, occasionally composed of vascular tissue, arises from episcleral connective tissue, corneal endothelium, or limbal stromal tissue[65–67] and extends through a wound gape over the posterior cornea, angle, and iris. In contrast to epithelial downgrowth, it is less progressive and less likely to cause devastating consequences. On the surface of the iris, the fibrous tissue may appear as a thick enveloping membrane or a thin gray sheet (Fig. 14–20). The pupil may be displaced or peaked toward the wound through which the proliferation initiated. Argon laser burns placed on areas of affected iris do not show a characteristic reaction like that seen in epithelial downgrowth. Glaucoma associated with fibrous downgrowth can be secondary to inflammation, PAS, fibrous obliteration of the angle, or recurrent hemorrhage from fibrovascular tissue. IOP may be controlled with medical therapy or surgical intervention, and other ocular complications may be managed with various surgical procedures as needed.

Examination of an eye with later stages of *neovascular glaucoma* may reveal loss of normal iris architecture. The invisible fibrous component of the fibrovascular membrane covering the iris in this condition is composed of contractile myofibroblasts[68] capable of flattening the iris surface (Fig. 14–21). This altered appearance persists even if the anterior segment neovascularization has regressed.

A "slick" iris surface observed in a patient who has

TABLE 14–7. CAUSES OF ABNORMAL IRIS ARCHITECTURE AND ASSOCIATED GLAUCOMA

Obscuration of iris details or loss of iris crypts
Epithelial downgrowth
Fibrous ingrowth
Later stages of neovascular glaucoma
Anterior chamber filled with silicone oil
Congenital ectropion uveae
Congenital glaucoma
Thick, velvety iris
Developmental glaucoma
Marfan's syndrome

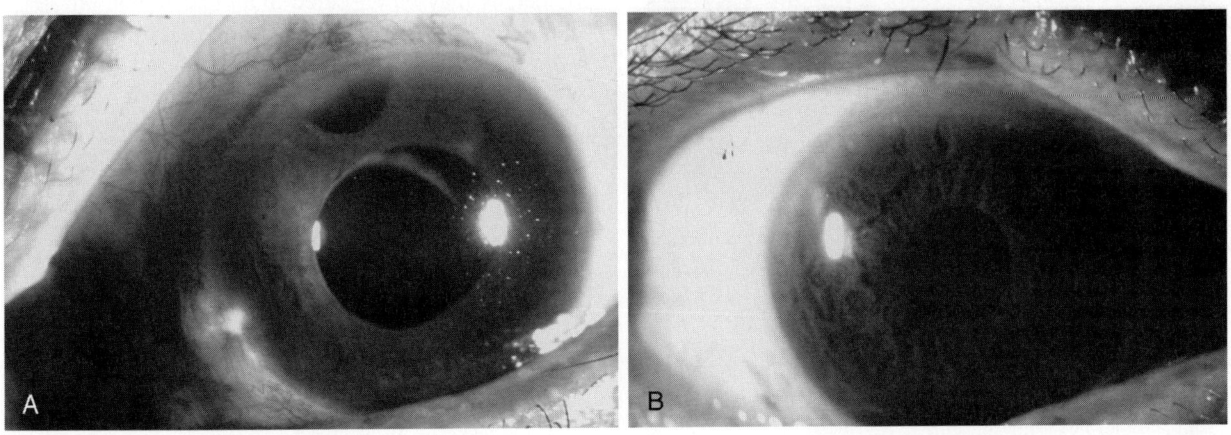

FIGURE 14–21. Slit-lamp views of the eyes of a patient with a history of neovascular glaucoma in the right eye. *A*, Smooth iris surface and loss of iris crypts in the affected (right) eye. *B*, Normal iris architecture of the left eye.

TABLE 14–8. CAUSES OF ECTROPION UVEAE AND ASSOCIATED GLAUCOMA

Congenital ectropion uveae
Isolated
Associated with systemic disorders
Disorders in which iris surface membranes pull iris pigment epithelium around pupillary margin
Epithelial downgrowth
Iridocorneal endothelial syndromes
Iris neovascularization

undergone a vitreoretinal procedure with adjunctive instillation of *silicone oil* should lead one to suspect that the oil has filled the anterior chamber. Although anterior migration of large amounts of silicone is uncommon, it may result in obstruction of trabecular meshwork outflow or may occlude the pupillary opening with resultant increased IOP. This condition may be managed with placement of an inferior peripheral iridotomy or removal of the silicone oil.

Finally, a reduction or absence of iris crypts may be observed in cases of congenital ectropion uveae (see later) or *congenital glaucoma.* In the latter condition, the abnormality of the iris crypts is related to anterior stromal hypoplasia and is associated with the finding of a malformed iris collarette.

THICK, VELVETY APPEARANCE OF IRIS

A rare finding of iris stromal hyperplasia with a thick, velvety iris has been noted in developmental glaucoma by Dickens and Hoskins.[69] The anterior iris surface in Marfan's syndrome (see Chapter 8), which can include an associated glaucoma, may exhibit a decreased number of crypts, furrows, and ridges, giving the iris a smooth, velvety appearance.[70]

ECTROPION UVEAE

Ectropion uveae refers to the presence of iris pigment epithelium on the anterior surface of the iris stroma. This may be a congenital anomaly[71–74] or may be acquired as in neovascular glaucoma (Table 14–8). Congenital ectropion uveae, a rare and nonprogressive anomaly of variable extent, may be an isolated finding or may be associated with systemic disorders (Fig. 14–22*A*). It is most typically found in neurofibromatosis but may also occur in primary facial hemihypertrophy, Prader-Willi syndrome, chromosome 15 abnormalities, and Axenfeld-Rieger syndrome (see Chapter 8 for a discussion of the systemic presentations of these syndromes).[72, 74–77]

Congenital ectropion uveae is usually unilateral and is associated with glaucoma (88%) and ptosis on the affected side.[76] The mechanism of compromised aqueous outflow in this disorder is uncertain. Although glaucoma usually begins in infancy or childhood, it may develop in adulthood, and all patients should be closely monitored for this complication.

Iris pigment epithelium may become pulled around the pupillary margin to create an ectropion uveae–like picture in various ocular disorders characterized by growth of membranes over the iris surface. In epithelial downgrowth, the ICE syndromes (see Fig. 14–22*B*), and anterior segment neovascularization, all described elsewhere in this chapter, ectropion uveae may occur along with other progressive iris findings and associated glaucoma. Areas of ectropion uveae in these conditions tend to occur in quadrants corresponding to the development of PAS.

Abnormal Iris Configuration or Position

IRIDOCORNEAL ADHESIONS

Synechiae between the iris and the corneal endothelium may be responsible for a malpositioned iris (Table 14–9). Many of these are best detected with gonioscopic examination and are more fully discussed in Chapter 13, but some are readily visible on slit-lamp examination. In the patient with Axenfeld-Rieger syndrome, in addition to other iris abnormalities already described, obvious tissue strands may extend from the peripheral iris to a prominent, anteriorly displaced Schwalbe's line (Fig. 14–23).

Another congenital disorder, Peters' anomaly, is characterized by a central corneal leukoma overlying a defect in Descemet's membrane and the posterior stroma, with

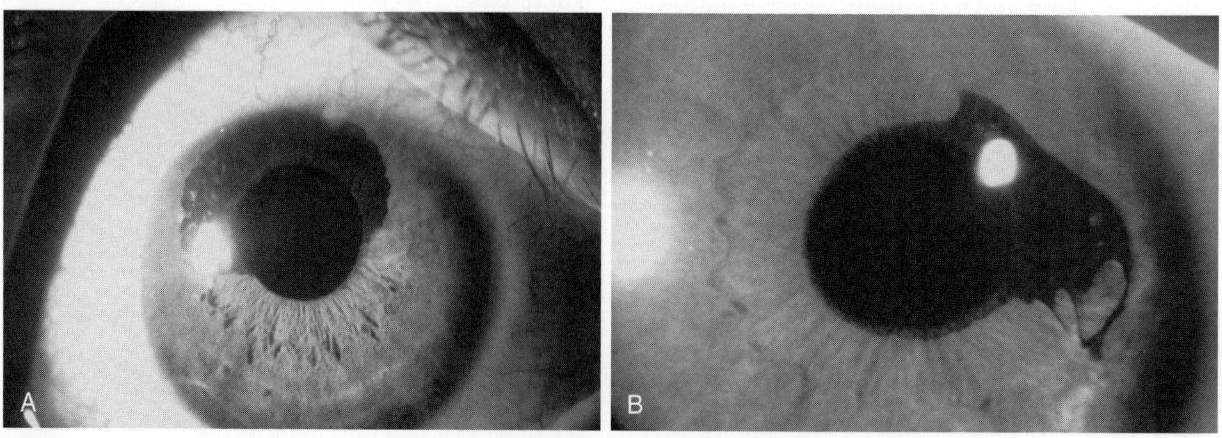

FIGURE 14–22. *A,* Congenital ectropion uveae in a patient with neurofibromatosis. *B,* Acquired ectropion uveae in a patient with iridocorneal endothelial syndrome. (*A* courtesy of Dr. James Richard.)

TABLE 14–9. CAUSES OF IRIDOCORNEAL ADHESIONS (VISIBLE ON SLIT-LAMP EXAMINATION) AND ASSOCIATED GLAUCOMA

Axenfeld-Rieger syndrome
Peters' anomaly
Prior shallowing or flattening of the anterior chamber

associated adhesions between the central iris and periphery of the corneal opacity (Fig. 14–24). These synechiae usually occur in the area of the iris collarette, more commonly in its temporal aspect, and cause a shallow anterior chamber by drawing the iris anteriorly toward the central posterior corneal surface. Frequently, the corneal opacity is so dense as to preclude observation of the typical iris findings. Fifty percent to 70% of cases of Peters' anomaly are reported to include associated glaucoma.[78, 79] Various other ocular and systemic anomalies may be found in Peters' anomaly but are not common.

Gonioscopically visible PAS can result from anterior chamber flattening or shallowing after penetrating trauma or surgical procedures, or from anterior segment inflammation from a number of causes. The same causes may lead to very anteriorly positioned focal iridocorneal adhesions or to widespread areas of iridocorneal contact seen without gonioscopic examination. In the presence of increased IOPs, these findings suggest compromise of the trabecular meshwork from the adhesion itself, its underlying cause, or both. Significant, prolonged shallowing or flattening of the anterior chamber in particular may result in high or broad adhesions.

ABNORMAL IRIS CONFIGURATION
(Table 14–10)

An unusual iris configuration noted on slit-lamp examination should prompt gonioscopic examination to further elucidate the anatomy of the anterior chamber angle and provide clues as to the cause of increased IOPs, if present.

Iris bombé, in which the flexible peripheral iris bows forward because of the impedance of aqueous flow from the posterior chamber to anterior chamber, may occur with

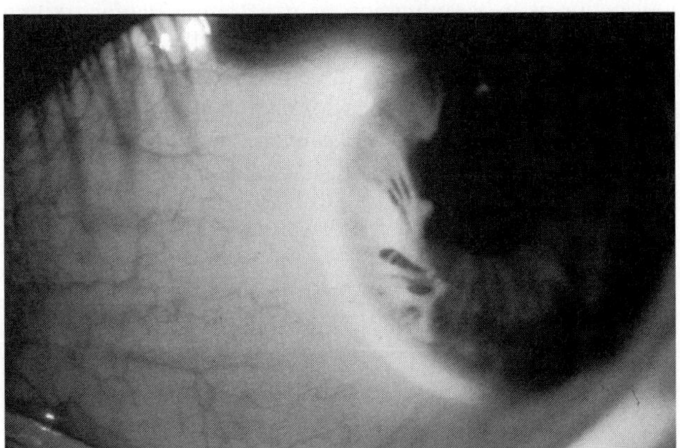

FIGURE 14–23. Iridocorneal adhesions visible on slit-lamp examination, extending to an anteriorly displaced Schwalbe's line, in a patient with Axenfeld-Rieger syndrome.

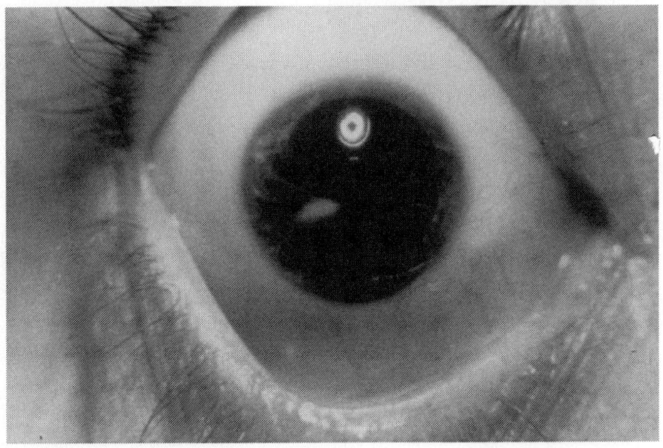

FIGURE 14–24. Slit-lamp view of the eye of a patient with Peters' anomaly, showing iris adhesions to a corneal leukoma.

the functional pupillary block of primary angle closure. It also occurs with pupillary block due to formation of posterior synechiae to the lens, pseudophakos, or anterior hyaloid face (Fig. 14–25). In the latter presentation, glaucoma may result from angle closure, from the primary inflammation which promoted the synechiae, or both.

Another, rarer type of primary angle closure may occur with the iris plateau configuration, wherein the mechanism of closure is crowding of the peripheral iris into the angle.[80, 81] Unlike in pupillary block angle closure, the contour of the plateau iris is flat to its periphery, where it abruptly angulates into a deep slit-like outlet.

An iris that bows forward centrally as well as peripherally, such that the central anterior chamber is shallow rather than deep as in the previously described entities, suggests possible angle closure due to anterior displacement of the lens-iris diaphragm. Further description of these conditions and their associated gonioscopic findings and management may be found in Chapter 13.

A concave contour may sometimes be detected with slit-lamp illumination of the iris surface in PDS. This configuration is believed to increase contact between the posterior surface of the iris and the zonules of the lens, thereby exacerbating the release of the pigment in this condition. It may be due to a "reverse pupillary block" phenomenon, in which a relatively higher aqueous pressure in the anterior chamber bows the iris posteriorly, toward the lower pressure in the posterior chamber.[14, 15] The iris

TABLE 14–10. CAUSES OF ABNORMAL IRIS CONFIGURATION AND ASSOCIATED GLAUCOMA

Iris bombé
Primary angle closure
Pupillary block from posterior synechiae
Plateau iris configuration
Angle closure from anterior rotation of iris-lens diaphragm
Concave iris contour
Pigment dispersion syndrome
Displaced silicone oil overfilling anterior chamber
Irregular, lumpy iris contour
Malignant melanoma of ciliary body
Cysts of the iris or ciliary body

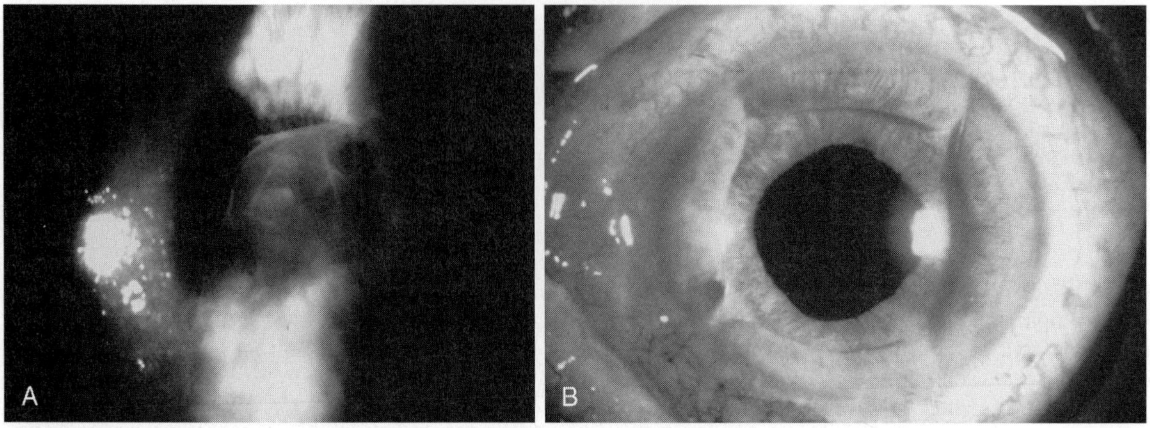

FIGURE 14–25. Slit-lamp views of iris bombé. *A,* Posterior synechiae to the crystalline lens in a patient with sarcoid uveitis. *B,* Pupillary block after placement of an anterior chamber intraocular lens implant.

may also be pushed posteriorly if the anterior chamber is inadvertently filled with displaced silicone oil utilized for retinal detachment repair. This may result in an unusually deep central chamber and occlusion of the trabecular meshwork.

Elevated IOP may occasionally be seen in conjunction with an irregular, lumpy iris contour. This contour should lead one to suspect a mass posterior to the iris. A malignant melanoma of the ciliary body, for example, may manifest as a smooth-domed elevation of overlying iris. This neoplasm may cause outflow obstruction of an open angle by tumor cells, pigment, or macrophages, or may cause angle closure by pushing the peripheral iris forward into the angle.[82–86] Cysts of the iris and ciliary body can result in an irregular iris and angle configuration and rarely may lead to angle closure glaucoma. These conditions are described more fully later in the chapter.

Synechiae of the Iris

POSTERIOR SYNECHIAE

Adhesions between the iris and the crystalline lens, an intraocular lens implant, or the anterior hyaloid face of the vitreous may occur at the pupillary border. They are promoted by intraocular inflammation of any cause and, if extensive, can result in pupillary block, iris bombé, and angle closure. With or without pupillary block, the finding of posterior synechiae may suggest an ongoing or previous inflammatory process (see Figs. 14–19 and 14–25*A*). The inflammation may compromise trabecular meshwork function such that synechial angle closure or a secondary open-angle glaucoma may result. Posterior synechiae and coincident glaucoma may also be observed after ocular trauma or various ophthalmic laser or surgical procedures.

Periphal Anterior Synechiae

Causes of PAS visible on slit-lamp examination were discussed previously along with iridocorneal adhesions. Conditions associated with PAS visible on gonioscopic examination are discussed in Chapter 13.

Cysts and Associated Glaucoma

(Table 14–11)

IRIS AND CILIARY BODY CYSTS

Iris and ciliary body cysts occasionally can produce acute or chronic angle-closure glaucoma.[87] They are sometimes seen protruding through the pupil or a peripheral iridectomy or, as mentioned previously, may give the iris a lumpy appearance. Most such cysts are congenital; they usually arise from the epithelial layers of the iris or ciliary body. Although generally benign and nonprogressive, multiple cysts within an eye may push the peripheral iris forward and subsequently occlude the chamber angle. Less commonly, the cysts are secondary to trauma or neoplasm; these are more likely than the primary type to cause inflammation and glaucoma. Administration of cholinesterase inhibitors may also produce iris epithelial cysts (Fig. 14–26). If the cysts cause glaucoma or other complications, they may be punctured with laser therapy.[88, 89]

EPITHELIAL DOWNGROWTH CYSTS

Although they do not arise from the iris itself, epithelial downgrowth or implantation cysts may be seen on the iris surface. Similar to epithelial downgrowth, epithelial cysts may occur as a complication of penetrating ocular trauma or surgical procedures.[64, 90, 91] They generally are connected with the wound from which the epithelial tissue originated, and they balloon into the anterior chamber against the front of the iris (Fig. 14–27). However, such cysts may be discontinuous with the wound, having presumably resulted from implanted epithelial cells. More rarely, they may

TABLE 14–11. ANTERIOR SEGMENT CYSTS WITH ASSOCIATED GLAUCOMA

Iris and ciliary body cysts
Congenital cysts
Cysts secondary to trauma or neoplasm
Iris epithelial cysts due to cholinesterase inhibitor administration
Epithelial downgrowth cysts
Pearl tumors

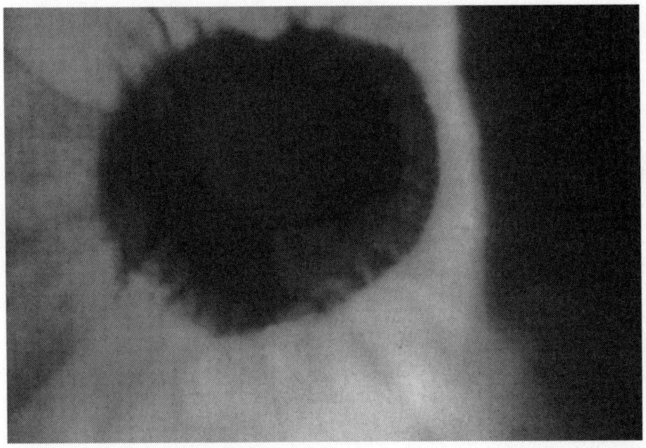

FIGURE 14–26. Iris epithelial cysts seen in the pupillary opening of a patient receiving topical cholinesterase inhibitor therapy.

extend through a peripheral iridectomy into the posterior chamber and can erode through the iris with the appearance of having arisen from the iris stroma.

Epithelial downgrowth cysts vary considerably in appearance and progression but are usually gray or translucent and have no pigment, unlike cysts actually arising from the iris pigment epithelium. Congenital iris stromal cysts (1) are similar in appearance to downgrowth cysts but are extremely rare, (2) usually occur before 1 year of age,[92, 93] and (3) are not associated with a penetrating ocular wound.

Another type of implantation cyst, pearl tumor, may occur as a result of traumatic seeding of skin or hair follicles into the anterior chamber.[91, 94] These appear as opaque cysts implanted on the iris surface and, in contrast to epithelial downgrowth cysts, tend to remain small. They are effectively managed with excision, if needed.

Complications of epithelial downgrowth cysts include occlusion of the visual axis, inflammation, and glaucoma. Management of the secondary glaucoma consists of medications to control ocular hypertension and control of the inflammation. Photocoagulation puncture of the cysts may be attempted[95–97] but has limited success, as does surgical excision utilizing various approaches.[98–100]

TABLE 14–12. CAUSES OF HETEROCHROMIA OF THE IRIS AND ASSOCIATED GLAUCOMA

Fuchs' heterochromic iridocyclitis
Posner-Schlossman syndrome (not typical)
Intraocular inflammation
Systemic disorders
Neurofibromatosis
Marfan's syndrome
Klippel-Trenaunay-Weber syndrome

Abnormal Iris Pigmentation and Pigmented Iris Lesions

ABNORMAL IRIS PIGMENTATION

Heterochromia of the irides, in which one eye manifests hypochromia or, more rarely, hyperchromia compared with the fellow eye, may be seen in a number of ocular and systemic conditions that may also be associated with glaucoma (Table 14–12).

One such condition is a primary ocular disorder known as Fuchs' heterochromic iridocyclitis, which classically comprises a triad of heterochromia, cyclitis, and cataract in the affected eye. A secondary glaucoma may also develop. The syndrome has no gender predilection and is usually unilateral, but in 3.5% to 13% of cases, it may be bilateral.[101, 102] It involves an insidious, chronic, mild nongranulomatous uveitis, most commonly presenting in the third or fourth decade of life. Cataract formation is frequent but tends to occur rather late in the course of the disease. Ipsilateral hypochromia is not absolutely necessary for diagnosis of the syndrome but is typically present (Fig. 14–28). The disorder may begin in infancy, increases slowly with time, and is more noticeable in patients with brown irides. It is the result of iris stromal atrophy, which begins at the pupillary border and then extends peripherally. The iris surface develops a thinned, mottled, fibrillar appearance, and normal radial vessels become evident (Fig. 14–29). It is described as having a translucent appearance on retroillumination. The affected eye may occasionally be hyperchromic (exhibiting "heterochromia inversa") if the iris stroma thins enough to expose the pigment epithelium.

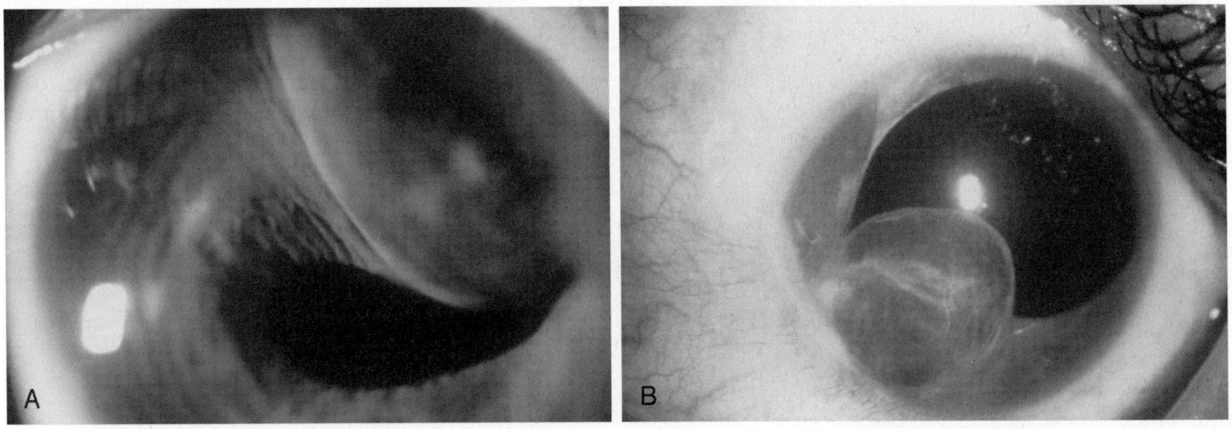

FIGURE 14–27. *A* and *B*, Slit-lamp views of epithelial downgrowth cysts.

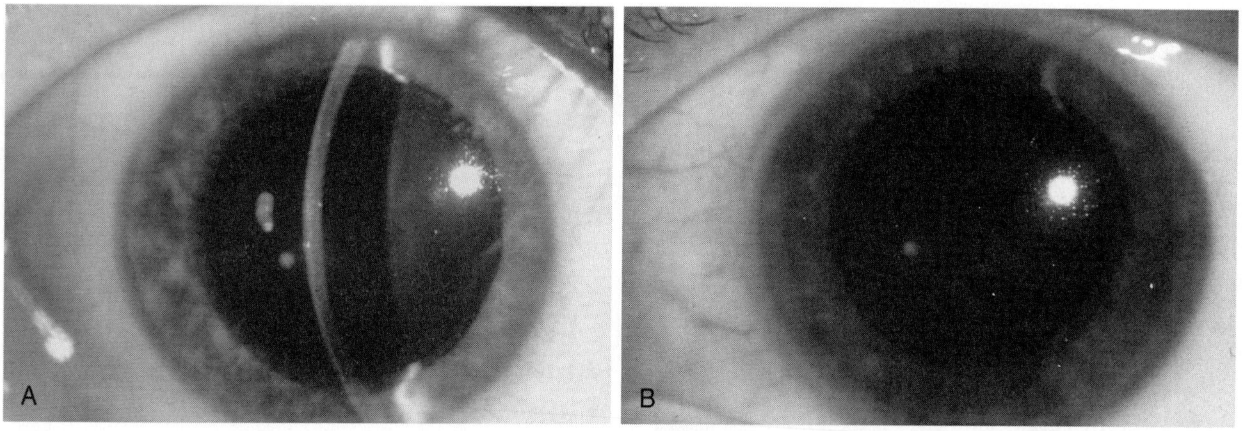

FIGURE 14–28. Slit-lamp views of the eyes of a patient with Fuchs' heterochromic iridocyclitis. *A*, Hypochromic iris of the affected eye. *B*, The normal other eye.

In some patients, iris nodules are found in association with the uveitis.[102–104] Other ocular findings characteristic of this disorder are discussed elsewhere in this book (see Chapters 11, 12, and 15).

The prevalence of glaucoma in Fuchs' heterochromic iridocyclitis is reported to be 6.3% to 59%.[104–109] Glaucoma is more common in patients who are black[109] or in whom Fuchs' heterochromic iridocyclitis is bilateral.[106] Increased IOP generally results from the chronic iritis in this syndrome, and the likelihood of associated glaucoma increases with the duration of the inflammation.[108, 110] Glaucoma may also be secondary to removal of the cataract typically associated with this disorder. Infrequently, iris neovascularization with neovascular glaucoma (discussed later) develops.[111] Aqueous suppressant therapy can be given initially to control the IOP, although medical control of the glaucoma typically is not satisfactory. Because of the associated inflammation, the use of miotics and laser trabeculoplasty is not advised. Moreover, corticosteroid administration is not recommended because it is not helpful in treating the iritis and may promote cataract formation and elevated IOP. Incisional filtration surgery with adjunctive antifibrotics is often indicated.

Although not so typically as Fuchs' heterochromic iridocyclitis, other ocular inflammatory conditions may result in enough diffuse or focal iris stromal thinning to cause heterochromia, and glaucoma may develop secondary to any type of uveitis. Of mention is that the original reports of the Posner-Schlossman syndrome, characterized by unilateral recurrent episodes of glaucoma associated with uveitis (see Chapter 12), noted heterochromia in some of the cases. This finding is not expected in Posner-Schlossman syndrome, however, and some speculate that these patients actually had Fuchs' heterochromic iridocyclitis.

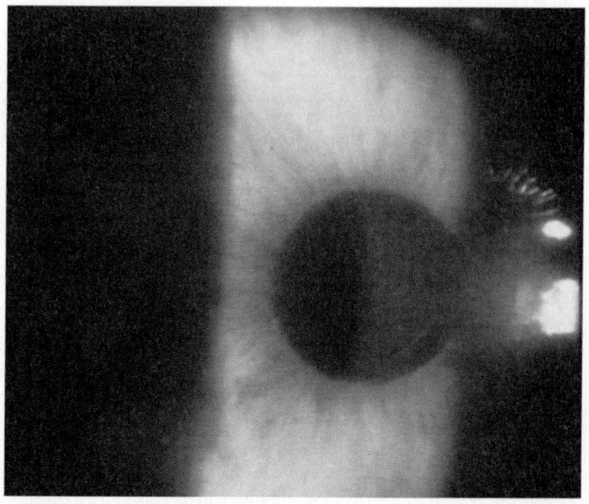

FIGURE 14–29. Normal radial iris vessels evident in thinned iris stroma of an eye with Fuchs' heterochromic iridocyclitis.

Some systemic disorders are also known to have ocular manifestations of both heterochromia of the iris and glaucoma. Examples are neurofibromatosis, Marfan's syndrome, and the Klippel-Trenaunay-Weber syndrome. These each may have a number of other iris and ocular findings, discussed elsewhere in this chapter and in other chapters. Associated nonocular findings are detailed in Chapter 8.

Unilaterally or bilaterally apparent increased pigmentation of the iris may be due to deposition of pigment particles associated with PDS or the exfoliation syndrome (Table 14–13). In the former condition, the pigment tends to collect in concentric furrows of the iris (Fig. 14–30) and is most easily observed in patients with blue eyes.[9, 112] An asymmetric deposition may result in heterochromia.[9, 113] In an eye with the exfoliation syndrome, pigment particles are observed on the iris sphincter and occasionally in a peripheral location (Fig. 14–31).[18] They tend to be larger and more evenly distributed than in PDS but are also more easily detected in light irides. These two syndromes have been described earlier.

The observation of a progressive diffuse pigmentation of the iris and late development of glaucoma after ocular trauma should lead the clinician to suspect a penetrating

TABLE 14–13. CAUSES OF INCREASED DIFFUSE IRIS PIGMENTATION AND ASSOCIATED GLAUCOMA

Pigment dusting of the iris
Pigment dispersion syndrome
Exfoliation syndrome
Siderosis and hemosiderosis
Diffuse iris melanoma
Administration of latanoprost

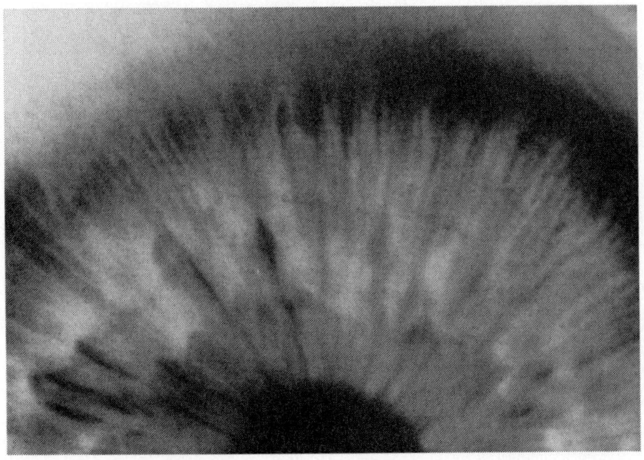

FIGURE 14–30. Pigment deposition in concentric furrows on the iris surface in a patient with pigment dispersion syndrome.

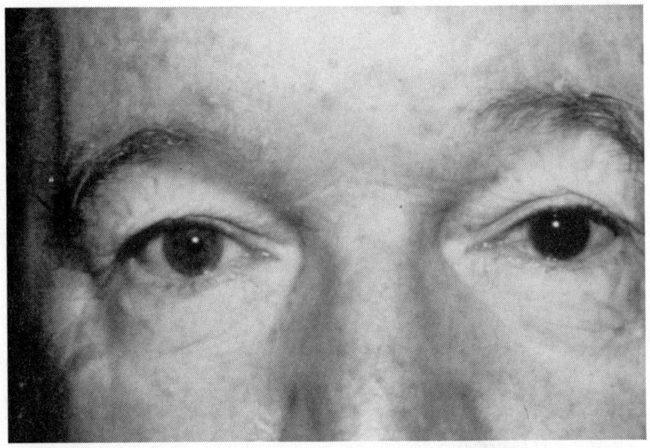

FIGURE 14–32. Iris heterochromia in a patient with an iris melanoma. Note the hyperchromia of the affected left eye.

injury with a retained ferrous-containing intraocular foreign body. In this setting, iron released from the foreign material can cause siderosis, in which toxic effects to various ocular tissues may occur.[114] The iris may be darkened by deposits of iron in the stroma, and discoloration in the lens and cornea may be noted as well. Retinal function may be altered, and it is believed that increased IOPs are the result of damage to the trabecular meshwork by the metal deposition. Hemosiderin from intraocular hemorrhage has the potential to produce an identical presentation, known as hemosiderosis. In either situation, glaucoma can also be secondary to other effects of the trauma or hemorrhage. Increased IOPs are managed with antiglaucoma medications or filtration surgery.

A progressively hyperchromic type of heterochromia may occur with development of a diffuse iris melanoma (Fig. 14–32). This uncommon tumor gives a unilateral patchy or diffuse pigmentation to the iris and may block aqueous outflow by invasion of the trabecular meshwork. Oculodermal melanocytosis, melanosis oculi, and the diffuse iris nodular nevus syndrome may each cause a unilateral iris hyperchromia and glaucoma (see later).

Worthy of special mention is the well-documented side effect of increased iris pigmentation seen with the topical administration of latanoprost.[115–117] This prostaglandin analogue, utilized for the management of glaucoma, lowers IOP by increasing uveoscleral outflow. It also has the potential to increase the number of melanosomes within the melanocytes of the iris stroma. This phenomenon is most likely to occur in irides of mixed colors, such as green-brown, yellow-brown, or blue/gray-brown, with brown pigmentation occurring in a concentric fashion to cause a darker-appearing iris. Unilateral instillation of the latanoprost may result in obvious heterochromia. Studies report up to a 23% incidence of this side effect, which develops gradually over a period of months.[115–117] The change in coloration is typically permanent but does not progress further once the medication is discontinued. Although no harmful effects to the eye are known to be associated with this phenomenon, patients in whom latanoprost is instituted must be warned of the possible cosmetic change, particularly if unilateral administration is planned.

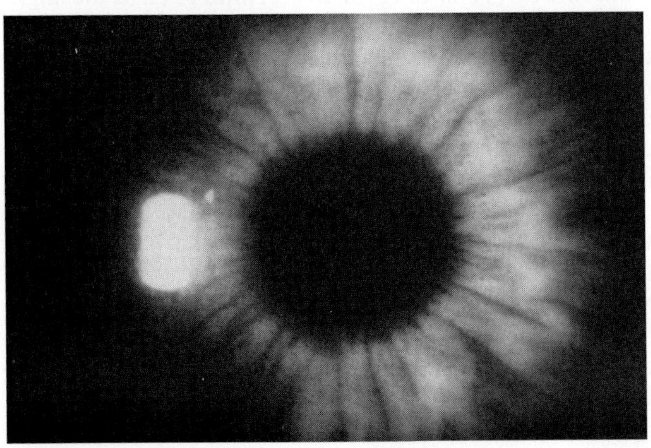

FIGURE 14–31. Pigment deposition on the surface of the iris sphincter in a patient with the exfoliation syndrome.

Iris Lesions with Associated Secondary Glaucoma

PIGMENTED IRIS LESIONS

Focal pigmented lesions of the iris are associated with a variety of conditions, in a number of which an associated glaucoma may also be present (Table 14–14). Uveal melanomas, the most common primary intraocular malignancy, may develop in the iris and typically present as well-circumscribed, brown, slightly elevated masses on the

TABLE 14–14. PIGMENTED IRIS LESIONS WITH ASSOCIATED GLAUCOMA

Uveal melanomas
Iris melanomas
Ciliary body melanomas with anterior extension into iris
Iris melanocytoma
Iris nevus syndrome
Cogan-Reese syndrome
Diffuse iris nodular nevus syndrome
Lisch's nodules
Oculodermal melanocytosis (nevus of Ota) and melanosis oculi
Juvenile xanthogranuloma

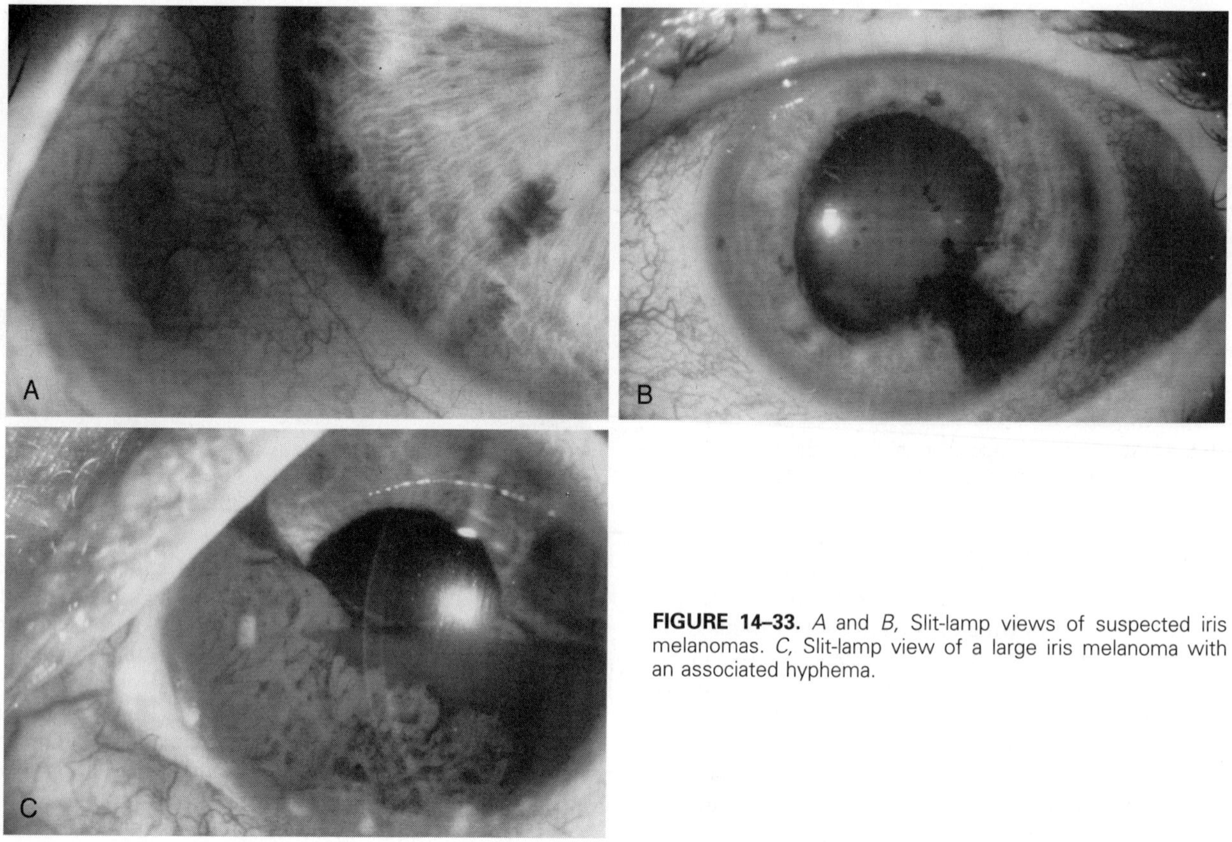

FIGURE 14–33. *A* and *B*, Slit-lamp views of suspected iris melanomas. *C*, Slit-lamp view of a large iris melanoma with an associated hyphema.

stroma (Fig. 14–33). Variation in pigmentation is possible (Fig. 14–34), however, with some iris melanomas being amelanotic or having a nodular appearance resembling tapioca (the so-called tapioca melanoma[118]). As mentioned previously, iris melanomas infrequently may also manifest in a diffuse distribution.

Iris melanomas are generally slow growing or stationary and have no associated complications, but at times may cause increased IOP. Tapioca melanomas in particular may have an associated glaucoma, in as many as one third of cases.[118] In any type of iris melanoma, the glaucoma is most commonly due to direct invasion of the trabecular meshwork by the tumor[83, 119–121] but occasionally may be secondary to a spontaneous hyphema originating from the neoplasm. In contrast to more posterior uveal melanomas, iris melanomas with associated glaucoma tend to be more benign and may be managed with observation and medical therapy for the increased IOP. For patients in whom glaucoma cannot be managed medically or growth of the tumor is noted, however, many authorities recommend local excision or enucleation and advise avoidance of invasive filtration surgery because of the potential of extrascleral seeding of the tumor.

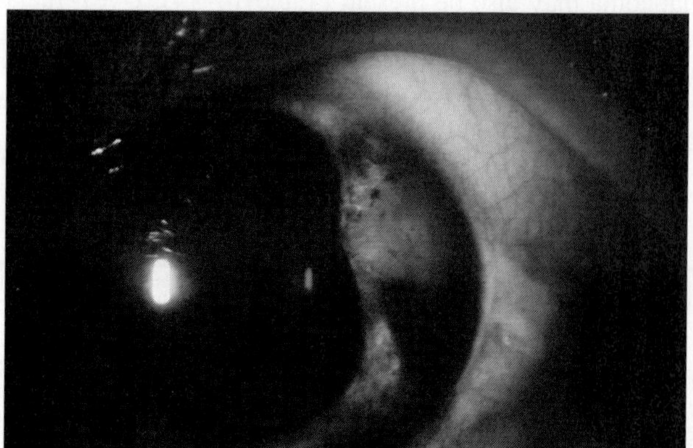

FIGURE 14–34. Slit-lamp view of an iris melanoma that has a pigmented component and an amelanotic, vascular component. (Courtesy of Dr. Robert Small.)

Primary melanomas of the ciliary body may be detected when they extend anteriorly and are seen eroding through the periphery of the iris (Fig. 14–35). They may cause glaucoma by (1) pushing the iris forward to close the angle, (3) obstructing the angle with direct tumor extension, or (3) seeding the trabecular meshwork with tumor cells or macrophages.[82, 83, 86, 120] Ciliary body tumors advanced enough to cause glaucoma are often managed with enucleation of the affected eye, but iridocyclectomy or plaque irradiation may also be considered.

A pigmented lesion of the iris that may be associated with glaucoma and simulate a melanoma is a particular type of uveal nevus known as a *melanocytoma*. It appears as a well-circumscribed, dark brown or black, irregular lesion.[121] This tumor has a propensity to undergo fragmentation and necrosis, with subsequent obstruction of the trabecular meshwork by the liberated material.

Another type of iris nevus sometimes associated with glaucoma is that found in the iris nevus syndrome, characterized by diffuse flat iris lesions. Although this entity is

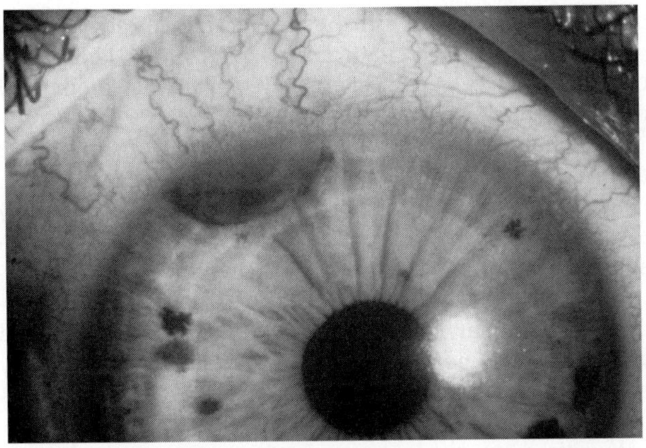

FIGURE 14–35. Slit-lamp view of a ciliary body melanoma that has eroded through the iris stroma. (Courtesy of Dr. Scott Sigler.)

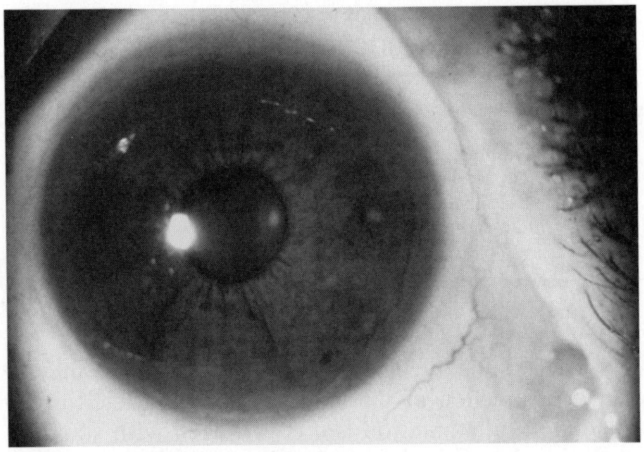

FIGURE 14–37. Slit-lamp photograph of Lisch's nodules found in a patient with neurofibromatosis.

sometimes believed to be synonymous with the Cogan-Reese syndrome, many writers believe that it is not in the spectrum of the ICE syndrome variants.[122] Eyes with the actual Cogan-Reese syndrome are at risk for development of glaucoma as well; they are characterized by pigmented, pedunculated nodules of the iris surface (see Fig. 14–12). In contrast to the lesions of the iris nevus syndrome, wherein the lesions have the histologic morphology of nevi, the nodules in Cogan-Reese syndrome are made up of tissue similar to that of the underlying iris stroma and are surrounded by the hallmark cellular membrane of the ICE variants (discussed earlier).

An additional separate entity occasionally involving glaucoma in the presence of ocular nevi is the diffuse iris nodular nevus syndrome. This familial or sporadic condition is characterized by multiple discrete nodular excrescences distributed diffusely on the surface of the iris, giving it the appearance of dotted swiss fabric (Fig. 14–36).[123–126] The disorder may be unilateral or bilateral. Its appearance on slit-lamp examination resembles that of the nodules in the Cogan-Reese syndrome, but histologically, diffuse iris nodular nevus syndrome is similar in appearance to the iris lesions in oculodermal or ocular melanocytosis (described later).[127] However, it differs from the latter disorder in that it has no associated pigmentation of other ocular structures. The nodules do not possess the excess pigmentation found in typical iris nevi. Associated open-angle glaucoma and ocular hypertension have been reported.[125] The nonfamilial form of the diffuse iris nodular nevus syndrome may also be associated with various other ocular and systemic disorders.[128]

Lesions sometimes confused with iris nevi are Lisch's nodules. These are found in patients with neurofibromatosis, one of the phakomatoses with which glaucoma may be associated. In contrast to the minimally elevated or flat iris nevi, Lisch's nodules are well-delineated, dome-shaped gelatinous elevations on the iris stroma and may be brown, yellowish, or clear (Fig. 14–37). They are composed of cells known to be melanocytic in origin.[129–131] They are bilateral in all patients with neurofibromatosis type 1 who are older than 16 years and are rare and unilateral in patients with neurofibromatosis type 2 (see Chapter 8).

Oculodermal melanocytosis, or the nevus of Ota, is another phakomatosis with a pigmented lesion of the iris and possible glaucoma. This condition (1) is characterized by pigmentation of the deep dermis and various tissues of the globe, (2) is usually unilateral, and (3) typically occurs in women of Asian descent. Involvement of the iris may be extensive. Both angle-closure and open-angle glaucomas

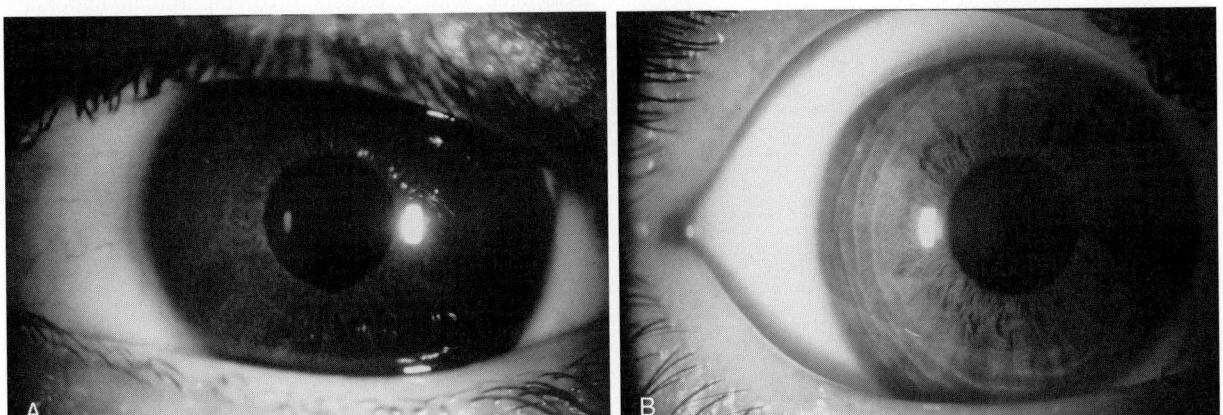

FIGURE 14–36. Slit-lamp photographs of the eyes of a child with diffuse iris nodular nevus syndrome in the right eye *(A)*; the left eye is normal *(B)*. This patient also has the Klippel-Trenaunay-Weber syndrome.

TABLE 14–15. NONPIGMENTED IRIS LESIONS WITH ASSOCIATED GLAUCOMA

Neoplasms
- Amelanotic iris melanomas
- Metastases from distant primary tumors
- Leukemic and lymphoid infiltrative tumors
- Medulloepithelioma

Inflammatory (Koeppe and Busacca) nodules
Nodules of Fuchs' heterochromic iridocyclitis

may occur in the affected eye.[132–135] The glaucoma may be due to obstruction of the angle by melanocytes[136] or by associated inflammation and is managed with standard medical and surgical therapy for glaucoma. Ocular melanocytosis, or melanosis oculi, is identical to the nevus of Ota except for the absence of skin involvement and can also be complicated by the development of glaucoma.

Lightly pigmented or salmon-colored iris lesions are a feature of juvenile xanthogranuloma, a benign disorder of infants and young children also characterized by yellow papular skin lesions on the head and neck.[137–139] The iris findings are usually unilateral and may cause a spontaneous hyphema. Glaucoma may occur in the affected eye secondary to the hyphema, associated inflammation, or invasion of the angle by the tumor cells, and may be managed with corticosteroids and antiglaucoma medications.

NONPIGMENTED IRIS LESIONS

Although less common than pigmented lesions, nonpigmented lesions of the iris are sometimes observed in the presence of a secondary glaucoma (Table 14–15). Some melanomas of the iris may be amelanotic and may have an associated vasculature (see Figs. 14–34 and 14–38). They behave much like their pigmented counterparts discussed previously. Metastatic tumors from distant primary sites, including the breast, lung, gastrointestinal tract, and kidney, may involve the iris and appear as focal, multifocal, or diffuse multinodular, nonpigmented lesions. Associated glaucoma is fairly common (64% in one series[120]) and is secondary to obstruction of the trabecular meshwork by tumor invasion or seeding of angle structures. Because the overall prognosis of a patient with this presentation is generally poor, glaucoma management should be conservative and may be ameliorated with palliative radiotherapy of the affected eye.

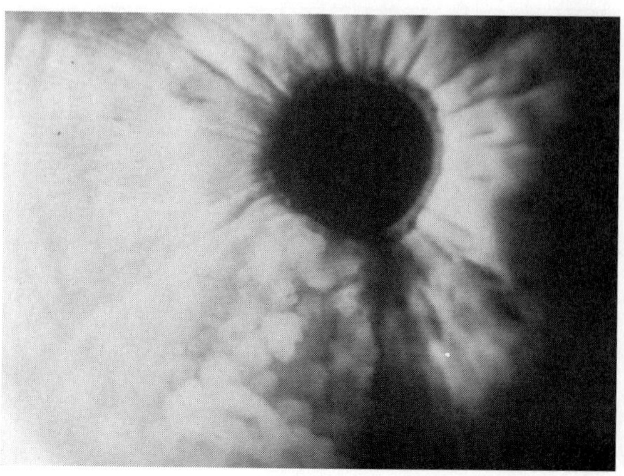

FIGURE 14–38. Slit-lamp view of an amelonotic melanoma of the iris. (Courtesy of Dr. Scott Sigler.)

Lymphoid tumors and leukemic cells may also infiltrate the iris and cause generalized thickening of the stroma. Glaucoma may result from obstruction of the angle by direct tumor involvement or the secondary iris thickening.[140, 141] Palliative treatment is recommended.

Secondary glaucoma may also be associated with a medulloepithelioma.[142] This uncommon tumor of childhood arises from the nonpigmented ciliary epithelium and may appear as a whitish gray mass or cyst of the iris. It is usually managed by resection or enucleaton.

Uveitis may also be a cause of nonpigmented iris nodules and glaucoma. Other findings typical of inflammation, such as synechiae and keratic precipitates, are often present as well. The nodules are focal accumulations of inflammatory cells, which appear as multiple, small white lesions on the iris surface at the pupillary border (Koeppe nodules) and in more peripheral locations (Busacca's nodules). This finding is most characteristic of a granulomatous uveitis, particularly that associated with sarcoidosis.[143] Corticosteroids should be utilized to control the inflammation, and IOP should be controlled with aqueous suppressant therapy. If IOP is inadequately controlled, filtration surgery with either a trabeculectomy with antifibrotic therapy or an aqueous shunt may be necessary. Fuchs' heterochromic iridocyclitis, discussed earlier, may also give rise to multiple translucent iris nodules[144]; glaucoma can also be associated with this disorder, distinguished from other forms of uveitis by the quiet appearance of the eye and the absence of synechiae.

Abnormal or Prominent Iris Vessels

(Table 14–16)

NEOVASCULARIZATION OF THE IRIS

One of the most striking iris findings with which glaucoma may be associated is that of neovascularization of the iris. Also known as *rubeosis iridis*, this condition is usually associated with disorders involving retinal hypoxia[145–147] and is believed to be incited by unknown angiogenesis

TABLE 14–16. CAUSES OF ABNORMAL OR PROMINENT IRIS VESSELS AND ASSOCIATED GLAUCOMA

Neovascularization of the iris
- Conditions with retinal hypoxia
- Exfoliation syndrome
- Fuchs' heterochromic iridocyclitis

Peripupillary vascular tufts
Prominent, normal iris vasculature
- Fuchs' heterochromic iridocyclitis
- Other intraocular inflammation with resultant iris atrophy and thinning
- Engorged iris vessels sometimes seen in acute iridocyclitis

Anomalous iris vessels of developmental glaucomas

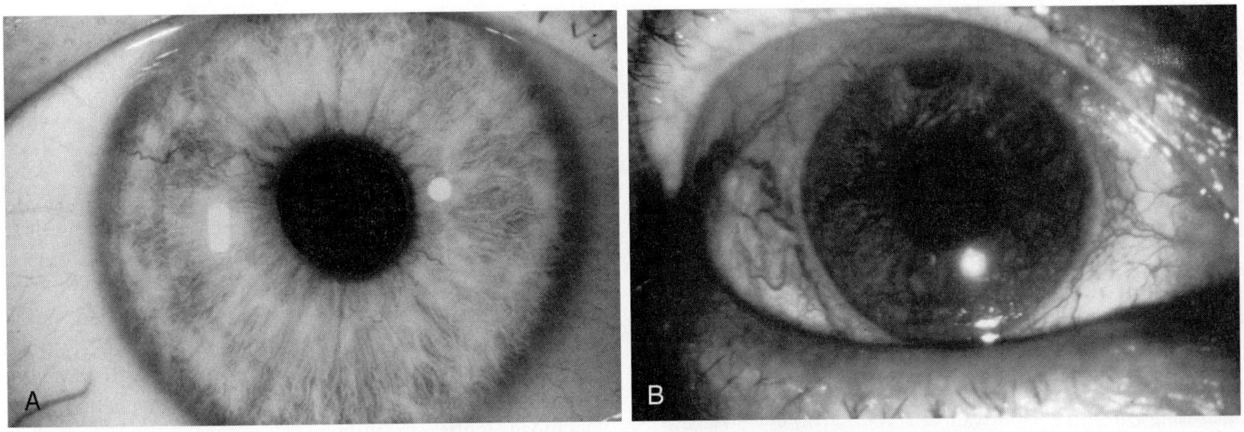

FIGURE 14–39. Slit-lamp views of two eyes with neovascularization of the iris. *A*, Peripupillary tufts of vessels and randomly arranged new vessels on the surface of the iris, extending toward the periphery. *B*, Florid neovascularization of the iris.

factors produced in the posterior segment.[148–151] The most common underlying causes are diabetic retinopathy (about a third of cases[152, 153]), central retinal vein occlusion (28% in one series[153]), and carotid occlusive disease (13% in one series[152]). Other causes are occlusive vascular diseases, central retinal artery occlusion, intraocular tumors, retinal detachment, and uveitis.

Iris neovascularization is capable of producing severe glaucoma; however, early detection of iris neovascularization may alert the clinician to the need to proceed with therapy designed to prevent glaucoma. In general, it first appears as tiny tufts of new vessels at the pupillary border (Fig. 14–39*A*),[154] although it may also first be detected elsewhere on the iris or in the angle.[155, 156] The initial, fine peripupillary vessels may be obscured by dilation of the pupil or collapsed by pressure from a goniolens.[154] From these tufts, other new vessels arise and extend peripherally over the surface of the iris in an irregular fashion (see Fig. 14–39), in contrast to normal iris vessels, which are arranged radially within the stroma. The rate of progression of the neovascularization varies widely. The neovascularization seen in association with a central retinal vein occlusion, for example, tends to be more fulminant with more engorged vessels.[157] Other iris findings, such as loss of iris crypts (see Fig. 14–21) and ectropion uveae (Fig. 14–40), may also be observed in rubeosis iridis and are discussed elsewhere in this chapter.

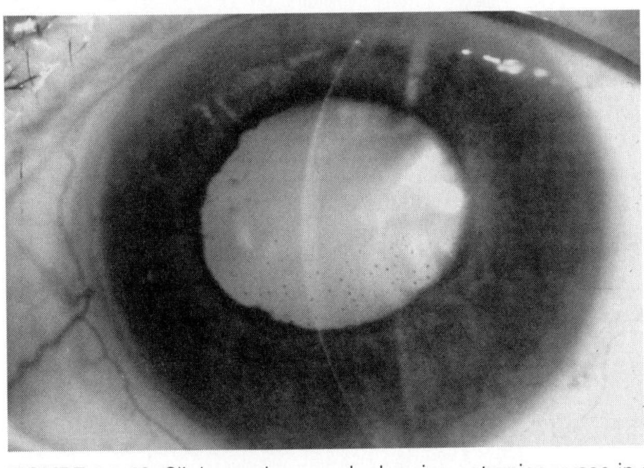

FIGURE 14–40. Slit-lamp photograph showing ectropion uveae in a patient with neovascular glaucoma.

Once the new rubeotic vessels involve the angle, increased IOPs may result from trabecular meshwork obstruction by a fibrovascular membrane (the earlier, open-angle glaucoma stage[158, 159]) or by PAS (the later, angle-closure glaucoma stage). A description of the appearance of the angle in neovascular glaucoma may be found in Chapter 13.

Management of iris neovascularization and neovascular glaucoma should begin with retinal ablation by panretinal photocoagulation[160–165] or, in the case of insufficient fundus visualization, transscleral cryotherapy[166] to achieve regression of the vessels. Resolution of the vessels may avert glaucoma altogether in neovascularization alone, allow control of IOP in the open-angle stage of glaucoma,[160, 162, 163] or decrease complications of any subsequently required intraocular surgery in the angle-closure stage.[167, 168] Initial treatment of increased IOP is attempted with aqueous suppressants. Topical corticosteroids and cycloplegics also help decrease resultant inflammation and pain. If advanced synechial angle closure ensues, medical therapy will likely become ineffective. Depending on the individual patient's visual prognosis and the status of anterior segment neovascularization, options for intervention in medically uncontrolled cases include filtration surgery with adjunctive antifibrotic therapy, implantation of an aqueous shunt, and cyclodestructive procedures.

Some ocular disorders that are not characterized by retinal hypoxia may also occasionally exhibit neovascularization of the iris. Iris neovascularization has been described in the exfoliation syndrome; it tends to be very fine neovascularization, is usually missed clinically, and is not known to have an associated neovascular glaucoma. Fuchs' heterochromic iridocyclitis is known sometimes to have an associated fine neovascularization in the angle, and although neovascularization of the iris surface with neovascular glaucoma has been observed in this entity (Fig. 14–41), it is rare.[110] Other inflammatory ocular conditions may develop iris neovascularization as well; in one series, 11% of eyes with rubeosis also had uveitis.[153]

A rather benign neovascular condition of the iris is that of peripupillary vascular tufts, also known as microhemangiomas of the iris (Fig. 14–42).[169] These are usually noted

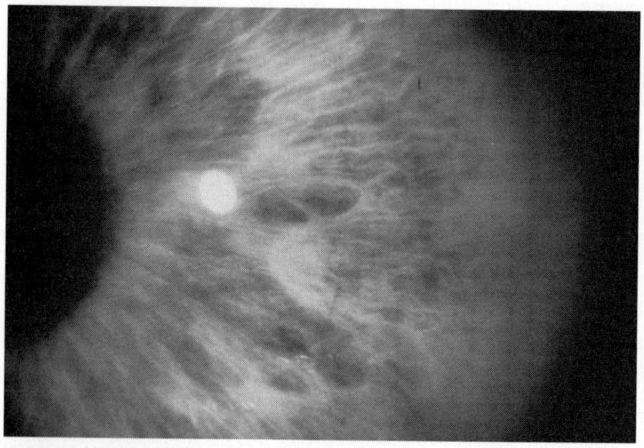

FIGURE 14–41. Neovascularization of the iris in an eye affected with Fuchs' heterochromic iridocyclitis.

in older patients, either as an isolated abnormality or in association with diabetes mellitus or myotonic dystrophy.[169–171] The vessels may be a source of spontaneous hyphema with transiently increased IOPs,[172, 173] but recurrent episodes and glaucomatous damage are uncommon. If repeated hemorrhages do occur, however, laser photocoagulation may be applied to the tuft to prevent further bleeding.[174]

PROMINENT IRIS VESSELS

Prominent normal iris vasculature may sometimes be confused with active neovascularization of the iris. For example, Fuchs' iridocyclitis may, as noted previously, cause an associated true neovascular glaucoma; more often, however, iris vessels observed in this disorder are actually normal vessels exposed because of stromal thinning (see Fig. 14–29), and associated glaucoma is secondary to other mechanisms. Other ocular inflammations and conditions may have a similar presentation, with iris vessels most easily observed in blue-eyed individuals. Normal iris vasculature can usually be differentiated from abnormal vessels by its regular, radial arrangement, in contrast to the random orientation of neovascularization. Acute iridocyclitis may also manifest as engorged normal iris vessels that can mimic rubeosis, but the former condition resolves with administration of corticosteroids.

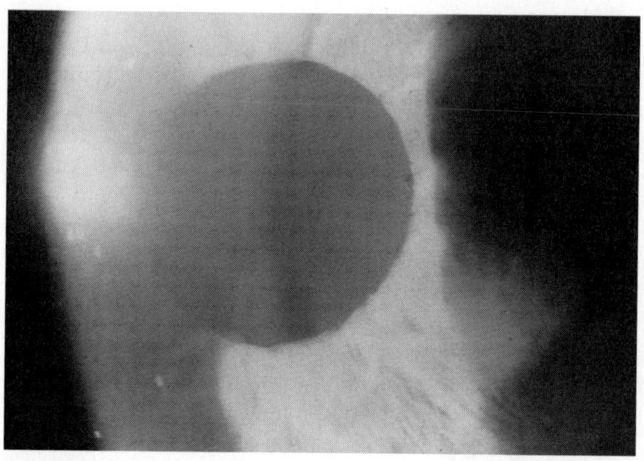

FIGURE 14–42. Slit-lamp view of microhemangiomas of the iris, seen as vascular tufts at the pupillary border.

DEVELOPMENTAL GLAUCOMAS WITH ANOMALOUS IRIS VESSELS

Although many cases of developmental glaucoma (i.e., glaucoma associated with developmental anomalies of the eye present at birth) are a result of an isolated malformation of the trabecular meshwork, some cases also exhibit iris anomalies. In addition to previously mentioned defects such as anterior stromal hypoplasia and aniridia, eyes with iridotrabeculodysgenesis may have associated anomalous iris vessels.[175] These may be part of a persistent tunica vasculosa lentis, in which prominent normal radial iris vessels are seen in association with vessels looping into the pupillary opening, or may be an irregular pattern of superficial vessels associated with an irregular pupil. The anomalous vascular findings are not a component of any defined ocular or systemic syndrome. Their presence is indicative of a more severe anterior segment malformation and portends a worse prognosis than for isolated trabeculodysgenesis. Associated glaucoma is usually present at birth. Management of elevated IOP in these cases includes goniotomy or trabeculotomy in patients less than 2 to 3 years old, antiglaucoma medications, and filtration or shunt procedures.

SUMMARY

The appearance of the iris and pupil may provide valuable clues to the underlying cause and mechanism of increased IOP or glaucoma. Decreased iris tissue due to developmental, traumatic, inflammatory, or other causes with associated glaucoma may cause full-thickness or partial-thickness transillumination defects. These defects may be focal or diffuse, or may involve near-total absence of the iris, as in aniridia. Examination of the anterior surface of the iris may reveal abnormal tissue responsible for decreased aqueous outflow or may produce findings indicative of various primary ocular or systemic causes of glaucoma. As in the case of iris bombé causing angle closure, the configuration of the iris can point to the mechanism of increased IOP. Unusual iris pigmentation, either increased or decreased, may be typical for various ocular and systemic disorders that can cause secondary glaucoma. Pigmented and nonpigmented iris lesions of malignant, inflammatory, and systemic entities may primarily or secondarily incite elevated IOP. Neovascular glaucoma is classically diagnosed from identification of iris neovascularization, but other disorders with unusual-appearing iris vessels and associated glaucoma may occur as well. Finally, the appearance of the pupil, whether abnormally large or small or unusual in shape or reaction, may give clues to the mechanism of increased IOP.

REFERENCES

1. Beauchamp GR: Anterior segment dysgenesis: Keratolenticular adhesion and aniridia. J Pediatr Ophthalmol Strabismus 1980;17:55.

2. Hamming NA, Miller MT, Rabb M: Unusual variant of familial aniridia. J Pediatric Ophthalmol Strabismus 1986;23:195.
3. Mondino BJ, Cohn HC: Corectopia with nystagmus, absent foveal reflexes, and cornea changes. Acta Ophthalmol (Copenh) 1981;59:85.
4. Elsas FJ, Maumenee IH, Kenyon KR, et al: Familial aniridia with preserved ocular function. Am J Ophthalmol 1977;88:718.
5. Hittner HM, Riccardi VM, Ferrell RE, et al: Variable expressivity in autosomal dominant aniridia by clinical, electrophysiologic and angiographic criteria. Am J Ophthalmol 1980;89:531.
6. Mapstone R: Pigment release. Br J Ophthalmol 1981;65:258.
7. Mauksch H: Uber idiopathischen Zerfall des retinalen Pigmentblattes der Iris bei zwei Brudern. Z Augenheilkd 1925;57:262.
8. Speakman JS: Pigmentary dispersion. Br J Ophthalmol 1981;65:249.
9. Sugar HS: Pigmentary glaucoma: A 25 year review. Am J Ophthalmol 1966;62:499.
10. Epstein DL, Boger WP II, Grant WM: Phenylephrine provocative testing in the pigmentary dispersion syndrome. Am J Ophthalmol 1978;85:43.
11. Richardson TM, Hutchinson BT, Grant WM: The outflow tract in pigmentary glaucoma: A light and electron microscopic study. Arch Ophthalmol 1977;95:1015.
12. Shimizu T, Hara K, Futa R: Fine structure of trabecular meshwork and iris in pigmentary glaucoma. Graefes Arch Clin Exp Ophthalmol 1981;215:171.
13. Campbell DG: Iridotomy and Pigmentary Glaucoma: Humphrey Lecture. Richmond, VA, University of Virginia, 1991.
14. Campbell DG: Pigmentary glaucoma: Past, Present and Future. San Diego, American Glaucoma Society, 1991.
15. Karickhoff JR: Pigment dispersion syndrome and pigmentary glaucoma: A new mechanism concept, a new treatment, and a new technique. Ophthalmic Surg 1992;23:269.
16. Aasved H: Incidence of defects in the pigmented pupillary ruff in eyes with and without fibrillopathia epitheliocapsularis. Acta Ophthalmol (Copenh) 1973;51:710.
17. Layden WE, Shaffer RN: Exfoliation syndrome. Am J Ophthalmol 1974;78:835.
18. Prince AM, Ritch R: Clinical signs of the pseudoexfoliation syndrome. Ophthalmology 1986;93:803.
19. Repo LP, Terasvirta ME, Tuovinen EJ: Generalized peripheral iris transluminance in the pseudoexfoliation syndrome. Ophthalmology 1990;97:1027.
20. Bergmanson JPG, Jones WL, Chu LW-F: Ultrastructural observations on (pseudo-) exfoliation of the lens capsule: A re-examination of the involvement of the lens epithelium. Br J Ophthalmol 1984;68:118.
21. Bertelsen TI, Drablos PA, Flood PR: The so-called senile exfoliation (pseudoexfoliation) of the anterior lens capsule: A product of the lens epithelium, fibrillopathia epitheliocapsularis: A microscopic, histochemical and electron microscopic investigation. Acta Ophthalmol 1964;42:1096.
22. Speakman JS, Ghosh M: The conjunctiva in senile lens exfoliation. Arch Ophthalmol 1976;94:1757.
23. Sugar HS: Onset of the exfoliation syndrome after intracapsular lens extraction. Am J Ophthalmol 1980;89:601.
24. Sugar HS: The pseudoexfoliation syndrome. Metab Pediatr Syst Ophthalmol 1983;6:227.
25. Prince AM, Streeten BW, Ritch R, et al: Preclinical diagnosis of pseudoexfoliation syndrome. Arch Ophthalmol 1987;105:1076.
26. Cashwell LF, Shields MB: Exfoliation syndrome prevalence in a southeastern United States population. Arch Ophthalmol 1988;106:335.
27. Hansen E, Sellevold OJ: Pseudoexfoliation of the lens capsule. I: Clinical evaluation with special regard to the presence of glaucoma. Acta Ophthalmol (Copenh) 1968;46:1095.
28. Hørvon I: Exfoliation syndrome. Arch Ophthalmol 1966;76:505.
29. Lemoine AN: Glaucoma: A statistical review of 816 patients with 1112 glaucomatous eyes. Am J Ophthalmol 1950;33:1353.
30. Brusini P, Tosoni C, Miani P: Increased prevalence of occludable angles and angle-closure glaucoma in patients with pseudoexfoliation (correspondence). Am J Ophthalmol 1994;118:540.
31. Gross FJ, Tingey D, Epstein DL: Increased prevalence of occludable angles and angle-closure glaucoma in patients with pseudoexfoliation. Am J Ophthalmol 1994;117:333.
32. Wishart PK, Spaeth GL, Poryzees EM: Anterior chamber angle in the exfoliation syndrome. Br J Ophthalmol 1985;69:103.
33. Campbell G, Shields MB, Smith TR: The corneal endothelium and the spectrum of essential iris atrophy. Am J Ophthalmol 1978;86:317.
34. Cogan DG, Reese AB: A syndrome of iris nodules, ectopic Descemet's membrane, and unilateral glaucoma. Doc Ophthalmol 1969;26:424.
35. Scheie HG, Yanoff M: Iris nevus (Cogan-Reese) syndrome: A cause of unilateral glaucoma. Arch Ophthalmol 1974;93:963.
36. Shields MB, Campbell DG, Simmons RJ, et al: Iris nodules in essential iris atrophy. Arch Ophthalmol 1976;94:406.
37. Wilson MC, Shields MB: A comparison of the clinical variations of the iridocorneal endothelial syndrome. Arch Ophthalmol 1989; 107:1465.
38. Cibis GW, Krachmer JH, Phelps CB, et al: Iridocorneal adhesions in posterior polymorphous dystrophy. Trans Am Acad Ophthalmol Otol 1978;81:770.
39. Cibis GW, Krachmer JH, Phelps CV, et al: The clinical spectrum of posterior polymorphous dystrophy. Arch Ophthalmol 1977;95:1529.
40. Grayson M: The nature of hereditary deep polymorphous dystrophy of the cornea: Its association with iris and anterior chamber dysgenesis. Trans Am Ophthalmol Soc 1974;72:516.
41. Gregor Z, Hitchings RA: Rieger's anomaly: A 42 year follow-up. Br J Ophthalmol 1980;64:56.
42. Judisch GF, Phelps CD, Hanson J: Rieger's syndrome: A case report with a 15 year follow-up. Arch Ophthalmol 1979;97:2120.
43. Shields MB: Axenfeld-Rieger syndrome: A theory of mechanism and distinctions from the iridocorneal endothelial syndrome. Trans Am Ophthalmol Soc 1983;81:736.
44. Alkemade PPH: Dysgenesis Mesodermalis of the Iris and the Cornea. Assen, The Netherlands, Van Corcum, 1969.
45. Henkind P, Friedman AG: Iridogoniodysgenesis with cataract. Am J Ophthalmol 1971;72:949.
46. Hodes BL, Noecker RJ, Prendiville KJ: Autosomal dominant inheritance of iridogoniodysgenesis and cataract. Ophthalmology 1993;100:168.
47. Spallone A: Retinal detachment in Axenfeld-Rieger syndrome. Br J Ophthalmol 1989;73:559.
48. Shields MB, Buckley E, Klintworth GK, Thresher R: Axenfeld-Rieger syndrome: A spectrum of developmental disorders. Surv Ophthalmol 1985;29:387.
49. Cross HE, Maumenee AE: Progressive spontaneous dissolution of the iris. Surv Ophthalmol 1973;18:186.
50. Rodrigues MC, Spaeth GL, Krahmer JH, et al: Iridoschisis associated with glaucoma and bullous keratopathy. Am J Ophthalmol 1983;95:73.
51. Shields MB, Campbell DG, Simmons RJ: The essential iris atrophies. Am J Ophthalmol 1978;85:749.
52. Shaw BR, Lewis RA: Intraocular pressure elevation after pupillary dilation in open angle glaucoma. Arch Ophthalmol 1987;104:1185.
53. Wand M, Grant WM, Simmons RJ, et al: Plateau iris syndrome. Trans Am Acad Ophthalmol Otol 1977;83:122.
54. Abramson DH, Chang S, Coleman DJ et al: Pilocarpine-induced lens changes: An ultrasonic biometric evaluation of dose response. Arch Ophthalmol 1974;92:464.
55. Abramson DH, Coleman DJ, Forbes, et al: Pilocarpine: Effect on the anterior chamber and lens thickness. Arch Ophthalmol 1972;87:615.
56. Poinoosawmy D, Nagasubramanian S, Brown NAP: Effect of pilocarpine on visual acuity and on the dimensions of the cornea and anterior chamber. Br J Ophthalmol 1976;60:676.
57. Bill A, Phillips CI: Uveoscleral drainage of aqueous humour in human eyes. Exp Eye Res 1971;12:275.
58. Bleiman BS, Schwartz AL: Paradoxical intraocular pressure response to pilocarpine: A proposed mechanism and treatment. Arch Ophthalmol 1979;97:1305.
59. Stark WJ, Michels RG, Maumenee AE, et al: Surgical management of epithelial ingrowth. Am J Ophthalmol 1978;85:772.
60. Weiner MJ, Trentacoste J, Pon DM, et al: Epithelial downgrowth: A 30-year clinicopathological review. Br J Ophthalmol 1989;73:6.
61. Bernardino VB, Kim JC, Smith TR: Epithelialization of the anterior chamber after cataract extraction. Arch Ophthalmol 1969;82:742.
62. Jenson P, Minckler DS, Chandler JW: Epithelial ingrowth. Arch Ophthalmol 1977;95:837.
63. Layden WE, Torczynski E, Font RL: Mucogenic glaucoma and goblet cell cyst of the anterior chamber. Arch Ophthalmol 1978;96:2259.

64. Terry TL, Chisholm JFJ, Schonberg AL: Studies on surface-epithelium invasion of the anterior segment of the eye. Am J Ophthalmol 1939;22:1083.
65. Friedman AH, Henkind P: Corneal stromal overgrowth after cataract extraction. Br J Ophthalmol 1970;54:528.
66. Sherrard ES, Rycroft PV: Retrocorneal membranes: Factors influencing their growth. Br J Ophthalmol 1967;51:387.
67. Swan KC: Fibroblastic ingrowth following cataract extraction. Arch Ophthalmol 1973;89:445.
68. John T, Sassani JW, Eagle RC: The myofibroblastic component of rubeosis iridis. Ophthalmology 1983;90:721.
69. Dickens CJ, Hoskins DH: Epidemiology and pathophysiology of congenital glaucoma. *In* Ritch R, Shields MD, Krupin T (eds): The Glaucomas, 2nd ed, vol 2. St. Louis, Mosby–Year Book, 1996, p 732.
70. Allen RA, Straatsma BR, Apt L, Hall MO: Ocular manifestations of the Marfan syndrome. Trans Am Acad Ophthalmol Otolaryngol 1967;71:18.
71. Dowling JL Jr, Albert DM, Nelson LB, et al: Primary glaucoma associated with iridotrabecular dysgenesis and ectropion uveae. Ophthalmology 1985;92:912.
72. Futterweit W, Ritch R, Teekhasaenee C, et al: Coexistence of Prader-Willi syndrome, congenital ectropion uveae with glaucoma, and factor XI deficiency. JAMA 1986;255:3280.
73. Gramer E, Krieglstein GK: Infantile glaucoma in unilateral uveal ectropion. Graefes Arch Clin Exp Ophthalmol 1979;211:215.
74. Ritch R, Forbes M, Hetherington J Jr, et al: Congenital ectropion uveae with glaucoma. Ophthalmology 1984;91:326.
75. Burke JP, Leitch RJ, Talbot JF, Parsons MA: Choroidal neurofibromatosis with congenital iris ectropion and buphthalmos: Relationship and significance. J Pediatr Ophthalmol Strabismus 1991;28:265.
76. Wilson ME: Congenital iris ectropion as a new classification for anterior dysgenesis. J Pediatr Ophthalmol Strabismus 1990;27:48.
77. Wolter JR, Butler RG: Pigment spots of the iris and ectropion uveae, with glaucoma in neurofibromatosis. Am J Ophthalmol 1963;56:964.
78. Kenyon KR: Mesenchymal dysgenesis in Peters' anomaly, sclerocornea and congenital endothelial dystrophy. Exp Eye Res 1974;21:125.
79. Waring GO, Bourne WM, Edelhauser HF, et al: The corneal endothelium: Normal and pathologic structure and function. Ophthalmology 1982;89:531.
80. Pavlin CJ, Ritch R, Foster FS: Ultrasound biomicroscopy in plateau iris syndrome. Am J Ophthalmol 1992;113:390.
81. Tornquist R: Angle-closure glaucoma in an eye with a plateau type of iris. Acta Ophthalmol (Copenh) 1958;36:413.
82. Hopkins RE, Carriker FR: Malignant melanoma of the ciliary body. Am J Ophthalmol 1958;45:835.
83. Shields MB, Klintworth GK: Anterior uveal melanomas and intraocular pressure. Ophthalmology 1980;87:503.
84. Van Buskirk EM, Leure-duPree AE: Pathophysiology and electron microscopy of melanomalytic glaucoma. Am J Ophthalmol 1978;85:160.
85. Yanoff M, Scheie HG: Melanomalytic glaucoma: Report of a case. Arch Ophthalmol 1970;84:471.
86. Yanoff M: Glaucoma mechanisms in ocular malignant melanomas. Am J Ophthalmol 1970;70:898.
87. Chandler PA, Braconier HE: Spontaneous intraepithelial cysts of iris and ciliary body with glaucoma. Am J Ophthalmol 196445:64.
88. Bron AJ, Wilson CB, Hill AR: Laser treatment of primary ring-shaped epithelial iris cyst. Br J Ophthalmol 1984;68:859.
89. Vela A, Rieser JC, Campbell DG: The heredity and treatment of angle-closure glaucoma secondary to iris and ciliary body cysts. Ophthalmology 1983;91:332.
90. Dvorak-Theobald G, Haas JS: Epithelial invasion of the anterior chamber following cataract extraction. Trans Am Acad Ophthalmol Otolaryngol 1948;52:470.
91. Maumenee AE, Shannon CR: Epithelial invasion of the anterior chamber. Am J Ophthalmol 1956;41:929.
92. Capó H, Palmer E, Nicholson DG: Congenital cysts of the iris stroma. Am J Ophthalmol 1993;116:228.
93. Shields JA: Primary cysts of the iris. Trans Am Ophthalmol Soc 1981;79:771.
94. Sitchevska, Payne BF: Pearl cysts of the iris. Am J Ophthalmol 1951;34:833.
95. Coston T: *In discussion of* Okun E, Mandell A: Photocoagulation treatment of epithelial implantation cysts following cataract surgery. Trans Am Ophthalmol Soc 1974;72:181.
96. L'Esperance FA: Ocular Photocoagulation: An Atlas. St. Louis, CV Mosby, 1975.
97. Okun E, Mandell A: Photocoagulation as a treatment of epithelial implantation cysts following cataract surgery. Trans Am Ophthalmol Soc 1974;74:170.
98. Bruner WE, Michels RG, Stark WJ, Maumenee AE: Management of epithelial cysts of the anterior chamber. Ophthalmic Surg 1981;12:279.
99. Farmer SG, Kalina RE: Epithelial implantation cyst of the iris. Ophthalmology 1981;88:1286.
100. Maumenee AE, Paton D, Morse PH, et al: Review of 40 histologically proven cases of epithelial downgrowth following cataract extraction and suggested surgical management. Am J Ophthalmol 1970;69:598.
101. Cantani A, Leonardi E: Bilateral Fuchs' syndrome of heterochromic cyclitis. Clin Oculist Patol Oculare 1982;3:91.
102. Franceschetti A: Heterochromic cyclitis: Fuchs' syndrome. Am J Ophthalmol 1955;39:50.
103. Jain IS, Gupta A, Gangwar DN, et al: Fuchs' heterochromic cyclitis: Some observations on clinical picture and on cataract surgery. Ann Ophthalmol 1983;15:640.
104. Jones NP: Fuchs' heterochromic uveitis: A reappraisal of the clinical spectrum. Eye 1991;5:649.
105. Dernouchamps JP: Fuchs' heterochromic cyclitis: An IUSG study of 550 cases. *In* Matti Saari K (ed): Uveitis Update. Amsterdam, Elsevier, 1984.
106. Huber A: Glaucoma as a complication in heterochromia of Fuchs'. Ophthalmology 1979;86:1270.
107. La Hey E, de Vries J, Langerhorst CT, et al: Treatment and prognosis of secondary glaucoma in Fuchs' heterochromic iridocyclitis. Am J Ophthalmol 1993;116:327.
108. Liesegang TF: Clinical features and prognosis in Fuchs' uveitis syndrome. Arch Ophthalmol 1982;100:1622.
109. Tabbut BR, Tessler HH, Williams D: Fuchs' heterochromic iridocyclitis in blacks. Arch Ophthalmol 1988;106:1688.
110. Jones NP: Glaucoma in Fuchs' heterochromic uveitis: Aetiology, management, and outcome. Eye 1991;5:662.
111. Lerman S, Levy C: Heterochromic iritis and secondary neovascular glaucoma. Am J Ophthalmol 1964;57:479.
112. Murrell WJ, Shihab Z, Lamberts DW, et al: The corneal endothelium and central corneal thickness in pigmentary dispersion syndrome. Arch Ophthalmol 1986;104:845.
113. Lichter PR: Pigmentary glaucoma: Current concepts. Trans Am Acad Ophthalmol Otolaryngol 1974;78:309.
114. Tawara A: Transformation and cytotoxicity of iron in siderosis bulbi. Invest Ophthalmol Vis Sci 1986;27:226.
115. Alm A, Stjernschantz J, the Scandinavian Latanoprost Study Group: Effects on intraocular pressure and side effects of 0.005% applied once daily, evening or morning: A comparison with timolol. Ophthalmology 1995;102:1744.
116. Watson P, Stjernschantz J, the Latanoprost Study Group: A six-month, randomized, double-masked study comparing latanoprost with timolol in open-angle glaucoma and ocular hypertension. Ophthalmology 1996;103:1.
117. Wistrand PJ, Stjernschantz J, Olsson K: The incidence and time-course of latanoprost-induced iridial pigmentation as a function of eye color. Surv Ophthalmol 1997;41:129.
118. Reese AB, Mund ML, Iwamoto T: Tapioca melanoma of the iris. Part 1: Clinical and light microscopy studies. Am J Ophthalmol 1972;74:840.
119. Shields CL, Shields JA, De Potter P, et al: Treatment of nonresectable, malignant iris tumors with custom-designed plaque radiotherapy. Br J Ophthalmol 1995;79:306.
120. Shields CL, Shields JA, Shields MB, et al: Prevalence and mechanisms of secondary intraocular pressure elevation in eyes with intraocular tumors. Ophthalmology 1987;95:839.
121. Shields JA, Sanborn GE, Augsberger JJ: The differential diagnosis of iris melanomas. Ophthalmology 198;90:716.
122. Sugar HS: The iris nevus and Cogan-Reese syndrome: Separate entities? Ann Ophthalmol 1981;13:405.
123. Coats G: Unilateral diffuse melanosis of the uvea, with small elevations on the surface of the iris. Trans Ophthalmol Soc UK 1912;32:165.
124. Collins ET: Unilateral melanosis of the uvea and sclera, with numerous small elevations on the surface of the iris. Trans Ophthalmol Soc UK 1912;32:171.

125. Joondeph BC, Goldberg MF: Familial iris melanosis—a misnomer? Br J Ophthalmol 1989;73:289.
126. Trabousli EI, Maumenee IH: Bilateral melanosis of the iris (letter). Am J Ophthalmol 1987;103:115.
127. Ticho BH, Rosner M, Mets M, et al: Bilateral diffuse iris nodular nevi: Clinical and histopathologic characterization. Ophthalmology 1995;02:419.
128. Bolande RP: The neurocristopathies: A unifying concept of disease arising in neural crest maldevelopment. Hum Pathol 1974;5:409.
129. Perry HD, Font RL: Iris nodules in von Recklinghausen's neurofibromatosis: Electron microscopic confirmation of their melanocytic origin. Arch Ophthalmol 1982;100:1635.
130. Ragge NK, Falk RE, Cohen WE, et al: Images of Lisch nodules across the spectrum. Eye 1993;7:95.
131. Williamson TH, Garner A, Moore AT: Structure of Lisch nodules in neurofibromatosis type 1. Ophthalmic Paediatr Genet 1991;12:11.
132. Fishman RFA, Anderson R: Nevus of Ota. Am J Ophthalmol 1962;54:453.
133. Foulks GN, Shields MB: Glaucoma in oculodermal melanocytosis. Ann Ophthalmol 1977;9:1299.
134. Liu JC, Ball ST: Nevus of Ota with glaucoma: Report of three cases. Ann Ophthalmol 1991;23:286.
135. Teekhasaenee C, Ritch R, Rutnin U, et al: Glaucoma in oculodermal melanocytosis. Ophthalmology 1990;97:562.
136. Weiss DI, Krohn DL: Benign melanocytic glaucoma complicating oculodermal melanocytosis. Ann Ophthalmol 1971;3:958.
137. Bruner WE, Stark WJ, Green WR: Presumed juvenile xanthogranuloma of the iris and ciliary body in an adult. Arch Ophthalmol 1982;100:457.
138. Schwartz LW, Rodrigues MM, Hallett JW: Juvenile xanthogranuloma diagnosed by paracentesis. Am J Ophthalmol 1974;77:243.
139. Zimmerman L: Ocular lesions of juvenile xanthogranuloma (nevoxanthoendothelioma). Trans Am Acad Ophthalmol Otol 1965; 69:412.
140. Duker JS, Shields JA, Ross M: Intraocular large cell lymphoma presenting as massive thickening of the uveal tract. Retina 1987;7:41.
141. Shields JA, Shields CL: Intraocular lymphoid tumors and leukemias. *In* Shields JA, Shields CL (eds): Intraocular Tumors: A Text and Atlas. Philadelphia, WB Saunders, 1992.
142. Broughton WL, Zimmerman LE: A clinicopathologic study of 56 cases of intraocular medulloepitheliomas. Am J Ophthalmol 1978;85:407.
143. Obenauf CD, Shaw HE, Sydnor CF, et al: Sarcoidosis and its ophthalmic manifestations. Am J Ophthalmol 1978;87:648.
144. Rothova A, La Hey E, Baarsma GS, et al: Iris nodules in Fuchs' heterochromic uveitis. Am J Ophthalmol 1994;118:338.
145. Bresnick GH, De Venecia G, Myers FL, et al: Retinal ischemia in diabetic retinopathy. Arch Ophthalmol 1975;93:1300.
146. Laatikainen L, Kohner EM: Fluorescein angiography and its prognostic significance in central retinal vein occlusion. Br J Ophthalmol 1976;60:411.
147. Wise GN: Retinal neovascularization. Trans Am Ophthalmol Soc 1956;54:729.
148. Federman JL, Brown GC, Felberg NT, et al: Experimental ocular angiogenesis. Am J Ophthalmol 1980;89:231.
149. Glaser BM, D'Amore PA, Michels RG, et al: The demonstration of angiogenic activity from ocular tissues: Preliminary report. Ophthalmology 1980;87:440.
150. Gu Xg, Fry GL, Lata GF, et al: Ocular neovascularization: Tissue cultures studies. Arch Ophthalmol 1985;103:111.
151. Patz A: Studies on retinal neovascularization. Invest Ophthalmol Vis Sci 1980;19:1133.
152. Brown GC, Magargal LE, Schachat A, et al: Neovascular glaucoma: Etiologic considerations. Ophthalmology 1984;91:315.
153. Hoskins HD Jr: Neovascular glaucoma: Current concepts. Trans Am Acad Ophthalmol Otol 1974;78:330.
154. Wand M, Ducker DK, Aiello LM, et al: Effects of panretinal photocoagulation on rubeosis iridis, angle neovascularization, and neovascular glaucoma. Am J Ophthalmol 1978;86:332.
155. Browning DJ: Risk of missing angle neovascularization by omitting screening gonioscopy in patients with diabetes mellitus. Am J Ophthalmol 1991;112:212.
156. Wand M, Madigan JC: Angle neovascularization as a marker for aqueous outflow after argon laser trabeculoplasty. Ophthalmic Surg 1991;22:114.
157. Jocson VL: Microvascular injection studies in rubeosis iridis and neovascular glaucoma. Am J Ophthalmol 1977;83:508.
158. Anderson DM, Morin JD, Hunter WS: Rubeosis iridis. Can J Ophthalmol 1971;6:183.
159. Schulze RR: Rubeosis iridis. Am J Ophthalmol 1967;63:487.
160. Jacobson DR, Murphy RP, Rosenthal AR: The treatment of angle neovascularization with panretinal photocoagulation. Ophthalmology 1979;86:1270.
161. Laatikainen L, Kohner EM, Khoury D, et al: Panretinal photocoagulation in central retinal vein occlusion: A randomised clinical study. Br J Ophthalmol 1977;61:741.
162. Laatikainen L: Preliminary report on effect of retinal photocoagulation on rubeosis iridis and neovascular glaucoma. Br J Ophthalmol 1977;61:278.
163. Little HL, Rosenthal AR, Dellaporta A, et al: The effect of panretinal photocoagulation on rubeosis iridis. Am J Ophthalmol 1976;81:804.
164. Murphy RP, Egbert PR: Regression of iris neovascularization following panretinal photocoagulation. Arch Ophthalmol 1979;97:700.
165. Pavan PR, Folk JC, Weingeist TA, et al: Diabetic rubeosis and panretinal photocoagulation: A prospective, controlled, masked trial using iris fluorescein angiography. Arch Ophthalmol 1983;101:882.
166. May DR, Bergstrom TJ, Parmet AJ, et al: Treatment of neovascular glaucoma with transscleral panretinal cryotherapy. Ophthalmology 1980;87:1106.
167. Flanagan DW, Blach RK: Place of panretinal photocoagulation and trabeculectomy in the management of neovascular glaucoma. Br J Ophthalmol 1983;67:526.
168. Wand M, Hutchinson BT: The surgical management of neovascular glaucoma. Pers Ophthalmol 1980;4:147.
169. Cobb B: Vascular tufts at the pupillary margin: A preliminary report on 44 patients. Trans Ophth Soc UK 1968;88:211.
170. Cobb G, Shilling JS, Chisholm IH: Vascular tufts at the pupillary margin in myotonic dystrophy. Am J Ophthalmol 1970;69:573.
171. Mason GI: Iris neovascular tufts: Relationship to rubeosis, insulin, and hypotony. Arch Ophthalmol 1979;97:2346.
172. Mason GI, Ferry AP: Bilateral spontaneous hyphema arising from iridic microhemangiomas. Ann Ophthalmol 1979;11:87.
173. Perry HD, Mallen FJ, Sussman W: Microhaemangiomas of the iris with spontaneous hyphaema and acute glaucoma. Br J Ophthalmol 1977;61:114.
174. Coleman SL, Green WR, Patz A: Vascular tufts of pupillary margin of iris. Am J Ophthalmol 1977;83:881.
175. Hoskins HD Jr, Shaffer RN, Hetherington J Jr: Anatomical classification of the developmental glaucomas. Arch Ophthalmol 1984; 102:1331.

CHAPTER 15

Crystalline Lens, Refractive Error, and Cataract Surgery

KARL J. SIEBERT

We are commonly confronted with a patient in whom the lens may be a consideration in the diagnosis of glaucoma. This may be a developmental or acquired association. Additionally, glaucoma and cataracts are more common in the elderly population. Therefore, the treatment of the cataract can lead to glaucoma. In this chapter, Karl Siebert discusses the impact of the lens on glaucoma. He begins with diagnostic signs of the crystalline lens that will aid in glaucoma diagnosis. He then describes conditions in which glaucoma and cataracts coexist alone or with other eye findings; the discussion includes the role of intraocular inflammation and abnormal lens size or position in the pathogenesis of glaucoma. Specific forms of glaucoma are then discussed with respect to the refractive state of the eye, either myopia or hyperopia. Finally, Dr. Siebert addresses the roles of cataract extraction and posterior capsulotomy and their relationship to glaucoma. The role of combined cataract and glaucoma surgery is specifically dealt with in Chapter 23.

Inspection of the crystalline lens is an important part of any ophthalmologic examination. Often this examination reveals characteristic lenticular findings that may aid the clinician in determining an etiology of elevated intraocular pressure (IOP) or assessing the risk of developing glaucoma in the future. This chapter reviews the clinical signs and pathogenesis of the more common conditions associated with glaucoma and abnormalities of the lens; they include diseases in which the lens is secondarily affected by the pathologic process (e.g., pseudoexfoliation syndrome) and those in which lens abnormalities may be directly or indirectly responsible for the associated glaucoma (e.g., pupillary block). Because the refractive state of the eye may be considered a clinical sign in the examination of patients with ocular hypertension or glaucoma, this chapter also addresses the association between the refractive state of the eye and different types of glaucoma.

With a population advancing in age, the coexistence of open-angle glaucoma and visually significant cataract has become an increasingly common phenomenon. Many of these patients require surgical intervention, so the decision-making process for managing patients with glaucoma and cataracts is explored. In addition, the clinical signs and pathogenesis of elevated postoperative IOP are reviewed. Finally, certain topics related to both cataract surgery and glaucoma are discussed, including aphakia, malignant glaucoma, and neodymium:yttrium-aluminum-garnet (Nd:YAG) laser posterior capsulotomy.

Clinical Signs of the Crystalline Lens and Their Role in Diagnosis and Management of Glaucoma

THE CRYSTALLINE LENS

Certain disease processes causing elevated IOP and glaucoma affect multiple components of the anterior segment, including the crystalline lens, iris, and anterior chamber angle. In the evaluation of patients who have elevated

TABLE 15–1. CONDITIONS ASSOCIATED WITH CHANGES IN THE ANTERIOR LENS AND GLAUCOMA

Pseudoexfoliation syndrome (material on anterior lens capsule)
Pigment dispersion syndrome (pigment on lens capsule)
Acute angle-closure glaucoma (glaukomflecken)
Uveitis (posterior synechiae)
Trauma (anterior subcapsular opacities)

IOP or who are at risk for glaucoma, a careful slit-lamp examination may reveal characteristic lenticular findings. The conditions discussed here represent clinical signs of diseases that, in addition to causing glaucoma, are frequently associated with pathology of the lens. In general, the abnormalities of the lens in these conditions are not responsible for the glaucoma, but they should be considered as important ancillary findings that may aid in proper diagnosis and management.

Conditions Associated with Glaucoma and Lens Capsular Changes (Table 15–1)

Certain disorders associated with elevated IOP and glaucoma demonstrate characteristic abnormalities of the anterior or posterior lens capsule. Close inspection may reveal these changes and aid in the diagnosis of the following conditions.

PSEUDOEXFOLIATION SYNDROME

Pseudoexfoliation (PXF) syndrome is an age-related disease of uncertain etiology in which abnormally produced basement membrane components accumulate in the anterior segment structures. The term *pseudoexfoliation* was coined by Dvorak-Theobold[1] in an attempt to avoid confusion with the condition of true lens capsule exfoliation seen in glassblowers.

The incidence of PXF syndrome is age-dependent, varies among ethnic populations, and seems to affect women two to three times more frequently than men. Numerous population studies have shown a significant increase in the occurrence of PXF syndrome with age. The prevalence of the disorder in the Framingham study was 2.6% for patients aged 65 to 74 years and 5% for those 75 years or older.[2] In Scandinavia, it is estimated that as much as 25% of the population older than 60 years have PXF syndrome.[3] Although less common than in Caucasian people, this disorder has been reported in most ethnic groups, including Middle Eastern, Mediterranean, Japanese, Chinese, and African-American people.[4–9]

The origin of pseudoexfoliation material is speculated to arise from a disorder of basement membrane production. Electron microscopy and immunohistochemical studies of PXF material have identified amyloid-like proteins and glycosaminoglycans consistent with abnormal production and altered metabolism of extracellular matrix components normally found in basement membranes.[10, 11]

Clinically, this material has been located on the lens capsule, zonular apparatus, iris, ciliary body, trabecular meshwork, and extraocular structures such as skin and kidneys.[6, 12, 13] Frequently, a central area of whitish, flaky material can be observed on the anterior lens capsule, surrounded by an intermediate clear zone where the material has been displaced by the posterior iris (Fig. 15–1).

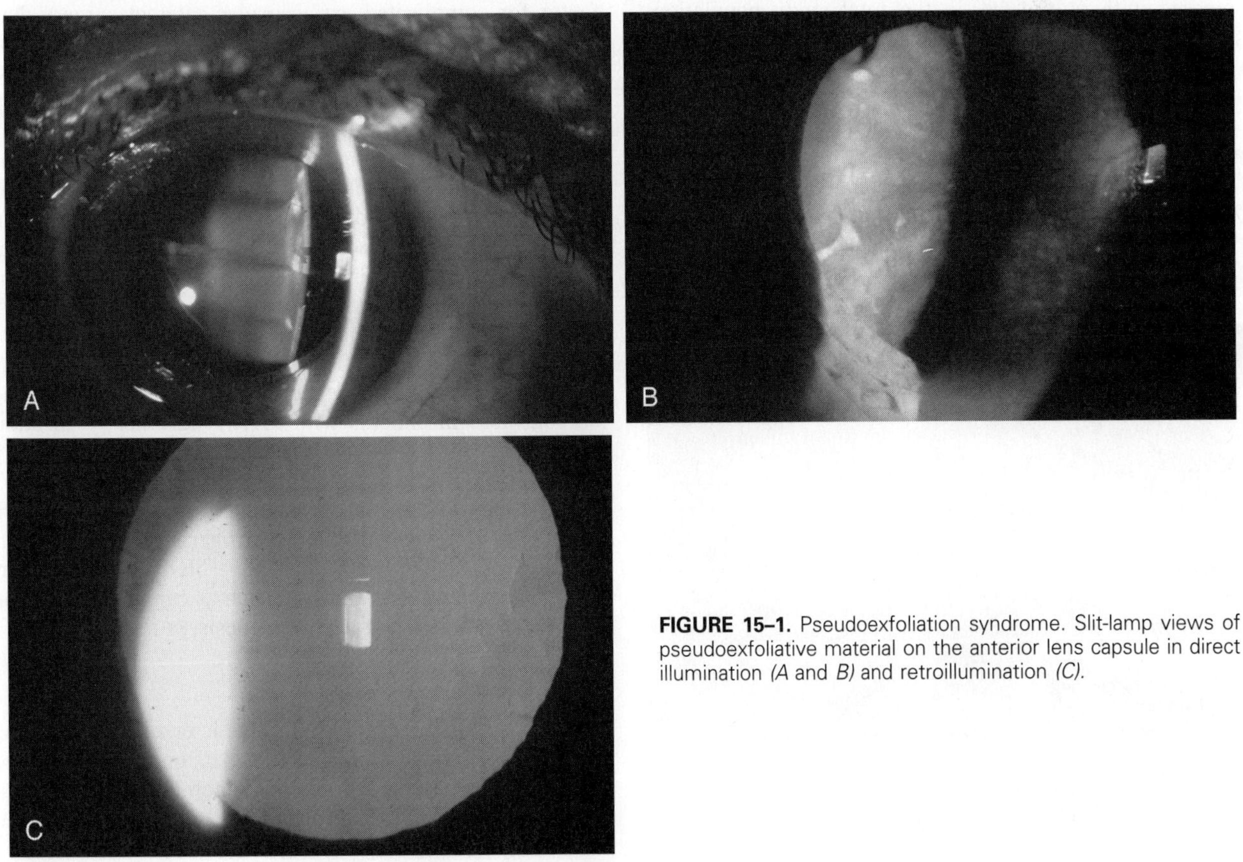

FIGURE 15–1. Pseudoexfoliation syndrome. Slit-lamp views of pseudoexfoliative material on the anterior lens capsule in direct illumination *(A* and *B)* and retroillumination *(C)*.

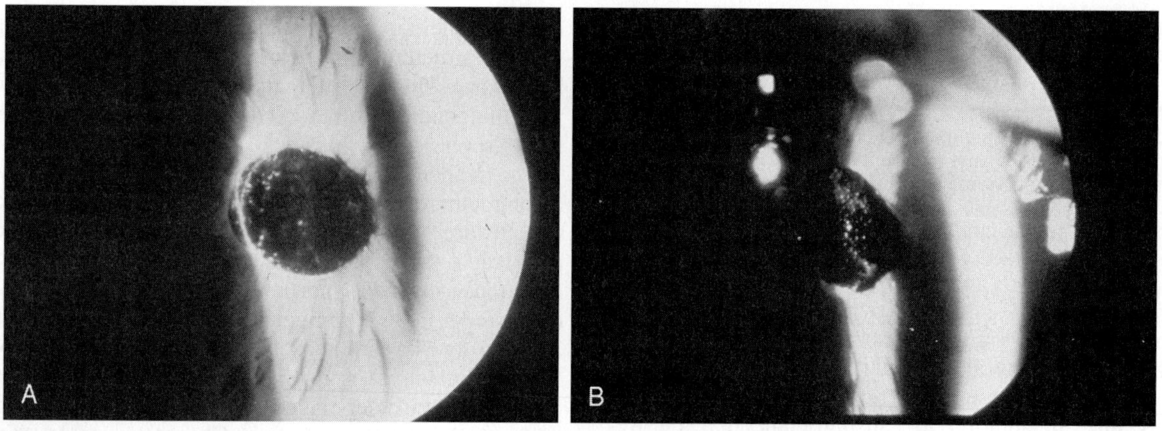

FIGURE 15–2. Pseudoexfoliation syndrome. Slit-lamp views of pseudoexfoliative material deposited on the anterior hyaloid face following intracapsular cataract extraction *(A)* and on a posterior chamber lens following extracapsular surgery *(B)*.

Deposits of PXF material on intraocular lens implants and the anterior hyaloid face after cataract extraction have been described[14] (Fig. 15–2). Peripupillary iris transillumination defects are a common finding. Accumulation of this material within the trabecular meshwork, noted clinically as an increased pigmentation, is hypothesized to cause an alteration in function of the meshwork and subsequent eventual elevation of IOP[15] (Fig. 15–3).

The association between PXF syndrome and open-angle glaucoma is well documented. Henry and associates[16] found the cumulative probability for elevated IOP in eyes with PXF syndrome was 5.3% at 5 years and 15.4% at 10 years. A prospective consecutive case series reported by Cashwell and Shields[17] found the prevalence of pseudoexfoliation to be 6.0% in patients with open-angle glaucoma compared with only 1.6% in the total study population. Pseudoexfoliation has been described in as many as 50% to 90% of patients with open-angle glaucoma in the Scandinavian countries.[3, 18]

Mounting evidence also supports an association between PXF syndrome and angle-closure glaucoma. Examination of the anterior chamber angle in patients with PXF syndrome by Wishart and colleagues[19] and Gross and coworkers[20] found occludable angles in 18% and 9%, respectively, compared with only 4% of the normal population. In a consecutive series of 60 patients with either acute angle closure or gonioscopically occludable angles, Ritch[21] found that 25% of patients demonstrated clinically evident PXF syndrome.

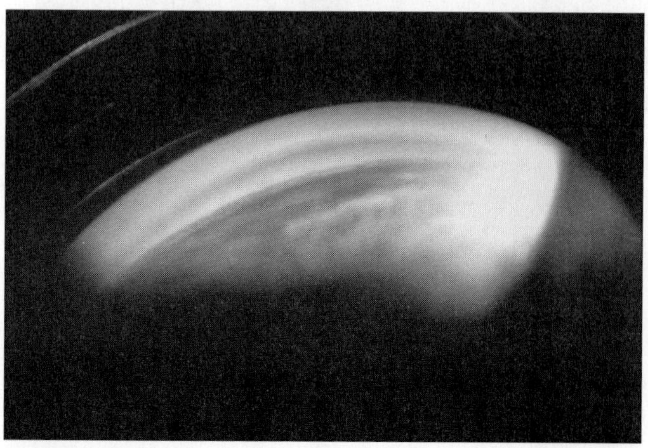

FIGURE 15–3. Gonioscopic view of the anterior chamber angle in a patient with pseudoexfoliation syndrome. Note the hyperpigmentation anterior to Schwalbe's line (Sampaolesi's sign).

A relationship between PXF syndrome and cataractous changes of the crystalline lens has been suggested. Comparing glaucomatous eyes with PXF syndrome to normal fellow eyes in patients with unilateral PXF syndrome, Puska[22] observed a significantly greater occurrence of subcapsular cataracts in the eyes with PXF syndrome. Using an opacity lens meter, Fama and associates[23] showed a higher lens opacity value for eyes with PXF syndrome than in normal eyes.

The presence of PXF syndrome is considered a risk factor for complicated extracapsular cataract surgery. Numerous case reports exist describing dislocation of the crystalline lens into the vitreous cavity during otherwise uncomplicated cataract surgery in patients with PXF syndrome.[5, 24] In a prospective study of extracapsular cataract surgery performed by seven different surgeons, Guzek and associates[4] found a four-fold risk of zonular breaks in patients with PXF syndrome compared with patients without evidence of the disease. Histopathologic examinations of eyes with PXF syndrome have demonstrated alterations in the zonular apparatus, including infiltration and apparent weakening of the zonular attachments to the pars plicata and capsular surface.[25] These findings likely explain the observed increased incidence of zonular dehiscence and vitreous loss in patients with PXF syndrome.[4, 26] In addition, eyes with PXF syndrome are predisposed to poorly dilating pupils and early postoperative pressure spikes.[27, 28]

Although PXF syndrome should be considered a risk factor for complicated cataract surgery, intraocular lens implantation is not contraindicated.[27, 29] Extra vigilance during the preoperative evaluation, such as careful observation of the crystalline lens for phacodenesis, is recommended.[24]

PIGMENTARY GLAUCOMA

Pigment dispersion syndrome is characterized by liberation of pigment from the iris, which deposits on the anterior and posterior lens capsule, corneal endothelium, and trabecular meshwork. When the amount of pigment accumulated

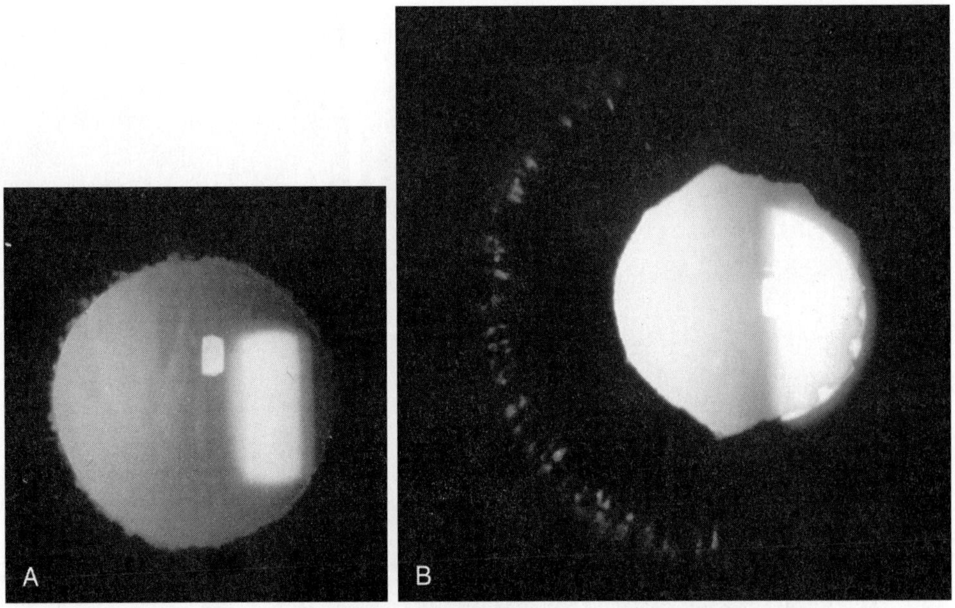

FIGURE 15–4. Iris transillumination defects. Note the difference between the peripupillary defects seen in pseudoexfoliation syndrome *(A)* and the midperipheral defects found in pigment dispersion syndrome *(B)*.

within the trabecular meshwork is sufficient to cause elevated IOP, presumably via obstruction of aqueous outflow, the term *pigmentary glaucoma* is often used. The etiology of pigment dispersion syndrome is an abnormal anatomic relationship between the midperipheral posterior iris and the lens zonules (Fig. 15–4). For a more detailed description of the etiology and treatment of pigmentary glaucoma see Chapter 14.

Clinical examination of the crystalline lens may reveal pigment deposition on the anterior and posterior lens capsule, frequently near the lens equator along the insertion of the lens zonules (Fig. 15–5).

GLAUKOMFLECKEN

Glaukomflecken is the term given to multiple, small, white opacities that develop in the central anterior subcapsular region of the crystalline lens following an acute attack of angle-closure glaucoma (Fig. 15–6). Histologically, glau-

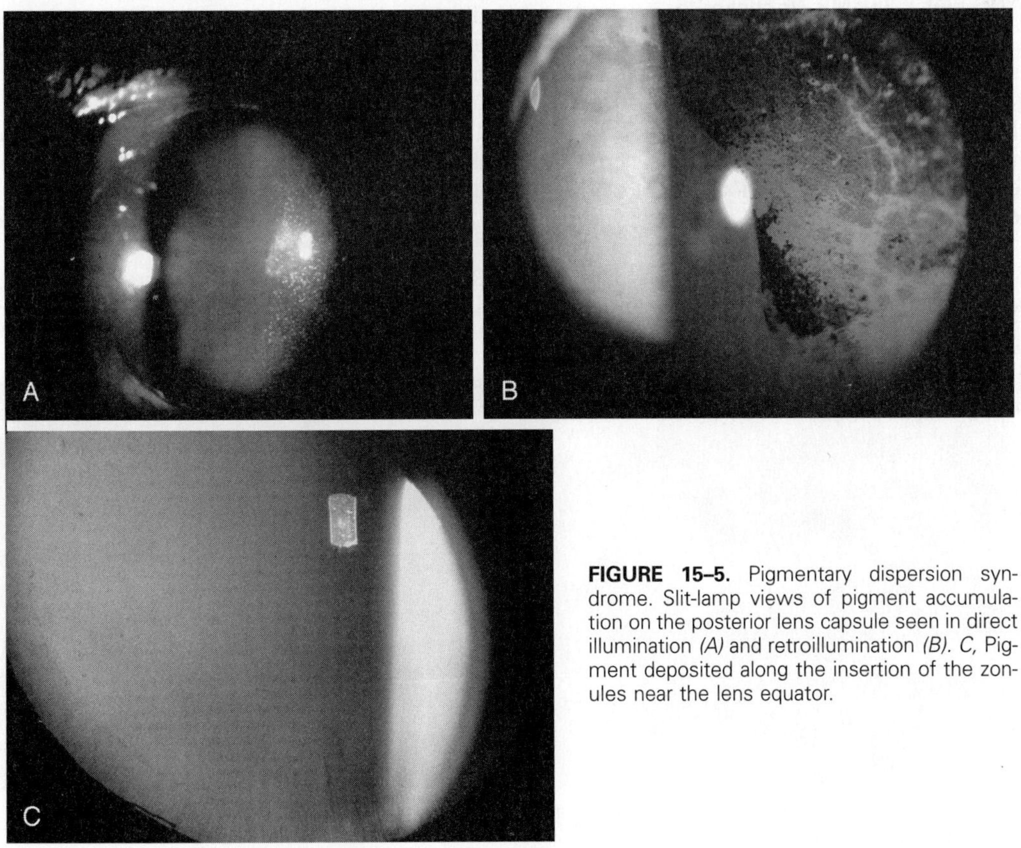

FIGURE 15–5. Pigmentary dispersion syndrome. Slit-lamp views of pigment accumulation on the posterior lens capsule seen in direct illumination *(A)* and retroillumination *(B)*. *C,* Pigment deposited along the insertion of the zonules near the lens equator.

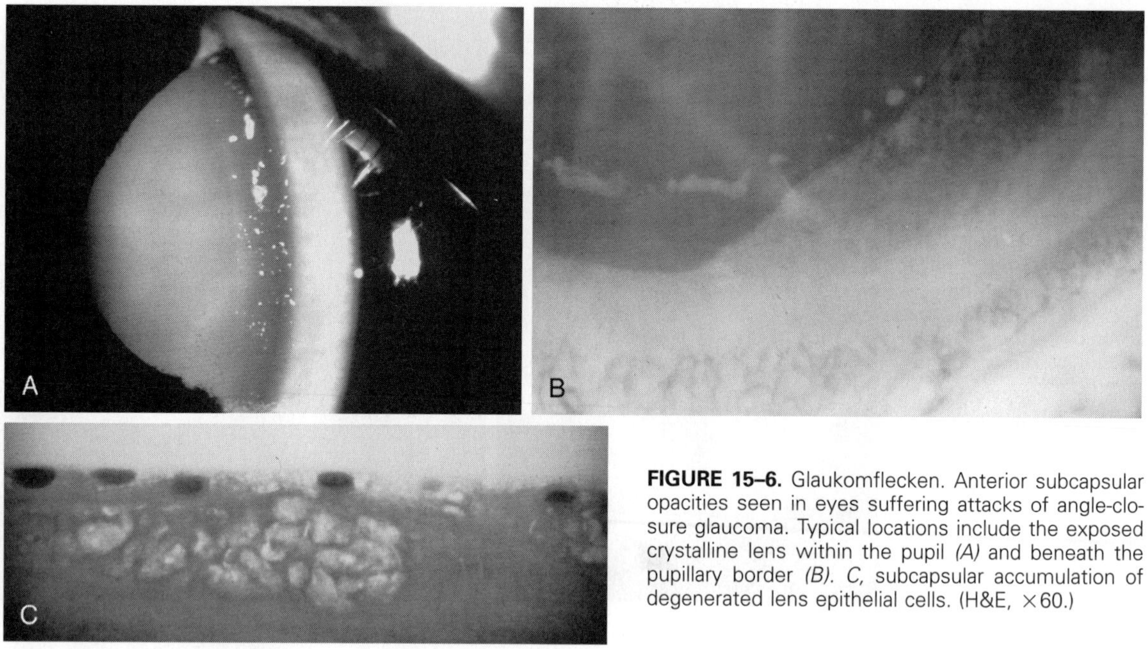

FIGURE 15–6. Glaukomflecken. Anterior subcapsular opacities seen in eyes suffering attacks of angle-closure glaucoma. Typical locations include the exposed crystalline lens within the pupil *(A)* and beneath the pupillary border *(B)*. *C,* subcapsular accumulation of degenerated lens epithelial cells. (H&E, ×60.)

komflecken represent focal necrosis of the anterior lens epithelium, presumably as a result of anoxia related to the acute elevation of IOP.[30, 31] As new lens fibers are formed, the opacities are displaced posteriorly, where they may coalesce into discrete plaques or may disappear completely.[32] Observation of glaukomflecken in an eye with a history of pain and redness should alert the clinician to the diagnosis of acute angle-closure glaucoma.

POSTERIOR SYNECHIAE (EVIDENCE OF PREVIOUS UVEITIS)

Glaucoma is a well-known complication of uveitis.[33, 34] Anterior segment inflammation may result in reduced trabecular meshwork outflow via obstruction by debris, release of humoral mediators, and formation of peripheral anterior synechiae. Evidence of previous anterior uveitis involving the crystalline lens includes posterior synechiae and anterior subcapsular cataracts (Figs. 15–7 and 15–8). When extensive, posterior synechiae may lead to pupillary block and acute angle closure (Fig. 15–9). Traditionally, filtration surgery in chronically inflamed eyes carries a guarded prognosis, although the use of antimetabolites may increase the success rate.[35, 36]

Conditions Associated with Glaucoma and Cataracts (Table 15–2)

Nonspecific age-related cataract is a common finding in patients with open-angle glaucoma. However, certain conditions associated with glaucoma demonstrate characteristic lenticular opacities that may aid in diagnosis and management. Although numerous syndromes and diseases have been associated with cataracts and glaucoma (see Table 15–2), this section reviews only those entities for which the clinical signs and pathogenesis have been extensively described.

RUBELLA CATARACT

Rubella virus is an RNA togavirus capable of both acquired and congenital human infection. If primary rubella infec-

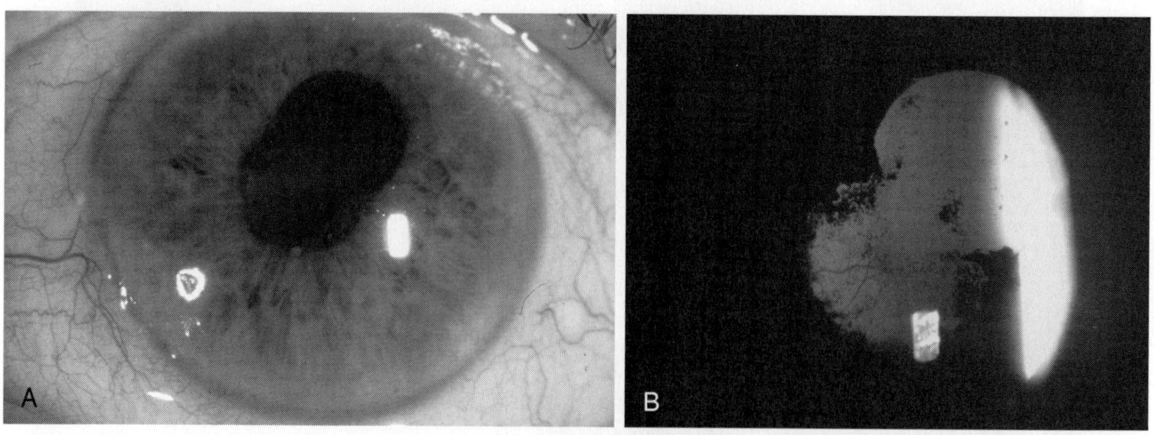

FIGURE 15–7. Evidence of intraocular inflammation. Slit-lamp view of posterior synechiae in a patient with ankylosing spondylitis. *A,* direct illumination; *B,* retroillumination.

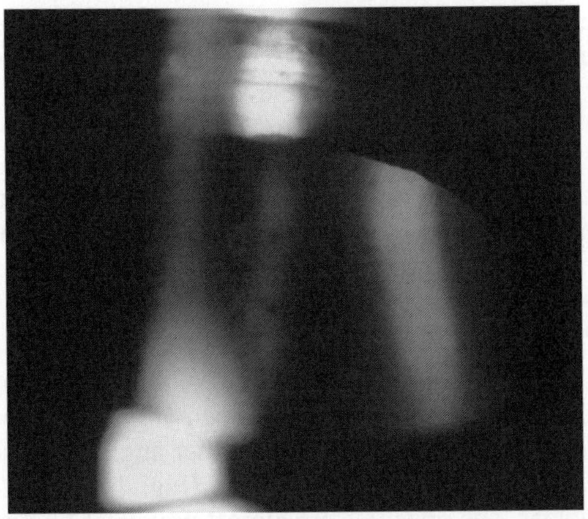

FIGURE 15–8. Slit-lamp view demonstrating anterior capsular remnants of broken posterior synechiae in a patient with idiopathic chronic anterior uveitis.

tion occurs in a mother during the first 12 weeks of pregnancy, there is a significant risk that the virus will cross the placenta and cause multisystem fetal infection.[37] The incidence of rubella-related defects decreases when maternal infection occurs between 13 and 16 weeks of pregnancy, and only rarely occurs with exposure after 16 weeks of gestation. Unlike acquired rubella infection, which is a short-lived process with clinically detectable viremia lasting only about 48 hours, congenital infection can persist throughout gestation. Live virus has been detected in the infant aqueous humor and lens material as late as 22 months after birth.[38]

Neonatal cataract and glaucoma are two clinically recognized features of the congenital rubella syndrome. Rubella-related cataract has been described either as a dense, central, white nuclear opacity with a relatively clear periphery or as a more uniform opacity involving the central and peripheral nucleus.[39, 40] The amount of cortical degeneration is variable, with some lenses assuming a spherophakic contour.

Glaucoma arising in the congenital rubella syndrome may result either from dysgenesis of the anterior chamber angle and trabecular meshwork or from postinflammatory

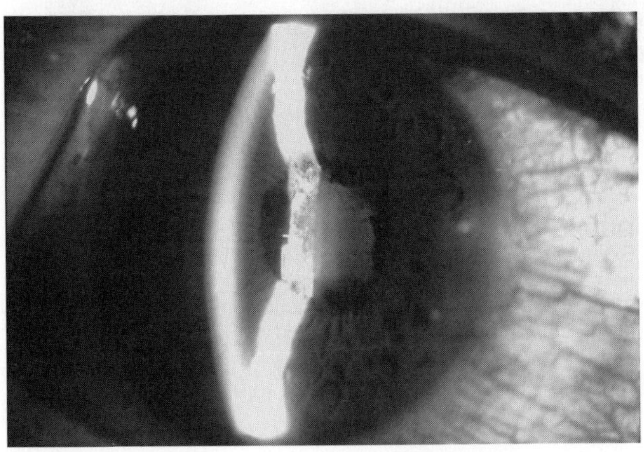

FIGURE 15–9. Slit-lamp view of iris bombé secondary to extensive posterior synechiae in a patient with sarcoid uveitis.

TABLE 15–2. SYNDROMES AND DISEASES ASSOCIATED WITH CATARACTS AND GLAUCOMA

Chromosome 13q partial deletion (long-arm) syndrome
Cockayne's syndrome (dwarfism with retinal atrophy and deafness)
Congenital rubella syndrome
Craniofacial dysostosis (Crouzon's syndrome)
Cretinism (congenital hypothyroidism)
Diabetes mellitus
Familial histiocytic dermatoarthritis syndrome
Fetal alcohol syndrome
Fuchs' heterochromic iridocyclitis
Gorlin-Goltz syndrome (multiple basal cell nevi syndrome)
Hallermann-Streiff syndrome (oculomadibulofacial dyscephaly)
Vogt-Koyanagi-Harada syndrome
Homocystinuria
Klippel-Trenaunay-Weber syndrome (angio-osteohypertrophy syndrome)
Krause's syndrome (congenital encephalo-ophthalmic dysplasia)
Lowe's syndrome (oculocerebrorenal syndrome)
Marfan's syndrome
Morquio's syndrome (mucopolysaccharidoses type IV syndrome)
Nieden's syndrome (telangiectasia-cataract syndrome)
Pierre Robin syndrome (micrognathia-glossoptosis syndrome)
Prader-Willi syndrome (hypogenital dystrophy with diabetic tendency)
Pseudoexfoliation syndrome
Rubinstein-Taybi syndrome (broad thumbs syndrome)
Stickler's syndrome (hereditary progressive arthro-ophthalmopathy)
Still's disease (juvenile rheumatoid arthritis)
Toxocariasis
Trisomy 13 syndrome (Patau's syndrome)
Trisomy 16 syndrome (Edwards' syndrome)
Trisomy 21 syndrome (Down's syndrome)
Turner's syndrome (gonadal dysgenesis)
Usher's syndrome (retinitis pigmentosa-deafness syndrome)
von Recklinghausen's syndrome (neurofibromatosis)
Wagner's syndrome (hyaloidoretinal degeneration)
Wilm's aniridia syndrome
Zellweger's syndrome (cerebrohepatorenal syndrome)

changes induced by anterior segment infection. Clinically, glaucoma associated with congenital rubella infection closely resembles primary congenital glaucoma. The diagnosis of congenital rubella syndrome should be considered in any child who presents with congenital cataracts and glaucoma. In such patients, an appropriate search should be undertaken for systemic involvement, including hearing loss and cardiac defects.

RETINITIS PIGMENTOSA CATARACT

Retinitis pigmentosa (RP) is an inherited retinal disease characterized by progressive retinal atrophy, nyctalopia, and visual field loss. Inheritance can be autosomal dominant, autosomal recessive, or X-linked. Cases without evidence of affected family members are termed *simplex.* Characteristic findings include pigment migration into the retina ("bone-spicule" appearance), attenuated retinal vasculature, and "waxy" pallor of the optic nerve.[41]

Characteristic posterior subcapsular cataracts are associated with RP.[41, 42] In an analysis of 345 eyes from 291 patients with RP, Heckenlively[42] found posterior subcapsular cataracts present in 41%. Although anatomically subcapsular in nature, the cataracts in patients with RP typically have a slightly different clinical picture from that of

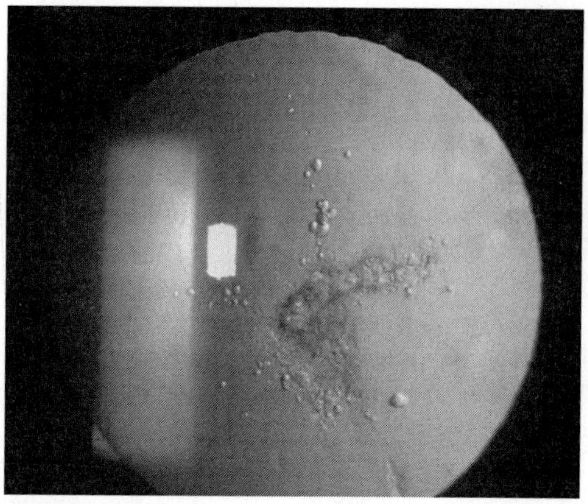

FIGURE 15–10. Retroillumination slit-lamp view of a posterior cortical cataract in a patient with retinitis pigmentosa. (Courtesy of Dr. Richard A. Lewis.)

age-related or corticosteroid-induced lens opacities. Generally, RP cataracts consist of focal, amorphous, yellow-white granular material that clusters in the posterior cortex slightly anterior to the posterior capsule (Fig. 15–10).

The association between RP and glaucoma is less well defined. Although the prevalence of open-angle glaucoma in patients with RP is estimated to be between 2% and 12%, these data rely on relatively small sample sizes with differing criteria for the diagnosis of glaucoma.[43–45] The diagnosis of glaucoma in the patient with RP can also be difficult, owing to the high frequency of optic atrophy and peripheral visual field changes caused by the primary retinal disease.

There have been reports of an association between RP and angle-closure glaucoma.[45–47] Badeeb and coworkers[45] found the prevalence of angle closure in 538 Canadian patients with RP to be approximately 1%, a number higher than expected when compared with a normal age-matched population. The reason for this apparent association is unclear, but it suggests that careful gonioscopy should be performed in all patients with RP.

FUCHS' HETEROCHROMIC IRIDOCYCLITIS

Fuchs' heterochromic iridocyclitis is a chronic, nongranulomatous uveitis associated with open-angle glaucoma, iris heterochromia, subtle anterior chamber angle neovascularization, and fine keratic precipitates (Fig. 15–11). Cortical and nuclear lens opacities are almost universal findings and occur at a younger age in the affected eye.[48, 49] Intraoperative anterior chamber hemorrhage and persistent postoperative uveitis are well-described complications of cataract surgery.[50, 51] For a more detailed description of the pathogenesis and clinical findings of Fuchs' heterochromic iridocyclitis, see Chapters 12 and 14.

CORTICOSTEROID-INDUCED CATARACT

Posterior subcapsular cataract (PSC) formation is a common side effect of corticosteroid use.[52–56] Depending on the dose, frequency, and route of administration of corticosteroids, the incidence of steroid-induced PSC is between 3% and 30%.[52, 55, 56] Young patients receiving high-dose, long-term systemic therapy for conditions such as juvenile rheumatoid arthritis and nephrotic syndrome or because they have undergone transplantation are more likely to experi-

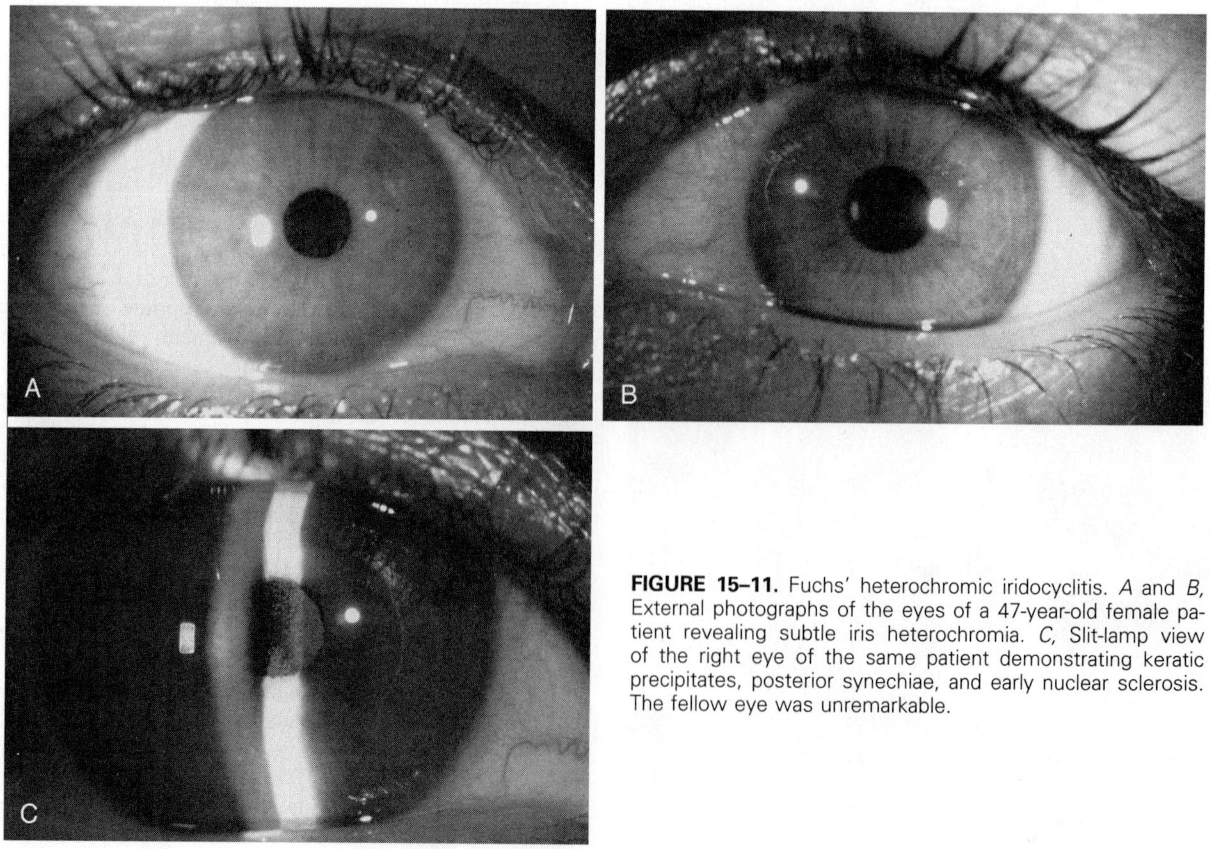

FIGURE 15–11. Fuchs' heterochromic iridocyclitis. *A* and *B*, External photographs of the eyes of a 47-year-old female patient revealing subtle iris heterochromia. *C*, Slit-lamp view of the right eye of the same patient demonstrating keratic precipitates, posterior synechiae, and early nuclear sclerosis. The fellow eye was unremarkable.

TABLE 15–3. CONDITIONS ASSOCIATED WITH IRIS ABNORMALITIES, GLAUCOMA, AND LENS CHANGES

Pseudoexfoliation syndrome
Pigment dispersion syndrome
Postoperative status
Trauma
Uveitis-glaucoma-hyphema (UGH) syndrome

TABLE 15–4. CONDITIONS ASSOCIATED WITH LENS-INDUCED INFLAMMATION AND GLAUCOMA

Phacolytic glaucoma
Phacoantigenic (phacoanaphylactic) uveitis
Retained cortical material (following cataract extraction)

ence PSC. Those patients receiving only intermittent treatment for diseases such as asthma are less likely to incur PSC.

Elevated IOP induced by systemic and topical corticosteroids is a well-described phenomenon, and concomitant steroid-induced cataract has been reported.[57–63] As much as 6% of a normal population may exhibit a marked increase in IOP following the administration of short-term topical ophthalmic corticosteroids.[64] The occurrence is even higher in patients with previously diagnosed open-angle glaucoma.[60, 64, 65] Persistently elevated IOP with loss of visual field has been described following the use of inhaled and topically applied facial corticosteroids.[66, 67] The IOP usually returns to pretreatment levels upon cessation of the steroids; however, persistently elevated IOP requiring medical and surgical intervention has been reported.[65, 68] Studies examining the response of human trabecular meshwork cells to glucocorticosteroids have helped identify the *TIGR* (trabecular meshwork inducible glucocorticoid response) gene in the GLC1A region of chromosome 1.[69–71]

Slit-lamp examination of corticosteroid-induced cataracts is similar to that of age-related PSC. The lens opacities frequently occupy the polar region of posterior cortex immediately anterior to the posterior capsule. The structure of the opacities consists of tiny whitish or yellow crystals, sometimes iridescent, often interspersed with small vacuoles, and surrounded by a sharp border. Retroillumination may demonstrate subtle PSC not easily seen with direct illumination.

The progression of steroid-induced PSC may halt with the cessation of steroid therapy.[61] If the cataracts become visually significant, good results with cataract extraction and intraocular lens implantation can be expected.

Conditions Associated with Iris Abnormalities, Glaucoma, and Lens Changes (Table 15–3)

Certain diseases and syndromes produce characteristic abnormalities of the iris in addition to glaucoma and lens changes. These entities are covered in detail elsewhere in this chapter.

ROLE OF CRYSTALLINE LENS IN PATHOGENESIS OF GLAUCOMA

Another set of diseases associated with glaucoma and lens changes are those wherein the lens contributes directly or indirectly to the elevated IOP. Unlike the previously described conditions, in which lenticular changes may be seen independent of glaucoma, elevated IOP in the following entities is due at least in part to abnormalities in lens position or integrity.

Conditions Associated with Glaucoma and Lens-Induced Inflammation (Table 15–4)

LENS-PROTEIN (PHACOLYTIC) GLAUCOMA

Phacolytic glaucoma is a form of secondary open-angle glaucoma in which soluble lens proteins leak from a mature or hypermature cataract, resulting in elevated IOP.[72, 73] Numerous histopathologic studies have identified lens proteins floating freely in the anterior chamber and in the trabecular meshwork of patients with phacolytic glaucoma.[74–77]

Lens proteins may contribute to intraocular inflammation and elevated IOP by several different mechanisms. These proteins, especially the gamma crystallin fraction, show high in vitro chemotactic stimulus for circulating blood monocytes.[78] This feature may explain the frequent finding

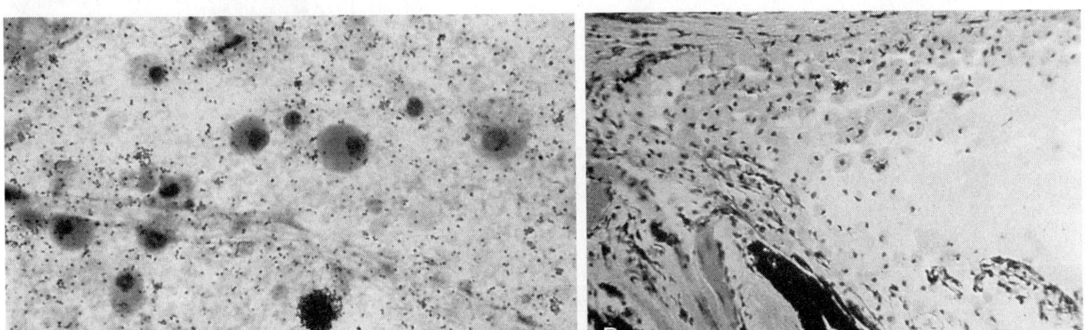

FIGURE 15–12. Phacolytic glaucoma. *A*, Cytologic specimen of an aqueous humor aspirate from a patient with phacolytic glaucoma reveals proteinaceous debris and numerous swollen macrophages (H&E, ×160.) *B*, Macrophages in the anterior chamber adjacent to the trabecular meshwork in another patient with phacolytic glaucoma. (H&E, ×150.) (Courtesy of Dr. Ramon L. Font.)

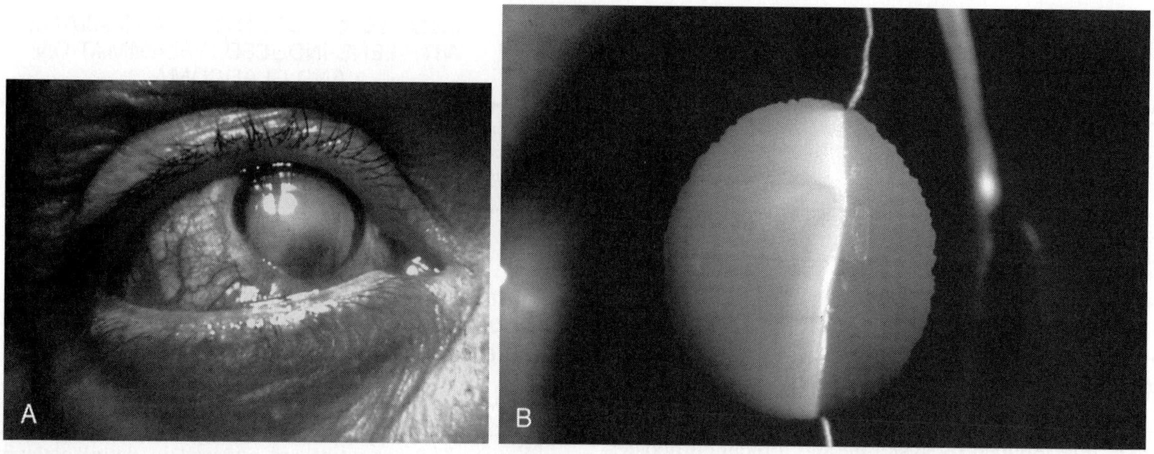

FIGURE 15–13. Phacolytic glaucoma. External picture *(A)* and slit-lamp view *(B)* of hypermature (morgagnian) cataracts prone to developing leakage of lens protein into anterior chamber. Note the inferior location of the lens nucleus within the capsular bag filled with liquefied cortex. (Courtesy of Dr. Ramon L. Font.)

of large numbers of macrophages, often with engulfed lens protein, in the trabecular meshwork of eyes with phacolytic glaucoma[74, 75, 77, 79, 80] (Fig. 15–12). Originally, the pathogenesis of phacolytic glaucoma centered on obstruction of the trabecular meshwork by these macrophages swollen with engulfed lens protein.[81, 82] Later work also supports direct blockage of trabecular outflow by soluble lens protein. Epstein and associates[83] have demonstrated the presence of high-molecular-weight (HMW) proteins large enough to mechanically obstruct the trabecular outflow system in the aqueous of eyes with phacolytic glaucoma.

Clinical examination commonly shows an eye with a hypermature cataract, often with a small dense nucleus floating in the capsular bag filled with liquefied cortex (Figs. 15–13 and 15–14). The anterior chamber is deep, but the aqueous may be filled with characteristic suspended iridescent particles and significant flare. Cells visible in the anterior chamber often appear larger than in other types of inflammation. Occasionally, the inflammatory debris may settle inferiorly and form a pseudohypopyon.

Initial treatment of phacolytic glaucoma consists of medical control of IOP and suppression of inflammation with corticosteroids. The definitive treatment of phacolytic glaucoma is extracapsular cataract extraction, which for many patients achieves good visual results and normalization of IOP.[84, 85]

PHACOANTIGENIC (PHACOANAPHYLACTIC) UVEITIS

Phacoantigenic uveitis is a severe sterile, inflammatory panuveitis that occurs after traumatic or surgical disruption of the lens capsule. The terms "phacoanaphylaxis" and "phacoanaphylactic endophthalmitis" have become entrenched in the ophthalmic literature; however, no evidence exists for an immunoglobulin E–mediated response, and the terms are used here only to describe the common clinical and pathologic findings. Experimental studies have revealed that phacoantigenic uveitis represents an immune complex–mediated response to the exposed lens material.[86–88] This response was seen more commonly following early techniques of extracapsular cataract extraction in which a relatively large amount of lens cortical material was left within the capsular bag.

Patients with phacoantigenic uveitis typically present within 1 to 14 days following disruption of the anterior lens capsule.[89, 90] However, cases have been reported months to years after the initial surgery or trauma.[91] The clinical picture usually demonstrates conjunctival hyperemia, corneal edema, severe anterior chamber reaction, often with a

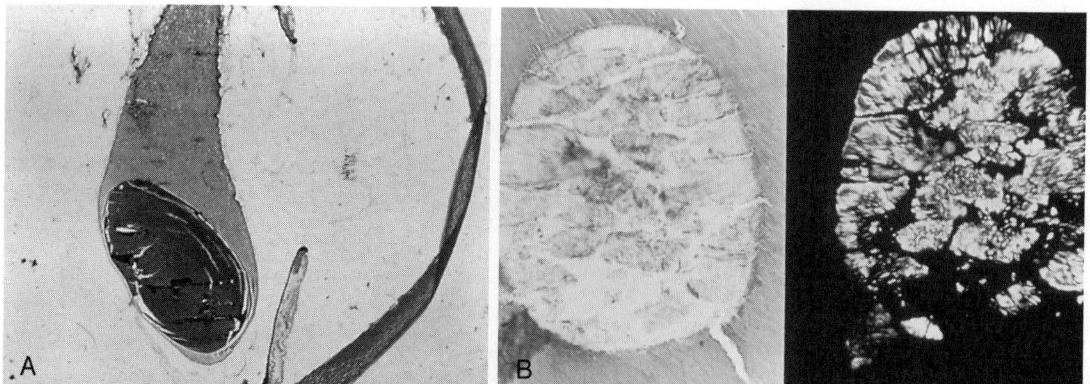

FIGURE 15–14. Phacolytic glaucoma. *A*, Histologic specimen of hypermature (morgagnian) cataract illustrating inferiorly displaced lens nucleus. (AMP, ×7.) *B*, Calcium oxalate crystals in a hypermature cataract demonstrating birefringence on examination with polarized light. (H&E, ×165.) (Courtesy of Dr. Ramon L. Font.)

hypopyon, and evidence of vitreal inflammation.[92–95] In contrast to lens protein–induced inflammation, significantly elevated IOP is uncommon in phacoantigenic uveitis. When glaucoma occurs, it is due to accumulation of inflammatory cells and HMW lens proteins within the trabecular meshwork as well as secondary cyclitic membranes and posterior synechiae. In cases of very severe inflammation, the eye may actually become hypotonous.

Pathologically, eyes suffering phacoantigenic uveitis demonstrate an Arthus-type autoimmune reaction. The classic histologic picture is a zonal, granulomatous reaction surrounding lens remnants.[86, 89, 94, 96] Neutrophils are found surrounding the remnants of lens fragments. Epithelioid cells, giant cells, and macrophages are typically observed around the periphery of the neutrophilic reaction.

Frequently, distinction between phacoantigenic uveitis and infectious endophthalmitis poses a diagnostic dilemma. Phacoantigenic uveitis should be suspected in cases of severe postoperative inflammation for which cultures are negative and that fail to respond to the administration of appropriate antimicrobial treatment.

The immediate treatment for phacoantigenic uveitis includes the frequent administration of high doses of corticosteriods.[89, 97] Definitive treatment involves the removal of any residual lens material from the eye.[92, 93] Modern techniques of cataract extraction, including phacoemulsification and meticulous cortical removal, have greatly reduced the incidence of phacoanaphylactic endophthalmitis.

TABLE 15–5. CONDITIONS ASSOCIATED WITH GLAUCOMA AND ABNORMAL LENS SIZE OR POSITION

Phacomorphic glaucoma
Dislocated crystalline lens
Adenoma of the nonpigmented ciliary body epithelium
Aspert's syndrome (sphenoacrocraniosyndactyly)
Ascariasis
Autosomal recessive or dominant forms
Cryptophthalmia syndrome (cryptophthalmos-syndactyly syndrome)
Dwarfism (genetic type)
Ectopia lentis et pupillae
Ehlers-Danlos syndrome
Gillum-Anderson syndrome (blepharoptosis, myopia, ectopia lentis)
Gorlin-Goltz syndrome
Hereditary ectodermal dysplasia syndrome
Homocystinuria
Hyperlysinemia
Mandibulofacial dysostosis (Franceschetti's syndrome)
Marfan's syndrome
Oculodental syndrome
Peters' syndrome
Pseudoexfoliation syndrome
Pseudoxanthoma elasticum
Retinal disinsertion syndrome
Retinoblastoma
Rieger's syndrome (neurocristopathies)
Spherophakia
Sulfite oxidase deficiency
Syphilis
Trauma
Weill-Marchesani syndrome

Conditions Associated with Glaucoma and Abnormal Lens Size or Position (Table 15–5)

PUPILLARY BLOCK (PHACOMORPHIC GLAUCOMA)

Phacomorphic glaucoma has been used to describe the condition whereby an intumescent cataractous lens causes pupillary block and angle-closure glaucoma.[72, 98] This may occur in eyes with both previously occludable and normal angles. This form of glaucoma is more common in developing countries, where access to ophthalmologic care is limited and advanced cataracts are more common.

As a dense nuclear cataract matures, the anterior to posterior diameter of the lens increases and the anterior lens surface becomes more convex. This causes greater contact between the anterior lens capsule and posterior iris surface, precipitating pupillary block and subsequent angle closure. In the early stages, the elevated IOP often responds favorably to medical therapy, including aqueous suppressants and mydriatic agents. Laser iridotomy has been advocated to reverse the pupillary block.[99] As the cataractous lens continues to swell, it may cause forward displacement of the peripheral iris. The pupillary block may be so extensive that it becomes refractory to treatment with peripheral iridotomy, because even the peripheral-most iris is in contact with the anterior capsule.

Examination of patients with phacomorphic glaucoma often reveals a dense mature cataract draped peripherally by the iris with a shallow anterior chamber. Evidence of acutely elevated IOP, consisting of decreased vision, hyperemia, and corneal edema, is usually present.

Regardless of the stage of phacomorphic glaucoma, the definitive treatment is cataract extraction.[72, 99, 100] In some cases, temporary relief may be obtained with vigorous pupillary dilation or peripheral iridotomy (Fig. 15–15). Unless permanent peripheral anterior synechiae have formed, cataract surgery may cure the glaucoma and dramatically improve vision.

SUBLUXATED LENS

Complete (luxation) or partial (subluxation) dislocation of the crystalline lens may produce glaucoma via a number of mechanisms. The most common etiology is anterior dislocation of the lens, which results in pupillary-block

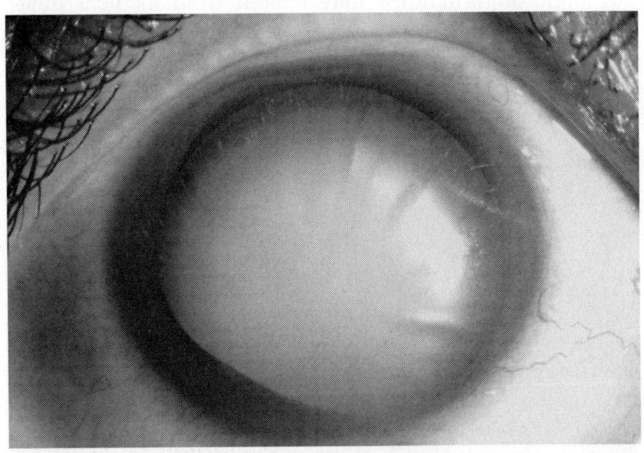

FIGURE 15–15. Phacomorphic glaucoma. Intumescent cataract in the right eye of a 75-year-old Latin-American female caused pupillary block that was temporarily relieved by peripheral iridotomy and maximum dilation. Cataract extraction was required to prevent recurrent pupillary block.

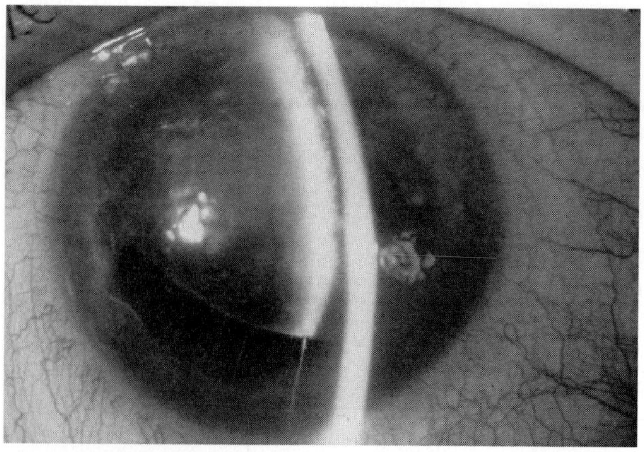

FIGURE 15–16. Traumatic lens subluxation into anterior chamber. Slit-lamp views of left eye of 57-year-old white male presenting with pain, decreased vision, corneal edema, and elevated intraocular pressure following blunt trauma.

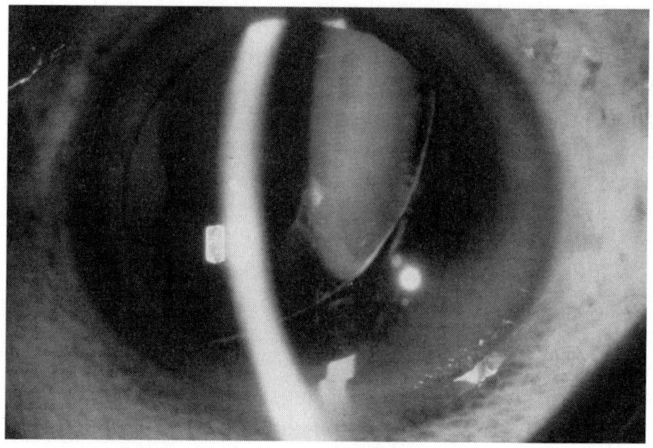

FIGURE 15–18. Subluxated lens in a patient with pseudoexfoliation syndrome. Note the vitreous prolapse into the anterior chamber.

angle closure. This phenomenon is well described in both traumatic and hereditary conditions.[101–104] Additional mechanisms leading to elevated IOP are pupillary block by vitreous, acute and chronic inflammation, and peripheral anterior synechiae formation. Post-traumatic patients and patients with Marfan's syndrome may also exhibit anatomic abnormalities of the anterior chamber angle predisposing to chronic IOP elevation.

Clinically, patients presenting with elevated IOP due to a subluxated lens demonstrate signs of pupillary block, such as a shallow anterior chamber, corneal edema, and conjunctival hyperemia (Figs. 15–16 and 15–17). The lens may be grossly displaced or even fully luxated into the anterior chamber. Occasionally, subtle phacodenesis may be detected by careful observation of the slit-lamp beam on the anterior and posterior lens capsule. Vitreous may be prolapsed into the anterior chamber (Fig. 15–18). After traumatic dislocation of the lens, hyphema, inflammation, and damage to the surrounding ocular structures may be evident.

Treatment of glaucoma secondary to a subluxated lens depends on the mechanism of elevated IOP. Inflammation and angle abnormalities may benefit from medical treatment, whereas pupillary block often requires surgical removal of the lens. In certain patients with a clear crystalline lens and good visual acuity, peripheral iridotomy may prevent pupillary block. Two iridotomies should be placed and should be separated by at least 90 degrees because a crystalline lens is capable of occluding both the pupil and a single iridotomy site. Care must be taken in planning the timing and type of surgery because such cases are prone to the development of surgical complications such as retinal detachment. Inflammation should be treated appropriately, and the anterior chamber examined carefully for evidence of vitreous prolapse and angle abnormalities. Following treatment, the final visual outcome of glaucomatous eyes with traumatic lens dislocation may not be as favorable as for those with dislocation from a hereditary cause because of associated ocular damage, including retinal detachment, traumatic maculopathies, and angle recession.

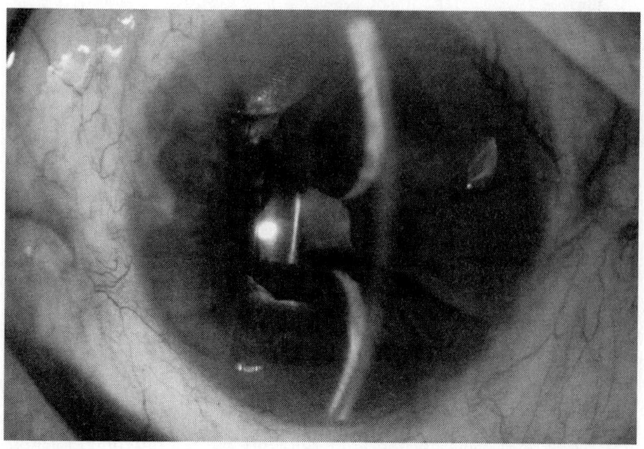

FIGURE 15–17. Slit-lamp view of iris bombé resulting from anterior subluxation of a crystalline lens.

Spontaneous subluxation of the lens without a history of antecedent trauma is frequently associated with characteristic systemic syndromes (see Table 15–5). In the absence of significant trauma, lens dislocation, especially when bilateral, should be assumed to be the result of a genetic abnormality, either inherited or a new mutation. Because dislocation of the crystalline lens, with or without glaucoma, may be the initial manifestation of these syndromes, a search for the underlying cause, including a thorough family history and physical examination, should be performed (Fig. 15–19). Such patients may benefit from treatment of their underlying systemic condition as well as genetic counseling. The clinical signs and pathogenesis of the syndromes most commonly associated with lens subluxation are described here.

TRAUMA. In a review of 166 cases of dislocation of the crystalline lens, Jarrett[101] found trauma to be the most common cause, accounting for more than 50% of cases. Of note, 27% of the patients with traumatic dislocation had positive syphilis serologic test results, an estimated incidence five times greater than that in the general population. Although corroborated by additional studies, the association of positive syphilis serologic test and traumatic dislocation of the lens is not universal, and the significance of positive syphilis test results as a risk factor remains unclear.[101, 102]

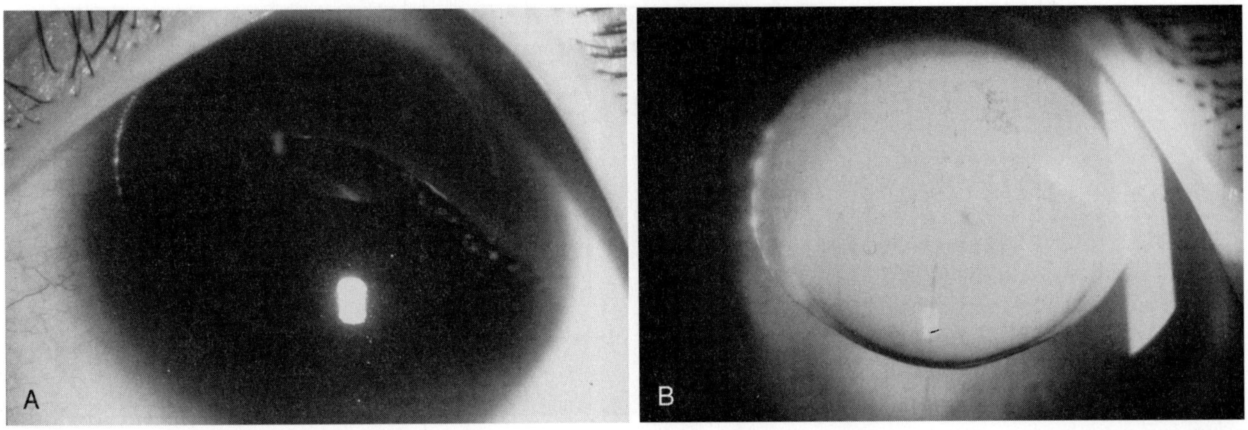

FIGURE 15–19. *A* and *B*, Dislocation of lens into the anterior chamber as the initial manifestation in a patient with microspherophakia and underlying connective tissue disease.

In a review of traumatic lens dislocations, Rodman[105] found the incidence of glaucoma to be between 31% and 93%, depending on the location of the crystalline lens, anterior luxation almost invariably being associated with pupillary block. However, a significant number of patients presenting with elevated IOP and a dislocated lens reported by Jarrett[101] and Rodman[105] demonstrated no actual pupillary block. This finding is explained by the high incidence of hemorrhage, inflammation, and angle abnormalities after concussive injury to the eye. Of 31 eyes with posterior luxation examined histologically, 30(97%) were found to have evidence of angle recession.[105]

MARFAN'S SYNDROME. The most common hereditary condition associated with spontaneous lens dislocation is Marfan's syndrome.[103, 106, 107] This syndrome is an autosomal dominantly inherited condition characterized by arachnodactyly, excessive joint laxity, cardiac valvular abnormalities, and spontaneous crystalline lens subluxation.[103] A proposed pathologic mechanism is the finding that patients with Marfan's syndrome exhibit a deficiency in the fibroblast microfibril system.[108, 109] The mean age at diagnosis of lens dislocation in patients with Marfan's syndrome is approximately 5 years; however up to 5% of such cases may not be diagnosed until the fourth decade or later. The most common location for subluxation in Marfan's syndrome is superotemporal, but it should be noted that hereditary dislocations may occur in any direction[103, 104] (Fig. 15–20). Anterior lens dislocation resulting in pupillary block can occur spontaneously, upon pharmacologic dilation, or after minimal ocular trauma. Although acute angle closure from pupillary block accounts for a higher percentage of cases of glaucoma than does traumatic dislocation, it has been suggested that structural abnormalities of the anterior chamber angle may predispose patients with Marfan's syndrome to primary open-angle glaucoma as well.[110–112]

HOMOCYSTINURIA. Homocystinuria is an autosomal recessive condition characterized by osteoporosis, coarse hair and pale skin with a malar flush, a predisposition to thromboembolic phenomenon, and spontaneous lens subluxation.[102, 103] Unlike Marfan's syndrome, in which mentation is usually normal, mental retardation is a common finding in homocystinuria. The biochemical basis of the disease is the virtual absence of the enzyme cystathionine β-synthetase, which catalyzes the conversion of homocysteine to cystathionine.[102, 113]

Lens subluxation is almost universal in patients with homocystinuria and is rarely diagnosed after the third decade.[102] The direction of dislocation is most often nasal or inferonasal (Fig. 15–21). The most common mechanism of elevated IOP is pupillary-block angle closure.[103] The incidence of primary open-angle glaucoma in this disorder

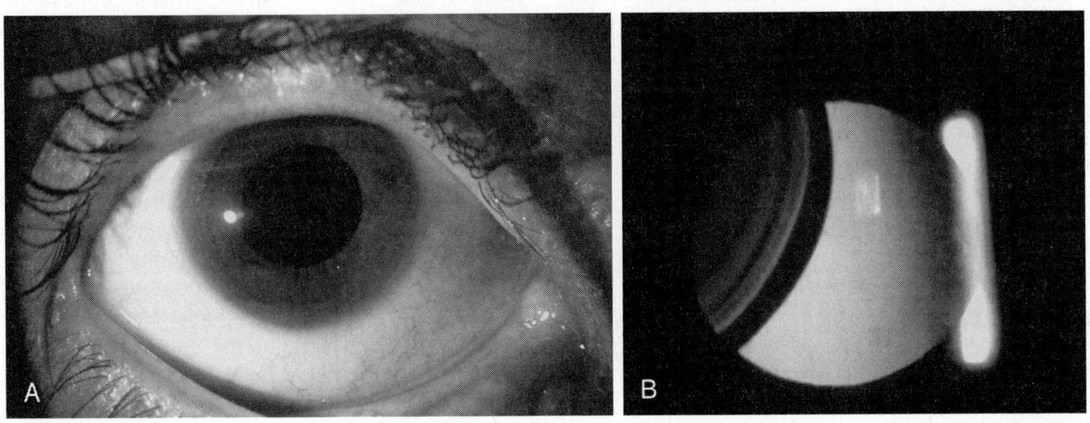

FIGURE 15–20. Subluxated lens in Marfan's syndrome. External *(A)* and slit-lamp *(B)* views of the right eye of a patient with Marfan's syndrome. Note the superotemporal position of the subluxated lens.

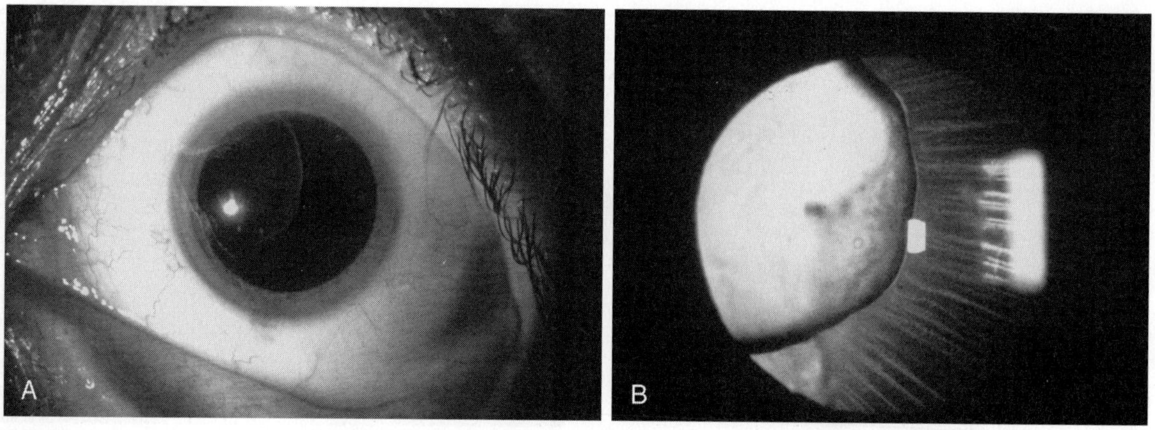

FIGURE 15–21. Subluxated lens in homocystinuria. External *(A)* and slit-lamp *(B)* views of the left eye of a patient with homocystinuria. Note the nasal position of the subluxated lens.

appears to be less common than in Marfan's syndrome. Care must be taken in planning surgery for patients with homocystinuria because they are prone to thromboembolic phenomena that may be exacerbated by general anesthesia.[114, 115]

WEILL-MARCHESANI SYNDROME. Another systemic disease associated with well-described musculoskeletal abnormalities and spontaneous lens subluxation is the Weill-Marchesani syndrome. The inheritance pattern is believed to be autosomal recessive, and to date, no biochemical or structural etiology has been demonstrated. Affected individuals manifest short, stubby fingers, short stature, leathery skin, and brachycephaly.[102, 116] The crystalline lens in patients with Weill-Marchesani syndrome is characteristically microspherophakic, with manifest refraction usually in the range of −7 to −21 diopters. Although case series are limited, the occurrence of lens subluxation in Weill-Marchesani syndrome is probably less common and is diagnosed at a later age than in Marfan's syndrome or homocystinuria. The majority of dislocations occur inferiorly. Glaucoma can occur with or without frank subluxation of the lens because the increased radius of curvature of the small lens predisposes the eye to pupillary block.[116] No association between the Weill-Marchesani syndrome and primary open-angle glaucoma has been documented.

OTHER DISORDERS. Other rare metabolic defects that have been described in association with spontaneous crystalline lens dislocation are hyperlysinemia and sulfite oxidase deficiency.[117–119] In addition, pedigrees have been described of families exhibiting dominantly inherited spontaneous subluxation of the lens that occurs without significant ocular or systemic abnormalities.[120] Lens dislocation in these families is typically diagnosed at an older age, usually after the second decade of life. The incidence of glaucoma in these syndromes has not been well documented.

Refractive State as a Clinical Sign of Glaucoma

Associations between the refractive state of an eye and glaucoma have been recognized for many years. Both epidemiologic data and anatomic studies have supported correlations between refraction and different types of glaucoma. Because refractive error and axial length are commonly assessed during evaluation of patients with cataracts, it is worthwhile to review the two most common of these associations, myopia with primary open-angle glaucoma and hyperopia with angle closure.

MYOPIA AND ITS ASSOCIATION WITH OPEN-ANGLE GLAUCOMA (Table 15–6)

There is epidemiologic evidence linking both increased axial length and myopia to primary open-angle glaucoma. In eyes with axial lengths between 21 and 26 mm, Tomlinson and Phillips[121] found a significant positive correlation between IOP and axial length. In addition, the mean IOP was significantly greater for patients with myopia (spherical refraction less than −0.5D) than those with hyperopia (spherical refraction greater than +0.5D). Abdalla and Hamdi[122] compared the difference in ocular tension between emmetropes (refractive error −2D to +2D) and myopes (greater than −2D). Although the differences failed to reach significance between all ages and refractive errors, these researchers were able to show a stepwise elevation in IOP with increasing myopic refraction. In a population survey of southern Israel, David and colleagues[123] also demonstrated a statistically significant positive relationship between IOP and increasing myopic refractive errors. Additionally, they found that myopia was a relative risk factor for ocular hypertension, defined as IOP greater than 21 mm Hg. Work by Lotufo and associates[124] demonstrated a much higher prevalence of myopia in patients with juvenile open-angle glaucoma (diagnosis of glaucoma between the ages of 10 and 35 years) than would be expected in a normal age-matched population.

In a retrospective study of patients treated at a glaucoma clinic, Perkins and Phelps[125] found that patients with myopia who had ocular hypertension were more likely to experience visual field loss than patients with emmetropia or hyperopia. On the basis of serial visual field testing in myopic and nonmyopic patients, Phelps[126] has suggested that myopia may facilitate the untoward effects of elevated IOP on the optic nerve head rather than cause an independent damaging effect.

Pathophysiologic theories attempting to explain the apparent correlation between myopia and open-angle glau-

TABLE 15–6. SUMMARY OF STUDIES RELATING MYOPIA AND OPEN-ANGLE GLAUCOMA

Study	Type of Study	n=	Population	Conclusions
Tomlinson and Phillips (1970)[121]	Cross-sectional	75 (axial length), 94 (refraction)	Normal subjects	Positive correlation between axial length and IOP Greater IOP in subjects with myopia (SE <−0.50D) than in those with hyperopia (SE >0.50D)
Abdalla and Hamdi (1970)[122]	Cross-sectional	760	Normal subjects	Greater IOP subjects with myopia (SE <−2D) than in those with emmetropia (SE <±2D)
Leighton and Tomlinson (1973)[132]	Cross-sectional	30	Patients with glaucoma	No correlation between axial length and IOP Greater axial length in patients with LTG than in those with POAG
Daubs and Crick (1981)[133]	Case-control	953	Patients with glaucoma and normal subjects	No correlation between refraction and IOP Increased relative risk of POAG with greater levels of myopia
Phelps (1982)[126]	Case-control	166	Patients with glaucoma	Myopic eyes (SE <−1D) more likely to have visual field loss than nonmyopic eyes
Perkins and Phelps (1982)[125]	Cross-sectional	411	Patients with glaucoma	Myopia (SE <−1D) more common in patients with OHT, POAG, and LTG than in normal population
David et al (1985)[123]	Population survey	2,403	Normal subjects	Positive correlation between increasing myopia and IOP
Wilson et al (1987)[131]	Case-control	535	Patients with glaucoma and normal subjects	Weak association between myopia (SE ≤−1D) and POAG
Lotufo et al (1989)[124]	Cross-sectional	68	Patients with juvenile glaucoma	Myopia (SE <1D) more common in patients with juvenile glaucoma and OHT than in patients without myopia

D, diopter; IOP, intraocular pressure; LTG, low-tension (normal-pressure) glaucoma; OHT, ocular hypertension; POAG, primary open-angle glaucoma; SE, spherical equivalent.

coma have centered on mechanical damage to the optic nerve head. Relationships between glaucomatous optic nerve damage and optic nerve head compliance,[127] as well as extracellular matrix changes,[128, 129] have been proposed. However, given conflicting data,[130] these theories remain speculative.

In contrast to the previously cited reports, not all studies confirm the correlation between myopia and primary open-angle glaucoma. In a case-control study of risk factors in open-angle glaucoma, Wilson and coworkers[131] found only a weak association between myopia and glaucoma. Other studies have debated the connection between IOP and axial length[132] as well as the increased risk of ocular hypertension in myopia.[133] In fact, it has been suggested that elevated IOP in a previously emmetropic eye may cause axial elongation of the globe and myopia, explaining the observed association.[134]

The following statements sum up the useful information regarding the association between myopia and primary open-angle glaucoma (see Table 15–6):

1. Patients with significant myopia (greater than 3D) should be followed carefully for the development of elevated IOP.
2. Patients with ocular hypertension and a similar level of myopia may be considered at an higher risk of visual field changes related to glaucomatous optic neuropathy than patients with emmetropia.

HYPEROPIA AND ITS RELATIONSHIP TO ANGLE-CLOSURE GLAUCOMA
(Table 15–7)

Much less debate surrounds the relationship between ocular anatomy and primary angle-closure glaucoma. Short axial lengths and hyperopia have long been recognized as risk factors for the development of angle-closure glaucoma.[135–137] In addition, numerous epidemiologic and anatomic studies have described characteristics of eyes predisposed to angle closure (see Table 15–7).

Anatomic studies support the concept that eyes at risk for angle-closure glaucoma have in common an abnormally shallow anterior chamber[138, 139] (Fig. 15–22). With advancing age, the depth of the anterior chamber steadily decreases.[140] In eyes with previously shallow chambers and narrow angles, the progressive shallowing poses a risk of pupillary block and angle-closure glaucoma.

One feature predisposing eyes to a shallow anterior chamber is an increased thickness of the crystalline lens. Biometric studies by Lowe[135, 141] and Tomlinson and Leighton[136] comparing normal eyes and those with angle-closure glaucoma demonstrate a statistically significant increase in lens thickness in eyes with a history of angle closure. Interestingly, this relationship also held true for the eyes of first-degree relatives of patients with angle closure.[136] Markowitz and Morin[142] noted that the ratio of lens thickness to axial length was significantly greater in patients

TABLE 15–7. SUMMARY OF STUDIES DESCRIBING ANATOMIC CHARACTERISTICS OF EYES AT RISK FOR ANGLE-CLOSURE GLAUCOMA

Anatomic Characteristic	Studies
Decreased anterior chamber depth	Sugar (1941),[137] Tornquist (1956),[138] Lowe (1970),[135] Alsbirk (1976),[147] Tomlinson and Leighton (1973),[136] Lee et al (1984),[139] Markowitz and Morin (1984)[144]
Anteriorly placed lens	Lowe (1969),[141] Tomlinson and Leighton (1973)[136]
Increased lens thickness	Lowe (1969),[141] Tomlinson and Leighton (1973),[136] Markowitz and Morin (1985)[142]
Increased anterior lens curvature	Lowe (1972),[145] Lowe and Clark (1973)[146]
Decreased axial length	Lowe (1969),[141] Tomlinson and Leighton (1973),[136] Markowitz and Morin (1984),[144] Markowitz and Morin (1985)[142]
Increased lens-thickness–to–axial-length ratio	Markowitz and Morin (1985),[142] Panek et al (1990)[143]

with primary angle-closure glaucoma than in age-matched normal subjects. Similarly, Panek and associates[143] found that eyes with a greater ratio of lens thickness to axial length were more likely to require a peripheral iridotomy due to angle closure. Because values for lens thickness and axial length are easily obtained with in-office ultrasonography, these researchers suggest that the ratio is an easily reproducible means of diagnosing and following patients with suspected angle-closure glaucoma.

The position of the crystalline lens is another morphologic feature predisposing to an abnormally shallow anterior chamber. The lens in patients undergoing attacks of angle-closure glaucoma has been found to be positioned more anteriorly compared to that in age-matched control subjects.[136, 141] A slow forward movement of the lens-iris diaphragm with increasing age has been attributed to progressive weakening of the zonular support and may help explain the correlation of angle closure with advancing age.[144]

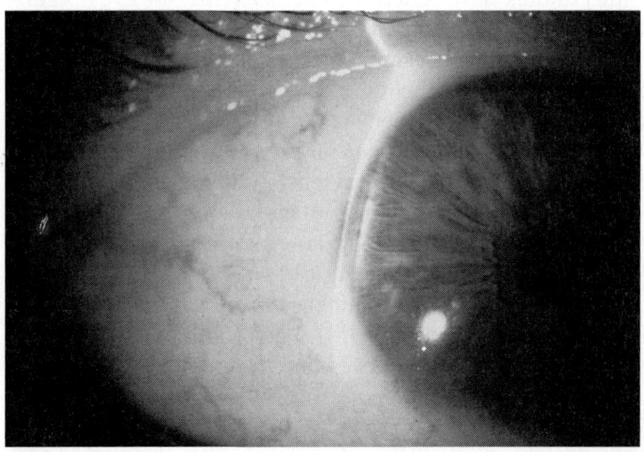

FIGURE 15–22. Slit-lamp view of a typical hyperopic eye at risk for developing angle-closure glaucoma. Note the close proximity of the peripheral iris to the cornea. Manifest refraction was +3.25 diopters.

In summary, the eye at risk for pupillary block and primary angle-closure glaucoma is a hyperopic eye with an abnormally shallow anterior chamber. Anatomically, this is secondary to a short axial length and an anteriorly placed crystalline lens with a proportionately greater thickness. Other morphologic features that have been proposed as risk factors for angle closure are a small corneal diameter and a decreased radius of curvature of the anterior lens surface.[136, 145–147] It should be kept in mind, however, that eyes of any axial length or refractive error may experience an attack of angle closure.

Cataract Surgery and Its Relationship to Glaucoma

DECISION-MAKING FOR PATIENTS WITH COEXISTING CATARACT AND GLAUCOMA (see also Chapter 23)

As the general population continues to age, the number of patients with coexistent open-angle glaucoma and visually significant cataracts will increase. Managing these patients often leads to confusion on the part of the operating surgeon. Depending on the extent of a patient's glaucoma and the level of the surgeon's experience with different techniques, three basic options are available:

- Cataract extraction with intraocular lens implantation alone
- A staged procedure with filtration surgery followed by cataract removal
- Combined glaucoma surgery with cataract extraction and intraocular lens placement (i.e., the "triple procedure")

The advantages and disadvantages of each technique are considered with respect to the decision-making process for individual patients.

Effect of Cataract Surgery on Intraocular Pressure

Before reviewing the surgical options available to patients with glaucoma and visually significant cataracts, it is worthwhile to briefly examine the evidence concerning the net effect of cataract surgery on IOP.

Numerous studies have shown either a decrease in IOP or no significant long-term change following extracapsular cataract extraction (including phacoemulsification) with intraocular lens implantation.[148–151] Steuhl and coworkers[152] revealed a statistically significant decrease in IOP at a mean of 12 months postoperatively in 33 glaucomatous eyes after extracapsular cataract extraction. In addition, no eye required additional antiglaucoma medication to achieve the same level of IOP control as was present preoperatively. Work by Cinotti and associates,[153] who examined 160 eyes with pre-existing glaucoma who underwent extracapsular cataract surgery, found that average IOP remained unchanged from preoperative levels at 2 years of follow-up.

At the end of the follow-up period, 48.1% of patients required less medication to achieve the preoperative IOP, 39.2% used the same amount, and only 12.6% required additional medications. Studies examining small-incision phacoemulsification cataract extraction have noted a long-term decrease in IOP of approximately 2 to 4 mm Hg in both glaucomatous and normal eyes.[154–156]

Although this evidence suggests that the long-term effect of modern cataract surgery on IOP is negligible or even beneficial, some important caveats must be considered in the planning of cataract surgery for patients with glaucoma. Extracapsular and phacoemulsification cataract procedures have been found to incur a significant incidence of elevated IOP in the immediate postoperative period. Gross and colleagues[157] found an IOP of 25 mm Hg or greater in 59% of 58 eyes at 2 to 3 hours after surgery. Other studies suggest that this postoperative IOP spike may be significantly more common in glaucomatous eyes than in normal eyes.[158, 159] It is possible that a brief postoperative pressure rise may lead to progression of optic nerve damage and visual field loss in some patients with glaucoma.[160] The incidence of persistently elevated IOP requiring additional medical or surgical treatment after routine cataract surgery in glaucomatous eyes has been estimated at between 1% and 20%.[148–151, 158] Patients with glaucoma and visually significant cataracts for whom cataract surgery is being planned should be counseled regarding the risks of loss of IOP control and progression of disease.

Cataract Extraction Alone

In general, cataract surgery alone is the treatment of choice for (1) patients whose glaucoma is adequately controlled by relatively few, well-tolerated medications and (2) patients with minimal glaucomatous damage that is unlikely to progress clinically if a postoperative IOP spike occurs. These patients may experience the benefits of visual rehabilitation from cataract extraction without the risk of potential complications from concurrent filtration surgery. Because it is not currently possible to predict whether a patient will require additional treatment postoperatively, careful and more frequent follow-up for the patient with glaucoma who has undergone cataract surgery is warranted. From a technique standpoint, a temporal approach for both clear corneal and scleral tunnel wound construction is a method of preserving the superior conjunctiva in case future filtering surgery is required.

Staged Procedure

A second scenario confronting the clinician is (1) the patient who has a visually significant cataract but whose glaucoma is uncontrolled by the maximum tolerable medical therapy or (2) the patient who has extensive glaucomatous disease that poses an immediate threat to the vision. In this case, a staged procedure of glaucoma filtering surgery followed by cataract extraction may be the preferred option. Although this approach subjects the patient to two separate surgical procedures, reported results suggest that the postoperative IOP following trabeculectomy alone is lower than with a combined glaucoma and cataract procedure.[160–163] In a series of 22 eyes treated with an initial filtering procedure followed by cataract extraction, Shields[160] found that glaucoma control was maintained in 21 eyes (95%). In addition, the presence of a definite postoperative filtering bleb was twice as likely for eyes undergoing the two-stage procedure than for those undergoing combined surgery. In patients with prior filtering surgery who underwent phacoemulsification cataract extraction, Park and colleagues[164] found no significant change in IOP 1 year postoperatively. These results suggest that filtering surgery performed alone and followed by cataract surgery at a later date results in the highest probability of long-term IOP control and bleb survival. Unless immediate visual rehabilitation is required, this is the procedure of choice for patients with severe or poorly controlled glaucoma.

Combined ("Triple") Procedure

A third group of patients with coexistent visually significant cataract and glaucoma includes (1) those with well-controlled IOP but moderate to severe glaucomatous damage, (2) those with borderline control of glaucoma by maximum treatment, and (3) those who cannot tolerate their current medical therapy. This group of patients may benefit from a combined glaucoma procedure at the time of cataract extraction. Numerous studies examining modified filtration surgery at the time of cataract removal and intraocular lens placement have shown a statistically significant decrease in IOP from preoperative levels.[154, 158, 165–167]

The combined procedure also reduces the risk of significant postoperative IOP spikes compared with cataract surgery alone. In a prospective study of eyes undergoing a combined procedure, Krupin and associates[158] measured a mean one-day postoperative IOP of 21.3 mm Hg compared with a 14.9 mm Hg preoperative IOP. In contrast, eyes undergoing cataract extraction and intraocular lens implantation alone had a mean postoperative IOP of 34.2 mm Hg, compared with 18.9 mm Hg before surgery. The number of eyes experiencing a postoperative pressure spike of more than 10 mm Hg above the preoperative level was also significantly reduced in the group undergoing the combined procedure.

In addition to an absolute reduction in IOP, most studies demonstrate a reduced requirement for pressure-lowering medications after combined filtration and cataract surgery. A retrospective review of combined procedures performed at the Mayo Clinic showed that the average number of medications needed to achieve adequate IOP control decreased from 2.6 preoperatively to 0.6 at 6 months postoperatively.[165] More than half of the patients remained free of the need for antiglaucoma medications at 6 months of follow-up. Similarly, 57% of the patients treated by McCartney and coworkers[167] required no postoperative medications to maintain control of IOP ($\leq$21 mm Hg) at 17 months of follow-up, and in 30%, IOP was controlled with fewer medications than required preoperatively.

Compared with cataract surgery alone, the combined procedure has a higher incidence of postoperative complications. Minor complications include transient bleb leaks, hyphema, increased inflammation, posterior synechiae, and earlier posterior capsular opacification.[165, 166] More serious, vision-threatening complications, such as persistent hypotony, choroidal detachment, and endophthalmitis, have also been described.[167, 168] In addition, long-term filtering bleb survival and the level of postoperative IOP control may be less with combined procedures compared with trabeculectomy alone.[162, 163, 169]

Conclusions

With the rapid advancement in cataract surgery techniques over the last few years, numerous variations on the standard technique of guarded sclerostomy or trabeculectomy combined with cataract extraction and intraocular lens implantation have been described. In general, these techniques are aimed at allowing better postoperative pressure control while attempting to avoid the complications seen with standard filtration surgery. They include the use of the small incision sizes allowed by phacoemulsification, implantation of foldable intraocular lenses, and clear corneal cataract extraction combined with a separate trabeculectomy site.[170–175] Although some researchers have also advocated combining cataract extraction with nonfiltering glaucoma surgery in an effort to achieve postoperative control of IOP, the reports consist mainly of small, uncontrolled case series with variable results. Described techniques include trabeculotomy, partial-thickness trabeculectomy, and intraoperative endoscopic ciliary process photocoagulation.[176–178]

Attention has also been focused on the use of antimetabolites to modulate the wound healing response after glaucoma filtration surgery.[179–183] Multiple prospective studies have shown a greater success rate following trabeculectomy with adjunctive 5-fluorouracil and mitomycin-C than in control subjects.[179, 180, 181, 184] However, the use of antimetabolites in combined procedures remains controversial. Prospective case-control studies have failed to show a significant difference in postoperative IOP control for combined filtration surgery and cataract extraction between those eyes receiving adjunctive 5-fluorouracil and control eyes.[185–187] Randomized, prospective studies evaluating the use of mitomycin-C in combined procedures have shown more promising results.[168, 188, 189] Work by Shin and colleagues[190, 191] has shown a beneficial effect of adjunctive mitomycin-C when it is used in patients who have certain risk factors for filtration failure including African-Americans, preoperative IOP greater than 20 mm Hg, diabetes, and use of more than two antiglaucoma medications preoperatively. It remains to be seen whether different intraoperative and postoperative regimens of antimetabolite application will be of benefit in the future when used for combined procedures.

In summary, for the patient who has both a visually significant cataract and coexistent glaucoma, three options are available to the surgeon: cataract surgery alone, glaucoma filtration surgery and later cataract extraction, or a combined procedure. The decision-making process should be undertaken with the following questions in mind:

1. What is the current level of IOP control?
2. What is the extent of glaucomatous damage?
3. How well does the patient tolerate the current medical regimen?
4. How important is the need for rapid visual rehabilitation?

The surgeon's experience with different types of procedures must also be considered. Recommended indications for each procedure have been described with respect to these issues. It remains to be seen how continued development in the areas of wound healing modulation and ocular surgical techniques will further alter the decision-making process in the future.

GLAUCOMA IN THE POSTOPERATIVE PERIOD (see also Chapter 12)

As noted in the discussion of surgical decision-making, elevated IOP following cataract surgery is a common occurrence. Depending on the level of IOP and the time elapsed since surgery, significant IOP spikes may occur in as many as 2% to 60% of cases.[157, 192–194] Cases of elevated IOP following cataract surgery can be divided into acute, those occurring in the early postoperative period (hours to weeks after surgery), and chronic, those occurring late postoperatively (typically, months to years later).

Acute Postoperative Rises in IOP (Table 15–8)

In the days when intracapsular cataract extraction (ICCE) was the standard of care, early postoperative IOP spikes were frequently attributed to enzymatic zonulolysis with alpha-chymotrypsin.[195] Today, extracapsular cataract extraction (ECCE), particularly phacoemulsification, has supplanted ICCE as the most common means of cataract removal. Currently, the most common causes of acute postoperative IOP rises after ECCE are the use of viscoelastic substances, hyphema, papillary block, retained cortical material, and inflammation.

RETAINED VISCOELASTIC SUBSTANCES

The use of viscoelastic substances during cataract surgery has become routine because they (1) facilitate capsulorrhexis,(2) maintain anterior chamber depth during surgery, and (3) protect the corneal endothelium from mechanical trauma. However, numerous studies have implicated sodium hyaluronate (Healon, Healon GV, Amvisc) and sodium chondroitin sulfate–sodium hyaluronate (Viscoat) as likely causes for elevated IOP in the first 24 hours after cataract extraction.[196–199]

Exactly how viscoelastic substances cause elevation of IOP is not known. Work done by Berson and colleagues[200] on enucleated human eyes suggests mechanical obstruction of the trabecular meshwork by these agents. Proposed

TABLE 15–8. CONDITIONS ASSOCIATED WITH ACUTE POSTOPERATIVE RISES IN INTRAOCULAR PRESSURE

Alpha-chymotrypsin used for zonulolysis
Ciliary block (malignant) glaucoma
Distortion of the anterior chamber angle by limbal sutures
Hyphema
Inflammation
Pupillary block
Retained lens cortex
Retained viscoelastic substance
Vitreous filling the anterior chamber

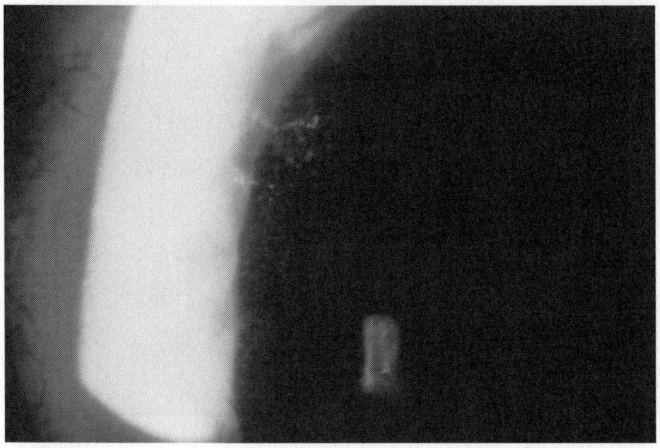

FIGURE 15–23. Slit-lamp view of anterior chamber following extracapsular cataract extraction. Pigment and inflammatory debris are seen suspended in residual viscoelastic material. Intraocular pressure was 52 mm Hg.

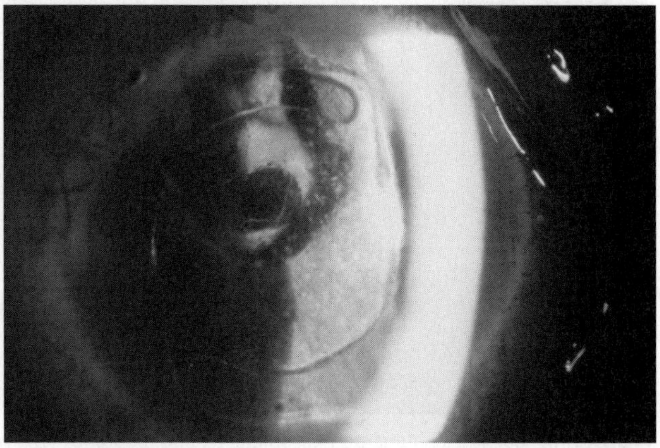

FIGURE 15–24. Slit-lamp view of right eye following complicated extracapsular cataract extraction with anterior chamber intraocular lens implantation. Note the retained cortical material and the inflammatory deposits on the intraocular lens.

techniques for decreasing the incidence of postoperative pressure spikes due to retained viscoelastic material are (1) use of the minimal amount necessary to maintain the anterior chamber and (2) thorough aspiration of the substance from the anterior chamber at the end of surgery (Fig. 15–23).

INFLAMMATION

Persistent inflammation is a common cause of acute postoperative IOP elevation. Often this inflammation results from cortical material retained within the anterior chamber or capsular bag (Fig. 15–24). Although retained cortical material was common after early techniques of extracapsular cataract surgery, modern methods of nucleus removal followed by automated irrigation-aspiration have resulted in a more complete removal of cortical material from the capsular bag with less resultant inflammation.

The mechanism of elevated IOP with inflammation due to retained cortical material is similar to that seen in phacolytic glaucoma, with a combination of direct trabecular obstruction and trabecular dysfunction due to inflammatory mediators. Additional evidence suggests that the surgical trauma of cataract surgery itself may transiently lead to a breakdown in the blood-aqueous barrier.[201] Whether this factor independently leads to transient rises in IOP is unknown.

The most effective technique for avoiding this type of postoperative inflammation is to perform meticulous cortical removal at the end of surgery. A postoperative medical regimen consisting of a topical corticosteroid and, possibly, a nonsteroidal anti-inflammatory agent is also recommended to suppress transient inflammatory changes that may lead to elevated IOP.

HYPHEMA

Hyphema is a well-known complication occurring in the immediate postoperative period after cataract surgery.[192, 193, 202] Usually, hyphema develops as a result of transient bleeding from the site of a peripheral iridectomy, inadequate hemostasis of a scleral tunnel incision, or intraoperative manipulation of the iris to enlarge the pupil. Fortunately, the majority of early postoperative hyphemas are self-limited and resolve in a few days. In some cases, however, significantly elevated IOP may necessitate aggressive treatment in order to avoid further damage to an already compromised optic nerve head or to prevent corneal blood staining. A rare cause of delayed postoperative hyphema is neovascularization of the surgical wound[203] (Fig. 15–25). If the bleeding site within the wound is visible on gonioscopy, argon laser photocoagulation or cryopexy may be attempted to prevent future hemorrhage.

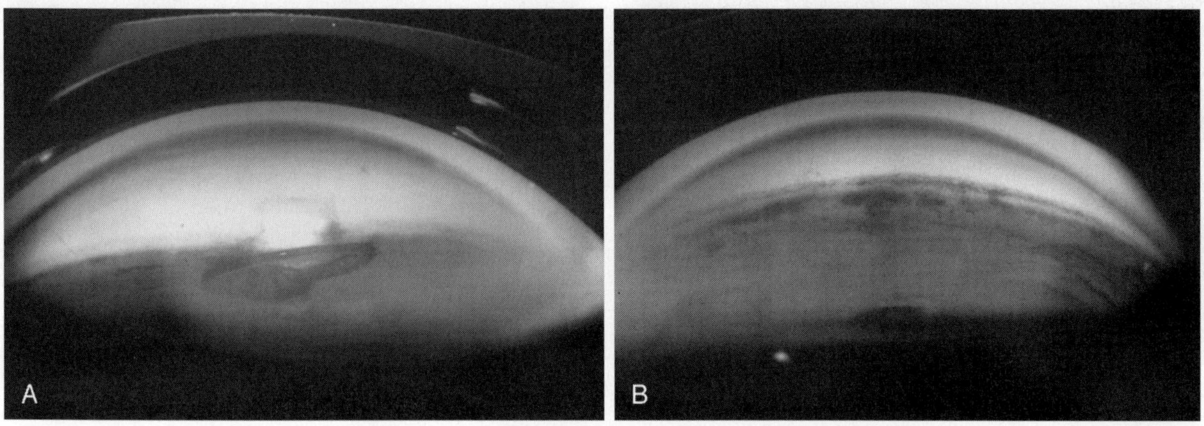

FIGURE 15–25. Neovascularization of a cataract incision. *A,* Superior gonioscopic view demonstrating neovascularization at the edge of a previous corneoscleral tunnel. *B,* Inferior gonioscopic view revealing hemorrhage in the inferior angle. (Courtesy of Dr. L. Jay Katz.)

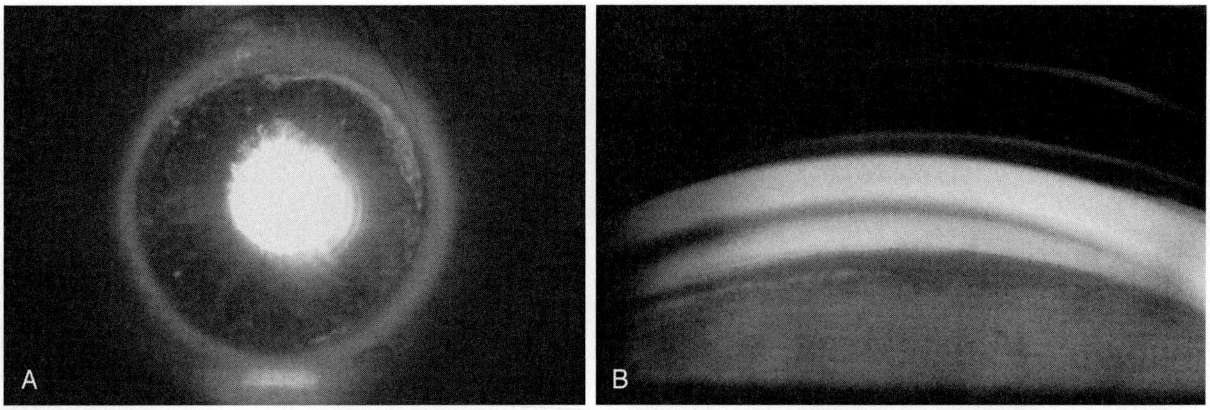

FIGURE 15–26. Iris chafing due to sulcus-fixated posterior chamber intraocular lens following phacoemulsification cataract extraction. *A,* Slit-lamp view of peripheral iris transillumination defects. *B,* Gonioscopic view revealing pigment deposition and distortion of anterior chamber angle overlying lens haptic.

Hyphema may also be associated with late postoperative IOP rises as part of the so-called UGH (uveitis-glaucoma-hyphema) syndrome. This syndrome, originally described by Ellington[204] as occurring with the use of the Choyce Mark VIII anterior chamber lens, consists of a spectrum of iris-pigment epithelial "window-defects," pigment dispersion, and transient microhyphemas. These phenomena are also, at least in part, responsible for the terms "sputtering hyphema syndrome" and "iris chafing syndrome" found in the literature.[192, 205]

Although more common with the early generation of anterior chamber lenses, this syndrome has also been well described for ciliary sulcus–fixated posterior chamber intraocular lenses (Fig. 15–26).[194, 205, 206] Apple and coworkers[207] have suggested that the haptics of the intraocular lens may chafe against the posterior surface of the iris when the lens is placed in the ciliary sulcus. The mechanism for elevated IOP in this scenario is probably multifactorial, with secondary pigment dispersion, chronic inflammation with blood-aqueous barrier breakdown, and recurrent hyphema all playing roles. Although the definitive treatment for this condition remains removal of the offending intraocular lens, many treatments, including miotic therapy, corticosteroids, and intraocular lens rotation, have been described as having variable success.[205, 208]

PUPILLARY BLOCK

Pupillary block with secondary angle-closure glaucoma is another recognized cause of early postoperative IOP rises. The mechanism of elevated IOP is lack of free access for aqueous humor from the posterior chamber into the anterior chamber, with resultant iris bombé and secondary angle closure. When the most common method of cataract surgery was ICCE without intraocular lens implantation, iridovitreal block became a well-described cause of pupillary block[209, 210] (Figs. 15–27 and 15–28). It was quickly noted that surgical or laser iridotomy could be used to prevent and treat angle closure from iridovitreal block.[211]

As anterior chamber intraocular lenses became popular for the correction of aphakia, pseudophakic pupillary block was recognized[209, 212] (Fig. 15–29). Factors leading to pupillary block in pseudophakic eyes with an anterior chamber lens include the omission of a patent iridectomy, an imperforate iridectomy, and occlusion of the iridectomy by the lens haptic, optic, or intact vitreous face. Pupillary block from a posterior chamber intraocular lens has also been described.[213] It is likely that in the majority of such cases,

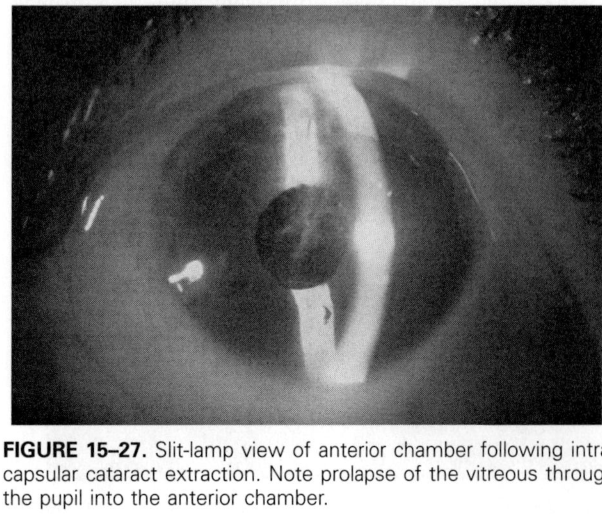

FIGURE 15–27. Slit-lamp view of anterior chamber following intracapsular cataract extraction. Note prolapse of the vitreous through the pupil into the anterior chamber.

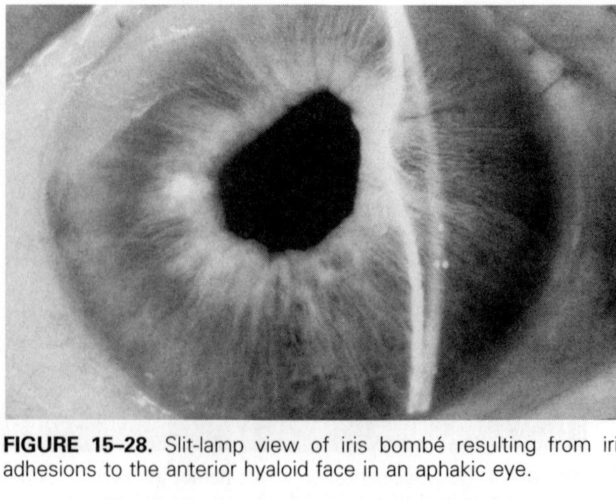

FIGURE 15–28. Slit-lamp view of iris bombé resulting from iris adhesions to the anterior hyaloid face in an aphakic eye.

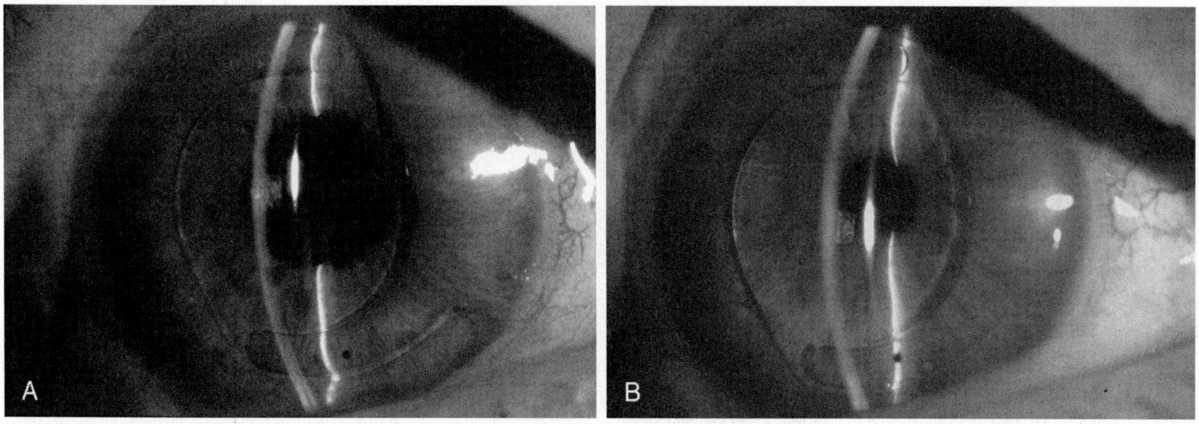

FIGURE 15–29. Pseudophakic pupillary block. *A,* Slit-lamp view of the left eye of a patient with an anterior chamber lens demonstrating temporal iris bombé. *B,* Relief of pupillary block following Nd:YAG laser peripheral iridotomy.

the lens was placed in the ciliary sulcus. The incidence of pupillary block from posterior chamber intraocular lenses with capsular bag fixation following continuous tear capsulorrhexis is extremely low.

Regardless of the type of pseudophakic pupillary block and secondary angle closure, the treatment of choice remains creation of a patent peripheral iridotomy.[209, 212, 213] The current availability of argon and Nd:YAG lasers has made this treatment a relatively easy in-office procedure. It should be noted that for the pseudophakic eye with a large-diameter optic intraocular lens or the aphakic eye with an intact vitreous face, multiple iridotomies may be required. The major long-term sequelae of secondary angle closure are the formation of peripheral anterior synechiae and persistently elevated IOP. In a case series reported by Shrader and associates,[209] 9 of 26 eyes (35%) treated for postoperative pupillary block required long-term antiglaucoma treatment.

Chronic (Delayed) Postoperative Rises in IOP (Table 15–9)

In contrast to acute postoperative IOP spikes, chronically elevated IOP is much less common after cataract extraction. For nonglaucomatous eyes undergoing uncomplicated cataract extraction with intraocular lens placement, the incidence of persistently elevated IOP greater than 6 months postoperatively is approximately 1%.[148, 150, 214] On the other hand, between 10% and 25% of glaucoma patients require additional medical or surgical treatment to maintain adequate IOP control after cataract surgery alone.[151, 153, 156] In many patients, the cause of elevated postoperative IOP is identifiable and treatable. However, it is worth considering that glaucoma is a chronic, progressive disease that may worsen during the postoperative period independent of the cataract surgery.

Postoperative inflammation and hyphema have been discussed as mechanisms of acute IOP rise, but their long-term sequelae may also lead to chronic pressure elevation (Table 15–10). Peripheral anterior synechiae, epithelial ingrowth, fibrous downgrowth, and corticosteroid-induced changes are causes of IOP elevation that may occur months to years following cataract extraction.

TABLE 15–9. CONDITIONS ASSOCIATED WITH CHRONIC (OR DELAYED) RISES IN INTRAOCULAR PRESSURE

Corticosteroid response
Degenerated intraocular blood
Ghost cell glaucoma
Hemolytic glaucoma
Hemosideric glaucoma
Epithelial downgrowth
Fibrous proliferation
Hyphema
Neovascularization of the internal corneal wound
Uveitis-glaucoma-hyphema syndrome
Peripheral anterior synechiae
Retained lens cortex
Vitreous filling the anterior chamber
Neodymium:YAG posterior capsulotomy

HAPTIC-ANGLE INTERACTIONS AND PERIPHERAL ANTERIOR SYNECHIAE

Numerous pathologic studies have demonstrated the development of peripheral anterior synechiae (PAS) associated with the haptics of both anterior and posterior chamber intraocular lenses.[215–217] Progressive, chronic angle closure and loss of IOP control have been associated with PAS related to intraocular lens haptics.[216, 218] Work by Hansen and colleagues[219] demonstrated progressive development of PAS over a 2.5 year period for eyes with implanted semi-flexible anterior chamber lens. Of the eyes in this study, 15.7% demonstrated an increase in IOP of at least 25% greater than the preoperative value, and 7.8% required the institution of antiglaucoma medication. A careful gonioscopic examination may reveal implantation of the lens

TABLE 15–10. CONDITIONS ASSOCIATED WITH BOTH ACUTE AND CHRONIC (OR DELAYED) RISES IN INTRAOCULAR PRESSURE

Hyphema
Inflammation
Retained lens cortex
Vitreous filling the anterior chamber

haptic within the substance of the iris, peripheral anterior synechiae, or iridodialysis (Fig. 15–30).

EPITHELIAL INGROWTH AND FIBROUS DOWNGROWTH
(see also Chapters 11 and 14)

Epithelial ingrowth is an uncommon cause of delayed glaucoma after cataract surgery.[220–223] Cases have been reported after both ICCE and ECCE procedures, including clear corneal phacoemulsification.[223, 224] Clinically, a sheet-like proliferation of epithelial tissue can be seen covering the posterior corneal surface, iris, and anterior chamber angle (for a full description, see Chapters 11 and 14). Diagnosis may be enhanced with the use of specular microscopy or anterior chamber paracentesis.[225–227] The source of the proliferating epithelium is most likely conjunctiva adjacent to the incision or wound.[223] Histopathologic examination reveals layers of stratified nonkeratinized squamous epithelium extending over the anterior segment structures.[220–222] In a retrospective review of 124 biopsy-proven cases of epithelial ingrowth, Weiner and associates[223] found glaucoma to be the presenting symptom in 43%. Although numerous surgical techniques have been described for the treatment of epithelial ingrowth, success is limited by a high recurrence rate.[228–230]

Fibrous downgrowth is a term used to describe the proliferation of fibroblastic tissue within the anterior chamber. The fibrous tissue, which is often vascularized, is believed to arise from subconjunctival tissue or the corneal stroma.[231–234] Access is gained into the anterior chamber via a break in Descemet's membrane caused by intraocular surgery or trauma. In one study, autopsy examination revealed fibrous downgrowth in 26 of 31 eyes with vitreous incarceration in the wound following cataract surgery.[235] Clinical examination demonstrates a white or tan fibrovascular membrane covering the iris, intraocular lens, or retrocorneal space (Fig. 15–31). Glaucoma may occur by means of direct obstruction of the trabecular meshwork with fibrous tissue or, more commonly, via progressive anterior synechiae formation.[232, 233] Fibrous downgrowth is usually less destructive and aggressive than epithelial ingrowth, and many cases can be treated with observation and medical antiglaucoma treatment. More progressive cases require surgical intervention.

CORTICOSTEROID RESPONSE
(see also Chapter 11)

As noted in the section on steroid-induced cataracts, elevated IOP is a well-described side effect of corticosteroid treatment. Although no characteristic clinical signs of steroid-induced ocular hypertension have been reported, it seems prudent to carefully examine postoperative patients for residual inflammation and continue corticosteroids only as needed. The topical glucocorticoids fluorometholone and rimexolone have been shown to be less likely to cause elevated IOP.[236] The substitution of topical nonsteroidal agents may be an alternative for patients with pre-existing glaucoma or a suspected steroid-induced IOP elevation.

Glaucoma in Aphakia

With the use of modern cataract surgical techniques, including phacoemulsification, and advances in intraocular lens design, aphakia is becoming an increasingly rare condition. However, aphakia poses unique problems related to IOP that warrant consideration; they include a preponderance for postoperative anterior chamber shallowing, a higher risk of pupillary block, an increased rate of glaucoma in aphakic children, and an increased failure rate with surgical filtration.

The large corneoscleral incisions used during intracapsular cataract surgery predispose to a shallow or flat chamber during the early postoperative period. Frequently, this is due to complications encountered in wound closure. In their review of 1,000 consecutive intracapsular cataract extractions using a 180-degree limbal incision with a Graefe's knife, Francois and Verbraeken[237] found nearly a 3% incidence of wound complications, including wound dehiscence, iris prolapse, and wound leak. A higher incidence of choroidal detachment, unrelated to a wound leak, has also been shown to predispose aphakic eyes to a postoperative shallow anterior chamber.[237–239] Anterior chamber shallowing during the early postoperative period may lead to the formation of peripheral anterior synechiae, chronic angle closure, and persistently elevated IOP.

As noted in the section on acute postoperative rises in IOP, aphakic eyes are at increased risk of pupillary block. Apposition of any surface with the pupillary aperture may

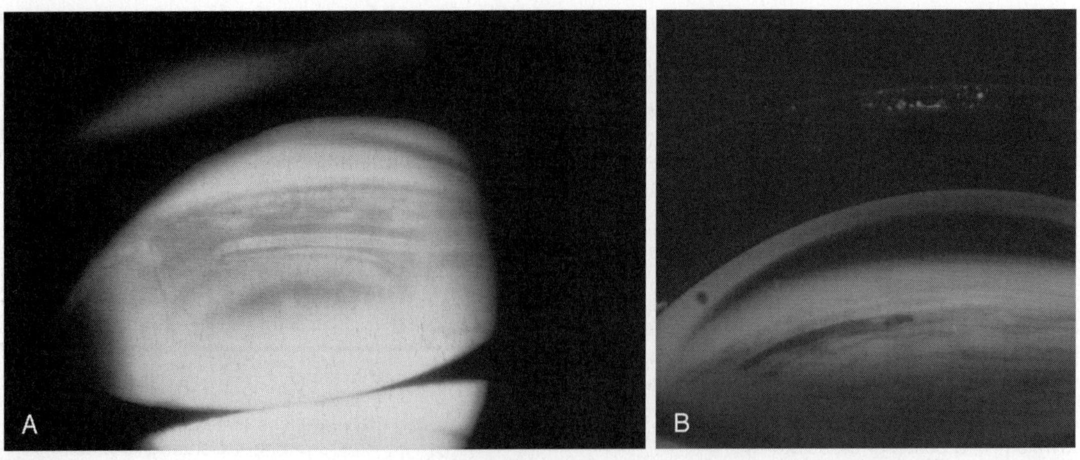

FIGURE 15–30. Haptic-angle interactions. *A*, Anterior chamber lens with angle distortion and peripheral anterior synechiae. *B*, Erosion of haptic into anterior chamber angle from ciliary sulcus-fixated intraocular lens.

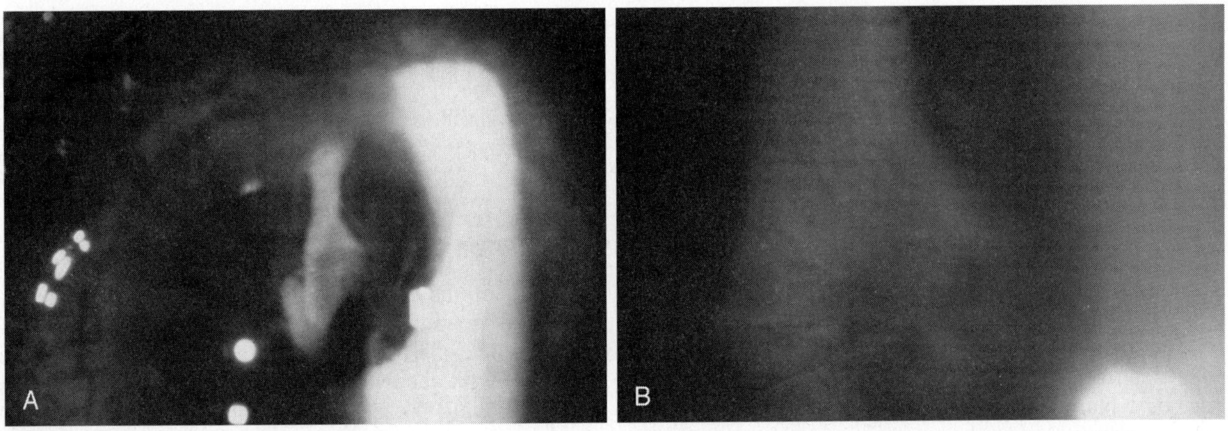

FIGURE 15–31. Fibrous downgrowth following cataract surgery. *A*, Slit-lamp view of left eye demonstrates a tan fibrovascular membrane extending from the superior corneoscleral incision. *B*, Greater magnification reveals extensive vascularization of the fibrous membrane.

lead to occlusion and resultant angle closure. Common forms of pupillary block encountered in aphakia are adhesions between the iris and anterior hyaloid face or to an intact posterior capsule.[238–241] A functioning iridotomy helps to prevent pupillary block but does not eliminate the risk completely. An often self-limited cause of pupillary block in aphakia is the presence of an air bubble behind the iris.[238, 239] When an expanding gas is used for retinal surgery, the pupillary block may persist until the gas is absorbed. Increased inflammation from vitreous loss may exacerbate these conditions and lead to seclusio pupillae.

The occurrence of glaucoma in aphakic children is alarmingly high. The incidence of glaucoma following surgery for congenital cataracts is estimated to be between 5% and 41% and may in fact be higher if long-term follow-up is examined.[242–244] Unlike in adults, pupillary block is an uncommon cause for the elevated pressure in children. In a case series of 65 pediatric patients who experienced glaucoma after lensectomy without intraocular lens implantation, pupillary block was the mechanism in only 5 of 90 eyes (6%).[243] Gonioscopy was performed in 80 of these eyes, 79 of which (98%) demonstrated an open angle. Seventy-six eyes (95%) were found to have angle "abnormalities," consisting of a circumferential repositioning of the iris insertion to the level of the middle or posterior trabecular meshwork. The high incidence of pediatric aphakic glaucoma has been related to pre-existing ocular abnormalities, the type of cataract, chronic postoperative inflammation, type of surgery, and length of follow-up.[243–248]

Regardless of the cause, glaucoma in the pediatric population may be difficult to diagnose, and the effects of treatment hard to evaluate. Measurements of IOP are often hard to obtain with variable reliability. Other means of assessing the progression of glaucomatous damage become extremely important, including appearance of the optic nerve, retinoscopy, and measurement of corneal diameter.[242, 243] Frequently, these measurements must be obtained by examination with the patient under anesthesia.

Finally, the treatment of glaucoma in aphakic patients is often less efficacious than in phakic or pseudophakic patients. Medical management of these patients is difficult, and numerous studies have demonstrated a lower success rate and a greater risk of complications with filtration surgery.[249–253]

Aqueous Misdirection (Malignant Glaucoma)

Although originally coined by von Graefe[254] in 1869 to describe acute shallowing of the anterior chamber with elevated IOP following peripheral iridectomy for angle-closure glaucoma, "malignant glaucoma" has now come to describe a spectrum of scenarios with a common clinical picture and a common response to treatment. Because *aqueous misdirection* represents the presumed etiology of the disease more precisely, it will be used here.

Classically, aqueous misdirection is characterized by a shallow or flat anterior chamber with an elevated IOP in spite of a patent peripheral iridotomy.[255–257] Other terms that have been used to describe this condition are ciliary block and ciliolenticular block. In contrast to pupillary-block glaucoma, in which the anterior chamber shallowing is usually greater in the periphery secondary to iris bombé, the shallowing observed in aqueous misdirection frequently involves the entire anterior chamber (Fig. 15–32).

Almost invariably, a history of previous intraocular surgery is found, but presentations resembling that of the classic condition have been described without antecedent surgery. It has been estimated that 2% to 4% of eyes undergoing surgery for angle-closure glaucoma may dem-

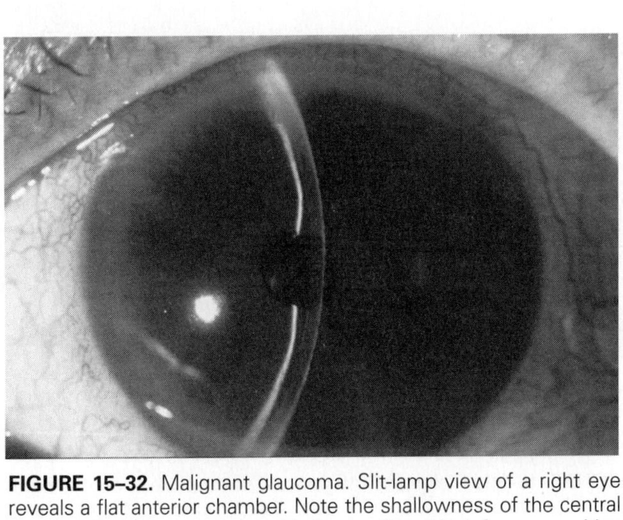

FIGURE 15–32. Malignant glaucoma. Slit-lamp view of a right eye reveals a flat anterior chamber. Note the shallowness of the central anterior chamber compared with the pupillary block form synechiae (see Fig. 15–9).

onstrate aqueous misdirection at some time during the postoperative period.[255] Aqueous misdirection has been reported following ICCE and ECCE with and without intraocular lens implantation, trabeculectomy, surgical and laser iridectomy, laser suture-lysis, and laser posterior capsulotomy (Fig. 15–33).[255, 257–263]

The universal theory describing aqueous misdirection is an alteration of the normal aqueous dynamics resulting in an abnormal accumulation of aqueous humor in the vitreous cavity.[255–257] The initial mechanism leading to the posterior diversion of aqueous has been theorized to occur from an obstruction of flow from the posterior chamber to the anterior chamber, usually occurring at the level of the ciliary body. Numerous studies have implicated a relative or absolute obstruction at almost every level of the anterior segment, including iridocapsular, iridovitreal, ciliovitreal, and ciliopseudophakos blocks.[255, 257–259]

Presumably, a pressure gradient across the peripheral anterior hyaloid and vitreous base is formed that drives the aqueous into the substance of the vitreous. Clinical and ultrasonographic reports supporting this theory have described what are believed to be collections of aqueous in the vitreous cavity.[255, 264] The aqueous continues to pool within the vitreous, possibly secondary to a resistance to outflow across the central anterior hyaloid. The vitreous volume consequently expands pushing the anterior segment structures forward. A form of angle-closure results often with markedly elevated IOP. Using biomicroscopic ultrasound to examine eyes with aqueous misdirection, Trope and associates[265] have shown forward displacement of the lens immediately behind the iris with forward rotation of the ciliary body. Clinically, Luntz and Rosenblatt[255] have noted congested, anteriorly rotated ciliary processes through a peripheral iridectomy in an eye with aqueous misdirection.

A hallmark of aqueous misdirection is its poor response to standard treatment. It may be worsened by miotic therapy, and filtration surgery has been shown to be of no benefit. Medical treatment is aimed at shrinking the vitreous volume, decreasing aqueous production, and promoting backward displacement of the lens-iris diaphragm. The Nd:YAG laser has been used to successfully treat aqueous misdirection in aphakic and pseudophakic eyes by means of posterior capsulotomy and disruption of the anterior hyaloid face.[261, 264] Current surgical treatment for phakic patients includes pars plana vitrectomy with possible lensectomy.[266, 267]

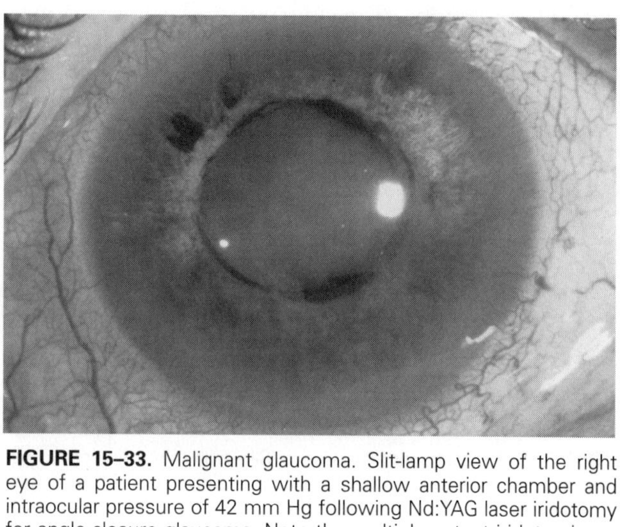

FIGURE 15–33. Malignant glaucoma. Slit-lamp view of the right eye of a patient presenting with a shallow anterior chamber and intraocular pressure of 42 mm Hg following Nd:YAG laser iridotomy for angle-closure glaucoma. Note the multiple patent iridotomies.

Intraocular Pressure and Nd:YAG Laser Capsulotomy

The use of the Nd:YAG laser constitutes a noninvasive means of treating visually significant opacification of the posterior capsule following cataract surgery. Extensive experience with the Nd:YAG laser has shown it to be an extremely safe procedure. Possible complications include an elevation of IOP, an increased risk of retinal detachment, cystoid macular edema, and damage to the intraocular lens.[268–271]

The 1985 report by the U.S. Food and Drug Administration[269] on the Nd:YAG laser found that 39% of patients experienced a 5-mm Hg or more elevation in IOP following posterior capsulotomy. In 28% of cases, the IOP reached a level of 30 mm Hg or higher. Slomovic and Parrish[272] described a 41% incidence of a pressure rise greater than 30 mm Hg following Nd:YAG posterior capsulotomy. Most studies have found that the peak IOP occurs within 2 hours after treatment.[269, 270, 272] In more than 90% of subjects, this rise is followed by a return to the pretreatment level within 24 hours. The incidence of persistently elevated IOP requiring surgery or long-term medical therapy is approximately 1%, and the development of typical glaucomatous optic neuropathy after Nd:YAG posterior capsulotomy has been reported.[269, 273–275]

Pre-existing glaucoma and the position of an intraocular lens have been suggested as risk factors for the development of a postcapsulotomy pressure spike.[268–270] Although Slomovic and Parrish[272] found a significantly lower mean IOP elevation in patients with glaucoma, this finding probably relates to the fact that the patients were instructed to continue their antiglaucoma medications until the time of treatment. Aphakic eyes are at greater risk than pseudophakic eyes, and work by Gimbel and associates[276] revealed a significantly higher incidence of substantial IOP rises for sulcus-fixated posterior chamber lenses than for lenses with capsular bag fixation.

The pathogenesis of elevated IOP following Nd:YAG posterior capsulotomy has been proposed as transient obstruction of trabecular meshwork by capsular, cortical, or vitreous particles liberated by laser photodisruption.[268, 270, 276] An intraocular lens within the capsular bag may act as a barrier to this material reaching the anterior chamber angle and may explain the lower incidence of IOP spikes observed with this type of lens fixation. The release of inflammatory mediators and shock-wave or pressure-induced mechanical trabeculopathy have also been proposed as causes.[276, 277]

Pretreatment with antiglaucoma medications has been shown to markedly decrease the rate of post–Nd:YAG laser IOP spikes. In a study of both glaucomatous and normal eyes, Silverstone and coworkers[278] showed the rate of IOP spikes greater than 5 mm Hg in eyes treated with apraclonidine 1.0% 1 hour prior to laser posterior capsulotomy was 7%, compared with 39% in patients treated with drug vehicle only. Other studies have shown similar efficacy with apraclonidine 0.5% and brimonidine 0.2%.[279–281] If a patient is using apraclonidine or bromonidine for long-term IOP control, prophylactic pretreatment with a different class of drug should be considered.

Although Nd:YAG laser posterior capsulotomy remains a safe and widely performed procedure, the risk of a significant and sustained rise in IOP following the treatment should be discussed with any patient who is to undergo the procedure. Prophylactic treatment may be warranted, and the IOP should be checked within a few hours after treatment to determine whether more aggressive antiglaucoma therapy is indicated.

SUMMARY

Examination of the crystalline lens may reveal many characteristic signs aiding in the diagnosis and management of elevated IOP. The lens capsule may demonstrate the deposition of pseudoexfoliation material or pigment from pigment dispersion syndrome. Distinct cataracts can be observed with certain conditions, such as retinitis pigmentosa and steroid-induced posterior subcapsular cataract. Inflammation and elevated IOP can be caused by hypermature cataracts or disruption of the lens capsule. Abnormalities in lens size and location may contribute to glaucoma. In addition, measurement of the refractive state of the eye can provide useful clinical information about the pathogenesis and risk of development of acute angle-closure or primary open-angle glaucoma.

Elevated IOP is common during the postoperative period after cataract extraction with or without intraocular lens. Careful clinical examination may assist in the management of both acute and delayed or chronic rises in IOP. Finally, certain conditions and procedures unique to the postoperative state, such as aphakia and Nd:YAG capsulotomy, are associated with acute and long-term IOP elevation.

REFERENCES

1. Dvorak-Theobald G: Pseudoexfoliation of the lens capsule: Relation to true exfoliation of the lens capsule as reported in the literature and role in the production of glaucoma capsulocuticulare. Trans Am Ophthalmol Soc 1953;51:385–407.
2. Hiller R, Sperduto RO, Krueger DE: Pseudoexfoliation, intraocular pressure, and senile lens changes in a population-based survey. Arch Ophthalmol 1982;100:1080–1082.
3. Forsius H: Exfoliation syndrome in various ethnic populations. Acta Ophthalmol 1988;66(suppl 184):71–85.
4. Guzek JP, Holm M, Cotter JB, et al: Risk factors for intraoperative complications in 1000 extracapsular cataract cases. Ophthalmology 1987;94:461–466.
5. Ota I, Miyake S, Miyake K: Dislocation of the lens nucleus into the vitreous cavity after standard hydrodissection. Am J Ophthalmol 1996;121:706–708.
6. Naumann GOH, Schlotzer-Schrehardt U, Kuchle M: Pseudoexfoliation syndrome for the comprehensive ophthalmologist: Intraocular and systemic manifestations. Ophthalmology 1998;105:951–68.
7. Moreno-Montanes J, Alcolea-Paredes A, Campos-Garcia S: Prevalence of pseudoexfoliation syndrome in the northwest of Spain. Acta Ophthalmol 1989;67:383–385.
8. Ye TC, Mao WS, Zhang J: Pseudoexfoliation syndrome in Chinese. Jpn J Ophthalmol 1989;33:300–310.
9. Krupin T, Patkin R, Kurata FK, et al: Argon laser trabeculoplasty in black and white patients with primary open-angle glaucoma. Ophthalmology 1986;93:811–816.
10. Dark AJ, Streeten BW, Cornwall CC: Pseudoexfoliation disease of the lens: A study in electron microscopy and histochemistry. Br J Ophthalmol 1977;61:462–472.
11. Schlotzer-Schrehardt U, Dorfler S, Naumann GO: Immunohistochemical localization of basement membrane components in pseudoexfoliation material of the lens capsule. Curr Eye Res 1992;11:343–355.
12. Sampaolesi R, Zarate J, Croxato O: The chamber angle in exfoliation syndrome: Clinical and pathological findings. Acta Ophthalmol 1988;66(suppl 184):48–53.
13. Seland JH: The ultrastructural changes in the exfoliation syndrome. Acta Ophthalmol 1988;66(suppl 184):28–34.
14. FitzSimon JS, Johnson DH: Exfoliation material on intraocular lens implants. Arch Ophthalmol 1996;114:355.
15. Puska P: The amount of lens exfoliation and chamber-angle pigmentation in exfoliation syndrome with or without glaucoma. Acta Ophthalmol 1995;73:226–232.
16. Henry JC, Krupin T, Schmitt M, et al: Long–term follow-up of pseudoexfoliation and the development of elevated intraocular pressure. Ophthalmology 1987;94:545–552.
17. Cashwell LF, Shields MB: Exfoliation syndrome in the southeastern United States. I: Prevalence in open-angle glaucoma and non-glaucoma populations. Acta Ophthalmol 1988;66(suppl 184):99–102.
18. Valle O: Prevalence of simple and capsular glaucoma in the central hospital district of Kotka. Acta Ophthalmol 1988;66(suppl 184):116–119.
19. Wishart PK, Spaeth GL, Poryzees EM: Anterior chamber angle in the exfoliation syndrome. Br J Ophthalmol 1985;69:103–107.
20. Gross FJ, Tingley D, Epstein DL: Increased prevalence of occludable angles and angle-closure glaucoma in patients with pseudoexfoliation. Am J Ophthalmol 1994;117:333–336.
21. Ritch R: Exfoliation syndrome and occludable angles. Trans Am Ophthalmol Soc 1994;92:845–944.
22. Puska P: Lens opacity in unilateral exfoliation syndrome with or without glaucoma. Acta Ophthalmol 1994;72:290–296.
23. Fama F, Castagna I, Salmeri G: Influence of pseudoexfoliation syndrome on human lens transparency. Ann Ophthalmol 1993;25:440–441.
24. Skuta GL, Parrish RK, Hodapp E: Zonular dialysis during extracapsular cataract extraction in pseudoexfoliation syndrome. Arch Ophthalmol 1987;105:632–634.
25. Schlotzer-Schrehardt U, Naumann GOH: A histopathologic study of zonular instability in pseudoexfoliation syndrome. Am J Ophthalmol 1994;118:730–743.
26. Naumann GOH, the "Erlanger Augenblatter-Group": Exfoliation syndrome as a risk factor for vitreous loss in extracapsular cataract surgery (preliminary report). Acta Ophthalmol 1988;66(supp 184):129–131.
27. Drolsum L, Haaskjold E, Davanger M: Pseudoexfoliation syndrome and extracapsular cataract extraction. Acta Ophthalmol 1993; 71:765–770.
28. Drolsum L, Haaskjold E, Davanger M: Results and complications after extracapsular cataract extraction in eyes with pseudoexfoliation syndrome. Acta Ophthalmol 1993;71:771–776.
29. Raitta C, Setala K: Intraocular lens implantation in exfoliation syndrome and capsular glaucoma. Acta Ophthalmol 1988;64:130–133.
30. Spencer WH: Lens. *In* Spencer WH (ed): Ophthalmic Pathology. Philadelphia, WB Saunders, 1985, pp 465–466.
31. Anderson DR: Pathology of the glaucomas. Br J Ophthalmol 1972;56:146.
32. Jones B: Dots in lens with glaucoma: Cataracta glaucomatosa and its role in the diagnosis of the acute glaucomas. Trans Ophthalmol Soc UK 1959;79:753.
33. Schlaegel TF: Complications of uveitis. Int Ophthalmol Clin 1977;17:65–74.
34. Kwon YH, Dreyer EB: Inflammatory glaucoma. Int Ophthalmol Clin 1996;36:81–89.
35. Jampel HD, Jabs DA, Quigley HA: Trabeculectomy with 5-fluorouracil for adult inflammatory glaucoma. Am J Ophthalmol 1990;109:168–173.
36. Skuta GL, Beeson CC, Higginbotham EJ, et al: Intraoperative mitomycin versus postoperative 5-fluorouracil in high-risk glaucoma filtering surgery. Ophthalmology 1992;99:438–444.

37. Best JM: Rubella. *In* Greenough A, Osborne J, Sutherland (eds): Congenital, perinatal and neonatal infections. Philadelphia, Churchill Livingstone, 1992, pp 171–184.
38. Boniuk M, Zimmerman LE: Ocular pathology in the rubella syndrome. Arch Ophthalmol 1967;77:455–473.
39. Zimmerman LE: Histopathologic basis for ocular manifestations of congenital rubella syndrome: The Eighth William Hamlin Wilder Memorial Lecture. Am J Ophthalmol 1968;65:837–862.
40. Spencer WH: Lens. *In* Spencer WH (ed): Ophthalmic Pathology. Philadelphia, WB Saunders, 1985, 471–473.
41. Merin S, Auerbach E: Retintits pigmentosa. Surv Ophthalmol 1976;20:303–345.
42. Heckenlively J: The frequency of posterior subcapsular cataract in the hereditary retinal degenerations. Am J Ophthalmol 1982;93:733–738.
43. Kogbe OI, Follmann P: Investigations into aqueous humor dynamics in primary pigmentary degeneration of the retina. Ophthalmologica 1975;171:165–75.
44. Gartner S, Schlossman A: Retinitis pigmentosa associated with glaucoma. Am J Ophthalmol 1949;32:1337–1350.
45. Badeeb O, Trope G, Musarella M: Primary angle closure glaucoma and retinitis pigmentosa. Acta Ophthalmol 1993;71:727–732.
46. Omphroy CA: Sector retinitis pigmentosa and chronic angle-closure glaucoma: A new association. Ophthalmologica 1984;189:12–20.
47. Fiore C, Reggiani FM, Buoncristiani U, et al: Familial nephropathy with retinitis pigmentosa and closed-angle glaucoma. Ophthalmic Paediatr Genet 1985;5:39–49.
48. La Hey E, de Jong PTVM, Kijlstra A: Fuchs' heterochromic cyclitis: Review of the literature on the pathogenetic mechanisms. Br J Ophthalmol 1994;78:307–312.
49. Jones NP: Fuchs' heterochromic uveitis: An update. Surv Ophthalmol 1993;37:253–272.
50. Jones NP: Cataract surgery in Fuchs' heterochromic uveitis: Past present, and future. J Cataract Refract Surg 1996;22:261–268.
51. O'Neill D, Murray PI, Patel BC, et al: Extracapsular cataract surgery with and without intraocular lens implantation in Fuchs' heterochromic cyclitis. Ophthalmology 1995;102:1362–1368.
52. Urban RC, Cotlier E: Corticosteroid-induced cataracts. Surv Ophthalmol 1986;31:102–110.
53. Skalka HW, Prchal JT: Effect of corticosteroids on cataract formation. Arch Ophthalmol 1980;98:1773–1777.
54. Karim AK, Jacob TJ, Thompson GM: The human lens epithelium: Morphological and ultrastructural changes associated with steroid therapy. Exp Eye Res 1989;48:215–224.
55. Cumming RG, Mitchell P, Leeder SR: Use of inhaled corticosteroids and the risk of cataracts. N Engl J Med 1997;337:8–14.
56. Spaeth GL, von Sallman L: Corticosteroids and cataracts. Int Ophthalmol Clin 1966;6:915–929.
57. Frandsen E: Glaucoma and posterior subcapsular cataract following topical prednisolone (ultracortenol) therapy. Acta Ophthalmol 1964;42:108–118.
58. Akduman L, Kolker AE, Black DL, et al: Treatment of persistent glaucoma secondary to periocular corticosteroids. Am J Ophthalmol 1996;122:275–276.
59. Weinreb RN, Polansky JR, Kramer SG, et el: Acute effects of dexamethasone on intraocular pressure in glaucoma. Invest Ophthalmol Vis Sci 1985;26:170–175.
60. Akingbehin AO: Corticosteroid-induced ocular hypertension. II: An acquired form. Br J Ophthalmol 1982;66:541–545.
61. Sowell JG, Levene RZ, Bloom J, et al: Primary open-angle glaucoma and sensitivity to corticosteroids in vitro. Trans Am Ophthalmol Soc 1977;75:339–351.
62. Lewis JM, Priddy T, Judd J, et al: Intraocular pressure response to topical dexamethasone as a predictor for the development of primary open-angle glaucoma. Am J Ophthalmol 1988;106:607–612.
63. Schwartz B: The response of ocular pressure to corticosteroids. Int Ophthalmol Clin 1966;6:929–989.
64. Becker B, Mills DW: Corticosteroids and intraocular pressure. Arch Ophthalmol 1963;70:500–507.
65. Urban RC, Dreyer EB: Corticosteroid-induced glaucoma. Int Ophthalmol Clin 1993;33:135–139.
66. Samiy N, Walton DS, Dreyer EB: Inhaled steroids: Effect on intraocular pressure in patients without glaucoma. Can J Ophthalmol 1996;31:120–123.
67. Aggarwal RK, Potamitis T, Chong NH, et al: Extensive visual loss with topical facial steroids. Eye 1993;7:664–666.
68. Spaeth GL, Rodrigues MM, Weinreb S: Steroid-induced glaucoma. A: Persistent elevation of intraocular pressure. Trans Am Ophthalmol Soc 1977;75:353–381.
69. Polansky JR, Kurtz RM, Alvarado JR, et al: Cellular production and glucocorticoid regulatory mechanisms in cultured human trabecular meshwork cells. Prog Clin Biol Res 1989;12:113–117.
70. Kee C, Ahn B: TIGR gene in primary open-angle glaucoma and steroid-induced glaucoma. Korean J Ophthalmol 1997;11:75–78.
71. Stone EM, Fingert JH, Alward WLM, et al: Identification of a gene that causes primary open angle glaucoma. Science 1997;275:668–670.
72. Epstein DL: Diagnosis and management of lens-induced glaucoma. Ophthalmology 1982;89:227–230.
73. Ellant JP, Obstbaum SA: Lens-induced glaucoma. Doc Ophthalmol 1992;81:317–338.
74. Yanoff M, Scheie HG: Cytology of human lens aspirate. Arch Ophthalmol 1968;80:166–170.
75. Ueno H, Tamai A, Iyota K, et al: Electron microscopic observation of the cells floating in the anterior chamber in a case of phacolytic glaucoma. Jpn J Ophthalmol 1989;33:103–113.
76. Brooks AM, Grant G, Gillies WE: Comparison of specular microscopy and examination of aspirate in phacolytic glaucoma. Ophthalmology 1990;97:85–89.
77. Avasthi P, Raizada VN, Agarwal MS, et al: Effect of cataract on intraocular pressure. Int Surg 1976;61:423–425.
78. Rosenbaum JT, Samples JR, Seymour B, et al: Chemotactic activity of lens proteins and the pathogenesis of phacolytic glaucoma. Arch Ophthalmol 1987;105:1582–1584.
79. Filipe JC, Palmares J, Delgado L, et al: Phacolytic glaucoma and lens-induced uveitis. Int Ophthalmol 1993;17:289–293.
80. Wei-rong S, Zhen-rong S, Ming-chen J: Histopathological observation of phacolytic glaucoma: Report of 5 cases. Chin Med J 1986;99:931–934.
81. Flocks M, Littwin CS, Zimmerman LE: Phacolytic glaucoma: A clinicopathologic study of one hundred thirty-eight cases of glaucoma associated with hypermature cataract. Arch Ophthalmol 1955;54:37–45.
82. Goldberg MF: Cytological diagnosis of phacolytic glaucoma utilizing Millipore filtration of the aqueous. Br J Ophthalmol 1967;51:847–853.
83. Epstein DL, Jedziniak JA, Grant WM: Identification of heavy-molecular-weight soluble protein in aqueous humor in human phacolytic glaucoma. Invest Ophthalmol Vis Sci 1978;17:398–402.
84. Lane SS, Kopietz LA, Lindquist TD, et al: Treatment of phacolytic glaucoma with extracapsular cataract extraction. Ophthalmology 1988;95:749-753.
85. Mandal AK: Endocapsular surgery and capsular bag fixation of intraocular lenses in phacolytic glaucoma. J Cataract Refract Surg 1996;22:288–293.
86. Thach AB, Marak GE, McLean IW, et al: Phacoanaphylactic endophthalmitis: A clinicopathologic review. Int Ophthalmol 1991; 15:271–279.
87. Marak GE, Font RL, Ward FP: Arthus-type panophthalmitis in rats sensitized to heterologous lens proteins. Ophthalmic Res 1977; 9:162–170.
88. Till GO, Lee S, Mulligan MS, et al: Adhesion molecules in experimental phacoanaphylactic endophthalmitis. Invest Ophthalmol Vis Sci 1992;33:3417–3423.
89. Apple DJ, Mamalis N, Steinmetz RL, et al: Phacoanaphylactic endophthalmitis associated with extracapsular cataract extraction and posterior chamber intraocular lens. Arch Ophthalmol 1984; 102:1528–1532.
90. Ellant JP, Obstbaum SA: Lens-induced glaucoma. Doc Ophthalmol 1992;81:317–338.
91. Perlman EM, Albert DM: Clinically unsuspected phacoanaphylaxis after ocular trauma. Arch Ophthalmol 1977;95:244–246.
92. Abrahams IW: Diagnosis and surgical management of phacoanaphylactic uveitis following extracapsular cataract extraction with intraocular lens implantation. J Cataract Refract Surg 1985;11:444–447.
93. Wohl LG, Lucier AC, Kline OR, et al: Pseudophakic phacoanaphylactic endophthalmitis. Ophthalmic Surg 1986;4:234–237.
94. McMahon MS, Weiss JS, Riedel KG, et al: Clinically unsuspected phacoanaphylaxis after extracapsular cataract extraction with intraocular lens implantation. Br J Ophthalmol 1985;69:836–840.
95. Smith RE, Weiner P: Unusual presentation of phacoanaphylaxis following phacoemulsification. Ophthalmic Surg 1976;7:65–68.

96. Allen JC: Sympathetic uveitis and phacoanaphylaxis. Am J Ophthalmol 1967;63:280–283.
97. Hodes BL, Stern G: Phacoanaphylactic endophthalmitis: Echographic diagnosis of phacoanaphylactic endophthalmitis. Ophthalmic Surg 1976;7:60–64.
98. Ellant JP, Obstbaum SA: Lens-induced glaucoma. Doc Ophthalmol 1992;81:317–338.
99. Tomey KF, Al-Rajhi AA: Neodymium:YAG laser iridotomy in the initial management of phacomorphic glaucoma. Ophthalmology 1992;99:660–665.
100. McKibbin M, Gupta A, Atkins AD: Cataract extraction and intraocular lens implantation in eyes with phacomorphic or phacolytic glaucoma. J Cataract Refract Surg 1996;22:633–636.
101. Jarrett WH: Dislocation of the lens. Arch Ophthalmol 1967;78:289–296.
102. Nelson LB, Maumenee IH: Ectopia lentis. Surv Ophthalmol 1982;27:143–160.
103. Cross HE, Jensen AD: Ocular manifestations in the Marfan syndrome and homocystinuria. Am J Ophthalmol 1973;75:405–420.
104. Hindle NW, Crawford JS: Dislocation of the lens in Marfan's syndrome. Can J Ophthalmol 1969;4:128–135.
105. Rodman HI: Chronic open-angle glaucoma associated with traumatic dislocation of the lens. Arch Ophthalmol 1963;69:445–454.
106. Seetner AA, Crawford JS: Surgical correction of lens dislocation in children. Am J Ophthalmol 1981;91:106–110.
107. Croxatto JO, Lombardi A, Malbran ES: Inflamed eye in Marfan's syndrome with posteriorly luxated lens. Ophthalmologica 1986; 193:23–26.
108. Godfrey M, Menashe V, Weleber RG, et al: Cosegregation of elastin-associated microfibrillar abnormalities with the Marfan phenotype in families. Am J Hum Genet 1990;46:652–660.
109. Hollister DW, Godfrey M, Sakai LY, et al: Immunohistologic abnormalities of the microfibrillar-fiber system in the Marfan syndrome. N Engl J Med 1990;323:152–159.
110. Burian HM, Allen L: Histologic study of the chamber angle of patients with Marfan's syndrome. Arch Ophthalmol 1961;65:323–333.
111. von Noorden GK, Schultz RO: A gonioscopic study of the chamber angle in Marfan's syndrome. Arch Ophthalmol 1960;64:929–934.
112. Maumenee IH, Izquierdo NJ, Traboulsi EI, et al: Glaucoma in the Marfan syndrome. Trans Am Ophthalmol Soc 1992;140:111–122.
113. Mudd SH, Skovby F, Levy HL, et al: The natural history of homocystinuria due to cystathionine beta-synthase deficiency. Am J Hum Genet 1985;37:1–31.
114. Regenbogen L, Ilie S, Elian I: Homocystinuria—a surgical and anaesthetic risk. Metab Pediatr Ophthalmol 1980;4:209–211.
115. Hayasaka S, Asano Y, Tateda H: Lens subluxation in homocystinuria: A case report. Acta Ophthalmol 1984;62:425–431.
116. Jensen AD, Cross HE, Paton D: Ocular complications in the Weill-Marchesani syndrome. Am J Ophthalmol 1974;77:261–269.
117. Smith TH, Holland MG, Woody NC: Ocular manifestations of familial hyperlysinemia. Trans Am Acad Ophthalmol Otolaryngol 1971;75:355–360.
118. Shih VE, Abroms IF, Johnson JL, et al: Sulfite oxidase deficiency: Biochemical and clinical investigations of a hereditary metabolic disorder in sulfur metabolism. N Engl J Med 1977;297:1022–1028.
119. Irreverre F, Mudd SH, Heizer WD, et al: Sulfite oxidase deficiency: Studies of a patient with mental retardation, dislocated ocular lenses, and abnormal urinary excretion of S-sulfo-L-cysteine, sulfite, and thiosulfate. Biochem Med 1967;1:187–217.
120. Malbran ES, Croxatto JO, D'alessandro C, et al: Genetic spontaneous late subluxation of the lens. Ophthalmology 1989;96:223–229.
121. Tomlinson A, Phillips CI: Applanation tension and axial length of the eyeball. Br J Ophthalmol 1970;54:548–553.
122. Abdalla MI, Hamdi M: Applanation ocular tension in myopia and emmetropia. Br J Ophthalmol 1970;54:122–125.
123. David R, Zangwill LM, Tessler Z, et al: The correlation between intraocular pressure and refractive status. Arch Ophthalmol 1985;103:1812–1815.
124. Lotufo D, Ritch R, Szmyd L, et al: Juvenile glaucoma, race, and refraction. JAMA 1989;261:249–252.
125. Perkins ES, Phelps CD: Open angle glaucoma, ocular hypertension, low-tension glaucoma, and refraction. Arch Ophthalmol 1982; 100:1464–1467.
126. Phelps CD: Effect of myopia on prognosis in treated primary open-angle glaucoma. Am J Ophthalmol 1982;93:622–628.
127. Zeimer RC, Ogura Y: The relation between glaucomatous damage and optic nerve head mechanical compliance. Arch Ophthalmol 1989;107:1232–1234.
128. Hernandez MR, Andrzejewska WM, Neufeld AH: Changes in the extracellular matrix of the human optic nerve head in primary open-angle glaucoma. Am J Ophthalmol 1990;109:180–188.
129. Quigley HA, Dorman-Pease ME, Brown AE: Quantitative study of collagen and elastin of the optic nerve head and sclera in human and experimental monkey glaucoma. Curr Eye Res 1991;10:877–888.
130. Quigley EN, Quigley HA, Pease ME, et al: Quantitative studies of elastin in the optic nerve heads of persons with primary open-angle glaucoma. Ophthalmology 1996;103:1680–1685.
131. Wilson MR, Hertzmark E, Walker AM, et al: A case-control study of risk factors in open angle glaucoma. Arch Ophthalmol 1987;105:1066–1071.
132. Leighton DA, Tomlinson A: Ocular tension and axial length of the eyeball in open-angle glaucoma and low tension glaucoma. Br J Ophthalmol 1973;57:499–502.
133. Daubs JG, Crick RP: Effect of refractive error on the risk of ocular hypertension and open angle glaucoma. Trans Ophthalmol Soc UK 1981;101:121–126.
134. Fong DS, Epstein DL, Allingham RR: Glaucoma and myopia: Are they related? Int Ophthalmol Clin 1990;30:215–218.
135. Lowe RF: Aetiology of the anatomical basis for primary angle-closure glaucoma. Br J Ophthalmol 1970;54:161–169.
136. Tomlinson A, Leighton DA: Ocular dimensions in the heredity of angle-closure glaucoma. Br J Ophthalmol 1973;57:475–486.
137. Sugar HS: The mechanical factors in the etiology of acute glaucoma. Am J Ophthalmol 1941;24:851–873.
138. Tornquist R: Chamber depth in primary acute glaucoma. Br J Ophthalmol 1956;40:421–429.
139. Lee DA, Brubaker RF, Ilstrup DM: Anterior chamber dimensions in patients with narrow angles and angle-closure glaucoma. Arch Ophthalmol 1984;102:46–50.
140. Fontana ST, Brubaker RF: Volume and depth of the anterior chamber in the normal aging human eye. Arch Ophthalmol 1980;98:1803–1808.
141. Lowe RF: Causes of shallow anterior chamber in primary angle-closure glaucoma: Ultrasonic biometry of normal and angle-closure glaucoma eyes. Am J Ophthalmol 1969;67:87–93.
142. Markowitz SN, Morin JD: The ratio of lens thickness to axial length for biometric standardization in angle-closure glaucoma. Am J Ophthalmol 1985;99:400–402.
143. Panek WC, Christensen RE, Lee DA, et al: Biometric variables in patients with occludable anterior chamber angles. Am J Ophthalmol 1990;110:185–188.
144. Markowitz SN, Morin JD: Angle-closure glaucoma: Relation between lens thickness, anterior chamber depth and age. Can J Ophthalmol 1984;19:300–302.
145. Lowe RF: Anterior lens curvature: Comparisons between normal eyes and those with primary angle-closure glaucoma. Br J Ophthalmol 1972;56:409–413.
146. Lowe RF, Clark BA: Radius of curvature of the anterior lens surface: Correlations in normal eyes and eyes involved with primary angle-closure glaucoma. Br J Ophthalmol 1973;57:471–474.
147. Alsbirk PH: Primary angle-closure glaucoma: Oculometry, epidemiology, and genetics in a high-risk population. Acta Ophthalmol 1976;54(suppl 127):5–31.
148. Kooner KS, Cooksey JC, Perry P: Intraocular pressure following ECCE, phacoemulsification, and PC-IOL implantation. Ophthalmic Surg 1988;19:643–646.
149. Smith JA, Anderson DR: Effect of the intraocular lens on intraocular pressure. Arch Ophthalmol 1976;94:1291–1294.
150. Radius RL, Schultz K, Sobocinski K, et al: Pseudophakia and intraocular pressure. Am J Ophthalmol 1984;97:738–742.
151. Obstbaum SA: Glaucoma and intraocular implantation. J Cataract Refract Surg 1986;12:257–261.
152. Steuhl KP, Marahrens P, Frohn C, et al: Intraocular pressure and anterior chamber depth before and after extracapsular cataract extraction with posterior chamber lens implantation. Ophthalmic Surg 1992;23:234–237.
153. Cinotti DJ, Fiore PM, Maltzman BA, et al: Control of intraocular pressure in glaucomatous eyes after extracapsular cataract extraction with intraocular lens implantation. J Cataract Refract Surg 1988;14:650–653.

154. Yalvac I, Airaksinen PJ, Tuulonen A: Phacoemulsification with and without trabeculectomy in patients with glaucoma. Ophthalmic Surg Lasers 1997;28:469–475.
155. Tong JT, Miller KM: Intraocular pressure change after sutureless phacoemulsification and foldable posterior chamber lens implantation. J Cataract Refract Surg 1998;24:256–262.
156. Perasalo R: Phaco-emulsification of cataract in eyes with glaucoma. Acta Ophthalmol 1997;75:299–300.
157. Gross JG, Meyer DR, Robin AL, et al: Increased intraocular pressure in the immediate postoperative period after extracapsular cataract extraction. Am J Ophthalmol 1988;105:466–469.
158. Krupin T, Feitl ME, Bishop KI: Postoperative intraocular pressure rise in open-angle glaucoma patients after cataract or combined cataract-filtration surgery. Ophthalmology 1989;96:579–584.
159. McGuigan LJ, Gottsch J, Stark WJ, et al: Extracapsular cataract extraction and posterior chamber lens implantation in eyes with preexisting glaucoma. Arch Ophthalmol 1986;104:1301–1308.
160. Shields MB: Combined cataract extraction and glaucoma surgery. Ophthalmology 1982;89:231–237.
161. Shields MB: Another reevaluation of combined cataract and glaucoma surgery. Am J Ophthalmol 1993;115:806–811.
162. Naveh N, Kottass R, Glovinsky J, et al: The long-term effect on intraocular pressure of a procedure combining trabeculectomy and cataract surgery, as compared with trabeculectomy alone. Ophthalmic Surg 1990;21:339–345.
163. Park HJ, Weitzman M, Caprioli J: Temporal corneal phacoemulsification combined with superior trabeculectomy. Arch Ophthalmol 1997;115:318–322.
164. Park HJ, Kwon YH, Weitzman M, et al: Temporal corneal phacoemulsification in patients with filtered glaucoma. Arch Ophthalmol 1997;115:1375–1380.
165. Johnson D: Extracapsular cataract extraction, intraocular lens implantation, and trabeculectomy: The combined procedure. Int Ophthalmol Clin 1990;30:209–214.
166. Longstaff S, Wormald RP, Mazover A, et al: Glaucoma triple procedures: Efficacy of intraocular pressure control and visual outcome. Ophthalmic Surg 1990;21:786–793.
167. McCartney DL, Memmen JE, Stark WJ, et al: The efficacy and safety of combined trabeculectomy, cataract extraction, and intraocular lens implantation. Ophthalmology 1988;95:754–763.
168. Shin DH, Simone PA, Song MS, et al: Adjunctive subconjunctival mitomycin C in glaucoma triple procedure. Ophthalmology 1995;102:1550–1558.
169. Murchison JF, Shields MB: An evaluation of three surgical approaches for coexisting cataract and glaucoma. Ophthalmic Surg 1989;20:393.
170. Allan BD, Barrett GD: Combined small incision phacoemulsification and trabeculectomy. J Cataract Refract Surg 1993;19:97–102.
171. Parker JS, Gollamudi S, John G, et al: Combined trabeculectomy, cataract extraction, and foldable lens implantation. J Cataract Refract Surg 1992;18: 582–585.
172. Williamson TH, Bacon AS, Flanagan DW, et al: Combined extracapsular cataract extraction and trabeculectomy using a separated corneal section. Eye 1989;3:547–552.
173. Tezel G, Kolker AE, Kass MA, et al: Comparative results of combined procedures for glaucoma and cataract. I: Extracapsular cataract extraction versus phacoemulsification and foldable versus rigid intraocular lenses. Ophthalmic Surg Lasers 1997;28:539–550.
174. Kosmin AS, Wishart PK, Ridges PJ: Long-term intraocular pressure control after cataract extraction with trabeculectomy: Phacoemulsification versus extracapsular technique. J Cataract Refract Surg 1998;24:249–255.
175. Wyse T, Meyer M, Ruderman JM, et al: Combined trabeculectomy and phacoemulsification: A one-site versus a two-site approach. Am J Ophthalmol 1998;125:334–339.
176. Gimbel HV, Meyer D, DeBroff BM, et el: Intraocular pressure response to combined phacoemulsification and trabeculotomy, ab externo versus phacoemulsification alone in primary open-angle glaucoma. J Cataract Refract Surg 1995;21:653–660.
177. Pasquale LR, Smith SG: Surgical outcome of phacoemulsification combined with the Pearce trabeculectomy in patients with glaucoma. J Cataract Refract Surg 1992;18:301–305.
178. Uram M: Combined phacoemulsification, endoscopic ciliary process photocoagulation, and intraocular lens implantation in glaucoma management. Ophthalmic Surg 1995;26:346–352.
179. Heuer DK, Parrish RK, Gressel MG, et al: 5-Fluorouracil and glaucoma filtering surgery. III: Intermediate follow-up of a pilot study. Ophthalmology 1986;93:1537.
180. Rockwood EJ, Parrish RK, Heuer DK, et al: Glaucoma filtration surgery with 5-fluorouracil. Ophthalmology 1987;94:1071.
181. Skuta GL: Antifibrotic agents in glaucoma filtering surgery. Int Ophthalmol Clin 1993;33:165–182.
182. Belyea DA, Dan JA, Lieberman MF, et al: Midterm follow-up results of combined phacoemulsification, lens implantation, and mitomycin-C trabeculectomy procedure. J Glaucoma 1997;6:90–98.
183. Joos KM, Bueche MJ, Palmberg PF, et al: One-year follow-up results of combined mitomycin-C trabeculectomy and extracapsular cataract extraction. Ophthalmology 1995;102:76–83.
184. Palmer SS: Mitomycin as adjunct chemotherapy with trabeculectomy. Ophthalmology 1991;98:317–321.
185. O'Grady JM, Juzych MS, Shin DH, et al: Trabeculectomy, phacoemulsification, and posterior chamber lens implantation with and without 5-fluorouracil. Am J Ophthalmol 1993;116:594–599.
186. Wong PC, Ruderman JM, Krupin T, et al: 5-Fluorouracil after primary combined filtration surgery. Am J Ophthalmol 1994; 117:149–154.
187. Hennis HL, Stewart WC: The use of 5-fluorouracil in patients following combined trabeculectomy and cataract extraction. Ophthalmic Surg 1991;22:451–454.
188. Cohen JS, Greff LJ, Novack GD, et al: A placebo-controlled, double-masked evaluation of mitomycin-C in combined glaucoma and cataract procedures. Ophthalmology 1996;103:1934–1942.
189. Carlson DW, Alward WL, Barad JP, et al: A randomized study of mitomycin augmentation in combined phacoemulsification and trabeculectomy. Ophthalmology 1997;104:719–724.
190. Shin DH, Hughes BA, Song MS, et al: Primary glaucoma triple procedure with or without adjunctive mitomycin. Ophthalmology 1996;103:1925–1933.
191. Shin DH, Ren J, Juzych MS, et al: Primary glaucoma triple procedure in patients with primary open-angle glaucoma: The effect of mitomycin C in patients with and without prognostic factors for filtration failure. Am J Ophthalmol 1998;125:346–352.
192. Goodman DF, Stark WJ, Gottsch JD: Complications of cataract extraction with intraocular lens implantation. Ophthalmic Surg 1989;20:132–140.
193. Bomer TG, Lagreze WD, Funk J: Intraocular pressure rise after phacoemulsification with posterior chamber lens implantation: Effect of prophylactic medication, wound closure, and surgeon's experience. Br J Ophthalmol 1995;79:809–813.
194. Lorusso V, Moramarco A, Pacella E, et al: Intraocular lens complications. Ann Ophthalmol 1990;22:377–381.
195. Rich WJ, Radtke ND, Cohan BE: Early ocular hypertension after cataract extraction. Br J Ophthalmol 1974;58:725.
196. Dada VK, Sindu N, Sachdev MS: Postoperative intraocular pressure changes with the use of different viscoelastics. Ophthalmic Surg 1994;25:540–544.
197. Fry LL: Postoperative intraocular pressure rises: A comparison of Healon, Amvisc, and Viscoat. J Cataract Refract Surg 1989;15:415–420.
198. Kohnen T, von Ehr M, Schutte E, et al: Evaluation of intraocular pressure with Healon and Healon GV in sutureless cataract surgery with foldable lens implantation. J Cataract Refract Surg 1996;22:227–237.
199. Shibasaki H, Kurome H, Hayasaka S, et al: Viscoelastic substance in the anterior chamber elevates intraocular pressure. Ann Ophthalmol 1994;26:10–11.
200. Berson FG, Patterson MM, Epstein DL: Obstruction of aqueous outflow by sodium hyaluronate in enucleated human eyes. Am J Ophthalmol 1983;95:668–672.
201. Sanders DR, Kraff MC, Lieberman HL, et al: Breakdown and reestablishment of blood-aqueous barrier with implant surgery. Arch Ophthalmol 1982;100:588–590.
202. Savage JA, Thomas JV, Belcher CD, et al: Extracapsular cataract extraction and posterior chamber intraocular lens implantation in glaucomatous eyes. Ophthalmology 1985;92:1506–1516.
203. Watzke RC: Intraocular hemorrhage from vascularization of the cataract incision. Ophthalmology 1980;87:19–23.
204. Ellington FT: Complications with the Choyce Mark VIII anterior chamber lens implant (uveitis-glaucoma-hyphema). J Cataract Refract Surg 1977;3:199–201.

205. Masket S: Pseudophakic posterior iris chafing syndrome. J Cataract Refract Surg 1986;12:252–256.
206. Johnson SH, Kratz RP Olson PF: Iris transillumination defect and microhyphema syndrome. J Cataract Refract Surg 1981;10:425–428.
207. Apple DJ, Mamalis N, Reidy JJ, et al: A comparison of ciliary sulcus and capsular bag fixation of posterior chamber intraocular lenses. J Cataract Refract Surg 1985;11:44–63.
208. John GR, Stark WJ: Rotation of posterior chamber intraocular lenses for management of lens-associated recurring hyphema. Arch Ophthalmol 1992;110:963–964.
209. Shrader CE, Belcher CD, Thomas JV, et al: Papillary and iridovitreal block in pseudophakic eyes. Ophthalmology 1984;91:831–837.
210. Chandler PA: Glaucoma from pupillary block in aphakia. Trans Am Ophthalmol Soc 1961;59:96.
211. Anderson DR, Forster RK, Lewis ML: Laser iridotomy for aphakic pupillary block. Arch Ophthalmol 1975;93:343–346.
212. Van Buskirk EM: Pupillary block after intraocular lens implantation. Am J Ophthalmol 1983;95:55–59.
213. Samples JR, Bellows AR, Rosenquist RC, et al: Pupillary block with posterior chamber intraocular lenses. Arch Ophthalmol 1987;105:335–337.
214. Smith JA: Glaucoma and intraocular lens implantation. Int Ophthalmol Clin 1984;24:61–77.
215. Poleski SA, Willis WE: Angle-supported intraocular lenses: A goniophotographic study. Ophthalmology 1984;91:838–840.
216. Evans RB: Peripheral anterior synechia overlying the haptics of posterior chamber lenses. Ophthalmology 1990;97:415–423.
217. Champion R, McDonnell PJ, Green R: Intraocular lenses: Histopathologic characteristics of a large series of autopsy eyes. Surv Ophthalmol 1985;30:1–32.
218. Van Buskirk EM: Late onset, progressive, peripheral anterior synechiae with posterior chamber intraocular lenses. Ophthalmic Surg 1987;18:115–117.
219. Hansen TE, Naeser K, Nissen JN, et al: Prospective study of intraocular pressure 21/2 years after intracapsular cataract extraction and implantation of a semiflexible anterior chamber lens. J Cataract Refract Surg 1987;13:554–556.
220. McAllister IL, Meyers SM, Meisler DM, et al: Epithelial downgrowth. Ophthalmic Surg 1988;19:713–714.
221. Jensen P, Minckler DS, Chandler JW: Epithelial ingrowth. Arch Ophthalmol 1977;95:837–842.
222. Ghosh M, McCulloch C: Epithelial downgrowth following cataract extraction. Can J Ophthalmol 1979;14:126–136.
223. Weiner MJ, Trentacoste J, Pon DM, et al: Epithelial downgrowth: A 30-year clinicopathological review. Br J Ophthalmol 1989;73:5–11.
224. Knauf HP, Rowsey JJ, Margo CE: Cystic epithelial downgrowth following clear-cornea cataract extraction. Arch Ophthalmol 1997;115:668–669.
225. Smith RE, Parrett C: Specular microscopy of epithelial downgrowth. Arch Ophthalmol 1978;96:1222–1224.
226. Holliday JN, Buller CR, Bourne WM: Specular microscopy and fluorophotometry in the diagnosis of epithelial downgrowth after a sutureless cataract operation. Am J Ophthalmol 1993;116:238–240.
227. Calhoun FP: An aid to the clinical diagnosis of epithelial downgrowth into the anterior chamber following cataract extraction. Am J Ophthalmol 1966;61:1055–1057.
228. Brown SI: Results of excision of advanced epithelial downgrowth. Ophthalmology 1979;86:321–331.
229. Costa VP, Katz LJ, Cohen EJ, et al: Glaucoma associated with epithelial downgrowth controlled with Molteno tube shunts. Ophthalmic Surg 1992;23:797–800.
230. Loane ME, Weinreb RN: Glaucoma secondary to epithelial downgrowth and 5-fluorouracil. Ophthalmic Surg 1990;21:704–706.
231. Allen JC: Epithelial and stromal ingrowths. Am J Ophthalmol 1968;65:179–182.
232. Friedman AH, Henkind P: Corneal stromal overgrowth after cataract extraction. Br J Ophthalmol 1970;54:528–534.
233. Kremer I, Zandbank J, Barash D, et al: Extensive fibrous downgrowth after traumatic corneoscleral wound dehiscence. Ann Ophthalmol 1991;23:465–468.
234. Bettman JW: Pathology of complications of intraocular surgery. Am J Ophthalmol 1969;68:1037–1050.
235. McDonnell PJ, de la Cruz ZC, Green WR: Vitreous incarceration complicating cataract surgery: A light and electron microscopic study. Ophthalmology 1986;93:247–253.
236. Akingbehin AO: Comparative study of the intraocular pressure effects of fluorometholone 0.1% versus dexamethasone 0.1%. Br J Ophthalmol 1983;67:661–663.
237. Francois J, Verbraeken H: Complications in 1,000 consecutive intracapsular cataract extractions. Ophthalmologica 1980;180:121–128.
238. Tomey KF, Traverso CE: The glaucomas in aphakia and pseudophakia. Surv Ophthalmol 1991;36:79–112.
239. Scheie HG, Ewing MQ: Aphakic glaucoma. Trans Ophthalmol Soc UK 1978;98:111–117.
240. Kessing SV, Rasmussen KE: Aphakic glaucoma. Acta Ophthalmol 1977;55:717–722.
241. Hitchings RA: Aphakic glaucoma: Prophylaxis and management. Trans Ophthalmol Soc UK 1978;98:118–123.
242. Wallace DK, Plager DA: Corneal diameter in childhood aphakic glaucoma. J Pediatr Ophthalmol Strabismus 1996;33:230–234.
243. Walton DS: Pediatric aphakic glaucoma: A study of 65 patients. Trans Am Ophthalmol Soc 1995;93:403–413.
244. Parks MM, Johnson DA, Reed GW: Long-term visual results and complications in children with aphakia. Ophthalmology 1993; 100:826–841.
245. Mills MD, Robb RM: Glaucoma following childhood cataract surgery. J Pediatr Ophthalmol Strabismus 1994;31:355–360.
246. Simon JW, Mehta N, Simmons ST, et al: Glaucoma after pediatric lensectomy/vitrectomy. Ophthalmology 1991;98:670–674.
247. Chrousos GA, Parks MM, O'Neill JF: Incidence of chronic glaucoma, retinal detachment and secondary membrane surgery in pediatric aphakic patients. Ophthalmology 1984;91:1238–1241.
248. Pressman SH, Crouch ER: Pediatric aphakic glaucoma. Ann Ophthalmol 1983;15:568-573.
249. Herschler J: Management of aphakic glaucoma. Int Ophthalmol Clin 1984;24:43–48.
250. Gross RL, Feldman RM, Spaeth GL, et al: Surgical therapy of chronic glaucoma in aphakia and pseudophakia. Ophthalmology 1988;95:1195–1201.
251. Heuer DK, Gressel MG, Parrish RK, et al: Trabeculectomy in aphakic eyes. Ophthalmology 1984;91:1045–1051.
252. Bellows AR, Johnstone MA: Surgical management of chronic glaucoma in aphakia. Ophthalmology 1983;90:807–813.
253. Herschler J: The effect of total vitrectomy on filtration surgery in the aphakic eye. Ophthalmology 1981;88:229.
254. von Graefe A: Beitrage zur pathologie und therapie des glaukoms. Graefes Arch Clin Exp Ophthalmol 1869;15:108–252.
255. Luntz MH, Rosenblatt M: Malignant glaucoma. Surv Ophthalmol 1987;32:73–93.
256. Ruben S, Tsai J, Hitchings R: Malignant glaucoma and its management. Br J Ophthalmol 1997;81:163–167.
257. Levene RZ: Current concepts of malignant glaucoma. Ophthalmic Surg 1986;17:515–520.
258. Reed JE, Thomas JV, Lytle RA, et al: Malignant glaucoma induced by an intraocular lens. Ophthalmic Surg 1990;21:177–180.
259. Duy TP, Wollensak J: Ciliary block (malignant) glaucoma following posterior chamber lens implantation. Ophthalmic Surg 1987;18:741–744.
260. Vajpayee RB, Talwar D: Pseudophakic malignant glaucoma in a child. Ophthalmic Surg 1991;22:266–267.
261. Halkias A, Magauran DM, Joyce M: Ciliary block (malignant) glaucoma after cataract extraction with lens implant treated with YAG laser capsulotomy and anterior hyaloidotomy. Br J Ophthalmol 1992;76:569–570.
262. Brooks AM, Harper CA, Gillies WE: Occurrence of malignant glaucoma after laser iridotomy. Br J Ophthalmol 1989;73:617–620.
263. DiScalafani M, Liebmann JM, Ritch R: Malignant glaucoma following argon laser release of scleral flap sutures after trabeculectomy. Am J Ophthalmol 1989;108:597–598.
264. Little BC: Treatment of aphakic malignant glaucoma using Nd:YAG laser posterior capsulotomy. Br J Ophthalmol 1994;78:499–501.
265. Trope GE, Pavlin CJ, Bau A, et al: Malignant glaucoma: Clinical and ultrasound biomicroscopic features. Ophthalmology 1994; 101:1030–1035.
266. Harbour JW, Rubsamen PE, Palmberg P: Pars plana vitrectomy in the management of phakic and pseudophakic malignant glaucoma. Ophthalmology 1996;114:1073–1078.
267. Byrnes GA, Leen MM, Wong TP, et al: Vitrectomy for ciliary block (malignant) glaucoma. Ophthalmology 1995;102:1308–1311.
268. Deutsch TA, Goldberg MF: Neodymium:YAG laser capsulotomy. Int Ophthalmol Clin 1985;25:87–100.

269. Stark WJ, Worthen D, Holladay JT, et al: Neodymium:YAG lasers: An FDA report. Ophthalmology 1985;92:209–212.
270. Gardner KM, Straatsma BR, Pettit TH: Neodymium:YAG laser capsulotomy: The first 100 cases at UCLA. Ophthalmic Surg 1985;16:24–28.
271. Jahn CE, Emke M: Long-term elevation of intraocular pressure after Neodymium:YAG laser posterior capsulotomy. Ophthalmologica 1996;210:85–89.
272. Slomovic AR, Parrish RK: Acute elevations of intraocular pressure following Nd:YAG laser posterior capsulotomy. Ophthalmology 1985;92:973–976.
273. Keates RH, Steinert RF, Puliafito CA, et al: Long-term follow-up of Nd:YAG laser posterior capsulotomy. J Cataract Refract Surg 1984;10:164–168.
274. Fourman S, Apisson J: Late-onset elevation in intraocular pressure after Neodymium-YAG laser posterior capsulotomy. Arch Ophthalmol 1991;109:511–513.
275. Demer JL, Koch DD, Smith JA, et al: Persistent elevation in intraocular pressure after Nd:YAG laser treatment. Ophthalmic Surg 1986;17:465–466.
276. Gimbel HV, Van Westenbrugge JA, Sanders DR, et al: Effect of sulcus vs. capsular fixation on YAG-induced pressure rises following posterior capsulotomy. Arch Ophthalmol 1990;108:1126–1129.
277. Adams EA, Verstraeten TC, Friberg TR, et al: Effect of Neodymium:YAG laser on sodium hyaluronate in vitro as a model for postcapsulotomy intraocular pressure change. J Cataract Refract Surg 1996;22:748–751.
278. Silverstone DE, Brint SF, Olander KW, et al: Prophylactic use of apraclonidine for intraocular pressure increase after Nd:YAG capsulotomies. Am J Ophthalmol 1992;113:401–405.
279. Rosenberg LF, Krupin T, Ruderman J, et al: Apraclonidine and anterior segment laser surgery. Ophthalmology 1995;102:1312–1318.
280. Barnebey HS, Robin AL, Zimmerman TJ, et al: The efficacy of brimonidine in decreasing elevations in intraocular pressure after laser trabeculoplasty. Ophthalmology 1993;100:1083–1088.
281. David R, Spaeth GL, Clevenger CE, et al: Brimonidine in the prevention of intraocular pressure elevation following argon laser trabeculoplasty. Arch Ophthalmol 1993;111:1387–1390.

CHAPTER 16

Retina and Vitreous

MARTHA M. WRIGHT and KIMBERLY A. NEELY

Although we would prefer not to admit it, the examination of the posterior segment plays a vital role in the diagnosis of many types of glaucoma. In this chapter, Martha Wright and Kim Neely guide us through this very extensive subject. They begin with the need for careful examination of anterior and posterior ocular structures that may provide important distinctive signs for diagnosis. They then describe the types of glaucoma specifically associated with abnormalities of the vitreous, retina, and uveal tract. Finally, they address the relatively common problem of elevated intraocular pressure following vitreoretinal surgery. The key points to be recognized are logically described to allow the proper identification of the cause of the elevation in intraocular pressure, allowing formulation of the proper therapeutic plan. Many of these problems are also addressed in Chapter 24, on the therapeutic interventions in the posterior segment.

Examination: Looking for the Cause of Elevated Pressure

The effective and rational treatment of glaucoma associated with diseases of the retina and vitreous requires an understanding of the pathophysiology of both glaucoma and vitreoretinal diseases. Although there may be many abnormalities in an eye with vitreoretinal disease, it is critical to distinguish the signs associated with the development of glaucoma in order to choose an appropriate approach to treatment. In addition to the typical history and examination, certain areas of the eye examination require particular attention and consideration.

IRIS

During the slit-lamp examination of a patient with vitreoretinal diseases, it is important to look carefully for neovascularization of the iris. This step is best performed before dilation of the pupil, because dilation may constrict the neovascular vessels or make them more difficult to see. The entire iris must be examined; even a small area of neovascularization is significant.

Neovascularization of the iris often begins at the pupillary margin but can be present across the entire iris. Neovascularization may also appear at the margins of a peripheral iridectomy. Normal iris vasculature is radial and can sometimes be seen running within the iris stroma in light-colored irides or in eyes with iris atrophy from a variety of causes. Neovascular vessels, however, are tortuous and are found on the surface of the iris, rather than in the iris stroma. They vary in size from tiny, spindly vessels that require a slit lamp and careful observation to detect to large vessels that give the iris a distinctively reddish cast, hence the name *rubeosis iridis* (Fig. 16–1).

Neovascularization of the iris usually indicates that ischemia is present in the eye, with the retina as the most common cause[1]; however, it may also be seen in some inflammatory diseases of the eye.

ANTERIOR CHAMBER ANGLE (GONIOSCOPY)

Gonioscopy is the simplest and easiest way to accurately assess the configuration of the angle. The depth of the anterior chamber does not always correlate with the depth of the angle. Hence, the only way to know whether the angle is open, partially open, or closed is to observe the

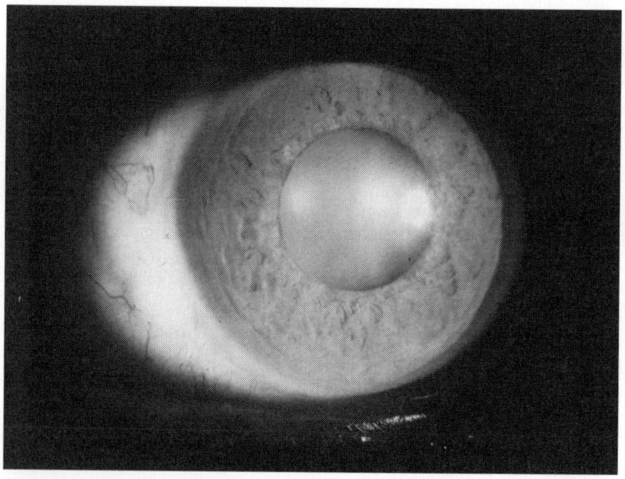

FIGURE 16–1. Rubeosis iridis. This patient with proliferative diabetic retinopathy experienced neovascular glaucoma. Neovascularization of the iris is present on the pupillary margin.

angle with gonioscopy. Gonioscopy may also make the ophthalmologist aware of neovascularization, pigmentation, inflammation, or debris in the angle. Neovascularization may be present in the angle before it is present on the iris[2]; therefore, one cannot assume that if there is no neovascularization of the iris, the angle is also free of new vessels. New vessels in the anterior chamber angle form irregular branching networks across the trabecular meshwork and should not be confused with normal circumferential vessels, which are sometimes visible posterior to the scleral spur.

VITREOUS AND RETINA

Examination of the vitreous may require a combination of examination techniques. The anterior vitreous may be seen with the slit lamp for determining the presence of inflammation or blood in the anterior vitreous. A 90-diopter or 78-diopter lens in conjunction with the slit lamp may help in the assessment of the posterior vitreous and retina. A Goldmann or other type of contact lens may give the best view of the posterior or peripheral vitreous, although the indirect ophthalmoscope may also provide a clear view of both the vitreous and the retina. The direct ophthalmoscope can provide a magnified view of the macula, optic nerve and posterior vitreous. Ultrasonography may provide information about the retina and vitreous in eyes with an opacity that precludes a direct view of the fundus.

OPTIC NERVE

Examination of the optic nerve constitutes an important assessment of the health of the nerve. A healthy nerve in the presence of elevated intraocular pressure (IOP) indicates ocular hypertension, whereas optic nerve damage associated with elevated IOP is glaucoma. The extent of optic nerve damage and the amount of IOP elevation help determine the aggressiveness and speed of pressure lowering required. Some acute, but transient, elevations of IOP may not require treatment, but extreme or chronic elevations often require treatment to prevent further damage to the optic nerve.

CAROTID ARTERIES

Because not all causes of ischemic retinal disease are within the eye itself, there are times when other sources of ischemia should be investigated. The ophthalmologist may examine the carotid arteries in the office by listening with a stethoscope at the point where the carotid arteries traverse the patient's neck. Presence of a bruit may indicate a partial occlusion of the artery and may require further evaluation. The absence of a bruit does not eliminate the possibility of a carotid occlusion. A carotid ultrasound or angiogram may be required if clinical suspicion of full or partial occlusion of the carotid is high.

Glaucoma Associated with Vitreoretinal Diseases

ABNORMALITIES OF THE VITREOUS

Ghost Cell Glaucoma (see also Chapter 12)

Ghost cells are red blood cells that have begun to degenerate with time. They may occur in the vitreous from a long-standing vitreous hemorrhage. Normal erythrocytes are red, biconcave, and pliable, but ghost cells are tan, spherical, and relatively rigid. The degeneration of red blood cells into ghost cells takes from 3 days to 3 weeks. Neither normal red blood cells nor ghost cells can cross an intact anterior hyaloid, so ghost cells enter the anterior chamber only if the anterior hyaloid face is disrupted. Once the cells are within the anterior chamber, their rigid structure prevents them from passing through the trabecular meshwork. Large numbers of ghost cells trapped in the trabecular meshwork impede the normal outflow of aqueous.

CLINICAL SETTING

The patient with ghost cell glaucoma may have a vitreous hemorrhage from a variety of causes, including trauma, surgery, and retinal diseases such as proliferative diabetic retinopathy. A disrupted anterior hyaloid face must be present and may be the result of previous surgery, trauma, or both.

FINDINGS

The cornea is usually clear unless extremely high IOPs have caused corneal edema. The anterior chamber has numerous khaki-colored cells in circulation, and some cells may have formed a layer in the inferior angle, causing a pseudohypopyon. These khaki-colored cells are smaller than white blood cells.[3] On gonioscopy, the angle has a layer of tan cells over the trabecular meshwork. The vitreous contains old vitreous hemorrhage, including many ghost cells.

DIFFERENTIAL DIAGNOSIS

Uveitis may also be confused with ghost cell glaucoma, but in uveitis, the cells in the anterior chamber are larger, white blood cells, whereas the cells in ghost cell glaucoma are smaller and tan or khaki-colored. Keratic precipitates may be seen in uveitis but are not seen in ghost cell glaucoma.

Vitreous hemorrhage may be associated with glaucomas other than ghost cell glaucoma.

Neovascular glaucoma from a central vein occlusion, diabetic retinopathy, or other ischemic process may also be associated with a vitreous hemorrhage. Neovascular glaucoma is distinguished from ghost cell glaucoma by the absence of ghost cells and the observation of neovascular vessels in the anterior chamber angle.

Aqueous Misdirection (Malignant Glaucoma) (see also Chapter 15)

Aqueous misdirection is an incompletely understood elevation in IOP that occurs only after surgery. In aqueous misdirection, aqueous humor does not follow its usual path from the posterior to the anterior chamber, but instead flows into the vitreous cavity, where it creates increasingly large pockets of aqueous in the formed vitreous. The vitreous expands, pushing the iris and lens (if present) forward and elevating the IOP.

CLINICAL SETTING

Patients with aqueous misdirection have almost always had recent intraocular surgery, although this disorder has also been reported following laser peripheral iridectomy.[4] The majority of patients have a history of acute angle-closure glaucoma, which may have been treated years ago. Aqueous misdirection may be precipitated or exacerbated by the use of miotics.

FINDINGS

Patients with aqueous misdirection typically have moderately to severely elevated IOP, although normal IOP has also been reported. The hallmark of aqueous misdirection is a shallow or flat anterior chamber that is shallow both peripherally and centrally (Fig. 16–2).

DIFFERENTIAL DIAGNOSIS

Pupillary block causing angle closure typically gives a bombé appearance to the iris, with a shallow peripheral chamber but a formed central chamber (Fig. 16–3), as opposed to aqueous misdirection, in which both the central

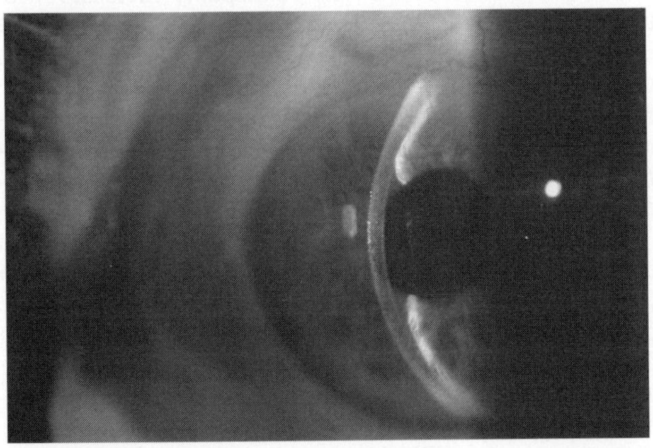

FIGURE 16–2. Aqueous misdirection. Both the central and peripheral anterior chambers are shallow.

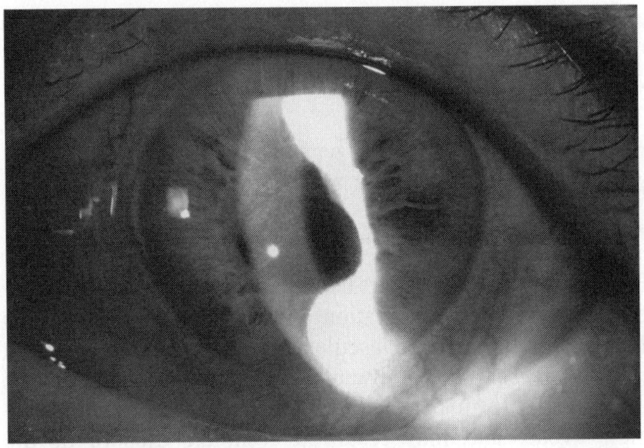

FIGURE 16–3. Pupillary block. The central chamber is deep but the peripheral anterior chamber is shallow with iris bombé.

and peripheral chamber areas are shallow. A patent peripheral iridectomy relieves pupillary block but not aqueous misdirection.

Peripheral shallowing of the anterior chamber may be seen with *choroidal effusions.*

A shallow anterior chamber may also result from *overfiltration* following trabeculectomy or from a *wound leak.* In either of these disorders, however, the IOP is low, but in aqueous misdirection, the IOP is elevated.

Stickler's Syndrome

Stickler's syndrome is an autosomal dominant connective tissue disease that may be due to a defect in collagen metabolism. It involves ocular, oral, facial, and skeletal abnormalities.

CLINICAL SETTING

The myopia seen in this disease is congenital and progresses in the first two decades of life. Retinal detachments usually occur by the second decade of life.

FINDINGS

Eye findings in Stickler's syndrome include cataracts, open-angle glaucoma, vitreous liquefaction, chorioretinal pigment changes, hypopigmentation of the fundus, and retinal detachments. The retinal breaks may be numerous, may be located posteriorly, and may include giant retinal tears.

Systemic findings include joint hyperextensibility, joint laxity, and premature degeneration. Dental abnormalities, cleft palate, midfacial flattening, and hearing loss are common.

DIFFERENTIAL DIAGNOSIS

High myopia, as an isolated finding, is more likely than Stickler's syndrome to be associated with lacquer cracks, staphyloma, and subretinal neovascular membranes.

Patients with *Wagner's disease* have myopia and cataracts, and have the same "optically empty" vitreous seen in those with Stickler's syndrome, but do not have the associated retinal detachments or the systemic findings of Stickler's syndrome.

In patients with Stickler's syndrome who have open-angle glaucoma, the visual field changes due to glaucoma may be difficult to distinguish from those due to the myopic degeneration associated with Stickler's syndrome.

GLAUCOMA ASSOCIATED WITH ABNORMALITIES OF THE RETINA

Neovascular Glaucoma

Both systemic and ocular diseases may result in the development of neovascularization of the iris and angle (Table 16–1). Initially, a fibrovascular membrane grows over the iris and trabecular meshwork. Over time, the membrane contracts to form peripheral anterior synechiae and ectropion uveae, and may result in complete closure of the angle.

CLINICAL SETTING

Retinal hypoxia and retinal capillary nonperfusion characterize the majority of diseases associated with neovascular glaucoma. Diabetic retinopathy and central retinal vein occlusion are the most common causes of neovascular glaucoma.

FINDINGS

The first sign of neovascular glaucoma is usually the appearance of small tufts of vessels at the pupillary margin. These enlarge and spread over the iris and often involve the angle. The IOP may remain normal until a significant portion of the trabecular meshwork is covered. Angle closure may progress slowly or rapidly. The patient with advanced neovascular glaucoma may have an inflamed, painful, and photophobic eye. Vision may be counts fingers or hand motion and the IOP is often as high as 60 mm Hg. Examination of the retina often reveals evidence of retinal hypoxia or poor perfusion: retinal hemorrhages, cotton-wool spots, neovascularization of the optic nerve or retina, and capillary dropout.

TABLE 16–1. FACTORS PREDISPOSING TO RUBEOSIS IRIDIS AND NEOVASCULAR GLAUCOMA

Diabetic retinopathy
Retinal vascular occlusive disorders
Central retinal vein occlusion
Central retinal artery occlusion
Branch retinal vein occlusion
Branch retinal artery occlusion
Other retinal disorders
Retinal detachment
Choroidal melanoma
Retinoblastoma
Hemorrhagic retinal disorders
Coats' exudative retinopathy
Retinopathy of prematurity
Sickle cell retinopathy
Syphilitic retinal vasculitis
Retinoschisis
Stickler's syndrome
Optic nerve glioma with subsequent venous stasis retinopathy
Photoradiation and helium ion radiation for uveal melanoma
Other ocular disorders
Uveitis
Intraocular lens implantation
Iris melanoma
Extraocular vascular disorders
Carotid artery obstructive disease
Carotid-cavernous fistula
Internal carotid artery occlusion

From Shields MB: Glaucoma associated with disorders of the retina, vitreous, and choroid. *In* Shields MB: Textbook of Glaucoma, 4th ed. Baltimore, Williams & Wilkins, 1998, p 270.

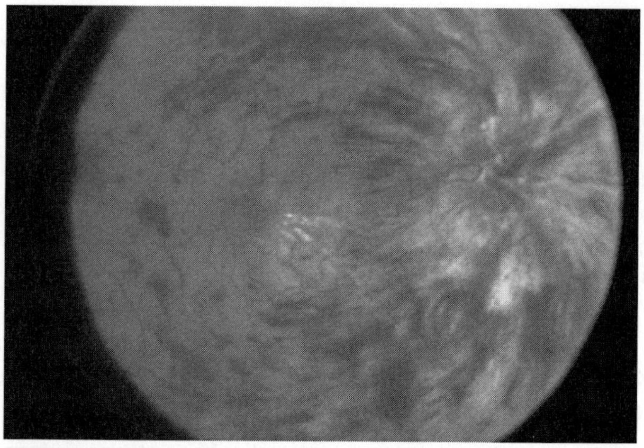

FIGURE 16–4. Central retinal vein occlusion with widely scattered hemorrhages, dilated veins, and swelling of the optic nerve.

DIFFERENTIAL DIAGNOSIS

The most common causes of neovascular glaucoma are central retinal vein occlusion, diabetes, and carotid artery occlusive disease.

Central retinal vein occlusion (CRVO) usually demonstrates dilated, tortuous veins, optic disc edema, retinal edema, cotton-wool spots, and intraretinal hemorrhages (Fig. 16–4). The vast majority of affected patients are older than 50 years. Many patients with CRVO have systemic hypertension. They may also have ocular hypertension or glaucoma. Diabetes mellitus, systemic vascular disease, the use of oral contraceptives, and hyperviscosity syndromes may also be associated with CRVO. Although CRVO may be either nonischemic or ischemic, those cases associated with neovascular glaucoma are usually of the ischemic variety. On fluorescein angiography, ischemic CRVO demonstrates at least 10 disc areas of nonperfusion in the posterior pole. Neovascularization usually occurs within 3 months of the onset of the vein occlusion.

The prevalence of *diabetic retinopathy* increases with the duration of the diabetes and with the patient's age. It is possible, although uncommon, for neovascular glaucoma to develop even though little or no proliferative diabetic retinopathy is noted on fundus examination. More commonly, in addition to a long-standing history of diabetes mellitus, the patient with neovascular glaucoma has proliferative diabetic retinopathy (Fig. 16–5).

Carotid artery occlusive disease (CAOD) may cause a clinical picture similar to that of CRVO (Fig. 16–6). In CAOD, hemorrhages are more commonly located in the midperiphery than in the posterior pole location seen with CRVO. The veins may be dilated in both entities; they are tortuous with CRVO, but not with CAOD. Ophthalmodynamometry will help to differentiate between the two entities; the patient with CRVO has a normal arterial pressure, whereas the patient with CAOD has low arterial pressure.

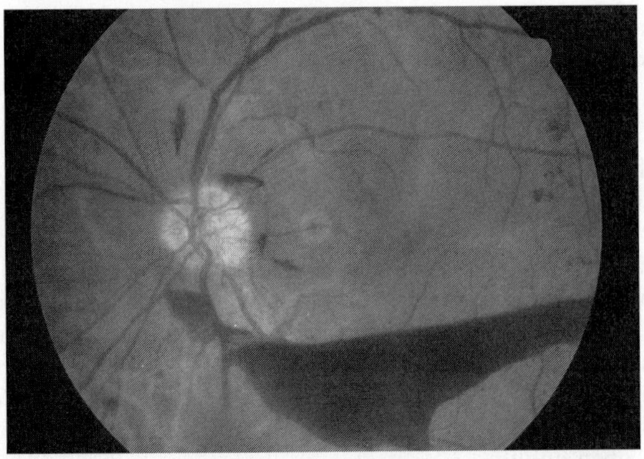

FIGURE 16–5. Proliferative diabetic retinopathy. Extensive neovascularization of the optic disc associated with preretinal hemorrhage along the inferotemporal arcade.

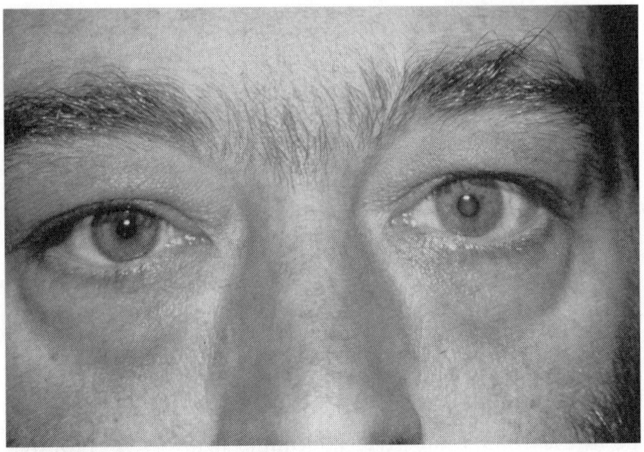

FIGURE 16–7. Fuchs' heterochromic iridocyclitis. The left (affected) eye has a lighter iris and a cataract.

Acute angle-closure glaucoma, like late neovascular glaucoma, may cause a red, painful eye with highly elevated IOP and corneal edema. In acute angle closure, however, there is no neovascularization of the iris. Even if severe corneal edema precludes examination of the angle and fundus in the affected eye, examination of the fellow eye reveals evidence of a narrow angle or diabetic retinopathy, both of which tend to be symmetric in the two eyes, a feature that helps in diagnosis of the eye in question.

Pseudoexfoliation syndrome is often associated with glaucoma, may be bilateral, and rarely demonstrates the development of new vessels on the iris. New vessels do not lead to neovascular glaucoma in pseudoexfoliation syndrome.

In *Fuchs' heterochromic iridocyclitis,* there may be cells in the anterior chamber and fine, stellate keratic precipitates, but the eye is otherwise white and quiet (Fig. 16–7). This disorder is unilateral and is frequently associated with heterochromia of the irides, glaucoma, and cataracts. There may be fine, new vessels in the angle, but they do not tend to arborize or close the angle as in neovascular glaucoma. These new vessels may bleed with manipulation of the eye during gonioscopy or surgery.

Glaucoma Associated with Retinopathy of Prematurity

Infants with retinopathy of prematurity (ROP) may have glaucoma in the more advanced stages (with partial or complete retinal detachment).

CLINICAL SETTING

The incidence of glaucoma has been reported to be as high as 30% among infants with stage IV or V ROP.[5] Glaucoma may occur also as a late complication in adults who had ROP during infancy.[6]

Some infants with ROP and glaucoma appear to have open but poorly developed angles[7]; however, the most common type of glaucoma among infants with ROP is angle closure,[8] which may occur via several mechanisms in these patients (Table 16–2).

Adults with late-onset glaucoma secondary to ROP generally have acute or chronic angle closure. In most patients, the responsible mechanism is pupillary block (often related to a thickened lens). In other adult patients with a history of ROP, angle closure may occur secondary to neovascularization of the angle.

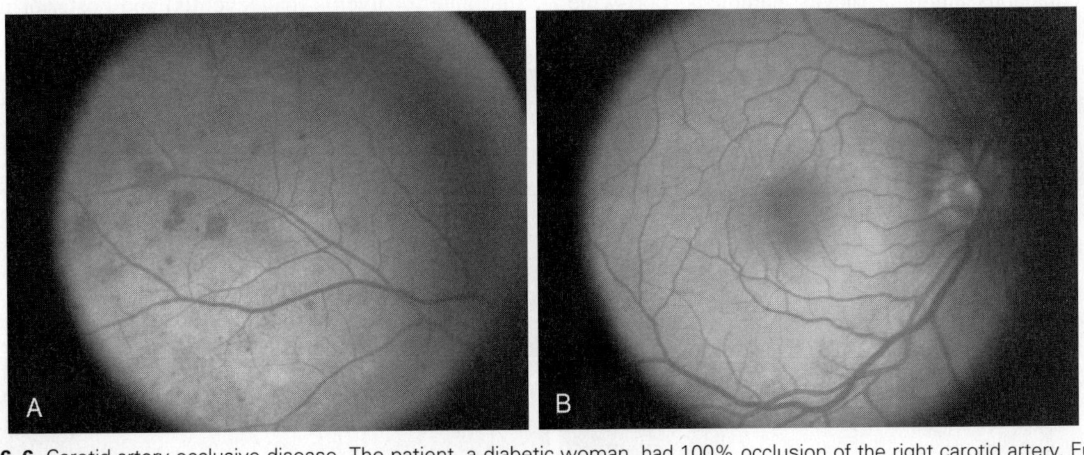

FIGURE 16–6. Carotid artery occlusive disease. The patient, a diabetic woman, had 100% occlusion of the right carotid artery. Funduscopic examination revealed intraretinal hemorrhages confined to the midperipheral retina *(A).* Rare microaneurysms were present in the macula *(B).* Three years later, iris neovascularization developed.

TABLE 16–2. MECHANISMS OF ANGLE CLOSURE WITH RETINOPATHY OF PREMATURITY

Pupillary block secondary to rotation of the ciliary body and/or anterior displacement of the iris-lens diaphragm by a contracting retrolental membrane
Pupillary block secondary to posterior synechiae, which may occur after surgical intervention or even in unoperated eyes
Peripheral anterior synechiae caused by inflammation or postoperative fibrin formation

FINDINGS AND EXAMINATION TECHNIQUES

The measurement of IOP in infants with ROP requires special consideration. First, IOP measurements in awake, struggling infants may be artificially elevated. Therefore, this parameter is most commonly measured during an examination with the patient under anesthesia. General anesthetics, however, can artificially lower IOP.

Second, the accuracy of the IOP measurement is related to the type of pressure-measuring instrument used. Applanation tonometry appears to give more accurate measurements than Schiøtz indentation tonometry.[5] Premature infants have variable scleral rigidity, which affects the accuracy of indentation tonometry, and their corneas have a steeper corneal curvature than adult corneas. The footplate of a Schiøtz tonometer, therefore, is too flat to yield an accurate IOP measurement in these infants.

Because of the difficulties in measuring IOP in premature infants, other clues, such as corneal diameter and refraction at sequential examinations, can signify the presence of glaucoma. Evaluation of the optic disc in premature infants with ROP may be of less use because retinal dragging over the disc alters the appearance of the disc.[8]

GLAUCOMA ASSOCIATED WITH ABNORMALITIES OF THE UVEAL TRACT (CILIARY BODY, CHOROID)

Sturge-Weber Syndrome (Encephalotrigeminal Angiomatosis) (see also Chapters 10 and 11)

Sturge-Weber syndrome is a phakomatosis causing the triad of facial cutaneous angioma (nevus flammeus, port-wine stain), leptomeningeal angioma, and ocular involvement. No hereditary pattern has been established.

CLINICAL SETTING

Glaucoma occurs in 30% to 60% of patients with Sturge-Weber syndrome.[9, 10] The onset of glaucoma is bimodal in occurrence: Glaucoma most commonly appears either in infancy or in preadolescence to early adolescence. Patients with a port-wine stain involving the trigeminal dermatomes of V_1 (ophthalmic division) and V_2 (maxillary division) have the highest incidence of glaucoma.[10] Episcleral hemangiomas may lead to elevated episcleral venous pressure, which may in turn cause elevated IOP in the presence of an open angle.

FINDINGS

The facial hemangioma of Sturge-Weber syndrome involves the distribution of the trigeminal nerve. It is often unilateral but may be bilateral. Ocular involvement may consist of dilated episcleral vessels from increased episcleral venous pressure, glaucoma, and choroidal hemangiomas. Choroidal hemangiomas, which are common, are usually flat and located in the posterior pole. If the choroidal hemangioma is diffuse, it may be detectable only through comparison of the redder color of the fundus in the involved eye ("tomato catsup fundus") with the normal-colored fundus in the uninvolved eye (Fig. 16–8). On gonioscopy, there may be blood in Schlemm's canal as a result of elevated episcleral venous pressure.

DIFFERENTIAL DIAGNOSIS

Klippel-Trenaunay-Weber Syndrome is similar to Sturge-Weber syndrome, but also involves a cutaneous hemangioma of one limb with varicosities and hypertrophy.[11] Ocular involvement is most common when the hemangioma involves the face.

Posterior Uveitis (see also Chapter 12)

Uveitis is a nonspecific term that refers to inflammation anywhere in the uveal tract. Uveitis is often subdivided into anterior uveitis (iridocyclitis) and posterior uveitis.

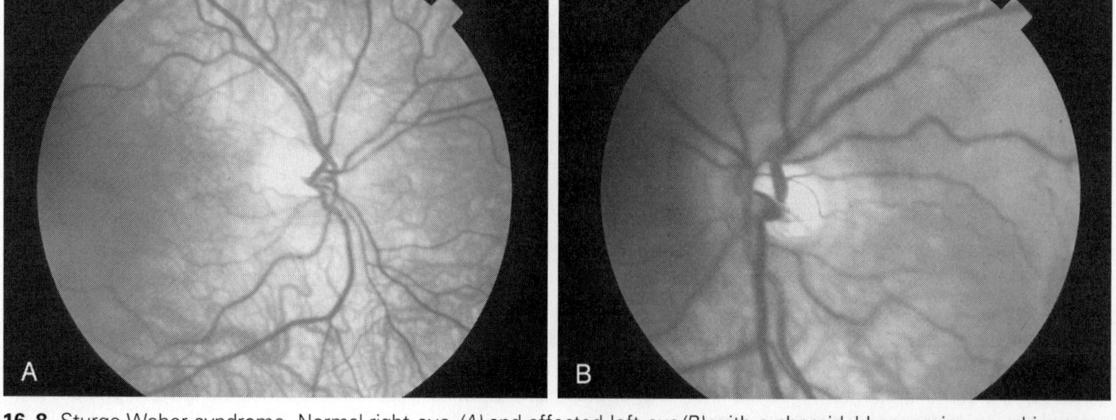

FIGURE 16–8. Sturge-Weber syndrome. Normal right eye *(A)* and affected left eye *(B)* with a choroidal hemangioma and increased cupping from glaucoma. (Courtesy of Dr. C. Gail Summers.)

CLINICAL SETTING

Inflammation may lead to lowered IOP when (1) ciliary body inflammation decreases aqueous production or (2) inflammation increases uveoscleral outflow. Uveitis may raise IOP through a variety of mechanisms: anterior or posterior synechiae may lead to angle closure; inflammation and inflammatory debris may decrease trabecular outflow; and corticosteroid-induced glaucoma may contribute to the elevated pressure.

Elevated IOP in the presence of uveitis may serve as a diagnostic clue. Uveitis secondary to toxoplasmosis or herpesviruses may cause an elevation of IOP, perhaps through an associated trabeculitis.

FINDINGS AND DIFFERENTIAL DIAGNOSIS

The onset of *pars planitis* is usually in the teens to early adulthood. It is characterized by cells in the anterior vitreous, exudation of the vitreous base along the inferior pars plana ("snow-banking"), peripheral retinal vasculitis, and cystoid macular edema. Vision loss is usually from chronic cystoid macular edema. Anterior segment findings include anterior chamber cell, posterior subcapsular cataract, and band keratopathy. Anterior and posterior synechiae, along with iris neovascularization, may contribute to the development of glaucoma.

Sarcoidosis is a systemic disease of noncaseating granulomas. It is seen more commonly in blacks than in whites, and most commonly presents in young adults. It may involve the lungs, liver, spleen, skin, central nervous system, and eye. Ocular involvement may consist of anterior uveitis, posterior uveitis, orbital disease, lacrimal gland involvement, and optic neuritis. The anterior uveitis is a chronic, granulomatous uveitis with mutton-fat keratic precipitates, synechiae, and iris nodules. The iris nodules are white, superficial, and located near the pupil (Koeppe nodules) or in the iris crypts (Busacca nodules) (Fig. 16–9). Posterior involvement is manifested by choroidal granulomas and retinal periphlebitis (Fig. 16–10). The chorioretinitis is not specific to sarcoidosis, but the "candle-wax drippings" of retinal periphlebitis seen with advanced cases is distinctive (Fig. 16–11). Inferior vitreous opacities occurring in chains ("string of pearls") are also characteristic of sarcoidosis. Cystoid macular edema is common.

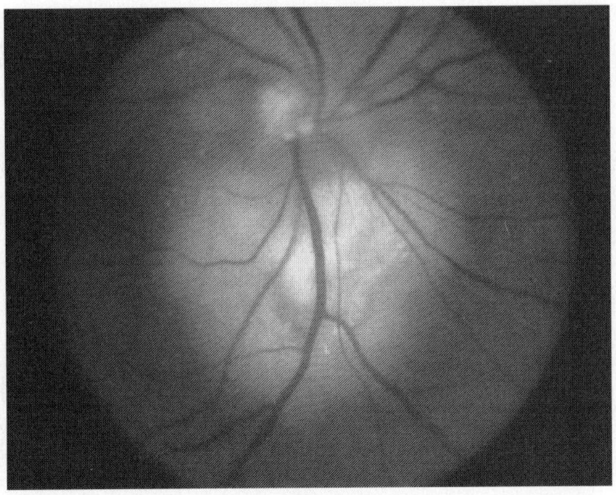

FIGURE 16–10. Peripapillary choroidal granuloma in a patient with pulmonary and ocular sarcoidosis.

Definitive diagnosis of sarcoidosis requires additional testing. A chest radiograph, biopsy of involved lymph nodes, or a conjunctival biopsy may lead to a diagnosis. Although a "blind" conjunctival biopsy is relatively simple and may yield the diagnosis in 10% to 28% of cases, biopsy of a conjunctival nodule produces the diagnosis 75% of the time[12] (Fig. 16–12). The serum concentration angiotensin-converting enzyme (ACE) may be elevated in sarcoidosis. The serum lysozyme concentration may also be elevated in sarcoidosis and other systemic inflammatory diseases.

Herpes simplex virus may cause viral keratitis, neurotrophic keratitis, anterior uveitis, or posterior uveitis. Because the uveitis may occur without concurrent corneal signs, diagnosis of this cause may be difficult.

Herpes zoster is less commonly associated with glaucoma than herpes simplex virus. The vesicular rash that develops in the distribution of the fifth cranial nerve with herpes zoster is preceded by pain in the area of the rash. The associated iridocyclitis demonstrates mutton-fat keratic precipitates, sector iris atrophy, and synechiae.

Acquired immune deficiency syndrome (AIDS) may affect the eye through direct infection by human immunodeficiency virus or through secondary infection by other agents (herpes, syphilis, toxoplasmosis). Uveitis is common, but

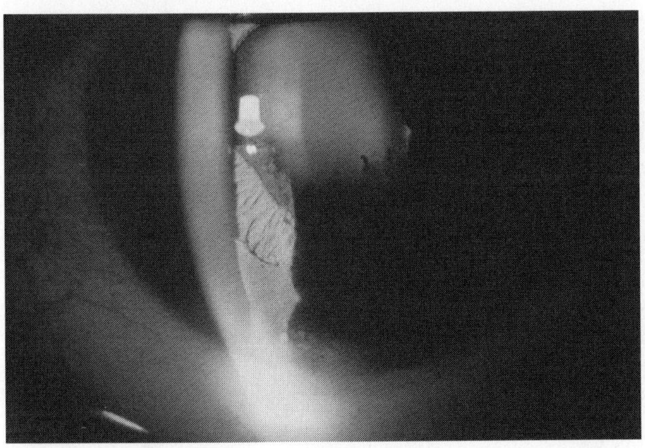

FIGURE 16–9. Iris nodules and posterior synechiae in a patient with pulmonary and ocular sarcoidosis.

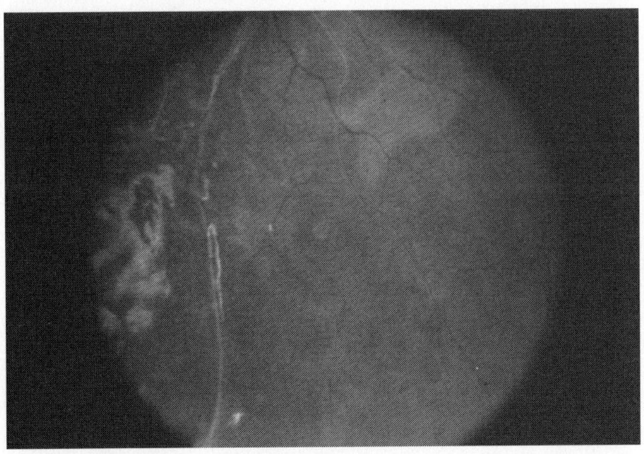

FIGURE 16–11. Retinal periphlebitis in a patient with ocular and systemic sarcoidosis.

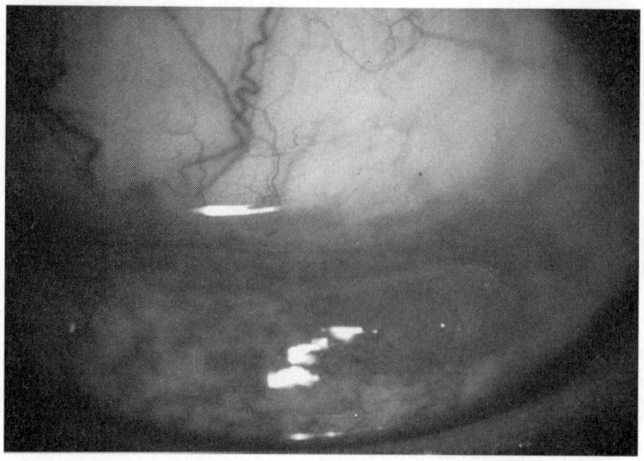

FIGURE 16–12. Conjunctival nodule in a patient with pulmonary and ocular sarcoidosis.

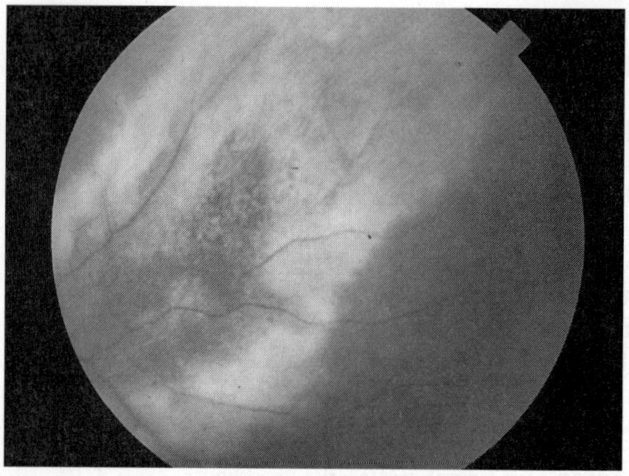

FIGURE 16–14. Active toxoplasmic retinochoroiditis in an immunosuppressed patient. This patient demonstrated yellow retinitis in the superotemporal periphery. In immunocompetent patients, toxoplasmic retinochoroiditis usually manifests as active retinitis on the border of an old chorioretinal scar and has an associated dense vitritis. In immunosuppressed patients, the vitreous inflammatory infiltrate may be mild and an old scar may be absent (possibly representing an acquired infection).

elevated IOP is rare. Bilateral angle closure due to choroidal effusions has been reported.

Syphilis, either congenital or acquired, may be associated with glaucoma. Patients with congenital syphilis may have interstitial keratitis and small anterior segments that predispose them to angle closure later on. Patients with normal-dimension anterior segments may have synechial angle closure from previous inflammation.

Toxoplasmosis is caused by an acquired or congenital infection with an intracellular protozoan. The ocular findings are characterized by vitritis and necrotizing retinochoroiditis. Active retinal lesions are often adjacent to atrophic, scarred areas indicative of previous retinal involvement (Fig. 16–13). Active retinal lesions have a white, fluffy appearance with surrounding retinal edema (Fig. 16–14). The retinal lesions are accompanied by overlying vitritis that creates the "headlight in the fog" appearance classically used to describe the clinical findings. Some patients with toxoplasmosis experience a chronic uveitis accompanied by cataract, glaucoma, and cystoid macular edema.

Behçet's disease is an occlusive vasculitis that affects multiple systems. It is characterized by uveitis and ulcers of the mouth and genitals (Fig. 16–15). The uveitis may be so severe that a sterile hypopyon results. Anterior and posterior uveitis develop late in the disease and are often bilateral. Necrotizing retinal vasculitis is common.

Vogt-Koyanagi-Harada (VKH) or *uveomeningitis syndrome* involves the eyes, ears, meninges, and skin. The ocular manifestations include anterior uveitis, severe vitritis, exudative retinal detachment, loss of the retinal pigment epithelium, and papilledema. Hearing loss, vitiligo, poliosis, and alopecia are common.

Sympathetic ophthalmia is similar in clinical appearance to (VKH) syndrome. It occurs weeks to years after penetrating trauma or surgery in the fellow eye.

Angle Closure from Forward Rotation of the Ciliary Body

Angle-closure glaucoma may occur through a variety of mechanisms, including pupillary block, contraction of a membrane or synechia that pulls the iris forward onto the trabecular meshwork, or a posterior pushing or rotating mechanism that pushes the iris forward over the trabecular meshwork.[13] Swelling and anterior rotation of the ciliary body may lead to angle closure by pushing the iris forward over the trabecular meshwork.

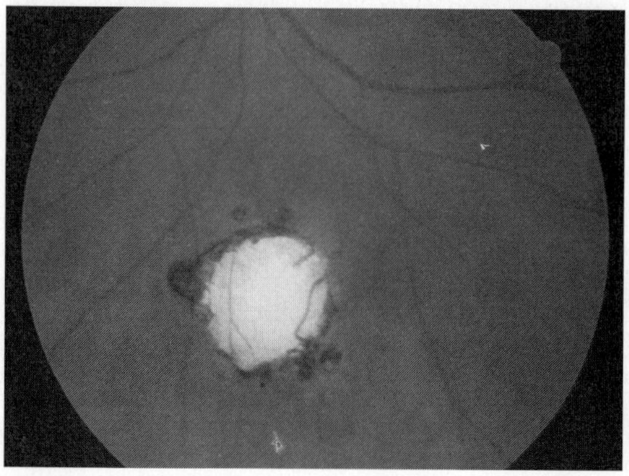

FIGURE 16–13. Old toxoplasmosis scar inferior to the optic disk. There is no active retinochoroiditis.

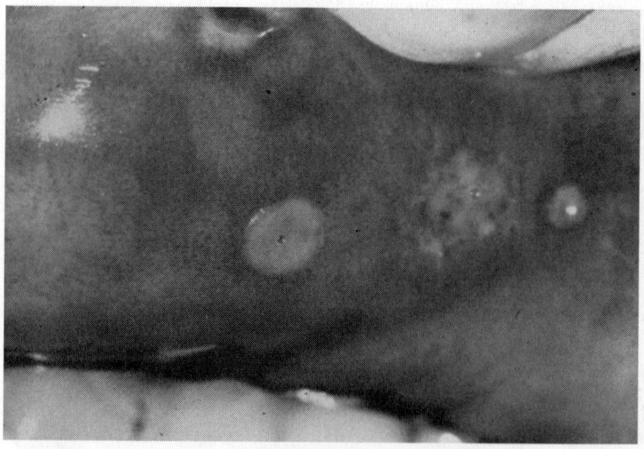

FIGURE 16–15. Ulcers on the mucous membranes of the mouth in a patient with Behçet's disease.

CLINICAL SETTING

Diseases that cause swelling and inflammation of the ciliary body that lead to choroidal effusions may result in angle closure through forward rotation of the ciliary body and anterior displacement of the lens-iris diaphragm.

FINDINGS AND DIFFERENTIAL DIAGNOSIS

Central retinal vein occlusion may be accompanied by choroidal effusion immediately after the onset of the vein occlusion. In addition to the findings of a vein occlusion (dilated, tortuous veins, retinal hemorrhages throughout the fundus, cotton-wool spots, and optic nerve swelling), one may also see a shallow anterior chamber and elevated IOP due to angle closure. It is not always possible to determine the sequence of events, since in some cases, angle-closure glaucoma leads to a central vein occlusion.

Scleral buckling or panretinal photocoagulation may lead to forward rotation of the ciliary body in the immediate postoperative period because of swelling of the ciliary body, choroidal effusions due to inflammation and obstruction of the venous outflow at the vortex veins, or both (see later discussion of postoperative IOP changes with scleral buckling).

Suprachoroidal hemorrhage may occur during or following intraocular surgery (Fig. 16–16). It is most common in eyes with a postoperative choroidal effusion. The rapidly expanding area of blood in the suprachoroidal space causes the sudden onset of severe pain, markedly elevated IOP, and a shallow anterior chamber. The suprachoroidal hemorrhage may be seen as a dark choroidal elevation in one or more quadrants.

Choroidal effusions appear as light brown elevations of the choroid on examination of the fundus (Fig. 16–17) and may be associated with hypotony or with a variety of conditions. *Nanophthalmos* is a bilateral condition with a short axial length but a normal-sized lens. Affected eyes have a tendency for spontaneous choroidal effusions, perhaps owing to an abnormally thick sclera and obstruction of outflow through the vortex veins. The diagnosis of nanophthalmos can be made by measuring an axial length of less than 20.5 mm.[14] *Drug reactions*,[15, 16] *HIV infection* or *AIDS*,[17] and *lymphoma* have all been reported, although rarely, to be associated with choroidal effusions.

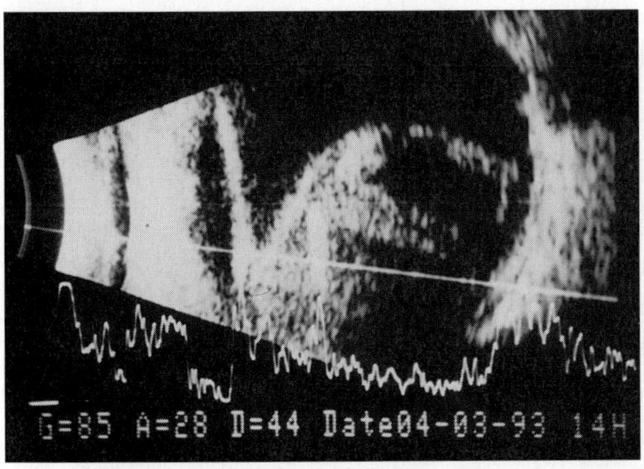

FIGURE 16–16. A large suprachoroidal hemorrhage demonstrated on ultrasonography. The internal reflections within the suprachoroidal space represent blood.

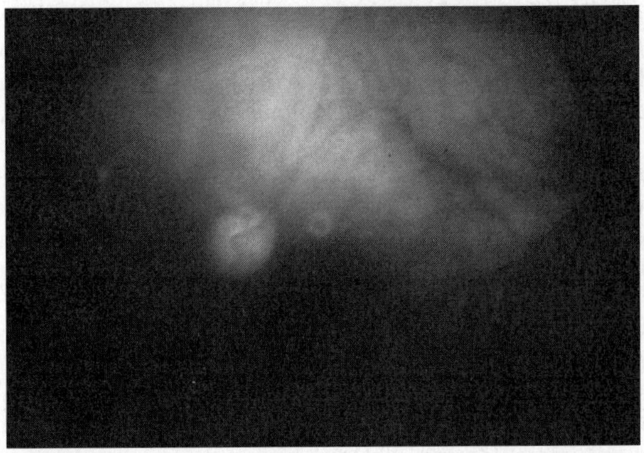

FIGURE 16–17. The two light brown, domed areas are choroidal effusions.

Ocular Hypotony

Hypotony is lower-than-normal IOP. There is no universally accepted definition of hypotony, but it is commonly defined as an IOP less than 6 mm Hg.

CLINICAL SETTING

Low IOP may lead to blurred vision or visual distortion due to hypotony maculopathy, retinal edema, choroidal effusions, corneal edema, and corneal folds (Fig. 16–18). The pressure level that leads to these problems varies from patient to patient. Some patients may experience blurred or distorted vision at pressures of 9 or 10 mm Hg, whereas others may have no visual complaints at IOPs of 1 or 2 mm Hg.

FINDINGS AND DIFFERENTIAL DIAGNOSIS

Retinal detachment may increase (uncommonly) or decrease (commonly) the IOP. With a small retinal break and limited retinal detachment, degenerating photoreceptor outer segments clog the trabecular outflow, resulting in elevated IOP and a clinical picture of uveitis. More commonly, a rhegmatogenous retinal detachment allows fluid to travel through the retinal break and exit the eye through nontrabecular outflow. This increase over the usual trabecu-

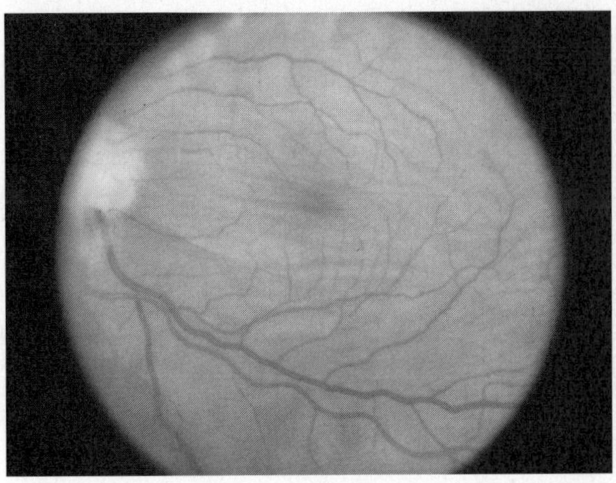

FIGURE 16–18. Folds in the macula in a patient with hypotony maculopathy.

lar outflow may result in a significant lowering of the IOP. Repair of the retinal detachment results in resolution of the hypotony. Patients with unexplained hypotony should undergo a thorough retinal examination.

Drugs that decrease aqueous production may be so effective that they cause hypotony. Drug-induced hypotony is rare unless there is a coexisting condition that may also lead to low eye pressure, such as intraocular inflammation, previous filtration or cyclodestructive surgery, or impaired circulation in the eye. Oral carbonic anhydrase inhibitors are the agents most commonly seen to cause hypotony in the aforementioned situations. Even if the eye in question is not being treated with medication to lower IOP, a beta-blocker applied to the contralateral eye may cause a "cross-over" effect, lowering the pressure in the untreated eye.

Cyclodestruction may have little effect on the IOP, may lower the pressure adequately, or may cause hypotony. Pressure that was initially well controlled may, with time, continue to decline to the point of hypotony. Eyes requiring cyclodestruction may also have a history of ocular inflammation or impaired circulation that causes variability in the rate of aqueous production and results in fluctuating IOP.

Inflammation within the eye, specifically, inflammation affecting the ciliary body, may cause a decrease in aqueous production and a low IOP.

Ischemia, including ischemia of the ciliary body, may result in decreased aqueous production and hypotony.

GLAUCOMA ASSOCIATED WITH INTRAOCULAR TUMORS

Intraocular tumors, whether primary or metastatic, may cause glaucoma through a variety of mechanisms, including angle closure, direct infiltration of the trabecular meshwork, and obstruction of aqueous outflow by liberated tumor cells.

CLINICAL SETTING

The glaucoma associated with intraocular tumors is almost always unilateral, although some cases of retinoblastoma and metastatic disease may be bilateral. The age of onset depends on the type of tumor: retinoblastoma, juvenile xanthogranuloma (JXG), and medulloepithelioma are usually seen in childhood, whereas melanomas and metastatic lesions are more common in older adults.

FINDINGS AND DIFFERENTIAL DIAGNOSIS

Melanoma of the uveal tract is the most common primary intraocular malignancy. Anterior melanomas are associated with glaucoma more commonly than posterior melanomas.

Iris melanomas usually have sharp borders, are variably pigmented, and are stationary or slow-growing. They are rarely associated with glaucoma unless tumor cells have significantly invaded the trabecular meshwork.

Ciliary body melanoma may extend through the iris and appear as a nodular mass on the peripheral iris stroma or may invade the anterior chamber angle (Fig. 16–19*A*). Sometimes a ciliary body melanoma manifests as a domed elevation of the iris, but it can be seen as a mass posterior to the iris and anterior to the lens on wide dilation of the pupil (Fig. 16–19*B*). Such a tumor may produce glaucoma by anterior displacement of the iris and angle closure, by neovascularization of the angle, or by tumor necrosis.

Choroidal melanoma, the most common melanoma of the uveal tract, is a pigmented mass that may be associated with a secondary, nonrhegmatogenous retinal detachment. The pigmentation of such lesions is variable. Some choroidal melanomas assume a mushroom shape, with a relatively thin "stalk" where the tumor broke through Bruch's membrane and a larger area of tumor between Bruch's membrane and the retina (Fig. 16–20). Choroidal melanomas are associated with glaucoma infrequently,[18] usually by causing neovascular glaucoma. A less common cause of glaucoma in patients with choroidal melanomas is inflammatory glaucoma from a necrotic tumor.

Metastatic tumors in the eye are most commonly found in the choroid. Breast and lung are the most common locations of primary tumors that metastasize to the eye. Metastatic tumors of the choroid are single, multiple and elevated, or diffuse lesions with an overlying nonrhegmatogenous retinal detachment. They are usually yellow or cream-colored, although metastatic melanomas may appear brown or gray. Glaucoma is not commonly seen with metastatic tumors; however, large metastatic tumors causing choroidal detachments, retinal detachments, or necrosis may be associated with the development of glaucoma.

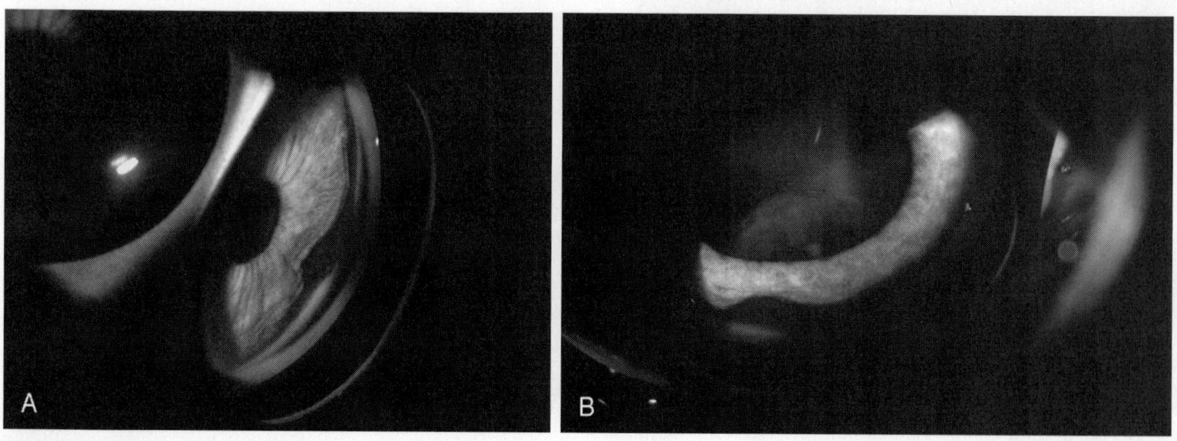

FIGURE 16–19. Ciliary body melanoma. *A,* Tumor seen on gonioscopy growing through the iris and into the angle. *B,* After dilation of the pupil.

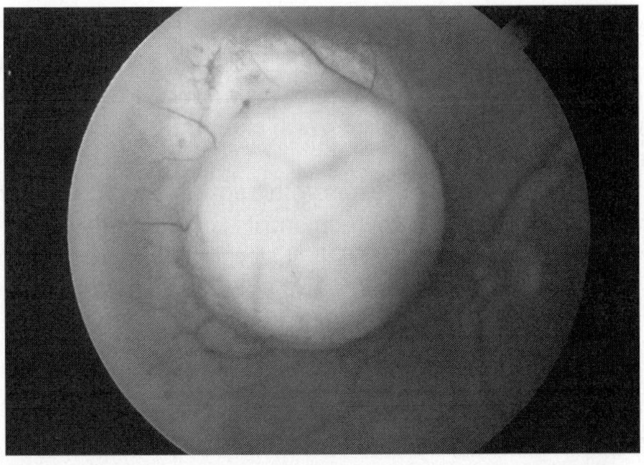

FIGURE 16–20. Choroidal melanoma, with a thin stalk through Bruch's membrane and the majority of the tumor mass under the retina (collar-button configuration).

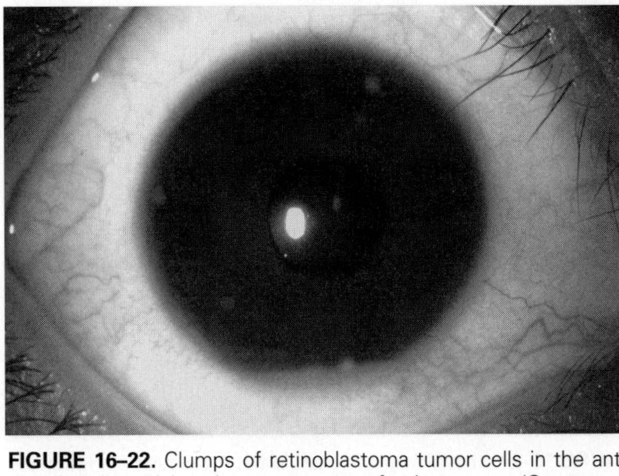

FIGURE 16–22. Clumps of retinoblastoma tumor cells in the anterior chamber, giving the appearance of a hypopyon. (Courtesy of Dr. C. Gail Summers.)

Retinoblastoma is the most common intraocular malignancy of children. Early lesions appear as elevated, white areas of the retina (Fig. 16–21). In the endophytic growth pattern, clumps of tumor cells may break free into the vitreous cavity or the anterior chamber (Fig. 16–22). In the exophytic growth pattern, the tumor cells grow outward in the subretinal space, causing a retinal detachment, but the vitreous remains clear. In advanced cases, leukocoria is noted. Glaucoma is seen in advanced cases and may develop from neovascularization of the iris and angle, angle closure, or tumor necrosis.

Medulloepithelioma (diktyoma) is a rare embryonal tumor that usually manifests in infancy or early childhood. It may appear as a solid or cystic, yellow or pink ciliary body mass extending into the anterior chamber (Fig. 16–23). It may cause leukocoria or hyphema. It is frequently associated with glaucoma due to angle closure, neovascularization of the angle, tumor seeding of the angle, or hyphema.

Juvenile xanthogranuloma (JXG) is a rare cutaneous disease of infancy. The skin lesions are yellow or orange nodules that regress over a period of years. Ocular findings most commonly consist of a singular or diffuse iris mass that manifests as vascular, salmon-colored lesions of the iris (Fig. 16–24). The ciliary body and trabecular meshwork may also be involved. Glaucoma is most commonly caused by spontaneous hyphema.

Glaucoma Associated with Vitreoretinal Surgery

IOP frequently becomes elevated after vitreoretinal procedures. The reported incidence of significant IOP elevation following vitrectomy ranges between 20% and 40%.[19, 20] In the majority of cases, the IOP elevation begins within the first day or two following surgery. Whether the IOP elevation occurs early or late in the postoperative period depends on the underlying mechanism of pressure elevation. A multitude of factors may cause IOP elevation after vitreoretinal procedures.

Patients with retinal disease sustain varying degrees of damage from elevated IOP, depending on the preoperative health of the optic nerve and retinal vasculature and on hematologic parameters such as blood viscosity. For example, patients with diabetes who have pre-existing poor

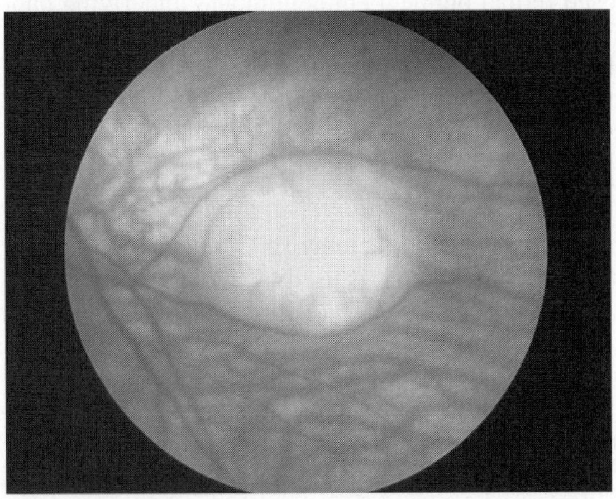

FIGURE 16–21. Retinoblastoma, appearing as an elevated white lesion in the retina of a 2-month-old girl with esotropia. (Courtesy of Dr. C. Gail Summers.)

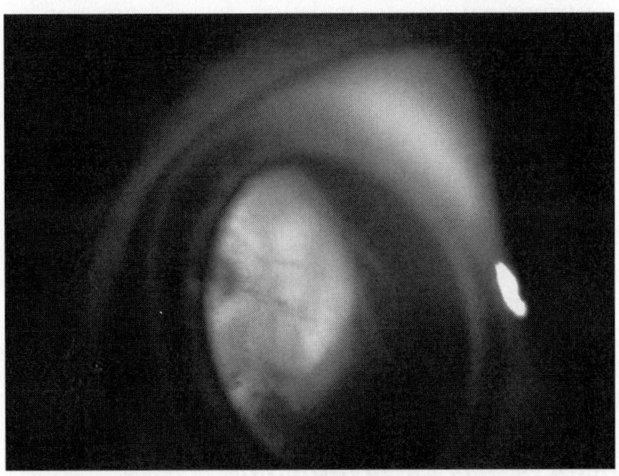

FIGURE 16–23. Although medulloepithelioma usually manifests in infancy or childhood, this yellow ciliary body mass was noted in a 50-year-old, asymptomatic patient. (Courtesy of Dr. Robert Letson.)

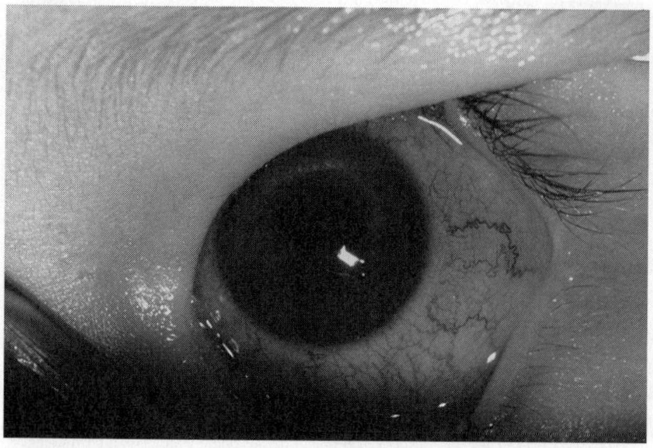

FIGURE 16–24. Juvenile xanthogranuloma. A vascular orange mass is present in the inferior iris. (Courtesy of Dr. C. Gail Summers.)

retinal vascular perfusion or those with sickle cell disease who are at risk for increased blood viscosity may experience visual loss, including loss of light perception, with even moderate IOP elevations. Because of the potential for visual loss, it is important to monitor IOP postoperatively in patients who have had retinal surgery.

Our discussion begins with an overview of vitreoretinal procedures that can produce postoperative IOP elevation, either transient or chronic. We then discuss the mechanisms by which these techniques cause IOP elevation in order to develop a framework for diagnostic assessment. From this information, the reader learns (1) to determine when and how often IOP should be checked after any given type of vitreoretinal procedure and (2) how to use the physical examination to arrive at a likely explanation for the IOP elevation.

BACKGROUND INFORMATION ON VITREORETINAL PROCEDURES

Panretinal Photocoagulation

Panretinal photocoagulation with the slit lamp, indirect ophthalmoscope, or endolaser is most commonly performed for neovascular retinopathies such as proliferative diabetic retinopathy (PDR). Patients with high-risk PDR have a 50% risk of severe visual loss over a 5-year interval; adequate panretinal photocoagulation causes regression of retinal and disc neovascularization, reducing this risk by about one-half. In diabetic patients who have vitreous hemorrhage or severe, progressive neovascularization, vitrectomy may be necessary, at which time scatter photocoagulation may be applied with the endolaser.

Another situation in which endophotocoagulation may be used is during vitrectomy and scleral buckling for proliferative vitreoretinopathy. In these patients, endophotocoagulation is applied around retinal breaks. If there are many small peripheral retinal breaks, endophotocoagulation may be applied to the involved retina over the scleral buckle in a scatter fashion for up to 360 degrees.

Peripheral Retinal Exocryotherapy

Cryotherapy can be applied to the peripheral retina in a panretinal fashion. With the retinal area to be treated viewed through the indirect ophthalmoscope, the cryoprobe is placed on the sclera with or without incision of the conjunctiva. Cryotherapy "spots" are applied to the retinal periphery in two or three rows extending from the ora serrata to the equator.

Panretinal peripheral exocryotherapy is most often performed for retinopathy of prematurity, in which the avascular peripheral retina is treated. Occasionally, exocryotherapy retinal ablation is useful in diabetic eyes with proliferative diabetic retinopathy in which laser treatment is not possible because of media opacity.

Scleral Buckling

Scleral buckles are used to treat rhegmatogenous retinal detachments. The adjective *rhegmatogenous* means that the retinal detachment results from a retinal break (either a tractional tear or an atrophic hole). The retinal break permits fluid from the vitreous cavity to enter the subretinal space, thus dissecting the neurosensory retina off the retinal pigment epithelium. Scleral buckles are silicone bands or sponges that are attached to the sclera with sutures or by passage through surgically created scleral tunnels. They may be oriented radially or circumferentially and serve to indent the sclera.

Essential to the repair of a rhegmatogenous retinal detachment is closure (tamponade) of the retinal break and relief of vitreous traction.[21] Scleral buckles provide tamponade by indenting the sclera and pushing the retinal pigment epithelium into apposition with the retinal breaks. The inward scleral indentation produced by scleral buckles also serves to reduce and counteract vitreous traction on the retinal break. Tamponade of the retinal break and relief of vitreous traction effectively reduce the flow of fluid through the break. As the flow of fluid into the subretinal space is reduced, the retinal pigment epithelium and choroid absorb subretinal fluid, and the retina reattaches. Cryotherapy is applied around the retinal break to promote formation of a scar and permanent adhesion between the retinal pigment epithelium and the neurosensory retina.

IOP is often lower than normal in patients with rhegmatogenous retinal detachments. The lower-than-normal IOP may result from the absorption of aqueous humor by the exposed retinal pigment epithelium and underlying choroid (which has a higher osmotic pressure than the aqueous). Reattachment of the retina permits the IOP to return to normal.

Pars Plana Vitrectomy

During pars plana vitrectomy, a 20-gauge guillotine-like instrument, the vitrector, is used to cut and aspirate vitreous from the closed eye. The vitrector and other instruments, such as tiny scissors and forceps, are placed through sclerotomies 3 to 4 mm posterior to the limbus. Placement of sclerotomies in this location ensures entry through the pars plana rather than through the neurosensory retina.

Vitrectomy is useful for removal of vitreous opacities, such as hemorrhage, and for peeling of tractional membranes on the retina, as in proliferative diabetic retinopathy and proliferative vitreoretinopathy.

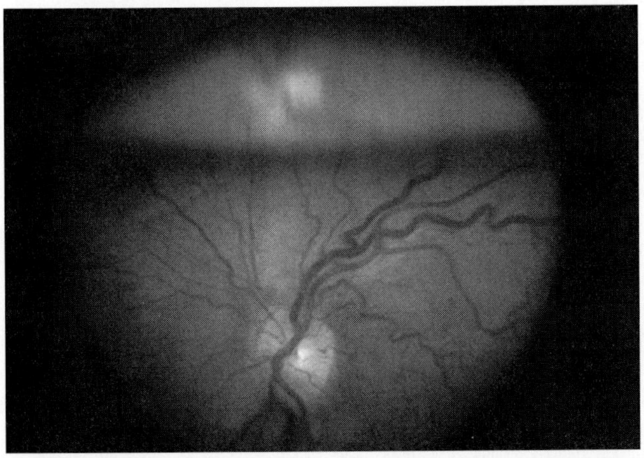

FIGURE 16–25. Gas bubble in vitreous cavity after fluid-gas exchange. The gas-fluid interface is seen at the top of the photograph. A reflection of the optic nerve is present on the undersurface of the gas bubble.

Adjuncts to Scleral Buckling and Vitrectomy Surgery

INTRAOCULAR GAS

USES. Air or perfluorocarbon gas can be injected into the vitreous cavity to provide tamponade to retinal breaks. The air or gas bubble closes the retinal break while subretinal fluid resorbs and holds the retina in place as the laser or cryotherapy scars form.

Intraocular gas is commonly used in three situations:

1. Air or gas can be injected into the vitreous cavity at the conclusion of scleral buckling surgery in order to provide tamponade to the retinal break in addition to that supplied by the buckle; this maneuver has been likened to "adding suspenders to the belt."
2. Gas may also be injected into the vitreous cavity as a primary treatment for rhegmatogenous retinal detachment. This technique, called *pneumatic retinopexy,* is appropriate for certain retinal detachments, generally with tears above the horizontal midline. The gas bubble provides tamponade to the retinal breaks. However, the issue of vitreous traction is not addressed by this technique.
3. At the conclusion of vitrectomy surgery, fluid in the eye may be exchanged for air or gas to provide tamponade as laser or cryotherapy scars form around retinal breaks. This procedure is called *fluid-gas exchange* (Fig. 16–25).

PHYSICAL PROPERTIES. The three most commonly used gases are air, sulfur hexafluoride (SF_6), and perfluoropropane (C_3F_8). Being less dense than physiologic saline and water, these gases exert an upward buoyant force on the retina when placed into the vitreous cavity. The patient's head can be positioned in such a way as to take advantage of this buoyancy to position the gas bubble over the retinal break.

The property of surface tension allows gas bubbles to function as tamponade to retinal breaks.[22] If a gas bubble is larger than a retinal break and the retina is mobile, the gas tends to close the break rather than move through it, because of surface tension between the gas bubble and the fluid under the retinal break.

Buoyancy helps the gas bubble to flatten the retina against the retinal pigment epithelium as laser or cryotherapy scars form.

EXPANSION AND DURATION. Air injected into the vitreous cavity has the same composition as room air. Therefore, there is no tendency for blood gases to diffuse into an intraocular air bubble, and the air bubble does not expand. Over 2 to 3 days, the gases composing the air bubble (mostly oxygen, carbon dioxide, and nitrogen) resorb because they are soluble in ocular tissues and blood.

The perfluorocarbon gases SF_6 and C_3F_8 are relatively insoluble in ocular tissues and blood. Therefore, they remain in the vitreous cavity longer than air. In clinical practice, after complete fluid-gas exchange, SF_6 and C_3F_8 remain in the vitreous cavity for about 2 and 4 weeks, respectively. The duration of a gas bubble in any given patient depends on the type of gas used, the concentration of the gas, and the extent of gas fill. Air is used when tamponade of a few days is desired, and perfluorocarbon gases are used for tamponade of several weeks (Table 16–3).

After a perfluorocarbon gas bubble is placed in the eye, blood gases initially diffuse into the bubble and reach an equilibrium. Oxygen and carbon dioxide are relatively soluble in the perfluorocarbon gases and diffuse in rather rapidly. Nitrogen, however, is relatively insoluble in these gases and diffuses into the gas bubble more slowly. As a result of this equilibration process, perfluorocarbon gas bubbles initially expand after placement in the eye. The maximal rate of expansion occurs during the first 6 hours after placement. Pure SF_6 bubbles expand to approximately twice their initial volume and reach maximal expansion 1 to 2 days after injection. Pure C_3F_8 bubbles expand to about four times their initial volume and reach maximal expansion at 3 to 4 days after injection. Perfluorocarbon gases, which are poorly soluble in tissue fluids and blood, diffuse slowly out of the eye over several weeks.

Pure perfluorocarbon gases initially expand when placed into the eye. However, concentrations of these gases may be chosen that are "nonexpansile," meaning that enough air is mixed into the gas that nitrogen influx and perfluoro-

TABLE 16–3. PROPERTIES OF INTRAOCULAR GASES

Gas	Expansile?	Reaches Maximal Expansion	Duration (Approximate)
Air	No	Nonexpansile	2–3 days
Sulfur hexafluoride (SF_6)	Yes; pure SF_6 expands to twice initial volume	1–2 days	2 weeks
Perfluoropropane (C_3F_8)	Yes; pure C_3F_8 expands to 4 times initial volume	3–4 days	4 weeks

carbon efflux are roughly equal. The nonexpansile concentration of SF_6 is 18%, and the nonexpansile concentration of C_3F_8 is 14%.

SILICONE OIL

USES. Silicone oil, like gas, can be used to provide intraocular tamponade for the treatment of rhegmatogenous retinal detachment. Because silicone oil does not resorb, it is used for complex retinal detachments complicated by proliferative vitreoretinopathy for which long-term tamponade is desired. Silicone oil is used also in patients who wish to have more rapid visual rehabilitation than is possible with gas or who wish to travel by air within several weeks of surgery; patients with intraocular gas bubbles must not fly.

PHYSICAL PROPERTIES. The silicone oil currently used in vitreoretinal surgery is a mixture of polymers composed of repeating dimethylsiloxane units. Silicone oil is less dense than physiologic saline and water, and therefore exerts a buoyant force on the retina. The upward pressure of silicone oil on the retina is less than that of a gas bubble.[23] As with gas bubbles, a silicone oil globule adopts the lowest energy configuration. This tends to be as nearly spherical as possible within the confines of the vitreous cavity (whose shape varies according to the size and location of the scleral buckle, if present).

The silicone oil–water interface has a relatively high surface tension, although it is less than that of a gas-water interface. As with gas bubbles, it is surface tension that allows silicone oil to effectively act as tamponade on retinal breaks.

Silicone oil does not expand after it is placed in the vitreous cavity. However, silicone oil can undergo emulsification, which will be discussed later.

PERFLUOROCARBON LIQUIDS

Perfluorocarbon liquids are more dense than physiologic saline and water. They are used as adjuncts during vitreoretinal surgery to drain subretinal fluid internally through pre-existing anterior retinal breaks. Their use obviates the need for posterior drainage retinotomies, which are required when fluid-gas exchange is used for internal drainage of subretinal fluid. Perfluorocarbon liquids are intraoperative tools only and are removed before the end of the procedure. Tiny droplets of perfluorocarbon liquid may remain in the eye postoperatively.

MEASUREMENT OF INTRAOCULAR PRESSURE IN GAS-FILLED AND SILICONE-FILLED EYES

It is important to monitor postoperative IOP after vitreoretinal procedures, especially if gas or silicone oil tamponade has been used. Both gas and silicone oil may affect measured IOP. A number of studies, as described here, have reported which types of tonometers yield the most accurate IOP measurements in this situation.

Indentation tonometry allows one to convert the extent of indentation of the cornea by the tonometer plunger to IOP in mm Hg by way of conversion tables. The standard conversion table for the Schiøtz tonometer, for example, is based on an average value for the coefficient of ocular rigidity (which is a measure of the elasticity of the corneoscleral outer ocular coat). If the actual coefficient of ocular rigidity is less or more than the average value, IOP is either underestimated or overestimated, respectively. Intravitreal air and gas, both of which are highly compressible, make the eye more elastic and cause the coefficient of ocular rigidity to be lower than normal. An experimental study in an enucleated eye in which 0.8 mL of vitreous was replaced with air confirmed that the Schiøtz tonometer underestimates IOP when the standard conversion table is used.[24]

Applanation tonometry is based on conversion of the force required to flatten a given area of cornea into IOP in mm Hg. Examples of applanation devices are the Goldmann tonometer, Perkins tonometer, Tono-Pen, and pneumatonometer. For practical purposes, applanation tonometer readings are independent of ocular rigidity. In a study of eye bank eyes, the Tono-Pen and pneumatonometer readings correlated well with manometric IOP, although both underestimated IOP at higher manometric pressures.[25] Compared with the manometer, the Tono-Pen underestimated IOP by approximately 8 mm Hg in the IOP range 30 to 50 mm Hg. This was true both in eye bank eyes after lensectomy, vitrectomy, and fluid-air exchange and in air-filled aphakic eyes at the time of surgery. At higher IOPs, the underestimation by the Tono-Pen increases.[26] The pneumatonometer, likewise, tends to underestimate IOP at higher manometric IOPs.[27]

Less information is available about the accuracy of various tonometers for silicone oil–filled eyes. A clinical study of eyes, both aphakic and phakic, after vitrectomy with silicone oil tamponade revealed a high degree of correlation between Tono-Pen and Goldmann tonometer readings.[28]

Practical considerations also affect the choice of tonometer for IOP measurement after vitreoretinal procedures. Often such eyes have an irregular or missing central corneal epithelium. The Tono-Pen is unaffected by this feature, whereas Goldmann or Perkins tonometer readings may be impossible because corneal irregularities distort the mires. The Tono-Pen has the advantage of using a clean cover over the plunger for each patient, which is especially important in patients with compromised corneal epithelium.

INTRAOCULAR PRESSURE ELEVATION DURING AND AFTER VITREORETINAL SURGERY

Intraoperative Intraocular Pressure Changes

Scleral buckles indent the sclera and reduce the volume of the eye. As a buckle is tightened, IOP rises, often dramatically. Gardner and coworkers[29] measured IOP continuously during scleral buckling surgery with a pars plana pressure transducer and found wide IOP fluctuations during application of the buckle. The maximum IOP of 210 mm Hg occurred during scleral depression and cryopexy. Scleral buckles may be performed with or without drainage of subretinal fluid. External drainage of subretinal fluid is performed before the buckle is tightened. This maneuver reduces the volume of the eye, and, therefore, diminishes the IOP elevation caused by tightening of the buckle.

Whether subretinal fluid is drained or not, the surgeon

must check the perfusion of the central retinal artery after tightening the scleral buckle. If IOP remains high enough to close the central retinal artery, an aqueous tap at the limbus may be performed to reduce IOP. Sometimes, multiple anterior chamber taps over several minutes are required to reduce IOP to a safe level. Generally, if aqueous outflow facility is normal, IOP normalizes fairly rapidly.

Postoperative Intraocular Pressure Changes

The causes of postoperative changes in IOP are summarized in Table 16–4.

ANGLE-CLOSURE GLAUCOMA

Angle Narrowing or Closure Secondary to Choroidal Effusions

SCLERAL BUCKLING. Aside from the immediate increase in IOP at the time of tightening, scleral buckles can cause postoperative IOP elevation secondary to narrowing or closure of the anterior chamber angle. Angle-closure glaucoma has been reported in up to 4% of patients undergoing scleral buckling surgery.

Choroidal effusions may form during or after scleral buckling procedures. The risk for choroidal detachment during scleral buckling is greatest when the eye becomes hypotonous after external drainage of subretinal fluid. Postoperatively, scleral buckling may cause compression of vortex veins and may impede venous drainage of the choroid. Suprachoroidal effusion and ciliary body swelling may result, leading to anterior rotation of the ciliary body about its muscular attachment at the scleral spur.[30] With anterior rotation of the ciliary body, the iris root moves anteriorly also, narrowing the entrance to the anterior chamber angle. With increased ciliary body swelling and larger amounts of suprachoroidal fluid, the ciliary body may come into contact with the iris, pushing it forward onto the cornea and resulting in complete angle closure and elevated IOP. Simultaneous forward movement of the lens-iris diaphragm may lead to pupillary block as well. IOP rises unless ciliary body detachment causes aqueous production to decline.

TABLE 16–4. SUMMARY OF CAUSES OF INTRAOCULAR PRESSURE ELEVATION AFTER VITREORETINAL SURGERY

INTRAOCULAR PRESSURE ELEVATION OCCURRING IN THE FIRST 24 HOURS AFTER SURGERY
Shallow anterior chamber and/or closed anterior chamber angle
Forward rotation of ciliary body with closure of anterior chamber angle
Choroidal effusion secondary to extensive panretinal photocoagulation
Choroidal effusion secondary to extensive exocryotherapy
Choroidal effusion complicating scleral buckling or vitrectomy
Pupillary block
Silicone oil
Intraocular gas
Posterior synechiae
Fibrin pupillary membrane
Open anterior chamber angle
Gas expansion
Viscoelastic substances
INTRAOCULAR PRESSURE ELEVATION OCCURRING AFTER THE FIRST POSTOPERATIVE DAY
Shallow anterior chamber and/or closed anterior chamber angle
Pupillary block
Posterior synechiae
Fibrin pupillary membrane
Peripheral anterior synechiae
Chronic postoperative inflammation
Neovascularization of anterior chamber angle
Open anterior chamber angle
Steroid-induced glaucoma
Intraocular gas expansion without angle closure
Silicone oil emulsification
Ghost cell glaucoma
Pre-existing glaucoma

VITRECTOMY. Choroidal detachments rarely form during pars plana vitrectomy but have been reported.[31] In a series of 683 consecutive pars plana vitrectomies, the incidence of hemorrhagic choroidal detachment was 1.9%, occurring in 13 eyes.[32] Risk factors that appear to increase the probability of choroidal hemorrhage during or immediately after pars plana vitrectomy are: greater patient age, scleral buckling at the time of vitrectomy, increased preoperative IOP, preoperative rhegmatogenous retinal detachment, pseudophakia or aphakia, and myopia.

Iatrogenic choroidal detachments may occur during vitrectomy from improper placement of the pars plana infusion line. If the pars plana infusion cannula is not inserted entirely through the pars plana epithelium, the cannula may infuse directly into the suprachoroidal space, creating a choroidal detachment.

PANRETINAL PHOTOCOAGULATION. Panretinal photocoagulation or peripheral scatter laser over a scleral buckle may cause fluid to collect in the suprachoroidal space. If extensive enough, the suprachoroidal fluid or effusion may cause the ciliary body to swell and rotate anteriorly. In turn, anterior rotation of the ciliary body pushes the peripheral iris forward, causing the anterior chamber angle to become narrow or closed over the trabecular meshwork. The anterior chamber angle appears narrow on slit-lamp examination. Iris bombé is present only if there is a component of pupillary block in addition to the anterior rotation of the ciliary body. Gonioscopy reveals a narrow or closed anterior chamber angle and, possibly, visible ciliary processes. Careful indirect ophthalmoscopy or ultrasonography may reveal choroidal detachments.

Angle closure may occur immediately after panretinal photocoagulation or 1 to 2 days later. Patients who undergo panretinal photocoagulation in several sessions are less likely to experience angle closure than those who receive panretinal photocoagulation in one session.[33]

Pupillary Block with Silicone Oil

Acute angle-closure glaucoma secondary to pupillary block may occur with silicone oil or gas tamponade. When using silicone oil for intraocular tamponade, the surgeon attempts to fill the entire vitreous cavity with oil. This results in a single large oil globule in the vitreous cavity with its anterior face at the pupillary plane. Contact between the anterior surface of the oil globule and the iris at the pupillary margin may produce pupillary block. Because aqueous cannot follow its usual route through the pupil to the anterior chamber in this situation, IOP rises, and angle-closure glaucoma may result. When silicone oil causes pupillary block, aqueous accumulates in the posterior chamber and vitreous cavity and may, in turn, force a portion of the silicone oil forward into the anterior chamber.

In 1985, Ando[34] published his method, the inferior iridectomy, for preventing pupillary block and forward migration of silicone oil. Placement of a peripheral iridectomy at the six o'clock position allows the more dense aqueous to flow under the silicone oil globule into the anterior chamber. Phakic eyes do not require inferior iridectomy because the intact lens-iris diaphragm prevents forward migration of oil into the anterior chamber. Lacking this barrier, aphakic eyes require an inferior iridectomy. Pseudophakic eyes do not necessarily require an inferior iridectomy unless the posterior capsule is open or otherwise unable to prevent forward migration of silicone oil.

In certain eyes, particularly those of diabetic patients, postoperative fibrin formation can occlude the inferior iridectomy, rendering it nonfunctional. Fibrin formation over the inferior iridectomy may contribute to the onset of pupillary block glaucoma and forward movement of the silicone oil. Although injection of tissue plasminogen activator into the anterior chamber can cause rapid fibrinolysis, fibrin occlusion of the inferior peripheral iridectomy can recur.

The supine position must be avoided in all postoperative patients with silicone oil tamponade. Silicone oil is less dense than physiologic saline. Therefore, the silicone oil globule exerts an upward force on the iris or lens-iris diaphragm in a supine patient, setting the stage for pupillary block and angle closure. During the evaluation of a patient with silicone oil and elevated IOP, it is wise to determine whether improper patient positioning may be a factor. (The same is true for intraocular gas bubbles, as discussed in the next section.)

When examining a postoperative patient with a silicone oil–filled eye, the physician must look for signs of pupillary block, including a shallow anterior chamber and iris bombé. If the anterior chamber appears shallow, gonioscopy is necessary to determine whether the anterior chamber angle is open or closed. The examiner must inspect the inferior iridectomy for signs of occlusion by blood, fibrin, or stray residual droplets of liquid perfluorocarbon.

The presence of silicone oil in the anterior chamber confirms the suspicion of pupillary block. Silicone oil in the anterior chamber can be overlooked easily because it appears optically empty. However, the optical emptiness can be used as a clue. Generally, the aqueous shows some cells or flare, especially in the postoperative eye. If the anterior chamber is optically empty, silicone oil may have replaced the aqueous. The presence of silicone oil in the anterior chamber is confirmed by the presence of an interface between the iris and silicone oil. When a slit-lamp beam is moved from side to side across the iris, the silicone oil–iris interface creates a characteristic sheen that is easy to see.

Pupillary Block with Intraocular Gas

Pupillary block with acute angle closure may occur with the use of intraocular gases under a variety of circumstances. Depending on the concentration of gas used, gas expansion may occur in the early postoperative period. Incorrect patient positioning or gas overfill may lead to pupillary block. Intraocular gas may expand with disastrous consequences during air travel and during general anesthesia with nitrous oxide. Each of these situations is described here.

GAS EXPANSION. Concentrations of SF_6 exceeding 18% and of C_3F_8 exceeding 14% expand in the eye postoperatively because of nitrogen equilibration, as explained previously. Gas expansion occurs most rapidly in the first 6 hours after instillation and may cause elevated IOP even in the absence of pupillary block, depending on the aqueous outflow facility of the eye. As the volume of gas expands further, gas overfill may result, with pupillary block and angle closure. On slit-lamp examination, a gas-filled eye with pupillary block has a shallow or flat anterior chamber. On indirect ophthalmoscopy, the vitreous cavity is completely or nearly completely filled with gas. In certain aphakic eyes with floppy irides, gas may flatten the superior anterior chamber even when the patient is in the upright position. Whether this closure of the superior angle results in elevated IOP depends on the outflow facility of the remaining open angle.

SUPINE POSITION. Gas in the vitreous cavity pushes the iris or lens-iris diaphragm forward when a patient assumes the supine position. This situation can lead to angle-closure glaucoma through a combination of posterior pushing and pupillary block (Fig. 16–26). For this reason, patients who have intraocular gas after vitreoretinal surgery must be warned to avoid the supine position. When a patient is taken to the recovery room after receiving intraocular gas, the recovery room nurses must be told to turn the patient to the side or stomach (whichever is feasible and more desirable given the location of the retinal breaks).

AIR TRAVEL. Intraocular gases (both air and perfluorocarbons) obey Boyle's law: Pressure $\times$ Volume $=$ Constant. Therefore, when the ambient pressure decreases at higher elevations, an intraocular gas bubble expands to occupy a larger volume. Air travel and mountain travel to higher elevations have caused painful episodes of angle-closure glaucoma (with loss of light perception in some instances) in patients with intraocular gas.[35]

An experimental study of IOP changes in air-filled eyes during conditions simulating commercial air travel was conducted in anesthetized monkeys.[36] At 35,000 feet with 0.5 mL of air in the eye, the IOP increased by approximately 150 mm Hg. This experiment demonstrates that IOP elevations resulting from air or mountain travel can be great enough to occlude the central retinal artery. No amount of intraocular air or long-acting gas can be considered to be definitely safe in postoperative patients who are considering travel to or at higher elevations.

GENERAL ANESTHESIA WITH NITROUS OXIDE. The solubility of nitrous oxide in water is 117 times greater than that of SF_6 in water. In addition, the diffusion coefficient of nitrous oxide in water is twice that of SF_6. When a patient under general anesthesia receives nitrous oxide, the nitrous oxide rapidly equilibrates with the intraocular SF_6 gas bubble. This rapid equilibration of nitrous oxide with the intraocular gas bubble causes the bubble to expand and IOP to increase.[37]

Patients with intraocular gas bubbles (whether of air or long-acting perfluorocarbon gas) must not receive nitrous

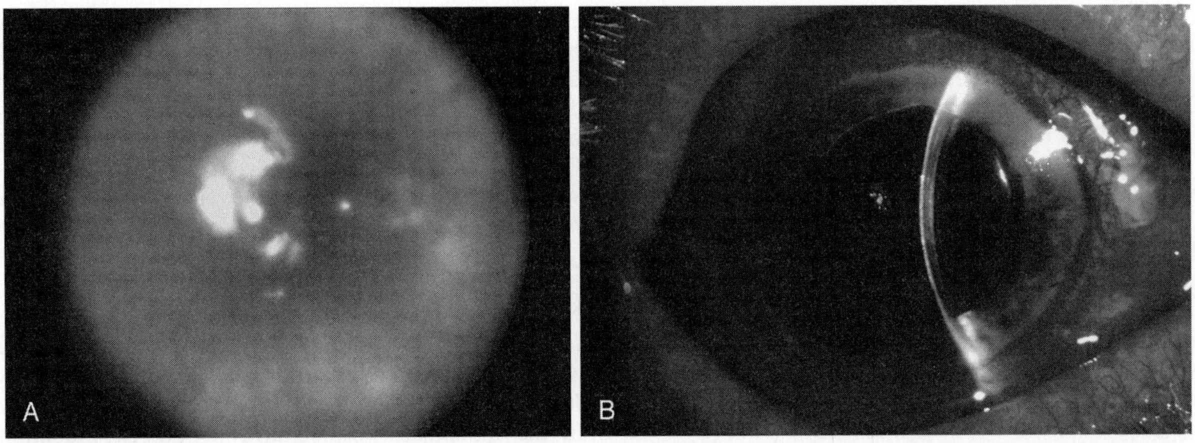

FIGURE 16–26. Gas-filled eye with pupillary block and angle-closure glaucoma. *A,* The fundus photograph demonstrates light reflections from the gas-retina interface in the temporal peripapillary area. Fresh laser scars surround a posterior drainage retinotomy nasal to the optic disc. *B,* The slit-lamp photograph reveals iridocorneal apposition and angle-closure glaucoma secondary to pupillary block by the gas bubble.

oxide. Those who have received nitrous oxide inadvertently have experienced IOP elevations with, in some cases, loss of light perception.

Pupillary Block Secondary to Posterior Synechiae and Occlusion of the Pupil

Intraocular fibrin formation after vitreoretinal procedures varies in severity. At times, it is severe enough to create posterior synechiae or to occlude the pupil. Posterior synechiae are adhesions of the iris around the pupil to the crystalline lens, to an intraocular lens, or to residual anterior hyaloid face. Extensive posterior synechiae or complete pupillary occlusion by fibrin may lead to pupillary block and angle-closure glaucoma. Intraocular fibrinolysis eventually removes fibrin membranes. Fibrin serves as a scaffold for cellular infiltration, however, and fibrin membranes may be transformed into permanent cellular pupillary membranes and posterior synechiae resistant to fibrinolysis.

Other situations in which severe intraocular fibrin formation occurs postoperatively are lensectomy in patients with uveitis and poorly controlled intraocular inflammation and vitrectomy in certain patients with proliferative diabetic retinopathy. Patients with endophthalmitis also are particularly prone to intraocular fibrin formation and may have pupillary membranes (which may cause pupillary block) or cyclitic membranes (which may detach the ciliary body, leading to hypotony).

On examination, pupillary membranes are visible with the slit lamp. If a pupillary membrane is present, it is necessary to determine its extent and to look for signs of pupillary block, such as shallowing of the anterior chamber and iris bombé.

Angle Closure Secondary to Peripheral Anterior Synechiae

Peripheral anterior synechiae (PAS) occur secondary to neovascularization of the anterior chamber angle or chronic intraocular inflammation. In these situations, contractile fibrovascular or fibrous membranes pull the iris toward the trabecular meshwork and peripheral cornea, creating adhesions, or synechiae. Extensive synechiae over the trabecular meshwork may block aqueous outflow and lead to chronic angle closure.

Peripheral anterior synechiae do not cause the anterior chamber angle to become shallow. However, if PAS are associated with posterior synechiae or a pupillary membrane, pupillary block may result, leading to a shallow anterior chamber and iris bombé. On gonioscopy, PAS appear as adhesions between the peripheral iris and trabecular meshwork. If extensive PAS are present, the gonioscopic appearance may be that of a "false angle."

OPEN-ANGLE GLAUCOMA

Intraocular Pressure Elevation without Angle Closure in Gas-Filled Eyes

Expanding intraocular gas may raise IOP even without causing angle closure. If IOP is not checked at appropriate times after surgery, significant IOP elevations may go unnoticed. As a general rule, appropriate times to check IOP in eyes with intravitreal perfluorocarbon gases are at 2 hours and at 6 hours after instillation. The 2-hour IOP check gives the physician an idea of how well the aqueous outflow mechanisms of the eye are responding to the gas bubble, and the 6-hour IOP check is performed because the rate of gas bubble expansion is greatest during the first 6 hours after instillation.

Silicone Oil Emulsification and Open-Angle Glaucoma

Emulsions arise from two immiscible liquids when tiny droplets of one liquid become suspended in the other liquid. Silicone oil may emulsify in the aqueous environment of the vitreous cavity and form tiny droplets, which then migrate into the anterior chamber. Proteins (such as fibrin) from postoperative breakdown of the blood-retina barrier act as emulsifiers, reducing the surface energy of tiny silicone droplets.[38] Saccadic eye movements probably impart the energy required to break off tiny droplets from the main silicone oil globule. Emulsification may be a more common problem in phakic than in aphakic oil-filled eyes, because more vitreous base (containing water) is left in phakic eyes after vitrectomy. Because of concern about possible damage to the crystalline lens, removal of the vitreous base cannot be as complete in phakic eyes as in aphakic eyes.

In its most obvious and least common form, silicone oil emulsification may result in a hyperoleon or "upside-down hypopyon" (Fig. 16–27). Emulsified silicone oil droplets may adhere to the iris stroma, where they cause no particular harm. However, they also may enter the trabecular meshwork and reduce aqueous outflow. Emulsified oil droplets can reach the anterior chamber angle in phakic as well as in aphakic and pseudophakic eyes. In most patients, gonioscopy is required to make the diagnosis of silicone oil emulsification.[39]

The incidence of late postoperative glaucoma following intraocular instillation of silicone oil has been reported to be as high as 48% in one series, in which *glaucoma* was defined as an IOP higher than 25 mm Hg and 10 mm Hg above the preoperative pressure.[40] In the Silicone Oil Study, the incidence of chronically elevated IOP among eyes randomly assigned to receive silicone oil was 8%.[41] The damage to the trabecular meshwork is permanent because removal of the silicone oil does not reverse the glaucoma.

Hyphema and Open-Angle Glaucoma

Two postoperative situations in which hyphema may occur are (1) after intraocular surgery in eyes with iris neovascularization and (2) after vitrectomy for fresh vitreous hemorrhage in aphakic or pseudophakic eyes. The fresh red blood cells may settle out in the anterior chamber, creating a hyphema. Fresh red blood cells generally do not obstruct the trabecular meshwork or cause pressure elevation. However, the following factors increase the likelihood of IOP elevation in the setting of postoperative hyphema: preexisting poor aqueous outflow facility, fibrinoid aqueous reaction accompanying the hyphema, and the presence of sickled red blood cells.

Viscoelastics and Open-Angle Glaucoma

In the past, viscoelastic substances were used to help unroll giant retinal tears. Fortunately, liquid perfluorocarbons have now replaced viscoelastics for this purpose. However, viscoelastic substances are still essential during vitreoretinal procedures for (1) protection of the corneal endothelium during pars plana lensectomy; (2) placement on the corneal endothelium in aphakic eyes during fluid-air exchange in order to create an optically smooth surface (otherwise, Descemet's folds in the air-filled eye impair the surgeon's view of the fundus; and (3) removal of water condensation on intraocular lenses during fluid-air exchange

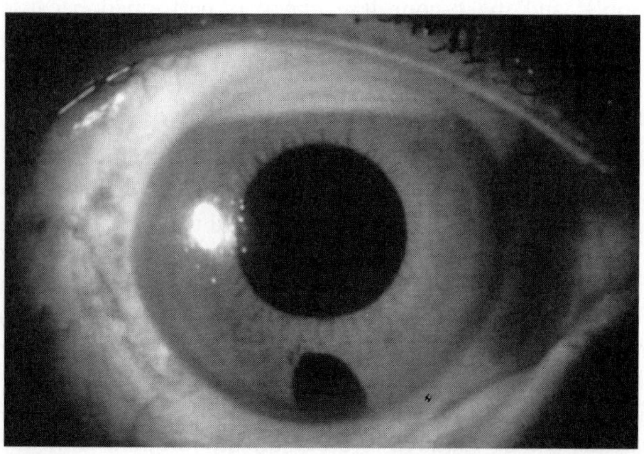

FIGURE 16–27. Emulsified silicone oil. The white material visible superiorly in the anterior chamber is emulsified silicone oil (hyperoleon). Aqueous fills the remainder of the anterior chamber, and silicone oil fills the vitreous cavity. This eye is aphakic. The inferior peripheral iridectomy helps to prevent pupillary block glaucoma secondary to silicone oil.

Corticosteroid-Induced Open-Angle Glaucoma

IOP may become elevated several weeks after surgery as a response to topical steroid drops. The steroid response of IOP is a delayed phenomenon and usually does not occur in the immediate postoperative period. Less commonly, IOP may rise in response to oral steroids. The injection of depot or long-acting steroids into the subconjunctival or sub-Tenon's space may result in months of elevated eye pressure.

What to Do When a Patient Who Has Had a Vitreoretinal Procedure Has Postoperative Intraocular Pressure Elevation

The diagnosis of postoperatively increased IOP in a patient who has undergone vitreoretinal surgery usually is made from a scheduled IOP check or during evaluation of specific complaints, such as increasing eye pain, nausea, or vomiting. A similar diagnostic approach may be used in all cases; the steps of the approach are as follows:

1. **DETERMINE WHAT MAJOR VITREORETINAL PROCEDURES WERE PERFORMED.** Risk factors for angle closure include: (a) scleral buckling, (b) intraocular gas, (c) silicone oil tamponade, (d) extensive peripheral scatter laser coagulation, and (e) possibly, extensive cryotherapy.

   Risk factors for IOP elevation in the presence of an open anterior chamber angle include: (a) lensectomy, because of enhanced postoperative fibrin formation and lens debris, (b) intraocular gas expansion not severe enough to cause angle closure but enough to raise IOP, (c) silicone oil emulsification, (d) postoperative use of steroids, (e) recurrent postvitrectomy vitreous hemorrhage, (f) postoperative fibrin formation, and (g) chronic postoperative intraocular inflammation.

   Compromised preoperative aqueous outflow facility also places the eye at greater risk for postoperative IOP elevation.
2. **CHECK FOR IMPROPER POSITIONING AFTER INTRAOCULAR GAS OR OIL.** If the patient has received intraocular gas or silicone oil, ask the patient or the nurses whether the patient has maintained face-down positioning. Lying in the supine position for several hours can lead to the development of pupillary block and angle closure in the presence of intraocular gas or oil. In any postoperative patient who received intraocular gas or silicone oil, face-down positioning should be included as part of the initial treatment plan.
3. **ALWAYS CHECK VISUAL ACUITY AT THE BEGINNING OF**

YOUR EXAMINATION. When possible, hold a +10.00-diopter to +12.00-diopter lens over an aphakic eye when checking postoperative visual acuity.

4. **PERFORM SLIT-LAMP EXAMINATION AND GONIOSCOPY.** Both of these examinations should be directed at determination of the mechanism of IOP elevation. Note anterior chamber depth, iris configuration (the presence or absence of iris bombé), and presence or absence of inflammatory cells, ghost cells, and fibrin.

   Gonioscopy may be performed in the operated eye with a corneal epithelial defect if the goniolens is carefully sterilized prior to use. Gonioscopy of the fellow eye may yield some clue as to whether the operated eye had a pre-existing occludable angle. In some cases, ciliary processes visible through the dilated pupil may indicate anterior rotation of the ciliary body which may be related to postoperative choroidal detachment or suprachoroidal effusion.
5. **PERFORM INDIRECT OPHTHALMOSCOPY.** Use this examination to confirm what procedures were performed (e.g., scleral buckling or extensive scatter laser treatment). Estimate the extent of gas or silicone oil fill, and look for choroidal detachments. Sometimes choroidal detachments are present only anterior to the scleral buckle.
6. **CHECK FOR PERFUSION OF THE RETINAL ARTERIES.** If you are unsure whether the retinal arteries are being perfused, press on the globe through the eyelid and see whether you can induce arterial pulsations. Central retinal artery occlusion is an emergency that requires rapid lowering of the IOP, often by aqueous tap or removal of some intraocular gas.
7. **REMEMBER THE MULTIFACTORIAL NATURE OF POSTOPERATIVE INTRAOCULAR PRESSURE ELEVATION.** Rises in IOP following vitreoretinal procedures can occur from many causes, as discussed in this chapter.

ACKNOWLEDGMENTS

Photography for this chapter was furnished by Timothy Bennett, COPRA (Department of Ophthalmology, The Milton S. Hershey Medical Center), and William C. McMichael (Department of Ophthalmology, University of Minnesota).

REFERENCES

1. Brown GC, Magargal LE, Schachat A, Shah H: Neovascular glaucoma: Etiologic considerations. Ophthalmology 1984;91:315–320.
2. Laatikainen L: Development and classification of rubeosis iridis in diabetic eye disease. Br J Ophthalmol 1979;63:150–156.
3. Campbell DG, Simmons RJ, Grant WM: Ghost cells as a cause of glaucoma. Am J Ophthalmol 1976;81:441–450.
4. Cashwell LF, Martin TJ: Malignant glaucoma after laser iridectomy. Ophthalmology 1992;99:651–659.
5. Hartnett ME, Hirose T, Richardson TM, et al: Intraocular pressure determination in infants with severe retinopathy of prematurity. Graefes Arch Clin Exp Ophthalmol 1992;230:406–410.
6. Michael AJ, Pesin SR, Katz LJ, et al: Management of late-onset angle-closure glaucoma associated with retinopathy of prematurity. Ophthalmology 1991;98:1093–1098.
7. Harnett ME, Gilbert MM, Richardson TM, et al: Anterior segment evaluation of infants with retinopathy of prematurity. Ophthalmology 1990;97:122–130.
8. Harnett ME, Gilbert MM, Hirose T, et al: Glaucoma as a cause of poor vision in severe retinopathy of prematurity. Graefes Arch Clin Exp Ophthalmol 1993;231:433–438.
9. Iwach AG, Hoskins HD, Hetherington J, Shaffer RN: Analysis of surgical and medical management of glaucoma in Sturge-Weber syndrome. Ophthalmology 1990;97:904–909.
10. Sujansky E, Conradi S: Sturge-Weber syndrome: Age of onset of seizures and glaucoma and the prognosis of affected children. J Child Neurology 1995;10:49–58.
11. Lindenauer SM: The Klippel-Trenaunay syndrome: Varicosity, hypertrophy and hemangioma with no arteriovenous fistula. Ann Surg 1965;162:303–314.
12. Krupin T, Feitl ME, Karalekas D: Glaucoma associated with uveitis. *In* Ritch R, Shields MB, Krupin T (eds): The Glaucomas, 2nd ed, vol 2. St. Louis, Mosby–Year Book, 1996, p 1243.
13. Hoskins HD, Kass MA: Angle closure glaucoma without pupillary block. *In* Hoskins HD, Kass MA: Becker-Shaffer's Diagnosis and Therapy of the Glaucomas, 6th ed. St. Louis, CV Mosby, 1989, p 238.
14. Byrne SF, Green RL: Axial length measurements. *In* Byrne SF, Green RL: Ultrasound of the Eye and Orbit. St. Louis, Mosby–Year Book, 1992, p 240.
15. Postel EA, Assalian A, Epstein DL: Drug-induced transient myopia and angle-closure glaucoma associated with supraciliary choroidal effusion. Am J Ophthalmol 1996;122:110–112.
16. Fan JT, Johnson DH, Burk RR: Transient myopia, angle-closure glaucoma, and choroidal detachment after oral acetazolamide. Am J Ophthalmol 1993;115:813–814.
17. Nash RW, Lindquist TD: Bilateral angle-closure glaucoma associated with uveal effusion: Presenting sign of HIV infection. Surv Ophthalmol 1992;36:255–258.
18. Shields CL, Shields JA, Shields MB, Augsburger JJ: Prevalence and mechanisms of secondary intraocular pressure elevation in eyes with intraocular tumors. Ophthalmology 1987;94:839–846.
19. Han DP, Lewis H, Lambrou FH, et al: Mechanisms of intraocular pressure elevation after pars plana vitrectomy. Ophthalmology 1989; 96:1357–1362.
20. Desai UR, Alhalel AA, Schiffman RM, et al: Intraocular pressure elevation after simple pars plana vitrectomy. Ophthalmol 1997;104: 81–786.
21. Machemer R: The importance of fluid absorption, traction, intraocular currents, and chorioretinal scars in the therapy of rhegmatogenous retinal detachments. Am J Ophthalmol 1984;98:681–693.
22. de Juan E, McCuen B, Tiedeman J: Intraocular tamponade and surface tension. Surv Ophthalmol 1985;30:47–51.
23. Petersen J: The physical and surgical aspects of silicone oil in the vitreous cavity. Graefes Arch Clin Exp Ophthalmol 1987;225:452–456.
24. Moses R A: Schiøtz tonometry with an air bubble in the eye. Am J Ophthalmol 1966;62:281–282.
25. Lim JI, Blair NP, Higginbotham EJ, et al: Assessment of intraocular pressure in vitrectomized gas-containing eyes. Arch Ophthalmol 1990; 108:684–688.
26. Badrinath SS, Vasudevan R, Murugesan R, et al: Intraoperative measurement of intraocular pressure in vitrectomized aphakic air-filled eyes using the Tono-Pen XL. Retina 1993;13:307–311.
27. Hines MW, Jost BF, Fogelman KL: Oculab Tono-Pen, Goldmann applanation tonometry, and pneumatic tonometry for intraocular pressure assessment in gas-filled eyes. Am J Ophthalmol 1988;106:174–179.
28. Alfaro DV, Tran VT: A clinical comparison of the Oculab Tono-Pen with the Goldmann applanation tonometer in eyes filled with silicone oil. Retina 1991;11:219–220.
29. Gardner TW, Quillen DA, Blankenship GW, Marshall WK: Intraocular pressure fluctuations during scleral buckling surgery. Ophthalmology 1993;100:1050–1054.
30. Pavlin CJ, Rutnin SS, Devenyi R, et al: Supraciliary effusions and ciliary body thickening after scleral buckling procedures. Ophthalmology 1997;104:433–438.
31. Lakhanpal V, Schocket SS, Elman MJ, et al: Intraoperative massive suprachoroidal hemorrhage during pars plana vitrectomy. Ophthalmology 1990;97:1114–1119.
32. Piper JG, Abrams GW, Mieler WF: Perioperative choroidal hemorrhage at pars plana vitrectomy: A case-control study. Ophthalmology 1994;100:699–704.
33. Doft BH, Blankenship GW: Single versus multiple treatment sessions of argon laser panretinal photocoagulation for proliferative diabetic retinopathy. Ophthalmology 1982;89:772–779.

34. Ando F: Intraocular hypertension resulting from pupillary block by silicone oil. Am J Ophthalmol 1985;99:87–88.
35. Hanscom TA, Diddie KR: Mountain travel and intraocular gas bubbles. Am J Ophthalmol 1987;104:546.
36. Dieckert JP, O'Connor PS, Schacklett DE, et al: Air travel and intraocular gas. Ophthalmol 1986;93:642–645.
37. Wolf GL, Capuano C, Hartung J: Nitrous oxide increases intraocular pressure after intravitreal hexafluoride injection. Anesthesiology 1983;59:547–548.
38. Heidenkummer HP, Kampik A, Thierfelder S: Emulsification of silicone oils with specific physicochemical characteristics. Graefes Arch Clin Exp Ophthalmol 1991;229:88–94.
39. Valone J, McCarthy M: Emulsified anterior chamber silicone oil and glaucoma. Ophthalmology 1994;101:1908–1912.
40. Nguyen QH, Lloyd MA, Heuer DK, et al: Incidence and management of glaucoma after intravitreal silicone oil injection for complicated retinal detachments. Ophthalmology 1992;99:1520–1526.
41. Barr CC, Lai MY, Lean JS, et al: Postoperative intraocular pressure abnormalities in the Silicone Oil Study: Silicone Study Report 4. Ophthalmology 1993;100:1629–1635.

SECTION IV

KEY THERAPEUTIC SIGNS

CHAPTER 17

Medical Considerations in the Management of Glaucoma

HOWARD S. BARNEBEY
and KATHY YANG-WILLIAMS

There is always a temptation to only consider the ocular manifestations of eye disease. In almost no disease must this be avoided more than in glaucoma. In this chapter Howard Barnebey and Kathy Yang-Williams take on a very complex but equally important task. They admirably review all of the key body systems, specifically addressing the three primary areas of interest: (1) the impact of specific systemic diseases and their treatment on glaucoma, (2) potential drug-drug interactions between medications used to treat systemic disorders and those used in glaucoma treatment, and (3) the systemic implications of glaucoma therapy. This chapter emphatically makes the point that the entire patient must be considered in the care of glaucoma and provides the necessary tools to accomplish this responsibility.

As physicians, we must be aware of the overall medical health of our patients with glaucoma in order to identify any conditions that may be affected by our treatment of the glaucoma. In addition, it is increasingly apparent that systemic factors can influence the potential for glaucoma to damage the eye. If side effects of therapy or possible systemic factors that exacerbate the disease are identified, they should be promptly addressed. This information needs to be communicated to the primary care physician as well as the patient to facilitate proper intervention. Open communication between the ophthalmologist, the patient, and all other physicians treating the patient is critical in optimizing the integration of eye care into the overall medical care of the patient. This dialogue is particularly important in patients with glaucoma, who often are elderly and have multiple medical problems for which they may seek the services of various medical specialists. It is incumbent upon all health care practitioners who are treating patients with glaucoma to be aware of the potential effect of the patient's medical status on the disease itself.

Since the realization that, despite initial claims to the contrary, topical β-blockers can provoke asthma[1] or contribute to complete heart block and even death, ophthalmologists have recognized the importance of identifying potential and actual systemic adverse effects of ophthalmic preparations. Optimizing the therapy of patients with glaucoma continues to challenge the best of physicians to identify potential contraindications to glaucoma medications prior to their introduction, as well as to provide constant surveillance for the development of medication-related side effects. This challenge is made more difficult because many patients do not regard eye drops as medications that have the potential for systemic effects as well as the numerous potential drug-drug interactions with systemic medications.

Tables 17–1 and 17–2 summarize the most important drug-drug interactions and adverse side effects related to glaucoma therapy.

Review of Systems

This chapter reviews the potential complications that can develop when patients with glaucoma who have specific

TABLE 17–1. POTENTIAL DRUG-DRUG INTERACTIONS FOR GLAUCOMA MEDICATIONS

Precipitant Drug: *"If I prescribe this medication . . ."*	**Object Drug:** *". . . for a patient taking this medication . . ."*	**Action:** *". . . then I should counsel my patient about . . ."*
β-Blocker (e.g., levobunolol, betaxolol, timolol, carteolol, metipranolol)	Oral β-blocker	Potential for additive systemic β-blockade,* exacerbation of Raynaud's syndrome
	Calcium channel blocker (e.g., verapamil)	Risk for bradycardia and asystole
	ACE inhibitors	Systemic hypotension
	Diuretics	Systemic hypotension
	Oral hypoglycemic	
	Insulin	
	Quinidine	Risk for sinus bradycardia
	Digoxin	Risk for cardiac arrest, bradycardia
	α-Adrenergic agonist	
	Levothyroxine	
	H_2-blocking agents	
	Phenobarbital	
	Phenothiazines	
	Xanthine derivative bronchodilators (e.g., theophylline, aminophylline)	Decreased activity of theophylline; can cause bronchospasm
	NSAID	Potential for reduced effect of β-blocker eye drops
α_2-Agonist (e.g., apraclonidine 0.5%, brimonidine 0.2%)	MAO inhibitor therapy	Exaggerated adrenergic response: tachycardia, cardiac arrhythmias, hypertension, tremor, sweating, fainting, pallor, collapse
	CNS depressants	Additive CNS depression
	Tricyclic antidepressants	Decreased effect of brimonidine
	Cardiac medications with potential to decrease pulse (e.g., β-blockers, antihypertensives, cardiac glycosides)	Risk for bradycardia and systemic hypotension
Nonselective adrenergic agonist (e.g., epinephrine 0.1–1%)	MAO inhibitor therapy	Exaggerated adrenergic response†
	Tricyclic antidepressant	As above†
	α_1-Antagonists	As above†
	Dopaminergic agents (e.g., methyldopa)	As above†
	Anticholinergic agents (e.g., scopolamine, atropine)	As above†
	Bretylium	As above†
	Cardiac glycosides	As above†
	Levothyroxine	As above†
	Antihistamines (e.g., chlorpheniramine)	As above†
	Sympathomimetics (e.g., isoproterenol)	As above†
Carbonic anhydrase inhibitor (e.g., methazolamide, acetazolamide, brinzolamide 1%, dorzolamide 2%)	NSAID	
	ASA	
	Cyclosporine	
	Digitalis	Toxic effects of digoxin
	Lithium	
	Quinidine	
	Diuretics	Hypokalemia
Prostaglandin analogue (e.g., latanoprost 0.005%)		
Miotic		
Direct-acting (e.g., carbachol, pilocarpine)	Topical NSAID	Decreased effect of miotic agent
Cholinesterase inhibitor (e.g., physostigmine, demecarium bromide, echothiophate)	Organophosphate insecticides and pesticides	
	Succinylcholine	
	Systemic anticholinesterase	

ACE, angiotensin-converting enzyme; ASA, acetylsalicylic acid; CNS, central nervous system; H_2, histamine$_2$; MAO, monoamine oxidase; NSAID, nonsteroidal anti-inflammatory drug.

*Features of systemic β-blockade include potential for systemic hypotension, bradycardia, heart block, depression, sexual dysfunction, and bronchospasm.

†Features of exaggerated adrenergic response include tachycardia, cardiac arrhythmias, hypertension, tremor, sweating, fainting, pallor, and collapse.

TABLE 17–2. POTENTIAL ADVERSE EFFECTS OF GLAUCOMA MEDICATIONS

Precipitant Drug: *"If I prescribe this medication . . ."*	**Medical Condition:** *". . . for a patient with this condition . . ."*	**Action:** *". . . then I should counsel my patient about . . ."*
β-Blocker	Asthma	Bronchospasm, (rarely) death
	Diabetes	Masked symptoms of hypoglycemia
	Depression	
	Bradycardia	
	Alopecia	
	Hyperthyroidism	Masked symptoms of thyrotoxicosis
	Heart block	
	Cardiac failure	Cardiac failure, (rarely) death
	Cerebrovascular insufficiency	↓ cerebral blood flow
	Impotence	↑ sexual dysfunction
	Myasthenia gravis	↑ muscle weakness
α_1-Agonist	Insulin-dependent diabetes	Hyperglycemia
	Depression	↑ depression
	Fatigue	↑ fatigue
	Bradycardia	
Adrenergic agonist	Hypertension	↑ blood pressure
	Diabetes	
	Hyperthyroidism	Exaggerated pressor response
	Heart disease	Heart block or heart failure
	Cerebral arteriosclerosis	↓ blood flow
	Asthma	Bronchospasm
	Headache	
	Arrhythmias	Palpitations, cardiac arrhythmias
Carbonic anhydrase inhibitors	Arthritis	Risk for interaction between CAI and NSAID or ASA
	Diarrhea	
	Urolithiasis	
	Sickle cell anemia	
	Sulfonamide allergy	Risk of Stevens-Johnson syndrome, toxic epidermal necrolysis
Prostaglandin analogue	Muscle pain	
	URI	
Direct-acting miotic (e.g., pilocarpine, carbachol)	Peptic ulcer	GI cramping
	Bronchial asthma	Bronchoconstriction
	Hyperthyroidism	
	Parkinson's disease	
	Headache	↑ headaches
	Diarrhea	
	Increased bladder tone	Urge to urinate
Cholinesterase inhibitors (e.g., echothiophate, demecarium bromide, physostigmine)	Myasthenias gravis	↑ symptoms of myasthenia gravis
	Bronchial asthma	Bronchoconstriction
	GI cramping	
	Parkinson's disease	
	Headache	
	Diarrhea	

ASA, acetylsalicylic acid; CAI, carbonic anhydrase inhibitor; GI, gastrointestinal; NSAID, nonsteroidal anti-inflammatory drug; URI, upper respiratory infection; ↑, increase in; ↓, decrease in.

organ- or disease-related health problems are treated for glaucoma. Possible drug contraindications, drug-drug interactions, and the effect of systemic diseases and their treatment on glaucoma are discussed where appropriate. Suggestions for alternative therapies or interventions are also offered.

EARS, NOSE, AND THROAT

Nasolacrimal flow is the primary means by which systemic absorption of topical medications occurs. Systemic absorption of these drugs can be markedly diminished by nasolacrimal occlusion or eyelid closure immediately after administration. These maneuvers have been shown to reduce systemic levels of timolol by more than 50%.[2] It is excellent practice to teach these techniques to all patients using topical ophthalmic medications and to reinforce their use on subsequent visits. An additional benefit of reducing nasolacrimal flow is increased absorption of the medication, presumably due to higher concentration and longer residence on the ocular surface, resulting in a longer duration of effect and reduced frequency of instillation of high-dose pilocarpine.[2]

Patients who are treated with any of the various classes

of topical glaucoma medications may complain of chronic postnasal drip or, alternatively, may have dryness of the nasal and oral mucosal membranes. Drainage of excess medication through the nasolacrimal system into the nasal passage has a direct effect on the nasal mucosa, including irritation and the development of typical symptoms. The vehicle and preservatives contained in the topical drop have been implicated as being potentially responsible for these effects. To confirm causality, the suspected irritant can be temporarily discontinued, possibly in a one-eyed therapeutic trial, and then reintroduced if the symptoms resolve or do not appear to be drop related.

Postnasal Drip

The symptoms of postnasal drip are often treated with medications. Many commercial preparations are available for this purpose, both by prescription and over the counter. Patients should be counseled as to the potential of such preparations for interaction or adverse effects. Most commonly, decongestants or antihistamines are used to alleviate the symptoms. In patients with occludable angles or plateau iris configuration, these medications have the potential to induce acute angle closure. Arylalkylamine decongestants, such as pseudoephedrine and phenylpropanolamine, and imidazoline decongestants, such as oxymetazoline and naphazoline, reduce nasal or sinus congestion by stimulating α-adrenergic receptors. As a side effect of adrenergic stimulation, the pupillary dilator activation results in mydriasis.

The effect is more pronounced with the use of combination products that also contain antihistamines. These compounds are H_1-histamine receptor blocking agents that relieve nasal congestion by decreasing mucus production as well as relaxing bronchial smooth muscle. Antihistamines can have anticholinergic effects, including mydriasis, through relaxation of the pupillary sphincter. Examples of antihistamines commonly used in combinations that contain decongestants are diphenhydramine (Benadryl), clemastine (Tavist), chlorpheniramine (Chlor-Trimeton), and brompheniramine (Dimetapp).

In a susceptible patient, an over-the-counter nasal decongestant, with or without antihistamine, may have substantial anticholinergic effects that can precipitate angle closure. Potash and Ritch[3] have described a case in which angle closure occurred in a 79-year-old woman after the use of a preparation containing chlorpheniramine maleate 4 mg and pseudoephedrine sulfate 60 mg (Chlor-Trimeton). Potentially serious interactions are also a risk if these medications are administered with a topical glaucoma medication, such as epinephrine or dipivefrin. The exaggerated pressor response that may result is discussed in detail in the cardiovascular section of this chapter.

Rhinitis

Other otorhinolaryngologic conditions may require the administration of similar medications to relieve nasal or sinus congestion. Patients with allergic rhinitis or vasomotor rhinitis may benefit from the use of oral decongestants to relieve the vasodilation and engorgement of the nasal mucosa vasculature or antihistamines to relieve rhinorrhea. Other conditions in which these medications would be indicated are acute otitis media, serous otitis media, and acute sinusitis. Antihistamines indicated for these problems, such as cyproheptadine (Periactin), hydroxyzine (Vistaril, Atarax), and tripelennamine (PBZ), possess anticholinergic properties that may cause pupillary dilation. The second-generation antihistamine agents, such as cetirizine, loratadine, astemizole, and terfenadine, have fewer anticholinergic effects. Sedation and dryness of the mucous membranes and respiratory pathway are less common with these medications.

Inner Ear Disorders

Medical treatment of inner ear conditions is also an important systemic consideration in the management of glaucoma. Specifically, medications used to alleviate symptoms related to vertigo can also precipitate angle closure in patients with anatomically narrow angles. Symptomatic relief from nausea can be obtained by the use of an anticholinergic agent, such as atropine or scopolamine. Antihistamine agents have also been shown to alleviate symptoms of vertigo, presumably through their anticholinergic effects. It has been reported that a combination of meclizine and scopolamine had additive effects.[4] Precipitation of an attack of acute angle closure is of concern.

Although the likelihood of acute angle closure secondary to the anticholinergic properties of α-agonist decongestants or H_1-histamine antagonists is low, the sequelae of such an event are serious. Therefore, it is important to evaluate the potential risk for each patient on the basis of gonioscopic observation, the need for treatment, the anticipated risk of angle closure, the patient's access to ophthalmologic care, and the implications for the patient's vision and life if an attack occurs. Given the long experience with laser peripheral iridotomy, the belief that the risk of an attack is excessive should prompt the performance of an iridotomy to minimize the risk.

Dry Mouth

Less serious but more frequent are patient complaints of dryness of mucous membranes related to the administration of histamine-blocking agents or α-agonist decongestants. These symptoms can be exacerbated by the concurrent administration of glaucoma medications, particularly β-adrenergic blocking agents and α-adrenergic agonists. In patients with dry eye as well, the loss of epithelial integrity increases both the absorption of topical medications and the risk of potential side effects. Tear substitutes, when appropriate, can be used to improve the symptoms of dry eye. Occasionally, drug therapy must be revised because of the severity of the symptoms. However, in all likelihood, the otorhinolaryngologic complaint will be relieved by a short course of therapy which will be discontinued once the acute symptoms have been resolved.

Dry mouth is also a frequently reported side effect of α_2-agonist therapy. It has been reported that approximately 30% of patients treated with brimonidine 0.2% twice daily experience symptoms of dry mouth.[5] Rarely, if ever, is it severe enough to necessitate discontinuation of the treatment. The symptoms can often be reduced with the use of nasolacrimal occlusion or eyelid closure, and they usually improve with time.

Summary

The considerations for management of otorhinolaryngologic conditions in patients with glaucoma are primarily related to the potential of systemic medications to induce angle closure in susceptible patients. Glaucoma medications can cause mild to moderate irritation of the mucousal membranes, but these effects are not vision threatening. Interactions between glaucoma medications and medications used to treat conditions of the ear, nose, and throat are less common now with the availability of newer glaucoma medications. Less serious effects include exacerbation of dryness of mucosal membranes, including the ocular surface, and the nasal and pharyngeal passages.

PULMONARY SYSTEM

Systemic considerations in the treatment of glaucoma include the potential for adverse pulmonary side effects related to topical and oral glaucoma medications and the potential for these medications to interact with other medications used to treat respiratory dysfunction. Furthermore, medications used to treat pulmonary disease can have adverse ocular effects, principally through pupillary mydriasis, with an increased risk of acute angle closure, and secondarily through open-angle mechanisms, as a result of a steroid response to oral or inhaled corticosteroids.

Pulmonary Side Effects of Glaucoma Medications

Of glaucoma medications prescribed, the topical nonselective β-adrenergic blocking agents have been the group of compounds most commonly associated with adverse pulmonary effects. In the lungs, stimulation of β_2-adrenergic receptors causes relaxation of the bronchiole smooth muscle tissue as well as reduction of mucus secretion. When these receptors are blocked, bronchospasm can occur. The β-blocking agents are not the only glaucoma medications implicated in respiratory side effects however. The stimulation of pulmonary parasympathetic innervation by cholinergic agents can be responsible for bronchospasm and increased bronchiole secretions. Further, blood-gas exchange can be affected by the pH of blood as well as the partial pressures of oxygen and carbon dioxide. Therefore, carbonic anhydrase inhibitors, particularly when orally administered, can have serious effects on respiratory function.

The highest-risk category of topical medications remains the nonselective β-blocking agents. Bronchospasm, airway obstruction, and interstitial lung disease have been directly attributed to the use of these topical medications.[6–15] These compounds have also been associated with fatal bronchospasm in susceptible patients and should be used with caution. Case reports have documented adverse reactions in patients with and without a prior history of asthma.

Patients susceptible to respiratory side effects of nonselective β-blockers may complain of wheezing, shortness of breath, coughing, or dyspnea. Everitt and Avorn[6] studied the medication history of patients receiving various topical glaucoma therapies.[6] These investigators found that elderly patients who had a history of a respiratory condition requiring either xanthine bronchodilators (e.g., theophylline) or inhaled corticosteroids and who received timolol maleate for glaucoma therapy were more likely to require an additional bronchodilator (e.g., sympathomimetic) than those patients without a history of bronchospasm.

Studies suggest that the β_1-selective blocking agent betaxolol may be safer for patients with respiratory conditions, although acute bronchospasm has been reported with this agent.[16, 17] In an earlier study involving patients with moderate chronic obstructive pulmonary disease (COPD) Schoene and associates[18] showed betaxolol 1% to behave no differently from a placebo as measured by spirometric measurements. In contrast, timolol 0.5% was found to reduce forced expiratory volume in 1 second (FEV_1) as well as the ratio of FEV_1 to vital capacity. These investigators suggested that timolol could have serious side effects for patients with a pre-existing lung condition. Weinreb and colleagues[16] prescribed betaxolol for patients with glaucoma who had a history of pulmonary dysfunction and evaluated the propensity of betaxolol to cause difficulties in breathing.[16] These patients had a previous diagnosis of COPD or asthma or had experienced bronchospasm with the use of timolol. Most of the patients suffered no ill effect from the use of betaxolol, and very few experienced symptoms of bronchospasm. Clinicians should weigh carefully the benefits of betaxolol against the possibility of adverse pulmonary reaction in susceptible patients.

Although topical β-blocking agents are most commonly associated with symptoms of bronchospasm or airway obstruction, it should be noted that other medications have this potential as well. In patients with severe COPD, oral carbonic anhydrase inhibitors can disrupt normal carbon dioxide transport and the acid-base balance. In addition to metabolic acidosis, these medications can precipitate respiratory acidosis or acute respiratory failure in susceptible patients with compromised alveolar surface area. Carbonic anhydrase inhibitors can increase peripheral concentrations of carbon dioxide as well as reduce the concentration of carobon dioxide in expired air. The risk of acute respiratory failure due to oral carbonic anhydrase inhibitors is lower for methazolamide than acetazolamide because metabolic acidosis is more severe, when it occurs, in patients treated with acetazolamide.[19] Therefore, methazolamide may be better tolerated in patients with significant pulmonary dysfunction.

Stimulation of muscarinic receptors in the pulmonary innervation reduces bronchiole secretions and stimulates bronchiole smooth muscles. In an animal model, bronchospasm occurred because of a decrease in pulmonary surfactant associated with high levels of pilocarpine.[20] The likelihood that this adverse effect would occur as a result of glaucoma therapy is low.

Careful consideration of medications is appropriate in the management of glaucoma for patients with a history of bronchial asthma. Topical medications to be considered include selective α-agonists, prostaglandin analogues, and topical carbonic anhydrase inhibitors. Patients who receive topical treatment with carbonic anhydrase inhibitors generally experience fewer serious side effects than patients who receive oral treatment.[21–24] Therefore, treatment with this route of administration would be less likely to induce metabolic acidosis in patients with serious respiratory dysfunction. The use of latanoprost was found to be safe in patients with asthma who were under treatment with steriod inhalers. Latanoprost did not decrease respiratory function in this patient population and may prove a safer alternative to topical β-blocker therapy.[25]

Glaucoma Medications and Respiratory Treatments

Patients with restrictive airway disease are also at risk for drug-drug interactions between topical β-blockers and the medications used to treat their pulmonary disease. Such patients generally should not be given topical nonselective β-blockers. Patients treated with theophylline therapy for their asthma are at higher risk for increased blood levels of theophylline when they are given nonselective β-blocking agents as glaucoma therapy. Another potential medication reaction is increased β-blockade, which could occur if a topical nonselective β-blocking agent is used in a patient taking systemic β-blockers. Although oral β-blockers are inappropriate for patients with a history of pulmonary dysfunction, the additional β-blockade from the topical agent could result in worsening respiratory function in patients who do not manifest pulmonary disease with oral therapy alone.

Reactive airway constriction can be managed by a number of modalities, including, but not limited to, (1) bronchodilating agents, (2) corticosteroids, (3) mast cell stabilizers, (4) decongestants, and (5) leukotriene receptor antagonists. Bronchospasm can be relieved by stimulating β_2-adrenergic receptors or antagonizing muscarinic receptors. Therefore, there exists a potential for acute angle closure to occur in response to inhaled medications via stimulation of the pupillary dilator or relaxation of the pupillary sphincter. Ipratropium bromide and salbutamol were reported to cause angle closure in a case report series of five patients.[26] Ipratropium bromide is an anticholinergic agent available in inhaled or nasal spray form as Atrovent. Salbutamol (albuterol, Proventil, Ventolin) is a sympathomimetic agent related to a number of other β_2-selective agonist compounds, including metaproterenol, terbutaline, and isoproterenol. Although inhaled antiasthmatic agents are believed to be site-specific, certain patients with occludable angles may need to be counseled about the risk of angle closure with use of such agents.

Current therapy for bronchial asthma may involve inhaled, nasal, or oral corticosteroids. Inflammation related to bronchial asthma can be treated with inhaled or nasal corticosteroids and, in more severe cases, by oral corticosteroid medications. The adverse side effects of corticosteroid administration include the risk of ocular hypertension and steroid-induced glaucoma. Side effects related to the various inhaled corticosteroids have been found to be dose-dependent and to occur at a lower rate than those related to oral corticosteroids.[27] Even so, physicians have been alerted to the very real risk of steroid-induced glaucoma as a response to inhaled and nasal corticosteroids. These investigators determined that patients treated with high-dose inhaled corticosteroids for 3 or more months were at greater risk for increased intraocular pressure or glaucoma compared with a normal population.[28]

Summary

Pulmonary side effects from glaucoma medications can occur and are more common in patients with a history of reactive airway disease who are treated with nonselective β-blocking agents. These medications can have serious and, rarely, fatal complications that can be easily avoided by screening of patients for whom the medications may pose a risk. A careful history and review of systems further reduces the risk of adverse complications secondary to the treatment of respiratory conditions. Clinicians should counsel their patients about the risks for (1) angle closure with use of certain bronchodilators and (2) elevated intraocular pressure (IOP) with long-term use of corticosteroids.

CARDIOVASCULAR SYSTEM

The importance of considering the effects of glaucoma therapy on the heart and circulatory system cannot be overemphasized. A number of cardiovascular disorders should be considered in the treatment of glaucoma. These conditions may preclude certain types of treatment; they may be treated with medications with a potential for serious interaction with glaucoma medications; or the optimization of their treatment may have a positive impact on the glaucoma.

Systemic Blood Pressure

Cardiac function is an important consideration in glaucoma treatment. The effect of blood pressure has long been debated, with conflicting reports about its importance in progression of visual field and optic nerve head changes. Some studies have documented a positive association between open-angle glaucoma and blood pressure,[29–32] whereas other investigations have found no significant relationship.[33, 34] Reports have also examined the effect of systemic hypotension on the progression of glaucoma as well as the impact of diurnal variation in blood pressure.[35, 36]

Tielsch and associates[29] performed The Baltimore Eye Survey, a population-based survey in patients 40 years of age and older. They reported a small but significant relationship between systolic and diastolic blood pressures and IOP. They reported that patients with systolic blood pressure greater than 130 mm Hg had a higher risk for open-angle glaucoma than patients with lower systolic levels. This relationship was even more significant for older patients. Dielemans and colleagues[32] found similar outcomes in the Rotterdam Study, reporting that systolic and diastolic blood pressures could be positively associated with elevated IOP and glaucoma. Wilson and coworkers[30] observed that elevated systolic blood pressure (>160 mm Hg) was more common in patients with open-angle glaucoma than in control subjects. It was also more common, although to a lesser degree, in patients in whom glaucoma was suspected. This study supported earlier findings by Leighton and Phillips,[31] who determined that both systolic and diastolic blood pressures were higher in patients with open-angle glaucoma than in normal patients or patients with normal-tension glaucoma (NTG).

Other studies, however, have found no particular relationship between IOP or the prevalence of glaucoma and blood pressure measurements. Leske[34] did not observe any difference between systolic blood pressure measurements in patients with manifest glaucoma and control subjects. Kahn and associates[33] reported similar findings as part of the Framingham Eye Study. Interestingly, a positive relationship was found relating ocular hypertension (IOP >20 mm Hg) and systolic blood pressure, but no such association was found for open-angle glaucoma. The investigators admit that the small number of patients with open-angle glaucoma in the study may have affected the ability to detect a significant relationship.[33]

Other aspects of circulatory function that may be of significance relating to blood pressure include a possible relationship between systemic hypotension and glaucoma and progression of visual field defects in patients who undergo a substantial decrease in systolic blood pressure during sleep—the "nocturnal dip" (see later in this chapter). Drance and colleagues[37] evaluated possible risk factors associated with NTG. They determined that patients with NTG had significantly lower systolic and diastolic blood pressures than their counterparts with ocular hypertension. This finding suggested that ocular perfusion had some role in the development of NTG, supporting a vascular theory for glaucomatous optic neuropathy. The data presented by Chumbley and Brubaker[38] in 1976 focused more closely on the small number of patients with NTG and with elevated diastolic pressures who demonstrated progressive visual field changes. Interestingly, further examination shows that twice as many patients with NTG (n = 8) with a diastolic blood pressure less than 100 mm Hg had progressive visual field defects as those with higher diastolic pressures (n = 4).[38] This finding was corroborated by the work of Richler and colleagues,[39] who determined that low diastolic blood pressure was more commonly associated with progressive visual field defects in a group that included both patients with primary open-angle glaucoma and patients with NTG. However, the Rotterdam study found no such relationship between systemic blood pressure and NTG.[32]

The Baltimore Eye Survey took a different approach, evaluating diastolic perfusion pressure in a group of patients with open-angle glaucoma.[29] The diastolic perfusion pressure was calculated as the difference between diastolic blood pressure and IOP. The investigators observed that a diastolic perfusion pressure of less than 50 mm Hg was significantly associated with open-angle glaucoma. Their data suggest that a relative decrease in blood flow to the optic nerve may be associated with greater vulnerability to the effects of IOP.

This possibility was also suspected by a number of other investigators who evaluated the impact of systemic hypotension and diurnal variation in blood pressure as factors related to primary open-angle glaucoma and NTG. Kaiser and associates[40] monitored blood pressure for 24 hours in a group of patients with poorly controlled open-angle glaucoma or NTG. The data demonstrated a significantly lower systolic blood pressure and slightly lower diastolic blood pressure in patient groups, including those with open-angle glaucoma and progressive nerve damage in whom IOP was well controlled, and those with NTG. The investigators suggested that in some patients, overly aggressive treatment of systemic hypertension should be avoided and that patients should be aware that hypotension might be associated with risk for optic nerve damage.

As previously mentioned, significant decrease in nocturnal blood pressure has been termed the "nocturnal dip." Patients have been further classified as those with a substantial change in blood pressure during sleep ("dippers"), and those without this reduction ("non-dippers"). This categorization used the criterion of a 10% decrease in both systolic and diastolic levels from day-time measurements.[41] Graham and colleagues[41] measured the ambulatory blood pressures in a group of patients with primary open-angle glaucoma or NTG and control patients over a 24-hour period. There was no significant difference in the overall blood pressure measurements between patients with NTG and primary open-angle glaucoma. Patients in these two groups who had progressive visual field loss, however, were found to experience a larger nocturnal dip. The researchers surmised that susceptibility to decreased perfusion pressure might be more important in patients with glaucoma and compromised autoregulation who were not able to compensate adequately for large changes in systemic blood pressure.

Other investigators have correlated episodes of nocturnal hypotension ("nocturnal dip") with visual field loss and focal ischemic glaucoma.[42] Collignon and associates[43] found similar results with "dippers" more commonly demonstrating progression than "non-dippers" among patients with primary open-angle glaucoma and NTG, although visual field progression was observed to occur in a significant number of patients in both groups with either an absence of or increase in nocturnal dip. Others have determined that groups of patients with either primary open-angle glaucoma or focal ischemic–type NTG did not necessarily differ in the proportion of "dippers," although visual field progression was not a primary outcome measure.

Systemic hypertension in patients with nocturnal hypotension was treated with a number of medications, including calcium channel blocking agents, oral β-blocking agents, angiotensin II-converting enzyme inhibitors, and diuretics. Some of these medications prompt particular concern about their potential for interactions with topical glaucoma medications. Recognition of a specific interaction of β-blockers with methyldopa is important. An exaggerated hypertensive response with tachycardia and arrhythmia can occur as a result of unopposed α-adrenergic stimulation. Conditions such as decompensated congestive heart failure, carotid artery insufficiency, and cardiac arrhythmias can potentially affect the course of glaucoma in all patients, but perhaps particularly in those with NTG. As a result of these concerns, it is reasonable to consider recommending to patients with hypertension or their internists that it may be preferable to administer systemic antihypertensive medications in the morning rather than in the evening or night to minimize the risk of exacerbating a "nocturnal dip."

Vascular Diseases

Beyond concerns about systemic blood pressure and its variations in glaucoma management, a number of other cardiovascular conditions may ultimately affect the diagnosis or management of glaucoma. For example, in a survey of patients with primary open-angle glaucoma, systemic hypertension was also present in 48%, and coronary artery disease and arteriosclerosis in 35%.[44] Any disease that reduces blood flow to the eye and in particular to the optic nerve can further compromise a susceptible nerve.

Carotid occlusive disease should be considered in the differential diagnosis of NTG. Carotid artery auscultation should be considered for patients in whom NTG is suspected. Ophthalmodynamometry can also be performed to determine whether there is significant compromise in ocular blood flow. Appropriate imaging studies and laboratory testing should be considered for those patients in whom carotid artery insufficiency is suspected.

Peripheral circulation abnormalities have also been implicated to play a role in glaucoma. Specifically, a higher incidence of Raynaud's phenomenon has been found in patients with NTG.[45, 46] When peripheral circulation was evaluated in normal patients and patients with open-angle glaucoma or NTG,[47] the investigators found that patients with NTG responded differently to cold and warm stimuli than both normal patients and those with open-angle glaucoma. The patients with NTG had a more significant decrease in blood velocity in response to cold stimuli that took longer to recover to baseline levels than either of the other groups. Even when other systemic conditions, such as migraine, vascular disease, and smoking, were excluded from the analysis, the results were unchanged. This finding suggested that patients with NTG were more susceptible to peripheral vasospasm. Additionally, Drance and associates[48] found that patients with a diagnosis of NTG were more likely to have a history of hemodynamic crisis. The alterations in blood flow included sudden change in blood pressure related to internal hemorrhage, cardiac arrest, and hypotension during anesthesia. Less significant but documented occurrences were also detected of postural hypotension, congestive heart failure, and episodes of cardiac arrhythmias.

Because perfusion and blood flow to the optic nerve have been implicated in the progressive nature of some cases of glaucoma, cerebrovascular studies have been undertaken to determine whether circulation was a factor in progression of glaucoma. An early study by Feldman and colleagues[49] evaluating patients with open-angle glaucoma by radiographic and neurologic testing, found that a large proportion of patients had a history of vascular disease, such as carotid, vertebrobasilar, or small vessel disorders, or of a hemodynamic crisis.

Later investigations have used magnetic resonance imaging (MRI) to evaluate patients with NTG. Ong and associates[50] determined that a small group of patients with NTG had a higher incidence of cerebral infarcts and atrophy of the corpus callosum. The cross-sectional area of the corpus callosum was inferred to reflect the number of nerve fibers present (similar to comparisons between neuroretinal rim area and optic nerve fiber layer density). These researchers suggest that neuronal degeneration may play a role in NTG and may manifest as a more rapid loss of neural tissue or, alternatively, may be related to a smaller number of nerve fibers at birth.

Other considerations in this area are the potential effects of systemic conditions primarily with ocular manifestations that could affect cardiovascular status. For example, pseudoexfoliation syndrome is predominantly observed in the eye as characteristic deposits along the pupillary ruff and anterior lens capsule. Electron miscroscopy study of tissues from patients with pseudoexfoliation demonstrates, however, that this condition may be more widespread than previously thought.[51, 52] Evidence of elastin and abnormal protein aggregates was found in many extraocular tissues, including the heart. The functional impact of this deposition has not been studied.

Aside from the causative effects of vascular disease on the pathophysiology of glaucoma, there is a significant comorbidity. As previously mentioned, patients treated for primary open-angle glaucoma (POAG) are likely to also have systemic hypertension (48%) and coronary artery disease (35%).[44] It is therefore quite likely and understandable that these patients are under treatment with calcium channel blockers, angiotensin II converting enzyme inhibitors, diuretics, and β-blockers. In fact, the Timolol Treatment Trial and Scandinavian Timolol Studies have demonstrated significant decrease in post–myocardial infarction mortality. On the basis of these clinical studies, the use of systemic β-blockers has become a constituent of coronary artery disease management.[53] These agents are now also frequently used in situations for which they were previously thought to be contraindicated (e.g., congestive heart failure).

Glaucoma Treatment and Cardiovascular Disorders

Because patients with glaucoma are likely to be using systemic cardiac and vascular medications, three questions must be considered during the planning of glaucoma treatment:

1. Does the systemic cardiovascular agent enhance or diminish the efficacy and side effect profile of the topical glaucoma medication?
2. What are the effects of the glaucoma medication on individual systems? (This issue has largely been discussed previously in this chapter.)
3. Is there a potential for drug-drug interactions between the topical glaucoma medication and the systemic cardiovascular agent?

EFFECTS OF SYSTEMIC CARDIOVASCULAR MEDICATION ON THE EYES

Schuman[54] found that oral β-blockers reduced the IOP-lowering effect of topical timolol in comparison with brimonidine. It is presumed that this effect is attributable to the systemic levels of orally administered medication. However, other studies found that less than 120 mg/day of propranolol had a minimal effect on IOP.[55] Additional systemic medication effects with which the ophthalmologist should be familiar include the risk for angle closure with class IA antiarrhythmia agents. This risk is greatest with disopyramide (Norpace), which has a greater anticholinergic effect than quinidine and procainamide.

Calcium channel blockers, which are class IV agents, may prove to be one of the novel drug classes of the new millennium. Although the potential adverse interaction with β-blockers has been identified (second- or third-degree heart block), there is also evidence that this class of agents may be beneficial in the treatment of glaucoma. The benefit has been suggested to result from potential neuroprotective effects and positive effects on ocular blood flow.[56, 59] In cardiac care, calcium channel blockers are used for control of angina, arrhythmias, hypertension, and some peripheral vascular disorders (peripheral vasodilation). Verapamil has greater cardiac depressant properties than nifedipine, whereas diltiazem has greater vasodilatory effects than verapamil. Nimodipine has the greatest ability to act in the central nervous system, but its routine use is limited.

EFFECTS OF TOPICAL GLAUCOMA MEDICATIONS ON THE CARDIOVASCULAR SYSTEM

As discussed previously in this chapter, topical glaucoma medications can have substantial effects on systemic function. This potential is particularly important with respect to topical β-blockers. Absolute contraindications to their topical use include conditions such as (1) decompensated congestive heart failure, (2) cardiac arrhythmias, (3) second- or third-degree atrioventricular block,[58] and (4) sinus bradycardia with a pulse less than 50 to 55 beats per minute.[8–15] There is concern about the use of β-blockers, particularly nonselective agents, in a patient who is susceptible to nocturnal hypotension or has vasospasm, in whom the use of medications such as topical timolol may be associated with exacerbation of Raynaud's phenomenon.[60] Effects are possible even in healthy patients in association with heavy exercise (e.g., reduction of exercise-induced tachycardia) and with testing of pulmonary function. Interestingly, one study found no increase in use of furosemide or digoxin in association with the use of glaucoma medications in patients for whom furosemide or digoxin was assumed to be associated with a diagnosis of congestive heart failure.[61]

Becker and associates[62] found that topical epinephrine significantly decreased IOP in patients with primary and secondary open-angle glaucoma; however, a large proportion of these patients also experienced adverse cardiac effects, most commonly, premature ventricular contractions.[62] Palpitations, hypertensive crisis, tachycardia, and cardiac arrhythmias also have been related to the use of topical epinephrine or dipivefrin.

Consideration for the administration of a nonspecific adrenergic agonist such as epinephrine or dipivefrin also includes the presence of hypertension. Kerr and colleagues[63] evaluated the potential cardiovascular side effects of both medications in a population with glaucoma. Although both medications were associated with an increase in pulse, epinephrine was more often associated with a significant increase in systolic or mean blood pressure. One patient even experienced ventricular ectopy after the administration of epinephrine. The investigators concluded that cardiovascular side effects are more likely with epinephrine than dipivefrin, although it would be difficult to predict which patients would be susceptible to these side effects. In a single-dose study in which epinephrine, dipivefrin, or a placebo was added to timolol maleate, there was no significant change in IOP.[64] The addition of epinephrine to timolol was associated with a slight change in diastolic blood pressure, but systolic blood pressure was unchanged. Although topical epinephrine has been associated with a number of adverse cardiovascular events, these concerns have not been confirmed with the α_2-selective agents. There have been no reported effects of apraclonidine or brimonidine on blood pressure and pulse.[65, 66] Both compounds, which are clonidine derivatives, have the potential to directly affect the central nervous system (CNS), resulting in lethargy and somnolence, although this effect appears more likely with brimonidine. For this reason, brimonidine is contraindicated in children, in whom it is believed to more easily cross the blood-brain barrier, increasing the incidence of side effects.

Atrioventicular (AV) block has been reported to be caused by pilocarpine eye drops used hourly for seven doses. The third-degree AV block resolved with discontinuation of pilocarpine.[67] This complication is highly unlikely to occur with normal therapeutic dosage.

INTERACTIONS BETWEEN GLAUCOMA AND SYSTEMIC CARDIOVASCULAR MEDICATIONS

Given the wide range of agents available to treat cardiovascular disorders and glaucoma, and the numerous potential interactions between them, a complete listing of all possible drug-drug interactions is beyond the scope of this discussion. However, a few potential interactions deserve mention. A common and very important potential problem involves the concomitant use of topical β-blockers and oral calcium channel blockers or β-blockers. For example, a topical nonselective β-blocker may potentiate the activity of calcium channel antagonists on the cardiac AV node. There are case reports of severe bradycardia involving topical timolol and oral verapamil.[68, 69] This interaction could potentially result in hypotension, bradycardia, and congestive heart failure. Therefore, prior to considering a topical β-blocker to treat glaucoma, the ophthalmologist should determine whether the patient is taking oral calcium channel blockers. Conversely, in the patients in whom the use of an oral calcium channel blocker for the treatment of glaucoma is considered, the ophthalmologist should determine whether the patient is taking either a topical or oral β-blocker. Unless such a patient has systemic hypertension, treatment of glaucoma with a calcium channel blocker should be avoided.

There is increased risk for decompensation of congestive heart failure when topical and oral β-blockers are combined. Topical timolol has been found to decrease IOP even when patients were already undergoing treatment for arterial hypertension with oral β-blocking agents,[70] although the magnitude of IOP lowering may be less than in patients who are not using oral β-blocking agents.[54] The ocular hypotensive effect of timolol may be in part determined by the dosage of oral β-blocking agent prescribed. One study found that timolol eye drops had minimal effect on IOP in patients who were treated with 160 mg of propranolol compared with those treated with 80 or 120 mg of propranolol.[71] Additional interactions of concern include (1) the additive cardiac effects of the combination of digoxin and β-blockade and (2) the risk of hypotension, bradycardia, or sinus arrest with amiodarone.

The use of quinidine for supraventricular arrhythmias has the potential to lead to bradycardia with the concomitant use of timolol.[72] Quinidine inhibits the enzyme responsible for timolol metabolism.

There is risk for patients taking β-blockers and epinephrine to experience an exaggerated pressor response owing to unopposed α-adenergic activity, in the form of hypertension and bradycardia.[73] This is a potential concern for patients treated with topical β-blockers who are then treated with epinephrine or for patients who are treated with epinephrine compounds who are then prescribed topical or oral β-blockers. The likelihood for an adverse experience to occur is low but possible in patients receiving polytherapy.

One specific interaction with serious potential is the concomitant use of oral carbonic anhydrase inhibitors and digoxin, because of the risk for digitalis toxicity. Nausea and vomiting, either due to acute glaucoma or related to the use of oral carbonic anhydrase inhibitors, can lead to potassium loss, encouraging the development of arrhythmias and digoxin toxicity. It is important to check electrolyte levels in patients at risk. Additionally, bone marrow suppression has been reported in patients who are taking both angiotensin-converting enzyme inhibitors and oral carbonic anhydrase inhibitors.

Finally, there is the potential for drug-drug interaction in patients who are being treated with catecholamines or similar medications to experience hypertensive crisis. This risk includes patients treated with monoamine oxidase (MAO) inhibitors and adrenergic agonists, such as epinephrine. Similar types of reactions have been reported as interactions between over-the-counter decongestants, especially phenylpropanolamine, and MAO inhibitors.[74]

GASTROINTESTINAL AND HEPATIC CONSIDERATIONS

Gastrointestinal and hepatic considerations in the management of glaucoma are primarily related to symptoms of nausea or signs such as diarrhea and cramping due to various glaucoma medications. There also exists the potential for medications used to treat these disorders to induce an acute angle-closure attack through pupillary dilation.

In general, patients with glaucoma do not have systemic symptoms of the disease unless the pressure rapidly increases to a level that causes pain, nausea, or vomiting. Administration of the appropriate oral glaucoma medications can be difficult if the patient is severely nauseated or vomiting. In these instances, adjunctive therapy with antiemetic agents would be appropriate to reduce these symptoms. An antidopaminergic drug such as prochlorperazine (Compazine) or an antihistamine such as promethazine (Phenergan) can be administered orally or rectally every 12 hours as needed. Suppositories are the generally preferred mode of administration because episodes of vomiting would reduce the effectiveness of the oral antiemetic. Once nausea and vomiting have been adequately controlled, treatment with oral carbonic anhydrase inhibitors or oral hyperosmotic agents can be initiated.

It is important to remember that even if glaucoma does not cause symptoms of nausea or vomiting, it is possible that its treatment may do so. This occurs most commonly with oral hyperosmotic agents such as glycerol (Osmoglyn) and isosorbide (Ismotic). Other antiglaucoma medications can also give rise to gastrointestinal distress or symptoms. Oral carbonic anhydrase inhibitors can cause nausea, vomiting, diarrhea and taste perversion. Other more serious complications can arise in patients with cirrhosis of the liver because carbonic anhydrase inhibitors cause ammonia originating in the kidneys to be redirected to the liver.[75] Patients with cirrhosis have substantially reduced liver function and cannot detoxify blood in the same manner as those with normal liver function. The toxins are therefore carried to the brain, where they can cause hepatic encephalopathy. This potential for toxicity when acetazolamide is used in patients with cirrhosis of the liver was reported by Margo[76] in 1986.

Gastrointestinal complications are also possible with topical carbonic anhydrase inhibitors[77] but are less likely to occur due to decreased systemic absorption and lower plasma levels with this mode of administration. Various studies have evaluated the effectiveness of dorzolamide and found that this agent, used topically, is less likely to cause serious adverse effects than oral carbonic anhydrase inhibitors.[78]

Of the topical glaucoma medications, the most significant potential for gastrointestinal side effects is associated with miotics. Because the smooth muscle of the gastrointestinal tract is innervated by muscarinic receptors, stimulation of these receptors by cholinergic agents can cause cramping or diarrhea. This effect occurs less frequently with direct-acting cholinergic agents such as pilocarpine, unless this medication is used frequently over a short period. Kushnick and associates[79] reported a case of pilocarpine toxicity related to excessive leakage from a pilocarpine wafer insert (Ocusert).[79] Indirect-acting cholinergic agents, such as echothiophate iodide, which inhibit cholinesterase activity, more commonly cause gastrointestinal symptoms. A case report by Wood and colleagues[80] has documented the adverse effects of echothiophate iodide that appeared after bilateral dacryocystorhinostomies. These investigators surmised that the complications developed secondary to increased systemic absorption of topical medications after surgery for canalicular stenosis. Wolfhagen and coworkers[81] have reported a case of gastrointestinal disturbance associated with topical timolol. Adverse effects related to other topical antiglaucoma agents have been reported to occur in association with topical β-blocking agents as well as selective α-agonists, but these effects are infrequently observed in clinical practice.

The risk of glaucoma associated with medications used to treat gastrointestinal system complaints is a particular concern for patients with occludable angles. Medications prescribed as antispasmodics generally have anticholinergic effects, blocking the muscarinic receptors that are responsible for smooth muscle contraction. The corresponding pupillary dilation poses a problem for patients at risk for angle closure. Substances such as atropine, scopolamine, hyoscyamine, and combination products containing diphenoxylate hydrochloride and atropine (Lomotil), or atropine, scopolamine, and hyoscyamine with phenobarbital (Donnatal) could precipitate such an attack. Other similar medications also present a risk, for example, glycopyrrolate (Robinul), clidinium (Quarzan), and propantheline bromide (Pro-Banthīne). Even given by alternative routes of administration, these medications can be associated with angle closure; transdermal scopolamine (Transderm-Scōp) has been associated with narrow-angle glaucoma.[82]

This effect may also occur with medications that are used to decrease gastric acid secretion, more specifically, through a histamine H_2-blocking pathway. These compounds have been used in the treatment of gastroesophageal reflux disorder, gastric ulcer, and duodenal ulcer. Several medications from this group have now become available as over-the-counter, lower-dose forms of their parent compounds. For example, cimetidine (Tagamet HB), famotidine (Pepcid AC), and ranitidine (Zantac 75) are now available without a prescription. This fact is of additional concern for physicians, because by using such products, patients with occludable angles may unknowingly place themselves at risk for angle closure.

ENDOCRINOLOGIC CONSIDERATIONS

Diabetes

Although there is no evidence directly linking open-angle glaucoma and diabetes, open-angle glaucoma and ocular hypertension are more prevalent among patients with diabetes.[83–91] The incidence of glaucoma in patients with newly diagnosed diabetes has been reported to be in threefold higher than in patients without diabetes. Therefore, it is likely that patients with glaucoma commonly have diabetes and are taking hypoglycemic agents.

The presence of diabetes appears to have a direct effect on glaucoma. Diabetes was found to be a risk factor for progression of visual field defects in a group of patients with open-angle glaucoma or NTG.[92] In another study,[91] a group of patients with a pre-existing diagnosis of diabetes was compared with a control group of patients and examined for elevated IOP. Armstrong and colleagues[91] found that a significantly higher number of patients with diabetes had elevated IOP than patients in the control group.[83] Interestingly, it has been shown that inferior visual field defects are more common in patients with diabetes and primary open-angle glaucoma (POAG)[92]; also, there is a higher number of patients with diabetes in POAG patients with inferior visual field defects.[93] It has been assumed that the vasculopathy associated with diabetes raises the risk for glaucomatous optic nerve damage. Lastly, given the risk of diabetic retinopathy, particularly of proliferative disease, the potential for neovascular glaucoma must always be considered in patients with diabetes.

INTERACTIONS BETWEEN GLAUCOMA MEDICATIONS AND SYSTEMIC DIABETES MEDICATIONS

The most likely effect reported of an interaction between agents used to treat glaucoma and diabetes has been the finding that nonselective β-blockers could increase the effects of oral hypoglycemic agents by decreasing gluconeogenesis. One theoretical concern is that both carbonic anhydrase inhibitors and oral hypoglycemic agents have the potential to cause the side effects seen with sulfa drugs, primarily an allergic response, but severe complications, such as Stevens-Johnson syndrome, are a risk.

EFFECTS OF GLAUCOMA MEDICATIONS ON ENDOCRINOLOGIC SYSTEM

The potentially most significant drug interaction concerns β-blockers and hypoglycemia. Patients who have diabetes that is under tight insulin control may become hypoglycemic. The effects of hypoglycemia become manifest via the sympathomimetic nervous system (tachycardia, peripheral vasoconstriction, diaphoresis). These symptoms may be blocked by topical or systemic β-blockers. This issue is of theoretical concern, but practically speaking, it is usually not significant. Studies demonstrated that the level of glucose capable of producing hypoglycemic symptoms was not significantly reduced when individuals were using β-blockers.

A case report has documented the change in a patient's reaction to hypoglycemia before and after topical timolol therapy.[94] Before the use of timolol maleate, this patient experienced perspiration and uneasiness that resolved by administration of glucose. Following the use of timolol maleate, more serious adverse reactions occurred in response to hypoglycemia, including alteration in mental status and even seizures. The resolution of the hypoglycemic episode was complicated by an apparent relative resistance to glucose therapy. Patients who are predisposed to hypoglycemic episodes should be counseled about the potential for altered symptomology if their glaucoma is being treated with a β-blocker.

The action of β-blockers can reduce glucose tolerance through release of greater amounts of glucose, by an increase in glycolysis of glycogen or through altered carbohydrate metabolism. In addition, these drugs can reduce peripheral circulation.

α-Agonists have the potential to decrease the effect of insulin by blocking insulin receptors and stimulating hyperglycemia. This potential effect has not been found clinically with the use of ophthalmic α-agonists.

Finally, in diabetic patients, there is risk to using some osmotic antiglaucoma agents in the treatment of acute glaucomas, particularly neovascular glaucoma, which is relatively common in patients with diabetes. Although the agents mannitol and isosorbide are not metabolized, the oral osmotic agent glycerol is metabolized, possibly resulting in marked increases in plasma glucose levels. Nonketotic hyperosmolar coma can develop, with diuresis and dehydration. It results from an increase in blood osmolarity associated with extreme hyperglycemia. There is a case report of this complication occurring in a 29-year-old diabetic patient who was treated with oral glycerol for acutely elevated IOP secondary to neovascular glaucoma.[95] The hyperosmolar nonketotic coma responded to medical therapy.

EFFECTS OF SYSTEMIC DIABETES MEDICATIONS ON THE EYES

There is a risk for angle-closure glaucoma with sulfa-based compounds, such as oral hypoglycemic agents, as a result of lens swelling and forward movement of lens-iris diaphragm. Conversely, diabetic therapy, for example, improper use of hypoglycemic agents, can actually trigger angle-closure glaucoma through osmotic swelling of the crystalline lens resulting from changes in the plasma glucose level.

Thyroid Dysfunction

The relationship between thyroid dysfunction and glaucoma is complex and poorly understood. Thyroid dysfunction has been implicated in the development of glaucoma. Both hypothyroidism and hyperthyroidism have been associated with elevated IOP albeit through varying mechanisms.

Hypothyroidism has been associated with a number of clinical signs, including intolerance to cold, dry skin, constipation, reduced energy, lethargy, and weakness. Hypothyroidism can be caused by (1) Hashimoto's disease (autoimmune), (2) surgical or radiation treatment for Graves' disease or goiter, or (3) medications such as lithium. A case report by Smith and coworkers[96] documented a possible link between hypothyroidism and open-angle glaucoma in a patient with poorly controlled IOP. This patient exhibited signs consistent with a diagnosis of hypothyroidism, including nonpitting periorbital edema and bilateral ptosis. Abnormal thyroid function test results required initiation of thyroxine therapy. The IOP decreased over the following 3 months and was kept low through the use of timolol eye drops. In a follow-up study evaluating aqueous outflow facility in hypothyroidism, the same investigators demonstrated a significant reduction in aqueous outflow that improved with management of the hypothyroidism.[97] The investigators believed that mucopolysaccharide accumulation in the periorbital tissues could occur in the trabecular meshwork with a corresponding decrease in aqueous outflow. This finding was supported by another investigation that found a statistically higher rate of hypothyroidism in patients with primary open-angle glaucoma than in normal patients.[98] This finding was clinically significant because a number of the cases of hypothyroidism were undiagnosed at the time of the investigation. Another group of researchers suggested that hypothyroidism is not linked to open-angle glaucoma, although their study was limited by the absence of a control group.[99]

There clearly is an association between hypothyroidism and glaucoma, hypothyroidism being common among patients with POAG. This relationship differs from that in Graves' thyroid eye disease, in which enlarged extraocular muscles either compress the optic nerve, causing compressive optic neuropathy, or compromise episcleral venous outflow, increasing episcleral venous pressure (EVP). Graves' disease is an autoimmune-related thyrotoxicosis in which the presence of high levels of thyroid hormone result in typical symptoms, including heat intolerance, weight loss, irritability, sweating, and increased basal metabolic rate. Caution should be used as the eye signs of Graves' disease can manifest without hyperthyroidism. Commonly, infiltration results in enlarged extraocular muscles, restricting gaze, and a change in IOP in different positions of gaze.[100] Abnormal scleral rigidity can also cause increased IOP.

In a study by Kalmann and associates,[101] some patients with increased IOP due to Graves' disease had decreased IOP after orbital decompression, and others had decreased IOP with inferior rectus muscle recession.[101] One study showed that the elevated IOP in patients with thyroid eye disease associated with high EVP improved with decompression surgery, which reduced IOP by decreasing EVP.[102] When evaluating possible visual loss in patients with Graves' disease, the ophthalmologist must distinguish between optic nerve damage secondary to elevated IOP and damage attributable to direct compressive optic neuropathy due to enlarged muscles. The compressive optic neuropathy can result in acquired visual field defects and is associated with color desaturation.

Potential drug-drug interactions between glaucoma medications and thyroid medications are rare. Theoretically, β-blockers may mask the symptoms of tachycardia associated with hyperthyroidism. The IOP-lowering effects of sympathomimetic medications may be reduced because the eye may be sensitized to the higher levels of catecholamines.

Sex Hormones

It has been shown that in normal eyes, increased levels of estrogen or progesterone are associated with decreased IOP.[103] Testosterone has been suggested to raise IOP.[104] Cushing's syndrome has been associated with increased IOP, but this effect is lost over time.[105, 106]

It is interesting that with the importance of sex in our culture, the role of drug-induced sexual dysfunction has been de-emphasized. It is not rare for impotence to be associated with the use of β-blockers.[107] It is sometimes uncomfortable to ask patients about decreased sex drive, impotence, and reduced libido, this issue is important to investigate with a patient being treated with β-blockers. Certainly, the use of newer drugs, such as Viagra, should clue the clinician into the potential for this interaction.

Medications used for sexual dysfunction may have ocular side effects. Viagra is one of the newer medications that act on the nitric oxide pathway to increase penile blood flow. Similar effects may simultaneously be occurring in the eye, compromising blood flow to the optic nerve. These potential effects remain theoretical at this time.

Hypercholesterolemia

Patients with hypercholesterolemia and an abnormal plasma lipid profile must first be examined as to their increased risk for carotid artery occlusive disease and fragmenting plaque formation that could result in central retinal artery occlusion or ocular ischemia. Carotid disease is a concern in all patients with glaucoma, particularly those with low-tension glaucoma, because it can result in diminished perfusion of the optic nerve. Abnormal lipoprotein findings have been shown to be more common in patients with NTG.[108] Retinal arterial emboli can cause visual field loss in the nerve fiber layer distribution, a process that may constitute an alternative explanation for typical glaucomatous visual field loss without a typical optic nerve appearance. If severe, ocular ischemia may result in neovascular glaucoma. Interestingly enough, prior to the development of elevated IOP, the IOP may actually be low because of decreased ocular perfusion.

The influence of glaucoma medications, most notably the β-blockers, on blood lipid high-density lipoprotein/low-density lipoprotein (HDL/LDL) profile has been demonstrated.[109, 110] Nonselective β-blockers (timolol) decrease the HDL/LDL ("good" cholesterol/"bad" cholesterol) ratio.[109] Unique is carteolol, a nonselective β-blocker with intrinsic sympathomimetic activity (ISA) that has a reduced effect on HDL and LDL in healthy men.[110] Timolol and carteolol are the only glaucoma agents that have been studied. However, betaxolol, a β_1-selective agent, was shown to have negligible effects on plasma lipids when given systemically.[111]

If a patient is being treated for elevations in serum cholesterol or plasma lipids, the clinician must be cognizant of the potential adverse effect of topical ophthalmic β-blockers. The risk of cardiac and peripheral vascular disease has been estimated theoretically to be increased as much as 21% with the use of topical timolol, although this estimate has not been confirmed.[110]

GENITOURINARY CONSIDERATIONS

Renal Calculi

Systemic carbonic anhydrase inhibitors are notorious for their systemic adverse effects, most notably, renal calculi.[111] This effect occurs with the renal metabolic acidosis and alkalinization of the urine. The pH of urine leads to precipitation of calcium in the form of calcium oxalate and calcium phosphate calculi. Ahlstrand and Tiselius[112] evaluated renal calculi from 12 patients who had been treated with acetazolamide. These researchers determined that calcium phosphate was the most significant component of the calculi and suggested that the reduced levels of urinary citrate may have had some role in the precipitation of calcium phosphate.[112] Increased risk of renal calculi formation occurs with both systemic acetazolamide and methazolamide. Shields and Simmons[113] reported a patient in whom renal calculi developed in response to both acetazolamide and methazolamide. In their patient with Paget's disease a calcium oxalate kidney stone developed in response to methazolamide, and a calcium phosphate kidney stone in response to acetazolamide. In this case, it was difficult to determine the exact role of the Paget's disease in the formation of renal calculi. The incidence of side effects can be diminished with the concomitant use of sodium bicarbonate, according to some investigators.

The advent of topical carbonic anhydrase inhibitors has reduced this side effect; however, case reports of renal calculi with topical dorzolamide use suggest that there may be some risk, in spite of the finding that topical agents have a negligible influence on renal acid-base metabolism.[114]

Impotence or Decreased Libido

Decreased libido has been reported to occur with the administration of several glaucoma medications, most commonly topical β-blocking agents and also with oral carbonic anhydrase inhibitors. Among glaucoma medications, β-blockers have the strongest association with impotence and decreased sex drive.[115] The mechanism appears to be CNS-linked, possibly in association with depression. Sexual dysfunction has been reported with the use of ocular timolol.[107]

Carbonic anhydrase inhibitors, both topical and systemic, have been reported to cause impotence. A report documented a reversible decrease in libido that was associated with an oral carbonic anhydrase inhibitor and that resolved or improved after the medication was discontinued.[116] The authors of the report proposed that malaise and depression associated with the patients' oral carbonic anhydrase inhibitor therapy caused a reducation in sex drive. A "symptom-complex," consisting of malaise, fatigue, weight loss, depression, and loss of libido, has been described as being associated with treatment by either acetazolamide or methazolmide.[117] These adverse effects were found to occur more frequently with metabolic acidosis and to decrease with the administration of sodium bicarbonate. Potassium concentration was unrelated to the onset of these symptoms, with the exception of patients taking thiazide diuretics for hypertension in whom hypokalemia developed.

Incontinence

The cause of incontinence is usually an anticholinergic medication that decreases bladder smooth muscle tone.

The more troublesome potential side effect is precipitating intermittent or frank angle closure in a patient with an anatomically narrow angle. The mechanism is the pupil dilation achieved, indirectly, by the anticholinergic blockade on the pupillary sphincter muscle. Antimuscarinic agents used for urgency incontinence, such as tolterodine tartrate (Detrol), can precipitate angle closure in patients with occludable angles. Other urinary antipasmotics, including flavoxate (Urispas) and oxybutinin (Ditropan), can have anticholinergic side effects.

Reduced Renal Function

Clinicians need to remember that dosage recommendations may require adjustment for the population being treated. Adverse systemic side effects may be reduced or eliminated by adjustment of the dosage and frequency of administration for each patient.

Chapron and associates[118] found that elderly patients treated with acetazolamide showed mean plasma and ultrafiltrate concentrations of acetazolamide far in excess of the therapeutic range. These investigators found that these measurements were significantly related to renal function and suggested that appropriate adjustments in dosage may help reduce the incidence of metabolic acidosis that may be associated with the use of acetazolamide.[118]

A case report demonstrates the potential for reduced renal function to ultimately affect the outcome of therapy with oral carbonic anhydrase inhibitors. Takeda and colleagues[119] reported a 66-year-old Japanese woman with a pre-existing diagnosis of chronic renal failure who died following acute hemorrhagic gastritis complicated by disseminated intravascular coagulation and septic shock due to bone marrow depression. She had previously been treated with acetazolamide 500 mg for glaucoma over a period of 11 days. The investigators suggested that dose modifications are necessary in patients with compromised renal function and that hemodialysis may be beneficial in acutely reducing elevated blood levels of acetazolamide.

Oral hyperosmotic agents have the potential for similar adverse effects and require similar individualization of dosages. Serious consideration of the side effects of hyperosmotic agents is imperative in patients with renal failure, in whom confusion, lethargy, stupor, and congestive heart failure may result from mannitol intoxication. There is a case report of acute oliguric renal failure following administration of mannitol for treatment of glaucoma.[120]

Finally, the effects of oral carbonic anhydrase inhibitors

on renal function must be addressed. As mentioned previously, these agents result in alkalinization of the urine with excretion of bicarbonate. Their diuretic effects result in obligatory loss of potassium. The potassium loss is exacerbated in the presence of non–potassium-sparing diuretics, such as thiazides. The side effects of carbonic anhydrase inhibitors have been shown to be greater in patients with reduced serum potassium levels. The risk of these effects is much lower with topical application.

NEUROLOGIC CONSIDERATIONS

Anxiety

Clearly, the psychologic impact of glaucoma is, in itself, anxiety provoking. The level of anxiety may be more problematic if the patient is monocular or has other diseases with the potential for visual loss, such as diabetic retinopathy or macular degeneration.

The salient point is not just whether anxiety can precipitate an episode of angle-closure glaucoma (it can); rather, patients already using antianxiety medication may be prone to additional emotional instability when informed of the diagnosis of glaucoma. This point needs to be conveyed to the primary caregiver as well as the psychiatric caregiver of such a patient.

As mentioned earlier, antianxiety medications have been associated with angle-closure glaucoma via pupillary mydriasis. Medications to be aware of in this regard include the benzodiazepines—clonazepam (Klonopin), diazepam (Valium), and lorazepam (Ativan)—and the antihistamine hydroxyzine. Benzodiazepines, which increase the effects of gamma-aminobutyric acid, can be used for anxiety disorders, panic attacks, and insomnia; in the management of alcohol withdrawal; and also as anticonvulsants. There is also a risk of angle-closure glaucoma with the use of antiepileptic medications such as carbamazepine (Tegretol) and clonazepam (Klonopin).

Depression

Clinical depression can also be exacerbated by the additional burden of a vision-threatening disease such as glaucoma. Numerous studies have demonstrated that the quality of life of patients with glaucoma is less than that of age-matched normal controls. When caring for the patient with glaucoma, one must always keep in mind the impact of social and occupational changes, stress, living conditions, family life, other medical problems, and medication. Such patients often have many reasons for depression, and if there is evidence of pre-existing depression, its impact must be taken into account in glaucoma therapy.

INTERACTIONS BETWEEN GLAUCOMA MEDICATIONS AND SYSTEMIC ANTIDEPRESSANTS

Brimonidine is contraindicated with concomitant use of MAO inhibitors because of the theoretical risk for hypertensive crisis from the increased sensitivity of adrenergic receptors. There are anecdotal reports of the safe use of brimonidine in patients in whom the use of an MAO inhibitor had not been identified. Additionally, there is concern for greater depression when both topical and oral β-blockers are used. Although one hopes this additional clinical effect is rare, transiently higher levels of β-blockade could follow use of a topical agent in a patient already using an oral agent.

GLAUCOMA MEDICATIONS AND DEPRESSION

Case reports have documented significant clinical depression associated with topical β-blocking agents.[121] Lynch and associates evaluated the adverse side effects associated with topical β-blocking agents,[122] including depression, emotional disturbances, and sexual dysfunction. Patients with CNS side effects attributed to timolol maleate were switched to betaxolol with the expectation that a selective β-blocker would be less likely to produce the side effects. A high proportion of patients in this group experienced a reduction in symptoms with the change.

A double-masked crossover study using a small patient population showed either a significant improvement or resolution of the nonselective β-blocker–induced CNS effects with selective β-blocker use. Duch and colleagues[123] found similar results in patients treated with either timolol or betaxolol. They concluded that depression in susceptible patients was more severe in assoication with timolol than with betaxolol. However, there are case reports documenting clinical depression with the use of betaxolol.[123]

Other topical medications can have CNS side effects, most notably the topical carbonic anhydrase inhibitors. Depression and dementia have been reported with the topical use of dorzolamide,[124] similar to the side effects seen with oral carbonic anhydrase inhibitors.[125, 126]

EFFECTS OF SYSTEMIC ANTIDEPRESSANTS ON THE EYES

It is recognized that oral antidepressants such as tricyclic and tetracyclic antidepressants can cause mydriasis,[127] which in turn may precipitate angle closure. Such agents include amitriptyline (Elavil), amoxapine (Asendin), desipramine (Norpramin), doxepin (Sinequan), imipramine (Tofranil), maprotiline (Ludiomil; tetracyclic), mirtazapine (Remeron; tetracyclic), nortriptyline (Pamelor), protriptyline (Vivactil), and trimipramine (Surmontil). They act as indirect adrenergic agents that inhibit the uptake of norepinephrine. Other antidepressants with anticholinergic effects are MAO inhibitors, such as phenelzine (Nardil), isocarboxazid (Marplan), tranylcypromine (Parnate), and nialamide (Miamid), that can be associated with mydriasis. Newer medications such as trazodone (Desyrel) have less anticholinergic effect and act as serotonin reuptake inhibitors. There is also risk for angle-closure glaucoma with paroxetine[128] and of mydriasis with fluoxetine (Prozac).

Parkinson's Disease

Parkinson's disease is an acquired neurologic disease manifesting as extrapyramidal defects, including tremor, rigidity, postural changes, loss of facial expression, and a decrease in blink rate (reptilian stare). It results from decreased dopaminergic activity related to the loss of the substantia nigra. From the standpoint of glaucoma therapy, it is important to use caution in the use of anticholinesterases in the patient with parkinsonism, which may be worsened by cholinergic stimulation. The medications often used to treat Parkinson's disease can increase the risk for angle closure due to mydriasis; they include trihexyphenidyl (Artane), benztropine (Cogentin), biperiden (Akineton), and procyclidine (Kemadrin).

Dementia

Glaucoma medications can be associated with other neurologic conditions, such as dementia. Reyes and colleagues[129] described three patients in whom the use of pilocarpine eye drops was associated with the onset of symptoms including confusion, irritability, agitation, and memory loss. Apparently, the change in mental status was observed shortly after treatment had been initiated with pilocarpine and resolved in two of three cases once the pilocarpine was withdrawn. These investigators suggested that decreased brain levels of acetylcholinesterase could potentiate a reaction to a direct-acting parasympathomimetic such as pilocarpine, causing confusion.

Another case report documented a case of delirium that was associated with another class of medications used for the treatment of glaucoma—carbonic anhydrase inhibitors.[130] Mental confusion was observed following the initiation of treatment using methazolamide for glaucoma. Other associated symptoms were sadness, weight loss, insomnia, incontinence, and disorientation. The symptoms appeared within 2 days after methazolamide treatment was initiated and resolved within 1 week after the medication was discontinued. In this particular case, appropriate management of a drug-related side effect allowed the patient to return to more normal daily function and avoid being institutionalized. Careful assessment of the neurologic status of any patient with glaucoma is recommended because elderly patients may be more susceptible to drug-related psychoses.

Psychosis

Glaucoma medications may have side effects that can be confused with symptoms of psychiatric disorders and certainly may contribute to symptoms of underlying diseases. Most notable are the β-blockers, but other classes of agents have been implicated as well.

Systemic medications, including anticholinergics, can contribute to pupillary mydriasis similar to the effect described with antidepressants. Such agents are antipsychotics in the phenothiazine class, including chlorpromazine (Thorazine), thioridazine (Mellaril), trifluoperazine (Stelazine), fluphenazine (Prolixin), mesoridazine (Serentil), perphenazine (Trilafon), prochlorperazine (Compazine), and promazine (Sparine). Similar effects have been described with chlorprothixene (Iaractan) and thiothixene (Navane).

Fatigue and Dizziness

Several classes of glaucoma medications have been associated with fatigue and dizziness. They include the β-blockers, oral carbonic anhydrase inhibitors[117] and the selective α_2-agonist brimonidine, the effect of which appears to be particularly of concern in children and is more common than with apraclonidine. In the evaluation of a patient for the presence of drug-related fatigue or dizziness, it is important to rule out the possibility that these symptoms are due to systemic hypotension. If decreased blood pressure is not present, the severity of the symptoms can be used to determine whether drug discontinuation is appropriate. If blood pressure is reduced, however, particularly with a narrowed perfusion pressure, drug discontinuation may be appropriate even with only mild symptoms. Other causes of fatigue, dizziness, or even light-headedness should be ruled out, even with evidence of improvement associated with drug discontinuation.

Headache, Including Migraine

The effect of headaches on the management of glaucoma is unclear. Patients may seek medical attention for symptoms related to eye pain or headache that may in fact be caused by acute elevations in IOP. Although the prescription of analgesics may relieve the symptoms, the underlying cause of the problem may not be addressed until more severe symptoms appear.

Other associations between glaucoma, specifically NTG, and migraine headache have been suggested. An evaluation of 27 patients with NTG with neurobehavioral testing, electroencephalography, computed tomography scan, neurologic history, and physical examination revealed no significant abnormalities. Interestingly, 12 of the patients volunteered a history of common or classic migraine in the neurologic history.[131] Phelps and Corbett[132] then surveyed patients with open-angle glaucoma, NTG, and ocular hypertension as well as normal patients as to the frequency and characteristics of headaches.[132] These investigators found that headaches were more common in patients with NTG than those with either open-angle glaucoma or ocular hypertension. Headaches associated with visual aura, nausea, or vomiting were more frequently described by patients with NTG than either open-angle glaucoma or normal patients.

The results of the Beaver Dam Eye Study did not reveal a significant relationship between open-angle glaucoma and migraine.[133] Klein and associates[133] found insufficient evidence of an association between NTG and migraine; however, the scarcity of this condition coupled with the difficulty in diagnosis under screening conditions may have limited the ability of this study to detect such a trend. A survey of Japanese patients comparing patients with open-angle or NTG with normal patients found no significant difference in frequency of headache with or without migraine features. Classic migraine was found to occur with equal frequency in all three groups.[134]

Vertigo and Motion Sickness

Use of medications to control motion sickness may have anticholinergic effects. These medications should be used with caution in the patient with occludable angles because they may precipitate acute angle-closure glaucoma through pupillary dilation.[135]

MUSCULOSKELETAL CONSIDERATIONS

Muscle Spasm

Use of muscle relaxants such as cyclobenzaprine (Flexeril), similar in chemistry to amitriptyline, can be used as a sedative and to treat back pain and muscle and tendon strain. This type of medication has anticholinergic effects, including mydriasis, which may be a concern in patients who are predisposed to angle-closure glaucoma.

Sjögren's Syndrome

Sjögren's syndrome manifests clinically as dryness of mucous membranes, including severe dry eyes (keratoconjunctivitis sicca) and dry mouth (xerostomia) with arthritis. It most often affects women and is more common in patients with rheumatoid arthritis. There is a lymphocytic infiltration of exocrine glands. Filamentary keratitis may complicate keratoconjunctivitis sicca. Diagnosis of Sjögren's syndrome is confirmed in a patient with dryness of mucous membranes, enlarged parotid gland, and a connective tissue disorder; two of these criteria are sufficient for diagnosis.

Dry mouth can be exacerbated by apraclonidine or brimonidine. The most common nonocular side effect of apraclonidine is dry mouth, which occurs in approximately 5% of patients when apraclonidine is added to maximal medical therapy.[136] The dry eye can be exacerbated by β-blockers, and any corneal epithelial irregularity may be made worse by the topical carbonic anhydrase inhibitors. In Sjögren's syndrome to a greater degree than in less severe tear deficiencies, residence time of medication in the preocular tear film is increased because of poor tear function and flow. As a result, medications instilled in the eye have longer contact time and greater potential for toxicity. Therefore, in these patients, one should consider decreasing the frequency of dosage.

Collagen-Vascular Diseases

There are several important issues to be aware of in relation to collagen-vascular diseases, including the association with ocular disease and the requirement for their treatment with potent anti-inflammatory medications, most notably corticosteroids, which can secondarily elevate IOP.

Sarcoidosis

A systemic inflammatory disorder, sarcoidosis is characterized by epithelial cells forming noncaseating granulomas in multiple organ systems, including the eye. Pulmonary signs and lymphadenopathy are common, and symptoms include malaise, weight loss, fever, and fatigue. Anterior uveitis is the most common ocular sign. Glaucoma is also common, with one study reporting secondary glaucoma in 22 of 202 patients who had anterior uveitis secondary to ocular sarcoid.[137] The mechanism is believed to be related to blockage of outflow in the trabeculum by inflammatory debris and nodules.[138]

Oral prednisone is used to treat the underlying disease as well as the symptoms. A loading dose followed by tapering dosage and then a minimum maintenance dose for 6 months is generally appropriate. As a result, there is the potential for secondary glaucoma related to steroid response in addition to the secondary inflammatory glaucoma.

Arthritis

From a practical point of view, arthritis affecting the fingers and hands can make instillation of eye drops difficult. This point should be considered and then discussed with the patient along with treatment options. There may be a time of day when eye drop instillation is manageable and other times when it is close to impossible. The patient may need to find a caregiver to give eye drop therapy. Alternatively, surgical options may be more desirable if use of eye drops is not practical in a patient with severe arthritis.

Arthritis is usually not linked with glaucoma among the elderly unless uveitis is present. Children with juvenile rheumatoid arthritis (JRA) have a significant incidence of glaucoma and severe vision loss.[139–141] One study found the incidence of glaucoma to be as high as 27% among patients with JRA and iridocyclitis.[142] Severe vision loss (i.e., <20/200 VA) is more common if the diagnosis of uveitis precedes that of JRA.[142]

INTERACTIONS BETWEEN GLAUCOMA MEDICATIONS AND SYSTEMIC ANTIARTHRITIS AGENTS

Oral indomethacin has been found to block the effects of epinephrine in a study conducted to test the theory that the epinephrine-mediated decrease in IOP is related to prostaglandins or other cyclo-oxygenase products.[143] Conversely, β-blockers do not appear to be influenced by nonsteroidal anti-inflammatory drugs (NSAIDs). Oral indomethacin, 25 mg TID, had no effect on the hypotensive effect of timolol maleate 0.5% BID in a randomized double-masked study of nine healthy patients.[144] It is not clear, at this time, whether systemic NSAIDs have any influence on the IOP-lowering response to prostaglandin analogues.

Patients who undergo long-term treatment with aspirin may demonstrate adverse side effects from the concurrent administration of acetazolamide.[145–149] Salicylates such as aspirin bind to plasma proteins and competitively prevent acetazolamide binding; this effect has been shown to occur in vitro in a concentration-dependent manner.[145] Unbound acetazolamide concentrations have been shown to be three times higher in the presence of salicylates.[148] Therefore, patients being treated with aspirin may be subject to higher plasma concentrations of acetazolamide that may predispose them to adverse side effects, including fatigue, lethargy, and confusion. This potential may be even greater in elderly patients, in whom the elimination of acetazolamide can be reduced. Furthermore, it has been shown that salicylate therapy may inhibit the renal secretion of acetazolamide in a population of patients that may already have diminished kidney function.[145]

Other case reports document the development of salicylate toxicity in response to the metabolic acidosis resulting from acetazolamide therapy. The combination of acetazolamide and aspirin led to salicylate intoxication. Salicylate intoxication may vary in severity with symptoms, including nausea, vomiting, drowsiness, perspiration, headache, tinnitus, and loss of hearing. More severe cases may manifest as CNS disturbances.[149]

Vogt-Koyanagi-Harada Syndrome

Vogt-Koyanagi-Harada syndrome is more common in Asians, and there is a greater tendency for symptoms to occur in spring and late fall. Systemic signs include vitiligo, alopecia, poliosis, headache, fever, nausea, scalp sensitivity, meningism, and hearing loss. Ocular signs include anterior and posterior granulomatous uveitis, chorioretinal scarring, vascular sheathing, and exudative retinal detachment. Glaucoma occurs in 20%[150] to 38%[151] of cases and may be due to inflammatory glaucoma or to angle closure[152] due to a swollen ciliary body with anterior rotation.[153]

In addition to the secondary glaucomas in this syndrome, the use of systemic corticosteroid therapy poses a risk for a steroid response, as described for arthritis.

DERMATOLOGIC CONSIDERATIONS

Topical glaucoma medications not infrequently can cause local as well as generalized dermatologic reactions. Dermatitis is particularly a concern with the use of sulfa-based medications. There are case reports of skin eruptions related to oral methazolamide.[154] However, severe and even life-threatening skin eruptions, including Stevens-Johnson sydrome,[155, 156] and toxic epidermal necrolysis have been reported.

Alopecia has been related to timolol usage. Latanoprost increases the number and thickness of eyelashes (hypertrichosis) as well as the pigmentation of the periocular skin. Unlike the increase in iris pigmentation that also occurs with latanoprost, the eyelash and skin changes may revert to normal with cessation of the medication because of tissue turnover. Contact dermatitis of the periocular skin is most common with the adrenergic agents, being more frequent with apraclonidine than with brimonidine. This finding can be present, however, with any topical ophthalmic antiglaucoma agent.

It is important to remember, the use of topical dermatologic corticosteroid preparations for a prolonged period on a large area of skin can rarely induce a steroid-related IOP response.

HEMATOLOGIC CONSIDERATIONS

The relationship between ocular blood flow and glaucomatous optic neuropathy remains controversial. There is increasing evidence linking the two. Drance and colleagues[37] evaluated a group of patients with NTG and determined that hematologic abnormalities were present in a significant number. Hypercoagulability was observed and was suggested to be a causal factor in the risk of microinfarcts at the optic nerve head, particularly in combination with hemodynamic events. Other studies found increased viscosity and hypercoagulability in patients with glaucoma.[157–161] Conversely, yet other investigators have not found any hematologic abnormalities.[48] In the medical treatment of glaucoma, factors that affect the systemic levels of drugs such as the oral carbonic anhydrase inhibitors have an impact on therapy. These factors include protein binding and free drug availability.

Anticoagulation Therapy

The role of anticoagulation in glaucoma remains unproven, although medications including *Ginkgo biloba* have been proposed to be beneficial. The science supporting these claims is currently lacking.

Of clinical relevance is the coagulability in the patient undergoing incisional ocular surgery, such as filtration surgery. It is generally recommended that anticoagulant agents be discontinued prior to surgery such that at surgery, the patient has normal coagulation capabilities. This recommendation requires the discontinuation of antiplatelet medications (aspirin, NSAIDs, dipyridamole) 5 to 7 days preoperatively. Warfarin should be discontinued (if it can be done safely) with a similar time frame, and confirmation of a normal blood clotting capability should be obtained preoperatively. Decreased coagulability during the perioperative period raises the risk of bleeding and, thereby, of excessive subconjunctival hemorrhage, hyphema, and suprachoroidal hemorrhage, each of which can decrease the chance of successful surgery and increase the potential for complications.

Anemia

Anemia is a pathologic reduction in blood cells. When severe enough, it can result in retinopathy that may manifest as visual field defects. Signs include enlargement of the spleen, bone pain, and bleeding. In patients with glaucoma, anemia may predispose the optic nerve to damage as a result of decreased perfusion.

The greatest hematologic concern in the patient treated for glaucoma, however, are the blood dyscrasias associated with oral carbonic anhydrase inhibitors.[162–169] Adverse hematologic events reported to the National Registry of Drug-Induced Ocular Side Effects related to the use of these agents included aplastic anemia, thrombocytopenia, and agranulocytosis. These complications were observed to develop within the first 6 months of treatment in a large number of cases and rarely with less than 14 days of use.

A case report of a series of patients taking acetazolamide reported that 10 of 11 died as a result of blood dyscrasias. The estimated incidence of aplastic anemia associated with use of acetazolamide is 1 in 18,000 patient years of use. Reports have also documented the association of blood dyscrasias, including aplastic anemia, agranulocytosis, and neutropenia, with the use of methazolamide.[168, 169] No association between topical carbonic anhydrase inhibitors and bone marrow aplasia has been noted to date. No blood test is currently available to identify patients at risk for this side effect because the majority of the events appear to be idiosyncratic. A survey of ophthalmologists in academic positions as well as private and glaucoma specialty practices found that relatively few practitioners supported routine blood testing. Regular follow-up and specific history-taking for symptoms related to adverse side effects were thought to be more beneficial.

Sickle Cell Anemia

This family of diseases encompasses five hemoglobulinopathies: sickle cell disease (SS), sickle cell trait (SA), sickle cell C disease (SC), sickle cell–thalassemia (S-Thal), and hemoglobin C trait (AC). Affected patients present with complaints of bone and joint pain. Abnormal hemoglobin results in increased rigidity of red blood cells, decreased flow through blood vessels, and a subsequent increase in blood viscosity and decrease in ability of the cells to carry oxygen. Ocular signs are due to vascular occlusions of small vessels and may result in neovascular glaucoma due to sickle cell retinopathy.[170]

Of special note is that in the patient with sickle cell anemia, acetazolamide can induce a crisis by creating systemic metabolic acidosis. Methazolamide may be a safer alternative. In addition, diuretics or hyperosmotics can induce a sickle cell crisis by increasing blood viscosity.

Treatment of the patient with both sickle cell anemia and glaucoma is particularly problematic. Most ophthalmologists believe that the optic nerve is more susceptible to glaucoma damage in sickle cell disease, possibly because of decreased perfusion. For that reason, for example, in a patient with sickle cell disease, traumatic hyphema, and elevated IOP, more aggressive therapy is warranted to lower the IOP than if the patient did not have sickle cell disease.

ONCOLOGIC CONSIDERATIONS

The most common metastases to the eye are from carcinomas of the breast and lung.[171, 172] Glaucoma is more common with metastasis to the anterior segment than to the posterior segment. The mechanism of increased IOP may be secondary open-angle glaucoma and clogging of the trabecular meshwork by abnormal cells[172, 173] or secondary angle closure due to an anteriorly pushing posterior mass or peripheral anterior synechiae.[172, 173] Glaucoma has been reported with other intraocular tumors, including leukemia,[174, 175] lymphoma,[176] multiple myeloma,[177] and metastatic malignant melanoma.[178]

EFFECTS OF SYSTEMIC ANTICANCER MEDICATIONS ON THE EYES

Alkylating agents, including nitrosurea and BCNU (carmustine) have been reported to result in elevation of IOP.[179, 180] Visual field loss (constriction and paracentral scotoma) has been reported with the antiestrogen tamoxifen.[181] Visual field abnormalities (paracentral scotoma, constriction, hemianopsia) have been reported with the vinca alkaloids (vinblastine, vincristine).[181]

SUMMARY

There are many systemic considerations in the management of glaucoma. Fortunately, with the advent of new medications and surgical alternatives for the treatment of glaucoma, the risk of systemic complications has been significantly reduced. In all cases, careful review of systems is essential before determination of the most appropriate medication. Furthermore, the potential for adverse side effects can be reduced if patients are taught simple maneuvers such as eyelid closure and punctal occlusion during administration of glaucoma medications. These techniques can reduce systemic absorption by up to 70%.[2]

There is no ideal medication for the treatment of glaucoma. Currently, the best outcome of management remains to help patients retain useful vision over the course of their lifetimes. We attempt to reach this goal by prescribing medications that we believe will be safest, most effective, and best tolerated. We try to anticipate possible side effects of these medications and provide alternative medications where appropriate. Patients must be actively involved in their management plan and adequately educated about the possible adverse effects of their medications.

REFERENCES

1. Jones FL Jr, Ekberg ML: Exacerbation of asthma by timolol [letter]. N Engl J Med 1979;301:270.
2. Zimmerman TJ, Kooner KS, Kandarakis AS, et al: Improving the therapeutic index of topically applied ocular drugs. Arch Ophthalmol 1984;102:551–553.
3. Potash SD, Ritch R: Acute angle-closure glaucoma secondary to Chlor-Trimeton. J Glaucoma 1992;1:258–259.
4. Schmitt LG, Shaw JE: Alleviation of induced vertigo. Therapy with transdermal scopolamine and oral meclizine. Arch Otolaryngol Head Neck Surg 1986;112:88–91.
5. Schuman JS, Horwitz B, Choplin NT, et al: A 1-year study of brimonidine twice daily in glaucoma and ocular hypertension. A controlled, randomized, multicenter clinical trial. Chronic Brimonidine Study Group [see comments]. Arch Ophthalmol 1997;115:847–852.
6. Everitt DE, Avorn J: Systemic effects of medications used to treat glaucoma. Ann Intern Med 1990;112:120–125.
7. Ostergaard Laursen S, Bjerrum P: Timolol eyedrop-induced severe bronchospasm. Acta Med Scand 1982;211:505–506.
8. Zimmerman TJ, Baumann JD, Hetherington J Jr: Side effects of timolol. Surv Ophthalmol 1983;28 Suppl:243–251.
9. Zimmerman TJ, Leader BJ, Golob DS: Potential side effects of timolol therapy in the treatment of glaucoma. Ann Ophthalmol 1981;13:683–689.
10. Diamond JP: Systemic adverse effects of topical ophthalmic agents. Implications for older patients. Drugs Aging 1997;11:352–360.
11. Cantor LB: Systemic side effects of glaucoma medications. Indiana Med 1995;82:105–107.
12. Fraunfelder FT, Meyer SM: Systemic adverse reactions to glaucoma medications. Int Ophthalmol Clin 1989;29:143–146.
13. Van Buskirk EM, Fraunfelder FT: Ocular beta-blockers and systemic effects. Am J Ophthalmol 1984;98:623–624.
14. Stewart WC, Garrison PM: Beta-blocker-induced complications and the patient with glaucoma. Newer treatments to help reduce systemic adverse events. Arch Intern Med 1998;158:221–226.
15. Rait JL: Systemic effects of topical ophthalmic beta-adrenoceptor antagonists. Aust N Z J Ophthalmol 1999;27:57–64.
16. Weinreb RN, van Buskirk EM, Cherniack R, Drake MM: Long-term betaxolol therapy in glaucoma patients with pulmonary disease. Am J Ophthalmol 1988;106:162–167.
17. Harris LS, Greenstein SH, Bloom AF: Respiratory difficulties with betaxolol. Am J Ophthalmol 1986;102:274–275.
18. Schoene RB, Abuan T, Ward RL, Beasley CH: Effects of topical betaxolol, timolol, and placebo on pulmonary function in asthmatic bronchitis. Am J Ophthalmol 1984;97:86–92.
19. Block ER, Rostand RA: Carbonic anhydrase inhibition in glaucoma: Hazard or benefit for the chronic lunger? Surv Ophthalmol 1978;23:169–172.
20. Curti PC, Renovanz HD: The effect of unintentional overdoses of pilocarpine on pulmonary surfactant in mice. [Die Wirkung akzidenteller Uberdosierung von Pilòcarpin auf den pulmonalen Surfaktant an der Maus.] Klin Monatsbl Augenheilkd 1981;179:113–115.
21. The MK-507 Clinical Study Group: Long-term glaucoma treatment with MK-507, dorzolamine, a topical carbonic anhydrase inhibitor. J Glaucoma 1995;4:6.
22. Adamsons IA, Polis A, Ostrov CS, Boyle JE: Two-year safety study of dorzolamide as monotherapy and with timolol and pilocarpine. Dorzolamide Safety Study Group. J Glaucoma 1998;7:395–401.
23. Maus TL, Larsson LI, McLaren JW, Brubaker RF: Comparison of dorzolamide and acetazolamide as suppressors of aqueous humor flow in humans. Arch Ophthalmol 1997;115:45–49.
24. Silver LH: Clinical efficacy and safety of brinzolamide (Azopt), a

new topical carbonic anhydrase inhibitor for primary open-angle glaucoma and ocular hypertension. Brinzolamide Primary Therapy Study Group. Am J Ophthalmol 1998;126:400–408.
25. Hedner J, Everts B, Moller CS: Latanoprost and respiratory function in asthmatic patients: randomized, double-masked, placebo-controlled crossover evaluation. Arch Ophthalmol 1999;117:1305–1309.
26. Shah P, Dhurjon L, Metcalfe T, Gibson JM: Acute angle closure glaucoma associated with nebulised ipratropium bromide and salbutamol [see comments]. BMJ 1992;304:40–41.
27. Mitchell P, Cumming RG, Mackey DA: Inhaled corticosteroids, family history, and risk of glaucoma. Ophthalmology 1999; 106:2301–2306.
28. Garbe E, LeLorier J, Boivin JF, Suissa S: Inhaled and nasal glucocorticoids and the risks of ocular hypertension or open-angle glaucoma [see comments]. JAMA 1997;277:722–727.
29. Tielsch JM, Katz J, Sommer A, Quigley HA, Javitt JC: Hypertension, perfusion pressure, and primary open-angle glaucoma. A population-based assessment. Arch Ophthalmol 1995;113:216–221.
30. Wilson MR, Hertzmark E, Walker AM, et al: A case-control study of risk factors in open angle glaucoma. Arch Ophthalmol 1987;105:1066–1071.
31. Leighton DA, Phillips CI: Systemic blood pressure in open-angle glaucoma, low tension glaucoma, and the normal eye. Br J Ophthalmol 1972;56:447–453.
32. Dielemans I, Vingerling JR, Wolfs RC, et al: The prevalence of primary open-angle glaucoma in a population-based study in The Netherlands. The Rotterdam Study. Ophthalmology 1994;101:1851–1853.
33. Leibowitz HM, Krueger DE, Maunder LR, et al: The Framingham Eye Study monograph: An ophthalmological and epidemiological study of cataract, glaucoma, diabetic retinopathy, macular degeneration, and visual acuity in a general population of 2631 adults, 1973–1975. Surv Ophthalmol 1980;24:Suppl:335–610.
34. Leske MC, Heijl A, Hyman L, Bengtsson B: Early Manifest Glaucoma Trial: design and baseline data. Ophthalmology 1999;106:2144–2153.
35. Drance SM, Schulzer M, Thomas B, Douglas GR: Multivariate analysis in glaucoma. Use of discriminate analysis in predicting glaucomatous visual field damage. Arch Ophthalmol 1981;99:1019–1022.
36. Graham SL, Drance SM, Wijsman K, et al: Ambulatory blood pressure monitoring in glaucoma. The nocturnal dip. Ophthalmol 1995;102:61–69.
37. Drance SM, Sweeney VP, Morgan RW, Feldman F: Studies of factors involved in the production of low tension glaucoma. Arch Ophthalmol 1973;89:457–465.
38. Chumbley LC, Brubaker RF: Low-tension glaucoma. Am J Ophthalmol 1976;81:761–767.
39. Richler M, Werner EB, Thomas D: Risk factors for progression of visual field defects in medically treated patients with glaucoma. Can J Ophthalmol 1982;17:245–248.
40. Kaiser HJ, Flammer J, Graf T, Stumpfig D: Systemic blood pressure in glaucoma patients. Graefes Arch Clin Exp Ophthalmol 1993;231:677–680.
41. Graham SL, Drance SM, Wijsman K, et al: Ambulatory blood pressure monitoring in glaucoma. The nocturnal dip. Ophthalmology 1995;102:61–69.
42. Bechetoille A, Bresson-Dumont H: Diurnal and nocturnal blood pressure drops in patients with focal ischemic glaucoma. Graefes Arch Clin Exp Ophthalmol 1994;232:675–679.
43. Collignon N, Dewe W, Guillaume S, Collignon-Brach J: Ambulatory blood pressure monitoring in glaucoma patients: The nocturnal systolic dip and its relationship with disease progression. Int Ophthalmol 1998;22:19–25.
44. Gottfredsdottir MS, Allingham RR, Shields MB: Physicians' guide to interactions between glaucoma and systemic medications. J Glaucoma 1997;6;377–383.
45. Drance SM, Douglas GR, Wijsman K, et al: Response of blood flow to warm and cold in normal and low-tension glaucoma patients. Am J Ophthalmol 1988;105:35–39.
46. Gasser P, Flammer J: Blood-cell velocity in the nailfold capillaries of patients with normal-tension and high-tension glaucoma. Am J Ophthalmol 1991;111:585–588.
47. O'Brien C, Butt Z: Blood flow velocity in the peripheral circulation of glaucoma patients. Ophthalmologica 1999;213:150–153.
48. Carter CJ, Brooks DE, Doyle PL, Drance SM: Investigations into a vascular etiology for low tension glaucoma. Ophthalmol 1990;97:49–55.
49. Feldman F, Sweeney VP, Drance SM: Cerebro-vascular studies in chronic simple glaucoma. Can J Ophthalmol 1969;4:358–364.
50. Ong K, Farinelli A, Bilson F, et al: Comparative study of brain magnetic resonance imaging findings in patients with low-tension glaucoma and control subjects. Ophthalmology 1995;102:1632–1638.
51. Schlotzer-Schrehardt UM, Koca MR, Naumann GO, Volkholz H: Pseudoexfoliation syndrome: Ocular manifestation of a systemic disorder? Arch Ophthalmol 1992;110:1752–1756.
52. Streeten BW, Li ZY, Wallan RN, et al: Pseudoexfoliative fibrillopathy in visceral organs of a patient with pseudoexfoliation syndrome. Arch Ophthalmol 1992;110:1757–1762.
53. Freemantle N, Cleland J, Young P, et al: Beta blockade after myocardial infarction: systematic review and meta regression analysis. BMJ 1999;318:1730–1737.
54. Schuman JS: Effects of systemic β-blocker therapy on the efficacy and safety of topical brimonidine and timolol. Ophthalmology 2000;107:1171–1177.
55. Wettrell K, Pandolfi M: Early dose response analysis of ocular hypotensive effects of propranolol in patients with ocular hypertension. Br J Ophthalmol 1976;60:680–683.
56. Kitayawa Y, Shirai H, Go FJ: The effect of calcium antagonist on visual field in low-tension glaucoma. Graefes Arch Clin Exp Ophthalmol 1989;227:408–412.
57. Netland PA, Chaturvedi N, Dreyer EB: Calcium channel blockers in the management of low-tension and open-angle glaucoma [see comments]. Am J Ophthalmol 1993;115:608–613.
58. Netland PA, Grosskrentz CL, Feke GT, Hart LJ: Color Doppler ultrasound analysis of ocular circulation after topical calcium channel blockers. Am J Ophthalmol 1995;119:694–700.
59. Kanellopoulos AJ, Erickson KA, Netland PA: Systemic calcium channel blockers and glaucoma. J Glaucoma 1996;5:357–362.
60. Meuche C, Heidrich H, Bleckmann H: Raynaud syndrome following the use of eyedrops containing timolol. Fortschr Ophthalmol 1990;87:45–47.
61. Monane M, Bohn RL, Burwitz JH, et al: Topical glaucoma medications and cardiovascular risk in the elderly. Clin Pharmacol Ther 1994;55:76–83.
62. Becker B, Montgomery SW, Kass MA, Shin DH: Increased ocular and systemic responsiveness to epinephrine in primary open angle glaucoma. Arch Ophthalmol 1977;95:789–790.
63. Kerr CR, Hass I, Drance SM, et al: Cardiovascular effect of epinephrine and dipivalyl epinephrine applied topically to the eye in patients with glaucoma. Br J Ophthalmol 1982;66:109–114.
64. Blondeau P, Cote M: Cardiovascular effects of epinephrine and dipivefrin in patients using timolol: A single-dose study. Can J Ophthalmol 1984;19:29–32.
65. Robin AL: Short-term effects of unilateral 1% apraclonidine therapy. Arch Ophthalmol 1988;106:912–915.
66. Coleman AL, Robin AL, Pollack IP, et al: Cardiovascular and intraocular pressure effects and plasma concentrations of apraclonidine. Arch Ophthalmol 1990;108:1264–1267.
67. Littmann L, Kempler P, Rohla M, Fenyvesi T: Severe symptomatic atrioventricular block induced by pilocarpine eye drops. Arch Intern Med 1987;147:586–587.
68. Pringle SD, MacEwen CJ: Severe bradycardia due to interaction of timolol eye drops and verapamil. BMJ 1987;294:155–156.
69. Sinclair NI: Timolol eyedrops and verapamil, a dangerous combination. Med J Aust 1983;1:548–549.
70. Maren N, Alvan G, Calissendorff BM, et al: Additive intraocular pressure reducing effect of topical timolol during systemic beta-blockade. Acta Ophthalmol (Copenh) 1982;60:16–23.
71. Blondeau P, Cote M, Tetrault L: Effect of timolol eye drops in subjects receiving systemic propranolol therapy. Can J Ophthalmol 1983;18:18–21.
72. Dinai Y, Sharir M, Navey N, Halkin H: Bradycardia induced by interaction between quinidine and ophthalmic timolol. Ann Intern Med 1985;103:890–891.
73. Gandy W: Severe epinephrine-propranolol interaction. Ann Emerg Med 1989;18:98–99.
74. Harrison WM, McGrath PJ, Stewart JW, Quitkin F: MAOIs and hypertensive crises: The role of OTC drugs (see comments). J Clin Psychiatry 1989;50:64–65.

75. Jackson EK: Diuretics. *In* Hardman JG, Limbird LE (eds): Goodman & Gilman's The Pharmacological Basis of Therapeutics, 9th ed. New York, McGraw-Hill, 1996, pp 685–713.
76. Margo CE: Acetazolamide and advanced liver disease. Am J Ophthalmol 1986;101:611–612.
77. Gillies WE, Brooks AM: A trial of dorzolamide for glaucoma. Ophthalmic Surg Lasers 1998;29:728–732.
78. Shields MB: Textbook of Glaucoma, 4th ed. Philadelphia, Lippincott–Williams & Wilkins, 1998, pp 433–434.
79. Kushnick H, Liebmann JM, Ritch R: Systemic pilocarpine toxicity from Ocusert leakage (letter). Arch Ophthalmol 1996;114:1432.
80. Wood JR, Anderson RL, Edwards JJ: Phospholine iodide toxicity and Jones' tubes. Ophthalmology 1980;87:346–349.
81. Wolfhagen FH, van Neerven JA, Groen FC, Ouwendijk RJ: Severe nausea and vomiting with timolol eye drops (letter) (see comments). Lancet 1998;352:373.
82. Fraunfelder FT: Transdermal scopolamine precipitating narrow-angle glaucoma (letter). N Engl J Med 1982;307:1079.
83. Armstrong JF, Daily RK, Dobson HL, Girard LJ: The incidence of glaucoma in diabetes mellitus. A comparison with the incidence of glaucoma in the general population. Am J Ophthalmol 1960;50:55–63.
84. Becker B: Diabetes mellitus and primary open-angle glaucoma. The XXVII Edward Jackson Memorial Lecture. Am J Ophthalmol 1971;71:1–16.
85. Klein BE, Klein R, Jensen SC: Open-angle glaucoma and older-onset diabetes. The Beaver Dam Eye Study. Ophthalmology 1994;101:1173–1177.
86. Tielsch JM, Katz J, Quigley HA, et al: Diabetes, intraocular pressure, and primary open-angle glaucoma in the Baltimore Eye Survey. Ophthalmology 1995;102:48–53.
87. Mitchell P, Smith W, Chey T, Healey PR: Open-angle glaucoma and diabetes: the Blue Mountains eye study, Australia. Ophthalmology 1997;104:712–718.
88. Dielemans I, de Jong PT, Stolk R, et al: Primary open-angle glaucoma, intraocular pressure, and diabetes mellitus in the general elderly population. The Rotterdam Study. Ophthalmology 1996; 103:1271–1275.
89. Nielsen NV: The prevalence of glaucoma and ocular hypertension in type 1 and 2 diabetes mellitus. An epidemiological study of diabetes mellitus on the island of Falster, Denmark. Acta Ophthalmol (Copenh) 1983;61:662–672.
90. Klein BE, Klein R, Moss SE: Incidence of self reported glaucoma in people with diabetes mellitus. Br J Ophthalmol 1997;81:743–747.
91. Schertzer RM, Wang D, Bartholomew LR: Diabetes mellitus and glaucoma. Int Ophthalmol Clin 1998;38:69–87.
92. Zeiter JH, Shin DH, Baek NH: Visual field defects in diabetic patients with primary open-angle glaucoma. Am J Ophthalmol 1991;111:581–584.
93. Zeiter JH, Shin DH: Diabetes in primary open-angle glaucoma patients with inferior visual field defects. Graefes Arch Clin Exp Ophthalmol 1994;232:205–210.
94. Velde TM, Kaiser FE: Ophthalmic timolol treatment causing altered hypoglycemic response in a diabetic patient. Arch Intern Med 1983;143:1627.
95. Oakley DE, Ellis PP: Glycerol and hyperosmolar nonketotic coma. Am J Ophthalmol 1976;81:469–472.
96. Smith KD, Tevaarwerk GJM, Allen LH: Reversal of poorly controlled glaucoma on diagnosis and treatment of hypothyroidism. Can J Ophthalmol 1992;27:345–347.
97. Smith KD, Tevaarwerk GJM, Allen LH: An ocular dynamic study supporting the hypothesis that hypothyroidism is a treatable cause of secondary open-angle glaucoma. Can J Ophthalmol 1992;27:341–344.
98. Smith KD, Arthurs BP, Saheb N: An association between hypothyroidism and primary open-angle glaucoma. Ophthalmology 1993;100:1580–1584.
99. Gillow JT, Shah P, O'Neill EC: Primary open angle glaucoma and hypothyroidism: Chance or true association? Eye 1997;11:113–114.
100. Buschmann W: Glaucoma and Graves' disease. Klin Monatsbl Augenheilkd 1986;188:138–140.
101. Kalmann R, Mourits MP: Prevalence and management of elevated intraocular pressure in patients with Graves' orbitopathy. Br J Ophthalmol 1998;82:754–757.
102. Dev S, Damji KF, DeBacker CM, et al: Decrease in intraocular pressure after orbital decompression for thyroid orbitopathy. Can J Ophthalmol 1998;33:314–319.
103. Treister G, Mannor S: Intraocular pressure and outflow facility: Effect of estrogen and combined estrogen-progestin treatment in normal human eyes. Arch Ophthalmol 1970;83:311–318.
104. Abdel-Aziz M, Labib MA: The relationship of the intra-ocular pressure to hormonal disturbance. Part IV: The gonads. Bull Ophthalmol Soc Egypt 1969;62:83–94.
105. Haas JS, Nootens RH: Glaucoma secondary to benign adrenal adenoma. Am J Ophthalmol 1974;78:497–500.
106. Robbin DS, Haas JS: A 16-year follow-up in a corticosteroid-sensitive patient with glaucoma secondary to a benign adrenal adenoma. Am J Ophthalmol 1989;107:293–295.
107. Flach AJ: Glaucoma and impotence [letter; comment]. JAMA 1990;264:3146.
108. Winder AF: Circulating lipoprotein and blood glucose levels in association with low-tension and chronic simple glaucoma. Br J Ophthalmol 1977;61:641–645.
109. Coleman AL, Diehl DL, Jampel HD, et al: Topical timolol decreases plasma high-density lipoprotein cholesterol level [see comments]. Arch Ophthalmol 1990;108:1260–1263.
110. Freedman SF, Freedman NJ, Sheilds MB, et al: Effects of ocular carteolol and timolol on plasma high-density lipoprotein cholesterol level [see comments]. Am J Ophthalmol 1993;116:600–611.
111. Kass MA, Kolker AE, Gordon M, et al: Acetazolamide and urolithiasis. Ophthalmology 1981;88:261–265.
112. Ahlstrand C, Tiselius HG: Urine composition and stone formation during treatment with acetazolamide. Scand J Urol Nephrol 1987;21:225–228.
113. Shields MB, Simmons RJ: Urinary calculus during methazolamide therapy. Am J Ophthalmol 1976;81:622–624.
114. Carlsen J, Durcan J, Zabriskie N, et al: Nephrolithiasis with dorzolamide. Arch Ophthalmol 1999;117:1087–1088.
115. Katz IM: Sexual dysfunction and ocular timolol. JAMA 1986;255:37–38.
116. Wallace TR, Fraunfelder FT, Petursson GJ, Epstein DL: Decreased libido—a side effect of carbonic anhydrase inhibitor. Ann Ophthalmol 1979;11:1563–1566.
117. Epstein DL, Grant WM: Carbonic anhydrase inhibitor side effects: Serum chemical analysis. Arch Ophthalmol 1997;95:1378–1382.
118. Chapron DJ, Gomolin IH, Sweeney KR: Acetazolamide blood concentrations are excessive in the elderly: Propensity for acidosis and relationship to renal function. J Clin Pharmacol 1989;29:348–353.
119. Takeda K, Nakamoto M, Yasunaga C, et al: Acute hemorrhagic gastritis associated with acetazolamide intoxication in a patient with chronic renal failure. Clin Nephrol 1997;48:266–268.
120. Weaver A, Sica DA: Mannitol-induced acute renal failure. Nephron 187;45:233–235.
121. Nolan BT: Acute suicidal depression associated with use of timolol (letter). JAMA 1982:247, 1567.
122. Lynch MG, Whitson JT, Brown RH, et al: Topical beta-blocker therapy and central nervous system side effects. A preliminary study comparing betaxolol and timolol. Arch Ophthalmol 1988;106:908–911.
123. Duch S, Duch C, Pasto L, Ferrer P: Changes in depressive status associated with topical beta-blockers. Int Ophthalmol 1992;16:331–335.
124. thoe Schwartzenberg GW, Trope GE: Anorexia, depression and dementia induced by dorzolamide eyedrops (Trusopt). Can J Ophthalmol 1999;34:93–94.
125. Stoudemire A, Houpt JL: Carbonic anhydrase inhibitors: an under-recognized cause of psychiatric symptoms. Psychiatr Med 1983;1:353–355.
126. Stoppe G, Schutze R, Kogler A, et al: Cerebrovascular reactivity to acetazolamide in (senile) dementia of Alzheimer's type: relationship to disease severity. Dementia 1995;6:73–82.
127. Ritch R, Krupin T, Henry C, Kurata F: Oral imipramine and acute angle closure glaucoma. Arch Ophthalmol 1994;112:67–68.
128. Lewis CF, DeQuardo JR, DuBose C, Tandon R: Acute angle-closure glaucoma and paroxetine (letter). J Clin Psychiatry 1997;58:123–124.
129. Reyes PF, Dwyer BA, Schwartzman RJ, Sacchetti T: Mental status changes induced by eye drops in dementia of the Alzheimer type. J Neurol Neurosurg Psychiatry 1987;50:113–115.
130. Cyr M, Laizure C, daCunha CM: Methazolamide-induced delirium. 1997;17:387–389.

131. Corbett JJ, Phelps CD, Eslinger P, Montague PR: The neurological evaluation of patients with low-tension glaucoma. Invest Ophthalmol Vis Sci 1985;26:1101–1104.
132. Phelps CD, Corbett JJ: Migraine and low-tension glaucoma: A case-control study. Invest Ophthalmol Vis Sci 1985;26:1105–1108.
133. Klein BE, Klein R, Neuer SM, Goetz LA: Migraine headache and its association with open-angle glaucoma: The Beaver Dam Eye Study. Invest Ophthalmol Vis Sci 1993;34:3024–3027.
134. Usui T, Iwata K, Shirakashi M, Abe H: Prevalence of migraine in low-tension glaucoma and primary open-angle glaucoma in Japanese. Br J Ophthalmol 1991;75:224–226.
135. Fraunfelder T: Transdermal scopolamine precipitating narrow-angle glaucoma (letter). N Engl J Med 1982;307:1079.
136. Robin AL, Ritch R, Shin DH, et al: Short-term efficacy of apraclonidine hydrochloride added to maximum-tolerated medical therapy for glaucoma: Apraclonidine Maximum-Tolerated Medical Therapy Study Group. Am J Ophthalmol 1995;120:423–432.
137. Obenauf CD, Shaw HE, Sydnor CF, Klintworth GK: Sarcoidosis and its ophthalmic manifestations. Am J Ophthalmol 1978;86:648–655.
138. Iwata K, Nanba K, Sobue K, Abe H: Ocular sarcoidosis: Evaluation of intraocular findings. Ann N Y Acad Sci 1976;278:445–454.
139. Chylack LT Jr, Bienfang DC, Bellows R, Stillman JS: Ocular manifestations of juvenile rheumatoid arthritis. Am J Ophthalmol 1975;79:1026–1033.
140. Kanski JJ: Anterior uveitis in juvenile rheumatoid arthritis. Arch Ophthalmol 1977;95:1794–1797.
141. Key SN 3d, Kimura SJ: Iridocyclitis associated with juvenile rheumatoid arthritis. Am J Ophthalmol 1975;80:425–429.
142. Wolf MD, Lichter PR, Ragsdale CG: Prognostic factors in the uveitis of juvenile rheumatoid arthritis. Ophthalmology 1987; 94:1242–1248.
143. Camras CB, Feldman SG, Podos SM, et al: Inhibition of the epinephrine induced reduction of intraocular pressure by systemic indomethacin in humans. Am J Ophthalmol 1985;100:169–173.
144. Lichter M, Felman F, Clark L, Cohen MM: Effect of indomethacin on the ocular hypotensive action of timolol maleate. Am J Ophthalmol 1984;98:79–81.
145. Sweeney KR, Chapron DJ, Brandt JL, et al: Toxic interaction between acetazolamide and salicylate: Case reports and a pharmacokinetic explanation. Clin Pharmacol Ther 1986;40:518–524; published erratum appears in Clin Pharmacol Ther 1987;41:67.
146. Rousseau P, Funtevilla-Clifton A: Acetazolamide and salicylate interaction in the elderly: A case report. J Am Geriatr Soc 1993;41:868–869.
147. Anderson CJ, Kaufman PL, Sturm RJ: Toxicity of combined therapy with carbonic anhydrase inhibitors and aspirin. Am J Ophthalmol 1978;86:516–519.
148. Sweeney KR, Chapron DJ, Antal EJ, Kramer PA: Differential effects of flurbiprofen and aspirin on acetazolamide disposition in humans. Br J Clin Pharmacol 1989;27:866–869.
149. Insel PA: Analgesic-antipyretic and antiinflammatory agents and drugs employed in the treatment of gout. *In* Hardman JG, Limbird LE (eds): Goodman & Gilman's The Pharmacological Basis of Therapeutics, 9th ed. New York, McGraw-Hill, 1996, pp 617–657.
150. Ohno S, Char DH, Kimura SJ, O'Connor GR: Vogt-Koyanagi-Harada syndrome. Am J Ophthalmol 1977;83:735–740.
151. Forster DJ, Rao NA, Hill RA, et al: Incidence and management of glaucoma in Vogt-Koyanagi-Harada syndrome. Ophthalmology 1993;100:613–618.
152. Shirato S, Hayashi K, Masuda K: Acute angle closure glaucoma as an initial sign of Harada's disease: Report of two cases. Jpn J Ophthalmol 1980;24:260.
153. Kishi A, Nao-I N, Sawada A: Ultrasound biomicroscopic findings of acute angle-closure glaucoma in Vogt-Koyanagi-Harada syndrome. Am J Ophthalmol 1996;122:735–737.
154. Gandham SB, Spaeth GL, Di Leonardo M, Costa VP: Methazolamide-induced skin eruptions. Arch Ophthalmol 1993;111:370–372.
155. Shirato S, Kagay F, Suzuki Y, Joukou S: Stevens-Johnson syndrome induced by methazolamide treatment. Arch Ophthalmol 1997;115:550–553.
156. Cotter JB: Methazolamide-induced Stevens-Johnson syndrome: A warning! [letter, comment] Arch Ophthalmol 1998;116:117.
157. Klaver JH, Greve EL, Goslinga H, et al: Blood and plasma viscosity measurements in patients with glaucoma. Br J Ophthalmol 1985;69:765–770.
158. Trope GE, Salinas RG, Glynn M: Blood viscosity in primary open-angle glaucoma. Can J Ophthalmol 1987;22:202–204.
159. Joist JH, Lichtenfeld P, Mandell AI, Kolker AE: Low tension glaucoma: A microvascular thrombotic disorder due to blood hypercoagulability? Bibl Anat 1977;16:105–108.
160. Garcia-Salinas P, Trope GE, Glynn M: Blood viscosity in ocular hypertension. Can J Ophthalmol 1988;12:305–307.
161. Wolf S, Arend O, Sponsel WE, et al: Retinal hemodynamics using scanning laser ophthalmoscopy and hemorheology in chronic open-angle glaucoma. Ophthalmology 1993;100:1561–1566.
162. Shapiro S, Fraunfelder FT: Acetazolamide and aplastic anemia. Am J Ophthalmol 1992;113:328–330.
163. Lubeck MJ: Aplastic anemia following acetazolamide therapy. Am J Ophthalmol 1970;69:684–685.
164. Keisu M, Wiholm BE, Ost A, Mortimer O: Acetazolamide-associated aplastic anemia. J Intern Med 1990;228:627–632.
165. Fraunfelder FT, Meyer SM, Bagby GC Jr, Dreis MW: Hematologic reactions to carbonic anhydrase inhibitors. Am J Ophthalmol 1985;100:79–81.
166. Wisch N, Fischbein FI, Siegel R, et al: Aplastic anemia resulting from the use of carbonic anhydrase inhibitors. Am J Ophthalmol 1973;75:130–132.
167. Fraunfelder FT, Bagby GC: Possible hematologic reactions associated with carbonic anhydrase inhibitors. JAMA 1989;261:2257.
168. Mogk LG, Cyrlin MN: Blood dyscrasias and carbonic anhydrase inhibitors. Ophthalmology 1988;95:768–771.
169. Werblin TP, Pollack IP, Liss RA: Blood dyscrasias in patients using methazolamide (Neptazane) for glaucoma. Ophthalmology 1980;87:350–354.
170. Bergren RL, Brown GC: Neovascular glaucoma secondary to sickle-cell retinopathy. Am J Ophthalmol 1992;113:718–719.
171. Ferry AP, Font RL: Carcinoma metastatic to the eye and orbit. I: A clinicopathologic study of 227 cases. Arch Ophthalmol 1974;92:276–286.
172. Ferry AP, Font RL: Carcinoma metastatic to the eye and orbit. II: A clinicopathological study of 26 patients with carcinoma metastatic to the anterior segment of the eye. Arch Ophthalmol 1974;93:472–482.
173. Shields CL, Shields JA, Shields MB, Augsburger JJ: Prevalence and mechanisms of secondary intraocular pressure elevation in eyes with intraocular tumors. Ophthalmology 1987;94:839–846.
174. Kincaid MC, Green WR: Ocular and orbital involvement in leukemia. Surv Ophthalmol 1983;27:211–232.
175. Rosenthal AR: Ocular manifestations of leukemia: A review. Ophthalmology 1983;90:899–905.
176. Saga T, Ohno S, Matsuda H, et al: Ocular involvement by a peripheral T-cell lymphoma. Arch Ophthalmol 1984;102:399–402.
177. Shakin EP, Augsburger JJ, Eagle RC Jr, et al: Multiple myeloma involving the iris. Arch Ophthalmol 1988;106:524–526.
178. Char DH, Schwartz A, Miller TR, Abele JS: Ocular metastases from systemic melanoma. Am J Ophthalmol 1980;90:702–707.
179. Shingleton BJ, Bienfang DC, Albert DM, et al: Ocular toxicity associated with high-dose carmustine. Arch Ophthalmology 1982;100:1766–1772.
180. Miller DF, Bay JW, Ledesman RJ, et al: Ocular and orbital toxicity following intracarotid injection of carmustine and cisplatinum for malignant glioma. Ophthalmology 1985;92:402–406.
181. Fraunfelder FT: Drug-Induced Ocular Side Effects and Drug Interaction (3rd ed). Philadelphia, Lea & Febiger, 1989, pp 402–403, 405–407.

CHAPTER 18

Filtration Surgery and Tube Shunts

LOUIS B. CANTOR

In the treatment of the patient with glaucoma, surgical intervention is often necessary. In this chapter, Lou Cantor addresses the issues involved in the therapy of glaucoma using incisional filtration surgery. This therapy most commonly involves guarded filtration surgery, but tube shunts are also discussed. Dr. Cantor begins with the indications for filtration surgery and its current place in the therapeutic regimen. Intrinsic to the indications are the expected rate of success and the need for patient education. The process then proceeds through the preoperative evaluation, anesthesia, and the actual surgical technique of guarded filtration surgery. Dr. Cantor describes his technique, with alternatives and modifications when available, including the use of antimetabolites. He then deals with the implications of the different types of glaucoma on filtration surgery. No surgery is without potential complications, including filtration surgery. The chapter therefore includes a section addressing the prevention, recognition, and treatment of some more common complications of this procedure. They are more extensively addressed in Chapters 20 to 22, and 24. Tube shunts are then discussed: the available devices as well as the indications, technique, modifications, and complications of their use. Overall, this chapter is a complete discussion of filtration surgery for glaucoma.

Guarded Filtration Surgery

First described by Sugar[1, 2] and later successfully performed by Cairns[3] and Watson,[4, 5] guarded filtration surgery has become the procedure of choice in the surgical reduction of the intraocular pressure (IOP). Guarded filtration surgery lowers the IOP through the creation of a corneal-scleral fistula, which permits passive diffusion of aqueous humor into the subconjunctival space. Through the fistula, aqueous humor bypasses conventional outflow through the trabecular meshwork, Schlemm's canal, and episcleral veins, potentially lowering IOP below the episcleral venous pressure. The surgical ostium is covered with partial-thickness sclera, potentially decreasing the risk of complications associated with full-thickness procedures (hypotony, flat anterior chambers, endophthalmitis) without significantly compromising long-term intraocular pressure control.[6]

Filtration of aqueous humor into the subconjunctival space in most cases elevates the conjunctiva over the sclerotomy; the elevated conjunctiva is referred to as a *filtering bleb*. From within the bleb, aqueous humor diffuses through conjunctiva into the tear film, egresses through the conjunctival lymphatic system,[7, 8] or is absorbed by conjunctival blood vessels and aqueous veins. Histologic evaluation of a functioning bleb demonstrates loosely arranged subepithelial connective tissue interspersed with fluid-filled spaces that appear as microcysts on the bleb surface.[9]

DECISION FOR SURGERY

The goal of filtration surgery is the preservation of visual function and quality of life. Multiple studies demonstrate that surgically lowering IOP slows and often stabilizes progressive damage in glaucoma.[10–13] Reversal of disc excavation and improvement in the visual field after IOP reduction can also occur in selected cases.[14–17]

Surgical intervention is indicated when, despite maximally tolerated medical and laser treatment, the expected rate of optic nerve damage with the current IOP is likely to produce loss of visual function and quality of life during the patient's lifetime. Several factors are important in the assessment of a patient's risk of losing functional vision within his or her estimated life expectancy.

Initially, it is important to determine whether the patient's glaucoma is worsening at the current IOP. Progressive glaucomatous damage can be assessed by serial ocular and visual field examinations to evaluate the rate and extent of optic nerve damage and visual field loss. Equally valuable and often more sensitive is the patient's own sense of visual function; this is especially true in very early and very advanced glaucoma, in which optic nerve and visual field assessment is difficult and the findings often nonspecific. Questions such as, "Is your vision getting worse?" and "How are you seeing compared with your last visit, or even last year?" should be asked. Patients with progression of glaucoma may complain of "cloudiness" in their vision or some other nonspecific change before optic nerve fiber loss or decrease in visual field sensitivity can be detected by standard testing.

An estimation of risk factors predisposing to progression is also important when one is assessing the need for intervention (Table 18–1). The risk factors are:

1. *Severity of optic nerve damage and visual field loss.* Early to moderate glaucoma progresses over months to years, and an estimated 85% of patients retain central vision in at least one eye for life with medical treatment alone.[18–20] It may be prudent, therefore, to defer surgery in a patient with a short life expectancy and moderate glaucoma. Patients with advanced glaucomatous damage experience optic nerve and visual field loss at an accelerated rate; having lost a significant number of optic nerve axons, such patients have fewer redundant axons and experience more rapid loss of vision.[21, 22]
2. *Black race.* Clinical and epidemiologic studies suggest that glaucoma may be a more severe disease in black patients. They have glaucoma at an earlier age, demonstrate more advanced disease at time of diagnosis, and may be more sensitive to a given level of IOP, experiencing greater optic nerve damage and more rapid visual field loss at lower IOP.[23–26] Earlier and more aggressive intervention is recommended in this population.
3. *Family history.* Patients with a family history of glaucoma and, especially, visual loss from glaucoma manifest a greater risk for progression independent of the IOP.[24, 27, 28]
4. *IOP > 30 mm Hg.* High IOP is the most consistent risk factor for disease progression, with the probability of glaucomatous damage increasing with higher pressures.[19, 22, 27, 28]
5. *Fellow eye response.* The response of the fellow eye to treatment is helpful in determining appropriate management of the eye in question. If the fellow eye demonstrated progressive glaucomatous damage despite maximal medical treatment, early surgical intervention may be warranted in the eye in question. However, if the fellow eye underwent surgical treatment that involved a complicated procedure or postoperative course, the eye in question may be approached with more caution.

An estimation of a patient's life expectancy in the context of the severity of the glaucoma, the patient's risk for progression, and the patient's own sense of visual function allows the surgeon to individualize medical and surgical management. A white, elderly patient with moderate glaucomatous damage, elevated IOP, and evidence of slow progression may best benefit from presumably conservative medical management. Conversely, a young black patient with moderate damage and a family history of visual loss from glaucoma may be a candidate for earlier surgery.

TABLE 18–1. RISK FACTORS FOR PROGRESSION OF GLAUCOMA

Severity of disease
Black or Hispanic
Family history
Intraocular pressure >30 mm Hg
Progression in the fellow eye
Long life expectancy

MAXIMALLY TOLERATED MEDICATION AND LASERS

For most surgeons, three or sometimes four different classes of antiglaucoma medications that are well-tolerated and proven effective would constitute maximal medical therapy. If a class of medication is ineffective or is not tolerated or if the patient is noncompliant with medical treatment, alternative therapy is considered.

Some surgeons attempt IOP reduction with an argon laser trabeculoplasty (ALT) before surgical intervention if it will achieve the target IOP. Maximal treatment consists of 360-degree treatment of the angle. An ALT can be efficacious in lowering IOP in primary open-angle glaucoma (POAG), especially pseudoexfoliative and pigmentary glaucoma. It is of questionable benefit in patients with secondary glaucoma or in glaucoma associated with closed or recessed angles. In addition, as evidenced by the Glaucoma Laser Trial (GLT), the ALT does not offer the degree of long-term IOP control seen with filtration surgery. In the GLT, 56% of patients who received initial treatment with an ALT were taking medication within 2 years, with the average duration of effect of the ALT being less than 5 years.[29, 30] Furthermore, ALT is often unable to achieve the low IOP necessary to maintain visual function, commonly required in patients with normal-tension or advanced open-angle glaucoma.[31–33] Foregoing ALT and proceeding to earlier surgery may be prudent in some cases.

GUARDED FILTRATION SURGERY AS THE INITIAL MANAGEMENT OF GLAUCOMA

Though currently my colleagues and I do not advocate filtration surgery in the initial management of glaucoma, evidence does suggest that the procedure achieves a high rate of glaucoma control. Migdal[34] and Sherwood and colleagues[35, 36] have reported exceptionally high success rates, up to 98.2% at 5 years, with guarded filtration surgery as the initial treatment for glaucoma.

Failure of filtration surgery in most cases is secondary to subconjunctival fibroblast proliferation and resultant bleb fibrosis.[7] Studies show that long-term treatment with multiple topical antiglaucoma medications, in particular the sympathomimetics and miotics, can increase subconjunctival inflammatory mediators, including fibroblastic cells, which deleteriously affect postoperative IOP control.[37–42] This theory is not universally supported.[43, 44] The Collaborative Initial Glaucoma Treatment Study (CIGTS) currently under way will attempt to assess the effectiveness of surgery in comparison with medical treatment in the initial management of newly diagnosed POAG.[45]

In patients with moderate to advanced disease who are unlikely to respond to or comply with medical treatment, earlier filtration surgery is a viable option.

SURGICAL SUCCESS RATE

Guarded filtration surgery is the procedure of choice as primary intervention in the surgical management of most cases of glaucoma. Success rates of the procedure (generally defined as IOP < 22 mm Hg without medications) range from 60% to 98%.[46–51] Studies with long-term follow-up report 75% and 67% rates of success at 10 years and 15 years, respectively.[14, 52]

Comparison of success rates among reports is difficult because of the variations in criteria for success, diagnostic categories, patient demographics, follow-up periods, and surgical abilities. More important is a qualitative understanding of which group of patients are at greatest risk for failure of filtration surgery (Table 18–2).

The ideal candidates for filtration surgery are phakic, elderly white patients with POAG. Filtration surgery is less successful in eyes with secondary glaucomas, previously failed filters, or previous intraocular surgery, including cataract extraction. Patients with active uveitic glaucoma and neovascular glaucoma have the worst prognosis. Even in these patients at high risk for surgical failure, guarded filtration surgery is for the most part safer and more efficacious than alternative treatments, such as cyclodestructive or tube shunt procedures.[53, 54] Utilization of antimetabolite therapy has markedly increased success rates in high-risk cases, although with more complications (see later discussion of Antimetabolites).

The role of youth and race in success of filtration surgery is controversial. Younger patients (< 50 years) have a more exuberant Tenon's capsule and produce a more vigorous postoperative inflammatory response. In these patients, a higher incidence of bleb failure is reported in some studies.[47, 55] Other studies report no decrease in the overall success rate.[56, 57] Filtration surgery, nevertheless, plays an important role in younger patients, including those with congenital and juvenile glaucoma (see discussion of "Pediatric Considerations").[58–60]

TABLE 18–2. FACTORS ASSOCIATED WITH FAILURE OF FILTRATION SURGERY*

LOWER RISK
Chronic angle closure
Young age
Black race
Filtration failure in contralateral eye
Pseudophakia
Angle recession
Congenital glaucoma (± trabeculotomy/goniotomy)
HIGHER RISK
Aphakia
Previous failed filtration procedure
Peripheral anterior synechia associated/uveitic inactive
Iridocorneal endothelial syndrome
Sturge-Weber syndrome
Nanophthalmos
Previous vitreoretinal surgery
Active neovascularization
Active uveitis

*Factors listed in order of ascending risk.

Black patients also demonstrate a marked inflammatory response. Histologic comparisons of conjunctivae from black and white patients reveal a greater number of conjunctival macrophages and fibroblasts in black patients.[61] Filtration surgery in these patients, in our experience and that of others, has a lower likelihood of success.[62–66] This statement is not universally accepted.[67]

INFORMED CONSENT AND PATIENT EDUCATION

A discussion with the patient to outline surgical goals and the associated risks is one of the most important aspects of preoperative preparation. Many patients expect to see better after filtration surgery. Patients must understand that the primary objective is not to restore vision but to preserve remaining visual function. Whenever possible, family members who will participate in postoperative care are included in the preoperative discussions. Vision-threatening complications, such as suprachoroidal hemorrhage, endophthalmitis, permanent loss of central fixation, and progressive cataract formation, are discussed openly, as is the possible failure of the procedure to control IOP. The risks of filtration surgery are balanced against the probability, and rate, of further glaucomatous damage if no intervention is made. Anesthesia techniques and complications are also discussed. The patient is informed that compared with recovery from cataract surgery, the recovery period after filtration surgery may be prolonged, often necessitating frequent postoperative visits.[68]

PREOPERATIVE EVALUATION

In preparation for surgery, certain ocular and systemic medications should be discontinued. Topical adrenergic agents, such as dipivefrin and apraclonidine, may be discontinued to decrease preoperative conjunctival inflammation and vascularity. Miotics, including pilocarpine and echothiophate, are associated with breakdown of the blood-aqueous barrier and may be discontinued to decrease postoperative inflammation. Echothiophate also inhibits pseudocholinesterase and is therefore discontinued 2 weeks before patients undergoing general anesthesia with succinylcholine. Discontinuation of aqueous suppressants, such as beta-blockers, 1 week preoperatively may reduce postoperative hypotony and promote postoperative aqueous flow through the bleb. Antiglaucoma medications are discontinued with caution in patients with advanced visual field loss or who may be at risk for a suprachoroidal hemorrhage.

If medically possible, oral anticoagulants such as aspirin are discontinued to decrease the risk of an intraoperative bleeding diathesis. Hypertensive patients are instructed to take their medications the morning of the surgery.

Preoperative ocular evaluation should note the presence and location of conjunctival scarring, the extent and location of peripheral anterior synechiae in the angle, and the possibility of posterior capsule compromise that can predispose to intraoperative vitreous prolapse. Blepharitis, if present, is treated to reduce the incidence of ocular infection.

Patients with marked elevations in IOP may benefit from preoperative hyperosmotic agents, such as intravenous mannitol, to prevent a large intraoperative fall in IOP with surgical entry into the eye. Intraoperative ocular decompression has been associated with expulsive hemorrhages, aqueous misdirection, and serous choroidal detachments.

Though not our current practice, preoperative subconjunctival depot corticosteroids (e.g., 40 mg triamcinolone) and topical corticosteroids have been reported to be beneficial in eyes at high risk for postoperative bleb failure.[69, 70] Preoperative systemic corticosteroids should be considered in patients with uveitic glaucoma. Antibiotic prophylaxis given several days preoperatively is also advocated by some glaucoma surgeons.

ANESTHESIA

Filtration surgery can be performed with the patient under local or general anesthesia.

Local

In cooperative patients, local anesthesia offers several advantages. Limited systemic absorption makes it preferable in patients with poor health, especially those with pulmonary or cardiac disease. Local anesthesia has a low risk of malignant hyperthermia and is not associated with the postoperative nausea and vomiting seen after general anesthesia. We prefer a 50:50 mixture of 2% lidocaine and 0.5% bupivocaine. Lidocaine has a rapid onset of action (4 to 6 minutes), whereas bupivocaine provides prolonged efficacy (4 to 12 hours).

Four methods of local anesthesia can be performed:

1. *Retrobulbar.* A retrobulbar block provides excellent anterior segment anesthesia and akinesia. Three to 5-mL of the anesthetic is injected across the inferior orbital rim into the muscle cone. Because this technique involves the blind insertion of a needle behind the globe, complications involving direct trauma to posterior ocular and orbital tissues can occur (Table 18–3).[71–75]
2. *Peribulbar.* Peribulbar anesthesia potentially decreases (but does not eliminate) some of the risks associated with retrobulbar blocks. The anesthetic is injected outside the muscle cone, presumably away from the extraocular muscles, optic nerve, and posterior globe.[76] This technique can result in suboptimal anesthesia and akinesia, and often, more than 7 mL of the anesthetic is required for maximal efficacy. The larger anesthetic volume in the retrobulbar space is reported in some cases to significantly elevate the IOP,[77, 78] an effect of particular concern in patients with glaucoma. In a patient with a bleeding diathesis, both peribulbar and retrobulbar injections should be used with caution to decrease the risk of a severe retrobulbar hemorrhage.
3. *Subconjunctival.* Subconjunctival anesthesia in filtration surgery has been advocated to avoid the complications of retrobulbar or peribulbar injection. Anesthesia comparable to that of a retrobulbar block is reported in multiple prospective randomized studies. Patients have only limited akinesia.

   Topical tetracaine 0.5% is applied to the eye. With the patient looking down, 2 mL of anesthetic is injected with a 30-gauge needle beneath Tenon's capsule, 8 mm posterior to the limbus and either over the superior rectus muscle or into the superotemporal quadrant.[79–81] A 19-gauge cannula directed posteriorly over bare sclera can be used to apply supplemental anesthetic, if necessary, during the procedure. A corneal traction suture is recommended, because a superior rectus bridle suture can be painful with this technique.
4. *Topical.* Topical anesthesia (tetracaine or proparacaine, 0.5%) without subconjunctival infiltration can be successfully used in fornix-based filtration surgery. In contrast to the partial akinesia caused by subconjunctival anesthesia, patients have complete eye movement with topical anesthesia. Although the iridectomy is surprisingly well tolerated, electrocautery can be painful.

General

General anesthesia is indicated in patients likely to cooperate poorly (i.e., children, demented or psychotic patients) or with strong patient preference. Systemic anesthetic agents can affect IOP. Inhalation anesthetics, in particular

TABLE 18–3. COMPLICATIONS OF RETROBULBAR AND PERIBULBAR ANESTHESIA

Globe perforation
Retrobulbar hemorrhage
Optic nerve injection[71]
Subarachnoid infiltration with brain stem paralysis
Extraocular muscle restriction
Systemic absorption (cardiopulmonary compromise)
Central retinal artery/vein occlusion

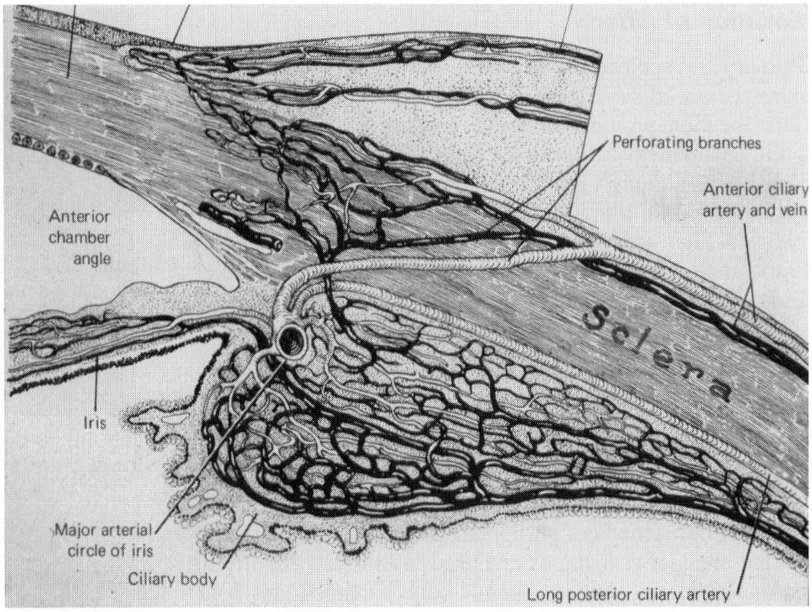

FIGURE 18–1. Anatomy of the surgical site. (From Kolker AE, Hethrington J (eds): Becker-Shaffer's Diagnosis and Therapy of the Glaucomas, 5th ed. St. Louis, CV Mosby, 1983.)

halothane, and amnestic agents, such as Diprivan, can reduce IOP. Succinylcholine, a depolarizing muscle relaxant, can transiently increase IOP secondary to sustained extraocular muscle contraction. Echothiophate, as already mentioned, can significantly prolong the action of succinylcholine and should be discontinued 2 weeks prior to surgery. General anesthesia is avoided in patients at risk for a suprachoroidal hemorrhage, as endotracheal intubation is associated with postoperative nausea and emesis.

ANATOMY

Conjunctiva and Tenon's Capsule

The conjunctiva begins posteriorly at the mucocutaneous junction of the eyelid and extends to the cornea, inserting anterior to the corneal-scleral sulcus. The junction between the cornea and sclera creates an indentation resulting from the difference in the radius of curvature between the two tissues (Fig. 18–1). Superiorly, the conjunctiva overhangs clear cornea, giving the cornea a horizontally elliptical shape. From limbus to limbus the adult cornea measures on average 11 mm vertically and 12 mm horizontally. The next-deeper tissue is Tenon's capsule, which although posteriorly a distinct layer, fuses with the conjunctiva and episclera at the limbus, inserting just posterior to the corneal-scleral sulcus. In children, Tenon's capsule is more prominent, becoming atrophic with age.

Limbus

The limbus represents the transition zone between the sclera and cornea. The surgical limbus is widest superiorly and inferiorly (~2 mm) and narrows nasally and temporally. Bluish white scleral tissue begins posteriorly over the iris root and scleral spur and extends anteriorly over Schlemm's canal and the trabecular meshwork. The blue-white scleral zone transitions anteriorly to a blue-gray translucent zone representing clear corneal tissue.

FILTRATION TECHNIQUE

It is important to follow certain general principles during a guarded filtration procedure:

- □ Achieve meticulous hemostasis to minimize fibroblast-inducing blood products.
- □ Use nontoothed instruments (e.g., straight dressing forceps) when holding the conjunctiva to prevent buttonholes.
- □ Minimize tissue manipulation to decrease fibroblast proliferation.
- □ Avoid multiplanar cuts or ragged edges when incising conjunctival or scleral tissue; sharp, linear cuts provide better wound apposition.

Our preferred technique for performing a superior guarded filtration procedure is presented here. The choice of suture material, blade type, forceps, and the like can vary according to the individual surgeon's preference and experience (Table 18–4).

Microscope

The operating microscope head is obliquely turned to reduce macular phototoxicity. The use of coaxial lighting should be minimized.

TABLE 18–4. PREFERRED TECHNIQUE OF GUARDED FILTRATION SURGERY

Traction suture
Conjunctival peritomy (limbus- or fornix-based)
Hemostasis
Antimetabolite application
Partial-thickness flap
Paracentesis
Formation of sclerotomy
Iridectomy
Suture flap
Closure of conjunctiva
Re-formation of anterior chamber

Location of Filter

Primary trabeculectomy in an eye without previous procedures is placed superiorly near the twelve o'clock position. This location provides adequate spacing for possible temporal cataract extraction in the future. Nasally placed filtration blebs, although successful, are associated with higher risk of discomfort and dellen formation.[82] Inferiorly placed blebs, which are prone to exposure and trauma and are associated with a several-fold greater incidence of bleb leaks and endophthalmitis, should be avoided.[83–86]

Assessing Conjunctival Scarring

Filtration surgery is most successful when performed in unscarred conjunctiva. The location and severity of conjunctival scarring ultimately determine the procedure site. Several techniques can be used to assess conjunctival mobility. A moistened cotton-tipped applicator applied to suspected areas of scarring can be used to estimate underlying conjunctival movement. Alternatively, balanced salt solution (BSS) can be injected beneath Tenon's capsule to "balloon up" the conjunctiva and Tenon's complex and to identify areas of scarring. In areas that do not elevate, tissue has been scarred down to the sclera. We employ this assessment technique in all eyes with previous ocular procedures.

TECHNIQUE

One to 2 mL of BSS is injected through a 30-gauge needle or cannula into sub–Tenon's space near the initial incision of a limbus-based flap (if possible, through the traction suture site), elevating the conjunctival and Tenon's capsule tissues (Fig. 18–2). Anesthetic can instead be injected, if necessary, to provide additional analgesia.

Traction Suture

The traction suture allows posterior conjunctival exposure and fixation of the globe.

SUPERIOR-RECTUS TENDON TRACTION SUTURE

A Lester or Elschnig forceps is brought from above with its teeth open and is pressed onto the conjunctiva, grasping

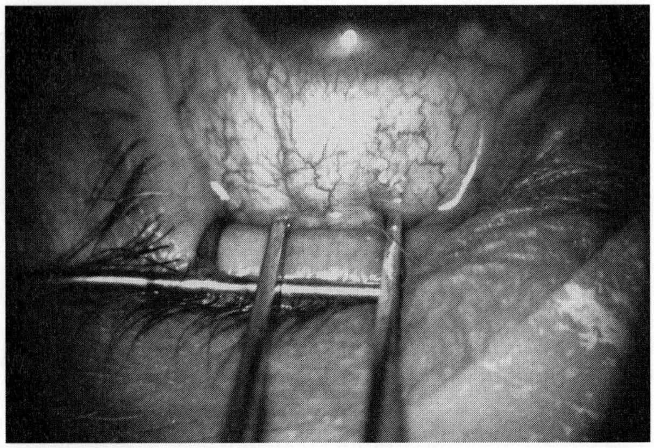

FIGURE 18–3. With a muscle hook depressing the inferior fornix, the superior rectus tendon is posteriorly grasped.

the superior rectus tendon at least 9 mm posteriorly (Fig. 18–3). Two large ciliary arteries signify the location of the tendon. The globe can be infraducted with a muscle hook by an assistant to provide greater posterior exposure. The tendon is lifted off the globe, and a 4-0 silk or similar suture on a tapered needle is passed under its belly (Fig. 18–4). The needle tip is directed away from the globe to minimize the risk of perforation. The suture is clamped on the forehead drape, rotating the eye down.

This technique allows isolation of the superior rectus tendon, decreasing the risk of tendon transection during conjunctival flap dissection. Its disadvantages include the risk of perforating a vascular tendon or the globe. The superior rectus tendon traction suture has also been implicated in the pathogenesis of postoperative ptosis.

CORNEAL FIXATION TECHNIQUE

Alternatively, a 7-0 Vicryl or similar suture on a cutting needle can be passed through the superior cornea at 50% depth. The suture is clamped onto the drape below to infraduct the globe. If the suture is placed too deep, inadvertent perforation of the cornea can occur. If placed too shallow, the suture can cheese-wire through the superficial cornea with complete loss of effect.

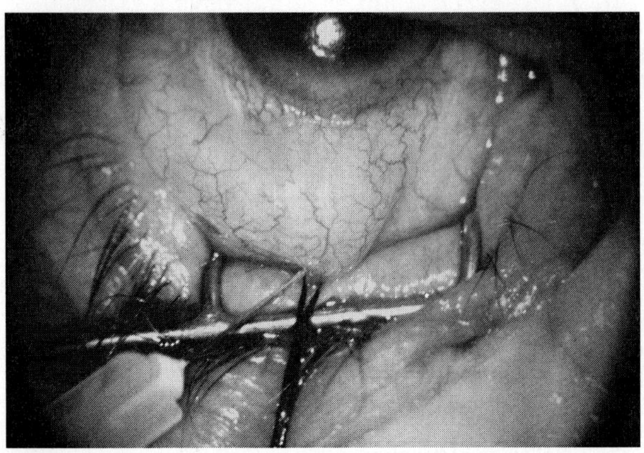

FIGURE 18–2. Injection of the subconjunctival and Tenon's space with a 30-gauge needle and balanced salt solution.

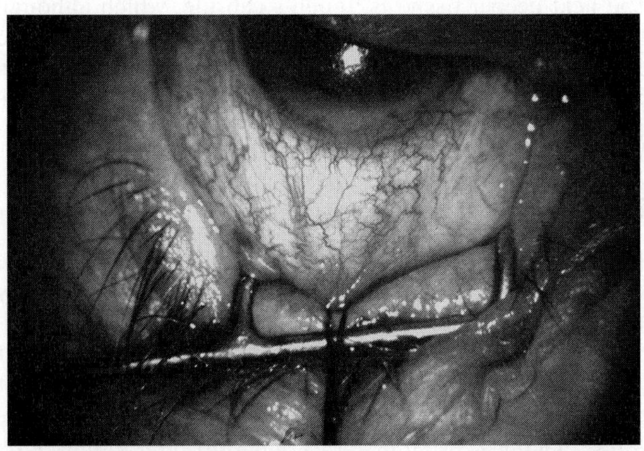

FIGURE 18–4. A 4-0 silk suture under the superior rectus tendon.

Conjunctival Flap

The initial step in filtration surgery is the dissection of conjunctival and episcleral tissues to expose bare corneal-scleral tissue. Limbus-based or fornix-based dissection can be performed. Limbus-based flaps are considered to have a lower risk of wound leak because of the posterior placement of the incision and are associated with a high focal bleb morphology. Fornix-based flaps may be associated with increased incisional leaks but in most studies are reported to have equal efficacy and complication rates.[87–91] The fornix-based approach is faster and less traumatic, providing excellent limbal exposure. Fornix-based flaps tend to produce low-lying, more diffuse blebs, because there is no posterior limiting incision line. We prefer the limbus-based approach for the theoretical security it offers for wound closure, especially in patients being treated with adjunctive antimetabolite agents.

LIMBUS-BASED INCISION TECHNIQUE

With nontoothed forceps, the conjunctiva is tented up over the tendon at least 8 mm posterior to the limbus. A buttonhole snip opening is made in the conjunctiva with Westcott scissors and extended one to two "clock hours" to either side with a sharp cut, parallel to the limbus and as high into the fornix as possible. This should be the last time the conjunctiva is grasped until incision closure (Fig. 18–5).

An incision is made into Tenon's capsule at the same site and extended the full length of the conjunctival incision. One to 2 mm anterior to the muscle insertion, the underlying episclera is then opened to bare sclera and extended the full length of the wound.

When incising tissues, the surgeon should ensure that both scissors blades are well visualized and are lifted up away from the superior rectus tendon to prevent sharp dissection into the tendon.

The Tenon's capsule–episcleral tissue flap is gently reflected and dissected anteriorly toward the cornea. Connective tissue adhesions to bare sclera can be broken by means of blunt dissection with a dry cellulose sponge (Fig. 18–6). Disinsertion of Tenon's capsule and episcleral tissue at the limbus often requires blade dissection, particularly in eyes with previous procedures. We prefer the dull edge of a No. 67 blade held perpendicular to the globe and swept sideways (as if strumming a guitar) to gently break these tight adhesions. A semilunar fold of tissue may appear on the undersurface of conjunctiva when the episcleral tissue–Tenon's capsule flap is disinserted (Fig. 18–7). Further dissection is performed with care to avoid conjunctival disinsertion. The end-point of dissection is visualization of the blue-gray of the limbal corneal tissue and the insertion of the conjunctiva into cornea.

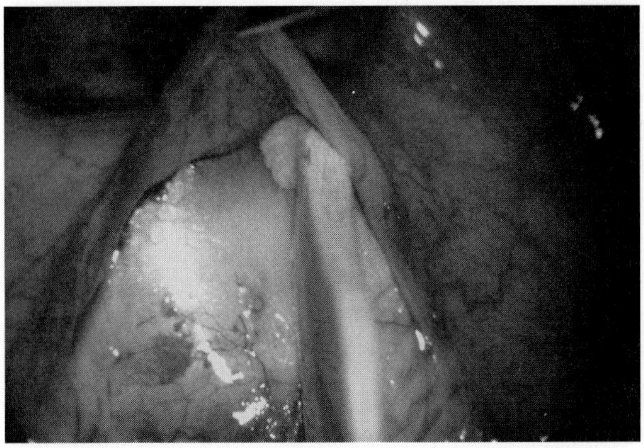

FIGURE 18–6. Blunt dissection with a dry cellulose sponge.

Hemostasis

Meticulous hemostasis is achieved throughout the procedure by means of fine-point electrocautery (Fig. 18–8). Blood, a stimulant for inflammatory factors, increases the risk of subconjunctival fibrosis. Vessels in the area of the scleral flap are lightly cauterized. Direct cautery to the conjunctiva is avoided except along the cut edge.

Scleral Flap

A partial-thickness scleral flap provides resistance to aqueous outflow through the sclerotomy, resulting in a more controlled reduction in IOP. Although many different flap shapes and sizes can be successful, all flaps should be

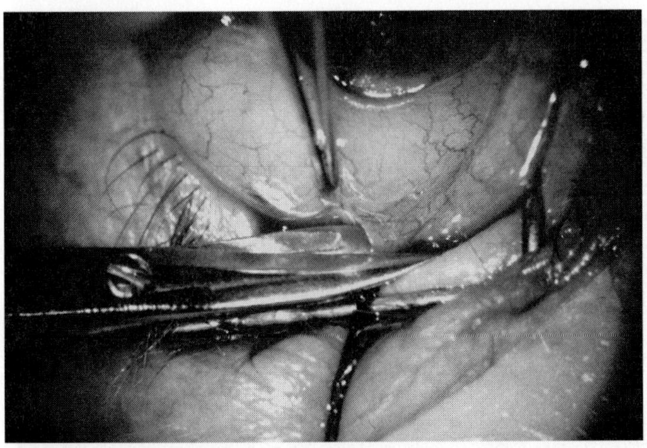

FIGURE 18–5. A conjunctival opening is made 8 mm posterior to the limbus. Note that the conjunctival tissue is lifted off the globe before the incision.

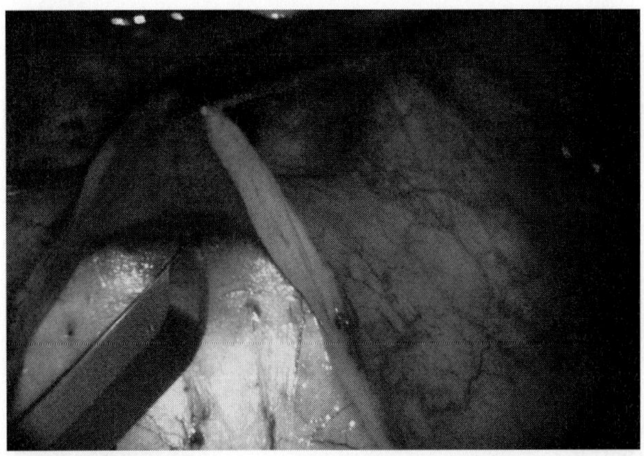

FIGURE 18–7. The blunt edge of a No. 67 blade performing tissue dissection. Note the semilunar fold on the conjunctiva with Tenon's tissue disinsertion.

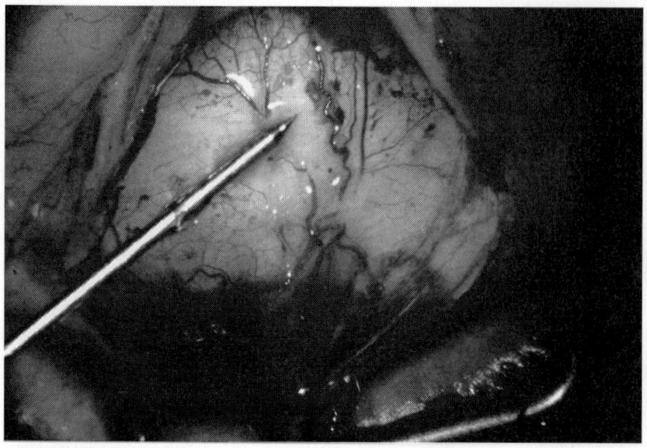

FIGURE 18–8. Fine-point electrocautery achieving hemostasis.

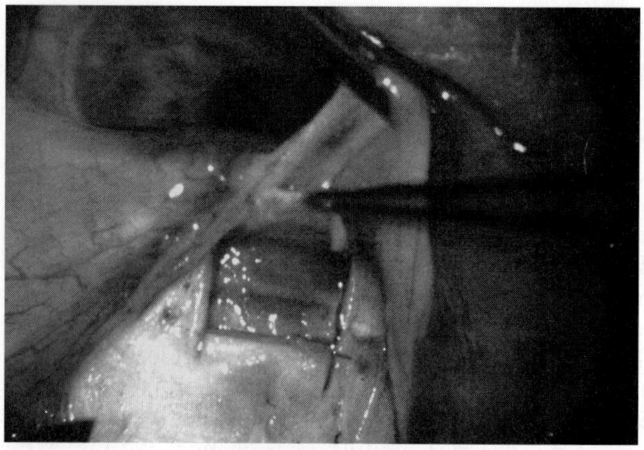

FIGURE 18–10. A dissected flap. Note that the anterior translucent corneal tissue is angled slightly upward.

approximately one half to two thirds of the scleral thickness and should be dissected into the perilimbal clear cornea. Thin flaps easily macerate and offer less resistance to aqueous outflow, increasing the incidence of hypotony. Posteriorly placed flaps can result in an opening over the ciliary body.

TECHNIQUE

Beginning as far anteriorly as possible, we use a No. 67 or similar size blade to incise an approximately 3 × 4-mm partial-thickness scleral flap to the desired depth. At a posterior corner, the sclera is lifted, and with the use of firm strokes, a lamellar dissection is performed. Firm strokes ensure sharper flap edges and better wound apposition (Fig. 18–9). As the flap is carried forward, the pearly white sclera transitions to a bluish white zone representing the area over the trabecular meshwork. Schlemm's canal resides at 90% depth in the junction between the opaque and blue-white sclera; if unroofed, the canal appears as a dark brown, narrow band.

The blue-white sclera transitions to a translucent zone representing the anterior clear cornea. The translucent cornea reflects the color of the underlying iris and is a dark blue-gray in patients with pigmented irides. The radius of curvature abruptly steepens at the corneal-scleral junction (Fig. 18–10). The dissecting blade should be angled upward to keep it parallel with the globe and prevent premature entry into the globe. The lamellar dissection is carried 1 to 2 mm into clear cornea. The sclera is kept dry during dissection to provide maximal visualization. Cautery, if necessary, is used judiciously to minimize shrinkage of the scleral bed and edges, thereby preventing wound gape.

Paracentesis

Before the fistula is created, a self-sealing paracentesis is made. The paracentesis provides access to the anterior chamber for both intraoperative and postoperative chamber re-formation.

TECHNIQUE

A 25-gauge needle (5/8-inch) on a tuberculin syringe is inserted at a plane parallel with the iris, 1 to 2 mm through clear cornea into the anterior chamber. It is directed inferiorly, away from the pupil margin, to prevent inadvertent lens trauma (Fig. 18–11). A sharp eye knife can also be used, particularly with soft eyes.

Internal Block Excision

Creation of the fistula involves the removal of corneal-scleral tissue. The sclerotomy should extend anteriorly

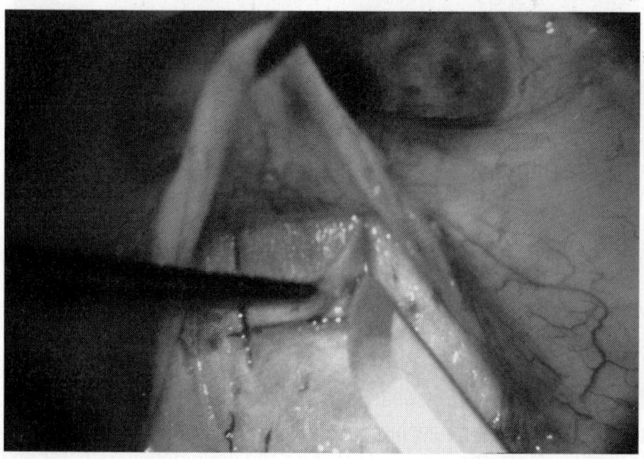

FIGURE 18–9. Dissection of the scleral flap with a No. 67 blade.

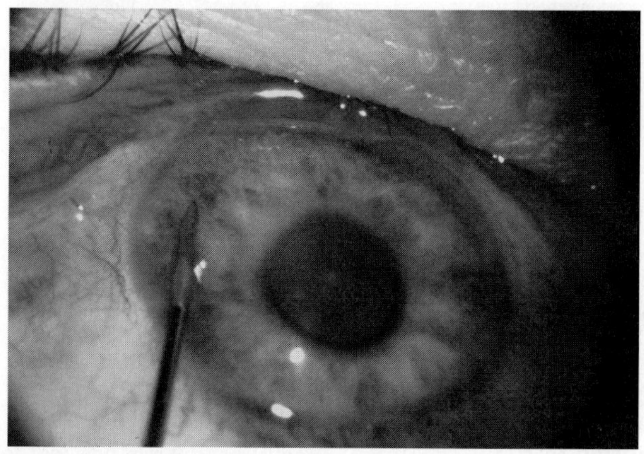

FIGURE 18–11. A 25-gauge needle creating a paracentesis. Note that the needle is directed away from the pupil margin.

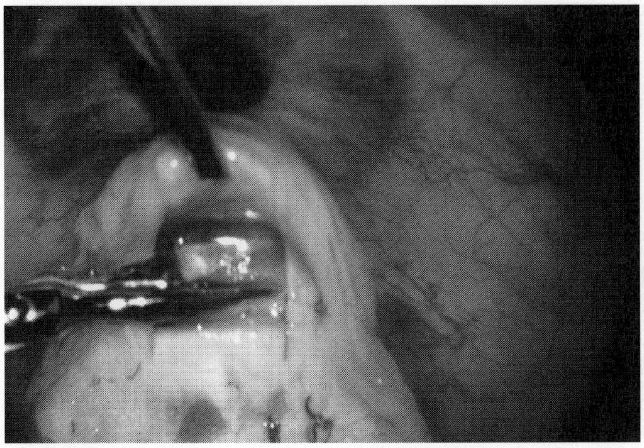

FIGURE 18–12. Excision of the scleral block by Vannas capsulotomy scissors. The blades should be turned perpendicularly prior to the incision.

from perilimbal clear cornea to the posterior blue-white scleral tissue of the limbus, so that it overlies trabecular meshwork. More posterior resection risks an opening over ciliary body and choroid, increasing the likelihood of ciliary body bleeding, cyclodialysis, or vitreous prolapse.

In addition, the flap size relative to sclerotomy size allows some control of outflow. The more the flap overlaps the sclerotomy, the less the flow. Maximal outflow occurs in a sclerotomy extended to the flap edge.

TECHNIQUE

A radial incision starting anteriorly in clear cornea is made with a sharp blade through one edge of the corneal-scleral bed. The blade should penetrate full-thickness through Descemet's membrane. One blade of Vannas capsulotomy scissors is introduced through the incision and slid to the posterior edge of the blue-white limbal zone (Fig. 18–12). Care is taken to avoid incorporation of iris between the blades. With the scissors positioned perpendicularly to avoid a beveled incision, a horizontal straight-edge cut is made. The remaining sclerotomy edges are similarly incised (Fig. 18–13). If prolapsing iris is encountered, a small iridotomy facilitates it to fall back into the anterior chamber.

Alternatively, a sclerotomy can be formed with the use of a Kelly–Descemet membrane punch. An iris plane incision is made into the anterior chamber through the anterior clear cornea with a sharp blade. The tip of the punch is inserted under the posterior internal edge of the corneal wound, avoiding incorporation of iris. With the instrument lifted toward the microscope to ensure that the tip is snug to the underlying tissue, a punch is made, creating a semicircular hole. Multiple similar bites are taken to create an adequate opening.

Iridectomy

A broad-based peripheral iridectomy is created wider than the sclerotomy to prevent iris from obstructing the ostium and prevent postoperative pupillary block.

TECHNIQUE

With toothed forceps, iris is pulled up gently through the sclerotomy. With scissors (e.g., Vannas or DeWecker) positioned parallel with the limbus, the iris is cut horizontally at its base (Fig. 18–14). The pupil is visualized to avoid an inadvertent sector iridectomy. Patients with large pupils can be given intracameral acetylcholine chloride (Miochol) or preoperative topical pilocarpine to decrease this risk. Elevating the iris too far out of the sclerotomy can result in an inadvertent resection of the highly vascularized ciliary body. Visualization of the iridectomy is important to ensure that it is patent and of adequate size relative to the sclerotomy. The iris is repositioned in the eye by gentle stroking on the cornea from the limbus centrally.

Suturing the Flap

The number of sutures and the tension on each suture determine the level of aqueous outflow and thus early postoperative IOP. Some surgeons prefer to avoid any hypotony and therefore place multiple, tight flap sutures, performing selective suture lysis postoperatively if necessary to achieve target IOP. We prefer a relatively low postoperative IOP and therefore place only two sutures to reappose the scleral flap in most patients. In patients with advanced disease that would be intolerant of any increase in IOP, fewer or looser sutures can be considered to reduce the risk of postoperative IOP elevations.

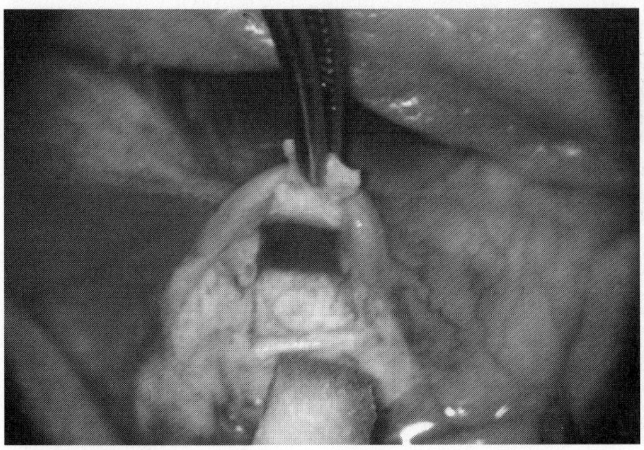

FIGURE 18–13. A completed sclerotomy. Note that the edge of the sclerotomy extends to the scleral flap margin in this patient.

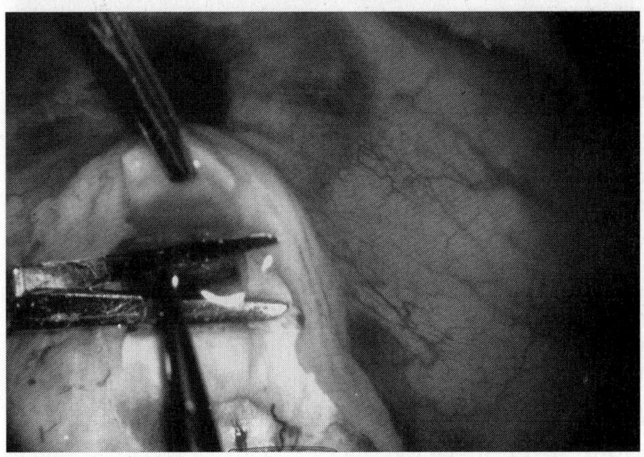

FIGURE 18–14. Dewecker scissors resecting the iris at its base.

TECHNIQUE

Nonabsorbable sutures (e.g., 10-0 nylon) are sutured into sclera diagonally, through the posterior corners of the flap (Fig. 18–15). Long suture tracts facilitate postoperative suture lysis. The tension in each suture should be just enough to lay the flap edge flat on the scleral bed. Suture knots are rotated into the sclera. BSS is injected through the paracentesis to assess flow through the filtration site. With this technique, filtration should occur through the anterior edges of the flap. A firm globe after chamber re-formation may indicate inadequate outflow. Electrocautery applied to the anterior edges of the scleral flap can induce scleral shrinkage and increase outflow. We find a 23-gauge cautery tip to be particularly effective in this regard. A recurrent flat anterior chamber and low IOP despite re-formation with BSS may indicate too great a flow through the sclerotomy, requiring tighter or additional flap sutures.

Conjunctival Closure

Essential in suturing of the conjunctiva is a watertight closure. We prefer closing Tenon's capsule and conjunctival tissue in separate layers to increase wound security. A tapered, rounded vascular needle (e.g., Ethicon BV-130) decreases the likelihood of leakage from suture tracts.

TECHNIQUE

Tenon's capsule is closed with the use of an 8-0 Vicryl or other absorbable suture on a vascular needle in a running fashion with locking bites. The suture is brought out through the conjunctiva. The conjunctiva is closed in a running fashion in the opposite direction without locking bites. The incision line in limbus-based flaps often demarcates the posterior extent of the bleb. Only a 1-mm bite at the anterior conjunctival edge is taken to avoid displacing the incision anteriorly toward the limbus (Fig. 18–16). The anterior chamber is re-formed with BSS, and a bleb should form (Fig. 18–17). If a bleb does not form, the scleral flap may be sutured too tightly (IOP high) or there may be a wound leak (IOP low). Fluorescein can be used to detect incisional or conjunctival buttonhole leaks.

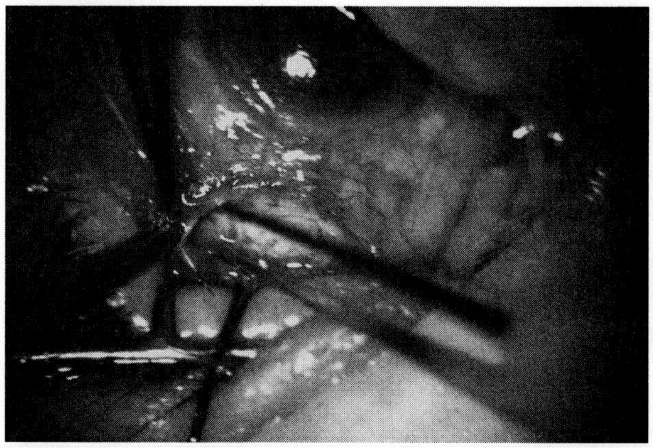

FIGURE 18–16. Conjunctiva is sutured closed with a tapered needle.

Intraoperative Medications

Topical atropine 1% is started after the flap is sutured to paralyze the pupillary sphincter and ciliary muscles and to stabilize the blood-aqueous barrier. Pupillary dilation decreases the formation of posterior synechiae, and ciliary muscle paralysis moves the lens iris diaphragm posteriorly, deepening the anterior chamber and decreasing the risk of aqueous misdirection. At the completion of the procedure, an antibiotic-steroid combination and atropine ointment are placed in the eye. If subconjunctival antibiotics or steroids are contemplated, the injection should be given with a small needle into the fornix, away from the surgical site, to prevent reflux into the eye or intrableb hemorrhages or leaks.

SURGICAL MODIFICATIONS

Fornix-Based Flaps

Fornix-based filtration surgery is reported to be equally effective in controlling IOP. Advantages of this technique include easier and less traumatic anterior conjunctival dissection, which is especially helpful in patients with conjunctival scarring. In addition, disinsertion of the conjunctiva provides excellent exposure of the corneal-scleral sulcus and anterior cornea.

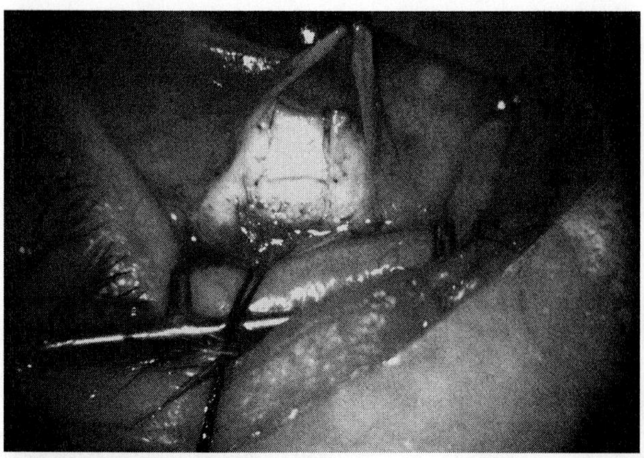

FIGURE 18–15. Scleral flap sutured down with two nylon sutures at each posterior corner.

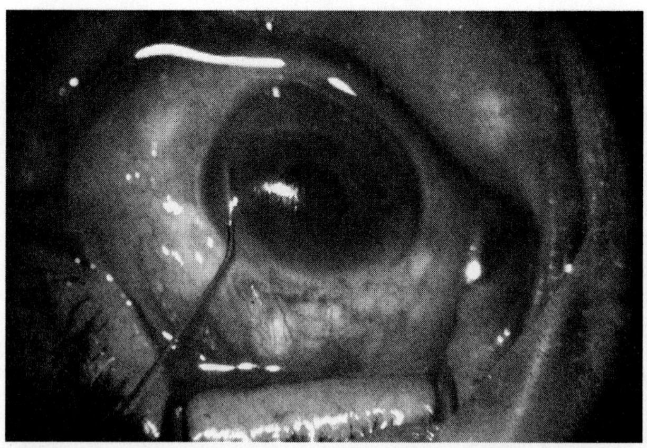

FIGURE 18–17. Re-formation of the anterior chamber, with the formation of a filtering bleb.

Traditionally, fornix-based flaps were thought to carry a greater risk of incisional leaks at the limbus, particularly in procedures utilizing topical antimetabolites. With modern suture techniques, the reported incidence of incisional leakage in these flaps compares favorably to that for limbus-based flaps.[87, 92]

INCISION OPENING

Nontoothed forceps and Wescott scissors are used to perform a conjunctiva–Tenon's capsule peritomy three to four "clock hours" wide at the limbus, exposing bare sclera. Radial relaxing incisions are made at each end to allow posterior reflection of the flap.

INCISION CLOSURE

The corneal epithelium at the limbus is removed with a sharp blade or cautery to prevent epithelium from obstructing the postoperative adhesion between conjunctiva and cornea. The conjunctival flap is pulled taut 2 to 3 mm over the anterior cornea. A Vicryl or similar suture is passed through the episclera parallel to the limbus and out through the conjunctiva at one edge of the flap. The suture is tied and the short end cut. The radial incision is then closed in a running fashion. The other flap edge is similarly closed. In procedures employing adjunctive antimetabolite therapy, vertical and running mattress suture techniques are reported to provide watertight closure.[92, 93]

Tenonectomy

The effectiveness of excising Tenon's capsule is controversial. Tenon's capsule, which is particularly exuberant in black and young patients, may induce fibroblast proliferation after surgical trauma. Its removal may therefore be beneficial in reducing postoperative bleb scarring. Removing Tenon's capsule can also facilitate postoperative suture lysis. However, two studies comparing guarded filtration surgery with and without a tenonectomy demonstrated no difference in postoperative IOP.[7, 94] Neither black, young, nor high-risk patients were studied, however. A tenonectomy in patients receiving adjunctive antimetabolites increases the risk of bleb leaks, hypotony, and wound gape and is considered with caution.

Antimetabolite Therapy

The topical antimetabolites mitomycin C (MMC) and 5-fluorouracil (5-FU) have significantly improved the success of filtration surgery in patients at risk for filtration failure.[95] Glaucoma surgery most commonly fails secondary to fibrosis of the episcleral, Tenon's capsule, and conjunctival tissue.[7, 96] Both 5-FU and MMC limit the conjunctival and scleral fibroblast proliferation associated with bleb fibrosis, albeit at the cost of increased complications.[7, 97]

5-FLUOROURACIL

A fluorinated pyrimidine analogue, 5-FU selectively inhibits the DNA synthesis phase of the fibroblast cell cycle, decreasing fibroblast proliferation.[98] The effect of 5-FU on cellular inhibition is temporary. Partial recovery of subconjunctival and scleral fibroblastic activity is seen in rabbit models within 30 days.[99, 100] This feature may limit the effectiveness of 5-FU and perhaps, correspondingly, its long-term complications. Complications reported with 5-FU include an increase in late-onset bleb leaks (9% vs. 2% without 5-FU),[101, 102] endophthalmitis (see later discussion), delayed suprachoroidal hemorrhage, and chronic hypotony.[103]

POSTOPERATIVE USE. Postoperative subconjunctival injection of 5-FU is reported in multiple studies to increase the success rate of filtration surgery.[104] The Fluorouracil Filtering Surgery Study Group reported that in patients at high risk for failure of the procedure, the overall success rate at 5 years increased two-fold with filtration and postoperative 5-FU (48%) compared with that of surgery without the adjunct (21%).[101, 105–108] High success rates (>95%) have been reported for the use of postoperative 5-FU in phakic patients with uncomplicated glaucoma.[109, 110]

Postoperative subconjunctival 5-FU injections are associated with a high incidence of corneal epithelial defects and risk of globe perforation and are labor-intensive, requiring frequent postoperative visits.[111–115, 116]

INTRAOPERATIVE USE. Animal and clinical studies have demonstrated that a single-exposure topical intraoperative application of 5-FU may be beneficial.[99, 100, 107, 117–120] Clinical investigations assessing filtration surgery using intraoperative topical 5-FU[121, 122] report efficacy equal to that of postoperative subconjunctival 5-FU in primary and complicated glaucoma.[123–125] Short-term prospective randomized studies comparing intraoperative applications of 5-FU and MMC report equal efficacy in low-risk[126] and high-risk[127] patients as well as potentially fewer complications. Clinically, blebs associated with the use of intraoperative 5-FU are not as avascular or thin-walled as those seen with the use of MMC.[117]

Advantages of applying 5-FU intraoperatively rather than postoperatively include ease of application and decreases in postoperative corneal toxicity and discomfort. The risks of hypotony, bleb leaks, and endophthalmitis remain. Supplemental injections of 5-FU can still be given postoperatively, with dosage titrated according to bleb appearance, IOP, and anterior chamber depth.

MITOMYCIN C

MMC, an antineoplastic antibiotic isolated from *Streptomyces caespitosus*, demonstrates long-lasting suppression of cellular activity in all cycles of fibroblast proliferation and collagen synthesis.[97, 128, 129] Animal studies show MMC to be 100 to 300 times more potent than 5-FU in inhibiting fibroblast synthesis and proliferation.[97, 130] Moreover, MMC-treated conjunctiva and sclera are devoid of fibroblasts on histopathologic analysis, indicating fibroblast cell death[96, 131] rather than just inhibition of proliferation. Marked disruption of tissue cytoarchitecture and epithelial acellularity is also noted.[132–135] These changes appear to be localized to the area treated.[136]

There is also evidence suggesting that MMC may penetrate intact sclera[137] and cornea. This agent has been found in aqueous humor after topical application and has been shown to be directly toxic to the ciliary body epithelium, perhaps resulting in persistent aqueous hyposecretion.[96, 97, 100, 134, 138–140] In addition, MMC may be toxic to blood vessel endothelium, rendering conjunctival tissue avascular.

Clinically, MMC-associated blebs are cystic, avascular,

and thin-walled with increased permeability, often with multifocal areas of transconjunctival aqueous "oozing" apparent on Seidel's testing (Fig. 18–18).

INTRAOPERATIVE MMC. Since its introduction by Chen and then Palmer as an adjunct to filtration surgery, intraoperative MMC has demonstrated superior IOP reduction,[141–143] and longer bleb survival in both low-risk[144, 145] and high-risk[146, 147] glaucoma with less corneal epithelial toxicity. Conversely, MMC has been reported to have significant complications.

Prolonged hypotony, hypotony maculopathy, increased rates of early and late bleb leaks, and endophthalmitis are well-documented.[85, 86, 146, 148] An accelerated rate of cataract formation[149, 150] and a higher risk of scleritis in inferiorly placed MMC blebs[151] are also reported.

MMC is also potentially devastating to intraocular contents. Rabbits receiving intraocular MMC demonstrate dense corneal edema with endothelial cell loss, iris and ciliary body necrosis, and damage to both the retinal pigment epithelium (RPE) and optic nerve.[152] Ciliary body necrosis and endothelial cell loss have been documented in humans.[150, 153, 154]

INDICATIONS FOR ANTIMETABOLITE THERAPY

The indications for adjunctive antimetabolite therapy in patients undergoing filtration surgery are as follows:

1. High risk of failure of filtration surgery[143, 155–159] (see Table 18–1).
2. Normal-tension glaucoma (NTG).
3. Advanced glaucoma. In patients with NTG or advanced POAG, a target IOP of less than 12 mmHg is often required for stabilization of visual function. Such patients would benefit from the low IOP offered by antimetabolite therapy.[31–33, 160–162]
4. Refractory congenital glaucoma. Success rates as high as 86.7% have been reported with MMC-associated filtration surgery in congenital glaucoma not responsive to previous goniotomy or trabeculotomy.[163, 164]
5. Secondary congenital glaucomas.[59, 60, 165]
6. Juvenile glaucoma (see "Pediatric Considerations").
7. Concurrent ocular surgery. Adjunctive antimetabolites (in particular MMC) have improved success of filtration surgery in patients undergoing other concurrent procedures (e.g., penetrating keratoplasty, vitreoretinal surgery).[166, 167]

TECHNIQUES OF 5-FU THERAPY

POSTOPERATIVE INJECTIONS. In general, 5 mg of 5-FU is injected subconjunctivally beginning on the first postoperative day, and dosage and frequency of administration are adjusted thereafter according to the patient's risk factors for surgical failure and bleb appearance (see later discussion on filtration surgery failure). The relationship between the total 5-FU dose and dosing schedule and the rates of success and complication is not clear. The 14-day duration of treatment used in the Fluorouracil Filtering Surgery Study was based in part on the timing of bleb fibrosis in monkey and rabbit animal models.[95, 97, 168, 169] The total dose of 105 mg of 5-FU administered in the study, although effective, was associated with a high rate of corneal complications. Fewer injections and a lower total dose are now advocated.[109, 110, 170, 171]

Four injections in low-risk cases and up to 10 injections in high-risk cases can be given over 2 weeks. Treatment should be deferred or discontinued in patients with conjunctival leaks or corneal epithelial defects.

SUBCONJUNCTIVAL INJECTION. A 0.1-mL dose is drawn into a tuberculin syringe from a vial concentration of 50 mg/mL. This 5-mg dose is injected with a 30-gauge needle subconjunctivally placed 180 degrees away from the filtration site. The entry site can be anesthetized with an anesthetic pledget to decrease discomfort. The needle is advanced 1 cm beyond the entry site to decrease reflux of 5-FU onto the cornea. Leakage from the entry site is the major cause of corneal epitheliopathy.

INTRAOPERATIVE APPLICATION. Intraoperative 5-FU is applied topically to bare sclera through the use of a cellulose sponge delivery system at a concentration of 50 mg/mL

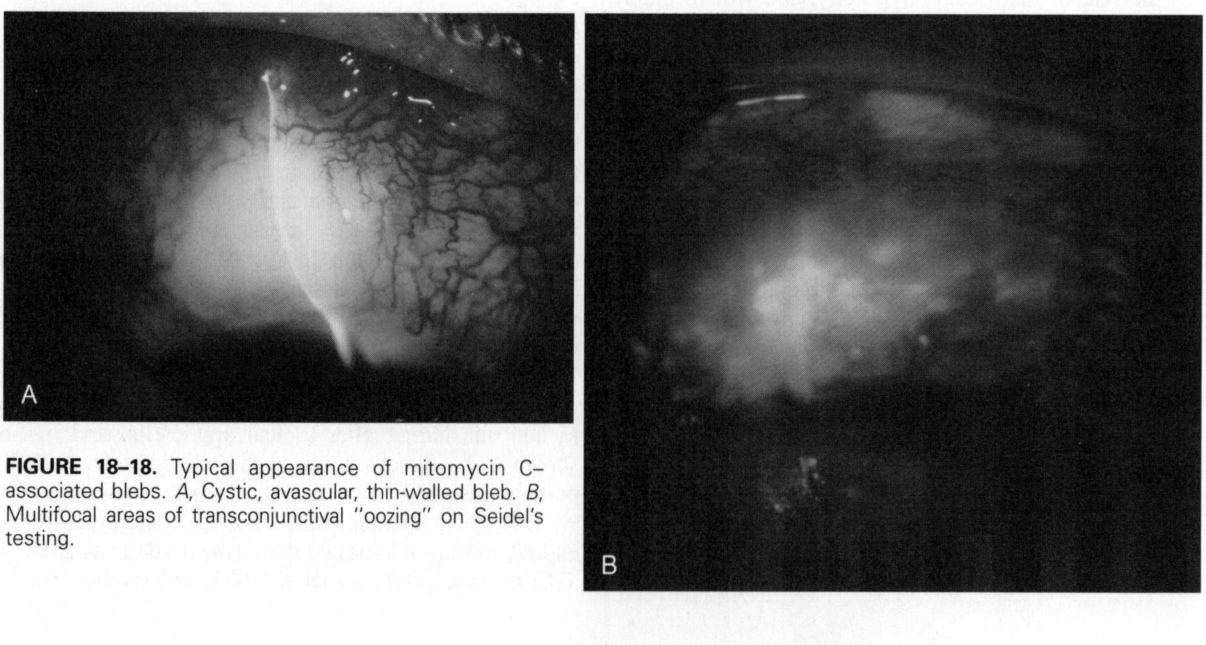

FIGURE 18–18. Typical appearance of mitomycin C–associated blebs. *A*, Cystic, avascular, thin-walled bleb. *B*, Multifocal areas of transconjunctival "oozing" on Seidel's testing.

for 5 minutes. The technique of delivery is similar to that described later for MMC.

TECHNIQUES OF MITOMYCIN C THERAPY

TITRATING DOSAGES. The dosage of MMC should be titrated according to the patient's risk for failure of filtration surgery and achievement of target IOP. There is no consensus in the literature about the ideal concentration of intraoperative MMC or the application time.[172] Prolonged application or high concentrations of MMC theoretically can result in thinner blebs with greater risks of hypotony and infections. Though MMC was initially used at a concentration of 0.5 mg/mL for 5 minutes, subsequent studies of filtration surgery with MMC report equal efficacy with lower concentrations and shorter exposure times.

Several studies suggest that varying the MMC concentration is more important in adjusting duration of application. Kitazawa and associates[173] have shown in randomized studies that varying MMC concentrations directly affects postoperative IOP control. Jampel[128] found a 68% inhibition of cultured human fibroblast during the first minute of exposure to MMC. Further exposure may therefore have only marginal incremental effects on fibrosis. Clinical studies by Megevand and colleagues[175] and Cohen and associates[174] reported no difference in success rates with varied MMC exposure times in filtration surgery.

Conversely, other studies support varied exposure time. In a prospective study by Robin and coworkers,[148] the duration of exposure appeared to be more important than MMC concentration in achieving the postoperative IOP target.

Currently, when titrating the application of MMC, we prefer a uniform exposure time of 2 minutes. We vary MMC concentration, using 0.2 mg/mL for our low-risk patients and 0.4 mg/mL in patients at higher risk for failure of filtration surgery.

Many factors (sponge type, area treated, and amount of irrigation) affect the actual dose of MMC delivered to tissue.[176] The inexperienced surgeon should initially consider using a lower concentration and shorter exposure time until individual technique results can be determined.

APPLICATION. Both fornix-based and limbus-based procedures are reported to be efficacious for the use of MMC. We believe the limbus-based approach provides a more secure closure. A fluid-retaining sponge (i.e., cellulose sponge) is put in a solution of MMC. The sponge then is placed most anteriorly (posteriorly in fornix-based flaps) onto bare sclera with conjunctiva, and Tenon's capsule is draped over it (Fig. 18–19). Care is usually taken to prevent wound edges from contacting the sponge. Constant pressure is applied to the sponge to allow continued egress of the MMC during exposure time, minimizing the variable release of solution that can occur with different sponges. We apply the MMC prior to flap dissection and irrigate the sclera copiously with two 30-mL bottles of BSS after its application to reduce intraocular penetration.[177] All disposable products that have come into contact with MMC are deposited in a toxic waste container.

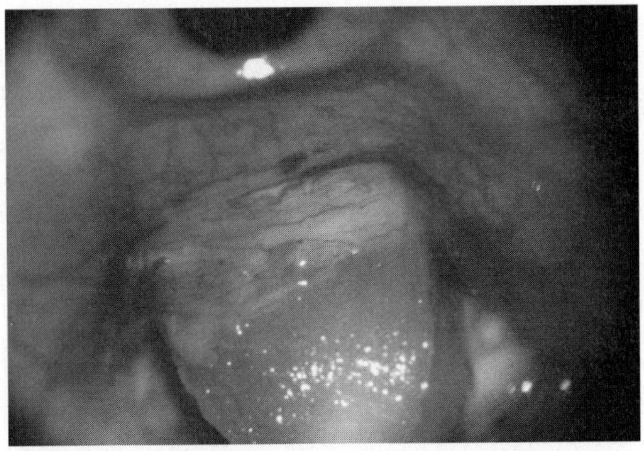

FIGURE 18–19. A cellulose sponge soaked with mitomycin C is placed under Tenon's tissue, onto bare sclera, advanced to the limbus.

Releasable Sutures

Postoperative removal of scleral flap sutures allows the surgeon to achieve tight flap closure intraoperatively with the assurance that filtration can be increased postoperatively. Multiple effective techniques, including externalized mattress sutures and slipknots, are reported and the reader is referred to the chapter references for the details of surgical methods.[178–182] Suture release is most effective in decreasing IOP if it is done within the first 2 weeks, although efficacy of this method is reported even when it is performed months after filtration surgery with antimetabolites. Patient cooperation is important for ease of suture removal. Sutures that are not released can be trimmed or removed.

The advantages of releasable sutures include ease of postoperative suture removal, especially if a laser is not available or if suture visualization is limited by exuberant or hemorrhagic conjunctival–Tenon's capsule tissue. However, placement of the sutures requires more intraocular manipulation and risks lens trauma and intraocular hemorrhage during suture passage. In addition, scleral flap tear and dehiscence can occur during both placement and removal of the sutures. Externalized sutures can produce discomfort and are potential wicks for intraocular infections.[183–185]

Viscoelastic Agents

Intracameral viscoelastics (e.g., sodium hyaluronate) applied intraoperatively can help maintain anterior chamber depth in the first 2 to 4 postoperative days. Presumably, during this time, ciliary body function increases and early conjunctival fibrosis occurs, reducing the risk of a shallow chamber. Higher-molecular-weight viscoelastics are cleared more slowly by the trabecular meshwork and may provide longer chamber maintenance.

Several studies recommend introduction of viscoelastics prior to excision of the internal scleral block, to avoid any intraoperative hypotony that can potentially initiate the pathophysiologic process of choroidal effusions.[186–188] Although the incidence of choroidal detachments and flat chambers is reportedly decreased with this technique, it renders an intraoperative assessment of aqueous outflow through the sclerotomy difficult.

Alternatively, viscoelastic agents can be injected into the anterior chamber at the conclusion of the procedure. Several studies report this method effective in decreasing the risk of postoperatively flat chamber,[47, 186, 189, 190] although the incidence of choroidal detachments and rate of long-term IOP control remain unchanged.[190, 191]

We prefer a relatively loose closure of the scleral flap, and we inject viscoelastic at the conclusion of surgery in the majority of cases. In our experience, the introduction of a higher-molecular-weight viscoelastic, such as Healon GV (5 million daltons), can be effective in maintaining anterior chamber depth during the immediate postoperative period.

Obstruction of the trabecular meshwork by sodium hyaluronate can result in significant postoperative elevations in IOP, most commonly within the first 24 hours.[192]

SURGICAL CONSIDERATIONS

Neovascular Glaucoma

In patients with neovascular glaucoma, panretinal photocoagulation should be applied to decrease the stimulus for fibrovascular proliferation and possibly to induce regression of angle neovascularization. The sclerotomy should be created more anteriorly to avoid vascularized trabecular meshwork tissue and synechiae. The use of adjunctive antimetabolites has significantly increased the success of filtration surgery. MMC minimizes the extensive scarring associated with fibrovascular proliferation and is reported to induce regression of rubeosis.[193]

Nonetheless, despite the best treatment, surgical treatment using any modality has a poor prognosis in neovascular glaucoma. Even with adequate IOP control, patients continue to lose visual function, commonly from retinal causes. Overall, it is our experience that in inflamed eyes with active rubeosis, tube shunt procedures provide the best chance for long-term IOP control and visual preservation, especially in young patients with neovascular glaucoma.[105]

PAS-Associated Glaucoma

Filtration surgery in glaucoma with peripheral anterior synechiae (PAS), such as primary angle-closure glaucoma and uveitic glaucoma, has a lower success rate than in POAG. In a patient with PAS, the scleral flap is dissected farther into clear cornea to avoid anteriorly displaced angle structures. In addition, the sclerotomy must open anterior to PAS to function maximally. Preoperative gonioscopy should be performed to identify areas of open angle. Filtration surgery should be directed toward these areas.

Primary Angle-Closure Glaucoma

Patients with shallow anterior chambers or narrow angles are at a greater risk for flat chambers and aqueous misdirection postoperatively.[194] Tighter flap sutures or use of anterior chamber viscoelastic can help maintain postoperative anterior chamber depth. Cycloplegic agents should be initiated early intraoperatively[129] and continued postoperatively. Suture lysis is performed judiciously to prevent the rapid IOP reductions associated with aqueous misdirection.

Uveitis

Antimetabolites have significantly improved success rates in patients with uveitic glaucoma, especially in perioperatively inflamed eyes.[155, 157] Uveitic eyes should be quieted with subconjunctival, topical, or oral corticosteroids, or a combination, as much as possible before surgery.[68] An adequate peripheral iridectomy should be performed to prevent inflammatory occlusion with pupillary block. Subconjunctival (dexamethasone, 4 mg) and even intraocular injection (dexamethasone, 400 μg/0.1 mL) of corticosteroids is considered at the end of the procedure. Postoperatively, the patient should be started on intensive topical and, for severely inflamed eyes, oral corticosteroids.

Aphakia

The success rate of filtration surgery in aphakic eyes, especially in younger patients, is notoriously poor, ranging from 5% to 62%.[195–197] Topical antimetabolites, especially MMC, have substantially increased the overall success rate. It is important to minimize vitreous prolapse and to perform an anterior vitrectomy on any presenting vitreous. Vitreous is believed to change the biochemical structure of aqueous humor, reducing its ability to inhibit fibroblasts[197] and thereby increasing conjunctival scarring. In addition, anterior chamber vitreous may obstruct the ostium. For these reasons, a pars plana vitrectomy has been advocated as a treatment option in several reports.

Intraoperative vitreous prolapse can be minimized by medical constriction of the pupil. Early and frequent use of a viscoelastic agent is recommended as well for tamponade of the vitreous face. Viscoelastic agents can also help maintain IOP, reducing hypotony and potentially decreasing the high risk of a suprachoroidal hemorrhage associated with aphakia.

Pediatric Considerations

Most surgeons reserve guarded filtration surgery for infants with congenital glaucoma for whom goniotomy or trabeculotomy has failed.[58, 60] Success rates reported in this group range from 50% (filtration without antimetabolites)[58, 60] to 94.7% (with adjunctive MMC).[164, 165] Several studies report a high rate of success (86.7% to 92%) with filtration surgery as primary treatment.[59, 163, 198] These studies for the most part do not provide long-term data, which are critically important in younger patients.

When operating on children, the surgeon must remember that the anterior chamber angle is not fully developed until age 12 months. Landmarks such as limbal coloration are less evident. In buphophthalmic eyes, the anatomy is further distorted. In addition, perilimbal infant sclera is fragile and thin, increasing the likelihood of premature entry into the anterior chamber.

INTRAOPERATIVE COMPLICATIONS

Suprachoroidal Hemorrhages

Patients undergoing filtration surgery are at increased risk for an intraoperative or delayed suprachoroidal hemorrhage (SCH). Rapid decompression of the globe during a paracentesis or formation of a sclerotomy may induce shearing forces that can tear the posterior ciliary arteries as they enter the suprachoroidal space.

The incidence of intraoperative SCH in glaucoma surgery is approximately 1.6%,[199, 200] and that of delayed SCH, 2% to 4.7%. History of aphakia especially with previous vitrectomy significantly increases the risk (6.6% to 33%).[199–201] An elevated preoperative IOP and postoperative hypotony are also major risk factors. Other reported ocular risk factors are increased axial length, SCH in the fellow eye, and disorders with elevated episcleral venous pressure, such as Sturge-Weber syndrome. The association of 5-FU and delayed SCH may be related to the hypotony seen after filtration surgery with antimetabolite therapy.[200, 202]

Systemic associations include hypertension, advanced atherosclerosis, advanced age, anticoagulant use, and intraoperative tachycardia.[203, 204] Perioperative and postoperative Valsalva maneuvers, such as during coughing and emesis, which are often associated with general anesthesia, can also increase the risk of hemorrhage.

Intraoperative signs of a SCH may initially be subtle. There may be loss of the red reflex. Patients may complain of increased pain despite previously adequate anesthesia. Persistent shallowing of the anterior chamber occurs in association with globe firmness, wound gape, and tissue prolapse.

Immediate closure of the incision is imperative. Tamponade can be applied to the wound with a finger until incision closure with a large-diameter, highly tensile suture can be accomplished. Shallow chambers are re-formed with viscoelastic or air (BSS can leak out the sclerotomy).

If wound closure is accomplished, drainage of the suprachoroidal space can be deferred to reduce the likelihood of further hemorrhaging.

Delayed SCH occurs more frequently and usually manifests within the first 2 postoperative weeks as acute severe ocular pain and marked decrease in vision. Slit-lamp examination reveals a shallow anterior chamber with increased IOP. Funduscopy demonstrates a dark-domed elevation of the choroid with high internal reflectivity on B-scan ultrasonography. SCH is often preceded by serous choroidal effusions.

SCH confined to one or two quadrants can be managed medically. Frequent topical corticosteroids are initiated to decrease inflammation and the risk of retinal adhesions.

Indications for surgical drainage of SCH are:

- Intractable pain
- Uncontrolled IOP
- Recurrent flat chamber
- Massive hemorrhage
- Retinal apposition

In general, one needs to allow 1 to 2 weeks for clot liquefication, as confirmed by B-scan ultrasonography.[205]

Preventive steps should be taken in patients at high risk for a SCH. Preoperatively, blood pressure and IOP should be maximally controlled; if medically possible, anticoagulants, including aspirin, are discontinued. Intraoperatively, local anesthesia should be used, scleral flap sutures placed before incising the trabeculectomy block, and a slow, controlled paracentesis performed to slowly decompress the globe. Tight flap sutures should be considered to reduce postoperative hypotony. Postoperatively, the patient is started on stool softeners and warned to avoid lifting heavy items and stooping. Nausea or coughing is aggressively treated.

Visual prognosis in an intraoperative SCH is best if the eye can be closed without extrusion of retina or uveal tissue.[206] Factors associated with poor visual prognosis are retinal detachment, 360-degree hemorrhage,[203] prolonged retinal apposition (>2 weeks),[207] vitreous incarceration, and vitreous or subretinal hemorrhage. Although the patient with a limited SCH, confined to one or two quadrants, can do well, only 29% to 40% of patients with appositional or massive SCH regain preoperative visual acuity.[203, 207, 208]

Conjunctival Buttonholes

Conjunctival buttonholes occur most commonly in older patients with thin tissue, though all patients are at risk. The conjunctiva should be examined intraoperatively under high magnification to identify holes or tears. Intraoperatively detected buttonholes should be closed immediately to prevent enlargement during further conjunctival manipulation. If a large buttonhole is identified early in the procedure, selecting a new surgical site may be prudent. Thought should be given to deferring antimetabolite therapy.

Methods of closure depend on the location of the tear. Initially, the conjunctiva is carefully examined to delineate the edges of the tear. Holes within the bleb are closed with a pursestring or mattress suture using a 10-0 monofilament nylon or similar suture on a vascular needle (e.g., Ethicon BV-130[209]) (Fig. 18–20). A large conjunctival opening can be managed with a compression suture technique.[210] If limbal disinsertion of the conjunctiva occurs in a limbus-based flap, the conjunctiva can be resutured to the cornea with interrupted buried mattress sutures. An intraoperative Seidel's test with fluorescein dye should be used to verify adequate closure. Conjunctival tissue distant from the surgical site can be harvested if needed as a patch graft.

Scleral Flap Complications

Scleral flap complications occur most commonly during flap dissection. Thin, superficial flaps can tear or avulse.

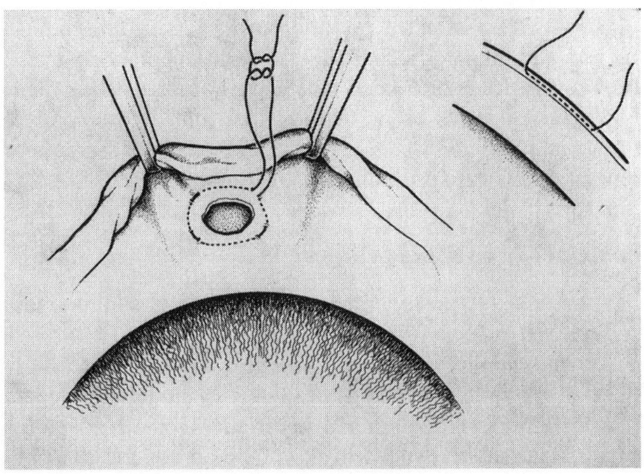

FIGURE 18–20. Pursestring suture closure of a conjunctival buttonhole. (From Sherwood MB, Spaeth GL (eds): Complications of Glaucoma Therapy. Thorofare, NJ, Slack, Inc., 1990, p 216.)

An avulsed flap can be repaired with the use of two horizontal mattress sutures passed from the scleral flap at each anterior corner and out through the cornea, creating a hinge.[211] Alternatively, donor sclera or cadaveric pericardium can be sutured over the sclerotomy to form a new flap.[212] Buttonholes within flaps are sutured closed or tamponaded with Tenon's capsule tissue.

Deeply dissected flaps can result in a premature entry into the anterior chamber or posterior perforation over the ciliary body. A superficial dissection of the overlying sclera can be performed, and the deeper scleral layer sutured back to the posterior lip of the sclerotomy.

Vitreous Through a Sclerotomy

Vitreous can protrude through a posteriorly placed sclerotomy, especially in eyes with a history of trauma, in aphakic patients, and in pseudophakic patients with compromised zonules or posterior capsular tears. Vitreous can mechanically obstruct a sclerotomy, increasing the risk of filtration failure.

Patients at risk for vitreous prolapse should be assessed preoperatively for the presence of anterior chamber vitreous or possible vitreous behind the iris in the intended iridectomy site. If this situation is anticipated, introduction of viscoelastic substance early in the procedure is recommended. Vitreous in the anterior chamber or prolapsed through the sclerotomy should be treated with a thorough mechanical vitrectomy.

POSTOPERATIVE MANAGEMENT

Postoperative Evaluation

Patients are examined on the first postoperative day. A complete anterior and posterior examination is performed with special attention given to the appearance of the bleb, the IOP, and the anterior chamber depth. The ideal bleb should appear elevated, diffuse, and relatively avascular with conjunctival microcysts. Though only corticosteroids have been proven efficacious in the postoperative management of the filtering bleb, we prefer to start our patients on a topical regimen of cycloplegic, anti-inflammatory, and anti-infectious agents.

Patients are instructed not to do any heavy lifting, bending, or straining, especially those with hypotonous eyes. They are instructed to keep protective coverings over their eyes (whether glasses or eye shields) and are seen in 1 week; intervals between visits are lengthened thereafter, depending on the appearance of the surgical site.

Postoperative Medications

Our regimen for postoperative medications is summarized in Table 18–5.

TABLE 18–5. POSTOPERATIVE MEDICATION REGIMEN FOR FILTRATION SURGERY

Medication	Daily Frequency	Duration
Atropine 1%	2	1–4 weeks
Phenylephrine 2.5%	2	1–2 weeks
Broad-spectrum antibiotic	4	4 weeks
Prednisolone acetate 1%	4	4 weeks, tapering thereafter

MYDRIATIC-CYCLOPLEGIC AGENTS

Postoperative cycloplegic and mydriatic agents help minimize inflammation by stabilizing the blood-aqueous barrier. These agents paralyze the ciliary body, thereby decreasing discomfort, and put the zonules on stretch to help maintain a deeper anterior chamber. In addition, dilating the pupil decreases posterior synechiae that can form in an inflamed eye. We currently prescribe atropine sulfate 1% twice daily postoperatively. For inflamed eyes or eyes with miotic pupils, we add phenylephrine 2.5% twice daily to enhance pupillary dilation. Discontinuation of these agents is performed judiciously on the basis of anterior chamber depth, intraocular inflammation, and level of patient discomfort.

CORTICOSTEROIDS

Postoperative use of topical corticosteroids is associated with a more cystic bleb morphology and greater long-term IOP control.[12, 213, 214] Corticosteroids inhibit factors involved in the early phases of inflammation and demonstrate a dose-dependent inhibition of fibroblast proliferation.[7] Oral prednisone does not appear to provide any additional benefit over topical steroids except perhaps in patients with uveitis. Topical cyclo-oxygenase inhibitors such as indomethacin and flurbiprofen have also not been proven beneficial.[215, 216] We recommend prednisolone acetate 1% four times per day for 2 to 4 weeks, tapering the dosage thereafter according to bleb appearance and degree of intraocular inflammation.

PROPHYLACTIC ANTIBIOTICS

A broad-spectrum antibiotic (i.e., trimethoprim–polymyxin B or fluoroquinolone) is recommended as prophylaxis for postoperative endophthalmitis.[217] No antibiotic has been proven more efficacious in preventing a bleb-related infection.[218] We prefer the fluoroquinolones because of their broad spectrum of activity and intraocular penetration.[217] Antibiotics are continued for 2 to 4 weeks.

EARLY POSTOPERATIVE COMPLICATIONS

Complications and bleb failure can occur at any time in the postoperative period, with diverse presentations. A failing bleb may have increasing IOP and may appear low-lying with few microcysts or, if encapsulated (Tenon's cyst), may have a high-domed shape. Conversely, a low IOP associated with bleb leakage can also predispose to failure. Appropriate postoperative diagnosis and management are essential in establishing long-term filtration.

High Postoperative IOP

High postoperative IOP can occur at any time and is usually due to decreased outflow through the filtration site. Bleb encapsulation, aqueous misdirection, SCH, and

TABLE 18–6. CAUSES OF ELEVATED INTRAOCULAR PRESSURE AFTER FILTRATION SURGERY

Bleb Height	Anterior Chamber	Diagnosis
High	Deep	Encapsulated bleb
Low or flat	Deep	Obstruction/fibrosis
High or low	Shallow	Aqueous misdirection Suprachoroidal hemorrhage Pupillary block

pupillary block can all be associated with elevated postoperative IOP (Table 18–6).

BLEB FIBROSIS OR OBSTRUCTION

NONPATENT SCLEROTOMY. The management of filtration failure early postoperatively depends on the location of aqueous outflow obstruction. Reduced filtration may be due to closure of the internal sclerotomy by iris, blood, fibrin, vitreous, or lens capsule. Gonioscopy should be performed to evaluate the sclerotomy site in all patients with increased IOP. Careful examination of the ostium is important because thin membranes can be easily missed.

Management. Intraocular inflammation, if present, should be treated with frequent use of topical corticosteroids. Adherent iris tissue and obstructing membranes can be opened with Nd:YAG laser therapy (2 to 7 mJ) applied to the internal ostium. Particular attention is given to the edges of the scleral flap, where the majority of filtration occurs.[219] Digital ocular massage may also be attempted.

Obstructing fibrin or blood can be dissolved with intracameral tissue plasminogen activator (tPA) (7 to 15 μg/0.1 mL), injected through a paracentesis under slit-lamp guidance.[220–222] Effects of tPA are usually seen within 1 to 3 hours, hyphema being the most common complication.

PATENT SCLEROTOMY. A more common cause of IOP elevation in the early postoperative period is bleb failure secondary to conjunctival and episcleral fibrosis. Failing blebs demonstrate denser, more compact collagenous tissue with increased fibroblasts and blood vessels on histologic examination.[7] Signs of early bleb failure include increasing IOP, diffuse conjunctival injection, anterior migration of the limbus-based incision line, and the presence of large rope-like vessels. The filtering bleb is often thickened and low-lying with reduced microcysts. Anterior chamber inflammation, subconjunctival hemorrhage, or an exposed suture, if present, can accelerate bleb fibrosis. The anterior chamber should be deep and the sclerotomy patent on gonioscopy.

Management. Topical corticosteroid therapy should be initiated or increased in frequency to reduce inflammation and fibroblast activity.[213] Subconjunctival injections of 5-FU (5 mg) may be given to suppress fibroblast proliferation, with treatment adjusted according to clinical signs of early bleb failure.[171] Although 5-FU is most effective during the first 2 postoperative weeks, improved bleb function is reported with 5-FU injections given 26 days postoperatively.[223]

Laser suture lysis or removal of releasable sutures can be performed to increase aqueous outflow. Laser suture lysis (or suture release) is usually effective only in the initial 2 to 4 postoperative weeks.[224–229] In MMC-enhanced filters, suture lysis is reported to be successful 6 months postoperatively.[230, 231] The longer the interval between surgery and suture lysis, the smaller the reduction in IOP.[232] Sustained hypotony with overfiltration has been reported with suture lysis following MMC-associated surgery.[233] Therefore, a single suture should be cut per session to minimize this risk.

We use a specially designed Hoskins lens or a Zeiss 4-mirror gonioscopy lens to flatten and blanch the overlying conjunctiva. An argon laser with a 50-μm spot size, 200 to 700 mW power, and 0.1-second duration is usually sufficient to cut the suture. If a subconjunctival hemorrhage is present over the suture, use of a krypton laser is recommended to decrease laser energy absorption by the blood, thereby reducing the risk of a conjunctival buttonhole.[234]

Ocular compression after suture lysis or release can further enhance aqueous outflow.[235] Pressure is applied to the scleral flap edge either with a finger through the eyelid or directly on the eye with a moistened cotton-tipped applicator, removing obstructing debris and elevating the bleb. If these maneuvers are not successful, needle puncture of the bleb and scleral flap in conjunction with supplemental 5-FU injections can in some cases improve filtration.[236–238] Revision of the fibrosed sclerotomy with a holmium:YAG laser or erbium laser is also reported successful.[239]

ENCAPSULATED BLEBS

An encapsulated filtering bleb or "Tenon's cyst" develops in 8% to 28% of patients after guarded filtration surgery without adjunctive antimetabolites. Predisposing risk factors are[240–243]:

- Male sex
- Previous use of topical sympathomimetics or beta-blockers
- Previous ocular procedures
- Prior ALT
- History of fellow eye bleb encapsulation
- Presence of surgical glove powder

Although the effect of 5-FU on bleb encapsulation is controversial, MMC-associated blebs appear to have a much lower incidence of encapsulation (2.4% in one report).[241, 244–246]

Bleb encapsulation usually occurs 2 to 4 weeks postoperatively, although it can manifest at any time after surgery. The mechanism of encapsulation is controversial. Histopathologic evaluation demonstrates a thickened connective tissue framework with collagen-secreting fibroblasts. The fibrous tissue is not lined with epithelium and therefore is not a true cyst. Slit-lamp examination typically reveals a high, thick-walled, localized bleb (Fig. 18–21) often associated with elevated IOP. The conjunctiva overlying a Tenon's capsule dome may be hyperemic and is usually freely mobile.

MANAGEMENT. The majority of encapsulated blebs either resolve spontaneously or respond to medical management within 2 to 4 months. Conservative management with topical aqueous suppressants (if IOP is elevated) and digital ocular massage can be effective in more than 90% of cases.[246, 247] After resolution, the antiglaucoma medication is discontinued. For a bleb encapsulation that is unrespon-

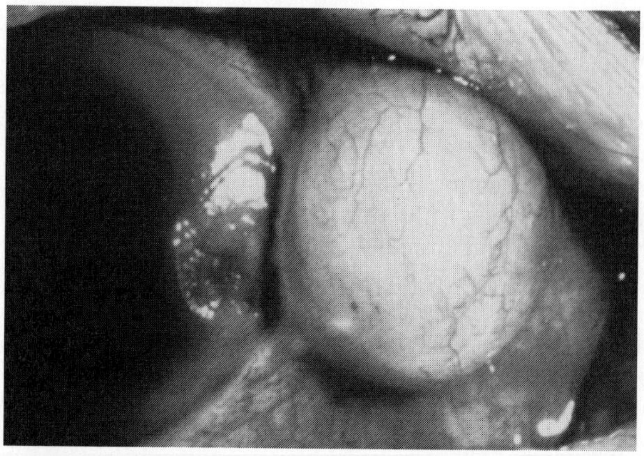

FIGURE 18–21. An encapsulated bleb. Note the high, focal bleb architecture. This patient has an associated corneal dellen.

sive to medical treatment or is associated with uncontrolled IOP, needle puncture of the bleb and, rarely, surgical excision of Tenon's capsule may be necessary.

AQUEOUS MISDIRECTION

Aqueous misdirection usually develops immediately after filtration surgery, although it can present at any time after surgery. Patients with a history of angle-closure glaucoma are at greatest risk, with a post–filtration surgery incidence of 2% to 4%.[248] Hyperopic and nanophthalmic eyes are also predisposed to this complication. Misdirection can also occur after scleral flap suture lysis or the cessation of postoperative cycloplegic therapy. The pathogenesis involves posterior diversion of aqueous humor into, behind, or beside the vitreous body, increasing vitreous volume and anteriorly rotating the ciliary body. Forward movement of the compressed vitreous and ciliary body shallows the anterior chamber.[129]

The affected patient presents with an elevated IOP in the presence of a uniformly shallow anterior chamber and patent iridectomy (Fig. 18–22). Pupillary block and SCH can have a similar presentation. Careful evaluation of the anterior and posterior segment, including the use of B-scan ultrasonography[249] if necessary, is imperative. Pupillary block can be differentiated by the presence of iris bombé with a more centrally deep anterior chamber.

MANAGEMENT. Initial therapy involves cycloplegic-mydriatic agents, such as atropine 1% and phenylephrine 2.5%, to relax the ciliary muscle, dilate the pupil, and help deepen the anterior chamber. Medications to suppress aqueous secretion (beta-blockers, carbonic anhydrase inhibitors) and decrease vitreous volume (20% intravenous mannitol 1–2 gm/kg over 30 to 40 minutes) are recommended. Miotic agents are contraindicated.[250]

Laser or surgical intervention may be necessary in cases unresponsive to medical treatment. Nd: YAG laser therapy to disrupt the anterior hyaloid face can be successful in pseudophakic or aphakic patients. Phakic eyes may require a pars plana vitrectomy.[248] Pars plana vitrectomy, lens extraction, and intraoperative capsulotomy can be considered if vitrectomy alone is not successful.[251]

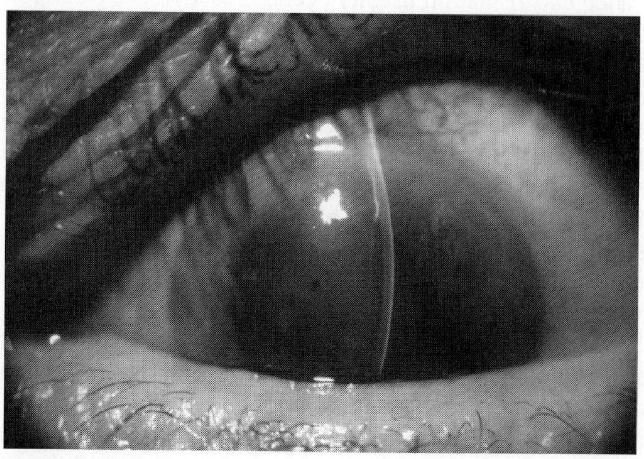

FIGURE 18–22. Patient in aqueous misdirection with a diffusely shallow anterior chamber. Note the proximity of the corneal slit beam to the iris slit beam.

Low Postoperative IOP

Early postoperative hypotony (IOP > 6 mm Hg) occurs most often secondary to decreased aqueous production, inadvertent cyclodialysis, overfiltration, or the presence of a wound leak. Hypotony (especially chronic hypotony) is more common after full-thickness filtration procedures and filtration with antimetabolites. Although most cases of hypotony in the immediate postoperative period resolve with usual postoperative management, chronic hypotony (longer than 3 months) can be associated with a high rate of visual loss. Eyes with low IOP can demonstrate intraocular inflammation, disc edema, retinal vascular tortuosity, ciliochoroidal effusions, hypotony maculopathy, Descemet's membrane folds, and progressive cataract formation. Early diagnosis and intervention are important for successful management (Table 18–7).

CILIARY BODY HYPOSECRETION

Postoperative reduction in aqueous secretion can develop in response to surgical trauma with resultant intraocular inflammation and typically lasts a few days to weeks. It is more frequent in eyes that have undergone previous cyclodestructive procedure(s). In addition, MMC has been demonstrated to be directly toxic to the ciliary body, perhaps causing prolonged hyposecretion. The anterior chamber depth, bleb morphology, and height can vary. Frequently, patients have ciliochoroidal effusions, which can further inhibit aqueous secretion, creating a ciliary shutdown–choroidal effusion cycle.

MANAGEMENT. Treatment involves frequent topical and, sometimes, systemic corticosteroids to aggressively quiet

TABLE 18–7. CAUSES OF LOW INTRAOCULAR PRESSURE AFTER FILTRATION SURGERY

Bleb Size	Seidel's Test Result	Diagnosis
High	Negative	Overfiltration
Low (or high)	Negative	Cyclodialysis cleft Ciliary shutdown
Low	Positive	Incision leak Conjunctival buttonhole

intraocular inflammation. Cycloplegic agents are indicated to improve the blood-aqueous barrier and help maintain anterior chamber depth. Topical and systemic aqueous suppressants, including oral beta-blockers and use of topical beta-blockers in the fellow eye, should be discontinued if possible.

CHOROIDAL DETACHMENT

In hypotonous eyes, transudation of fluid across choroidal capillaries collects in the potential space between choroid and sclera, elevating the choroid. Predisposing factors include:

- Hyperopia
- Systematic hypertension (especially if uncontrolled)
- Older age
- Atherosclerosis
- Ocular inflammation
- Aqueous suppressant therapy

Clinically, the IOP is below the episcleral venous pressure (usually < 6 mm Hg), and the anterior chamber can be shallow peripherally. Funduscopy reveals a whitish domed elevation of the retina-choroid that is acoustically hollow on B-scan ultrasonography (Fig. 18–23).

MANAGEMENT. Mild to moderate choroidal detachments are well-tolerated even after a few weeks, with minimal ocular morbidity. Most cases resolve once the IOP increases. Medical management of persistent ciliochoroidal effusions is similar to the treatment of ciliary body hyposecretion (see earlier discussion). Surgical drainage is indicated in eyes with corneal-lenticular touch and persistent flat chambers secondary to large effusions or prolonged (>2 weeks) retinal apposition in the macular area. Reformation of the anterior chamber with a viscoelastic agent can transiently elevate the IOP, which in some cases can decrease the effusion, stimulate aqueous secretion, and break the ciliary shutdown–choroidal effusion cycle.[252–254]

OVERFILTRATION

Excessive aqueous outflow through a sclerotomy can result in chronic postoperative hypotony. Although traditionally associated with full-thickness filtration procedures, excessive filtration has become more common with the use of antimetabolites. Patients often present with large thin-walled, avascular blebs.

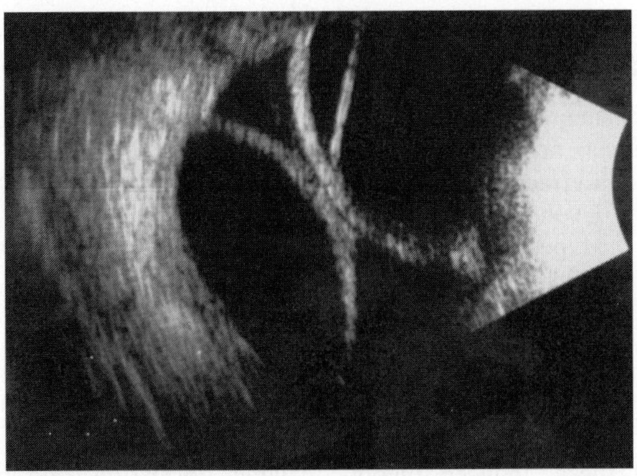

FIGURE 18–23. Acoustically hollow elevation seen on B-scan ultrasonography in a patient with a choroidal detachment. Note the bridging choroidal vessel on stretch, which can result in a suprachoroidal vessel if it ruptures.

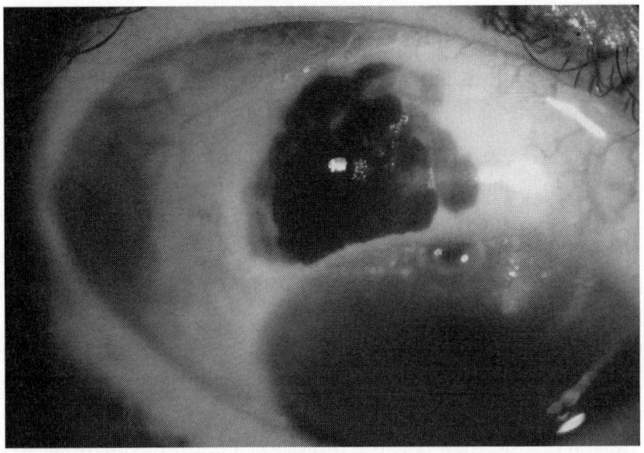

FIGURE 18–24. An autologous blood injection into an overfiltering bleb.

MANAGEMENT. In the management of overfiltration, the goal is to cause enough conjunctival and episcleral scarring to reduce aqueous outflow. Overfiltering blebs have been treated with cryotherapy, diathermy, trichloracetic acid, and focal argon and Nd: YAG laser treatment.[255]

We prefer intrableb injection of autologous blood. We inject approximately 0.5 mL of blood into the bleb through adjacent conjunctiva with a 30-gauge needle. Bleb height and function appear to decrease, perhaps through blood product–induced fibrosis, although the actual mechanism is unknown (Fig. 18–24). Acute bleb failure, hyphema, and marked elevations in IOP can occur after this injection.[253, 256–258]

Cataract extraction has also been reported to promote resolution of hypotony.[259] In severe cases of hypotony, intraoperative resuturing of the flap or a scleral patch graft may be necessary. Replacing thin permeable conjunctiva with thicker adjacent conjunctiva can also reduce aqueous outflow.

HYPOTONY MACULOPATHY

Persistent hypotony (usually IOP < 6 mm Hg[260]) can result in a maculopathy characterized by chorioretinal striae radiating from the fovea. The low IOP is thought to cause an inward bowing of the sclera with resultant macular choroidal and retinal folds. Although hypotony maculopathy was previously a rare occurrence, its incidence has dramatically increased with the use of MMC and 5-FU, now being reported as high as 15% to 35%.[47, 261–263] Increasing MMC concentration or exposure time may increase its occurrence.[262, 264] Other reported risk factors are young age, myopia, and high preoperative IOP.[265] The incidence in black patients, however, may be substantially lower. Clinically, patients complain of blurred and distorted vision.

MANAGEMENT. Treatment is directed at the cause of the hypotony in an attempt to increase the IOP. In our experience, hypotony maculopathy seems to be reversible if the IOP can be increased within 3 to 6 months.[256, 261, 266–269] Beyond this time, the maculopathy is more likely to be irreversible. In some cases, the anatomic change and the visual acuity do not improve even after successful elevation of IOP. Pars plana vitrectomy with heavy liquid tamponade is reportedly successful in reducing retinal and choroidal folds and improving visual function[260] in patients with persistent maculopathy despite successful elevation of IOP.

BLEB LEAKS

Filtration bleb leaks can occur early postoperatively, especially in eyes with the thin, avascular blebs seen after full-thickness or antimetabolite-associated filtration procedures. Leaks persist at the incision line or the limbus in fornix-based flaps and less frequently as buttonholes within the bleb, and are detected by Seidel's test. Clear aqueous humor can be seen within a pool of fluorescein using the cobalt blue filter (Fig. 18–25). The eyes are hypotonous, often with shallow or flat anterior chambers with a low-lying or flat bleb.

MANAGEMENT. The majority of early bleb leaks are managed conservatively to allow their spontaneous closure. Initial medical treatment involves manipulating postoperative medications. Corticosteroid dosages are decreased to allow wound healing. Conjunctiva-irritating topical antibiotics, such as gentamicin, may be started to promote fibrosis. If the eye is not hypotonous, agents to decrease aqueous secretion are initiated to reduce outflow, improving conjunctival adherence to underlying tissues.

In the patient with a persistent leak, applying a large-diameter bandage contact lens and leaving it undisturbed for several days may allow for conjunctival surface re-epithelialization. Alternatively, pressure can be applied over the filtration site with a tight (torpedo) patch. Other therapeutic modalities used to induce wound closure are application of fibrin adhesives onto and within the bleb, use of cyanoacrylate glue, cryotherapy, and argon laser treatment.[270–273]

We prefer to inject autologous blood in the same manner as described for the treatment of overfiltering blebs, to induce fibrosis.[256, 274, 275] In some cases, the bleb leak may require resuturing. Care must be taken in cases in which antimetabolite therapy has been used, as the conjunctiva may be friable and may leak from the additional suture tracts.

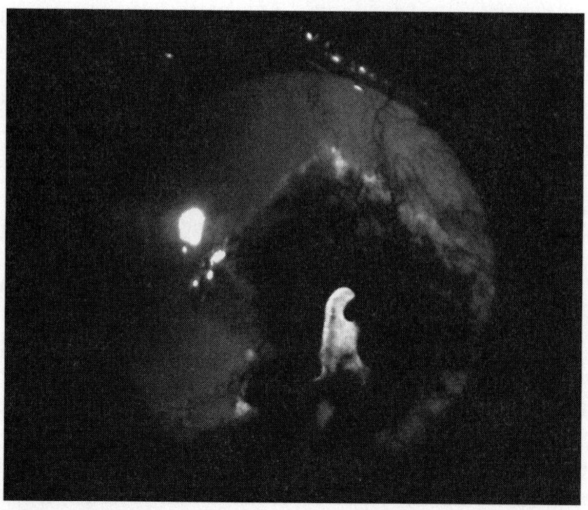

FIGURE 18–25. Clear aqueous is seen within a pool of fluorescein under cobalt-blue light in a patient with a bleb leak.

TABLE 18–8. GRADING ANTERIOR CHAMBER DEPTH

Grade	Anterior Chamber Findings
I	Peripheral iridocorneal touch
II	Pupillary border iridocorneal touch
III	Corneal-lenticular (or vitreous) apposition

SHALLOW OR FLAT ANTERIOR CHAMBER

A shallow or flat anterior chamber due to excessive aqueous outflow frequently occurs after filtration surgery, especially in patients with preoperatively shallow chambers. In cases of flat anterior chamber and elevated IOP, aqueous misdirection or SCH should be considered. In flat chambers associated with hypotony, bleb leaks should be ruled out before excessive filtration is concluded to be the cause. There are three grades of flat anterior chamber (Table 18–8).

MANAGEMENT. Anterior chamber shallowing in most cases resolves spontaneously (often within 2 weeks).[194] Initial treatment consists of observation, to allow the chamber to re-form as increasing aqueous production compensates for excess filtration. Frequent use of topical corticosteroid to minimize inflammation and maintenance of total cycloplegia with atropine 1% are initiated. Cycloplegic agents posteriorly displace the lens iris diaphragm and help maintain chamber depth. Focal compression of the filtration site with a pressure patch can decrease aqueous outflow and promote anterior chamber re-formation.

Patients with corneal-lenticular touch (grade III flat anterior chamber) are at a high risk for bleb failure, corneal edema, and cataract formation. Prompt re-formation of the anterior chamber is indicated in this group[276] and is accomplished with intraocular injection of air, BSS, viscoelastics, or expandable gases. We prefer injecting sodium hyaluronate (Healon) through a paracentesis tract,[277, 278] which can increase anterior chamber depth for up to 2 days.[279] A significant though transient elevation in IOP can occur with this technique. Anterior chamber re-formation with air is associated with formation of anterior subcapsular cataract and loss of endothelial cells.[280]

Visual Loss

Transient and permanent loss of visual acuity after filtration surgery occurs by a variety of mechanisms, including:

- Refractive shifts
- Uveitis
- Hypotony with maculopathy
- Lens opacification
- Loss of central fixation ("wipeout")
- Cystoid macular edema
- Endophthalmitis
- Suprachoroidal or vitreous hemorrhage
- Retinal detachment

Of these, induced myopia, cataract formation, and hypotony maculopathy are the most common. Progressive opacification of the lens after glaucoma surgery is reported to occur in 2% to 26% of eyes, with higher risk after filtration with MMC, in eyes with pre-existing cataract, and in eyes with postoperatively shallow or flat anterior chamber.[281]

Visual recovery even after uncomplicated filtration surgery can take several weeks. Patients with advanced preoperative visual field loss demonstrate a delay in postoperative visual recovery (2 to 8 months), especially if they also have postoperative hypotony.[282]

LOSS OF CENTRAL FIXATION

The loss of the central visual field ("snuff syndrome," "wipeout") after uncomplicated filtration surgery is a devastating postoperative complication. Although older studies reported up to a 13.6% incidence of central visual field loss in eyes with advanced glaucoma,[160] later reports suggest a much lower incidence, 1% to 2%[281–284] or less.[285] Predisposing factors reported include advanced glaucomatous defects within 5 degrees of fixation, older age, and severe postoperative hypotony (IOP < 2 mm Hg).[160, 281, 282] The greater the preoperative visual field constriction (especially if the field defect splits fixation), the greater the risk of postoperative central fixation loss.

Although the cause of this syndrome is not known, one possible mechanism is a transient elevation of postoperative IOP, reported to occur in 17% of eyes 4 to 6 hours after filtration surgery.[192] Eyes with advanced glaucomatous visual field loss may be less likely to tolerate any elevation in IOP. Optic nerve hypoperfusion due to low systemic blood pressure or epinephrine in the retrobulbar blocks and profound postoperative hypotony with resultant optic nerve hemorrhage or edema have also been proposed.[284, 285]

Steps to minimize the occurrence of central fixation loss are (1) avoidance of epinephrine in the anesthetic solution, (2) early and frequent monitoring of postoperative IOP in susceptible eyes, and (3) more controlled release of flap sutures to avoid postoperative hypotony.[284] Overall, the incidence of this complication is rare and should not preclude filtration surgery, even in predisposed eyes.

RETINAL DETACHMENT

The incidence of rhegmatogenous retinal detachment after filtration surgery is 1.2%.[6] This incidence is confounded by the larger number of patients with glaucoma who have a history of trauma, complicated intraocular procedures, and myopia.

ENDOPHTHALMITIS

Patients with filtering blebs are at a continuing risk for ocular infection. Two major types of infections occur, blebitis and bleb-associated endophthalmitis. Either can occur months to years after filtration surgery.

In *blebitis,* bacteria colonize the bleb and, in some cases, the anterior chamber without infiltrating the vitreous. Bleb-related *endophthalmitis* implies a bleb infection with intravitreal involvement. Blebitis may represent a prodrome or a limited endophthalmitis.

The reported incidence of bleb-related endophthalmitis ranges from 0.2% (no antimetabolite therapy)[286] to 13% (inferior bleb with adjunctive MMC),[85, 286] depending on surgical technique. Thin, cystic blebs associated with full-thickness procedures and adjunctive antimetabolite therapy are at a greater risk. Inferiorly placed blebs have up to a ten-fold greater incidence,[15, 16, 84, 85] perhaps owing to increased mechanical trauma from the lower eyelid, more contact to potential pathogens within the inferior tear lake, or greater bleb exposure.

The route of infection is presumed to be transconjunctival migration, often though not always through an area of focal conjunctival breakdown and aqueous leakage. Blepharitis, diabetes mellitus, a compromised immune system, contact lens wear, and eye rubbing increase the risk. Winter months and axial myopia may also be associated risks.[287]

Patients present with sudden onset of pain and decreased vision. Slit-lamp examination reveals conjunctival injection with a purulent, white infiltration of the bleb, anterior chamber inflammation, and, in severe cases, a hypopyon and intravitreal inflammation (Fig. 18–26). Patients with blebitis often have a more indolent course, complaining of a few days of ocular irritation and discomfort,[288, 289] perhaps indicating a less virulent pathogen.

MANAGEMENT. Although a wide range of bacteria are reported, the most common causative organisms in endophthalmitis are *Haemophilus* and streptococcal species. Blebitis is more commonly associated with staphylococcal species.[85, 86, 289, 290]

Treatment depends on the extent of the infection. Bleb infiltration in the presence of a clear vitreous should be managed aggressively with intensive topical and systemic broad-spectrum antibiotic therapy. We prefer the fluoroquinolones because of their level of intraocular penetration (e.g., topical ofloxacin every 1 to 2 hours while the patient is awake, supplemented with oral ofloxacin). Supplemental fortified topical and subconjunctival antibiotics (i.e., cefazolin and vancomycin) are considered for eyes with a severe anterior segment reaction (e.g., hypopyon) to improve coverage against staphylococcal and streptococcal species.[291] Patients should be monitored closely to allow for evaluation of the vitreous.

In cases with initial or subsequent involvement of the vitreous, rapid and aggressive management with intravitreal antibiotics (i.e., vancomycin 1 mg and amikacin 0.4 mg) is indicated. The use of systemic antibiotics was not proven beneficial in the Endophthalmitis Vitrectomy Study (EVS).[292] The EVS evaluated postcataract endophthalmitis and may not be directly applicable to bleb-associated endophthalmitis because of the difference in organisms and

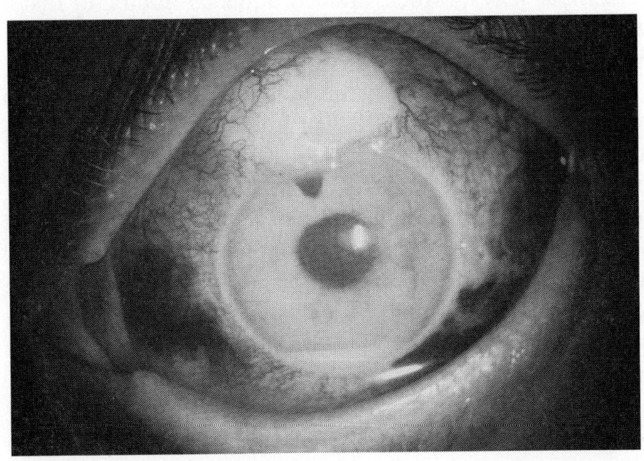

FIGURE 18–26. Bleb infiltration and a hypopyon in a patient with postfiltration endophthalmitis.

pathogenesis of infection. Only a low percentage of infections were caused by a *Streptococcus* species in the EVS. Intravenous vancomycin and ceftazidime or an oral fluoroquinolone provide excellent coverage for bleb-related infections and should be considered.[292]

Although vitreous cultures are recommended, the diagnostic yield from conjunctival cultures is controversial.

Visual outcome in culture-proven endophthalmitis is poor,[85, 290, 293] with most patients achieving less than 20/400 Snellen visual acuity. Blebitis, if appropriately treated, has a much better prognosis, with most patients recovering better than 20/200 Snellen visual acuity.[294] This difference may reflect less virulent pathogens in blebitis or early treatment success prior to progression of the disease to a fulminant endophthalmitis.

The best management is early diagnosis. Patients with filtering blebs should be instructed to report immediately any redness, discharge, pain, or decrease in vision. Prompt evaluation and treatment are necessary to ensure maximal visual recovery.

FUTURE DIRECTIONS IN GUARDED FILTRATION SURGERY

Although the guarded filtration procedure with adjunctive antimetabolite therapy is the current standard in the surgical management of most glaucomas, it is not without significant complications. Clinical investigations to develop alternative, safer procedures continue. Endoscopic cyclophotocoagulation and the trabeculotomy are being evaluated for the management of adult glaucoma. Nonpenetrating surgical techniques, such as the viscocanulostomy and the "glaucoma wick" procedure, are being evaluated. Whether these procedures will supplant modern filtration surgery has yet to be seen.[295–298]

Posterior Drainage Implants

Shunting of aqueous humor out of the anterior chamber via a foreign body conduit to treat glaucoma was reported as early as 1906, when Rollet and Moreau[298a] used horsehair to wick aqueous from the anterior chamber. Materials used since then include silk threads, plastic rods, and even lacrimal canalicular tissue. The subsequent development of translimbal tubes, which drained aqueous humor to distal sites such as the subconjunctival space, the lacrimal sac, and the superficial temporal vein, had limited success.

Molteno[299] introduced the prototype for the modern aqueous humor shunting implant in 1968. Molteno's objective was not only to shunt aqueous humor into the subconjunctival space but also to create a functioning filtering bleb. In his initial design, an acrylic tube allowed egress of aqueous humor from the anterior chamber onto a circular subconjunctival acrylic plate implanted at the limbus. The plate served as a stimulus for fibrovascular encapsulation, forming a collagenous reservoir into which the aqueous humor would drain.

The decades since then have brought surgical improvements in this initial design. Modern tube shunts, although differing in shape and size of tube and implant, share basic concepts. An anterior chamber tube inserted at the limbus functions as a nonsealing sclerotomy, shunting aqueous to an equatorially placed episcleral implant. The perilimbal location of Molteno's original 8.5-mm circular plate formed large anterior blebs, which were associated with discomfort, dellen formation, and implant extrusion. Moving the plate posterior to the muscle insertions alleviated some of these complications and allowed the implantation of larger plates, which formed large posterior blebs.[300]

Intraocular pressure reduction in drainage devices is proportional to the level of aqueous humor outflow. In the immediate postoperative period, aqueous flows unobstructed through the tube into the subconjunctival space over the plate. Four to 6 weeks postoperatively, collagen encapsulates the episcleral plate, creating resistance to aqueous outflow. From within the capsular bleb, aqueous humor is eventually absorbed by conjunctival capillaries and lymphatics.

The magnitude of IOP pressure reduction depends in part on the capsular wall resistance to aqueous outflow.[301] Greater resistance to aqueous diffusion from a thickened capsular wall or overlying conjunctival–Tenon's capsule fibrosis, raises IOP.[302, 303] Conversely, a thin or absent capsule offers no resistance to outflow and can result in a very low IOP.

TUBE SHUNT DESIGNS

Tube shunts are classified as shunts with no obstruction to flow (nonrestrictive or nonvalved) and shunts that limit flow (restrictive or valved) (Fig. 18–27).

Nonrestrictive shunts allow free flow of aqueous from the anterior chamber onto the surface of an episcleral implant. Aqueous outflow is limited only by the resistance of the fibrous capsule. Therefore, the risk of profound hypotony and flat anterior chamber is greater with these shunts than with valve shunts in the immediate postoperative period, prior to plate encapsulation.

Restrictive shunts have pressure-sensitive valves designed to impede aqueous outflow once IOP falls below a specified range, thereby decreasing the risk of hypotony and flat anterior chamber. The ability of the valves to function as designed is disputed.[304, 305] Prata and coworkers[305] found that these implants function as true valves when tested in air but not when immersed in liquid such

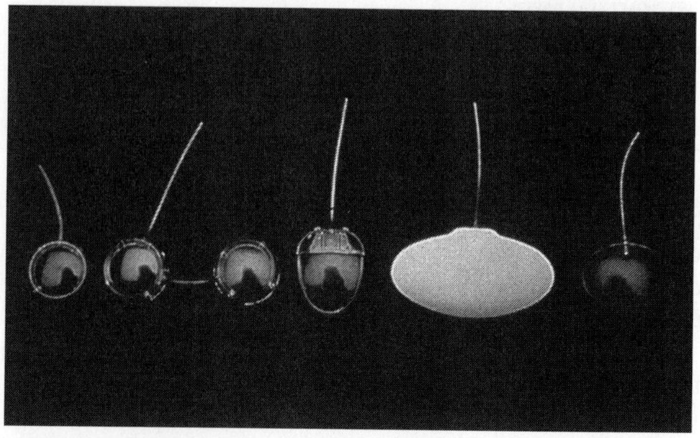

FIGURE 18–27. Modern posterior tube shunts. *Left* to *right:* A single-plate Molteno implant, a double-plate Molteno implant, an Ahmed valve, a Baerveldt implant, and a Krupin valve.

as BSS or plasma. These researchers concluded that although the "valves" in vivo increase resistance to aqueous outflow, they do not open and close with varying IOP as designed.

Nonrestrictive Implants

MOLTENO IMPLANT

The Molteno implant is the most widely used posterior drainage device. A nonvalved silicone tube opens onto the surface of a single 13.0-mm circular polypropylene plate with a surface area of 134 mm^2. A double-plate variation allows two plates (total surface area 268 mm^2) to be placed in separate quadrants; they are connected by a 10-mm silicone tube. Left or right eye styles are used, depending on the location of the tube insertion. An available dual-chamber implant contains a dividing pressure ridge on the upper surface of the proximal plate designed to decrease the risk of early postoperative hypotony.[306] An 8-mm circular plate with a surface area of 50 mm^2 is available for pediatric use.

BAERVELDT IMPLANT

The Baerveldt implant is a nonvalved silicone tube attached to a barium-impregnated, oval, silicone plate. With single-plate surface areas of 250, 350, and 425 mm^2, the Baerveldt implant offers single-quadrant placement of implants with large surface areas. The silicone plate can be trimmed to fit into a tight quadrant. The plate is fenestrated to allow fibrovascular ingrowth from the sclera to adhere to the overlying capsule, minimizing bleb height and reducing the risk of ocular motility disturbance. A tube with a 105-degree bend has been introduced with the Baerveldt implant to facilitate pars plana insertion.

SCHOCKET IMPLANT

The Schocket implant is a No. 20 or a No. 220 silicone encircling band with a central groove. A silicone lacrimal intubation tube passes through a notch cut in one wall and is secured with interrupted 9-0 nylon or similar sutures onto the groove.[307] The band can be placed 180 to 360 degrees. When placed 360 degrees, the No. 20 band has approximately 900 mm^2 in total surface area.[308–310]

Restrictive Implants

KRUPIN IMPLANT

The Krupin valve uses a silicone tube with horizontal and vertical slits in its distal end (over the plate) to create a pressure-sensitive valve designed to open at an IOP greater than 12 mm Hg and close when IOP fails below 8 mm Hg.[311] The tube is connected to a 13 × 18–mm oval, Silastic disc with a surface area of 183 mm^2. The disc has a 1.75-mm-high sidewall to increase the inner surface area of the encapsulating bleb. Alternatively, the tube can be sutured into the groove of an available No. 220 Silastic-encircling band.[312]

AHMED IMPLANT

The Ahmed glaucoma valve implant uses a silicone tube to shunt aqueous humor into a 13 × 16–mm oblong polypropylene plate with a surface area of 184 mm^2. The valve mechanism consists of two sheets of a silicone elastomer membrane on the upper plate surface that create a venturi-shaped chamber. The membranes are tensioned to separate when the IOP rises above 8 to 12 mm Hg, draining aqueous from the eye through the use of Bernoulli's principle.[313, 314]

Shunt Selection

Factors involved in the selection of a tube shunt are:

- □ Size and shape of the shunt
- □ Number of available quadrants
- □ Previous or concurrent ocular procedures
- □ Severity of the patient's glaucoma
- □ Surgeon's preference or experience

Studies comparing implants with varying surface areas demonstrate that increasing the implant surface area may improve postoperative IOP control. Prata and coworkers[315] demonstrated a direct relationship between the plate surface area and the surface area and filtering capacity of the overlying fibrous capsule in rabbit eyes.[315] Heuer and associates[316] reported that in aphakic and pseudophakic patients, IOP was controlled at 2 years in more patients receiving double-plate than single-plate Molteno implants (71% vs. 46%).[316]

There does appear to be an upper limit on implant size above which there is no further contribution to IOP control and possibly an increased complication rate (i.e., hypotony, diplopia). Neither the 900-mm^2 Schocket nor a 350-mm^2 Baerveldt implant demonstrates greater IOP control than the 268-mm^2 double-plate Molteno implant.[309, 310, 317, 318] Similarly, equivalent levels of IOP control are obtained with 350-mm^2 and 500-mm^2 Baerveldt implants.[319]

IOP control in patients with drainage devices also depends on the level of resistance to aqueous outflow. Nonvalved implants allow unobstructed outflow of aqueous humor into the reservoir over the episcleral plates, permitting low postoperative IOP, albeit with a higher rate of initial hypotony and flat anterior chamber.

Valved shunts, whether functioning as true valves or as resistance devices, impede aqueous outflow. Although valved implants may minimize the risk of profound hypotony in the early postoperative period, it is our experience that their resistance to outflow may also limit the amount of IOP reduction. The increase in resistance to flow may also raise the likelihood of tube occlusion and of a higher overall IOP. Nonetheless, numerous reports document the success of valved implants in the management of complicated glaucoma.[311, 314, 320, 321]

The shape of the implant in relation to the anatomy of the operative eye also plays a major role in shunt selection. If only a single quadrant is viable for implantation in an eye at high risk for failure, a Baerveldt implant with a large surface area may be indicated. Patients with ocular motility disturbances may benefit from the oblong Ahmed valve, which does not require fixation under adjacent rectus muscles. Conversely, in patients with posterior scarring or an encircling element, the oblong Ahmed implant may be difficult to insert.

Currently we use the valved Ahmed implant for our patients at low risk for failure, when we want to use less aggressive therapy, or when only a single quadrant for implantation is available. We reserve the double-plate Molteno implant for high-risk patients such as those with neovascular glaucoma or complicated, uncontrolled, or advanced glaucoma.

SURGICAL INDICATIONS

Before the advent of antimetabolite therapy, aqueous shunting procedures were widely used for the management of complicated glaucoma. The use of MMC as an adjunct to guarded filtration surgery has greatly improved the success of this procedure and should be considered before tube implantation in the surgical management of most cases of glaucoma[322] in children and adults.

Indications for aqueous shunting procedures are as follows:

- Implantation in infants, children, and adults with uncontrolled glaucoma in whom previous filtration surgery with adjunctive antimetabolites has failed.
- Primary-implantation in patients in whom marked conjunctival scarring or recession makes a trabeculectomy technically difficult and likely to fail.
- Patients with very anterior PAS that can prevent communication into the anterior chamber through a standard filtration sclerotomy.
- Primary implantation in patients at high risk for failure of a trabeculectomy with adjunctive antimetabolite agents, such as those with active neovascular or uveitic glaucoma.
- Primary implantation in patients with previous or concomitant ocular surgery, such as keratoplasty or pars plana vitrectomy.[313, 323, 324]

Comparing relative success rates among surgical reports is difficult, as previously mentioned (see discussion of success rate of trabeculectomy), especially with the variety of shunts available. Although the overall success rate in tube shunt procedures is greatest in eyes with POAG, uveitic and other secondary glaucomas have also been successfully managed.[314, 325–331] Tube shunts can be successful in lowering IOP in pediatric glaucoma not responsive to alternative surgical treatments, although with a high long-term complication rate.[332–334] Several researchers suggest caution regarding prognosis in the pediatric population.[59, 335]

In active neovascular glaucoma, tube shunts appear to have better long-term IOP control with a lower incidence of phthisis bulbi than either guarded filtration surgery with antimetabolite therapy or transscleral cyclodestructive procedures.[307, 335–341]

SURGICAL TECHNIQUE

Although tube shunt designs vary in size and shape, implantation techniques are fundamentally the same for all but the encircling bands. Surgery can be performed with the patient under general, peribulbar, or retrobulbar anesthesia. Our technique for superior quadrant tube shunt implantation is presented here. Instrumentation, suture size, and suture type for the most part depend on the individual surgeon's preference and comfort level.

Location

A tube shunt is preferably placed in the superotemporal quadrant. The distance from the limbus to the optic nerve is greatest superotemporally (~33 mm), providing maximal exposure and decreasing the likelihood of oblique muscle involvement and ocular motility disturbance. Tube shunts, however, can be placed in any quadrant. Unlike in filtration surgery, even inferiorly placed shunts are well-tolerated. In addition, implants may be positioned such that the tube enters nasally or temporally, depending on anterior chamber anatomy or other considerations.

Ultimately, the mobility of the conjunctiva and fornices is the most important in determining shunt placement. There must be sufficient space to fixate the plate approximately 10 mm posterior to the limbus. The conjunctiva should be able to be brought easily to the limbus over the implant without significant tension.

Conjunctival Incision

In the initial step, a conjunctival–Tenon's capsule peritomy is performed flush to the limbus with radial relaxing incisions (Fig. 18–28). The incision size is determined by the implant type (Table 18–9). Although a 100-degree peritomy is sufficient for a single-quadrant device, a 180-degree peritomy is needed for a double-plate Molteno implant.

Blunt dissection is performed posteriorly into the chosen quadrants, breaking any adhesions that would prevent posterior placement of the plates.

TABLE 18–9. POSTERIOR DRAINAGE IMPLANTS FOR TREATMENT OF GLAUCOMA

	Plate Size (mm)	Type	Surface Area (mm^2)	Peritomy Size
NONVALVED				
Molteno				
Single-plate	13	Polypropylene	134	100
Double-plate	13 × 2	Polypropylene	268	180
Baerveldt	350: 32 × 14	Silicone	250, 350, 425	100
Schocket	No. 20 No. 220	Silicone	900	360
VALVED				
Ahmed	13 × 16	Polypropylene	184	100
Krupin	18 × 13	Silastic	180	100

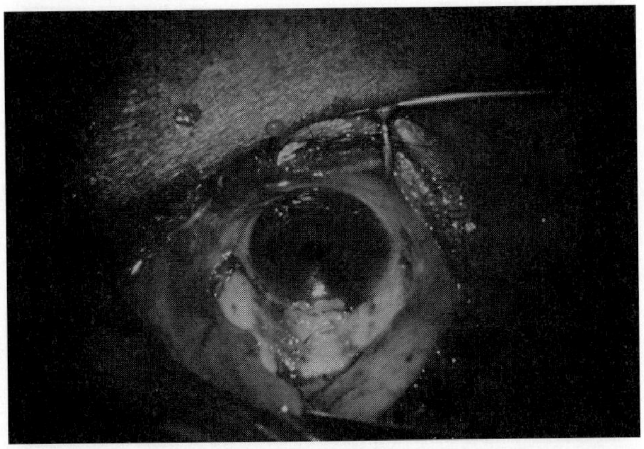

FIGURE 18–28. A 180-degree conjunctival peritomy in a patient undergoing placement of a double-plate Molteno implant.

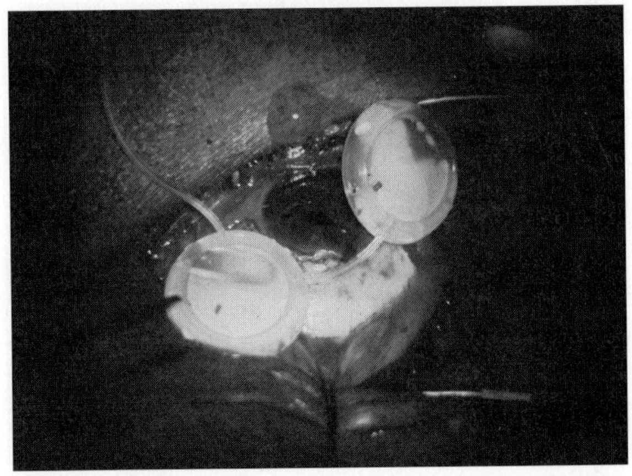

FIGURE 18–30. A double-plate Molteno implant being placed posteriorly. In this case, the distal plate will be passed under the previously isolated superior rectus suture.

Posterior Placement and Fixation of the Episcleral Plate

An implant previously soaked in an antibiotic solution is positioned posteriorly over bare sclera between adjacent rectus muscles in a quadrant. The anterior plate edge should be behind the muscle insertions, approximately 8 to 10 mm posterior to the limbus. For a double-plate Molteno implant, the distal plate is passed beneath the rectus muscle separating the two quadrants. Isolating the muscle with a suture tie (we prefer a 4-0 silk suture) or placing the muscle on traction with a muscle hook allows easier passage of the plate (Figs. 18–29 and 18–30). If necessary, the distal plate can be placed over the muscle. The large single-quadrant Baerveldt plate extends and fixates under the adjacent rectus muscles. Sweeping under these muscles with a muscle hook allows the surgeon to identify any obstructions to fixation. The conjunctiva should be drawn forward over the implant toward the limbus to ensure adequate conjunctival mobility.

Nonabsorbable sutures (we prefer 4-0 to 6-0 silk) on a spatulated needle are then placed through the eyelets or anterior platform of the plate or plates and sutured securely into sclera (Fig. 18–31).

Tube Entry Site in Anterior Chamber

A surgical blade or electrocautery is used to remove conjunctival epithelium from the intended tube entry site to prevent epithelial ingrowth into the anterior chamber or over the inner bleb wall of the episcleral plate.[342, 343] Removal of epithelium also allows better adherence of the conjunctival flap to the cornea.

The tube is laid over the cornea and trimmed in a beveled-up fashion to a size extending 3 to 4 mm into the anterior chamber (Fig. 18–32). In eyes with rubeosis iridis, the tube should extend further toward the pupillary margin and away from the large neovascular iris vessels that can occlude the tube.

With a 23-gauge needle, an entry track is made approximately 1 mm posterior to the edge of the limbal blue line. The needle is directed parallel to the plane of the iris (Fig. 18–33). Prior to the sclerotomy formation, the anterior chamber can be inflated with a viscoelastic agent, posteriorly displacing the iris and preventing it from obstructing passage of the needle. Viscoelastic can also be used to tamponade any bleeding that may occur. However, the viscoelastic artificially deepens the anterior chamber, possibly contributing to inaccurate tube positioning. Anterior chamber depth should be noted prior to introduction of viscoelastic.

Using nontoothed forceps or tube introducer forceps to prevent tube perforation the surgeon inserts the tube

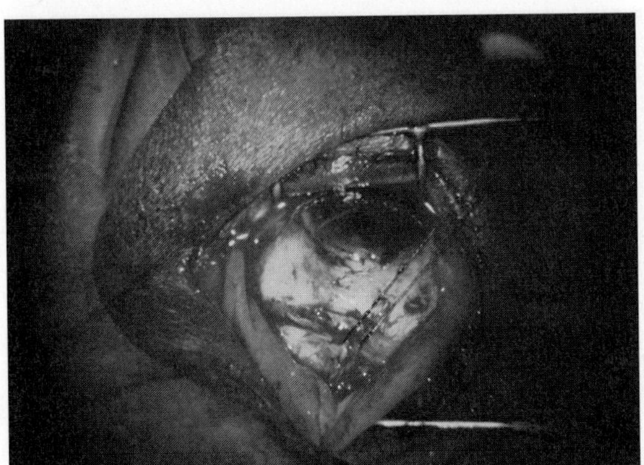

FIGURE 18–29. 4-0 silk suture isolating the superior rectus tendon.

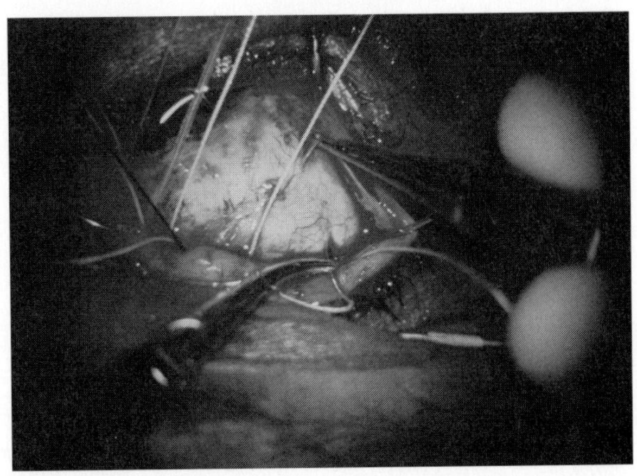

FIGURE 18–31. A 4-0 white silk suture on a spatulated needle is used in this case to secure the plates posteriorly to the sclera.

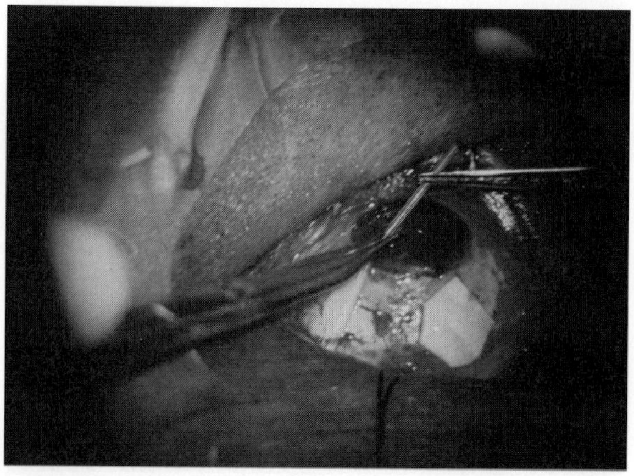

FIGURE 18–32. Westcott scissors are used to trim the tube to an appropriate size.

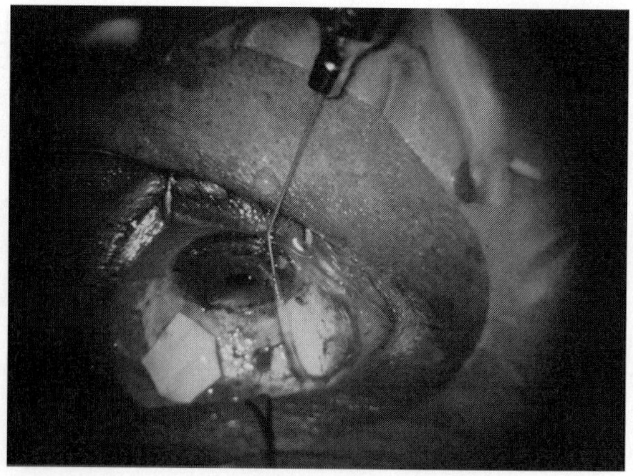

FIGURE 18–34. Irrigation of the tube with balanced salt solution on a 30-gauge cannula.

through the tract.[344] Viscoelastic can be injected into the entry site to facilitate passage of the tube. The tube should be positioned well below the cornea but above the plane of the iris. It should lie flat on the globe without kinks or sharp turns that could impede aqueous flow and increase the likelihood of progressive tube straightening, migration, or retraction. If necessary, the tube can be sutured to the sclera to reduce this risk. With valved implants, it is important to irrigate the tube with BSS before inserting it into the eye to ensure free flow of fluid through the valve leaflets (Figs. 18–34 and 18–35).

Tube Coverage

Tubes that are left uncovered can erode through the overlying conjunctiva, raising the risk of endophthalmitis.[345] Initially, tubes were inserted under partial-thickness scleral flaps. This procedure remains the least expensive method of tube coverage and avoids the risk of cadaveric transmission of infections. It is often complicated, however, by erosion of the tube through the thin overlying sclera.

We prefer the placement of grafts over the anterior aspect of the tube, adjacent to the limbus. Glycerin-preserved donor sclera can be placed over the tube and sutured at each of its corners with interrupted sutures (e.g., 9-0 nylon) (Fig. 18–36). Alternatively, similarly secured human cadaveric pericardium has been used successfully,[346] with a low incidence of tube erosion. Human pericardium has a low profile, allowing easier coverage with conjunctiva while maintaining excellent tensile strength. Coverage of the tube with human dura mater as well as cadaveric fascia lata has also been reported.[347, 348]

Conjunctival Closure

The conjunctiva is brought down to the limbus with non-toothed forceps. It is important that the limbus be de-epithelialized to ensure conjunctival adherence anterior to the tube and scleral graft. Using an 8-0 Vicryl suture, we place a mattress suture with scleral fixation at each end of the peritomy and close the radial incision in a running fashion. Care is taken to avoid inadvertently creating conjunctival buttonholes over the tube (Fig. 18–37).

SURGICAL MODIFICATIONS

Tube Insertion Through the Pars Plana

Placement of the tube into the posterior segment through the pars plana, concurrent with or subsequent to a pars

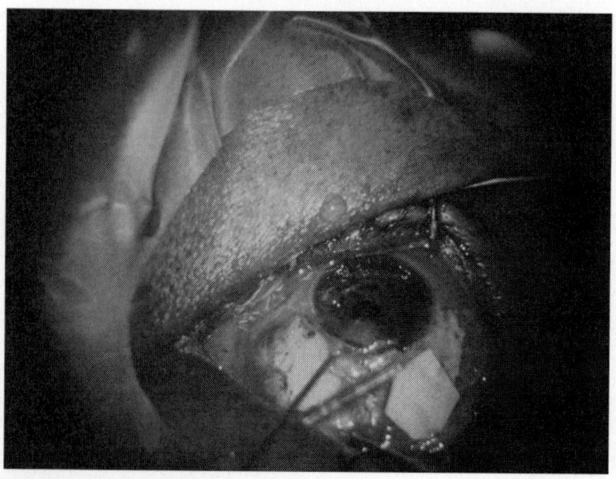

FIGURE 18–33. A 23-gauge needle passed parallel to the iris plane to create a paracentesis tract.

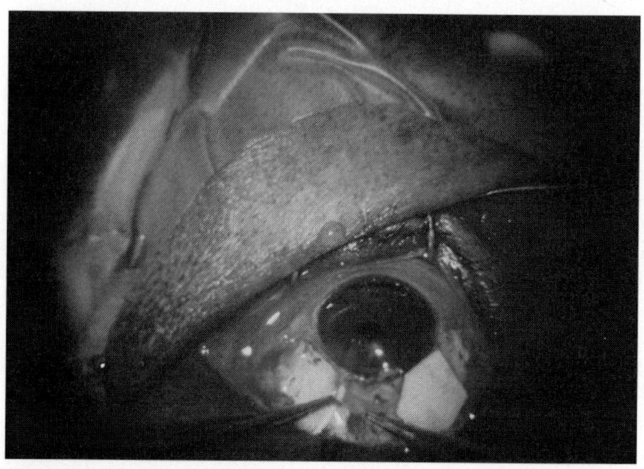

FIGURE 18–35. Tube insertion into the anterior chamber.

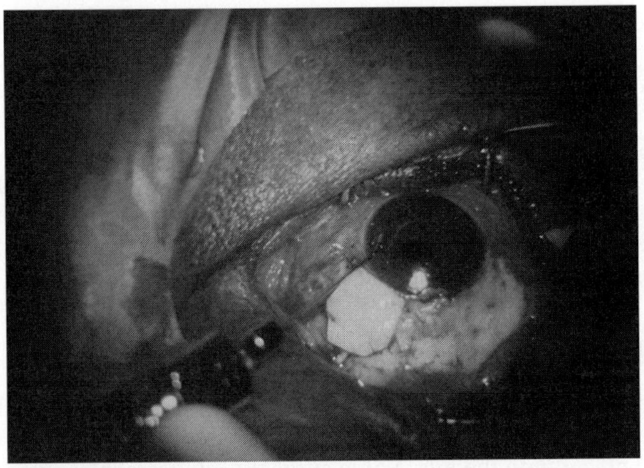

FIGURE 18–36. Bank sclera covering the tube to prevent conjunctival erosion by the tube.

plana vitrectomy, can be effective in controlling IOP.[323, 349] Surgical indications for such a procedure include a very shallow or obliterated anterior chamber, trauma, and eyes with conjunctival foreshortening such as after chemical burns. Pars plana tube implantation avoids the anterior segment complications of corneal decompensation and progressive tube straightening with corneal erosion. Disadvantages of this technique include higher risk of retinal detachment, vitreous base dialysis, and vitreous obstruction of the tube lumen.

The tube is inserted through a sclerotomy performed approximately 3 mm posterior to the limbus in aphakic or pseudophakic patients and 4 mm in phakic patients. The tube is trimmed to allow 3 to 4 mm of extension into the posterior chamber and is beveled up to prevent vitreous plugging. Care is taken to avoid subchoroidal placement. Patients should undergo complete vitrectomy to decrease risks of vitreous traction and tube obstruction. A Baerveldt implant with an appropriately sized, posteriorly directed tube is available. Postvitrectomy intravitreal gas tamponade is reported to limit aqueous humor outflow through the tube and reduce the risk of postoperative hypotony.[323, 339]

Adjunctive Antimetabolite Therapy

The success of aqueous drainage implants depends on the level of aqueous diffusion through the fibrous plate capsule. MMC has been shown in rabbit models to increase the aqueous permeability of the encapsulating plate capsule.[350] Several nonrandomized studies (most uncontrolled) suggest that the application of MMC to bare sclera prior to plate implantation may be associated with a lower final IOP.[351–353] In randomized, controlled studies comparing the use of double-plate Molteno implants with and without MMC, no significant difference in outcome has been found.[354] Currently, we do not use adjunctive antimetabolite therapy when implanting aqueous shunts.

SURGICAL MODIFICATIONS TO PREVENT HYPOTONY

Many of the complications associated with aqueous drainage implants are related to early postoperative hypotony, which occurs prior to the establishment of aqueous outflow resistance by the fibrous plate encapsulation. Multiple methods have been devised to reduce early postoperative overfiltration, as described here.

SHUNT DESIGN

As previously discussed, valved tube shunts (Krupin and Ahmed) are, by their design, associated with greater resistance to aqueous outflow and therefore perhaps a lower incidence of postoperative hypotony. The nonvalved Molteno dual-chamber implant contains an anterior pressure ridge designed to limit postoperative hypotony. Fibrovascular tissue forms a small capsule over the ridge in the early postoperative period, increasing resistance to aqueous outflow[306, 355] (Figs. 18–38 and 18–39). Although several studies report the ridge to be effective,[356] others suggest that it has variable effectiveness in preventing hypotony.[355]

TWO-STAGED PROCEDURE

In an effort to prevent hypotony, glaucoma surgeons have attached the plate in the subconjunctival space and, in 4 to 6 weeks, presumably after plate encapsulation, returned the patient to the operating room to insert the tube into the anterior chamber. This procedure is not commonly used, because the IOP reduction is not achieved until the completion of the second stage. An adjacent trabeculectomy can be considered at the time of the first stage, with the second stage being performed only if the filtration surgery fails.

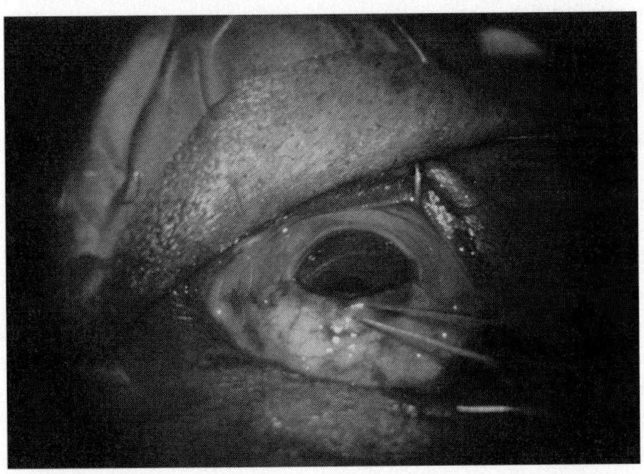

FIGURE 18–37. Conjunctival tissue brought down over the anterior cornea.

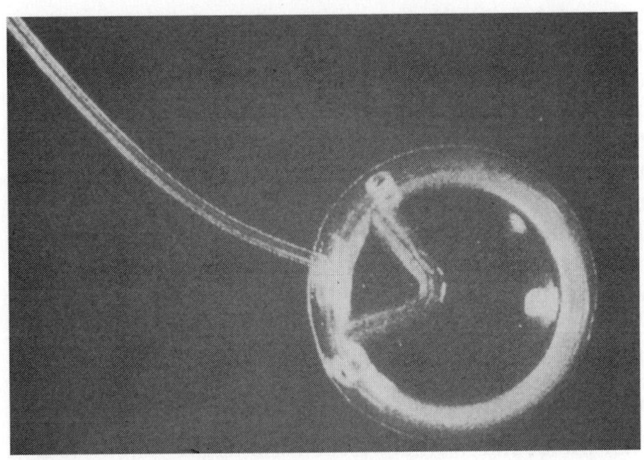

FIGURE 18–38. A pressure ridge on a single-plate Molteno implant.

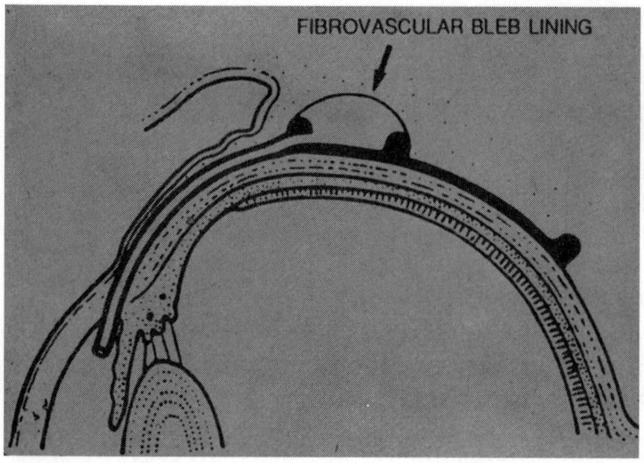

FIGURE 18–39. A fibrovascular bleb formed over the pressure ridge of a Molteno plate in the early postoperative period.

TUBE LIGATURE

A nonabsorbable suture with a releasable slipknot (i.e., 7-0 nylon)[357] or an absorbable suture (e.g., 7-0 Vicryl or chromic)[355, 358] can be tied around the tube near the tube-plate junction to reduce tube lumen size and restrict aqueous outflow. Absorbable Vicryl sutures in general take 4 weeks to dissolve. Nonabsorbable sutures either are exposed externally for future release or are internalized and later cut with an argon laser. These sutures can be released after plate encapsulation or earlier in patients with uncontrolled IOP.

Disadvantages of suture ligature include (1) elevated IOP in the early postoperative period, (2) variable dissolution of the absorbable suture, and (3) the occasional inability to cut or remove nonabsorbable sutures, especially if the suture is encapsulated by surrounding fibrous tissues. A full-thickness slit can be made along the axis of the tube anterior to the ligature to provide some aqueous outflow flow prior to suture removal.[359]

Nylon suture ligature of the tube inside the anterior chamber can also be done. The suture is released, if necessary, with argon laser suture lysis.[358, 360]

TUBE OCCLUSION

Occlusion of the lumen of the tube by 3-0 or 4-0 chromic or polypropylene suture has also been reported to be effective in temporarily limiting aqueous flow.[362–364] The suture is threaded from the fornix through the tube and is positioned a few millimeters from the tube opening in the anterior chamber to obstruct the tube lumen. An exposed tip of suture can be a nidus for infection; the external suture end is therefore placed subconjunctivally in an adjacent quadrant. The suture is then removed under slit-lamp guidance within 2 weeks, before suture degradation. Removal of the suture has been associated with a severe inflammatory response, including sterile hypopyon, and with endophthalmitis.[361]

Attempts to occlude the tube lumen with biodegradable materials such as collagen have had only limited success.[365]

VISCOELASTIC AGENTS

High-molecular-weight viscoelastic agents (e.g., Healon GV) can be injected into the anterior chamber at the conclusion of the implantation procedure to maintain chamber depth and prevent hypotony in the first few postoperative days. Viscoelastic flows poorly through the tube lumen and is slowly absorbed by the trabecular meshwork. Although this technique is our preferred method to prevent postoperative hypotony, its disadvantages include a short duration of resistance to aqueous outflow and variability in the rate of viscoelastic absorption among patients. Direct injection of the viscoelastic into the tube can prolong its effect.

PERIOPERATIVE MEDICATIONS

At the conclusion of the implantation procedure, topical atropine 1% and an antibiotic and corticosteroid ointment are placed into the eye. Some surgeons advocate intraoperative subconjunctival injections of corticosteroids and antibiotics, but this is not our current practice.

INTRAOPERATIVE COMPLICATIONS

Scleral Perforation

Perforation of the sclera may occur during suture fixation of the plate. Evidence of retinal penetration on indirect ophthalmoscopy and the presence of vitreous through the perforation site are indications for retinal cryotherapy. Surgery can continue in the same quadrant. A thorough postoperative retinal evaluation is recommended.

Improper Entry Incision

A poorly directed tube can be redirected through a new incision site 1 to 2 mm to either side of the first incision. There is no need to suture close the initial entry site unless frank leakage occurs through the opening. Leakage around the tube due to too large an opening generally decreases with scarring. Excessive leakage is reduced with suture closure of the opening.

Suprachoroidal Hemorrhage

Intraoperative SCH is a rare complication with an incidence after implantation similar to that after filtration surgery (see earlier). Delayed SCH occurs in 5% to 8% of cases, most often in patients with systemic hypertension or postoperative hypotony.[366, 367]

POSTOPERATIVE MANAGEMENT

Postoperative care and medications are similar to those after filtration surgery, utilizing prophylactic topical antibiotics, corticosteroids, and cycloplegic agents (see earlier discussion of postoperative medications after filtration surgery). Most surgeons no longer adhere to the postoperative regimen of oral prednisone, colchicine, and flufenamic acid initially advocated by Molteno, because of the associated systemic side effects.[299, 300] One caveat is that postoperative intraocular inflammation after a tube shunt procedure can be intense, in part owing to the severity and nature of glaucoma in patients selected for this procedure. Intense topical corticosteroid therapy (every 1 to 2 hours) may be necessary in some patients. All patients, but especially those with profound hypotony, should be instructed about taking precautions to prevent SCH.

EARLY POSTOPERATIVE COMPLICATIONS

Low IOP

As mentioned, profound hypotony can occur in the immediate postoperative period secondary to excessive aqueous outflow through the tube shunt prior to plate encapsulation. It is not uncommon to observe large ciliochoroidal detachments and a flat anterior chamber in this situation. Modifications of surgical technique can reduce, but often does not eliminate, this complication. Patients who have a shallow anterior chamber without corneal-lenticular touch can be managed conservatively either with observation or, in more severe cases, with anterior chamber re-formation with a viscoelastic agent under slit-lamp visualization. Eyes with prolonged flat anterior chambers, with ciliochoroidal apposition (>2 weeks), or with corneal-lenticular touch may require intraoperative drainage of choroidal effusions, re-formation of anterior chamber, and possible shunt revision with the use of surgical modifications to prevent hypotony as described earlier. Persistent hypotony refractory to these maneuvers may necessitate removal of the shunt.

As in filtration surgery, ciliary body hyposecretion can contribute to early postoperative hypotony. The frequent use of topical corticosteroids to decrease inflammation associated with ciliary body hyposecretion should be weighed against the detrimental effects of corticosteroids on wound healing and fibrosis, which are important components of plate encapsulation.

High IOP

TUBE OBSTRUCTION

Obstruction of the anterior chamber tube opening by iris, blood, fibrin, lens capsule, or vitreous can prevent aqueous outflow (Figs. 18–40 and 18–41). Methods for removing the obstructing agents include the use of argon or Nd: YAG laser,[368] and intracameral tPA to dissolve obstructing blood or fibrin clots.[369] Irrigation of the tube through a paracentesis with a small cannula under slit-lamp visualization is

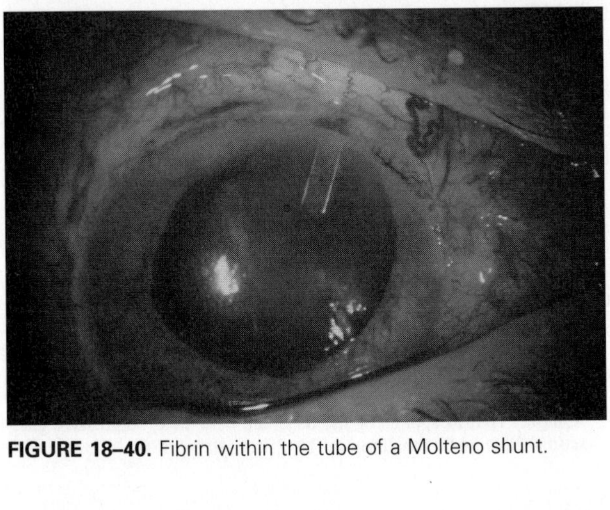

FIGURE 18–40. Fibrin within the tube of a Molteno shunt.

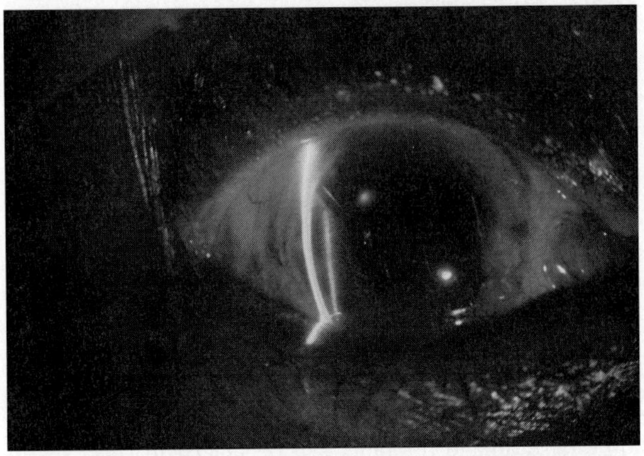

FIGURE 18–41. A blood clot within the tube of a Molteno shunt.

often successful in flushing debris from within the tube or between valve leaflets.[370] Intraoperative removal of the obstruction may be necessary if conservative management is not successful.

The eye with a suture-ligated or suture-occluded tube and a high IOP uncontrolled by topical antiglaucoma medications may require early release of sutures, although this procedure can result in hypotony and a flat anterior chamber.

HYPERTENSIVE PHASE

Two to 6 weeks postoperatively, IOP in an eye with a glaucoma drainage device can increase, when fibrous encapsulation of the episcleral plate increases the resistance to aqueous outflow. In most cases, the elevation in IOP is temporary. Over time, aqueous humor dissects the fibrous capsule off the plate and creates outflow channels, reducing IOP. Antiglaucoma medications can be used to treat marked elevations in IOP during this phase, which in some cases can persist for several months.[311]

LATE POSTOPERATIVE COMPLICATIONS

High IOP

Late elevation of IOP is most commonly due to decreased shunt function, which is most often secondary to one of the following mechanisms:

1. The tip of the tube may be obstructed by inflammation or fibrous debris, which if visible can be managed as previously described.
2. Obstruction may occur within the tube; though less likely, this obstruction may respond to irrigation with slit-lamp visualization.
3. More commonly, subconjunctival fibrosis and encapsulation of the bleb may overlie the plate and prevent egress of aqueous humor.

Slit-lamp evaluation will demonstrate either a low-lying bleb over the plate or absence of a bleb. The presence of a bleb over the proximal plate but not the distal plate of a double-plate Molteno implant may indicate an obstruction in the tube connecting the two plates. Although needle revision of fibrosed plate blebs with slit-lamp visualization can be successful, we prefer surgical revision of a tube-

TABLE 18–10. MECHANISMS OF STRABISMUS AFTER TUBE SHUNT IMPLANTATION

A posterior fixation (Faden) effect from the bleb's adherence to the rectus muscles
Direct trauma to muscle
A large bleb crowding the muscle and limiting ocular rotation in any direction[375–379]
Fat adherence syndrome producing a progressive restrictive strabismus

shunt bleb, dissecting the conjunctiva over the plate and removing fibrous tissue. Alternatively, in our experience, additional drainage implants can be placed in other available quadrants to provide additional IOP control.

Ocular Motility Disturbance

Postoperative ocular motility disturbance after tube shunt implantation is not rare, with a reported incidence of 3% (Krupin valve)[311] to 77%[371] (350-mm^2 nonfenestrated Baerveldt implant) in retrospective studies. In a prospective study at our institution, 47% of patients receiving double-plate Molteno implants experienced motility disturbance. Multiple mechanisms for the strabismus with varying clinical presentations are proposed (Table 18–10).[372–374]

The incidence of ocular motility disturbance increases with greater bleb and implant height and the extent of rectus muscle involvement. Oblique muscle disturbance may be greatest with nasally placed implants.[377–379] Baerveldt implants have the highest reported incidence,[371, 373] prompting the introduction of fenestrations within the implant to allow fibrovascular ingrowth, which decreases bleb height and associated motility disturbance. The Ahmed implant is shaped so as not to require fixation under rectus muscles, perhaps decreasing the strabismus risk.

Diplopia in most patients improves without treatment in several months. Intractable diplopia may require surgical correction or, in recalcitrant cases, removal of the implant.

Plate and Tube Migration

Poorly secured episcleral plates with slippage or loss of anchoring sutures can lead to plate dislocation with resultant tube migration and anterior displacement of the encapsulated bleb, which cause discomfort and dellen formation. The episcleral plate may also extrude through conjunctiva, necessitating revision or removal of the shunt.[380]

The tube can migrate anteriorly into the anterior chamber or posteriorly out of the anterior chamber.[381] Poorly positioned tubes with kinks or bends and short tubes are more likely to retract out of the anterior chamber. Progressive straightening of the tube with corneal erosion and transcorneal tube exposure is also reported. Tube repositioning may require intraoperative dissection of the tube and episcleral plate followed by repositioning and anchoring of both tube and plate to the sclera with nonabsorbable sutures (e.g., 10-0 nylon).

Corneal Decompensation

Corneal decompensation can occur with anterior chamber tube implants even in patients without evident tube-endothelium contact. The cause of endothelial cell loss is probably multifactorial. In eyes with obvious tube-cornea contact, direct trauma to the endothelium likely produces a focal decrease in endothelial cells. In patients without obvious tube-endothelium contact, intermittent contact between the tube and the peripheral cornea, perhaps due to eye rubbing, may produce repeated endothelial trauma. Endothelial cells may then migrate from the center to the periphery to compensate for the peripheral cell loss, thereby producing progressive diffuse endothelial cell loss.[382]

Although tube shunts can be successful in controlling IOP in patients with penetrating keratoplasty, they are associated with reduced graft survival. It is not clear whether graft failure is secondary to the tube or to the natural history of eyes with multiple previous procedures, intraocular inflammation, and uncontrolled glaucoma.

REFERENCES

1. Sugar HS: Course of successfully filtering blebs: A followup study. Ann Ophthalmol 1971;3:485–487.
2. Sugar HS: Complications, repair and reoperation of antiglaucoma filtering blebs. Am J Ophthalmol 1967;63:825–833.
3. Cairns JE: Trabeculectomy: Symposium: Microsurgery of the outflow channels. Trans Am Acad Ophthalmol Otolaryngol 1972;76:384–388.
4. Scorcia G, Balestrazzi E, Del Bene P, Cusumano A: Preliminary results of original modifications to Cairns's trabeculectomy technique. Glaucoma 1987;9:81–83.
5. Watson P: Trabeculectomy—a modified ab externo technique. Ann Ophthalmol 1970;2:199.
6. Sastry SM, Street DA, Javitt JC: National outcomes of glaucoma surgery: Complications following partial and full-thickness filtering procedures. J Glaucoma 1992;1:137–140.
7. Skuta GL, Parrish RK II: Wound healing in glaucoma filtering surgery. Surv Ophthalmol 1987;32:149–170.
8. Galin MA, Baras I, McLean JM: How does a filtering bleb work? Trans Am Acad Ophthalmol Otolaryngol 1965;69:1082–1091.
9. Addicks EM, Quigley HA, Green WR, Robin AL: Histologic characteristics of filtering blebs in glaucomatous eyes. Arch Ophthalmol 1983;101:795–798.
10. Shirakashi M, Iwata K, Sawaguchi S, et al: Intraocular pressure-dependent progression of visual field loss in advanced primary open-angle glaucoma: A 15-year follow-up. Ophthalmologica 1993; 207:1–5.
11. Roth SM, Spaeth GL, Starita RJ, et al: The effects of postoperative corticosteroids on trabeculectomy and the clinical course of glaucoma: Five-year follow up study. Ophthalmic Surg 1991;22:724–729.
12. Chauhan BC, Drance SM: The relationship between intraocular pressure and visual field progression in glaucoma. Graefes Arch Clin Exp Ophthalmol 1992;230:521–526.
13. Akafo SK, Goulstine DB, Rosenthal AR: Long-term post trabeculectomy intraocular pressures. Acta Ophthalmol (Copenh) 1992; 70:312–316.
14. Yassur Y, Lusky M, Grunewald E, Ben-Sira I: Regression of optic disc excavation and visual field damage following glaucoma surgery in eyes with long-standing glaucoma. Glaucoma 1984;6:202–207.
15. Gandolfi SA: Improvement of visual field indices after surgical reduction of intraocular pressure. Ophthalmic Surg 1995;26:121–126.
16. Tsai CS, Shin DH, Wan JY, Zeiter JH: Visual field global indices in patients with reversal of glaucomatous cupping after intraocular pressure reduction. Ophthalmology 1991;98:1412–1419.
17. Katz LJ, Spaeth GL, Cantor LB, et al: Reversible optic disk cupping and visual field improvement in adults with glaucoma. Am J Ophthalmol 1989;107:485–492.
18. Quigley HA: Open angle glaucoma. N Engl J Med 1993;328:1097–1106.
19. Quigley HA: Reappraising the risks and benefits of aggressive glaucoma therapy. Ophthalmology 1997;104:1985–1986.

20. Quigley HA, Tielsch JM, Katz J, Sommer A: Rate of progression in open-angle glaucoma estimated from cross-sectional prevalence of visual field damage. Am J Ophthalmol 1996;122:355–363.
21. Wilson R, Walker AM, Dueker DK, Crick RP: Risk factors for rate of progression of glaucomatous visual field loss. Arch Ophthalmol 1982;100:737–741.
22. Kolker AE: Visual prognosis in advanced glaucoma: A comparison of medical and surgical therapy for retention of vision in 101 eyes with advanced glaucoma. Trans Am Ophthalmol Soc 1977;75:539–555.
23. Wilson R, Richardson TM, Hertzmark E, Grant WM: Race as a risk factor for progressive glaucomatous damage. Ann Ophthalmol 1985;17:653–659.
24. The AGIS Investigators: The Advanced Glaucoma Intervention Study (AGIS) 3: Baseline characteristics of black and white patients. Ophthalmology 1998;105:1137–1145.
25. Sommer A, Tielsch JM, Katz J, et al: Relationship between intraocular pressure and primary open angle glaucoma among white and black Americans: The Baltimore Eye Survey. Arch Ophthalmol 1991;109:1090–1095.
26. Tielsch JM, Sommer A, Katz J, et al: Racial variations in the prevalence of primary open-angle glaucoma: The Baltimore Eye Survey. JAMA 1991;266:369–374.
27. Kass MA, Hart WM Jr, Gordon M, Miller JP: Risk factors favoring the development of glaucomatous visual field loss in ocular hypertension. Surv Ophthalmol 1980;25:155–162.
28. Hart WM Jr, Yablonski M, Kass MA, Becker B: Multivariate analysis of the risk of glaucomatous visual field loss. Arch Ophthalmol 1979;97:1455–1458.
29. Glaucoma Laser Trial Research Group: The Glaucoma Laser Trial (GLT). 6: Treatment group differences in visual field changes. Am J Ophthalmol 1995;120:10–22.
30. Glaucoma Laser Trial Research Group. The Glaucoma Laser Trial and Glaucoma Laser Trial Follow-up Study. 7: Results. Am J Ophthalmol 1995;120:718–731.
31. Koseki N, Araie M, Shirato S, Yamamoto S: Effect of trabeculectomy on visual field performance in central 30 degree field in progressive normal-tension glaucoma. Ophthalmology 1997; 104:197–201.
32. Bhandari A, Crabb DP, Poinoosawmy D, et al: Effect of surgery on visual field progression in normal-tension glaucoma. Ophthalmology 1997;104:1131–1137.
33. Abedin S, Simmons RJ, Grant WM: Progressive low-tension glaucoma: Treatment to stop glaucomatous cupping and field loss when these progress despite normal intraocular pressure. Ophthalmology 1982;89:1–6.
34. Migdal C: What is the appropriate treatment for patients with primary open-angle glaucoma: Medicine, laser, or primary surgery? Ophthalmic Surg 1995;26:108–109.
35. Sherwood MB, Migdal CS, Hitchings RA, et al: Initial treatment of glaucoma: Surgery or medications. I: Filtration Surgery. II: Medical therapy. III: Editorial: Chop or Drop? Surv Ophthalmol 1993;37:293–305.
36. Sherwood MB, Migdal CS, Hitchings RA: Therapeutics and techniques: Filtration surgery as the initial therapy for open-angle glaucoma. J Glaucoma 1993;2:64–67.
37. Broadway D, Hitchings R, Grierson I: Topical antiglaucomatous therapy: Adverse effects on the conjunctiva and implications for filtering surgery. J Glaucoma 1995;4:136–148.
38. Ariturk N, Oge I, Baris S, et al: The effects of antiglaucomatous agents on conjunctiva used for various durations. Am J Ophthalmol 1997;124:272.
39. Sherwood MB, Grierson I, Millar L, Hitchings RA: Long-term morphologic effects of antiglaucoma drugs on the conjunctiva and Tenon's capsule in glaucomatous patients. Ophthalmology 1989;96:327–335.
40. Young TL, Higginbotham EJ, Zou X, Farber MD: Effects of topical glaucoma drugs on fistulized rabbit conjunctiva. Ophthalmology 1990;97:1423–1427.
41. Broadway D, Grierson I, Hitchings R: Adverse effects of topical antiglaucomatous medications on the conjunctiva. Br J Ophthalmol 1993;77:590–596.
42. Batterbury M, Wishart PK: Is high initial aqueous outflow of benefit in trabeculectomy? Eye 1993;7:109–112.
43. Johnson DH, Yoshikawa K, Brubaker RF, Hodge DO: The effect of long-term medical therapy on the outcome of filtration surgery. Am J Ophthalmol 1994;117:139–148.
44. Smith DL, Skuta GL, Kincaid MC, et al: The effects of glaucoma medications on Tenon's capsule and conjunctiva in the rabbit. Ophthalmic Surg 1991;22:336–340.
45. Wilson MR: The myth of "21". J Glaucoma 1997;6:75–77.
46. Gressel MG, Heuer DK, Parrish RK II: Trabeculectomy in young patients. Ophthalmology 1984;91:1242–1246.
47. Vesti E, Raitta C: A review of the outcome of trabeculectomy in open-angle glaucoma. Ophthalmic Surg Lasers 1997;28:128–132.
48. Chen TC, Wilensky JT, Viana MAG: Long-term follow-up of initially successful trabeculectomy. Ophthalmology 1997;104:1120–1125.
49. Shields MB: Trabeculectomy vs full-thickness filtering operation for control of glaucoma. Ophthalmic Surg 1980;11:498–505.
50. D'Ermo F, Bonomi L, Doro D: A critical analysis of the long-term results of trabeculectomy. Am J Ophthalmol 1979;88:829–835.
51. Tornqvist G, Drolsum LK: Trabeculectomies: A long-term study. Acta Ophthalmol (Copenh) 1991;69:450–454.
52. Chen TC, Wilensky JT, Viana MA: Long-term follow-up of initially successful trabeculectomy. Ophthalmology 1997;104:1120–1125.
53. Mermoud A, Salmon JF, Barron A, et al: Surgical management of post-traumatic angle recession glaucoma. Ophthalmology 1993; 100:634–642.
54. Katz LJ, Spaeth GL: Surgical management of the secondary glaucomas: Part I. Ophthalmic Surg 1987;18:826–834.
55. Vesti E: Filtering blebs: Follow up of trabeculectomy. Ophthalmic Surg 1993;24:249–255.
56. Costa VP, Katz LJ, Spaeth GL, et al: Primary trabeculectomy in young adults. Ophthalmology 1993;100:1071–1076.
57. Sturmer J, Broadway DC, Hitchings RA: Young patient trabeculectomy: Assessment of risk factors for failure. Ophthalmology 1993;100:928–939.
58. Cadera W, Pachtman MA, Cantor LB, et al: Filtering surgery in childhood glaucoma. Ophthalmic Surg 1984;15:319–322.
59. Wallace DK, Plager DA, Snyder SK, et al: Surgical results of secondary glaucomas in children. Ophthalmology 1998;105:101–111.
60. Khaw P: What is the best primary surgical treatment for the infantile glaucomas? Br J Ophthalmol 1996;80:495–496.
61. Broadway D, Grierson I, Hitchings R: Racial differences in the results of glaucoma filtration surgery: Are racial differences in the conjunctival cell profile important? Br J Ophthalmol 1994;78:466–475.
62. Shingleton BJ, Distler JA, Baker BH: Filtration surgery in black patients: Early results in a West Indian population. Ophthalmic Surg 1987;18:195–199.
63. McMillan TA, Stewart WC, Hennis HL, et al: Histologic differences in the conjunctiva of black and white glaucoma patients. Ophthalmic Surg 1992;23:762–765.
64. Stewart WC, Reid KK, Pitts RA: The results of trabeculectomy surgery in African-American versus white glaucoma patients. J Glaucoma 1993;2:236–240.
65. Glaucoma Laser Trial, GLT: The Glaucoma Laser Trial (GLT) 5: Subgroup differences at enrollment. Ophthalmic Surg 1993;24:232–240.
66. Stone RT, Herndon LW, Allingham RR, Shields MB: Results of trabeculectomy with 0.3 mg/mL mitomycin C titrating exposure times based on risk factors for failure. J Glaucoma 1998;7:39–44.
67. Levene RZ: Glaucoma filtering surgery: Factors that determine pressure control. Ophthalmic Surg 1984;15:475–483.
68. Parrish RK II: Filtering procedures in patients predisposed to failure. Curr Ther Ophthalmic Surg 1989;182–186.
69. Giangiacomo J, Dueker DK, Adelstein E: The effect of preoperative subconjunctival triamcinolone administration on glaucoma filtration. Arch Ophthalmol 1986;104:838–841.
70. Giangiacomo J, Dueker DK, Adelstein EH: Histopathology of triamcinolone in the subconjunctiva. Ophthalmology 1987;94:149–153.
71. Morgan CM, Schatz H, Vine AK, et al: Ocular complications associated with retrobulbar injections. Ophthalmology 1988;95:660–665.
72. Ahn JC, Stanley JA: Subarachnoid injection as a complication of retrobulbar anesthesia. Am J Ophthalmol 1987;103:225–230.
73. Brookshire GL, Gleitsmann KY, Schenk EC: Life-threatening complications of retrobulbar block. Ophthalmology 1986;93:1476–1478.
74. Javitt JC, Addiego R, Friedberg HL, Libonati MM: Brain stem anesthesia after retrobulbar block. Ophthalmology 1987;94:718–724.

75. Castillo A, Lopez-Abad C, Macias JM, Diaz D: Respiratory arrest after 0.75% bupivacaine retrobulbar block. Ophthalmic Surg 1994;25:628–629.
76. Hagan JC III: Retrobulbar versus peribulbar anesthesia. Ophthalmic Surg 1988;19:143–144.
77. Stevens J, Giubilei M, Lanigan L, Hykin P: Sub-tenon, retrobulbar and peribulbar local anaesthesia: The effect upon intraocular pressure. Eur J Implant Refract Surg 1993;5:25–28.
78. O'Donoghue E, Batterbury M, Lavy T: Effect on intraocular pressure of local anaesthesia in eyes undergoing intraocular surgery. Br J Ophthalmol 1994;78:605–607.
79. Petersen WC, Yanoff M: Subconjunctival anesthesia: An alternative to retrobulbar and peribulbar techniques. Ophthalmic Surg 1991;22:199–201.
80. Buys YM, Trope GE: Prospective study of sub-Tenon's versus retrobulbar anesthesia for inpatient and day-surgery trabeculectomy. Ophthalmology 1993;100:1585–1589.
81. Azuara-Blanco A, Moster MR, Marr BP: Subconjunctival versus peribulbar anesthesia in trabeculectomy: A prospective, randomized study. Ophthalmic Surg Lasers 1997;28:896–899.
82. Sanders R, MacEwen CJ, Haining WM: Trabeculectomy: Effect of varying surgical site. Eye 1993;7:440–443.
83. Tabbara KF: Late infections following filtering procedures. Ann Ophthalmol 1978;8:1228–1231.
84. Wolner B, Liebmann JM, Sassani JW, et al: Late bleb-related endophthalmitis after trabeculectomy with adjunctive 5-fluorouracil. Ophthalmology 1991;98:1053–1060.
85. Greenfield DS, Suner IJ, Miller MP, et al: Endophthalmitis after filtering surgery with mitomycin. Arch Ophthalmol 1996;114:943–949.
86. Higginbotham EJ, Stevens RK, Musch DC, et al: Bleb-related endophthalmitis after trabeculectomy with mitomycin c. Ophthalmology 1996;103:650–656.
87. Levkovitch-verbin H, Goldenfeld M, Melamed S. Fornix-based trabeculectomy with mitomycin-C. Ophthalmic Surg Lasers 1997;28:818–821.
88. Shuster JN, Krupin T, Kolker AE, Becker B: Limbus-v fornix-based conjunctival flap in trabeculectomy. Ann Emerg Med 1984;361–362.
89. Traverso CE, Tomey KF, Antonios S: Limbal-vs fornix-based conjunctival trabeculectomy flaps. Am J Ophthalmol 1987;104:28–32.
90. Brincker P, Kessing SV. Limbus-based versus fornix-based conjunctival flap in glaucoma filtering surgery. Acta Ophthalmol (Copenh) 1992;70:641–644.
91. Reichert R, Stewart W, Shields MB: Limbus-based versus fornix-based conjunctival flaps in trabeculectomy. Ophthalmic Surg 1987;18:672–676.
92. Wise JB: Mitomycin-compatible suture technique for fornix-based conjunctival flaps in glaucoma filtration surgery. Arch Ophthalmol 1993;111:992–997.
93. Liss RP, Scholes GN, Crandall AS: Glaucoma filtration surgery: New horizontal mattress closure of conjunctival incision. Ophthalmic Surg 1991;22:298–300.
94. Miller KN, Blasini M, Shields MB, Ho CH: A comparison of total and partial tenonectomy with trabeculectomy. Am J Ophthalmol 1991;111:323–326.
95. Ophir A, Ticho U: A randomized study of trabeculectomy and subconjunctival administration of fluorouracil in primary glaucomas. Arch Ophthalmol 1992;110:1072–1075.
96. Bergstrom TJ, Wilkinson WS, Skuta GL, et al: The effects of subconjunctival mitomycin-C on glaucoma filtration surgery in rabbits. Arch Ophthalmol 1991;109:1725–1730.
97. Nguyen KD, Reyes MR, Lee DA: Control of wound healing following glaucoma surgery. J Glaucoma 1995;4:130–135.
98. Jampel HD: Therapeutics and techniques: Impact of adjuvant chemotherapy on glaucoma filtration surgery. J Glaucoma 1993;2:58–63.
99. Khaw PT, Sherwood MB, Doyle JW, et al: Intraoperative and post operative treatment with 5-fluorouracil and mitomycin-c: Long term effects in vivo on subconjunctival and scleral fibroblasts. Int Ophthalmol 1992;16:381–385.
100. Khaw PT, Sherwood MB, MacKay SLD, et al: Five-minute treatments with fluorouracil, floxuridine, and mitomycin have long-term effects on human Tenon's capsule fibroblasts. Arch Ophthalmol 1992;110:1150–1154.
101. Fluorouracil Filtering Surgery Study Group: Three-year follow-up of the fluorouracil filtering surgery study. Am J Ophthalmol 1993;115:82–92.
102. Van Buskirk EM: Five-year follow-up of the Fluorouracil Filtering Surgery Study. Am J Ophthalmol 1996;122:751–752.
103. Ticho U, Ophir A: Late complications after glaucoma filtering surgery with adjunctive 5-fluorouracil. Am J Ophthalmol 1993; 115:506–510.
104. Heuer DK, Parrish RKC II, Gressel MG, et al: 5-Fluorouracil and glaucoma filtering surgery III: Intermediate follow-up of a pilot study. Ophthalmology 1986;93:1537–1546.
105. Tsai JC, Feuer WJ, Parrish RK II, Grajewski AL: 5-Fluorouracil filtering surgery and neovascular glaucoma: Long-term follow-up of the original pilot study. Ophthalmology 1995;102:887–893.
106. The Fluorouracil Filtering Surgery Study. Fluorouracil filtering surgery study one-year follow-up. Am J Ophthalmol 1989;108:625–635.
107. Khaw PT, Grierson I, Hitchings RA, Rice NS: 5-Fluorouracil and beyond. Br J Ophthalmol 1991;75:577–578.
108. Fluorouracil Filtering Surgery Study Group: Five-year follow-up of the Fluorouracil Filtering Surgery Study. Am J Ophthalmol 1996;121:349–366.
109. Liebmann JM, Ritch R, Marmor M, et al: Initial 5-fluorouracil trabeculectomy in uncomplicated glaucoma. Ophthalmology 1991;98:1036–1041.
110. Goldenfeld M, Krupin T, Ruderman JM, et al: 5-Fluorouracil in initial trabeculectomy: A prospective, randomized, multicenter study. Ophthalmology 1994;101:1024–1029.
111. Franks WA, Hitchings RA: Complications of 5-fluorouracil after trabeculectomy. Eye 1991;5:385–389.
112. Knapp A, Heuer DK, Stern GA, Driebe WT: Serious corneal complications of glaucoma filtering surgery with postoperative 5-fluorouracil. Am J Ophthalmol 1987;103:183–187.
113. Lee DA, Hersh P, Kersten D, Melamed S: Complications of subconjunctival 5-fluorouracil following glaucoma filtering surgery. Ophthalmic Surg 1987;18:187–190.
114. Ando H, Ido T, Kawai Y, et al: Inhibition of corneal epithelial wound healing: A comparative study of mitomycin C and 5-fluorouracil. Ophthalmology 1992;99:1809–1814.
115. Hurvitz LM: Corneal opacification after 5-fluorouracil injections. Ophthalmic Surg 1994;25:130.
116. Hickey-Dwyer M, Wishart PK: Serious corneal complication of 5-fluorouracil. Br J Ophthalmol 1993;77:250–251.
117. Khaw PT, Doyle JW, Sherwood MB, et al: Effects of intraoperative 5-fluorouracil or mitomycin C on glaucoma filtration surgery in the rabbit. Ophthalmology 1993;100:367–372.
118. Doyle JW, Sherwood MB, Khaw PT, et al: Intraoperative 5-fluorouracil for filtration surgery in the rabbit. Invest Ophthalmol Vis Sci 1993;34:3313–3319.
119. Pablo LE, Larrosa JM, Ronchera JM, et al: Effectiveness of intraoperative versus subconjunctival mitomycin C on glaucoma filtering surgery in the rabbit. Ann Ophthalmol 1996;28:35–39.
120. Occleston NL, Daniels JT, Tarnuzzer RW, et al: Single exposures to antiproliferatives: Long-term effects on ocular fibroblast wound-healing behavior. Invest Ophthalmol Vis Sci 1997;38:1998–2007.
121. Lanigan L, Sturmer J, Baez KA, et al: Single intraoperative applications of 5-fluorouracil during filtration surgery: Early results. Br J Ophthalmol 1994;33–37.
122. Dietze PJ, Feldman RM, Gross RL: Intraoperative application of 5-fluorouracil during trabeculectomy. Ophthalmic Surg 1992;23:662–665.
123. Smith MF, Sherwood MB: Results of intraoperative 5-fluorouracil supplementation on trabeculectomy for open-angle glaucoma. Am J Ophthalmol 1992;114:737–741.
124. Mora JS, Nguyen N, Iwach AG, et al: Trabeculectomy with intraoperative sponge 5-fluorouracil. Ophthalmology 1996;103:963–970.
125. Hugkulstone CE, Vernon SA: Low-dose perioperative 5-fluorouracil in trabeculectomy. Ophthalmic Surg Lasers 1996;27:910–916.
126. Smith MF, Doyle JW, Nguyen QH, Sherwood MB: Results of intraoperative 5-fluorouracil or lower dose mitomycin C administration on initial trabeculectomy surgery. J Glaucoma 1997;6:104–110.
127. Singh K, Egbert PR, Byrd S, et al: Trabeculectomy with intraoperative 5-fluorouracil vs. mitomycin C. Am J Ophthalmol 1997;123:48–53.
128. Jampel HD: Effect of brief exposure to mitomycin C on viability and proliferation of cultured human Tenon's capsule fibroblasts. Ophthalmology 1992;99:1471–1476.

129. Trope GE, Pavlin CJ, Bau A, et al: Malignant glaucoma: Clinical and ultrasound biomicroscopic features. Ophthalmology 1994; 101:1030–1035.
130. Mattox C: Glaucoma filtration surgery and antimetabolites. Ophthalmic Surg Lasers 1995;26:473–480.
131. Crowston JG, Akbar AN, Constable PH, et al: Antimetabolite-induced apoptosis in Tenon's capsule fibroblasts. Invest Ophthalmol Vis Sci 1998;39:449–454.
132. Shields MB, Scroggs MW, Sloop CM, Simmons RB: Clinical and histopathologic observations concerning hypotony after trabeculectomy with adjunctive mitomycin C. Am J Ophthalmol 1993; 116:673–683.
133. Khaw PT: Antiproliferated agents and the prevention of scarring after surgery: Friend or foe? Br J Ophthalmol 1995;79:627.
134. Nuyts RMMA, Felten PC, Pels E, et al: Histopathologic effects of mitomycin C after trabeculectomy in human glaucomatous eyes with persistent hypotony. Am J Ophthalmol 1994;118:225–237.
135. Mietz H, Brunner R, Addicks K, Krieglstein GK: Histopathology of an avascular filtering bleb after trabeculectomy with mitomycin C. J Glaucoma 1993;2:266–270.
136. Khaw PT, Doyle JW, Sherwood MB, et al: Prolonged localized tissue effects from 5-minute exposures to fluorouracil and mitomycin C. Arch Ophthalmol 1993;111:263–267.
137. Seah SKL, Prata JA Jr, Minckler DS, et al: Mitomycin C concentration in human aqueous humour following trabeculectomy. Eye 1993;7:652–655.
138. Sarraf D, Eezzuduemhoi RD, Cheng Q, et al: Aqueous and vitreous concentration of mitomycin C by topical administration after glaucoma filtration surgery in rabbits. Ophthalmology 1993;100:1574–1579.
139. Yaldo MK, Stamper RL: Long-term effects of mitomycin on filtering blebs: Lack of fibrovascular proliferative response following severe inflammation. Arch Ophthalmol 1993;111:824–826.
140. Gandolfi SA, Vecchi M, Braccio L: Decrease of intraocular pressure after subconjunctival injection of mitomycin in human glaucoma. Arch Ophthalmol 1995;113:582–585.
141. Kitazawa Y, Kawase K, Matsushita H, Minobe M: Trabeculectomy with mitomycin: A comparative study with fluorouracil. Arch Ophthalmol 1991;109:1693–1698.
142. Skuta GL, Beeson CC, Higginbotham EJ, et al: Intraoperative mitomycin versus postoperative 5-fluorouracil in high-risk glaucoma filtering surgery. Ophthalmology 1992;99:438–444.
143. Lamping KA, Belkin JK: 5-Fluorouracil and mitomycin C in pseudophakic patients. Ophthalmology 1995;102:70–75.
144. Kupin TH, Juzych MS, Shin DH, et al: Adjunctive mitomycin C in primary trabeculectomy in phakic eyes. Am J Ophthalmol 1995;119:30–39.
145. Katz GJ, Higginbotham EJ, Lichter PR, et al: Mitomycin C verses 5-fluorouracil in high risk glaucoma filtering surgery. Ophthalmology 1995;102:1263–1269.
146. Singh J, O'Brien C, Chawla HB: Success rate and complications of intraoperative 0.2mg/cc mitomycin C in trabeculectomy surgery. Eye 1995;9:460–466.
147. Liang LL, Epstein DL: Comparison of mitomycin C and 5-fluorouracil on filtration surgery success in rabbit eyes. J Glaucoma 1992;1:87–93.
148. Robin AL, Ramakrishnan R, Krishnadas R, et al: A long-term dose-response study of mitomycin in glaucoma filtration surgery. Arch Ophthalmol 1997;115:969–974.
149. Higginbotham EJ: Adjunctive use of mitomycin in filtration surgery: Is it worth the risk (editorial)? Arch Ophthalmol 1997;115:1068–1069.
150. Dreyer EB, Chaturvedi N, Zurakowski D: Effect of mitomycin C and fluorouracil-supplemented trabeculectomies on the anterior segment. Arch Ophthalmol 1995;113:578–580.
151. Fourman S: Scleritis after glaucoma filtering surgery with mitomycin C. Ophthalmology 1995;102:1569–1571.
152. Derick RJ, Pasquale L, Quigley HA, Jampel H: Potential toxicity of mitomycin C. Arch Ophthalmol 1991;109:1635.
153. Pastor SA, Williams R, Hetherington J, et al: Corneal endothelial cell loss following trabeculectomy with mitomycin C. Glaucoma 1993;2:112–113.
154. McDermott ML, Wang J, Shin DH: Mitomycin and the human corneal endothelium. Arch Ophthalmol 1994;112:533–537.
155. Prata JA Jr, Neves RA, Minckler DS, et al: Trabeculectomy with mitomycin C in glaucoma associated with uveitis. Ophthalmic Surg 1994;25:616–620.
156. Mermoud A, Salmon JF, Murray ADN: Trabeculectomy with mitomycin C for refractory glaucoma in blacks. Am J Ophthalmol 1993;116:72–78.
157. Wright MM, McGehee RF, Pederson JE: Intraoperative mitomycin C for glaucoma associated with ocular inflammation. Ophthalmic Surg Lasers 1997;28:370–376.
158. Parrish RK II: Who should receive antimetabolites after filtering surgery? Arch Ophthalmol 1992;110:1069–1071.
159. Prata JA Jr, Minckler DS, Lee PP, et al: Trabeculectomy in pseudophakic patients: Postoperative 5-fluorouracil versus intraoperative mitomycin C antiproliferative therapy. Ophthalmic Surg 1995; 26:73–77.
160. Kolker AE: Visual prognosis in advanced glaucoma: A comparison of medical and surgical therapy for retention of vision in 101 eyes with advance glaucoma. Trans Am Ophthalmol Soc 1977;75:539–555.
161. Yamamoto T, Ichien M, Suemori-Matsushita H, Kitazawa Y: Trabeculectomy with mitomycin C for normal-tension glaucoma. J Glaucoma 1995;4:158–163.
162. Costa VP, Comegno PEC, Vasconcelos JPC, et al: Low-dose mitomycin C trabeculectomy in patients with advanced glaucoma. J Glaucoma 1996;5:193–199.
163. Agarwal HC, Sood NN, Sihota R, et al: Mitomycin C in congenital glaucoma. Ophthalmic Surg Lasers 1997;28:979–985.
164. Mandal AK, Walton DS, John T, Jayagandan A: Mitomycin C–augmented trabeculectomy in refractory congenital glaucoma. Ophthalmology 1997;104:996–1003.
165. Susanna R Jr, Oltrogge EW, Carani JCE, Nicolela MT: Mitomycin as adjunct chemotherapy with trabeculectomy in congenital and developmental glaucomas. J Glaucoma 1995;4:151–157.
166. Schuman JS: Surgical management of coexisting cataract and glaucoma. Ophthalmic Surg Lasers 1996;27:45–59.
167. Figueiredo RS, Araujo SV, Cohen EJ, et al: Management of coexisting corneal disease and glaucoma by combined penetrating keratoplast and trabeculectomy with mitomycin C. Ophthalmic Surg Lasers 1996;27:903–909.
168. Desjardins DC, Parrish RK II, Folberg R, et al: Wound healing after filtering surgery in owl monkeys. Arch Ophthalmol 1986;104:1835–1839.
169. Hever D, Gressel M, Parrish R, et al: Topical fluorouracil—postoperative administration in an animal model of glaucoma filtering surgery. Arch Ophthalmol 1986;104:132–136.
170. Yamamoto T, Varani J, Soong HK, Lichter PR: Effects of 5-fluorouracil and mitomycin C on cultured rabbit subconjunctival fibroblasts. Ophthalmology 1990;97:1204–1210.
171. Hefetz L, Keren T, Naveh N: Early and late postoperative application of 5-fluorouracil following trabeculectomy in refractory glaucoma. Ophthalmic Surg 1994;25:715–719.
172. Cheung JC, Wright MM, Murali M, Pederson JE: Intermediate-term outcome of variable dose mitomycin C filtering surgery. Ophthalmology 1997;104:143–179.
173. Kitazawa Y, Suemori-Matsushita H, Yamamoto T, Kawase K: Low-dose and high-dose mitomycin trabeculectomy as an initial surgery in primary open-angle glaucoma. Ophthalmology 1993;100:1624–1628.
174. Cohen JS, Novack GD, Li Li Z: The role of mitomycin treatment duration and previous intraocular surgery on the success of trabeculectomy surgery. J Glaucoma 1997;6:3–9.
175. Megevand GS, Salmon JF, Schultz RP, Murray ADN: The effect of reducing the exposure time of mitomycin C in glaucoma filtering surgery. Ophthalmology 1995;102:84–90.
176. Mietz H, Addicks K, Krieglstein GK: A scleral shield for the application of mitomycin C during trabeculectomy: A rabbit model. Ophthalmic Surg 1994;25:466–470.
177. Kawase K, Matsushita H, Yamamoto T, Kitazawa Y: Mitomycin concentration in rabbit and human ocular tissues after topical administration. Ophthalmology 1992;99:203–207.
178. Prevezas DC, Melissurgos ID: Adjustable temporal suture in trabeculectomy with scleral flap. Ophthalmic Surg Lasers 1997;28:745–750.
179. Maberley D, Apel A, Rootman DS: Releasable U suture for trabeculectomy surgery. Ophthalmic Surg 1994;25:251–255.
180. Hsu CT, Yarng SS: A modified removable suture in trabeculectomy. Ophthalmic Surg 1993;24:579–585.

181. Johnstone MA, Wellington DP, Ziel CJ: A releasable scleral-flap tamponade suture for guarded filtration surgery. Arch Ophthalmol 1993;111:398–403.
182. Chopra H, Goldenfeld M, Krupin T, Rosenberg LF: Therapeutics and techniques: Early postoperative titration of bleb function: Argon laser suture lysis and removable sutures in trabeculectomy. J Glaucoma 1992;1:54–57.
183. Cohen JS, Osher RH: Endophthalmitis associated with releasable sutures. Arch Ophthalmol 1997;115:292.
184. Rosenberg LF, Siegfried CJ: Endophthalmitis associated with a releasable suture. Arch Ophthalmol 1996;114:767.
185. Burchfield JC, Kolker AE, Cook SG: Endophthalmitis following trabeculectomy with releasable sutures. Arch Ophthalmol 1996; 114:766.
186. Wand M: Intracameral sodium hyaluronate before fistulization. Ophthalmic Surg 1995;26:289.
187. Wand M: Viscoelastic agent and the prevention of post-filtration flat anterior chamber. Ophthalmic Surg 1988;19:523–524.
188. Wand M: Intraoperative intracameral viscoelastic agent in the prevention of postfiltration flat anterior chamber. J Glaucoma 1994;3:101–105.
189. Yusuf S, Collins R, Peto R: Why do we need some large, simple randomized trials? Stat Med 1984;3:409–420.
190. Raitta C, Lehto I, Puska P, et al: A randomized, prospective study on the use of sodium hyaluronate (Healon) in trabeculectomy. Ophthalmic Surg 1994;25:536–539.
191. Wilson RP, Lloyd J: The place of sodium hyaluronate in glaucoma surgery. Ophthalmic Surg 1986;17:30–33.
192. Liebmann JM, Ritch R, DiSclafani M, Stock L: Early intraocular pressure rise after trabeculectomy. Arch Ophthalmol 1990; 108:1549–1552.
193. Gaspar AZ, Flammer J, Hendrickson P: Regression of rubeosis iridis after trabeculectomy combined with mitomycin C. Ophthalmic Surg Lasers 1996;27:709–712.
194. Kao SF, Lichter PR, Musch DC: Anterior chamber depth following filtration surgery. Ophthalmic Surg 1989;20:332–336.
195. Bellows AR, Johnstone MA: Surgical management of chronic glaucoma in aphakia. Ophthalmology 1983;90:807–813.
196. Gross RL, Feldman RM, Spaeth GL, et al: Surgical therapy of chronic glaucoma in aphakia and pseudophakia. Ophthalmology 1988;95:1195–1201.
197. Herschler J: The effect of total vitrectomy on filtration surgery in the aphakic eye. Ophthalmology 1981;88:229–232.
198. Fulcher T, Chan J, Lanigan B, et al: Long term follow up of primary trabeculectomy for infantile glaucoma. Br J Ophthalmol 1996;80:499–502.
199. Givens K, Shields MB: Suprachoroidal hemorrhage after glaucoma filtering surgery. Am J Ophthalmol 1987;103:689–694.
200. Ruderman JM, Harbin TS Jr, Campbell DG: Postoperative suprachoroidal hemorrhage following filtration procedures. Arch Ophthalmol 1986;104:201–205.
201. Whitehouse GM, Filipic M, Francis IC: Expulsive choroidal hemorrhage: A clinical and pathologic review. Aust N Z J Ophthalmol 1990;17:225–232.
202. Frenkel REP, Shin DH: Prevention and management of delayed suprachoroidal hemorrhage after filtration surgery. Arch Ophthalmol 1986;104:1459–1463.
203. Reynolds MG, Haimovici R, Flynn HW Jr, et al: Suprachoroidal hemorrhage: Clinical features and results of secondary surgical management. Ophthalmology 1993;100:460–465.
204. Speaker MG, Guerriero PN, Met JA, et al: A case-control study of risk factors for intraoperative suprachoroidal expulsive hemorrhage. Ophthalmology 1991;98:202–210.
205. Cantor LB: Suprachoroidal hemorrhage. *In* Spaeth GL, Katz LJ, Parker KW (eds): Current Therapy in Ophthalmic Surgery. Philadelphia, BC Decker, 1989, pp 325–327.
206. Maumenee AE, Schwartz MF: Acute intraoperative choroidal effusion. Am J Ophthalmol 1985;100:147–154.
207. Scott IU, Flynn HW, Schiffman J, et al: Visual acuity outcomes among patients with appositional suprachoroidal hemorrhage. Ophthalmology 1997;104:2039–2046.
208. The Fluorouracil Filtering Surgery Study Group: Risk factors for suprachoroidal hemorrhage after filtering surgery. Am J Ophthalmol 1992;113:501–507.
209. Petursson GJ, Fraunfelder FT: Repair of an inadvertent buttonhole or leaking filtering bleb. Arch Ophthalmol 1978;97:926–934.
210. Furgason TG, Perkins TW: A "clothesline" suture technique for the repair of a conjunctival tear during trabeculectomy. Ophthalmic Surg Lasers 1997;28:772–773.
211. Riley SF, Smith TJ, Simmons RJ: Repair of a disinserted scleral flap in trabeculectomy. Ophthalmic Surg 1993;24:349–350.
212. Rumelt S, Rehany U: A donor corneal patch graft for an incompetent scleral flap following trabeculectomy. Ophthalmic Surg Lasers 1996;27:878–880.
213. Starita RJ, Fellman RL, Spaeth GL, et al: Short- and long-term effects of postoperative corticosteroids on trabeculectomy. Ophthalmology 1985;92:938–946.
214. Araujo SV, Spaeth GL, Roth SM, Starita RJ: A ten-year follow-up on a prospective, randomized trial of postoperative corticosteroids after trabeculectomy. Ophthalmology 1995;102:1753–1759.
215. Cantor LB, Phillips CA, Kramer D, et al: Effect of topical flurbiprofen on trabeculectomy. J Glaucoma 1995;4:98–102.
216. Gwin TD, Stewart WC, Gwynn DR: Filtration surgery in rabbits treated with diclofenac or prednisolone acetate. Ophthalmic Surg 1994;25:245–250.
217. Sunaric-Mégevand G, Pournaras CJ: Current approach to postoperative endophthalmitis. Br J Ophthalmol 1997;81:1006–1015.
218. Wand M, Quintiliani R, Robinson A: Antibiotic prophylaxis eyes with filtration blebs: Survey of glaucoma specialists, microbiological study, and recommendations. J Glaucoma 1995;4:103–109.
219. Oh Y, Katz LJ: Indications and technique for reopening closed filtering blebs using the Nd:Yag laser—a review and case series. Ophthalmic Surg 1993;24:617–622.
220. Piltz JR, Starita RJ: The use of subconjunctivally administered tissue plasminogen activator after trabeculectomy. Ophthalmic Surg 1994;25:51–53.
221. Johnson MW, Olsen KR, Hernandez E: Tissue plasminogen activator thrombolysis during surgical evacuation of experimental subretinal hemorrhage. Ophthalmology 1992;99:515–521.
222. Olivier MM, Kupin TH, McDermott ML, Shin DH: Intracameral tissue plasminogen activator in neovascular glaucoma. Arch Ophthalmol 1993;111:586.
223. Krug JH Jr, Melamed S: Adjunctive use of delayed and adjustable low-dose 5-fluorouracil in refractory glaucoma. Am J Ophthalmol 1990;109:412–418.
224. Singh J, Bell RWD, Adams A, O'Brien C: Enhancement of post trabeculectomy bleb formation by laser suture lysis. Br J Ophthalmol 1996;80:624–627.
225. Chopra H, Goldenfeld M, Krupin T, Rosenberg LF: Early postoperative titration of bleb function: Argon laser suture lysis and removable sutures in trabeculectomy. J Glaucoma 1992;1:54–57.
226. Asamoto A, Yablonski ME, Matsushita M: A retrospective study of the effects of laser suture lysis on the long-term results of trabeculectomy. Ophthalmic Surg 1995;26:223–227.
227. Savage JA, Khan KA: Fine-tuning the filter: Adjusting aqueous humor dynamics. Clin Signs Ophthalmol 1990;11:1–15.
228. Melamed S, Ashkenazi I, Glovinski J, Blumenthal M: Tight scleral flap trabeculectomy with postoperative laser suture lysis. Am J Ophthalmol 1990;109:303–309.
229. Savage J, Lytle R, Condon GP, Simmons R: Laser suture lysis after trabeculectomy. Ophthalmology 1988;95:1631–1638.
230. Kasahara N, Smith TJ, Sibayan SA, et al: Midterm reversible failure in trabeculectomies with adjunctive mitomycin C. Ophthalmic Surg Lasers 1997;28:986–991.
231. Pappa KS, Derick RJ, Weber PA, et al: Late argon laser suture lysis after mitomycin C trabeculectomy. Ophthalmology 1993;100:1268–1271.
232. Morinelli EN, Sidoti PA, Heuer DK, et al: Laser suture lysis after mitomycin C trabeculectomy. Ophthalmology 1996;103:306–314.
233. Geijssen HC, Greve EL: Mitomycin, suture lysis and hypotony. Int Ophthalmol 1992;16:371–374.
234. Kumar H, Talwar D: Is krypton red better than argon blue-green for laser suturotomy? Ophthalmic Surg 1991;22:303–304.
235. Schwartz LW, Traverso C, Spaeth GL, Greenidge KC: Variation of techniques on the results of argon laser trabeculoplasty. Ophthalmology 1983;90:781–784.
236. Greenfield DS, Miller MP, Suner IJ, Palmberg PF: Needle elevation of the scleral flap for failing filtration blebs after trabeculectomy with mitomycin C. Am J Ophthalmol 1996;122:195–204.
237. Mardelli PG, Lederer CM, Murray PL, et al: Slit-lamp needle revision of failed filtering blebs using mitomycin C. Ophthalmology 1996;103:1946–1955.

238. Shin DH, Juzych MS, Khatana AK, et al: Needling revision of failed filtering blebs with adjunctive 5-fluorouracil. Ophthalmic Surg 1993;24:242–248.
239. Schuman JS, Stinson WG, Hutchinson T, et al: Holmium laser sclerectomy: Success and complications. Ophthalmology 1993; 100:1060–1065.
240. Feldman RM, Gross RL, Spaeth GL, et al: Risk factors for the development of Tenon's capsule cysts after trabeculectomy. Ophthalmology 1989;96:336–341.
241. Oh Y, Katz LJ, Spaeth GL, Wilson RP: Risk factors for the development of encapsulated filtering blebs: The role of surgical glove powder and 5-fluorouracil. Ophthalmology 1994;101:629–634.
242. Feldman RM, Gross RL, Wilson RP, et al: Encapsulated filtering blebs. Arch Ophthalmol 1987;105:1589.
243. Gross RL, Wilson RP, Feldman RM: Encapsulated bleb after trabeculectomy: A frequent complication. Clin Signs Ophthalmol 1987;9:1–12.
244. Azuara-Blanco A, Bond JB, Wilson RP, et al: Encapsulated filtering blebs after trabeculectomy with mitomycin C. Ophthalmic Surg Lasers 1997;28:805–809.
245. Ophir A, Ticho U: Encapsulated filtering bleb and subconjunctival 5-fluorouracil. Ophthalmic Surg 1992;23:339–341.
246. Costa VP, Correa MM, Kara-Jose N: Needling versus medical treatment in encapsulated blebs: A randomized, prospective study. Ophthalmology 1997;104:1215–1220.
247. Shingleton BJ, Richter CU, Bellows AR, Hutchinson BT: Management of encapsulated filtration blebs. Ophthalmology 1990;97:63–68.
248. Byrnes GA, Leen MM, Wong TP, Benson WE: Vitrectomy for ciliary block (malignant) glaucoma. Ophthalmology 1995;102:1308–1311.
249. Dugel PU, Heuer DK, Thach AB, et al: Annular peripheral choroidal detachment simulating aqueous misdirection after glaucoma surgery. Ophthalmology 1997;104:439–444.
250. Ruben S, Tsai J, Hitchings R: Malignant glaucoma and its management. Br J Ophthalmol 1997;81:163–167.
251. Harbour JW, Rubsamen PE, Palmberg P: Pars plana vitrectomy in the management of phakic and pseudophakic malignant glaucoma. Arch Ophthalmol 1996;114:1073–1078.
252. Schubert HD: Postsurgical hypotony: Relationship to fistulization, inflammation, chorioretinal lesions, and the vitreous. Surv Ophthalmol 1996;41:97–125.
253. Liebmann JM, Sokol J, Ritch R: Management of chronic hypotony after glaucoma filtration surgery. J Glaucoma 1996;5:210–220.
254. Berke SJ, Bellows AR, Shingleton BJ, et al: Chronic and recurrent choroidal detachment after glaucoma filtering surgery. Ophthalmology 1987;94:154–162.
255. Lynch MG, Roesch M, Brown RH: Remodeling filtering blebs with the neodymium:YAG laser. Ophthalmology 1996;103:1700–1705.
256. Leen MM, Moster MR, Katz LJ, et al: Management of overfiltering and leaking blebs with autologous blood injection. Arch Ophthalmol 1995;113:1050–1055.
257. Shingleton BJ: Management of the failing glaucoma filter. Ophthalmic Surg Lasers 1996;27:445–451.
258. Choudhri SA, Herndon LW, Damji KF, et al: Efficacy of autologous blood injection for treating overfiltering or leaking blebs after glaucoma surgery. Am J Ophthalmol 1997;123:554–555.
259. Sibayan SAB, Igarashi S, Kasahara N, et al: Cataract extraction as a means of treating postfiltration hypotony maculopathy. Ophthalmic Surg Lasers 1997;28:241–243.
260. Duker JS, Schuman JS: Successful surgical treatment of hypotony maculopathy following trabeculectomy with topical mitomycin C. Ophthalmic Surg 1994;25:463–465.
261. Nuyts RMMA, Greve EL, Geijssen HC, Langerhorst CT: Treatment of hypotonous maculopathy after trabeculectomy with mitomycin C. Am J Ophthalmol 1994;118:322–331.
262. Suner IJ, Greenfield DS, Miller MP, et al: Hypotony maculopathy after filtering surgery with mitomycin C. Ophthalmology 1997;104:207–215.
263. Jampel HD, Pasquale LR, Dibernardo C: Hypotony maculopathy following trabeculectomy with mitomycin C. Arch Ophthalmol 1992;110:1049–1050.
264. Zacharia PT, Deppermann SR, Schuman JS: Ocular hypotony after trabeculectomy with mitomycin C. Am J Ophthalmol 1993;116: 314–326.
265. Stamper RL, McMenemy MG, Lieberman MF: Hypotonous maculopathy after trabeculectomy with subconjunctival 5-fluorouracil. Am J Ophthalmol 1992;114:544–553.
266. Wise JB: Treatment of chronic postfiltration hypotony by intrableb injection of autologous blood. Arch Ophthalmol 1993;111:827–830.
267. Cohen SM, Flynn HW, Palmberg PF, et al: Treatment of hypotony maculopathy after trabeculectomy. Ophthalmic Surg Lasers 1995;26:435–441.
268. Haynes WL, Alward WLM: Rapid visual recovery and long-term intraocular pressure control after donor scleral patch grafting for trabeculectomy-induced hypotony maculopathy. J Glaucoma 1995;4:200–201.
269. Costa VP, Wilson RP, Moster MR, et al: Hypotony maculopathy following the use of topical mitomycin C in glaucoma filtration surgery. Ophthalmic Surg 1993;24:389–394.
270. Asrani S, Wilensky JT: Management of bleb leaks after glaucoma filtering surgery. Ophthalmology 1996;103:294–298.
271. Wright MM, Brown EA, Maxwell K, et al: Laser-cured fibrinogen glue to repair bleb leaks in rabbits. Arch Ophthalmol 1998;116:199–202.
272. Graham SL, Goldberg I: Cyanoacrylate adhesive closure of wound leaks following fornix-based trabeculectomy with adjunct 5-fluorouracil. J Glaucoma 1993;2:297–302.
273. Hennis HL, Stewart WC: Use of the argon laser to close filtering bleb leaks. Graefes Arch Clin Exp Ophthalmol 1992;230:537–541.
274. Smith MF, Magauran RG III, Betchkal J, Doyle JW: Treatment of postfiltration bleb leaks with autologous blood. Ophthalmology 1995;102:868–871.
275. Graham SL, Murray B, Goldberg I: Closure of fornix-based posttrabeculectomy conjunctival wound leaks with autologous fibrin glue. Am J Ophthalmol 1992;114:221–222.
276. Stewart WC, Shields MB: Management of anterior chamber depth after trabeculectomy. Am J Ophthalmol 1988;106:41–44.
277. Gerber SL, Cantor LB: Slit lamp reformation of the anterior chamber following trabeculectomy. Ophthalmic Surg 1990;21:404–406.
278. Osher RH, Cionni RJ, Cohen JS: Re-forming the flat anterior chamber with healon. J Cataract Refract Surg 1996;22:411–415.
279. Liesegang TJ: Viscoelastic substances in ophthalmology. Surv Ophthalmol 1990;34:268–293.
280. Asamoto A, Yablonski ME: Posttrabeculectomy anterior subcapsular cataract formation induced by anterior chamber air. Ophthalmic Surg 1993;24:314–319.
281. Costa VP, Smith M, Spaeth GL, Gandham S, Markovitz B: Loss of visual acuity after trabeculectomy. Ophthalmology 1993;100:599–612.
282. Seah SKL, Prata JA Jr, Minckler DS, et al: Visual recovery after trabeculectomy. J Glaucoma 1995;4:228–233.
283. Levene RZ: Central visual field, visual acuity, and sudden visual loss after glaucoma surgery. Ophthalmic Surg 1992;23:388–394.
284. Henry JC: Therapeutics and techniques: Snuff syndrome. J Glaucoma 1994;3:92–95.
285. Martinez JA, Brown RH, Lynch MG, Caplan MB: Risk of postoperative visual loss in advanced glaucoma. Am J Ophthalmol 1993;115:332–337.
286. Katz LJ, Cantor LB, Spaeth GL: Complications of surgery in glaucoma—early and late bacterial endophthalmitis following glaucoma filtering surgery. Ophthalmology 1985;92:959–963.
287. Ashkenazi I, Melamed S, Avni I, et al: Risk factors associated with late infection of filtering blebs and endophthalmitis. Ophthalmic Surg 1991;22:570–574.
288. Palmberg R, Gutierrez YS, Miller D, et al: Potential bacterial contamination of eyedrops used for tonometry. Am J Ophthalmol 1994;117:578–582.
289. Ayyala RS, Bellows AR, Thomas JV, Hutchison BT: Bleb infections: Clinically different courses of "blebitis" and endophthalmitis. Ophthalmic Surg Lasers 1997;28:452–460.
290. Mandelbaum S, Forster RK, Gelender H, Culbertson W: Late onset endophthalmitis associated with filtering blebs. Ophthalmology 1985;92:964–972.
291. Donnenfeld E, Katz LJ, Cantor LB: A new way to manage infected blebs. Rev Ophthalmol 1997;8:140–145.
292. Endophthalmitis Vitrectomy Study Group: Results of the endophthalmitis vitrectomy study. Arch Ophthalmol 1995;113:1479–1496.
293. Kangas TA, Greenfield DS, Flynn HW, et al: Delayed-onset endophthalmitis associated with conjunctival filtering blebs. Ophthalmology 1997;104:746–752.

294. Brown RH, Yang LH, Walker SD, et al: Treatment of bleb infection after glaucoma surgery. Arch Ophthalmol 1994;112:57–61.
295. Sanchez E, Schnyder CC, Sickenberg M, et al: Deep sclerotomy: Results with and without collagen implant. Int Ophthalmol 1997;20:157–162.
296. Hara T, Hara T: Deep sclerectomy with trabeculotomy ab externo: One-stage procedure (DS 1). Ophthalmic Surg 1989;20:406–409.
297. Tanihara H, Negi A, Akimoto M, et al: Surgical effects of trabeculotomy ab externo on adult eyes with primary open angle glaucoma and pseudoexfoliation syndrome. Arch Ophthalmol 1993;111:1653–1661.
298. Mora JS, Iwach AG, Gaffney MM, et al: Endoscopic diode laser cyclophotocoagulation with a limbal approach. Ophthalmic Surg Lasers 1997;28:118–123.
298a. Rollet M, Moreau M: Traitement de le hypopyon por de drainage capillaire de la chambre anterieure. Rev Gen Ophthalmol 1906;25:481.
299. Molteno ACB: New implant for drainage in glaucoma: Animal trial. Br J Ophthalmol 1969;53:161–168.
300. Molteno ACB, Straughan JL, Ancker E: Long tube implants in the management of glaucoma. S Afr Med J 1976;50:1062–1066.
301. Wilcox MJ, Minckler DS, Ogden TE: Pathophysiology of artificial aqueous drainage in primate eyes with Molteno implants. J Glaucoma 1994;3:140–151.
302. Classen L, Kivela T, Tarkkanen A: Histopathologic and immunohistochemical analysis of the filtration bleb after unsuccessful glaucoma seton implantation. Am J Ophthalmol 1996;122:205–212.
303. Rubin B, Chan CC, Burnier M, et al: Histopathologic study of the Molteno glaucoma implant in three patients. Am J Ophthalmol 1990;110:371–379.
304. Porter JM, Krawczyk CH, Carey RF: In vitro flow testing of glaucoma drainage devices. Ophthalmology 1997;104:1701–1707.
305. Prata JA Jr, Mermoud A, LaBree L, Minckler DS: In vitro and in vivo flow characteristics of glaucoma drainage implants. Ophthalmology 1995;102:894–904.
306. Molteno ACB: The dual chamber single plate implant—its use in neovascular glaucoma. Aust N Z J Ophthalmol 1990;18:431–436.
307. Minckler DS, Shammas A, Wilcox M, Ogden TE: Experimental studies of aqueous filtration using the Molteno implant. Trans Am Ophthalmol Soc 1987;85:368–392.
308. Hitchings RA, Joseph NH, Sherwood MB, et al: Use of one-piece valved tube and variable surface area explant for glaucoma drainage surgery. Ophthalmology 1987;94:1079–1084.
309. Wilson RP, Cantor L, Katz LJ, et al: Aqueous shunts: Molteno versus Schocket. Ophthalmology 1992;99:672–678.
310. Smith MF, Sherwood MG, McGorray SP: Comparison of the double-plate Molteno drainage implant with the Schocket procedure. Arch Ophthalmol 1992;110:1246–1250.
311. Krupin Eye Valve Filtering Surgery Study Group: Krupin eye valve with disk for filtration surgery. Ophthalmology 1994;101:651–658.
312. Krupin T, Ritch R, Camras CB, et al: A long Krupin-Denver valve implant attached to a 180 degree scleral explant for glaucoma surgery. Ophthalmology 1988;95:1174–1180.
313. Coleman AL, Mondino BJ, Wilson MR, Casey R: Clinical experience with the Ahmed glaucoma valve implant in eyes with prior or concurrent penetrating keratoplasties. Am J Ophthalmol 1997;123:54–61.
314. Coleman AL, Hill R, Wilson MR, et al: Initial clinical experience with the Ahmed glaucoma valve implant. Am J Ophthalmol 1995;120:23–31.
315. Prata JA Jr, Santos RCR, LaBree L, Minckler DS: Surface area of glaucoma implants and perfusion flow rates in rabbit eyes. J Glaucoma 1995;4:274–280.
316. Heuer DK, Lloyd MA, Abrams DA, et al: Which is better? One or two? A ramdomized clinical trial of a single-plate versus double plate Molteno implantation for glaucomas in aphakia and pseudophakia. Ophthalmology 1992;99:1512–1519.
317. Smith MF, Doyle JW, Sherwood MB: Comparison of the Baerveldt glaucoma implant with double-plate Molteno drainage implant. Arch Ophthalmol 1995;113:444–447.
318. Fitzgerald-Shelton K, Higginbotham EJ: Comparison of the Baerveldt implant with the double-plate Molteno implant. Arch Ophthalmol 1996;114:1030–1031.
319. Lloyd MA, Baerveldt G, Fellenbaum PS, et al: Intermediate-term results of a randomized clinical trail of the 350- versus the 500-mm^2 Baerveldt implant. Ophthalmology 1994;101:1456–1464.
320. Fellenbaum PS, Almeida AR, Minckler DS, et al: Krupin disk implantation for complicated glaucomas. Ophthalmology 1994; 101:1178–1182.
321. Krupin T, Podos SM, Becker B, Newkirk JB: Valve implants in filtering surgery. Am J Ophthalmol 1976;81:232–235.
322. Sayyad FE, Helal M, Elsherif Z, El-Maghraby A: Molteno implant versus trabeculectomy with adjunctive intraoperative mitomycin C in high-risk glaucoma patients. J Glaucoma 1995;4:80–85.
323. Varma R, Heuer DK, Lundy DC, et al: Pars plana Baerveldt tube insertion with vitrectomy in glaucomas associated with pseudophakia and aphakia. Am J Ophthalmol 1995;119:401–407.
324. Beebe WE, Starita RJ, Fellman RL, et al: The use of Molteno implant and anterior chamber tube shunt to encircling band for the treatment of glaucoma in keratoplasty patients. Ophthalmology 1990;97:1413–1422.
325. Lloyd MAE, Baerveldt G, Heuer DK, et al: Initial clinical experience with the Baerveldt implant in complicated glaucomas. Ophthalmology 1994;101:640–650.
326. Siegner SW, Netland PA, Urban RC, et al: Clinical experience with the Baerveldt glaucoma drainage implant. Ophthalmology 1995;102:1298–1307.
327. Hodkin MJ, Goldblatt WS, Burgoyne CF, et al: Early clinical experience with the Baerveldt implant in complicated glaucomas. Am J Ophthalmol 1995;120:32–40.
328. Price FW Jr, Wellemeyer M: Long-term results of Molteno implants. Ophthalmic Surg 1995;26:130–135.
329. Mills RP, Reynolds A, Emond MJ, et al: Long-term survival of Molteno glaucoma drainage devices. Ophthalmology 1996;103:299–305.
330. Lloyd MA, Sedlak T, Heuer DK, et al: Clinical experience with the single-plate Molteno implant in complicated glaucomas: Update of a pilot study. Ophthalmology 1992;99:679–687.
331. Mermoud A, Salmon JF, Straker C, Murray ADN: Use of the single-plate Molteno implant in refractory glaucoma. Ophthalmologica 1992;205:113–120.
332. Coleman AL, Smyth RJ, Wilson R, Tam M: Initial clinical experience with the Ahmed glaucoma valve implant in pediatric patients. Arch Ophthalmol 1997;115:186–191.
333. Fellenbaum PS, Sidoti PA, Heuer DK, et al: Experience with the Baerveldt implant in young patients with complicated glaucomas. J Glaucoma 1995;4:91–97.
334. Netland PA, Walton DS: Glaucoma drainage implants in pediatric patients. Ophthalmic Surg 1993;24:723–729.
335. Eid TE, Katz LJ, Spaeth GL, Augsburger JJ: Long-term effects of tube-shunt procedures on management of refractory childhood glaucoma. Ophthalmology 1997;104:1011–1016.
336. Folberg R, Hargett NA, Weaver JE, McLean IW: Filtering valve implant for neovascular glaucoma in proliferative diabetic retinopathy. Ophthalmology 1982;89:286–289.
337. Krupin T, Kaufman P, Mandell A, et al: Filtering valve implant surgery for eyes with neovascular glaucoma. Am J Ophthalmol 1980;89:338–343.
338. Krupin T, Kaufman P, Mandell A, et al: Long-term results of valve implants in filtering surgery for eyes with neovascular glaucoma. Am J Ophthalmol 1983;95:775–782.
339. Sidoti PA, Dunphy TR, Baerveldt G, et al: Experience with the Baerveldt glaucoma implant in treating neovascular glaucoma. Ophthalmology 1995;102:1107–1118.
340. Schocket SS, Lakhanpal V, Richards RD: Anterior chamber tube shunt to an encircling band in the treatment of neovascular glaucoma. Ophthalmology 1982;89:1188–1194.
341. Mermoud A, Salmon JF, Alexander P, et al: Molteno tube implantation for neovascular glaucoma: Long-term results and factors influencing the outcome. Ophthalmology 1993;100:897–902.
342. Sidoti P, Minckler DS, Baerveldt G, et al: Epithelial ingrowth and glaucoma drainage implants. Ophthalmology 1994;101:872–875.
343. Costa VP, Katz LJ, Cohen EJ, Raber IM: Glaucoma associated with epithelial downgrowth controlled with Molteno tube shunts. Ophthalmic Surg 1992;23:797–800.
344. Fechtner RD, Acland RD: Tubing introducer forceps for glaucoma drainage-tube implants. J Glaucoma 1994;3:79–80.
345. Krebs DB, Liebmann JM, Ritch R, Speaker M: Late infectious endophthalmitis from exposed glaucoma setons. Arch Ophthalmol 1992;110:174–175.
346. Raviv T, Greenfield DS, Liebmann JM, et al: Pericardial patch grafts in glaucoma implant surgery. J Glaucoma 1998;7:27–32.

347. Brandt JD: Patch grafts of dehydrated cadaveric dura mater for tube-shunt glaucoma surgery. Arch Ophthalmol 1993;111:1436–1439.
348. Tanji TM, Lundy DC, Minckler DS, et al: Fascia lata patch graft in glaucoma tube surgery. Ophthalmology 1996;103:1309–1312.
349. Smiddy WE, Rubsamen PE, Grajewski A: Vitrectomy for pars plana placement of a glaucoma seton. Ophthalmic Surg 1994;25:532–535.
350. Prata JA Jr, Minckler DS, Mermoud A, Baerveldt G: Effects of intraoperative mitomycin C on the function of Baerveldt glaucoma drainage implants in rabbits. J Glaucoma 1996;5:29–38.
351. Perkins TW, Cardakli UF, Eisele JR, et al: Adjunctive mitomycin C in Molteno implant surgery. Ophthalmology 1995;102:91–97.
352. Susanna R Jr, Nicolela MT, Takahashi WY: Mitomycin C as adjunctive therapy with glaucoma implant surgery. Ophthalmic Surg 1994;25:458–462.
353. Azuara-Blanco A, Moster MR, Wilson RP, Schmidt CM: Simultaneous use of mitomycin C with Baerveldt implantation. Ophthalmic Surg Lasers 1997;28:992–997.
354. Lee D, Shin DH, Birt CM, et al: The effect of adjunctive mitomycin C in Molteno implant surgery. Ophthalmology 1997;104:2126–2135.
355. Gerber SL, Cantor LB, Sponsel WE: A comparison of postoperative complications from pressure-ridge Molteno implants versus Molteno implants with suture ligation. Ophthalmic Surg Lasers 1997;28:905–910.
356. Freedman J: Clinical experience with the Molteno dual-chamber single-plate implant. Ophthalmic Surg 1992;23:238–241.
357. El-Sayyad F, El-Maghraby A, Helal M, Amayem A: The use of releasable sutures in Molteno glaucoma implant procedures to reduce postoperative hypotony. Ophthalmic Surg 1991;22:82–84.
358. Price FW Jr, Whitson WE: Polypropylene ligatures as a means of controlling intraocular pressure with Molteno implants. Ophthalmic Surg 1989;20:781–783.
359. Brooks SE, Dacey MP, Lee MB, Baerveldt G: Modifications of the glaucoma drainage implant to prevent early postoperative hypertension and hypotony: A laboratory study. Ophthalmic Surg 1994;25:311–316.
360. Liebmann J, Ritch R: Intraocular suture ligature to reduce hypotony following Molteno seton implantation. Ophthalmic Surg 1992; 23:51–52.
361. Ball SF, Loftfield K, Scharfenberg J: Molteno rip-cord suture hypopyon. Ophthalmic Surg 1990;21:407–412.
362. Hoare Nairne JEA, Sherwood D, Jacob JSH, Rich WJCC: Single stage insertion of the Molteno tube for glaucoma and modifications to reduce postoperative hypotony. Br J Ophthalmol 1988;72:846–851.
363. Egbert PR, Lieberman M: Internal suture occlusion of the Molteno glaucoma implant for the prevention of postoperative hypotony. Ophthalmic Surg 1989;20:53–56.
364. Sherwood MB, Smith MF: Prevention of early hypotony associated with Molteno implants by a new occluding stent technique. Ophthalmology 1993;100:85–90.
365. Stewart W, Feldman RM, Gross RL: Collagen plug occlusion of Molteno tube shunts. Ophthalmic Surg 1993;24:47–48.
366. Law SK, Kalenak JW, Connor TB, et al: Retinal complications after aqueous shunt surgical procedures for glaucoma. Arch Ophthalmol 1996;114:1473–1480.
367. Paysse E, Lee PP, Lloyd MA, et al: Suprachoroidal hemorrhage after Molteno implantation. J Glaucoma 1996;5:170–175.
368. Tessler Z, Jluchoded S, Rosenthal G: Nd:YAG laser for Ahmed tube shunt occlusion by the posterior capsule. Ophthalmic Surg Lasers 1997;28:69–70.
369. Lundy DC, Sidoti P, Winarko T, et al: Intracameral tissue plasminogen activator after glaucoma surgery. Ophthalmology 1996;103:274–282.
370. Krawitz PL: Treatment of distal occlusion of Krupin eye valve with disk using cannular flush. Ophthalmic Surg 1994;25:102–104.
371. Smith SL, Starita RJ, Fellman RL, Lynn JR: Early clinical experience with the Baerveldt 350mm glaucoma implant and associated extraocular muscle imbalance. Ophthalmology 1993;100:914–918.
372. Christmann LM, Wilson ME: Motility disturbances after Molteno implants. J Pediatr Ophthalmol Strabismus 1992;29:44–48.
373. Munoz M, Parrish RK II: Strabismus following implantation of Baerveldt drainage devices. Arch Ophthalmol 1993;111:1096–1099.
374. Frank JW, Perkins TW, Kushner BJ: Ocular motility defects in patients with the Krupin valve implant. Ophthalmic Surg 1995;26:228–232.
375. Kooner KS, Cavanagh HD, Zimmerman CF, Itani KM: Eye movement restrictions after Molteno implant surgery (letter). Ophthalmic Surg 1993;24:498–499.
376. Cardakli UF, Perkins TW: Recalcitrant diplopia after implantation of a Krupin valve with disc. Ophthalmic Surg 1994;25:256–258.
377. Dobler AA, Sondhi N, Cantor LB, Ku S: Acquired Brown's Syndrome after a double-plate Molteno implant. Am J Ophthalmol 1993;116:641–642.
378. Ball SF, Ellis GS Jr, Herrington RG, Liang K: Brown's superior oblique tendon syndrome after Baerveldt glaucoma implant. Arch Ophthalmol 1992;110:1368.
379. Prata JA Jr, Minckler DS, Green RL: Pseudo-Brown's syndrome as a complication of glaucoma drainage implant surgery. Ophthalmic Surg 1993;24:608–611.
380. Billson F, Thomas R, Grigg J: Resiting Molteno implant tubes. Ophthalmic Surg Lasers 1996;27:801–803.
381. Cantor LB: Tube migration after glaucoma shunt procedure. Am J Ophthalmol 1989;108:334–335.
382. McDermott ML, Swendris RP, Shin DH, Juzych MS: Corneal endothelial cell counts after Molteno implantation. Am J Ophthalmol 1993;115:93–96.

CHAPTER 19

Cyclodestructive Procedures

SAI B. GANDHAM and L. JAY KATZ

Despite our best efforts, the treatment of some patients with glaucoma may require ciliary body ablation. Although this measure is generally reserved until the end of the treatment regimen, it is important to understand the available techniques. In this chapter, Sai Gandham and Jay Katz discuss the history, mechanism of action, treatment options, technique, results, and complications of this type of surgery. A narrow therapeutic window often limits the clinical usefulness of these procedures, but understanding their limitations allows us to better utilize them appropriately.

Medical and surgical therapies in glaucoma involve increasing aqueous outflow or decreasing aqueous production. Filtration procedures resulting in an increase in the aqueous outflow are typically the first line of surgical treatment. However, in some cases, glaucoma is refractory to such treatment, and in others, filtration surgery is undesirable because of patient-specific characteristics such as poor visual potential or patient choice. In these cases, ciliary body ablation may represent a reasonable alternative for successful control of intraocular pressure (IOP).

Historical Aspects

The destruction of the ciliary body was first reported in 1933 by Weve,[1] who used diathermy. The principle was the ablation of ciliary body by the heat caused by diathermy. Penetrating diathermy was reported by Vogt[2] in 1936 and later by Stocker[3] in 1945. Subsequently, Walton and Grant[4] reported low success rates for the procedure as well as a significant risk of hypotony. These results led to abandonment of the procedure. Nonpenetrating diathermy was studied by others.[5] However, both penetrating and nonpenetrating procedures appeared to cause significant scleral damage in addition to the ablative effect on the ciliary body.

Freezing to destroy the ciliary body (cyclocryotherapy [CCT]) was suggested first by Bietti[6] in 1950, and its long-term effectiveness was shown by de Roetth.[7, 8] CCT was adopted quickly, and it was found to be less destructive and more predictable than cyclodiathermy. Bellows and Grant[9] reported that CCT was especially effective in lowering IOP in advanced uncontrolled glaucoma, particularly in aphakic eyes. A major complication noted with CCT was phthisis bulbi, particularly with neovascular glaucoma (NVG), with the frequency reported to be from 0–12%; visual loss occurred in up to 67% of the treated eyes.[10]

Ultrasound was also used to cause focal ciliary body destruction, as initially reported by Purnell in 1964.[11, 12] Freyler and Scheimbauer[13] noted that partial surgical cyclectomy could control end-stage glaucoma in some cases; however, the rate of phthisis bulbi was 10% to 15%.

More recently, laser cyclophotocoagulation has become a common method of ciliary body ablation. Several different types of lasers as well as different techniques of application have been described. These will be addressed in greater detail later in this chapter.

Mechanism

Cyclocryotherapy and cyclophotocoagulation destroy the epithelial and capillary elements of the ciliary processes, which are replaced by fibroblast-like cells. The loss of the ciliary epithelium results in a reduction of IOP by decreasing the aqueous production.[14] As an alternative mechanism, Schubert and colleagues[15–17] showed that transscleral pars plana lesions reduce the IOP by enhanced outflow through a presumed neuroepithelial defect. Lesions up to 6 mm posterior to the limbus have been associated with a reduction of IOP. Additionally, intraocular inflammation combined with decreased aqueous production also has been suggested as a possible mechanism of reduction of IOP.[17]

Ciliary body ablation is usually a therapeutic procedure of last resort. Because such eyes often have compromised outflow, the therapeutic window may be relatively narrow. Aggressive treatment can result in hypotony, whereas an insufficient treatment may not produce adequate control of the IOP, necessitating additional treatment. Other risks include pain, inflammation, hypotony with macular edema, and phthisis bulbi.

Indications

In general, the usual indications for cyclodestructive procedures are:

1. Patients needing further reduction of IOP despite maximally tolerated medical therapy and following unsuccessful filtration surgery.
2. Poor visual potential, such that the eye is being treated with cyclophotocoagulation to maintain comfort and prevent visual loss.
3. Unsuitability of the patient as a surgical candidate for filtration surgery (e.g., general medical reasons or patient preference).

Preoperative Treatment

Because cyclodestruction is not expected to result in an immediate decrease in IOP, treatment with osmotic agents may be appropriate in some patients to immediately reduce IOP (this statement assumes that patients are already receiving maximally tolerated medical therapy).

General Principles

Intrinsic to cyclodestructive procedures is that the effectiveness of lowering IOP from a single treatment session is unpredictable. There is always a risk that with the same treatment parameters it is possible to achieve an excellent result in one patient, hypotony in a second patient, and have no effect on IOP at all in a third patient. Therefore, it is important to inform the patient of this unpredictability and prepare him or her for the possibility that additional procedures may be needed for adequate IOP control.

In general, it is better to err on the side of slight undertreatment because the effects of overtreatment are usually irreversible. To this end, it is often appropriate not to treat the entire circumference of the ciliary body in a single session. Leaving one quadrant untreated may also minimize the risk of anterior segment ischemia.

If additional treatment appears necessary because IOP control is still inadequate, it is best deferred for at least 4 to 6 weeks after the first procedure to allow the full effect of the ablation to become manifest and to decrease the chance of overtreatment.

Anesthesia

Local anesthesia with a retrobulbar injection of a long-lasting anesthetic, such as 0.75% bupivacaine with hyaluronidase, provides perioperative anesthesia in most cases. In children and uncooperative adults, general anesthesia should be used. Even with general anesthesia it is often desirable to perform a retrobulbar injection of anesthetic to provide postoperative pain control.

Postoperative Treatment

Postoperatively, topical cycloplegic agents and corticosteroids are continued for at least 1 month. Pain medication, including narcotics, may be needed in the early postoperative period. In addition, all glaucoma medications except miotics and prostaglandins, which may enhance post-treatment inflammation, should be continued until IOP reduction is obtained. Postoperatively, patients are usually seen at 1 day to 1 week, and 1 month.

Specific Procedures

CYCLOCRYOTHERAPY

TECHNIQUE

CCT has been described in detail by Prost.[45] All the glaucoma medications are continued until the day of the procedure. Because no incision is made, the procedure does not require sterile technique.

The cryotherapy unit consists of nitrous oxide with a cryoprobe tip 2.5 mm in diameter. The cryoprobe is placed with its anterior edge 1 mm from the limbus. The cryoprobe temperature should be −80° C. A lid speculum is placed before the procedure. Each application should last 60 seconds. The ice ball created by the cryotherapy may extend 1 to 2 mm into the peripheral cornea. Maximum therapy would be three to four cryolesions per quadrant for 360 degrees during a single session. A 180 degree area of treatment reduces the incidence of phthisis bulbi but at the expense of lower success rate. Light pressure with the cryoprobe facilitates penetration of the ice ball to the tips of the ciliary processes.

The ice ball should be allowed to thaw slowly. Removal of the cryoprobe while it is still adherent to the conjunctiva may cause damage to the underlying tissue. At the end of the procedure, 0.5 mL (1 mg) dexamethasone is injected subconjunctivally.

The precise optimal duration of application is not known. Some advocate a shorter duration (20–30 sec) with a freeze-thaw-refreeze technique.

COMPLICATIONS

Marked pain in the early postoperative period is common. Retrobulbar alcohol injection can be combined with CCT when patients have severe pain and poor vision prior to the procedure. Postoperative inflammation is common, and its sequelae, extensive posterior synechiae, pupillary block, and cataract, may occur. Choroidal and retinal detachments occur infrequently. Hyphema is common. Brindley[48] re-

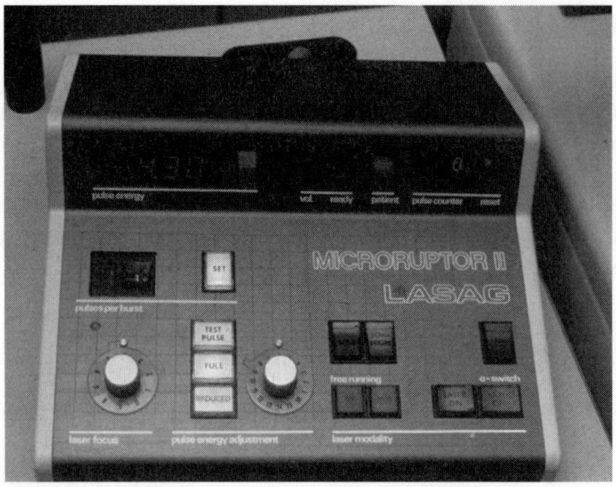

FIGURE 19–1. The Microruptor II (MR II) (Lasag AG, Thun, Switzerland) is a Nd:YAG laser that provides slit-lamp delivery in a free-running thermal mode with 20-millisecond pulses. It is capable of delivering energy up to 8 to 9 joules.

ported a 52% reduction in postoperative visual acuity. Reduction of visual acuity may be due to a postoperative rise of IOP and cystoid macular edema. Phthisis bulbi remains the most feared complication: in one study, 14% percent of all patients and 24% of patients with NVG experienced phthisis bulbi.[47]

RESULTS

Better IOP control with retention of visual acuity was reported in patients with glaucoma after penetrating keratoplasty[46, 47] and in patients with aphakia[48, 49] who underwent cyclocryotherapy. West and coworkers[46] reported satisfactory IOP control with CCT in 19 of 23 eyes with penetrating keratoplasty that demonstrated uncontrolled glaucoma in the preoperative or postoperative period. Binder and colleagues[47] obtained IOP control with CCT in 30 of 36 patients (83%) who had glaucoma after penetrating keratoplasty, and 23 of 28 grafts (82%) remained clear. Bellows and associates[49] reported that CCT in 24 of 26 eyes (92%) with aphakic glaucoma achieved IOP control. However, patients with NVG had a poorer prognosis in most series.[50, 51] Krupin and colleagues[51] reported IOP control in 17 of 50 eyes (34%) with NVG, and 24 of 41 eyes in their series lost light perception.

LASER CYCLOPHOTOCOAGULATION

Transscleral Cyclophotocoagulation

The Nd:YAG laser consists of a medium of neodymium atoms in a crystal of yttrium, aluminum, and garnet. When the Nd:YAG laser is used in the free-running thermal mode (10^{-3} sec), it creates energy levels approximately 1000-fold greater than those used for routine photodisruptive applications (Q-switched). Brancato and associates[58] used contact Nd:YAG transscleral cyclophotocoagulation (TSCPC) in rabbits. In the immediate postoperative period, ciliary body destruction consisted of damage to the pigmented and nonpigmented epithelium and stroma without evidence of damage to the overlying sclera.[58]

TECHNIQUES

NONCONTACT Nd:YAG TRANSSCLERAL CYCLOPHOTOCOAGULATION. After retrobulbar injection, the patient is positioned at the laser slit-lamp. The eyelids are separated, usually with a wire speculum[18] or a Shields contact lens.[19] With the Microruptor II (Fig. 19–1), cyclophotocoagulation is performed in the free-running thermal mode, which is preset at 20-msec single pulses.[20, 18] The maximum posterior offset is used by setting the focusing dial at the number "9" position,[18, 21, 22] which provides separation between the HeNe aiming beam focus and the therapeutic beam of approximately 3.6 mm in air. Laser applications are placed after the aiming beam is focused on the conjunctival surface (Fig. 19–2).

Eyes are usually treated in the primary position, with the laser energy applied parallel to the visual axis[21–25] or perpendicular to the sclera.[26] In one study, patients treated 1.5 mm posterior to the limbus had a significantly lower IOP and less visual loss than those treated 3 mm from the limbus.[23] Thirty to 40 applications evenly placed 360 degrees around the limbus are recommended[23, 24] (Fig. 19–3).

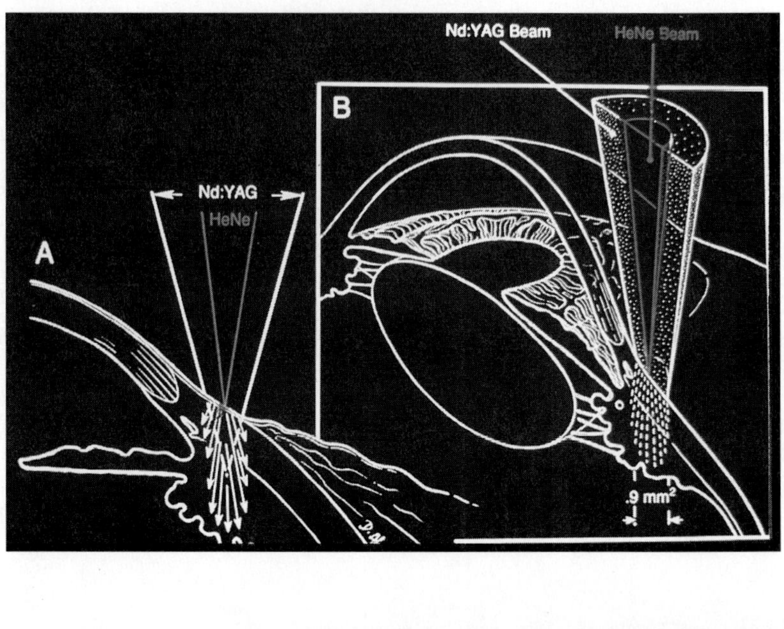

FIGURE 19–2. Noncontact transscleral Nd:YAG cyclophotocoagulation through a contact lens, showing HeNe aiming beam focused on conjunctiva with therapeutic Nd:YAG beam offset deep into ocular tissues and producing disruption of the ciliary epithelium.

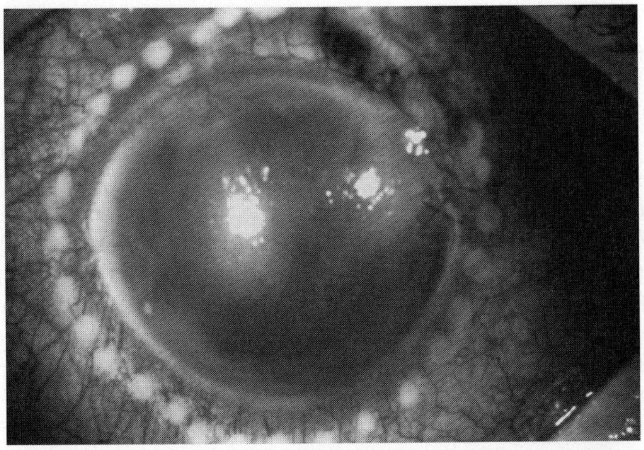

FIGURE 19–3. Slit-lamp view of conjunctival burns immediately after noncontact, free-running transscleral Nd:YAG cyclophotocoagulation.

The three o'clock and nine o'clock positions are avoided so as not to damage the long posterior ciliary arteries.

The distance from the limbus to the laser site can be measured in several ways: with calipers, with the slit beam of the biomicroscope, or with the Shields contact lens, which has 1-mm marks (Fig. 19–4). The Shields lens has an opaque disc of 8 mm in diameter that helps to prevent transpupillary entrance of laser light into the eye. The limbal portion of the lens helps to compress the conjunctiva and blanch blood vessels, thereby helping with focus and limiting thermal damage to these tissues.[19, 27] The contact lens also helps to control the eye movements and keep the eyelids separated. Four to 8 joules (J) of pulse energy per shot is suggested in most studies.

CONTACT Nd:YAG TRANSSCLERAL CYTOPHOTOCOAGULATION. Contact Nd:YAG TSCPC is performed with a fiberoptic probe placed on the conjunctiva.[29, 30] Surgical Laser Technologies (SLT) CL60 provides contact probe delivery of Nd:YAG laser in a continuous wave mode of 0.12 to 10 seconds (Fig. 19–5). A wire speculum is used to separate the lids, and 30 to 40 applications are placed using 4 to 6 J of energy with a duration of 0.5 to 1.0 second. The anterior edge of the probe is placed 1.0 mm from the limbus. The probe should be held perpendicular to the sclera (Fig. 19–6).

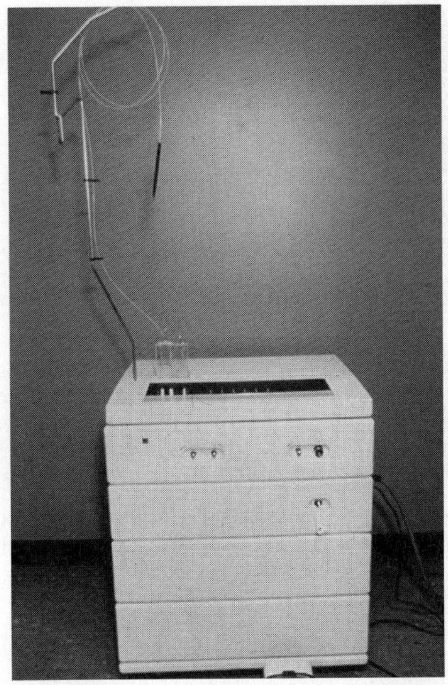

FIGURE 19–5. Surgical Laser Technologies (SLT) CL60 (Surgical Laser Technologies, Oaks, PA) provides contact probe delivery of Nd:YAG laser in a continuous-wave mode for 0.12 to 10 seconds.

COMPLICATIONS

Iritis and conjunctival burns are common. Uveitis is variable, is usually mild, and subsides with the first week. Conjunctival burns heal without sequelae. Mild pain is to be expected for 1 to 3 days. Less common anterior segment complications include corneal epithelial defects, focal scleral thinning, corneal graft failure, hyphema, hypopyon, and

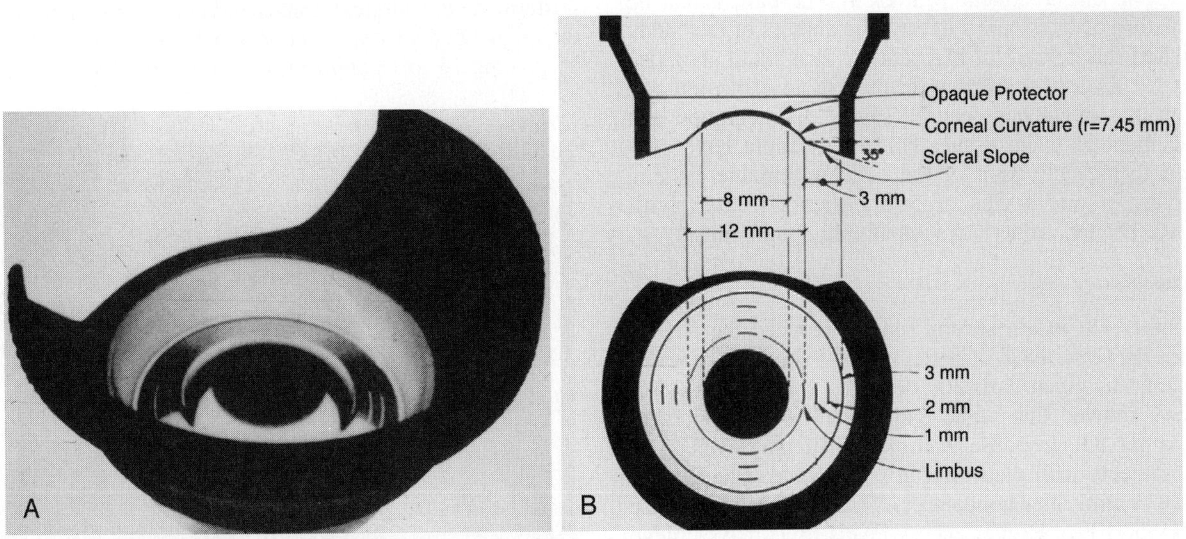

FIGURE 19–4. *A,* Noncontact, transscleral Nd:YAG cyclophotocoagulation, which utilizes the Microruptor II (Lasag AG, Thun, Switzerland), can be performed with or without a contact lens. This photograph shows a lens that has been developed for this procedure. *B,* The advantages of using a contact lens are compressing and blanching of the conjunctiva, maintaining lid separation, and providing measurements of distance from the limbus.

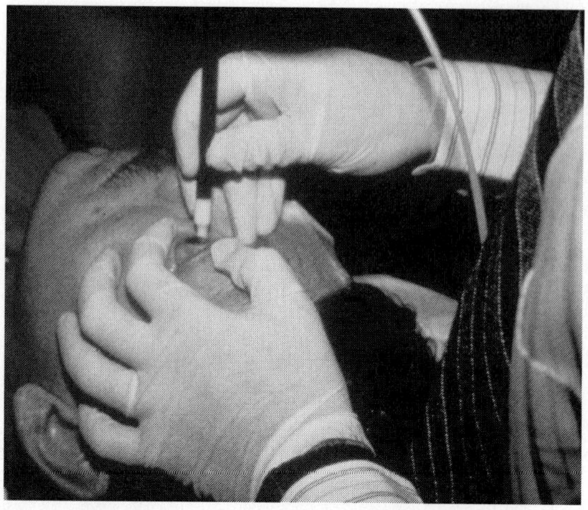

FIGURE 19–6. Contact, transscleral Nd:YAG cyclophotocoagulation is being performed with the SLT CL60 (Surgical Laser Technologies, Oaks, PA). The lids are separated by a speculum, and the tip of the fiberoptic probe is applied perpendicular to the surface of the sclera at a measured site 1.0 to 1.5 mm away from the limbus.

posterior capsule fibrosis. Forty percent of patients who had clear corneal grafts preoperatively were reported to experience corneal edema.[22] Uncommon posterior segment complications include serous and choroidal effusions, vitreous hemorrhage, hypotony, malignant glaucoma, and cystoid macular edema.

Sympathetic ophthalmia has been reported in several patients after Nd:YAG TSCPC.[38–43] In one institution, the incidence of sympathetic ophthalmia was reported as 5.8% (4 of 69) after noncontact Nd:YAG TSCPC and 0.67% (1 of 150) after contact Nd:YAG TSCPC.[41] All the patients had undergone previous incisional surgical procedures, and the sympathizing eyes responded promptly to steroid therapy. Later in 1994, Bechrakis and coworkers[43] reported that sympathetic ophthalmia occurred in a patient with Coats' disease who had undergone cyclodestructive therapy. The patient underwent three treatments with contact Nd:YAG TSCPC and one treatment with CCT. The patient had no prior history of incisional surgery. The authors of this study speculated that release of high energy in a small spot size during Nd:YAG cyclotherapy resulted in an explosion-like reaction that might have caused severe disintegration and displacement of uveal tissue. This event could have contributed to the activation of the cellular immune system. However, in one series of 500 patients treated with Nd:YAG TSCPC, none had sympathetic ophthalmia.[44]

RESULTS

Noncontact TSCPC in several reports reduced the IOP in between 44% and 68% of patients.[21, 32–34] In most patients, treatment was given over 360 degrees. Simmons and colleagues[35] showed that white patients (60 of 81, or 74%) had a better IOP response than black patients (9 of 19, or 47%). Patients with glaucoma in pseudophakia had better pressure control after noncontact TSCPC (76%) than those with NVG (10%). Higher energy levels (8 J) may achieve a better response than lower levels (4 J).[36] Age, gender, and preoperative IOP were not associated with postoperative IOP control. Results of primary contact TSCPC were similar to those of the noncontact technique.[37]

Most investigators found that Nd:YAG TSCPC is as effective as CCT in reducing IOP with fewer complications.[53, 54] Nd:YAG TSCPC has been compared with tube shunt implantation in clinical trials. One year after surgery, patients who had undergone tube implantation required fewer medications and had IOP less than 21 mm Hg (87%, or 39 of 45) more often than those who had undergone Nd:YAG TSCPC (69%, or 31 of 45).[32] Eid and coworkers,[55] in a study comparing tube shunt implantation with cyclophotocoagulation, observed a satisfactory IOP control with less hypotony and less visual loss with tube shunts. Satisfactory IOP control was achieved in 38% (9 of 24) of eyes undergoing TSCPC, versus 67% (16 of 24) receiving tube shunts. Loss of light perception occurred in 46% (11 of 24) of the patients receiving TSCPC compared with 17% (4 of 24) of the patients receiving tube shunts.

Semiconductor Diode Laser TSCPC

INSTRUMENTATION

The diode laser incorporates two light-emitting diodes with a combined wavelength of 810 nm. Laser energy at this wavelength has the potential advantage over the Nd:YAG laser wavelength of greater melanin absorption. The semiconductor diode laser attempts to maximize the ciliary body destruction while minimizing the scleral absorption of the energy delivered. Commercial units for performing noncontact diode laser TSCPC are the DC-3000 (Nidek, Inc, Palo Alto, CA), OcuLight SLX (IRIDEX, Mountain View, CA) (Fig. 19–7), and Microlase (Keeler Instruments, Broomall, PA). These instruments are less expensive and more available than the Nd:YAG lasers used for contact TSCPC.

TECHNIQUE

Diode laser cyclophotocoagulation was first reported by Hennis and Stewart.[74] Investigators have used 1200 to 1500 mW of power, a 1-second duration, and a 100- to 400-μm spot size.[70] Applications were placed 0.5 mm to 1.0 mm posterior to the surgical limbus and defocused 1 mm toward the ciliary body. Contact diode TSCPC has been performed by placing 16 to 18 applications around the limbus, sparing

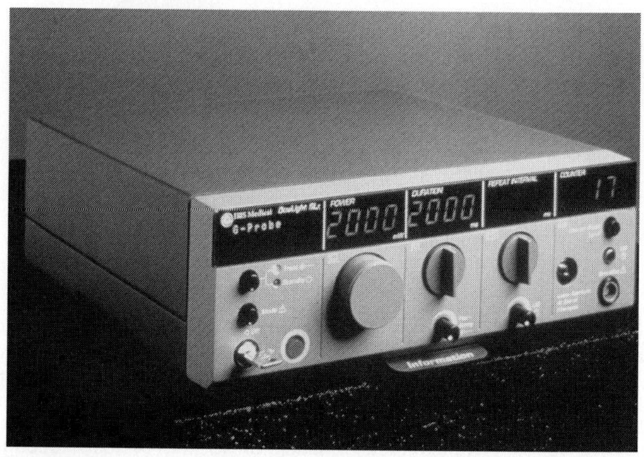

FIGURE 19–7. Semiconductor diode laser (OcuLight SLX) which provides continuous-wave, contact delivery of the diode laser at a wavelength of 810 nm. (Courtesy of IRIDEX Corporation, Mountain View, CA.)

the three o'clock and nine o'clock positions. The G probe (IRIDEX, Mountain View, CA) is designed so that the distance from the surgical limbus need not be measured (Fig. 19–8). The anterior edge of the probe approximates the surgical limbus, and the laser beam is directed at a distance of 1 to 1.5 mm posteriorly so that the ciliary processes are ablated. One to 2 seconds of duration and 1.5 to 2.5 W of power were used for each application.[56] A mean IOP reduction of 30% at 6 months was reported after single treatment with a noncontact technique. Similar results were reported by Brancato and associates.[56–58]

OTHER TECHNIQUES

Several cilioablative techniques are less frequently used today because of inconvenience or relatively poor results. They include transpupillary cyclophotocoagulation, intraoperative intraocular cyclophotocoagulation with direct visualization, transpupillary cyclophotocoagulation, and therapeutic ultrasound.

Intraoperative Intraocular Cyclophotocoagulation with Transpupillary Visualization

During lensectomy or during pars plana vitrectomy (PPV), the endolaser probe is inserted through the pars plana. Under direct visualization of the ciliary processes through the pupil and with use of a scleral depression, the ciliary processes can be photocoagulated with the endoscopic laser.[75–78] Encouraging results were reported by Patel and associates[63] and Zarbin and coworkers.[64] Complications included vitreous hemorrhage, retinal dialysis, transient choroidal detachment, hypotony, and decreased vision.[64]

Because this intraocular cyclophotocoagulation procedure must be combined with pars plana vitrectomy, the complications related to PPV may also occur with this procedure. In appropriate cases, intraocular cyclophotocoagulation can be considered an adjunct to PPV, but a PPV would rarely be indicated for the purpose of allowing intraocular cyclophotocoagulation to be performed.

Transpupillary Cyclophotocoagulation

The argon laser may be used to photocoagulate the ciliary processes when they can be visualized gonioscopically. The procedure is performed by placing a Goldmann contact lens to visualize the ciliary processes. Typical parameters are a 50- to 100-μm spot size, 700 to 1500 mW of power, and 0.1 to 0.2 second of duration. Adequate reaction is a dark pit with a surrounding white area on the ciliary process. All the visible portions of ciliary processes can be photocoagulated, a goal that requires three to four applications per process.

Lee and coworkers[59–61] showed an average reduction of IOP of 50% in 15 of 22 patients. They also suggested that at least 25% of all the ciliary processes needed to be photocoagulated to achieve a hypotensive effect. However, Shields and associates[62] reported that only 6 of their 27 patients maintained an IOP lower than 21 mm Hg, and half of these patients had an elevated IOP within the first month postoperatively. The results of transpupillary cyclophotocoagulation are unpredictable and often disappointing. In addition, the procedure is technically more difficult, requiring direct visualization of ciliary processes.

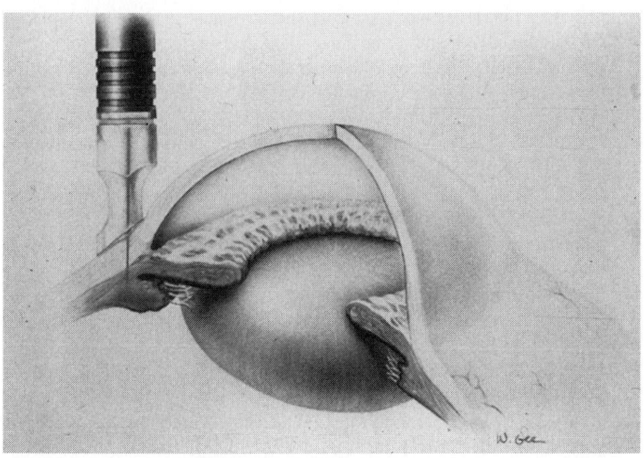

FIGURE 19–8. The G-Probe is shown in position during transscleral diode cyclophotocoagulation. (Courtesy of IRIDEX Corporation, Mountain View, CA.)

Intraocular Cyclophotocoagulation with Endoscopic Visualization

Endoscopic technique combined with laser treatment was first described by Shields and colleagues[65] in 1985. An argon laser fiberoptic probe was attached to an ocular endoscope. Laser energy could be successfully applied to the ciliary processes in a monkey study.

In a later report, Uram[66] described a semiconductor diode laser attached to an endoscope with videomonitoring that showed favorable results when used for intraocular cyclophotocoagulation. When the laser endoscope was 1 to 4 mm from the target, the aiming beam was positioned on the surface of a ciliary process, and the laser was activated. The power settings were 400 to 600 mW in a continuous-wave mode. The end-point of the treatment was whitening and shrinkage of the ciliary processes. Six of the 10 eyes treated had IOPs of less than 21 mm Hg without medications, and three eyes had similar IOP control with medications. Hypotony with a chronic retinal detachment was observed in two eyes. Intraocular inflammation was not prominent. Five of the 10 eyes were described as being very quiet following the treatment.[66]

Therapeutic Ultrasound

Therapeutic ultrasound is the use of transscleral ultrasonic radiation to produce localized destruction of the ciliary body. It was introduced in 1964 by Purnell and associates.[11]

TECHNIQUE

After a retrobulbar block, the transducer is placed in a water bath and focused on the sclera 1.5 to 3.0 mm from the limbus; three to 12 exposures have been used, each lasting 5 seconds. The probe is a ceramic shell with a diameter of 50 mm.[67] Initial studies showed an IOP reduction to less than 25 mm Hg in 65% to 72% of patients.[68, 69] However, patients may have an elevated IOP in the first few hours after treatment. Visual acuity was decreased in 39% of the patients. Other complications were uveitis, phthisis bulbi, choroidal detachment, scleral thinning, and scleral perforation, occurring in less than 10% of patients.[68] Therapeutic ultrasound is a cumbersome system with a relatively poor success rate.

SUMMARY

Cyclodestructive procedures as a group are limited by their narrow therapeutic window. The goal has been to develop a cyclodestructive procedure that predictably lowers aqueous production to a level that controls the IOP with a low complication rate. A number of current cilioablative techniques are clinically useful for IOP reduction in patients who have refractory glaucoma or who are not candidates for surgery. . Although the incidence of sympathetic ophthalmia is low after cyclodestructive procedures, the patients should be alerted to the possibility of this complication.

REFERENCES

1. Weve H: Die Zyklodiatermie das Corpus ciliare bei Glaukom. Zentralbl Ophthalmol 1933;29:562.
2. Vogt A: Versuche zur intrakularen Druckherabsetzung mittels Diatermieschadigung des Corpus cilare (Zyklodiatermiestichelung). Klin Monatsbl Augenheilkd 1936;97:672.
3. Stocker F: Response of chronic simple glaucoma to treatment with cyclodiathermy puncture. Arch Ophthalmol 1945;34:181.
4. Walton D, Grant W: Penetrating cyclodiathermy for filtration. Arch Ophthalmol 1970;83:47.
5. Pham L, Wang Y, Wang N, et al: Experimental nonpenetrating transscleral cyclodiathermy in rabbits. Ophthalmic Surg Lasers 1996; 27:301.
6. Bietti G: Surgical intervention on the ciliary body: New trends for the relief of glaucoma. JAMA 1950;142:889.
7. de Roetth A: Cryosurgery for the treatment of glaucoma. Trans Am Ophthalmol Soc 1965;63:189.
8. de Roetth A: Cryosurgery for the treatment of advanced simple glaucoma. Am J Ophthalmol 1968;66:1034.
9. Bellows AR, Grant WM: Cyclocryotherapy in advanced inadequately controlled glaucoma. Am J Ophthalmol 1973;75:679.
10. Bellows AR, Grant WM: Cyclocryotherapy of chronic open angle glaucoma in aphakic eyes. Am J Ophthalmol 1978;85:615.
11. Purnell E, Sokollu A, Torchia R, et al: Focal chorioretinitis produced by ultrasound. Invest Ophthalmol 1964;3:657.
12. Coleman D, Lizzi F, Driller J, et al: Therapeutic ultrasound in the treatment of glaucoma: Experimental model. Ophthalmology 1985;92:339.
13. Freyler H, Scheimbauer I: Excision of the ciliary body (Sautter procedure) as a last resort in secondary glaucoma. Klin Monatsbl Augenheilkd 1981;179:473.
14. van der Zypen E, England C, Frankhauser F, Kwasniewska S: The effect of transscleral laser cyclophotocoagulation on rabbit ciliary body vascularization. Graefes Arch Clin Exp Ophthalmol 1989;227:172.
15. Schubert HD, Agarwala A, Arbizo V: Changes in aqueous outflow after in vitro neodymium:yttrium aluminum garnet laser cyclophotocoagulation. Invest Ophthalmol Vis Sci 1990;31:1834.
16. Schubert HD, Agarwala A: Quantitative CW Nd:YAG pars plana transscleral photocoagulation in postmortem eyes. Ophthalmic Surg 1990;21:835.
17. Schubert HD, Federman JL: The role of inflammation in CW Nd:YAG contact transscleral photocoagulation and cryopexy. Invest Ophthalmol Vis Sci 1989;30:543.
18. Klapper RM, Wandel T, Donnenfeld E, Perry HD: Transscleral neodymium:YAG thermal cyclophotocoagulation in refractory glaucoma. A preliminary report, Ophthalmology 95:719,1988.
19. Shields MB, Blasini M, Simmons R, Erickson PJ: A contact lens for transscleral Nd:YAG cyclophotocoagulation (letter). Am J Ophthalmol 1989;108:457.
20. Blasini M, Simmons R, Shields MB: Early tissue response to transscleral neodymium:YAG cyclophotocoagulation. Invest Ophthalmol Vis Sci 1990;31:1114.
21. Balazsi G: Noncontact thermal mode Nd:YAG laser transscleral cyclocoagulation in the treatment of glaucoma. Ophthalmology 1991;98:1858.
22. Cohen EJ, Schwartz LW, Luskind RD, et al: Neodymium:YAG laser transscleral cyclophotocoagulation for glaucoma after penetrating keratoplasty. Ophthalmic Surg 1989;20:713.
23. Crymes BM, Gross RL: Laser placement in noncontact Nd:YAG cyclophotocoagulation. Am J Ophthalmol 1990;110:670.
24. Hampton C, Shields MB, Miller KN, Blasini N: Evaluation of a protocol for trans-scleral neodymium:YAG cyclophotocoagulation in one hundred patients. Ophthalmology 1990;97:910.
25. Kalenak JW, Oarkinson JM, Kass MA, Kolker AE: Transscleral neodymium:YAG laser cyclocoagulation for uncontrolled glaucoma. Ophthalmic Surg 1990;21:346.
26. Badeeb O, Trope GE, Mortimer C: Short-term effects of neodymium-YAG transscleral cyclocoagulation in patients with uncontrolled glaucoma. Br J Ophthalmol 1988;72:615.
27. Simmons RB, Blasini M, Shields MB, Erickson PJ: Comparison of transsscleral neodymium:YAG cyclophotocoagulation with and without a contact lens in human autopsy eyes. Am J Ophthalmol 1990;109:174.
28. Fiore PM, Latina MA: A technique for precise placement of laser applications in transscleral Nd:YAG cyclophotocoagulation (letter). Am J Ophthalmol 1989;107:292.
29. Federman JL, Ando F, Schubert HD, Eagle RC: Contact laser for transscleral photocoagulation. Ophthalmic Surg 1987;18:183.
30. Krasnov MM, Naumidi LP: Contact transscleral laser cyclocoagulation in glaucoma. Ann Ophthalmol 1990;22:354.
31. Schuman JS, Puliafito CA: Laser cyclophotocoagulation. Int Ophthalmol Clin 1990;30:111.
32. Noureddin BN, Wilson-Holt N, Lavin M, et al: Advanced uncontrolled glaucoma: Nd:YAG cyclophotocoagulation or tube surgery. Ophthalmology 1992;99:430.
33. Trope GE, Ma S: Mid-term effects of neodymium:YAG transscleral cyclophotocoagulation in glaucoma. Ophthalmology 1992;99:1823.
34. Wright MM, Grajewski AL, Feuer WJ: Nd:YAG cyclophotocoagulation: Outcome of treatment for uncontrolled glaucoma. Ophthalmic Surg 1991;22:279.
35. Simmons RB, Shields MB, Blasini M, et al: Comparison of transscleral neodymium:YAG cyclophotocoagulation with a contact lens. Am J Ophthalmol 1991;112:671.
36. Shields MB, Wilkerson MH, Echelman DA: A comparison of two energy levels for non contact transscleral neodymium-YAG cyclophotocoagulation. Arch Ophthalmol 1993;111:484.
37. Brancato R, Giovanni L, Trabucchi G, Pietroni C: Contact transscleral cyclophotocoagulation with Nd:YAG laser in uncontrolled glaucoma. Ophthalmic Surg 1989;20:547.
38. Brown SVL, Higginbotham E, Tessler H: Sympathetic ophthalmia following Nd:YAG cyclotherapy (letter). Ophthalmic Surg 1990; 21:736.
39. Edward DP, Brown SVL, Higginbotham E, et al: Sympathetic ophthalmia following neodymium:YAG cyclotherapy. Ophthalmic Surg 1989;20:544.
40. Minckler DS: Does Nd:YAG cyclotherapy cause sympathetic ophthalmia (editorial)? Ophthalmic Surg 1989;20:543.
41. Lam S, Tesler HH, Lam BL, Wilensky JT: High incidence of sympathetic ophthalmia after contact and non contact neodymium:YAG cyclotherapy. Ophthalmology 1992;99:1818.
42. Pastor SA, Iwach A, Nozik RA: Presumed sympathetic ophthalmia following Nd:YAG transscleral cyclophotocoagulation. J Glaucoma 1993;2:30.
43. Bechrakis NE, Mullerstolzenburg NW, Helbig H, Foerster MH: Sympathetic ophthalmia following laser cyclocoagulation. Arch Ophthalmol 1994;112:80.
44. Shields MB, Shields SE: Noncontact transscleral Nd:YAG cyclophotocoagulation: A long-term follow-up of 500 patients. Trans Am Ophthalmol Soc 1994;92:271.
45. Prost M: Cyclocryotherapy for glaucoma: Evaluation of techniques. Surv Ophthalmol 1983;28:93.
46. West CE, Wood TO, Kaufman HE: Cyclocryotherapy for glaucoma pre- or post penetrating keratoplasty. Am J Ophthalmol 1973;76:485.
47. Binder PS, Abel R Jr, Kaufman HE: Cyclocryotherapy for glaucoma after penetrating keratoplasty. Am J Ophthalmol 1975;79:489.

48. Brindley G, Shields MB: Value and limitations of cyclocryotherapy. Graefes Arch Clin Exp Ophthalmol 1986;224:545.
49. Bellows AR, Grant WM: Cyclocryotherapy of chronic open angle glaucoma in aphakic eyes. Am J Ophthalmol 1978;85:615.
50. Faulborn J, Birnbaum F: Cyclocryotherapy of hemorrhagic glaucoma: Clinical long term and histopathologic results. Klin Monatsbl Augenheilkd 1977;170:651.
51. Krupin T, Mitchell KB, Becker B: Cyclocryotherapy in neovascular glaucoma. Am J Ophthalmol 1978;86:24.
52. Shihab ZM, Fu YA, Lee P-F: Cyclocryotherapy in advanced glaucoma. Glaucoma 1982;4:146.
53. Stewart WC: Clinical Practice of Glaucoma. Thorofare, NJ, Slack, 1990.
54. Suzuki Y, Araie M, Yumita A, Yamamoto T: Transscleral Nd:YAG laser cyclophotocoagulation versus cyclocryotherapy. Graefes Arch Clin Exp Ophthalmol 1991;229:33.
55. Eid TE, Katz LJ, Spaeth GL: Tube-shunt surgery versus Nd:YAG cyclophotocoagulation in the management of neovascular glaucoma. Ophthalmology 1997;104:1692.
56. Brancato R, Carassa RG, Bettin P, et al: Contact transscleral cyclophotocoagulation with diode laser in refractory glaucoma. Eur J Ophthalmol 1995;5:32.
57. Brancato R, Carassa R, Trabucchi G: Contact transscleral cyclophotocoagulation with diode laser. Ophthalmology 1993;100(suppl):110.
58. Brancato R, Leoni G, Trabucchi E, et al: Histopathology of continuous wave neodymium:yttrium, garnet and diode laser contact transscleral lesions in rabbit ciliary body: A comparative study. Invest Ophthalmol Vis Sci 1991;32:1586.
59. Lee P-F: Argon laser photocoagulation of the ciliary processes in cases of aphakic glaucoma. Arch Ophthalmol 1979;97:2135.
60. Lee P-F, Pomeranzeff O: Transpupillary cyclophotocoagulation of rabbit eyes: An experimental approach to glaucoma surgery. Am J Ophthalmol 1971;71:911.
61. Lee P-F, Shihab Z, Eberle M: Partial ciliary process laser photocoagulation in the management of glaucoma. Laser Surg Med 1980;1:85.
62. Shields S, Stewart WC, Shields MB: Transpupillary argon laser cyclophotocoagulation in the treatment of glaucoma. Ophthalmic Surg 1988;19:171.
63. Patel A, Thompson JT, Michels RG, Quigley HA: Endolaser treatment of the ciliary body for uncontrolled glaucoma. Ophthalmology 1986;93:825.
64. Zarbin MA, Michels RG, de Bustros S, et al: Endolaser treatment of the ciliary body for severe glaucoma. Ophthalmology 1988;95:1639.
65. Shields MB, Chandler DB, Heckingbotham D, Klintworth GK: Intraocular cyclophotocoagulation: Histopathologic evaluation in primates. Arch Ophthalmol 1985;103:1731.
66. Uram M: Ophthalmic laser microendoscope ciliary process ablation in the management of neovascular glaucoma. Ophthalmology 1992;99:1823.
67. Polack PJ, Iwamoto T, Silverman RH, et al: Histologic effects of contact ultrasound for the treatment of glaucoma. Invest Ophthalmol Vis Sci 1991;32:2136.
68. Burgess SEP, Silverman RH, Coleman DJ, et al: Treatment of glaucoma with high intensity focused ultrasound. Ophthalmology 1986;93:831.
69. Harmon GK, Yablonski ME: Ultrasound in the treatment of glaucoma. *In* Caldwell DR (ed): Mediguide to Ophthalmology. New York, Lawrence Dellacort, 1988.
70. L'Esperance FA Jr: Ophthalmic Lasers. Photocoagulation, Photoradiation, and Surgery, 2nd ed. St. Louis, CV Mosby, 1983.
71. Shields MB: Textbook of Glaucoma, 3rd ed. Baltimore, Williams & Wilkins, 1992.
72. Brancato R, Leoni F, Trabucchi G, Cappellini A: Histopathology of continuous wave neodymium:yttrium aluminum garnet and diode laser contact transscleral lesions in rabbit ciliary body: A comparative study. Invest Ophthalmol Vis Sci 1991;32:1586.
73. Schuman JS, Puliafito CA, Allingham RR, et al: Contact transscleral continuous wave neodymium:YAG laser cyclophotocoagulation. Ophthalmology 1990;97:571.
74. Hennis HL, Stewart WC: Semiconductor diode laser transscleral cyclophotocoagulation in patients with glaucoma. Am J Ophthalmol 1992;113:81.
75. Charles S: Endophotocoagulation. Retina 1981;1:117.
76. Fleischman JA, Swartz M, Dixon JA: Argon laser endophotocoagulation: An intraoperative trans pars plana technique. Arch Ophthalmol 1981;99:1610.
77. Landers MB 3rd, Trese MT, Stefansson E, Bessler M: Argon laser intraocular photocoagulation. Ophthalmology 1982;89:785.
78. Peyman GA: A bent-tipped endolaser probe. Ophthalmic Surg 1987;18:185.

CHAPTER 20

Eyelids, Lacrimal Apparatus, Orbit, Motility

J. BRENT BOND

In the determination of the proper therapy for glaucoma or the possible implications of therapy, the examination of the external ocular signs plays an important role. These signs are easy to overlook, and Brent Bond addresses them to facilitate better decisions. He begins with the possible impact of eyelid abnormalities, including infection and inflammation, on medical and surgical therapy. Next, he addresses abnormal eyelid position and function. Lacrimal function is also discussed, including the lacrimal apparatus and abnormal tear production. He then considers motility disturbances following tube shunt implantation and the impact of suspected exophthalmos. A wide variety of subjects are covered, many of which are very common. Recognizing and addressing these problems can substantially improve patient quality of life.

The examination of the eyelids and orbits must not be ignored when therapeutic decisions are being made for the patient with any of the various types of glaucoma. Certain systemic diseases diagnosable on external examination of the lids can cause glaucoma or may have significant impact on the way that glaucoma should be managed. Also, abnormalities limited to the eyelids or orbits that either are present prior to glaucoma treatment or occur as a result of treatment must be noted and treated appropriately if one is to provide the optimal care for the patient with glaucoma. The purpose of this chapter is to elucidate these external examination findings and recommend glaucoma management strategies based on them.

Eyelid Erythema and Swelling

Examination of the eyelids and eyelashes can reveal findings that must be taken into account prior to institution of treatment, especially any incisional surgical treatment. One of the key considerations, especially prior to surgery, is eliminating any erythema or swelling of the eyelids. It is crucial to define and address these external eyelid diseases because many can incite an inflammatory reaction that can affect the ocular surface, including the conjunctiva. Potentially this low-grade inflammation can decrease the likelihood of successful glaucoma surgery.

INFECTIONS

Often, periorbital skin erythema is due to acute or chronic infection of the eyelids. Eradicating this abnormality may also be important prior to beginning medical treatment, to prevent the diagnostic uncertainty of not knowing whether inflammation is due to allergy, to topical glaucoma medications, or to the eyelid disease. The infectious and inflammatory lesions most commonly seen are hordeola, chalazion, meibomitis, and blepharitis.

Hordeola and chalazia both manifest as focal erythematous swelling just above the eyelid margin (Fig. 20–1). *Hordeolum* is the term commonly used for nodular suppurative inflammation of the anterior lamella of the eyelid. Hordeola are often infectious, due to *Staphylococcus aureus*, and require treatment with topical antibiotics and warm compresses, with incision and drainage infrequently required. A *chalazion* is a chronic nonsuppurative granu-

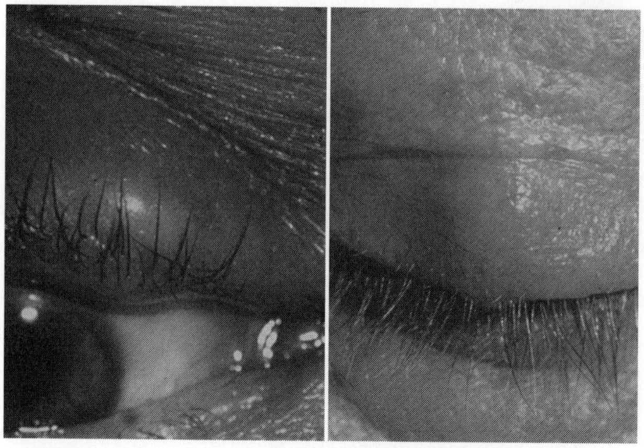

FIGURE 20–1. Swelling of upper eyelids representative of hordeola and chalazia. (© American Academy of Ophthalmology, San Francisco, CA, 1994.)

loma occurring from extrusion of lipid from an obstructed meibomian gland. It may be in the more posterior lamella of the eyelid and may require curettage. In some cases, however, the chalazion resolves spontaneously within 1 or 2 weeks. Warm compresses may hasten the resolution. Both hordeolum and chalazion should be treated and eradicated prior to glaucoma surgery.

Meibomitis is often due to secretory dysfunction of the meibomian glands at the eyelid margins. The dysfunction results in swelling and erythema localized to the eyelid margin, and is further manifested by whitish or yellowish thick discharge at the meibomian orifices along the eyelid margin. If the examiner applies digital pressure, thick secretions extrude. Meibomian gland inflammation may be treated with oral tetracycline, with or without warm compresses and eyelid scrubs.

Blepharitis is perhaps the most common erythematous eyelid abnormality that will be identified in the glaucoma population. It is evidenced by chronic erythema along the eyelid margins and at the base of the eyelashes, with the patient often complaining of foreign body sensation, itching, or tearing. On slit-lamp examination, fibrin collarettes may be noted adherent to the base of the eyelashes with scaling and crusting of the eyelid margin (Fig. 20–2). The most effective treatment is daily scrubbing of the eyelid margins with cotton-tipped applicators that have been moistened with baby shampoo or other eyelid scrub preparation. Antibiotic ointment (e.g., bacitracin, erythromycin) may also be applied in a similar fashion.

Bacterial infection commonly associated with these entities must be eliminated or reduced prior to glaucoma filtration surgery to lessen the chance of a potentially devastating postoperative intraocular infection.

ALLERGIC DERMATITIS

Another common cause of eyelid erythema is dermatitis, which is often seen as a result of allergy to topical antiglaucoma medications. This allergic response is not uncommon and is due either to the medication itself, most commonly adrenergic agents, or to vehicles or preservatives, especially benzalkonium chloride. This toxicity may result in significant erythema localized to the eyelids, with swelling and scaling of the eyelid skin (Fig. 20–3). A follicular conjunctivitis is often present.

The offending medication must be stopped, even if it has been effective in lowering the intraocular pressure (IOP). One may be tempted to reduce the frequency of the antiglaucoma medication and add topical anti-inflammatory medication. However, this approach does not provide long-term resolution of the problem; therefore, the medication must simply be discontinued. After resolution of the inflammation, the patient can be rechallenged with the medication, perhaps with a monocular trial, to confirm the cause of the allergic response. If the allergy is confirmed, one must proceed with either another type of antiglaucoma medication or with surgical treatment. If the allergy is environmental rather than medicinal, it will not improve with cessation of medication and can be treated with topical antihistamines, mast-cell stabilizers, or topical steroids for a short duration.

Abnormal Eyelid Position or Function

Other eyelid abnormalities apparent on external examination that have impact on appropriate glaucoma management are those resulting in abnormal positioning of the eyelids or abnormal functioning of the eyelids.

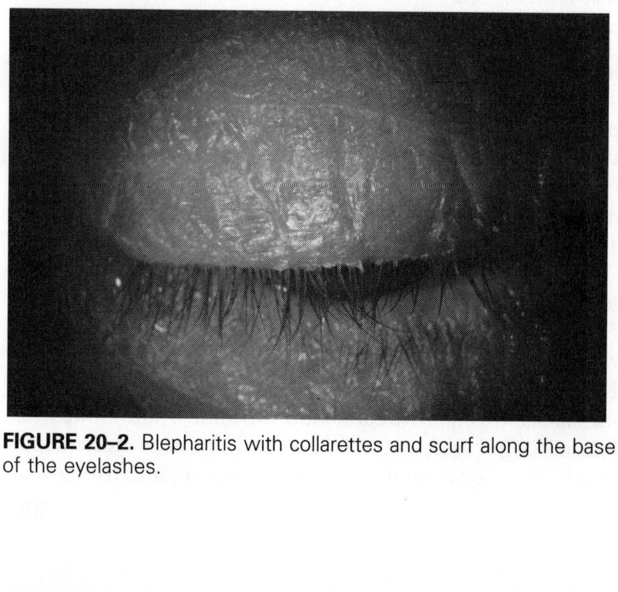

FIGURE 20–2. Blepharitis with collarettes and scurf along the base of the eyelashes.

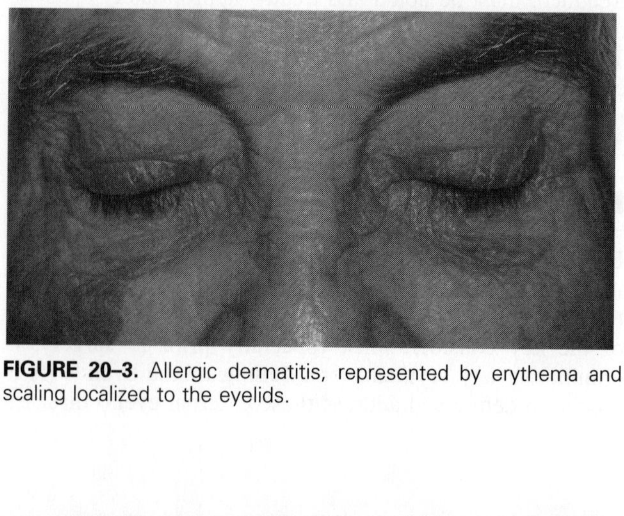

FIGURE 20–3. Allergic dermatitis, represented by erythema and scaling localized to the eyelids.

Lagophthalmos, or poor eyelid closure of any cause resulting in exposure and drying of the ocular surface, is especially important to recognize in the patient who has a filtering bleb. Poor eyelid closure may put the patient at risk for bleb trauma or dellen formation with or without drying of the bleb and associated problems if the bleb is exposed and does not receive proper tear film coverage. Copious artificial tears and nocturnal ointment may be required to prevent or treat these problems.

Entropion and *ectropion* may also result in similar effects and may require correction before any glaucoma surgery is undertaken. The clinician should be wary of intermittent entropion, also commonly referred to as spastic entropion, in the patient with glaucoma. This may be especially likely to occur in the elderly population if the eye is inflamed as in uveitic glaucoma or neovascular glaucoma. Also, ocular irritation as a side effect of topical antiglaucoma medication or postoperative inflammation after glaucoma filtration surgery may result in spastic entropion.

Abnormal positioning of the eyelashes, *distichiasis* or *trichiasis*, which may be primary or related to other abnormalities, is also particularly of concern in the patient with glaucoma who has had filtration surgery. If the eyelashes abrade or otherwise injure the filtration bleb, the patient will be at risk of bleb leak and bleb infection, with potentially disastrous complications, including endophthalmitis. Such eyelash abnormalities must be recognized and addressed as thoroughly as possible prior to any glaucoma filtration surgery. Eyelash abnormalities have been reported with the use of latanoprost (Xalatan). Some patients have been noted to have an increase in length, thickness, and number of eyelashes on the eyelids of the eye treated with latanoprost.[1] Abnormal morphology of these eyelashes occurs, with aberrant positioning and texture.

Ptosis is fairly commonly encountered after any intraocular surgery, including glaucoma filtration surgery and tube shunt surgery. This ptosis is due to trauma to the levator muscle apparatus in a predisposed elderly patient in whom a superior rectus muscle traction suture was placed at the time of surgery. Positioning of the eye with a clear cornea traction suture rather than a rectus suture may decrease, but not completely alleviate, the risk of ptosis. In patients whose postoperative ptosis is related to poor levator muscle function, ptosis repair surgery should not be performed for at least 3 to 4 months after the initial surgery as some patients have experienced slow spontaneous resolution. Also, many patients have a transient ptosis related to steroid treatment. Topical steroids are known to cause a transient ptosis, and intensive topical steroid treatment is often needed after filtration surgery for glaucoma.

SYSTEMIC PHAKOMATOSES

Two systemic phakomatoses with prominent findings on external examination of the eyelids are particularly likely to be associated with glaucoma. The presence of both neurofibromatosis and Sturge-Weber syndrome can affect the management of the glaucoma.

Neurofibromatosis has multiple well-known systemic manifestations but also frequently affects the eyelids and the globe. The classic eyelid defect is a temporal ptosis with a characteristic S-shaped contour of the upper eyelid resulting from a plexiform neurofibroma (Fig. 20–4). Besides the significant ptosis that may result, this finding is of importance, because the risk of glaucoma seems to be much higher in patients who have upper eyelid neurofibromas. As many as 50% of patients who have upper eyelid neurofibromas may eventually have glaucoma on that side.[2] When glaucoma does result, it is usually congenital and may occur early in the development of the neurofibromatosis. This glaucoma is difficult to control, with a poor prognosis for vision.

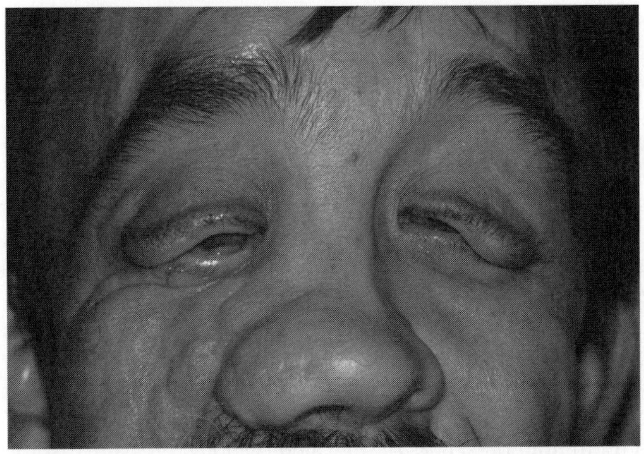

FIGURE 20–4. Severe plexiform neurofibroma producing classic S-shaped eyelid ptosis.

The classic sign of *Sturge-Weber syndrome* is a unilateral nevus flammeus of the face resulting from capillary angiomatosis (Fig. 20–5). The nevus flammeus usually corresponds to a portion of the distribution of the trigeminal nerve (another name for Sturge-Weber syndrome is "encephalotrigeminal angiomatosis"). The nevus flammeus (also known as port-wine stain) is usually unilateral and present at birth.[3] Glaucoma occurs in 30% of patients, but it is not unusual for the glaucoma to be delayed until late childhood or early adulthood. The increased IOP is secondary to elevated episcleral venous pressure related to the angiomatosis. Nearly always this occurs when the angiomatosis involves not only the eyelids but also the conjunctiva and episclera. The glaucoma is nearly always ipsilateral to the nevus flammeus, although contralateral or bilateral glaucoma has been reported. When the port-wine

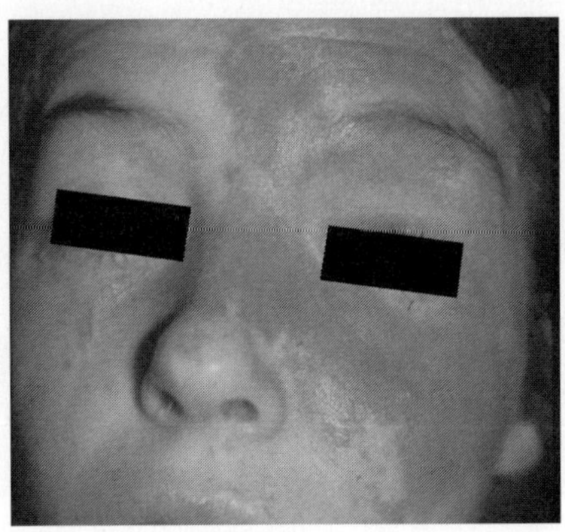

FIGURE 20–5. Unilateral nevus flammeus representative of Sturge-Weber syndrome.

stain is bilateral, the glaucoma may be either unilateral or bilateral.

Unfortunately, the glaucoma is frequently difficult to control. Medical management often fails. Furthermore, when proceeding with surgery, one must be aware, both for preoperative surgical planning and in discussion with the patient or family, that patients with Sturge-Weber syndrome are at increased risk of postoperative complications after filtration surgery. If a choroidal hemangioma is present, expulsive choroidal hemorrhage may occur intraoperatively. The IOP should be lowered as much as possible preoperatively, often with the use of hyperosmotic agents. These patients are also more likely to have severe choroidal effusions postoperatively because of sudden lowering of IOP in the presence of elevated venous pressure. Some surgeons have suggested performing a prophylactic posterior sclerotomy before entry into the anterior chamber.[4]

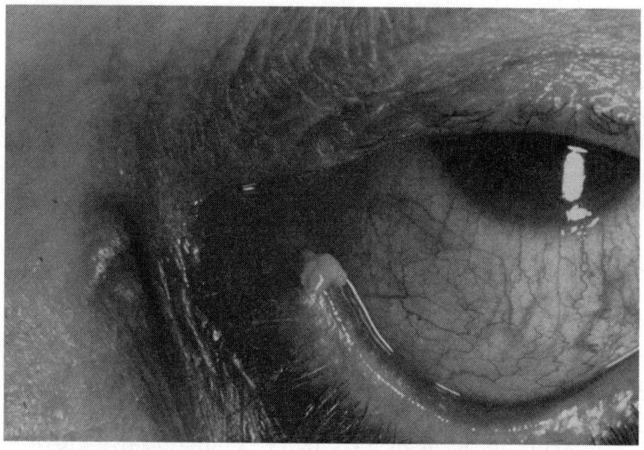

FIGURE 20–7. Retrograde extrusion of material after pressure over lacrimal sac in patient with low-grade chronic obstruction of the nasolacrimal duct. (© American Academy of Ophthalmology, San Francisco, CA, 1994.)

Lacrimal Duct Erythema or Swelling

Prior to proceeding with any incisional glaucoma surgery, the surgeon should make certain that no dacryocystitis is present (Fig. 20–6). If there is any question of duct obstruction, digital pressure over the lacrimal sac may produce reflux through the lacrimal punctum (Fig. 20–7). Eradication of any obstruction is necessary before intraocular surgery is performed, since the increased bacteria potentially present in the tear film can raise the risk of postoperative infection.

Punctal Occlusion for Medical Therapy

Temporally occluding the tear drainage system after instilling topical antiglaucoma medications can both increase the efficacy of the medication and decrease the incidence and severity of systemic side effects. Any patient being started on topical antiglaucoma medication should be taught the technique of punctal occlusion. After installation of the eyedrop, the patient should be instructed to close the eyelids for 2 to 5 minutes without squeezing. This prevents the pumping mechanism of blinking, which drives the tear film nasally and down the lacrimal punctum. While the eyes are closed, the patient should (1) place the index finger over the medial canthus (using the pad of the finger rather than the fingertip, the patient can often feel the caruncle as a landmark for correct placement) and (2) press with firm but gentle, steady pressure for 2 to 3 minutes (Fig. 20–8). This procedure costs the patient nothing, is easily performed, and may significantly increase the amount of medication absorbed through the cornea while decreasing the amount absorbed systemically.

Abnormal Tearing

In patients with glaucoma who have been receiving strong miotic agents for a number of years, epiphora may occur as a result of stenosis or closure of the lacrimal punctum. This disorder should be suspected in the evaluation of any patient with epiphora who has been receiving long-term miotic therapy.

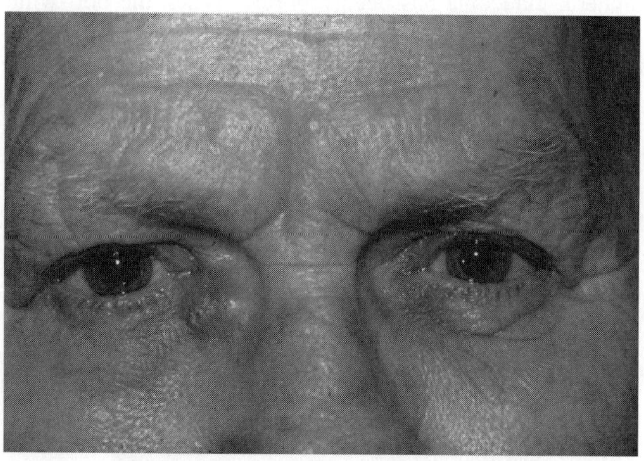

FIGURE 20–6. Focal erythematous swelling over the lacrimal sac representative of dacryocystitis in an adult. (© American Academy of Ophthalmology, San Francisco, CA, 1994.)

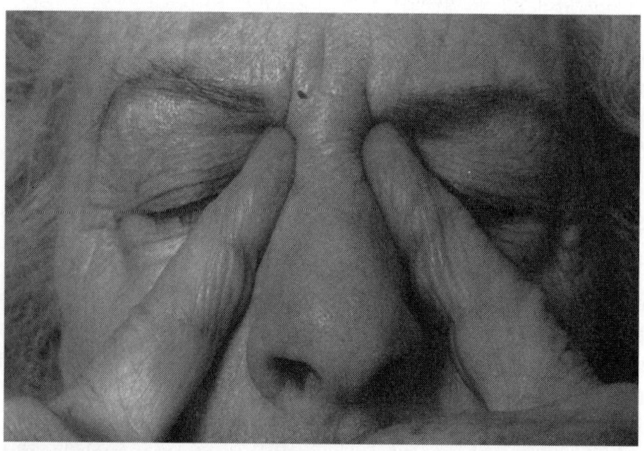

FIGURE 20–8. Positioning of index fingers over lacrimal puncta for punctal occlusion after instillation of topical glaucoma medication. (© American Academy of Ophthalmology, San Francisco, CA, 1994.)

Excess tearing is a common complaint of patients with glaucoma, both those receiving medical therapy and those who have undergone surgery. Most often, because such patients are often elderly, this complaint is related to dry eye syndrome. Patients who require long-term topical antiglaucoma medications often have a low-grade keratitis or ocular allergy, which may cause reflex tear production. In the postoperative patient, abnormal tear production often occurs as a response to foreign body sensation from an elevated ischemic filtration bleb. Especially in patients who have extremely elevated blebs after filtration surgery performed with application of mitomycin, the irritation and reflex tearing may be severe.

In some patients, the excess tearing is associated with dellen located along the base of highly elevated blebs. *Dellen* are areas of focal peripheral keratitis due to drying. A highly elevated filtration bleb prevents lid apposition to the base of the bleb and restricts normal tear film lubrication. Severe dellen may result in corneal thinning, but most do not have severe sequelae. In these instances, patients require copious artificial tears and nocturnal application of ointment for comfort and to prevent reflex tearing. In some severe cases, dellen are not corrected by tears and ointment, and the discomfort and reflex tearing may be severe enough to mandate surgical revision of the bleb. This often is a technically demanding procedure and certainly can threaten the continued functioning of the filtration site. Increasingly, with earlier filtration surgery and use of antiproliferative agents, the potential complication of bleb dysesthesia must be discussed with the patient, recognized, and treated.

Exophthalmos

A variety of disease processes associated with a secondary glaucoma may result in exophthalmos that is noticeable on external examination. Thyroid-related orbitopathy is a common cause of exophthalmos and may result in a secondary open-angle glaucoma. The thyroid abnormality leads to swelling and infiltration of orbital tissue, which may elevate the episcleral venous pressure (Fig. 20–9). IOP may also be increased in specific directions of gaze when ocular movement is attempted away from a fibrosed or infiltrated rectus muscle. Classically, this finding occurs in attempted upgaze in the presence of inferior rectus restriction.

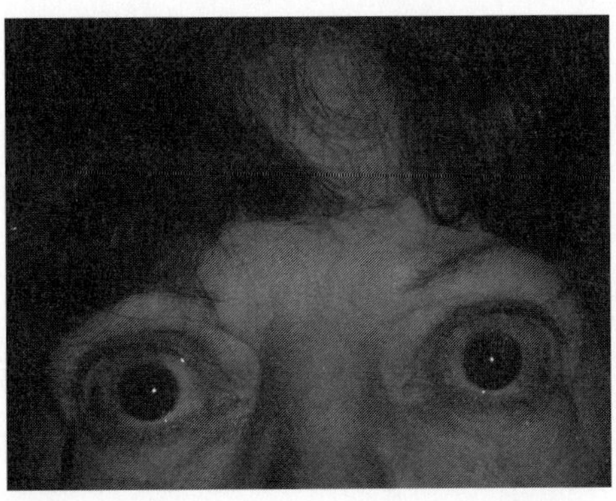

FIGURE 20–9. Exophthalmos with eyelid retraction due to thyroid-related orbitopathy.

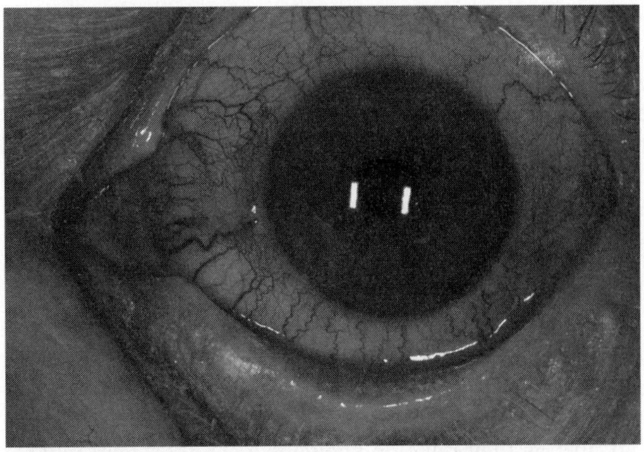

FIGURE 20–10. Dilated tortuous episcleral plexus characteristic of elevated episcleral venous pressure, in this case due to carotid cavernous fistula.

A pulsating exophthalmos may be seen in a patient with neurofibromatosis who has orbital wall defects. A nonpulsating proptosis commonly also occurs from a mass effect of orbital neurofibromas. Glaucoma associated with neurofibromatosis was previously discussed.

Intraoperative, postoperative, or traumatic retrobulbar hemorrhage may result in severe exophthalmos with marked elevation of pressure and compromise of ocular blood flow as manifested by pulsations of the central retinal artery. This is an ocular emergency requiring emergent lateral canthal lysis with emergent medical treatment to lower IOP.

Another cause of exophthalmos associated with glaucoma is carotid artery–cavernous sinus fistula. As the carotid artery runs through the cavernous sinus, fistulas may develop, most often after significant head trauma but also spontaneously. This shunting of blood from the high-pressure carotid arterial system into the low-pressure venous system within the cavernous sinus results in engorgement of the venous system with dilation of orbital and ocular veins. Episcleral venous pressure may be markedly elevated, and the dilated, tortuous conjunctival and episcleral veins may take on a "caput medusa" appearance (Fig. 20–10). The novice examiner may misdiagnose and treat this presentation as conjunctivitis (Fig. 20–11). The orbital vascular engorgement may result in exophthalmos that may

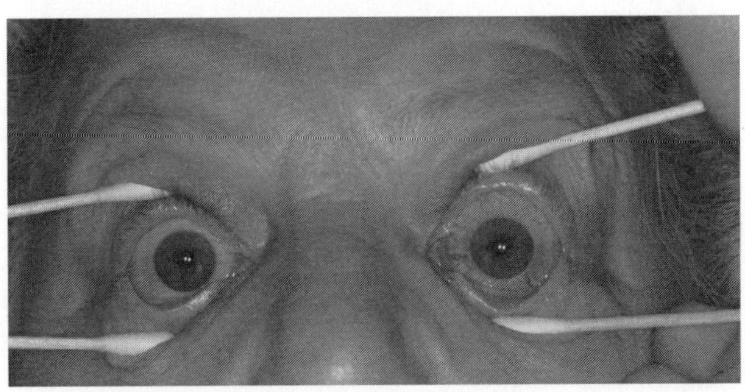

FIGURE 20–11. Hyperemic appearance of conjunctiva related to increased vascularity secondary to carotid cavernous fistula, which may be erroneously diagnosed as conjunctivitis.

pulsate.[5] The patient may subjectively be aware of a bruit, which may be audible to the examiner on auscultation of the orbit. The IOP is elevated in the majority of cases via an open-angle mechanism with elevated episcleral venous pressure.[6] Patients may experience spontaneous choroidal detachments and have a narrow or closed angle with elevated pressure via that mechanism. Rarely, a neovascular glaucoma develops because of ocular ischemia resulting from decreased ocular perfusion due to the venous stasis and decreased arterial perfusion.

Spontaneous dural shunts may result from rents in branch arteries from the carotid, shunting blood into the cavernous sinus. These fistulas may have a more subtle presentation than the traumatic carotid cavernous fistulas and, just as they develop spontaneously, they may resolve spontaneously.

Diagnosis of either type of fistula may be made clinically and may be confirmed with computed tomography scanning of the cavernous sinus and orbits. Cerebral angiography with digital subtraction techniques and selective catheterization may be done by an experienced interventional radiologist.[7] A variety of occluding elements have been used via catheterization to close the fistulas. Initially, glaucoma control should be attempted medically, as surgery in patients with fistulas may be complicated by bleeding and choroidal detachment due to engorgement of choroidal vessels.

Strabismus

External examination of ocular motility may reveal restriction of range of motion in the operative eye after tube shunt implantation. Motility disturbances have been reported with many different types of tube shunt implants, regardless of the extent of extraocular muscle manipulation required to position the implant. The resulting strabismus is usually due to restriction of movement in the direction of the tube shunt. This is more common in shunts placed in the superonasal quadrant. Most often, the restriction is due to capture of the muscle sheath or tendon within scar tissue encapsulating the tube shunt plate or to stretching and displacement of the muscle over a significant capsule.[8] When heterotropia develops postoperatively, it appears not to lessen over time. Patients with binocular functioning have been treated with glasses with prisms, strabismus surgery, or removal of the tube shunt.

SUMMARY

Key signs of disease processes affecting the appearance or function of the eyes that are visible on external examination have been discussed. Given the adage, "you only see what you look for, and you only look for what you know," it is crucial to know of these signs. Their presence may significantly affect the choice of optimal treatment for patients with glaucoma.

REFERENCES

1. Wand M: Latanoprost and hyperpigmentation of eyelashes. Arch Ophthalmol 1997;115:1206.
2. Mattox C: Glaucoma in the phakomatoses. *In* Epstein DL, Allingham RR, Schuman JS (eds): Chandler and Grant's Glaucoma, 4th ed. Baltimore, Williams & Wilkins, 1997, p 438.
3. Weiss JS, Ritch R: Glaucoma in the phakomatoses. *In* Ritch R, Shields MB, Krupin T (eds): The Glaucomas. St. Louis, CV Mosby, 1989.
4. Bellows AR, Chylack LT, Epstein DL, Hutchinson T: Choroidal effusion during glaucoma surgery in patients with prominent episcleral vessels. Arch Ophthalmol 1979;97:493.
5. Henderson JW, Schneider RC: The ocular findings of carotid-cavernous fistula in a series of 17 cases. Am J Ophthalmol 1959;48:585.
6. Weinreb RN, Jeng S, Goldstick BJ: Glaucoma secondary to elevated episcleral venous pressure. *In* Ritch R, Shields MB, Krupin T (eds): The Glaucomas. St. Louis, CV Mosby, 1989.
7. Kupersmith MJ, Berenstein A, Flamm E, Ransohoff J: Neuro-ophthalmologic abnormalities and intravascular therapy of traumatic carotid-cavernous fistula. Ophthalmology 1986;93:906.
8. Smith SL, Starita RT, Fellman RL, Lynn JR: Early clinical experience with the Baerveldt 350mm glaucoma implant and associated extraocular muscle imbalance. Ophthalmology 1993;100:914.

CHAPTER 21

Cornea, Conjunctiva, and Bleb

DAVID P. CAMPBELL, JOHN D. GROSS,
and MARK B. SHERWOOD

The effect of glaucoma treatment on the ocular surface is one of the most common problems we confront in taking care of patients with glaucoma. This chapter logically addresses all of these possible concerns. The authors begin with the possible effects of glaucoma medications: Is this reaction toxic or allergic? How common is it? They then move to the controversial area, the effect of the use of these medications on subsequent glaucoma filtration surgery. Another medication effect associated with surgery is that of the use of antimetabolites. The authors also consider the issue of how the status of the conjunctiva and cornea initially affects the choice of surgical procedure.

Finally, and almost mystical in its importance, is the bleb after filtration surgery. The authors describe the favorable and unfavorable signs and appearance of the bleb in detail. Unfortunately, bleb complications are more common than any of us would desire. The chapter authors identify and address such complications, from bleb leaks and overfiltration to excessive scarring, bleb encapsulation with inadequate filtration, or infection. The extensive amount of information the authors provide will enable the reader to correctly manage the ocular surface in patients with glaucoma.

Effects of Topical Antiglaucoma Medications on the Conjunctiva and Cornea

Currently, most patients in the United States who are identified as having glaucoma or are considered to be at risk for glaucomatous damage to the optic nerve head are treated initially with topical medical therapy.[1, 2] The recent expansion of available pressure-lowering agents for glaucoma has enabled the ophthalmologist to select the most effective medication or combination of medications for each patient. All of these medications, however, have the potential for adverse effects on the cornea and conjunctiva.

β-BLOCKERS

β-blockers decrease aqueous production, are generally well tolerated, and are widely accepted as first-line antiglaucoma drugs. Nevertheless, as many as 43.6% of patients report ocular discomfort upon instillation of β-blockers, and approximately 3% of patients experience blepharoconjunctivitis after their long-term use.[3–6] Changing to a different topical β-blocker or to a preservative-free form may alleviate these problems.

Isolated cases of corneal anesthesia and epithelial changes have been reported. Such effects can be more of a problem in older patients who have decreased tear production and are using higher-concentration forms of β-blockers.[3, 4, 7–9] The integrity of the precorneal tear film may be adversely affected by timolol therapy, as reflected by a shortened tear break-up time (BUT).[3, 10, 11] Switching to a preservative-free form has been shown to improve this condition and is recommended in patients with dry eyes.[9, 10] Examination of conjunctival biopsy specimens has revealed a minimal effect of β-blockers on the conjunctival cell profile.[12–14]

ADRENERGIC AGONISTS

Adrenergic agonists, which decrease intraocular pressure by increasing aqueous outflow, can cause stinging and irritation and a blepharoconjunctivitis with or without periocular skin involvement. The conjunctivitis is typically a toxic follicular type and generally manifests as follicles (most prominent in the lower tarsal conjunctiva), redness, and a mucoid discharge. This effect can appear weeks to years after initiation of therapy with an adrenergic agonist. After discontinuation of the drug, the follicular reaction may take months to fully resolve.[15, 16]

Patients almost universally notice red eyes while using topical *epinephrine.* This effect is due to initial blanching of the conjunctiva because of vasoconstriction, followed by a reactive hyperemia, which can persist for several hours. Ocular pigment deposition has also been reported with the use of epinephrine. Infrequently, long-term epinephrine therapy can produce dense brown deposits in the stroma and Bowman's layer of the cornea as well as staining of contact lenses.[15] Conjunctival deposits have been reported in up to 30% of patients treated for more than 9 months. Tarsal conjunctival deposits have been linked to recurrent erosions of the underlying cornea.[15–17] Also, it is recommended that epinephrine use be avoided in patients with a history of ocular herpes simplex infection because animal studies have shown a potential for reactivation of the infection.[17]

Dipivefrin, an epinephrine prodrug, has pressure-lowering properties similar to those of epinephrine but is associated with a lower incidence of burning and stinging upon instillation. Reported rates of blepharoconjunctivitis attributed to dipivefrin use range from 11.1% to 28.6%, and the effect occurred 4 to 26 months after initiation of treatment.[17–19] Examination of conjunctival cell profiles has shown an increase in the number of subepithelial fibroblasts, lymphocytes, macrophages, and epithelial lymphocytes in patients treated with sympathomimetics alone.[12–14]

Apraclonidine, an α-adrenergic agonist, is associated with a 11% to 17% rate of conjunctival blanching and a 24% rate of burning-stinging.[20] Allergic reactions, some of which may be severe, occur in as many as 48% of patients treated with 1% solutions of apraclonidine, and less commonly with lower concentrations. The mean time to reaction development is 4.7 months.[7] A switch to brimonidine in patients with such an allergy has been shown to be safe and efficacious.[21] *Brimonidine* is associated with an allergic reaction rate ranging from 4.8% to 11.5%, and burning and stinging was reported in 28% of patients who used it.[22–24]

MIOTIC AGENTS

Miotics have been reported to cause burning on instillation and a transient conjunctival hyperemia due to vasodilation.[25] Rare cicatricial pemphigoid has been reported in patients treated with regimens that included pilocarpine.[26] Local allergic sensitivity, typically affecting the conjunctiva and eyelids, has been reported uncommonly. If it occurs, a drop containing a different preservative can be tried. In 20% of patients who use pilocarpine gel for longer than 8 weeks, a diffuse superficial corneal haze develops.[25] Miotics alone were found to raise the numbers of conjunctival subepithelial fibroblasts, macrophages, lymphocytes, mast cells, and epithelial macrophages and lymphocytes and to decrease the number of goblet cells.[12–14]

CARBONIC ANHYDRASE INHIBITORS

Topical carbonic anhydrase inhibitors, such as *dorzolamide* and *brinzolamide,* block the formation of bicarbonate in the ciliary body, thus decreasing the production of aqueous and, subsequently, intraocular pressure (IOP). Ocular side effects include some degree of discomfort upon instillation and occasional follicular conjunctivitis.[27–31] One study has reported superficial punctate keratitis in 12% of patients; however, this finding may be a response to the vehicle, which provides the proper tonicity, buffering, and preservative, because 10.5% of the patients receiving placebo in the study also experienced the keratitis.[27, 32] Brinzolamide has been shown to produce less ocular discomfort than dorzolamide (1.8% to 3.0% versus 16.4%, respectively).[33] Permanent corneal edema was reported in a small series of patients who had a history of corneal endothelial compromise.[34]

PROSTAGLANDIN ANALOGUES

The prostaglandin analogue latanoprost reduces IOP by increasing uveoscleral outflow. Controlled clinical trials of latanoprost, 0.005% drops used once daily, have revealed irritative symptoms and a typically mild conjunctival hyperemia in 30% to 36% of patients that diminishes with continued use of the drops. Greater iris pigmentation was noted in 5% to 18% of patients being treated with latanoprost.[35, 36] An association between the use of latanoprost and the development of herpes simplex keratitis has also been reported.[37]

CORTICOSTEROIDS

Topical steroids, which are used to decrease inflammation following trabeculectomy, have been shown to thin bleb tissue and significantly improve the surgical success rate.[38, 39] There is the danger that underlying ocular infection may be encouraged or may proceed uncontrolled and undetected with topical steroid use.[40] Also, corneal wound healing has been shown to be inhibited by topical steroids.[40, 41]

CHRONIC MEDICATION USE

Several studies have shown that long-term administration of topical glaucoma medications induces a subclinical inflammation in the conjunctiva and Tenon's capsule.[31, 32, 42–44] This inflammation has been demonstrated by comparison of conjunctival biopsy specimens from medically treated patients and patients undergoing primary glaucoma surgery without prior medical therapy. Studies revealed significantly more inflammatory cells and fibroblasts in the conjunctiva and Tenon's capsule with long-term therapy. There was also a decrease in the number of conjunctival goblet cells and some epithelial metaplasia with ultrastructural changes. This effect was more pronounced in patients who had received multiple-drug regimens, especially those that included pilocarpine or sympathomimetic agents. One study described histopathologic and inflammatory changes in the deeper tissues of the trabeculum in addition to the effect on the ocular surface tissues in patients who had been using β-blocker eyedrops for years.[43] The cell infiltrates were found to be markedly increased in the trabecular meshwork of patients receiving multiple-drug treatment regardless of the topical regimen. It was also shown, through a companion animal study, that the preservative benzalkonium contributes significantly to these effects.[14]

It is clear the status of the conjunctiva and Tenon's capsule in the region of the drainage fistula is critical in patients undergoing filtration surgery. These vascularized tissues likely contribute the most to fibroblast proliferation, and it is the postoperative fibrotic process that most often leads to failure of filtration surgery.[12, 44] There is growing evidence that prior antiglaucoma medication treatment may negatively influence the outcome of filtration surgery by enhancing external bleb fibrosis.[44] One study showed higher surgical success rates in patients who initially underwent primary trabeculectomy (98%) than in patients who underwent trabeculectomy after medical therapy failed (79%).[42] The only identifiable difference in the two groups was the duration of glaucoma eyedrop treatments. A study of filtration surgery in 24 patients who used four different long-term antiglaucoma topical regimens found the success rates for trabeculectomy to be the same in patients undergoing primary surgery (90%) and patients receiving β-blockers alone (93%), to be lower in patients receiving β-blockers and miotics (72%), and to be lowest in patients receiving a combination of β-blockers, miotics, and sympathomimetics (45%). Failure of surgery was closely correlated with the extent of subclinical conjunctival inflammation as assessed by preoperative conjunctival biopsy.[45] A similar study concluded that the largest single influence on outcomes was the number of preoperative glaucoma medications used, particularly exposure to sympathomimetics. However, β-blockers seem to have no significant adverse effect.[13]

It is possible to reverse medication-induced conjunctival subclinical inflammation and improve surgical success by instituting preoperative treatment with topical steroids and discontinuing sympathomimetics 1 month prior to the procedure. One study conducted to examine this concept compared biopsy findings and surgical outcomes in two groups of patients with a history of medical multiple-drug treatment. The group that had undergone "reversal" treatment had an 81% trabeculectomy success rate, compared with a 50% rate in the matched group of control patients, after at least 1 year of follow-up.[46]

Effects of Antimetabolites on the Conjunctiva and Cornea

Use of adjunctive antimetabolite agents increases the success rate of glaucoma filtration surgery by inhibiting fibroblast proliferation. The fibroblast appears to play a central role in the postoperative scarring process, which is the major determinant of long-term IOP control and surgical success.

The use of postoperative subconjunctival 5-fluorouracil (5-FU) became accepted in the late 1980s for the treatment of eyes at high risk for or showing early signs of bleb failure. 5-FU is a pyrimidine analogue that has been shown to inhibit fibroblast proliferation.[47, 48] Initial studies, which involved daily subconjunctival injections of 5 mg of 5-FU for 7 to 14 days, confirmed the ability of 5-FU to improve the success of filtering surgery in high-risk cases.[49–52]

Significant complications are associated with the use of 5-FU, however, including wound leaks, corneal epithelial defects,[49, 53–59] and late-onset bleb leaks.[50, 60–64] There is no consensus about the lowest effective dose that can be applied to the individual patient.

The use of mitomycin C (MMC), an antineoplastic antibiotic that almost completely inhibits fibroblast proliferation in tissue culture, has also been advocated.[65] Multiple studies have confirmed the efficacy of MMC as an adjunct to trabeculectomy.[66–71] When compared with postoperative subconjunctival 5-FU, intraoperative MMC has been proved in many studies to have superior efficacy in lowering IOP following trabeculectomy.[58, 62, 63, 72] MMC may also have some direct effect on lowering IOP by disrupting the ciliary body epithelium.[73–75]

Like 5-FU, MMC is associated with uncommon but serious postoperative complications. Along with wound leaks, MMC has been associated with hypotony maculopathy, which is probably related to excessive filtration or aqueous hyposecretion.[73, 74, 76, 77] Intraocular MMC has been shown to cause anterior chamber inflammation and toxicity to rabbit,[78] bovine, and human donor,[79] endothelial cells.[80, 81] Mitomycin C should be applied prior to entry into the anterior chamber, but contact of the agent with edges of the conjunctival flap should be avoided. The area of application should be thoroughly irrigated after treatment.

Preoperative Factors Involved in the Selection of Surgical Procedure

When medical therapy fails to keep IOP at an acceptable level, surgical therapy is indicated. Close examination of the superficial ocular structures can be very helpful in the selection of the most appropriate surgical procedure to give the patient the greatest chance of surgical success.

CONJUNCTIVA

Previous ocular surgery is a well-known risk factor for failure of trabeculectomy.[82, 83] The physician can easily identify previous surgery at the slit-lamp by simply observing the mobility of the anesthetized conjunctiva when it is moved with a sterile cotton-tipped applicator. Some surgeons advocate ballooning the tissues by injecting balanced salt solution (BSS) beneath the conjunctiva with a needle at the beginning of surgery, allowing for direct visualization of scarred areas. Using this information, the surgeon can formulate a strategy to place the new surgical site in the best possible location. For example, significant perilimbal scarring with recessed tissues from previous cataract surgery would probably preclude use of a limbus-based conjunctival flap. Trabeculectomy may be a less successful procedure in eyes with significant conjunctival scarring because of the greater chance of intraoperative complications, such as conjunctival buttonholes. Conjunctival scarring may also reduce the total obtainable bleb surface area, thus limiting the final reduction in IOP.[82–85]

As previously discussed, patients who have received topical antiglaucoma medications for many years also may have poorer surgical outcomes than those who have not.[42–44] This difference may be due to greater vascularity of the tissues that contributes to the inflammatory response and subsequent scarring in patients who have used such agents.

The use of antimetabolites has significantly raised success rates for trabeculectomy in high-risk cases as well as in patients undergoing primary surgery.[82, 84–88] Many surgeons, however, place a glaucoma drainage tube when the amount of conjunctival scarring is substantial and the risk of surgical complications or bleb failure is excessively high. Of course, this decision lies with the surgeon and is based on individual experience and skill. Other surgical options are laser surgery and cyclodestructive procedures.

CORNEA (See also Chapter 11)

Post–Penetrating Keratoplasty Glaucoma

Glaucoma occurring after penetrating keratoplasty (PKP) has a reported incidence ranging from 10% to 53%.[89–93] Risk factors for the development of post-keratoplasty glaucoma are (1) pre-existing glaucoma, (2) either aphakia or pseudophakia (either pre-existing or incurred at the time of PKP), (3) repeated keratoplasty, and (4) the presence of an early postoperative rise in pressure.[94–96] One large study found that 80% of patients with pre-existing glaucoma experienced post-keratoplasty glaucoma versus 8% of patients with no prior glaucoma history.[97] The mechanics of the keratoplasty surgery itself may aggravate glaucoma in patients with pre-existing disease.[94, 98]

The management of glaucoma in patients who have undergone PKP is often difficult; however, effective control of IOP is very important. The post-keratoplasty eye with glaucoma is particularly at risk of significant visual impairment, and effective treatment is necessary to maintain graft integrity.[89] Medical treatment of post-keratoplasty glaucoma with aqueous suppressants such as β-blockers, α_2-adrenergic agonists, and carbonic anhydrase inhibitors may be successful initially, but surgical intervention is required in a high percentage of cases. After failure of medical therapy, it is necessary to select the most appropriate surgical intervention for the patient. Unfortunately, no glaucoma procedure stands out clearly as the most effective for both lowering IOP and maintaining graft integrity.

TRABECULECTOMY

Failure rates for traditional trabeculectomy have been reported to be as high as 90% in the first 6 to 9 months following keratoplasty.[99] It was found that patients with a second or further graft or those with closed-angle post-PKP glaucoma have a significantly reduced chance of successful trabeculectomy.[99] Attempts to maintain a filtering bleb with antimetabolites, such as 5-FU and mitomycin, may risk graft failure from epithelial or wound toxicity. Some studies, however, have reported 77% (n = 17) to 87% (n = 16) success rates at a mean follow-up of 14.6 to 26 months after trabeculectomy using MMC.[100–102]

CYCLOCRYOTHERAPY

Cyclocryotherapy has been widely used in the past to treat intractable secondary glaucoma following keratoplasty. Small studies have reported successful IOP control in 83% (n = 36) to 88% (n = 17) of patients.[90] Complications have limited its use; they include significant visual loss, phthisis, chronic uveitis, severe pain, hemorrhage, hypotony, macular edema, and graft failure. Making conservative applications over just a portion of the ciliary body and repeating applications if necessary may help to reduce these complications.[90]

TRANSSCLERAL LASER CYCLODESTRUCTION

Transscleral neodymium:yttrium-aluminum-garnet (Nd:YAG) laser cyclodestruction may be a useful technique for controlling IOP in patients with post-keratoplasty glaucoma, but loss of visual acuity in these patients is a common complication. Reported success rates range from 68% (n = 13) to 85% (n = 33) with significant lowering of IOP.[102–108] Complications include (1) decrease in vision of 2 or more lines (22% to 56% of patients), (2) graft failure (11% to 39%), and (3) hypotony (12% to 22%). It is recommended the total energy of the initial session should not exceed 256 joules in order to avoid hypotony, particularly in eyes with a history of prior cyclocryotherapy.[108]

DRAINAGE TUBE IMPLANTATION

A drainage tube implant, our treatment of choice, has proved to be useful in the control of IOP in patients with post-keratoplasty glaucoma. Successful IOP control was achieved in 69% (n = 45) to 96% (n = 26) of patients with average follow-up of 13 months to more than 30 months. Visual acuity remained stable or improved in 70% to 94% of eyes after drainage implant surgery for post-keratoplasty glaucoma.[92, 109–114] The success rates for the grafts in these cases ranged from 56% to 80%.

The prevention of PKP graft rejection is a major issue, but aggressive topical corticosteroid therapy can often reverse this complication. Close attention to the placement of the tube in the anterior chamber is important to avoid undue loss of endothelial cells by direct trauma from the tube and subsequent graft decompensation. Graft failure may occur at a significant rate when eyes with clear grafts undergo any additional surgical procedure associated with anterior segment inflammation. The use of either a tube-occluding suture or stent with a nonvalved implant or a valved implant helps prevent certain hypotony-associated complications, such as flat anterior chamber, kissing choroidal effusions, and suprachoroidal hemorrhage.[115] Further experience in the use of aqueous drainage implants offers some optimism for the future of treatment of post-keratoplasty glaucoma.

Post-Trabeculectomy Evaluation of the Bleb and Conjunctiva

The postoperative assessment of bleb function is an extremely valuable tool in ensuring the successful outcome of filtering surgery. Like preoperative evaluation, careful postoperative examination of the involved tissues can give clues as to whether additional therapies should be employed to improve the chance of surgical success.[116]

FAVORABLE SIGNS

Initially, a well-functioning bleb is elevated and has a diffuse surface area, covering at least one quadrant of the globe, and preferably two quadrants. A larger bleb area provides a greater surface area for aqueous absorption and, subsequently, lower IOP. Additionally, a larger surface area also allows the aqueous pressure to be distributed among the tissues and may prevent distention of the conjunctival and subconjunctival tissues.[117] Blebs with smaller surface areas sometimes become either hypervascular or very thin-walled and function poorly. This outcome may be related to the effects of tension on the tissues, which some surgeons suspect to result in a vicious circle of additional fibroblast stimulation, further collagen deposition, bleb encapsulation, closure of drainage channels, and further elevation of pressure and tissue distention.[117–119]

Relatively quiet, or minimally injected, conjunctiva and episclera suggest that there is adequately controlled inflammation and that the dosage frequency for the topical anti-inflammatory medication is probably sufficient.[38–40] If antimetabolites have been used, especially MMC, there will be evidence of early avascular changes whereby the conjunctival vessels become attenuated and eventually disappear.[117]

A very promising sign of bleb function, in regard to transconjunctival filtration, is the appearance of microcystic changes in the superficial conjunctiva overlying the bleb. These changes can be readily observed adjacent to a broad slit-lamp beam, with the use of retroillumination, as confluent areas of microcysts in the conjunctival epithelium. This characteristic, also referred to as *succulence*, confirms that there is established aqueous flow both into and through the bleb.[117]

POTENTIALLY UNFAVORABLE SIGNS AND COMPLICATIONS AND THEIR MANAGEMENT (See Chapter 22)

Bleb or Wound Leak

Bleb leak can occur in the early days after trabeculectomy surgery or many years later (Fig. 21–1). Particularly in the initial postoperative period, the presence of a leak can be very detrimental to the long-term survival of the bleb. If the bleb does not look well-elevated on the first postoperative day, either flow through the scleral flap is inadequate (secondary to tight suturing, internal ostium occlusion by hemorrhage, iris, vitreous, etc., or aqueous shutdown) or there is a leak.[116, 117, 120] The leak may be occurring either through the overlying conjunctival tissues or at the conjunctival incision line.

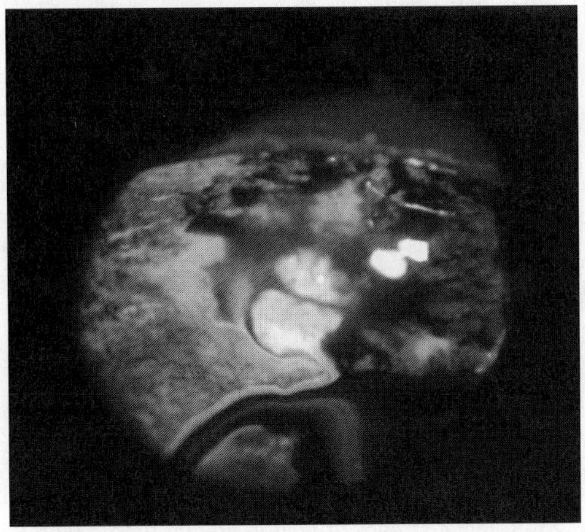

FIGURE 21–1. Bleb leak.

One may test for a leak by using a fluorescein strip or drop of fluorescein to paint the entire area of the bleb and the incision line after applying a topical anesthetic to the eye (Fig. 21–2). Under the cobalt blue light at the slit-lamp, the painted area appears a uniform dark green to black. If there is a hole in the tissues, a stream of brighter and paler green in the fluorescein-painted area identifies it and, by gravity, tracks dependently (Figs. 21–3 and 21–4). In contrast, in areas where the bleb wall is thin but still intact, one or more bright green spots are highlighted in the painted zone after a brief delay. These spots represent transudation through the conjunctival tissues and can sometimes, when brisk, be difficult to distinguish from leaks confirmed by a positive response to Seidel's test.

Occasionally, if the bleb is completely flat or if there is secondary aqueous shutdown because of hypotony, it may be hard to detect a true Seidel's test–positive hole in the tissues. Because of the lack of aqueous flow through the defect, no dilution is created in the fluorescein, and it remains dark. If the presence or absence of a hole is still in doubt, mild pressure can be applied to the eye (if the anterior chamber is deep) to elevate its pressure and force fluid into the bleb and through any hole that may be present; this procedure is called a positive-pressure Seidel's

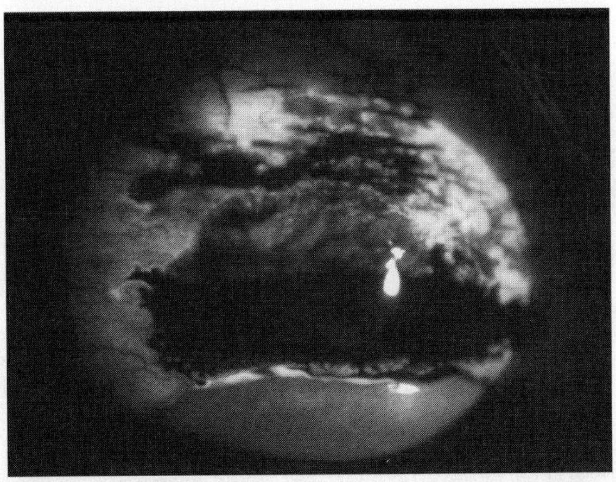

FIGURE 21–2. Uniform color of an eye painted with fluorescein and viewed under a cobalt blue light. This figure demonstrates the absence of a hole in the ocular tissues.

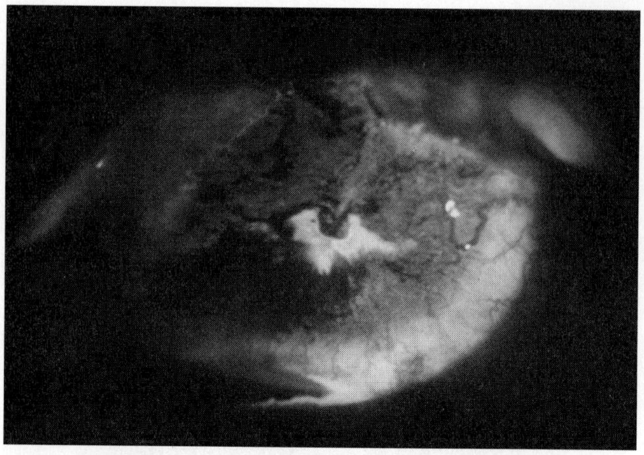

FIGURE 21–3. Initial stream of fluid in an eye with a bleb leak.

test.[120] It is important to consider the possibility of a bleb leak and to diligently search for one, particularly in the presence of thin or previously scarred conjunctival–Tenon's capsule tissues.

MANAGEMENT OF EARLY BLEB LEAK

The management of a bleb leak is influenced by several factors[116]:

- Size and site of the leak
- Depth of the anterior chamber
- Residual height of the bleb
- Degree of inflammation of the bleb tissues
- Prior or desired use of antimetabolites and other drugs

If the leak is at the wound margin in a limbus-based or fornix-based conjunctival flap, additional suturing of the incision line is generally recommended. An alternative management option for the fornix-based flap is to consider a trial with a bandage soft contact lens (BSCL) for a few days, with the intention of proceeding to suturing if the Seidel's test–positive leak does not heal or, especially, if the bleb appears low, the anterior chamber's shallow, or a choroidal effusion is developing.[121] The BSCL, even if oversized, usually docs not reach a well-placed limbus-based incision line.

For closure of a fornix-based conjunctival wound leak with sutures, it is helpful to pull the conjunctival tissue anteriorly, beyond the limbus. The epithelium should be removed from the underlying peripheral cornea to aid adhesion of the conjunctiva. Horizontal tension on the leading edge of the conjunctival flap to slightly indent the underlying cornea creates a mechanically watertight seal.[122]

If the leak is in the body of the bleb, management options are (1) use of a BSCL, (2) injection of autologous blood, and (3) suture closure of the hole.[122] Intraoperative use of antimetabolites may limit or delay the spontaneous healing that is required for a BSCL to be effective. Contact lenses, however, can achieve closure of a small leak even following application of MMC.

Autologous blood may promote leak closure but has the disadvantage of increasing inflammatory response to the whole bleb at the same time in the early postoperative phase, when the efforts of the surgeon are generally directed toward reducing such inflammation. There is a risk of later bleb scarring and failure.[123–125]

If the hole is small, an external 10-0 or 11-0 nylon pursestring suture, with the needle bite being passed intrastromally through the conjunctiva in a nonpenetrating fashion, is often helpful.[126] However, when the tissues are very thin, this suture may be extremely difficult to place. Penetration of the tissues runs the risk of creating an even larger hole from the needle track or from erosion of the suture.

For large holes or if the tissue is particularly thin, a two-layer suture closure may provide the best result. This requires reopening the conjunctival–Tenon's capsule incision, reflecting the tissues back to allow an initial running suture closure on the deep side of Tenon's capsule, and then separately suturing the overlying conjunctival tear. The closed leak site should be checked by forcible irrigation with BSS to ensure that the hole is fully sealed before the incision line is closed again. If the Tenon's capsule is too thin in the area of the leak for suturing, rotation of a Tenon's capsule pedicle or a Tenon's capsule patch graft from another part of the eye could be considered.[127, 128]

MANAGEMENT OF LATE BLEB LEAK

Late blcb lcaks arc becoming more common with the growing use of antimetabolites and are particularly common in thinned, avascular, often somewhat localized blebs.[120] They may be recurrent and are associated with higher risk of blebitis and endophthalmitis,[129–136] with an additional increased risk in blebs created inferiorly.[137] In many cases, the surgeon is torn between the desire to maintain good IOP control in an eye with already damaged and compromised tissues (which may limit further surgical options if the bleb subsequently fails) and the need to heal the bleb leak.

A conservative approach to late bleb leaks is often preferred for this reason. This approach consists of (1) the use of a BSCL (Fig. 21–5) together with aqueous suppressants to reduce fluid flow through the hole and (2) antibiotic coverage with agents that are effective against a broad spectrum of gram-positive and gram-negative organisms, especially *Streptococcus* and *Haemophilus* species. Careful assessment of the bleb, anterior chamber, and vitreous should be performed regularly to ensure that there is no evidence of blebitis or endophthalmitis, that the bleb area is being maintained, and that choroidal effusions or macu-

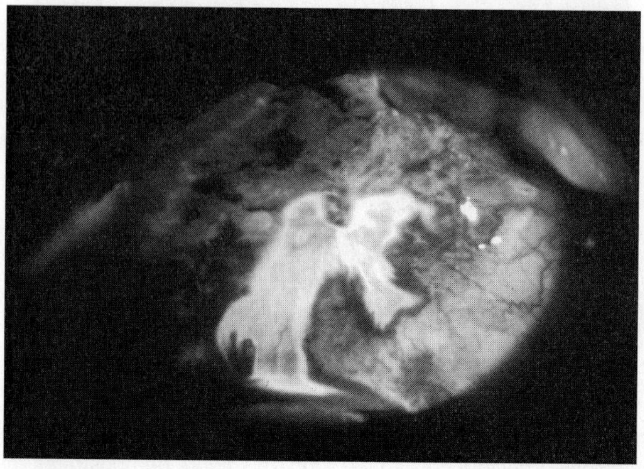

FIGURE 21–4. Gravity-dependent flow of leakage from a bleb.

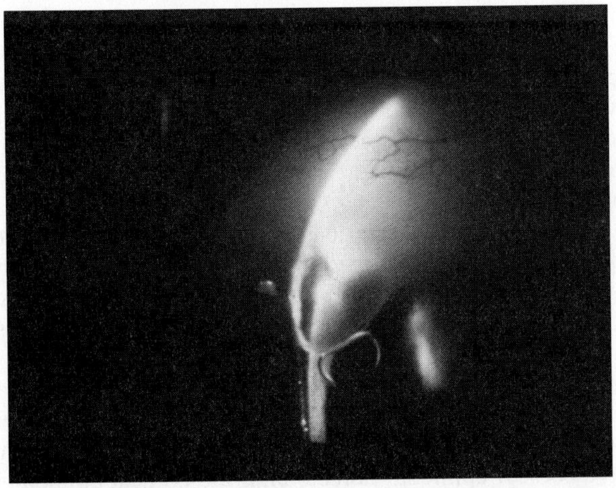

FIGURE 21–5. Application of a bandage soft contact lens (BSCL).

lar edema is not developing. It is reasonable to continue this conservative management and to monitor for several weeks or longer, provided that these parameters are stable and that the patient understands the need to seek urgent care if ocular discharge, decreased vision, pain, or greater redness of the eye develops. We routinely see patients with bleb leaks at least twice a week to remove and re-sterilize the BSCL, to check the eye for the earliest signs of blebitis and endophthalmitis, and to perform Seidel's test to determine whether the bleb leak has resolved.

Many other techniques have been proposed short of surgical revision to help resolve late bleb leaks. The mere fact that there are so many techniques indicates the partial nature of their success. Wise has suggested injection of autologous blood into the bleb (Fig. 21–6).[125] The clotting of the blood can serve to occlude the leak, and factors in the blood are thought to enhance healing and fibrosis.[123–125] Success rates between 58% and 75% have been described. There is a small risk of total loss of bleb function, and unless a viscoelastic agent is injected into the anterior chamber prior to the blood injection, backflow of the blood into the anterior chamber can occur, leading to visual disturbance until the hyphema settles. Subconjunctival injection of the blood around the bleb rather than into it has been shown to be effective and does not pose the risk of hyphema (Fig. 21–7).[123]

The use of autologous fibrinogen in combination with thrombin or application of cyanoacrylate glue to create a temporary seal at the leak site, following which healing and natural repair can more rapidly occur, has also been explored. There is a risk that if the glue plug is traumatized and knocked off, a larger hole in the bleb tissue may result. Covering the glue plug with a BSCL or collagen shield is usually recommended.[138, 139]

Argon and thermal-mode Nd:YAG lasers have also been employed to close bleb leaks by creating inflammation and collagen contraction.[140, 141] With the use of an argon laser, the external surface of the bleb tissue is painted with a dye to enhance the absorption of laser energy.

Cryotherapy can be a very useful mode of therapy, particularly for a bleb that has dissected anteriorly to form a cornealized bleb or a leak that is in the cornealized portion of the bleb structure.[142] The aim is to create an adhesion between the two bleb surfaces and eliminate aqueous flow to this area. The corneal extension of the bleb is often paper-thin, consisting primarily of epithelium, and the leak frequently is seen on the sloping sidewall of the bleb close to the bleb-cornea junction. Cryotherapy can be performed as an office procedure. After topical anesthesia is achieved, a freeze lasting a few seconds can be applied with the standard retinal cryoprobe to create an iceball that involves both the superficial and deep surfaces of the bleb. A freeze-thaw-freeze technique can be employed. This is generally not a painful procedure, but the patient must be carefully instructed to keep the other eye fixated on a chosen target to prevent tearing of the fragile bleb by inadvertent eye movement while the probe is attached to the eye by the iceball. Antibiotic ointment without corticosteroid and a compression patch are applied overnight.

Compression sutures can also be placed in an office procedure. A 9-0 polypropylene (Prolene) stitch is placed externally over the bleb, with an anchoring moderate-depth bite passed through the peripheral cornea anterior to the bleb and another through the episcleral tissues posterior to the bleb (Fig. 21–8). These sutures can be left in place for several weeks to indent the bleb. Bleb leak closure has been achieved in 69% of patients with this procedure.[120, 143]

When all else fails, surgical revision of the bleb may be

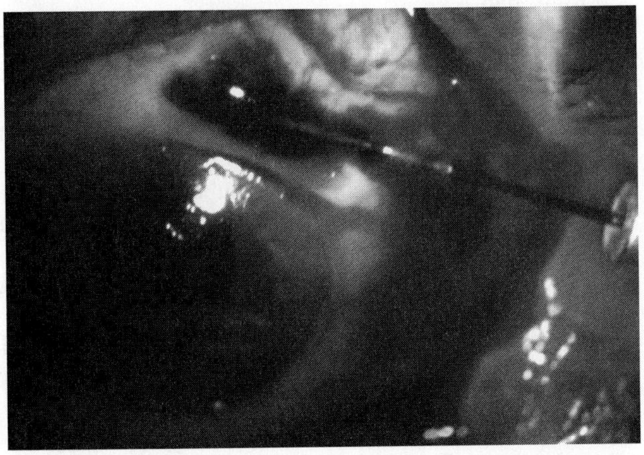

FIGURE 21–6. Injection of autologous blood into leaking bleb, and subsequent clotting.

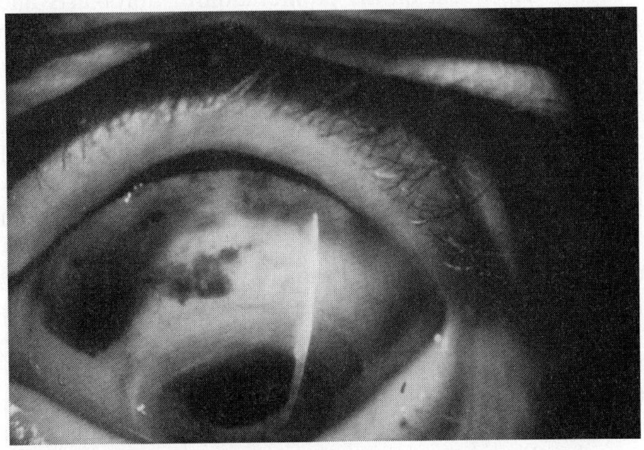

FIGURE 21–7. Subconjunctival injection of autologous blood, rather than direct injection into the leaking bleb.

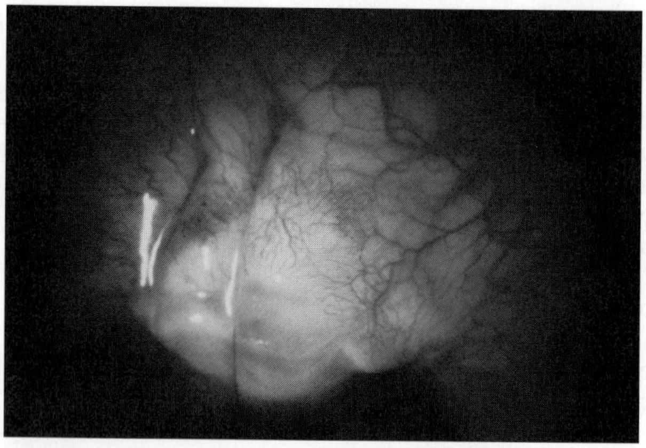

FIGURE 21–8. Compression suture of a bleb.

indicated. Several different techniques are described, but common to them all is the excision or covering of the thinned generally avascular bleb tissues with fresh conjunctival tissue from surrounding, often more posterior, areas.[126–128] The front edge of this fresh tissue is sutured anteriorly to lie well forward over the peripheral cornea (as has previously been described for the closure of a fornix-based conjunctival flap). It is frequently difficult to free up sufficient superior conjunctiva–Tenon's capsule tissue to fully cover the old bleb site, and a posterior relaxing incision is sometimes required in the upper fornix to sufficiently advance the tissues. Separating the conjunctiva from the underlying Tenon's capsule and pulling this layer alone forward to cover the bleb often allows the closure to be made without recourse to a relaxing incision. It is generally wise not to treat this fresh tissue with antimetabolites; late thinning of the new bleb conjunctiva can occur even without their use. Occasionally, the revised bleb may fail or may function poorly. If so, medical therapy may be reintroduced or a new trabeculectomy may be performed if medical therapy proves inadequate to control IOP.

Control of Inflammation and Scarring

Scarring of the filtering bleb is the most common cause of bleb failure in filtering surgery.[144] Postoperative inflammation and wound healing constitute a complex process that is highly dependent on the proliferation of fibroblasts and the laying down of collagen.[147] Therefore, measures to modulate the inflammatory response in order to limit postoperative fibrosis of tissues and increase the chance for long-term bleb function have been increasingly studied. First-line therapy against inflammation consists of topical corticosteroids. These agents are uniformly used postoperatively to decrease inflammation, and their efficacy has been proved in several clinical studies.[38, 145, 146] Corticosteroids are known to inhibit cell attachment and proliferation.[147, 148]

Persistent inflammation of tissues is evident when the conjunctiva and episcleral tissues remain injected. Untreated, this inflammation eventually leads to hypervascularity of the bleb, with a decrease in bleb height and area, loss of succulence of the tissues, and bleb failure. To control inflammation, we routinely give a subconjunctival injection of corticosteroid (Solu-Medrol) at the conclusion of surgery and have the patient use topical corticosteroids at least four times a day beginning on the first postoperative day. Higher-risk eyes, including those with a history of uveitis or neovascularization, frequently require a more intensive regimen. If excessive inflammation is evident, the frequency of topical corticosteroid applications may be increased.

If the bleb appearance does not improve with corticosteroid therapy, careful consideration should be given to the use of subconjunctival 5-FU. Multiple studies have reported that the adjunctive use of 5-FU increases the success rate of filtering surgery.[49–53, 56] The long-term complication rate, however, is higher with the use of antimetabolites than for trabeculectomy without 5-FU. In addition, we avoid using postoperative antimetabolites in patients who have corneal epithelial defects until the corneal epithelium is healed. In patients who have only superficial keratopathy, subconjunctival 5-FU may still be used, but the eye should be watched closely for the development of frank epithelial defects. Postoperative antimetabolites should be used with care in patients who have a history of intraoperative complications, such as conjunctival buttonholes and wound leaks.

Usually, 5 mg (0.1 mL of 50 mg/mL concentration) of 5-FU is given via subconjunctival injection with a 30-gauge needle on a tuberculin syringe. Care should be taken to inject the 5-FU a sufficient distance from the trabeculectomy site so as not to inject the antimetabolite directly into the anterior chamber. Historically, 5-FU has been injected 180 degrees from the trabeculectomy site in order to avoid the seepage of 5-FU into the anterior chamber. However, several studies have shown the localized nature of tissue effects from 5-FU, and we now routinely inject the antimetabolite relatively adjacent to the scleral flap.[51, 53] It is also important to try to avoid perforation of conjunctival and subconjunctival vessels with the needle in order to prevent bleeding into the bleb tissues, which could lead to increased inflammation. This goal can be most easily achieved by performing the injection under slit-lamp illumination with an assistant, as follows:

1. Topical anesthetic is instilled.
2. The conjunctiva is inspected under the slit-lamp in order to locate an appropriate area to penetrate the conjunctiva, usually an area devoid of large vessels and several millimeters away from the trabeculectomy flap.
3. A cotton-tipped applicator soaked with anesthetic is applied to the area for several seconds to further anesthetize the tissues.
4. A lid speculum may be utilized if the help of an assistant is not available.
5. The needle is passed into the subconjunctival space and tracked for several millimeters, with care taken to directly observe the tip of the needle so as not to perforate any vessels or create a buttonhole through the conjunctiva.
6. The 5-FU is slowly injected into the subconjunctival space while ballooning of the surrounding tissues is observed.
7. The needle is withdrawn, and a cotton-tipped applicator is immediately placed over the 30-gauge wound, effectively preventing the reflux of 5-FU back

through it. (A longer needle track also helps in preventing inadvertent exposure of the corneal surface to an antimetabolite.)

8. The applicator is held in place for several seconds, and the eye is flushed with several drops of topical antibiotic in order to dilute any seepage of 5-FU onto the corneal and conjunctival surface.
9. The wound should be checked under the slit-lamp to ensure a negative Seidel's test result.

Postoperative subconjunctival administration of 5-FU may be repeated several times on subsequent visits. We frequently repeat injections four or five times on subsequent visits, even in patients who have received intraoperative antimetabolites (5-FU or MMC).

The Low Bleb

Guarded filtration procedures are designed to limit excessive flow through the sclerotomy during the early postoperative period, and many surgeons deliberately tie their scleral flaps down fairly tightly during surgery. We recommend BSS infusion into the anterior chamber through the paracentesis tract at the end of surgery to demonstrate appropriate aqueous flow through the scleral flap and to separate the conjunctival–Tenon's capsule tissues from the underlying sclera. Tissues in the bleb area are inflamed after surgery, and fibroblasts are stimulated to produce collagen, leading to scar formation and bleb failure. If the bleb becomes flat or very low, the inflamed tissues are approximated, greatly enhancing scar development and adhesion.

As discussed earlier, Seidel's test should first be performed to confirm that there is no bleb leak. If there is a leak, the eye is usually soft. The anterior chamber may be deep or shallow. Treatment is directed at closure of the leak.

The most common cause of a low bleb, however, is inadequate aqueous flow through the scleral flap. The IOP is moderate to high, and the anterior chamber is full depth. Laser lysis of sutures or pulling of a releasable suture, if it has been placed at surgery, can be performed in the office. Either maneuver both rapidly elevates the bleb and decreases the IOP.[117, 149–154]

We examine the patient 1 day after suture release to confirm that an adequate, but not excessive, effect has been achieved. Further suture lysis or pulling of releasable sutures can be performed if little change in the bleb or IOP is seen. Close monitoring or even placement of an oversized BSCL to give mild external bleb compression may be required if hypotony, anterior chamber shallowing, or choroidal effusion is observed. If severe overdrainage occurs following suture release, with corneolenticular touch, then either anterior chamber re-formation with a viscoelastic agent or resuturing of the scleral flap in the operating room, possibly with drainage of choroidal effusions if present, may need to be performed.

LASER LYSIS

Laser lysis of sutures is undertaken to increase aqueous flow through the scleral flap. A Hoskins lens or the edge of a Zeiss four-mirror lens is used to blanch the tissues overlying the scleral flap suture. A 50-μ spot size is usually selected, with pulse time of 0.1 to 0.2 sec. A relatively low power setting, about 0.2 to 0.4 mW, is recommended initially; the power is then increased if required. Generally, the suture can be cut in one or two shots. Precise focusing of the laser spot is essential. Care must be taken if there is overlying hemorrhage, pigmentation, or vascularity of the conjunctiva–Tenon's capsule, because the laser energy may be taken up in these tissues and a buttonhole created.

RELEASABLE SUTURES

We prefer the use of releasable sutures because, even though they take a few minutes longer at surgery to place, time is saved postoperatively because there is no need to use the laser. Further, in patients in whom superior subconjunctival hemorrhage or thick tissues are present or who have difficulty keeping their eyes stationary, there is never any visualization difficulty that may prevent suture release at the appropriate time, as may be present in laser lysis. Many different releasable suture techniques are described in the literature[149, 152–154]; we describe only our preferred technique here:

1. A 10-0 nylon suture on a cutting needle is passed in standard fashion through the corner of the scleral flap, and exits through the adjacent sclera.
2. The short, trailing end of the suture is grasped with the suture-tying forceps, and a quadruple throw is made around the forceps.
3. A loop of the long end of the suture, which has the needle attached, is pulled through the quadruple throws to form a bow-like knot.
4. A small superficial scleral bite is taken opposite the end of the corner of the scleral flap to create a tangential direction of pull at the bowed knot (i.e., acts like a pulley).
5. The needle is then passed, partial-thickness, through the sclera at the limbus to emerge at the peripheral cornea. Great care is taken not to allow the needle to emerge prematurely, to avoid conjunctival perforation in the area of the bleb.
6. An additional partial-thickness corneal bite is passed to bury the suture in the superficial stroma of the cornea. This maneuver prevents "windshield wiper" effects on the corneal epithelium.

Only the small exit point between the two corneal bites is exposed on the corneal surface, and it generally epithelializes in a week or so, providing cover for the entire suture length.

Releasable sutures can be removed at any time postoperatively by elevation of the buried end of the suture at this previously exposed point and pulling of the loop, which releases the slipknot. If adequate IOP control has already been achieved, the suture end can be cut flush. If gentle traction was applied (insufficient to loosen the knot), the suture end will retract and will be immediately buried. Multiple releasable sutures can be placed, and the amount of initial flow through the scleral flap can be controlled during the surgery by tightening the knots or by placing extra sutures if the aqueous flow is excessive. If more flow is desired before surgical closure, the looped knots may be loosened somewhat. Thus, there is a great deal of flexibility for the surgeon in controlling the aqueous outflow, both at the time of surgery and subsequently in the early postoperative period, with the use of releasable sutures.

Later in the postoperative course, a low bleb in the presence of elevated IOP and normal depth anterior chamber results from excessive scarring and bleb failure. Some advocate needling of these blebs in an attempt to restore function.[155]

Large or Cystic Blebs and Dellen

LARGE BLEB WITH HYPOTONY

Frequently, a patient with a large intact bleb demonstrates hypotony that is not due to a bleb leak. Other factors that might contribute to hypotony and are unrelated to the bleb are (1) aqueous hyposecretion from intraocular inflammation, (2) ciliary body detachment, (3) cyclodialysis cleft, (4) undetected retinal detachment, and (5) severe anterior ocular ischemia.[117, 120] If none of these factors is identified, overfiltration or aqueous hyposecretion is most likely the cause of the hypotony, and treatment should be directed at decreasing aqueous outflow.

A large BSCL can be used to slightly increase pressure within the bleb and slow the flow of aqueous from the anterior chamber. We also decrease or discontinue topical steroids for the patient in whom hypotony appears within the early postoperative period, in order to hasten some scarring of the tissues and limit aqueous absorption. If the anterior chamber shallows and there is a possibility for corneolenticular touch, re-formation of the anterior chamber with a viscoelastic agent should be performed and then repeated when necessary.[156]

With time, most overfiltering blebs resolve without the need for surgical intervention. However, if hypotony remains prolonged or other complications, such as hypotony maculopathy and kissing choroidal effusions, develop, early surgical intervention is warranted.[75, 76, 157]

LARGE CYSTIC BLEB

Large, thin-walled, cystic blebs may occur after filtration surgery and are now more common because of the use of antimetabolites.[60, 117] The thinness of these blebs also predisposes to the sight-threatening complication of bleb-related endophthalmitis.[158] Therefore, affected patients must be educated and continually reminded about the signs and symptoms of bleb-related infections.

Some patients with large cystic blebs experience intolerable symptoms that necessitate intervention (Fig. 21–9). These symptoms include foreign body sensation, irritation, disturbances in blinking, monocular diplopia, and change in peripheral visual field.[140, 159]

Surgical excision of large, overhanging blebs is the definitive treatment for blebs in which function is to be maintained. Some blebs become large enough to overhang the cornea but do not dissect into the tissue planes. The redundant tissue can be freed from the underlying cornea with blunt dissection and excised parallel to the limbus. The cut edges of the conjunctiva are then sutured to each other. Usually, the area overhanging the cornea is nonfunctional, so the anterior chamber is not lost during the procedure, and no leak occurs at the cut bleb surface.[159]

Argon and Nd:YAG laser therapy, cryotherapy, and cauterization (heat or chemical) have been used to shrink large cystic blebs in symptomatic patients.[140, 159–161] These

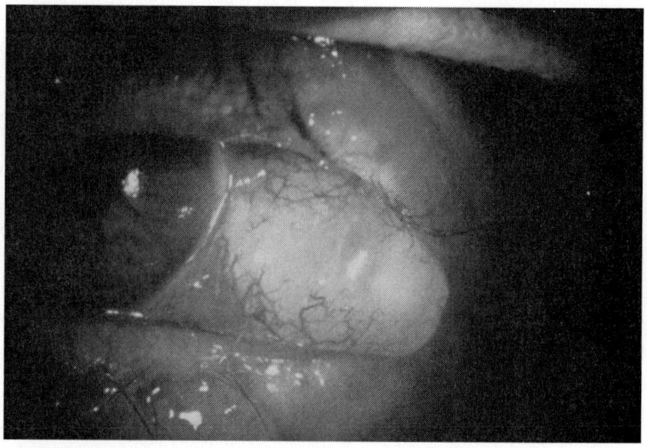

FIGURE 21–9. A large, cystic bleb.

procedures rely on the creation of collagen contraction and inflammation within the bleb tissues, with subsequent scarring and shrinkage of the bleb. Of course, given the intent of the intervention, complete loss of bleb function is an uncommon but possible complication of all of the described procedures.[140]

SUPERFICIAL PUNCTATE KERATOPATHY

Superficial punctate keratopathy and erosions are commonly found adjacent to blebs postoperatively. These areas usually resolve without complication and are secondary to poor tear coverage during blinking. The patient is sometimes symptomatic and complains of pain. Treatment consists of the frequent use of artificial tears and application of an ocular lubricant at night, if needed. Occasionally, temporary punctal occlusion may be required.

DELLEN

Dellen are saucer-shaped indentations with stromal thinning at the peripheral cornea. They occur in approximately 10% of eyes with trabeculectomy filtering blebs (Fig. 21–10).[140, 162] Dellen may be stained or may be covered by an intact epithelium, but there should be no corneal infiltrate, which distinguishes dellen from ulcers. Dellen are probably due to a localized disruption of the precorneal tear film caused by the adjacent bleb. The eyelid blink is unable to

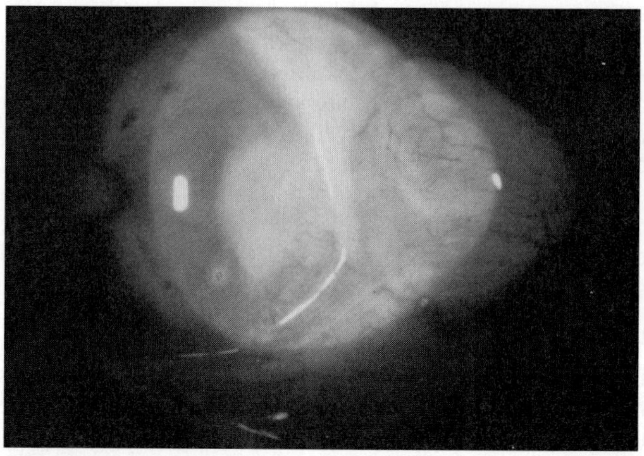

FIGURE 21–10. Dellen formed following the establishment of a filtering bleb.

spread the tear film in a normal fashion, and the resulting corneal dehydration causes stromal thinning. The problem is believed to be exacerbated by pooling of topical steroids within the depression, where they inhibit epithelial wound healing.[162]

A review of 97 trabeculectomies revealed nine cases in which dellen developed (9%).[162] Most (7 of 9) occurred within the first postoperative week. Therapy aimed at prompt hydration and re-expansion of the locally compacted stromal lamellae should result in rapid resolution of the dellen. In two of the nine cases in the study, deep corneal ulceration occurred; it resolved over several months, leaving a vascularized scar with localized stromal thinning. The recommended treatment is frequent use of artificial tears and application of an ocular lubricant at bedtime. If a deep erosion or persistent dellen occur, it may be necessary to discontinue or reduce postoperative steroids in order to promote epithelial wound healing.[162] Rarely, a temporary tarsorrhaphy may be required to cover the involved corneal area, or the bleb may be surgically revised in order to improve spreading of tear film over the surface.

Bleb Encapsulation

Encapsulated blebs, or Tenon's cysts, are not uncommon, occurring in approximately 13% of eyes in the early postoperative period after trabeculectomy.[163, 164] These blebs appear highly elevated, tense, and localized and are most commonly seen 2 to 5 weeks after surgery (Fig. 21–11). Adhesions between Tenon's capsule and the episcleral tissues create a fibrotic, avascular cystic capsule that becomes a barrier to aqueous outflow (Fig. 21–12). The overlying conjunctiva is usually freely mobile over the cyst, and there is absence of the intraepithelial microcystic changes, signifying loss of transconjunctival aqueous filtration.[117] Accompanying this change in bleb architecture is an elevation of IOP that usually necessitates re-introduction of antiglaucoma medications.

Conservative therapy with ocular hypotensive agents is typically used in this hypertensive phase, with a success rate of 70% to 90%.[165–167] Some surgeons advocate increased topical steroids and ocular massage, whereas others favor reducing or stopping topical steroid therapy. We typically start the patient on a β-blocker and add aqueous

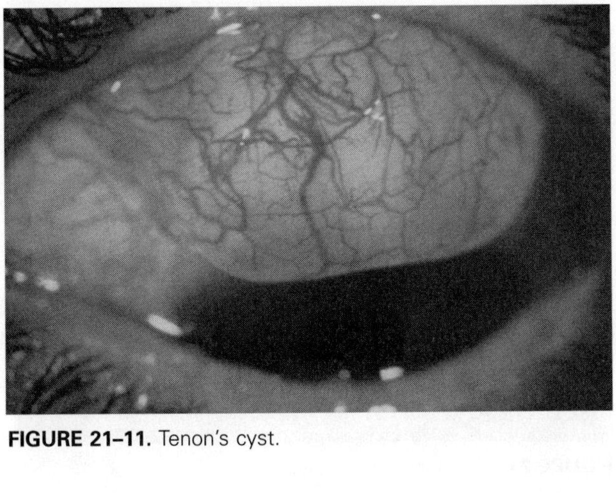

FIGURE 21–11. Tenon's cyst.

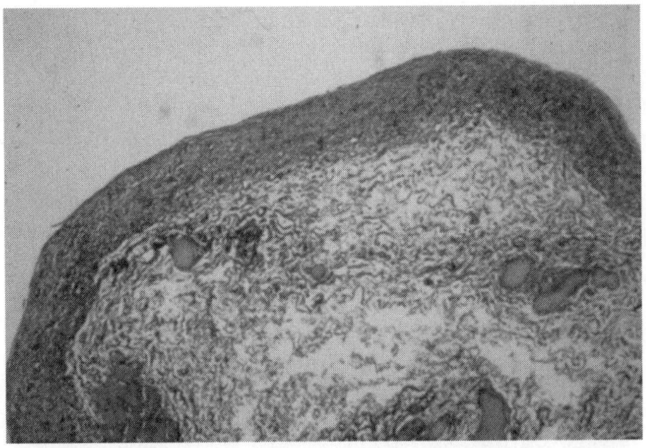

FIGURE 21–12. Histopathology of adhesions between a Tenon's cyst and episcleral tissues.

suppressants as needed to control the pressure. Ocular massage may also be prescribed, but gonioscopy should be performed first to ensure that the internal sclerostomy is not at risk of becoming blocked. If vitreous or iris is near the sclerostomy, it can be pushed into the sclerostomy by massage.[168] We usually recommend that the patient (1) perform ocular compression through the lower eyelid while looking up for 5 to 10 seconds, (2) relax for 5 seconds, and then (3) repeat the compression for 5 to 10 seconds; this sequence is performed 4 or more times per day. With time, most of the blebs remodel, adequate IOP control is achieved, and medications can be reduced as necessary. Generally, some long-term medical therapy is required to maintain appropriate IOP control.

For blebs that do not respond to conservative therapy or in eyes that cannot tolerate a short-term pressure elevation, some form of surgical therapy is required. Most recently, injection of the bleb cyst with 5-FU has been favored as the initial approach, with success rates ranging from 73% to 91%.[155, 163, 169–171] Complications of 5-FU therapy include decreased vision, conjunctival buttonholes and leaks, bleeding, infection, hypotony, choroidal detachment, and the corneal epithelial defects associated with 5-FU.[172]

The procedure is performed at the slit-lamp as follows:

1. Topical anesthetic is instilled.
2. A lid speculum is placed, and the patient is instructed to look down.
3. A 27-gauge needle attached to a tuberculin syringe and containing sterile BSS is used to enter the subconjunctival space 8 to 10 mm from the bleb cyst.
4. The needle is advanced carefully with intermittent instillation of BSS to inflate the surrounding tissues. This technique helps prevent inadvertent buttonholing of the conjunctiva but can make the needle tip more difficult to visualize.
5. As the cyst is encountered, the needle is used to perforate the wall of the cyst and then is moved from side to side, parallel to the sclera, to enlarge the perforation in the cyst wall (Fig. 21–13). If the wall is perforated, aqueous is seen to further elevate the surrounding tissues and bleb.
6. The needle is slowly withdrawn, and the wound is covered momentarily with a sterile cotton-tipped applicator.

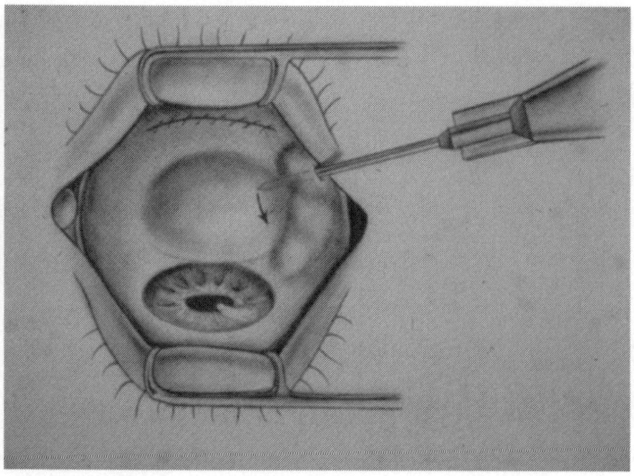

FIGURE 21–13. Enlargement of the perforation in the cyst wall.

7. Once Seidel's test has confirmed the wound no longer to be open, a subconjunctival injection of 5 mg (0.1 mL of 50 mg/mL) of 5-FU is given, through a new 30-gauge needle and syringe adjacent and superior to the bleb. This wound is also covered momentarily with a cotton-tipped applicator.
8. A broad-spectrum antibiotic solution is instilled into the eye to flush and dilute any refluxed antimetabolite, and Seidel's test is performed to confirm wound sealing.

Ocular hypotensive agents are discontinued, and topical dexamethasone is prescribed. The patient is evaluated the following day. Needling of the cyst and subconjunctival 5-FU can be repeated as the appearance, and relative function, of the bleb dictates. In some blebs, re-encapsulation with return of elevated IOP occurs despite the use of 5-FU.

An alternative surgical technique that requires returning the patient to the operating room is complete excision of Tenon's cyst.[159] The original surgical incision is opened, and the conjunctiva is bluntly dissected from the underlying cyst wall and reflected forward. Once the cyst is exposed, it is dissected free of the sclera and removed with the use of nontoothed forceps and Vannas scissors (Fig. 21–14). Aqueous should then freely flow from the visible trabeculectomy site. If not, the flap should be revised, or a new sclerostomy made. The conjunctiva and Tenon's layers are then closed again in a watertight fashion with a two-layer closure. Antimetabolites may be used if there is no risk of reflux into the anterior chamber.

Although most blebs with cysts respond to medical therapy, they usually function suboptimally and continue to require topical antiglaucoma treatment. Surgical intervention carries added risks, and cysts can recur in up to 30% of cases treated with needling with 5-FU and in 9% of cases treated with excision.[159, 171]

Bleb-Related Infections

Every patient who undergoes trabeculectomy should be cautioned preoperatively and postoperatively about the risk of bleb infections (blebitis) and bleb-related endophthalmitis. The use of adjunctive antimetabolites probably increases the risk of blebitis and bleb-related endophthalmitis because of the relative avascularity and thinness of the treated tissues.[132] This thinning may cause spontaneous bleb leaks, permitting direct inoculation of the bleb with organisms or transconjunctival spread of organisms. Blebitis and bleb-related endophthalmitis can occur months to years after the original procedure.[129–132, 135, 136] The patient should be educated about signs and symptoms of bleb infection and should be encouraged to seek immediate attention if any such symptoms arise. Accordingly, any patient with a history of filtering surgery, especially one in whom antimetabolites were used intraoperatively or postoperatively, should be examined immediately if he or she notices symptoms of decreased vision, eye pain, redness, or discharge.

BLEBITIS

Infection in filtering blebs generally begins as a blebitis. The bleb becomes white or opaque and is surrounded by an intense conjunctival inflammation (Fig. 21–15). Commonly, the conjunctiva is chemotic, and there is some purulent discharge. The patient may have only mild to moderate discomfort, usually associated with an accompanying anterior uveitis. Frequently the bleb is Seidel's test–positive and the eye hypotonus. Elevated pressure may occur as well, presumably in response to blockage of the sclerostomy by inflammatory debris. There can be varying

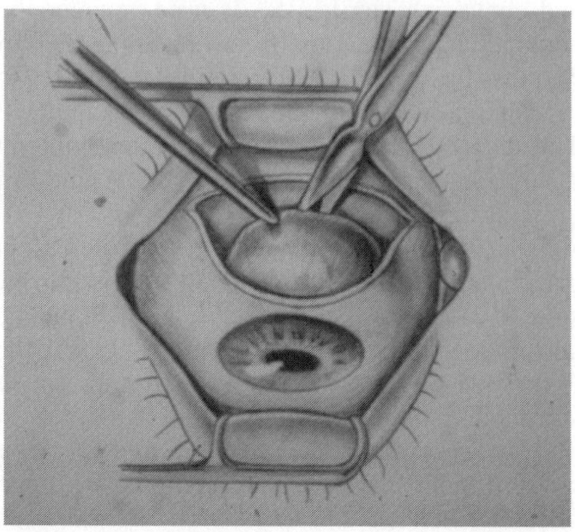

FIGURE 21–14. Complete excision of a Tenon's cyst.

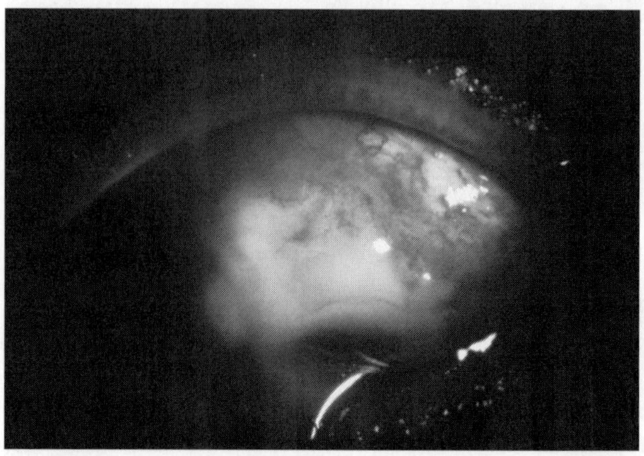

FIGURE 21–15. An infected filtering bleb.

amounts of anterior chamber inflammation, but no vitreous inflammation.[130, 133, 135, 136]

Typically, culture specimens are taken from the surface of the bleb and the fornices. We order a Gram's stain and culture on multiple media, including blood agar, chocolate agar, Sabouraud's medium, and thioglycolate broth. The common ocular flora are responsible for most bleb-related infections, especially *Haemophilus influenzae, Streptococcus* species, and *Staphylococcus* species. One study showed, in cases of early bleb-related endophthalmitis (before 6 weeks), that *Staphylococcus epidermidis* was the most likely organism.[136] In late infections, *Streptococcus* and gram-negative organisms made up the majority of offending organisms. Unfortunately, cultures frequently show no growth or do not correlate with the intraocular organisms found after vitreous tap.[136]

We routinely start the patient on a rigorous regimen of either fortified vancomycin (25 mg/mL) or fortified cefazolin (50 mg/mL) and fortified tobramycin (14 mg/mL), alternating the drops every half hour (initially around the clock), and a cycloplegic agent. Once the infection begins to show signs of improvement, usually within 48 hours, we add topical steroids to help control anterior chamber inflammation and, one hopes, prevent scarring of the bleb. Initial culture results are generally available after 48 hours, and antibiotic therapy may be adjusted accordingly. If the patient does not show relatively rapid improvement after using the fortified antibiotics for 24 to 48 hours, or if the symptoms become worse with increasing eye pain or the development of vitreous inflammation, the patient should be treated for endophthalmitis.

BLEB-RELATED ENDOPHTHALMITIS

If blebitis is not treated or is inadequately treated, it usually progresses to full-blown endophthalmitis. Any bleb-related infection that has associated vitreous inflammation should be aggressively treated through collection of a vitreous sample for culture and administration of intravitreal antibiotics.[173] Many surgeons also obtain an aqueous sample in hopes of increasing the yield of the culture. Subconjunctival antibiotics are given, and fortified topical antibiotics, given every 30 minutes around the clock, are begun. Some have also suggested adding oral ofloxacin.[117, 131, 173]

After the infection has resolved, bleb function is usually impaired, requiring additional antiglaucoma medication to obtain pressure control. In cases that are detected and treated early, during the initial blebitis, visual recovery is usually good. Once the infection enters the posterior segment, however, the visual prognosis is often poor.[173]

Perhaps more important is the prevention of infection in post-trabeculectomy eyes. Blepharitis and conjunctivitis should be treated aggressively, and patients should be discouraged from the use of contact lenses.[117] Long-term antibiotic prophylaxis has not been shown to have any effect on resident ocular flora, although in selected cases, such as recurrent or chronic uncomplicated bleb leaks, many surgeons use long-term topical antibiotics for prophylaxis.[117, 174]

Management After Drainage Implant Surgery

In some high-risk patients and in patients who are not candidates for trabeculectomy (e.g., because of extensive conjunctival scarring), long-term IOP control may be achieved with a glaucoma drainage tube. The postoperative management after tube implantation is similar to that after filtering surgery in regard to control of inflammation and prophylaxis against infection. We routinely have the patient use a topical corticosteroid and a broad-spectrum topical antibiotic four times a day. We discontinue the antibiotic after 10 to 14 days and then begin to taper the steroid dosage over a few weeks.

The management of postoperative IOP is quite different from that after trabeculectomy. With both valved and nonvalved implants, the IOP in the early postoperative period is not always predictable. There may be an elevation in IOP, or the eye may be hypotonus. In nonvalved implants, some form of occlusion of the drainage tube is used to prevent hypotony. Eventually, after a few weeks, sufficient scarring and capsule formation have occurred over the plate, and the iatrogenic occlusion is removed. The surgeon must be prepared to provide IOP control during this healing period before the tube can be made functional.

We routinely use nonvalved implants modified intraoperatively with a removable stent.[175, 176] Venting slits are made in the tube during the procedure to allow some control of IOP while the eye is given a chance to form a capsule around the plate.[176] The stent is typically removed 3 to 6 weeks postoperatively, after formation of a capsule around the implant plate that will limit the amount of aqueous outflow. Early postoperative management requires topical antiglaucoma medications to help control IOP until the stent can be removed.

CONJUNCTIVA

Careful surgical technique for wound closure is important in avoiding postoperative complications associated with dehiscence and subsequent tube exposure. The size and placement of the conjunctival incision depend on the type of implant, the amount of conjunctival scarring, and the preferences of the surgeon. If a limbus-based incision is used, it is recommended that the wound not be located over the area where the plate is to be fixed to the sclera. This location may help prevent erosion of the plate through the conjunctiva. Erosion of the tube itself is a more common problem. Originally, tubes were covered with a trabeculectomy-type scleral flap. This procedure, however, was associated with a significant number of tube erosions.[177–179] Now tubes are routinely covered with a piece of donor sclera or of rehydrated preserved pericardium or dura. Nevertheless, melting of the graft may occasionally occur. If the conjunctiva over the tube remains intact, close observation is sufficient. Tube exposure requires placement of a new graft and mobilization of conjunctiva to cover it.

With a well-functioning tube, a bleb is located over the drainage plate. When the tube is occluded, either intentionally by a stent or by an unanticipated problem such as iris, vitreous, or inflammatory material, no bleb is present, and the pressure is elevated.[175, 176]

A significant complication that usually occurs in the late postoperative period is encapsulation of the drainage-plate bleb. This is probably similar to encapsulation of filtering blebs and may involve compression of bleb tissues and closure of outflow channels through the capsule tissues.[178, 180] Often, a hypertensive phase is encountered 2 to 5 weeks postoperatively or after the stent is removed. This hypertensive phase is usually self-limited and resolves with the institution of aqueous suppressants and subsequent thinning of the capsule. Sometimes topical therapy alone is inadequate, and some surgeons have suggested needling of the bleb.[178, 181]

If IOP is uncontrolled after additional topical medications or needling of the bleb capsule, placement of a second tube may be indicated to increase the surface area for drainage. Alternatively, a ciliodestructive procedure to reduce aqueous production may be considered. No studies have reported on the effectiveness of IOP reduction through placement of an additional drainage plate. One study showed little difference in final IOP between the 500-mm^2 and 350-mm^2 Baerveldt implants at initial surgery.[182] However, another study showed that the double-plate Molteno implant provides better IOP control than the single-plate implant.[183]

CORNEA

Tube-cornea contact may cause corneal decompensation and may have to be surgically corrected by repositioning or removal of the offending tube.[184, 185] Rarely, the tube may migrate anteriorly toward the cornea. Tube migration is mainly a problem during growth of the globe in early childhood. A well-placed tube in an infant may migrate out of the anterior chamber entirely or may end up touching the cornea as the child ages. If this occurs, the tube may require repositioning.[177] We routinely perform endothelial cell counts in children with glaucoma drainage tubes to monitor for development of corneal compromise related to the drainage tube. Tube retraction can also occur in adults and may be related to cicatricial changes or poor fixation of the tube or plate during surgery.

SUMMARY

The conjunctival and Tenon's capsule tissues play a critical role in the success of glaucoma surgery and, with the cornea, in the long-term comfort and visual function of the patient with glaucoma. Careful examination of these tissues, and early intervention if problems are detected, can play an important role in the successful management of these challenging cases.

REFERENCES

1. Alward W: Medical management of glaucoma. N Engl J Med 1998;339:1298–1307.
2. Serle J: Pharmocological advances in the treatment of glaucoma. Drugs Aging 1994;5:156–170.
3. Van Buskirk E: Adverse reactions from timolol administration. Ophthalmology 1980;87:447–450.
4. Novack G: Ophthalmic beta-blockers since timolol. Surv Ophthalmol 1987;31:307–327.
5. Fellman R, Starita R: Ocular and systemic side effects of topical beta adrenergic antagonists. *In* Sherwood M, Spaeth G (eds): Complications of Glaucoma Therapy. Thorofare, NJ, Slack Inc, 1990, p 38.
6. Gross R, Pineyro A: Current use of ophthalmic beta blockers. J Glaucoma 1997;6:188–191.
7. Stewart WC, Laibovity R, Horwitz B, et al: A 90-day study of the efficacy and side effects of 0.25% and 0.5% apraclonidine vs. 0.5% timolol: Apraclonidine Primary Therapy Study Group. Arch Ophthalmol 1996;114:938–942.
8. Van Buskirk E: Corneal anesthesia after timolol malate therapy. Am J Ophthalmol 1979;88:739–743.
9. Weissman S, Asbell P: Effects of topical timolol (0.5%) and betaxolol (0.5%) on corneal sensitivity. Br J Ophthalmol 1990;74:409–412.
10. Kuppens E, de Gang CA, Stolwijk TR, et al: Effect of timolol with and without preservative on the basal tear turnover in glaucoma. Br J Ophthalmol 1995;79:339–342.
11. Marquardt R, Schubert T: Modification of tear film break-up time by beta blocker eyedrops without preservatives. Klin Monatsbl Augenheilkd 1991;199:75–78.
12. Broadway D, Grierson I, O'Brien C, et al: Adverse effects of topical antiglaucoma medication I. The conjunctival cell profile. Arch Ophthalmol 1994;112:1437–1445.
13. Baudoin C, Pisella PJ, Fillacier K, et al: Ocular surface inflammatory changes induced by topical antiglaucoma drugs. Ophthalmology 1999;106:556–562.
14. Burstein N: Corneal toxicity of topically applied drugs, vehicles and preservatives. Surv Ophthalmol 1980;25:15–30.
15. Starita R, Fechtner R, Fellman R: Ocular and systemic side effects of topical epinephrine and dipivefrin. *In* Sherwood M, Spaeth G (eds): Complications of Glaucoma Therapy. Thorofare, NJ, Slack Inc, 1990, p 23.
16. Wilson F: Adverse external ocular effects of topical ophthalmic medications. Surv Ophthalmol 1979;24:57–88.
17. Kass M, Mandell AI, Goldberg I, et al: Dipivefrin and epinephrine treatment of elevated intraocular pressure: A comparative study. Arch Ophthalmol 1979;97:1865–1866.
18. Wandel T, Spinak M: Toxicity of dipivalyl epinephrine. Ophthalmology 1981;88:259–260.
19. Liesegang, T: Bulbar conjunctival follicles associated with dipivefrin therapy. Ophthalmology 1985;92:228–233.
20. Stewart W, Ritch R, Shin D, et al: The efficacy of apraclonidine as an adjunct to timolol therapy. Arch Ophthalmol 1995;113:287–292.
21. Shin D, Glover BK, Cha SC, et al: Long-term brimonidine therapy in glaucoma patients with apraclonidine allergy. Am J Ophthalmol 1999;127:511–515.
22. Schuman J, Horwitz B, Choplin NT, et al: A 1-year study of brimonidine twice daily in glaucoma and ocular hypertension: A controlled, randomized, multicenter clinical trial: Chronic Brimonidine Study Group. Arch Ophthalmol 1997;115:847–852.
23. Katz L: Brimonidine tartrate 0.2% twice daily vs timolol 0.5% twice daily: 1 year results in glaucoma patients: Brimonidine Study Group. Am J Ophthalmol 1999;127:20–26.
24. Serle J: A comparison of the safety and efficacy of twice daily brimonidine 0.2% in subjects with elevated intraocular pressure: The Brimonidine Study Group III. Surv Ophthalmol 1996;41:S39–S47.
25. Fellman R, Starita R: Ocular and systemic side effects of topical cholinergic and anticholinergic drugs. *In* Sherwood M, Spaeth G (eds): Complications of Glaucoma Therapy. Thorofare, NJ, Slack Inc, 1990, p 11.
26. Butt Z, Kaufman D, McNab A, et al: Drug-induced ocular cicatricial pemphigoid: A series of clinico-pathological reports. Eye 1998; 12:285–290.
27. Strahlman E, Tipping R, Vagel R: A six week dose-response study of the ocular hypotensive effect of dorzolamide with a one year extension. Am J Ophthalmol 1996;122:183–194.
28. Strahlman E, Tipping R, Vagel R: A double-masked, randomized 1-year study comparing dorzolamide (Trusopt), timolol, and betaxolol. Arch Ophthalmol 1995;113:1009–1016.
29. Adamsons IA, Polis A, Ostrov CS, et al: Two-year safety of dorzolamide as monotherapy and with timolol and pilocarpine: Dorzolamide Safety Study Group. J Glaucoma 1998;7:395–401.
30. Pfeiffer N: Dorzolamide: Development and clinical application of a topical carbonic anhydrase inhibitor. Surv Ophthalmol 1997;42:137–151.
31. Nuzzi R, Finazzo C, Cerruti A: Adverse effects of topical antiglaucomatous medications on the conjunctiva and the lachrymal (Brit Engl) response. Int Ophthalmol 1998;22:31–35.
32. Mietz H, Niesen V, Krieglstein GK: The effect of preservatives and antiglaucoma medication on the histopathology of the conjunctiva. Graefes Arch Exp Ophthalmol 1994;232:561–565.

33. Silver L: Clinical efficacy and safety of brinzolamide (Azopt), a new topical carbonic anhydrase inhibitor for primary open-angle glaucoma and ocular hypertension: Brinzolamide Primary Therapy Study Group. Am J Ophthalmol 1998;126:400–408.
34. Konowal A, Morrison JC, Brown SV, et al: Irreversible corneal decompensation in patients treated with topical dorzolamide. Am J Ophthalmol 1999;127:403–406.
35. Camras CB, Wax MB, Ritch R, et al: Latanoprost treatment for glaucoma: Effect of treating for 1 year and of switching from timolol. United States Latanoprost Study Group. Am J Ophthalmol 1998;126:390–399.
36. Watson P: Latanoprost: Two years' experience of its use in the United Kingdom. Latanoprost Study Group. Ophthalmology 1998; 105:82–87.
37. Wand M, Gilbert CM, Liesegang TJ: Latanoprost and herpes simplex keratitis. Am J Ophthalmol 1999;127:602–604.
38. Duke-Elder S, Ashton N: Action of cortisone on tissue reactions of inflammation and repair with special reference to the eye. Br J Ophthalmol 1951;35:695–707.
39. Starita RJ, Fellman RL, Spaeth GL, et al: Short- and long-term effects of postoperative corticosteroids on trabeculectomy. Ophthalmology 1985;92:938–946.
40. Rubin B, Palestine A: Complications of corticosteroids and immunosuppresive drugs. Int Ophthalmol Clin 1989;29:137–211.
41. Ashton N, Cook C: Effect of cortisone on healing of corneal wounds. Br J Ophthalmol 1951;35:708–717.
42. Sherwood MB, Migdal CS, Hitchings RA, et al: Initial treatment of glaucoma: Surgery or medications. Surv Ophthalmol 1993;37:293–305.
43. Sibayan SA, Latina MA, Sherwood ME, et al: Apoptosis and morphologic changes in drug-treated trabecular meshwork cells in vitro. Exp Eye Res 1998;66:521–529.
44. Sherwood MB, Grienson I, Millar L, et al: Long-term morphologic effects of antiglaucoma drugs on the conjunctiva and Tenon's capsule in glaucomatous patients. Ophthalmology 1989;96:327–335.
45. Broadway D, Grierson I, O'Brien C, Hitchings R: Adverse effects of topical antiglaucoma medication. II. The outcome of filtration surgery. Arch Ophthalmol 1994;112:1446–1453.
46. Broadway DC, Grierson I, Sturmer J, et al: Reversal of topical medication effects on the conjunctiva. Arch Ophthalmol 1996; 114:262–267.
47. Blumenkranz MS, Claflin A, Hajek AS: Selection of therapeutic agents for intraocular proliferative disease: Cell culture evaluation. Arch Ophthalmol 1984;102:598–604.
48. Khaw PT, Ward S, Porter A, et al: The long-term effects of 5-fluorouracil and sodium butyrate on human tenon's fibroblasts. Invest Ophthalmol Vis Sci 1992;33:2043–2052.
49. The Fluorouracil Filtering Surgery Study Group: Fluorouracil filtering surgery study one-year follow-up. Am J Ophthalmol 1989; 108:625–635.
50. The Fluorouracil Filtering Surgery Study Group: Three Year Follow-Up of the Fluorouracil Filtering Surgery Study. Am J Ophthalmol 1993;115:82–92.
51. Weinreb R: Adjusting the dose of 5-fluorouracil after filtration surgery to minimize side effects. Ophthalmology 1987;94:564–570.
52. Ruderman JM, Welch DB, Smith MF, et al: A randomized study of 5-fluorouracil and filtration Surgery. Am J Ophthalmol 1987; 104:218–224.
53. Heuer DK, Parrish RK 2d, Gressel MG, et al: 5-fluorouracil and glaucoma filtering surgery. Ophthalmology 1986;93:1537–1546.
54. Singh KN, Egbert PR, Byrd S, et al: Trabeculectomy with intraoperative 5-fluorouracil vs mitomycin C. Am J Ophthalmol 1997; 123:48–53.
55. Prata Jr JA, Minckler DS, Baerveldt G, et al: Postoperative complications and short-term outcome after 5-fluorouracil or mitomycin C trabeculectomy. J Glaucoma 1995;4:25–31.
56. Smith MF, Sherwood M, Doyle JW, et al: Results of intraoperative 5-fluorouracil supplementation on trabeculectomy for open-angle glaucoma. Am J Ophthalmol 1992;114:737–741.
57. Liebmann JM, Ritch R, Marmor M, et al: Initial 5-fluorouracil trabeculectomy in uncomplicated glaucoma. Ophthalmology 1991; 98:1036–1041.
58. Katz J, Higginbotham EJ, Lichter PR, et al: Mitomycin C versus 5 fluorouracil in high-risk glaucoma filtering surgery. Ophthalmology 1995;102:1263–1269.
59. Rockwood EJ, Parrish RK 2d, Hever DK, et al: Glaucoma filtering surgery with 5-fluorouracil. Ophthalmology 1987;94:1071–1078.
60. Costa VP, Moster MR, Wilson RP, et al: Effects of topical mitomycin C on primary trabeculectomies and combined procedures. Br J Ophthalmol 1993;77:693–697.
61. Mizra G, Karakucek S, Dogan H, et al: Filtering surgery with mitomycin-C in uncomplicated (primary open angle) glaucoma. Acta Ophthalmol 1994;72:155.
62. Kitazawa Y, Kawase K, Matsushita H, et al: Trabeculectomy with mitomycin: A comparative study with fluorouracil. Arch Ophthalmol 1991;109:1693–1698.
63. Skuta GL, Beeson CC, Higginbotham EJ, et al: Intraoperative mitomycin versus postoperative 5-fluorouracil in high-risk glaucoma filtering surgery. Ophthalmology 1992;99:438–444.
64. El Sayyad F, El-Rashood A, Helal M, et al: Fornix-based versus limbal-based conjunctival flaps in initial trabeculectomy with postoperative 5-fluorouracil: Four year follow-up findings. J Glaucoma 1999;8:124–128.
65. Jampel H: Effect of brief exposure to mitomycin C on viability and proliferation of cultured human Tenon's capsule fibroblasts. Ophthalmology 1992;99:1471–1476.
66. Mermoud A, Salmon JF, Murray AD: Trabeculectomy with mitomycin C for refractory glaucoma in blacks. Am J Ophthalmol 1993;116:72–78.
67. Palmer SS: Mitomycin as adjunct chemotherapy with trabeculectomy. Ophthalmology 1991;98:317–321.
68. Prata JA Jr, Neves RA, Minckler DS, et al: Trabeculectomy with mitomycin C in glaucoma associated with uveitis. Ophthalmic Surg 1994,25:616–620.
69. Susanna R, Oltragge E, Carani J, et al: Mitomycin as adjunct chemotherapy with trabeculectomy in congenital and developmental glaucoma. J Glaucoma 1995;4:151.
70. Yamamoto T, Ichien M, Suemori-Matsushita H, et al: Trabeculectomy with mitomycin C for normal-tension glaucoma. J Glaucoma 1995;4:158.
71. Kupin TH, Juzych MS, Shin DH, et al: Adjunctive mitomycin C in primary trabeculectomy in phakic eyes. Am J Ophthalmol 1995; 119:30–39.
72. Lamping K, Belkin J: 5-Fluorouracil and mitomycin C in pseudophakic patients. Ophthalmology 1995;102:70–75.
73. Nuyts RM, Felten PC, Pels E, et al: Histopathologic effects of mitomycin C after trabeculectomy in human glaucomatous eyes with persistent hypotony. Am J Ophthalmol 1994;118:225–237.
74. Mietz H, Addicks K, Diestehorst M, et al: Extraocular application of mitomycin C in a rabbit model: Cytotoxic effects on the ciliary body epithelium. Ophthalmic Surg 1994;25:240–244.
75. Shields M, Addicks K, Diestelhorst M, et al: Clinical and histopathologic observations concerning hypotony after trabeculectomy with adjunctive mitomycin C. Am J Ophthalmol 1993;16:673.
76. Costa VP, Wilson RP, Moster MR, et al: Hypotony maculopathy following the use of topical mitomycin C in glaucoma filtration surgery. Ophthalmic Surg 1993;24:389–394.
77. Hietz H, Brunner R, Addicks K, et al: Histopathology of an avascular filtering bleb after trabeculectomy with mitomycin C. J Glaucoma 1993;2:266.
78. Morrow GL, Stein RM, Heathcote JG, et al: Ocular toxicity of mitomycin C and 5-fluorouracil in the rabbit. Can J Ophthalmol 1994;29:268–273.
79. McDermott ML, Wang J, Shin DH: Mitomycin and the human corneal endothelium. Arch Ophthalmol 1994;112:533–537.
80. Smith S, D'Amore PA, Dreyer EB: Comparative toxicity of mitomycin C and 5-fluorouracil in vitro. Am J Ophthalmol 1994;118:332–337.
81. Derick RJ, Pasquale L, Guigley HA, et al: Potential toxicity of mitomycin C. Arch Ophthalmol 1991;109:1635.
82. Broadway DC, Grierson I, Hitchings RA: Local effects of previous conjunctival incisional surgery and the subsequent outcome of filtration surgery. Am J Ophthalmol 1998;125:805–818.
83. Sturmer J, Broadway D, Hitchings R, et al: Young patient trabeculectomy: Assessment of risk factors for failure. Ophthalmology 1993;100:928–939.
84. The Fluorouracil Filtering Surgery Study Group: Five year follow-up of the fluorouracil filtering surgery study. Am J Ophthalmol 1996;121:349–366.
85. Honjo M, Tanihara H, Inatani M, et al: Mitomycin C trabeculectomy

in eyes with cicatricial conjunctiva. Am J Ophthalmol 1998; 126:823–824.
86. Watts P, McAllister J: Is the single use of 5-fluorouracil in filtering surgery for high-risk cases enough? Eye 1998;12:374–378.
87. Mattox C: Glaucoma filtration surgery and antimetabolites. Ophthalmic Surg Lasers 1995;26:473–480.
88. Patitsas C, Rockwood EJ, Meisler DM, et al: Glaucoma filtration surgery with postoperative 5-FU in patients with intraocular inflammatory disease. Ophthalmology 1992;99:594–599.
89. Muenzler WS, Harms WK: Visual prognosis in aphakic bullous keratopathy treated by penetrating keratoplasty: A retrospective study of 73 cases. Ophthalmic Surg 1981;12:210–212.
90. Thoft RA, Gordon JM, Folman CH: Glaucoma following keratoplasty. Trans Am Acad Ophthalmol Otolaryngol 1974;78:352–364.
91. Heuer D, Gressel MG, Parrish RK 2nd, et al: Trabeculectomy in aphakic eyes. Ophthalmology 1984;91:1045–1051.
92. Sherwood MB, Smith MF, Driebe WT, et al: Drainage tube implants in the treatment of glaucoma following penetrating keratoplasty. Ophthalmic Surg 1993;24:185–189.
93. Ing JJ, Ing HH, Nelson LR, et al: Ten-year postoperative results of penetrating keratoplasty. Ophthalmology 1998;105:1855–1865.
94. Karesh JW, Nirankari VS: Factors associated with glaucoma after penetrating keratoplasty. Am J Ophthalmol 1983;96:160–164.
95. Gross RL, Feldman RM, Spaeth GL, et al: Surgical therapy of chronic glaucoma in aphakia and pseudophakia. Ophthalmology 1988;95:1195–2001.
96. Sihota R, Sharma N, Panda A, et al: Post-penetrating keratoplasty glaucoma: Risk factors, management and visual outcome. Aust N Z J Ophthalmol 1998;26:305–309.
97. Foulks GN: Glaucoma associated with penetrating keratoplasty. Ophthalmology 1987;94:871–874.
98. Irvine AR, Kaufmann HE: Intraocular pressure following penetrating keratoplasty. Am J Ophthalmol 1969;68:835–844.
99. Gilvarry AME, Kirkness CM, Steele AD, et al: The management of postkeratoplasty glaucoma by trabeculectomy. Eye 1989;3:713–718.
100. Sharma A, Kumar S, Ram J, et al: Trabeculectomy with mitomycin-C for postkeratoplasty glaucoma: A preliminary study. Ophthalmic Surg Lasers 1997;28:891–895.
101. WuDunn D, Alfonso E, Oalmberg PF: Combined penetrating keratoplasty and trabeculectomy with mitomycin C. Ophthalmology 1999;106:396–400.
102. Ayyala R, Pieroth L, Vinals AF, et al: Comparison of mitomycin C trabeculectomy, glaucoma drainage device implantation, and laser neodymium: YAG cyclophotocoagulation in the management of intractable glaucoma after penetrating keratoplasty. Ophthalmology 1998;105:1550–1556.
103. Munoz F, Rebolleda G: Cyclophotocoagulation for glaucoma after penetrating keratoplasty. Ophthalmology 1999;106:644–645.
104. Threlkeld AB, Shields, MB: Non-contact transscleral Nd:YAG cyclophotocoagulation for glaucoma after penetration keratoplasty. Am J Ophthalmol 1995;120:569–576.
105. Levy NS, Bonney RC: Transcleral YAG cyclocoagulation of the ciliary body for persistently high intraocular pressure following penetrating keratoplasty. Cornea 1989;8:178–181.
106. Wheatcroft S, Singh A, Casey T, et al: Treatment of glaucoma following PKP with transscleral YAG cyclophotocoagulation. Int Ophthalmol Vis Sci 1992;16:397–400.
107. Hardten D, Brown J, Holland E, et al: Results of neodymium:YAG laser transscleral cyclophotocoagulation for postkeratoplasty glaucoma. J Glaucoma 1993;2:241–245.
108. Noureddin BN, Wilson-Holt N, Lavin M, et al: Advanced uncontrolled glaucoma: Nd:YAG cyclophotocoagulation or tube surgery. Ophthalmology 1992;99:430–436.
109. McDonnell PJ, Robin JB, Schanglin DJ, et al: Molteno implant for control of glaucoma in eyes after penetrating keratoplasty. Ophthalmology 1988;95:364–369.
110. Beebe WE, Starita RJ, Fellman RL, et al: The use of Molteno implant and anterior chamber tube shunt to encircling band for the treatment of glaucoma in keratoplasty patients. Ophthalmology 1990;97:1414–1422.
111. Kirkness CM, Ling Y, Rice NS: The use of silicone drainage tubing to control post-keratoplasty glaucoma. Eye 1988;2:583–590.
112. Hodkin MJ, Goldblatt WS, Burgoyne CF, et al: Early clinical experience with the Baerveldt implant in complicated glaucomas. Am J Ophthalmol 1995;120:32–40.
113. Coleman AL, Mondino BJ, Wilson MR, et al: Clinical experience with the Ahmed glaucoma valve implant in eyes with prior or concurrent penetrating keratoplasties. Am J Ophthalmol 1997; 123:54–61.
114. Kirkness CM, Steele AD, Ficker LA, et al: Coexistent corneal disease and glaucoma managed by either drainage surgery and subsequent keratoplasty or combined drainage surgery and penetrating keratoplasty. Br J Ophthalmol 1992;76:146–152.
115. Sherwood MB, Smith MF: Prevention of early hypotony associated with Molteno implants by a new occluding stent technique. Ophthalmology 1993;100:85–90.
116. Haynes WL, Alward WL: Control of intraocular pressure after trabeculectomy. Surv Ophthalmol 1999;43:345–355.
117. Azura-Blanco A, Katz L: Dysfunctional filtering blebs. Surv Ophthalmol 1998;42:93–121.
118. Sugar H: Current successfully filtering blebs. Ann Ophthalmol 1971;3:485–487.
119. Sugar H: The course of change in size of successful filtering cicatricies. Am J Ophthalmol 1960;49:795–800.
120. Liebmann JM, Sopol J, Pitch R: Management of chronic hypotony after glaucoma filtration surgery. J Glaucoma 1996;5:210–220.
121. Smith M, Doyle J: Use of oversized bandage soft contact lenses in the management of early hypotony following filtration surgery. Ophthalmic Surg Lasers 1996;27:417–421.
122. Spaeth G: Glaucoma surgery. *In* Spaeth G (ed): Ophthalmic Surgery: Principles and Practice. WB Saunders, 1990, p 272.
123. Smith M, Magauran R, Betchkal J, et al: Treatment of postfiltration bleb leak by bleb injection of autologous blood. Ophthalmology 1995;102:868–871.
124. Leen MM, Master MR, Katz LJ, et al: Management of overfiltering and leaking blebs with autologous blood injection. Arch Ophthalmol 1995;113:1050–1055.
125. Wise J: Treatment of chronic postfiltration hypotony by intrableb injection of autologous blood. Arch Ophthalmol 1993;111:827–830.
126. Spaeth G: Glaucoma surgery. *In* Spaeth G (ed): Ophthalmic Surgery: Principles and Practice. WB Saunders, 1990, p 238.
127. O'Connor DJ, Tressler CS, Caprioli J: A surgical method to repair leaking filtering blebs. Ophthalmic Surg 1992;23:336–338.
128. Wilson R, Neumann R: Free conjunctival patch for repair of persistent late bleb leak. Am J Ophthalmol 1994;117:569–574.
129. Higginbotham E, Stevens R, Musch D, et al: Bleb-related endophthalmitis after trabeculectomy with mitomycin C. Ophthalmology 1996;103:650–656.
130. Mochizuki K, Jikihara S, Ando Y, et al: Incidence of delayed onset infection after trabeculectomy with adjunctive mitomycin C or 5-fluorouracil treatment. Br J Ophthalmol 1997;81:877–883.
131. Phillips WB 2d, Wong TP, Beraren RL, et al: Late onset endophthalmitis associated with filtering blebs. Ophthalmic Surg 1994;25:88–91.
132. Greenfield DS, Suner IJ, Miller MP, et al: Endophthalmitis after filtering surgery with mitomycin. Arch Ophthalmol 1996;114:943–949.
133. Aaberg TM Jr, Flynn HW Jr, Schiffman J, et al: Nosocomial acute-onset postoperative endophthalmitis survey: A 10 year review of incidence and outcome. Ophthalmology 1998;105:1004–1010.
134. Waheed S, Ritterband DC, Greenfield DS, et al: Bleb-related ocular infection in children after trabeculectomy with mitomycin C. Ophthalmology 1997;104:2117–2120.
135. Akova YA, Bulut S, Dabil H, et al: Late bleb-related endophthalmitis after trabeculectomy with mitomycin C. Ophthalmic Surg Lasers 1999;30:146–151.
136. Ciulla TA, Beck AD, Tapping TM, et al: Blebitis, early endophthalmitis, and late endophthalmitis after glaucoma-filtering surgery. Ophthalmology 1997;104:986–995.
137. Caronia RM, Liebmann JM, Friedman R, et al: Trabeculectomy at the inferior limbus. Arch Ophthalmol 1996;114:387–391.
138. Asrani S, Wilensky JT: Management of bleb leaks after glaucoma filtering surgery: Use of autologous fibrin tissue glue as an alternative. Ophthalmology 1996;103:294–298.
139. Zalta AH, Weder RH: Closure of leaking filtering blebs with cyano-acrylic tissue adhesive. Br J Ophthalmol 1991;75:171–173.
140. Geyer O: Management of large, leaking, and inadvertent filtering blebs with the neodymium:YAG laser. Ophthalmology 1998; 105:983–987.
141. Baum M, Weiss HS: Argon laser closure of conjunctival bleb leak. Arch Ophthalmol 1993;111:438.

142. Cleasby GW, Fung WE, Webster RG Jr: Cryosurgical closure of filtering blebs. Arch Ophthalmol 1972;87:319–323.
143. Palmberg P, Zacchei AC: Compression sutures: A new treatment for leaking or painful filtering blebs. Invest Ophthalmol Vis Sci 1996;37:S444.
144. Maumenee A: External filtering operations for glaucoma: The mechanism of function and failure. Trans Am Ophthalmol Soc 1960; 58:319.
145. Roth SM, Spaeth GL, Starita RJ, et al: The effects of postoperative corticosteroids on trabeculectomy and the clinical course of glaucoma: Five year follow-up study. Ophthalmic Surg 1991;22:224–729.
146. Araujo SV, Spaeth GL, Roth SM, et al: A ten year follow-up on a prospective, randomized trial of postoperative corticosteroids after trabeculectomy. Ophthalmology 1995;102:1753–1759.
147. Schultz G, Khaw PT, Olford K, et al: Growth factors and ocular wound Healing. Eye 1994;8:184–187.
148. Nguyen K, Lee D: Effect of steroids and nonsteroidal antiinflamatory agents on human ocular fibroblast. Inv Ophthalmol Vis Sci 1992;33:2693–2701.
149. Shin D: Removable suture closure of the lamellar scleral flap in trabeculectomy. Am J Ophthalmol 1987;19:51–53.
150. Savage JA, Condon GP, Jytle RA, et al: Laser suture lysis after trabeculectomy. Ophthalmology 1988;95:1631–1638.
151. Melamed S, Ashbenaye I, Glovinski J, et al: Tight scleral flap trabeculectomy with postoperative laser suture lysis. Am J Ophthalmol 1990;109:303–309.
152. Johnstone MA, Wellington DP, Ziel CJ: A releasable scleral-flap tamponade suture for guarded filtration surgery. Arch Ophthalmol 1993;111:398–403.
153. Kolker AE, Kass MA, Rait JL: Trabeculectomy with releasable sutures. Arch Ophthalmol 1994;112:62–66.
154. Cohen J, Cohen JS, Osher RH, et al: Releasable scleral flap suture. Ophthalmol Clin North Am 1988;1:187–197.
155. Greenfield DS, Miller MP, Suner IJ, et al: Needle elevation of the scleral flap for failing filtration blebs after trabeculectomy with mitomycin C. Am J Ophthalmol 1996;122:195–204.
156. Stewart WC, Shields MB: Management of anterior chamber depth after trabeculectomy. Am J Ophthalmol 1988;106:41–44.
157. Suner IJ, Greenfield DS, Miller MP, et al: Hypotony maculopathy after filtering surgery with mitomycin C: Incidence and treatment. Ophthalmology 1997;104:207–214.
158. Hattenhauer JM, Lipsich MP: Late endophthalmitis after filtering surgery. Am J Ophthalmol 1971;72:1097–1101.
159. Sherwood M: Complications and management of large cystic blebs. *In* Sherwood M, Spaeth G (eds): Complications of Glaucoma Therapy. Thorofare NJ, Slack Inc, 1990, p 283.
160. Scheie HG, Guehl JJ 3d: Surgical management of overhanging blebs after filtering procedures. Arch Ophthalmol 1979;97:325–326.
161. Fitzgerald J, et al: Surgery of the filtering bleb. Arch Ophthalmol 1962;68:453–467.
162. Soong HK, Quigley HA: Dellen associated with filtering blebs. Arch Ophthalmol 1983;101:385–387.
163. Azuara-Blanco A, Bond JB, Wilson RP, et al: Encapsulated filtering blebs after trabeculectomy with mitomycin-C. Ophthalmic Surg Lasers 1997;28:805–809.
164. Sherwood M: Tenon's cysts (encapsulated filtering blebs). *In* Sherwood M, Spaeth G (eds): Complications of Glaucoma Therapy. Thorofare, NJ, Slack Inc, 1990, p 296.
165. Shingleton BJ, Richter CU, Bellows AR, et al: Management of encapsulated filtration blebs. Ophthalmology 1990;97:63–68.
166. Sherwood MB, Spaeth GL, Simmons ST, et al: Cysts of Tenon's capsule following filtration surgery: Medical management. Arch Ophthalmol 1987;105:1517–1521.
167. Scott DR, Quigley HA: Medical management of a high bleb phase after trabeculectomies. Ophthalmology 1988;95:1169–1173.
168. Wieland M, Spaeth G: Use of digital compression following glaucoma surgery. Ophthalmic Surg 1988;19:350–352.
169. Pederson JE, Smith SG: Surgical management of encapsulated filtering blebs. Ophthalmology 1985;92:955–958.
170. Allen LE, Manuchehri K, Coridan PG: The treatment of encapsulated trabeculectomy blebs in an out-patient setting using a needle technique and subconjunctival 5-fluorouracil injection. Eye 1998; 12:119–123.
171. Ewing R, Stamper RL: Needle revisions with and without 5-fluorouracil for the treatment of failed filtering blebs. Am J Ophthalmol 1990;110:254–259.
172. Howe LJ, Bloom P: Delayed suprachoroidal haemorrhage following trabeculectomy bleb needling. Br J Ophthalmol 1999;83:757.
173. Verbaken H: Treatment of postoperative endophthalmitis. Ophthalmologica 1995;209:165–171.
174. Wand M, Quintiliani R, Robinson A, et al: Antibiotic prophylaxis in eyes with filtration blebs: Survey of glaucoma specialists, microbiological study, and recommendations. J Glaucoma 1995;4:103–109.
175. Egbert PR, Lieberman MF: Internal suture occlusion of the Molteno glaucoma implant for the prevention of postoperative hyopotony. Ophthalmic Surg 1989;20:53–56.
176. Sherwood MB, Smith MF: Prevention of early hypotony associated with Molteno implants by a new occluding stent technique. Ophthalmology 1993;100:85–90.
177. Molteno AC, Ancker E, Van Biljon G: Surgical technique for advanced juvenile glaucoma. Arch Ophthalmol 1984;102:51–57.
178. Sherwood MB, Joseph NH, Hitchings RA: Surgery for refractory glaucoma: Results and complications with a modified Schocket technique. Arch Ophthalmol 1987;105:562–569.
179. Traverso C, et al: The Molteno implant for the treatment of refractory glaucomas. Invest Ophthalmol Vis Sci 1987;28:271.
180. Freedman J, Rubin B: Molteno implants as a treatment for refractory glaucoma in black patients. Arch Ophthalmol 1991;109:1417–1420.
181. Chen PP, Palmberg PF: Needling revision of glaucoma drainage device filtering blebs. Ophthalmology 1997;104:1004–1010.
182. Lloyd MA, Baerveldt G, Fellenbaum PS, et al: Intermediate-term results of a randomized clinical trial of the 350- versus the 500-mm^2 Baerveldt implant. Ophthalmology 1994;101:1456–1463.
183. Heuer DK, Lloyd MA, Abrams DA, et al: Which is better? One or two? A randomized clinical trial of single-plate versus double-plate Molteno implantation for glaucomas in aphakia and pseudophakia. Ophthalmology 1992;99:1512–1519.
184. Zalloum JN, Ahuja RM, Shin D, et al: Assessment of corneal decompensation in eyes having undergone Molteno shunt procedures compared to eyes having undergone trabeculectomy. CLAO J 1999;25:57–60.
185. Lotufo D: Postoperative complications and visual loss following Molteno implantation. Ophthalmic Surg 1991;22:650–656.

CHAPTER 22

Anterior and Posterior Chambers, Iris and Pupil, and Lens

SILVIA ORENGO-NANIA

In the assessment of glaucoma therapy, one of the most exciting aspects of the examination is the anterior chamber. Nothing is so worrisome as the flat anterior chamber. This chapter, by Silvia Orengo-Nania, takes the fear out of seeing the patient who has undergone a filtration procedure. Once you identify the key factors—intraocular pressure, chamber depth, and bleb height—you can easily decide on the proper course of action. On the basis of your findings, excessive or inadequate resistance to outflow, reduced aqueous production, hypotony, choroidal effusions, and aqueous misdirection can all be successfully diagnosed and then treated. Other treatment regimens needed in this area are the medical and surgical treatment of angle-closure glaucoma. The author addresses the indications, technique, and complications of peripheral iridotomy. Next, she discusses how the presence of blood, inflammatory cells and debris, vitreous, gas, and silicone oil in the anterior segment can modify glaucoma treatment. This information enables the physician to provide postoperative care to all patients with glaucoma, particularly those who have undergone filtration surgery, with much less anxiety.

The *anterior chamber* is the space formed by the cornea anteriorly, the iris and lens posteriorly, and the trabecular meshwork in its angular junction (Fig. 22–1). Its depth is approximately 2 mm centrally but can vary. It is filled with aqueous humor produced by the ciliary body at a rate of 2 μL/min for a total volume of approximately 200 μL.[1] The *posterior chamber* is the space bordered by the iris diaphragm anteriorly and the zonules posteriorly; it contains the processes of the ciliary body muscle. In this relatively small space, the ciliary epithelium secretes aqueous humor, which then flows through the zonules between the iris and lens, then through the pupil into the anterior chamber. The aqueous humor exits primarily through the trabecular meshwork to rejoin the systemic circulation via the episcleral veins (Fig. 22–2).

A record of anterior chamber content, depth, and shape is critical to the diagnosis and management of glaucoma. Although physicians tend to focus on the anterior chamber in postoperative patients, careful documentation of its properties is also helpful in monitoring patients receiving medical therapy for glaucoma. This chapter begins with a discussion of the effects of anterior segment surgery on the anterior chamber and proceeds to discuss the effects of medicines. The chapter concludes with a discussion of potential problems originating in the posterior chamber.

Anterior Chamber

Glaucoma filtering surgery is challenging, partly because of the technique itself but largely because of the follow-up

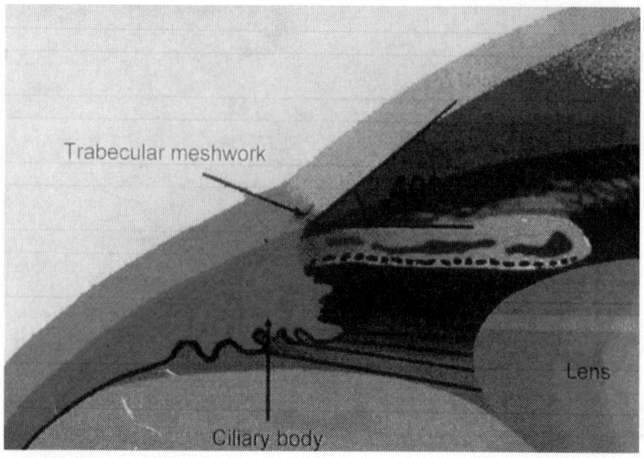

FIGURE 22–1. Schematic of anterior chamber anatomy.

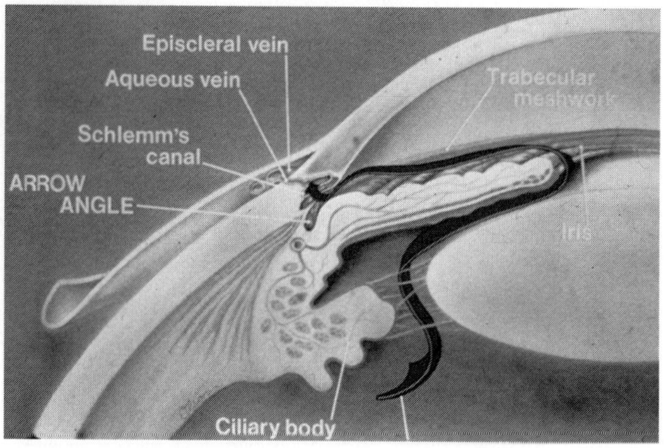

FIGURE 22–2. Schematic showing the path of the aqueous humor through the anterior chamber.

care.[2] A surgeon can perform apparently identical operations on different patients, but the results can be quite different and can vary according to the age and health of the patient or treatment history. There is a variety of potential outcomes of glaucoma filtering surgery (Table 22–1); for each outcome, three important characteristics must be evaluated: anterior chamber depth, intraocular pressure (IOP), and bleb height. The clinical appearance of each possibility, the etiology of each diagnosis, and possible ways to prevent adverse outcomes are detailed. Additionally, specific treatment individualized to the characteristics of the postoperative state of the eye is discussed.

CAUSES OF A POSTOPERATIVELY SHALLOW CHAMBER WITH LOW IOP

A shallow anterior chamber after glaucoma filtering surgery can be either temporary and benign or chronic and disastrous. The goal is to prevent a benign shallow anterior chamber from becoming chronic and visually debilitating. The first step is to clinically assess the appearance of the anterior chamber. Because evaluation can be somewhat subjective, the following grades of anterior chamber depth are helpful in follow-up and treatment decisions (Fig. 22–3)[3]:

- *Grade I*: There is contact between the peripheral iris (up to but not including the iris collarette) and the corneal endothelium.
- *Grade II:* The iris touches the posterior surface of the cornea, including the periphery and pupillary collarette, but there is space between the lens (crystalline or intraocular), iris crypts and iridotomy, if present, and the corneal endothelium.
- *Grade III:* The entire surface of the iris and part or

TABLE 22–1. ETIOLOGY AND CHARACTERISTICS OF THE ANTERIOR CHAMBER FINDINGS AFTER SURGERY FOR GLAUCOMA

Findings	Anterior Chamber	Intraoccular Pressure	Bleb	Postoperative Time Course
Normal or desirable result	Normal	6–18 mm Hg	High	Early or late
CAUSED BY INADEQUATE RESISTANCE TO OUTFLOW				
Overfiltration	Normal to shallow	Low	High	
Large sclerostomy				Early or late
Large, thin ischemic bleb				Late
Cyclodialysis cleft	Normal to shallow	Low	Low	Early
Conjunctival buttonhole or wound leak	Normal to shallow	Low	Low	Early or late
CAUSED BY INADEQUATE AQUEOUS PRODUCTION				
Ciliary body shutdown	Normal to shallow	Low	Low	Early
Choroidal effusion	Normal to shallow	Low	High or low	Early
Suprachoroidal hemorrhage, hemorrhagic choroidals	Shallow	Normal to high	High or low	Early
Previous cyclodestructive procedure	Shallow	Low	Low	Early or late
Uveitis	Normal to shallow	Low	Low	Early
CAUSED BY INADEQUATE FLOW				
Blockage of internal sclerostomy	Normal	High	Low	Early
Too tightly secured flap	Normal	High	Low	Early
OTHER CAUSES				
Aqueous misdirection (ciliary block glaucoma)	Shallow peripherally and centrally	High	Low	Early or late
Angle-closure glaucoma	Shallow peripherally	High	Low	Early or late
Plateau iris syndrome	Shallow peripherally	High	N/A	N/A
Failed bleb	Normal	High	Low	
Episcleral fibrosis				Late
Encapsulated bleb				Late

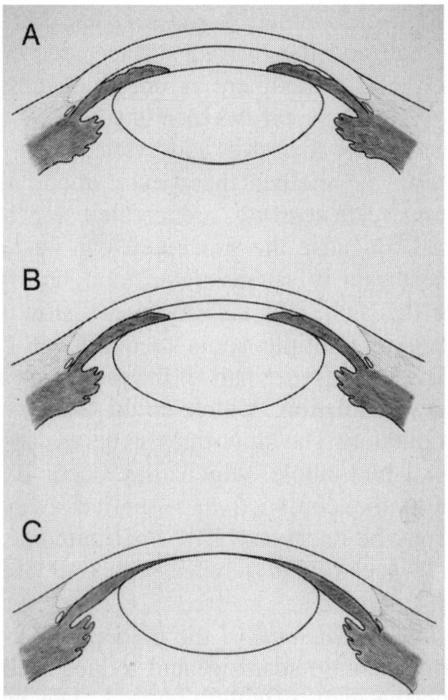

FIGURE 22–3. Schematic of the various grades of shallowness of the anterior chamber. *A,* grade I; *B,* grade II; *C,* grade III.

all of the lens (or vitreous in aphakic patients) is in contact with the posterior cornea. Chambers that are grade III shallow are sometimes referred to as "flat chambers" (Fig. 22–4).

Detailed examination of the anterior chamber depth in postoperative patients is important because each grade behaves differently and requires different management. For example, in a grade I or II shallow anterior chamber, the urgency for intervention is not as immediate as for a grade III chamber. In most circumstances, a grade I or II shallow anterior chamber spontaneously resolves. After a tube shunt procedure, however, intervention is required quickly to prevent corneal decompensation if the anterior chamber has shallowed so that the tube touches the corneal endothelium.

In developing a treatment plan, the physician must determine the cause of the postoperatively shallow or flat anterior chamber, which can arise from a variety of causes, either alone or in combination. Three diagnostic features should be examined:

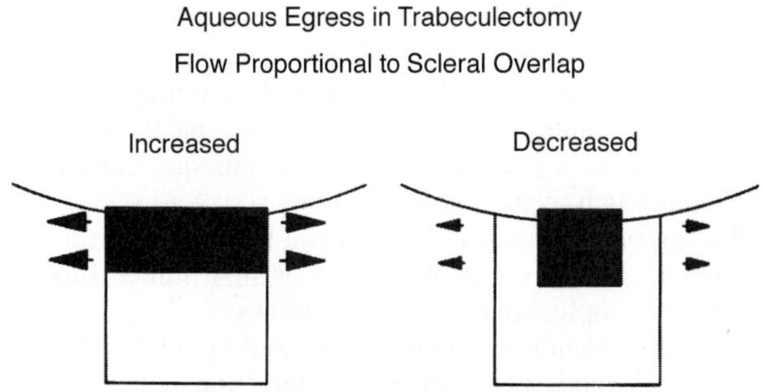

FIGURE 22–5. Schematic showing a large sclerostomy with little overlap and a small sclerostomy with a lot of overlap.

1. IOP.
2. Nature of the filtering bleb (high vs. low, ischemic vs. injected, thick vs. thin).
3. Patency of the pupil and iridectomy.

In general, the causes of a shallow chamber with hypotony (IOP lower than 6 mm Hg) can be divided into two groups: inadequate resistance to outflow and inadequate aqueous production.

Inadequate Resistance to Aqueous Outflow

OVERFILTRATION

Inadequate resistance to aqueous outflow is probably the most common cause of a shallow anterior chamber. In the early postoperative period, overfiltration is usually secondary to a large sclerostomy with little or no overlap by the scleral flap (Fig. 22–5).[3] In the late postoperative period, overfiltration commonly results from a large, thin, ischemic bleb (Fig. 22–6).

Clinically, the patient with overfiltration presents with a high bleb and low IOP. Early postoperative overfiltration, in many cases, resolves over time as scar tissue develops and creates resistance to outflow. If hypotony and a shallow chamber persist or a flat chamber develops and the bleb decreases in height or develops excessive blood vessel injection, more aggressive treatment is initiated.

EARLY POSTOPERATIVE MANAGEMENT. For early postoperative overfiltration in a patient in whom the anterior chamber is flat (grade III), intervention initially involves immediate reformation of the anterior chamber with a

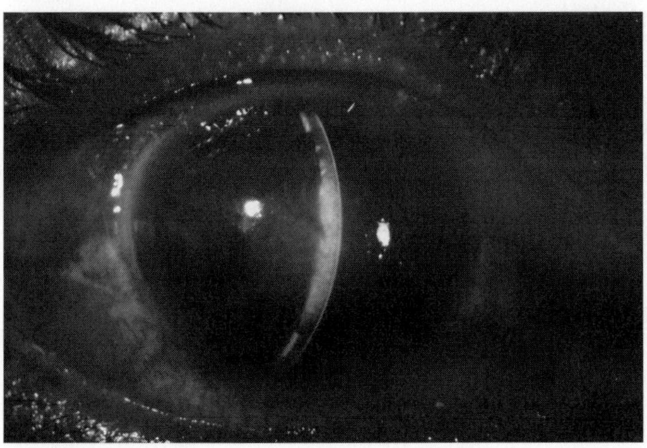

FIGURE 22–4. Flat anterior chamber (grade III).

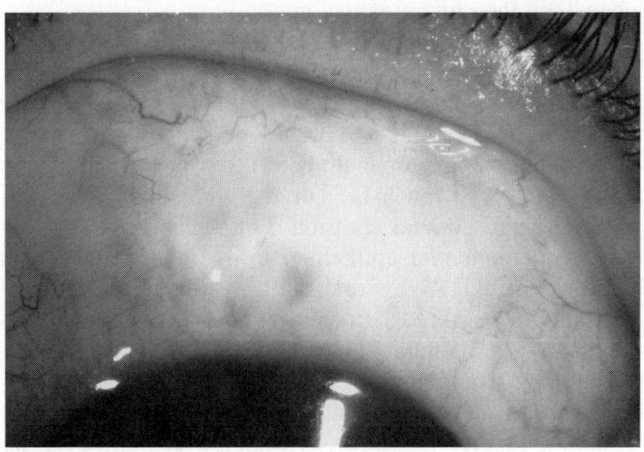

FIGURE 22–6. Large, thin succulent bleb.

viscoelastic substance, air, or balanced saline solution (BSS). This procedure provides time for the reduction of aqueous egress through the normal scarring process, allowing the anterior chamber to deepen and minimizing the destructive corneal and lenticular consequences of endothelial touch to the lens or vitreous.

Filling of the anterior chamber can be done with the use of topical anesthesia in the office or in a minor surgery suite under topical anesthesia, as follows:

1. A lid speculum is placed, followed by administration of antibiotic drops to prevent infection.
2. A 30-gauge blunt cannula on a viscoelastic-filled syringe is used to enter the paracentesis site previously placed during surgery.
3. Prior to viscoelastic agent injection, the cannula tip must be confirmed to be located completely in the anterior chamber; otherwise, Descemet's membrane might be dissected away from the corneal stroma, leading to corneal decompensation.
4. The anterior chamber is then filled slowly until it is completely formed and an intraocular pressure of approximately 25 mm Hg is obtained.

If needed, the procedure may be repeated several times. If a flat anterior chamber recurs or if the procedure fails to resolve the shallowed anterior chamber and overfiltration, choroidal effusion drainage with anterior chamber reformation may be necessary; this procedure is discussed in detail later in the chapter. If this is unsuccessful, surgical revision of the filter with additional sutures placed in the scleral flap to decrease flow may be necessary. In the circumstance that the structure of the scleral flap is insufficient to limit flow, a patch graft may be used.

LATE POSTOPERATIVE MANAGEMENT. For a patient with overfiltration 8 weeks postoperatively who has an IOP of less than 6 mm Hg with large serous choroidal effusions, shallow anterior chamber, hypotony maculopathy, and decreased vision, the surgeon should institute therapy. If overfiltration persists or becomes manifest during the late postoperative period, treatment options are aimed at reducing the size and/or function of the filtering bleb. Modalities used (in order of increasing aggressiveness) are: (1) treatment of the bleb with trichloroacetic acid (TCA), (2) cryotherapy, (3) neodymium:yttrium-aluminum-garnet (Nd:YAG) laser treatment, (4) blood injection, and (5) surgical revision of the sclerostomy or the conjunctiva. Which modality is chosen and when it is implemented depends on the clinical situation.

Trichloroacetic acid treatment is a form of chemical cauterization to induce scar formation.[4] Topical anesthesia is required. A supersaturated solution is applied to the entire surface of the bleb with the wooden end of a sterile, cotton-tipped applicator, with care taken not to allow any of the solution to touch the corneal epithelium, thus preventing a large corneal abrasion. Following TCA application, the conjunctival epithelium turns white. The eye is then rinsed with BSS. Several months and multiple applications may be required before the final effects can be observed. On the average, TCA treatment may achieve a 3 or 4 mm Hg rise in IOP.

This noninvasive treatment can be performed easily and painlessly in the office. Its effects are presumed to be secondary to protein coagulation in the conjunctival epithelium, leading to inflammation and scarring that reduce the size of the bleb and the overall surface area of filtration. Unfortunately, TCA treatment is not as successful as we would like. It works best if the bleb is succulent and diffuse in appearance rather than thin and cystic.

Cryotherapy[5] is another therapeutic mode to increase inflammation, create scarring, reduce bleb size, and thicken the bleb wall. Because the procedure can be painful, retrobulbar anesthesia is usually required. The cryoprobe is placed over the bleb, and a short freeze–slow thaw technique is used in multiple spots to confluently cover the bleb area. The short-freeze part of the procedure is required to prevent cycloablation, which could lead to decreased aqueous production. The slow-thaw is necessary to prevent a conjunctival buttonhole, which may occur if the probe, still frozen to the conjunctiva, is pulled away. Multiple treatments may be necessary. The final outcome is evident within 2 to 4 weeks. If it is successful, IOP rises approximately 3 to 4 mm Hg.

Nd:YAG laser treatment[6] of the bleb can likewise create inflammation, increase scarring, and reduce bleb size. Retrobulbar anesthesia is usually required. The approximate laser setting is 3 joules in the thermal mode with an offset of 3. The number of applications depends on the size of the bleb; the entire bleb should be treated (Fig. 22–7). As treatment proceeds, visible whitening of the conjunctival epithelium is noted. IOP is measured 1 hour postoperatively. An effect, if treatment is successful, is noted within 2 to 4 weeks as an approximate rise in IOP of 3 to 4 mm Hg. One must take care not to be too overaggressive in this form of treatment, that is, use too much energy, because a conjunctival buttonhole can occur.

Autologous blood injection also can be used to reduce the size of an overfiltering bleb.[7, 8] This treatment potentially decreases overfiltration by two mechanisms: (1) the red blood cells themselves or the clot occludes the sclerostomy and (2) plasma supplies fibroblast-transforming growth factors that can increase healing and scar tissue formation, thus increasing resistance to outflow. The procedure can be performed at the slit lamp, as follows:

1. A lid speculum is placed in the eye following instillation of topical antibiotics and a topical anesthetic agent.
2. Approximately 1 mL of blood is withdrawn from the patient's antecubital vein with a tuberculin syringe.

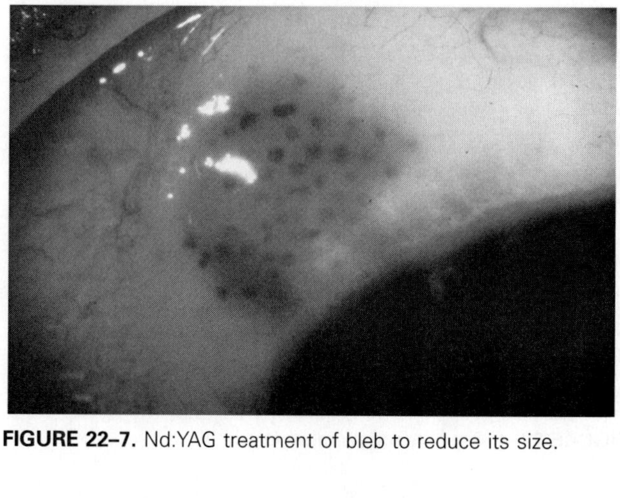

FIGURE 22–7. Nd:YAG treatment of bleb to reduce its size.

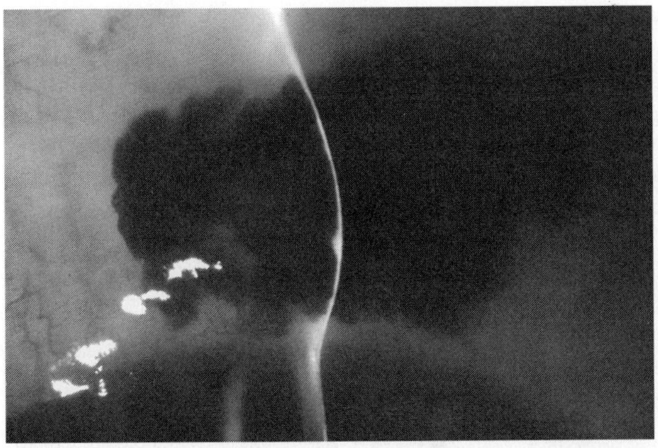

FIGURE 22–8. Blood in bleb injection immediately after injection.

3. A 30-gauge needle is quickly placed on the syringe.
4. The needle tract penetrates the conjunctiva in a site as far away from the bleb as possible and is slowly advanced into the center of the bleb, where blood is injected. Care is taken not to penetrate the conjunctiva over the bleb, to avoid creating a buttonhole.
5. If the bleb is loculated, the needle is retracted and placed in each loculus in order to fill all areas of the bleb.
6. Blood is injected until the bleb is filled or blood begins to enter the anterior chamber. To help prevent blood from entering the globe, a viscoelastic substance can be injected into the anterior chamber via the surgically placed paracentesis prior to injection of the blood.
7. The patient is treated postoperatively with antibiotics for 1 week.

Re-injection may be necessary if there is some effect but the hypotony has not resolved completely after blood clears from the subconjunctival space (Figs. 22–8 and 22–9).

Surgical revision[9, 10] of the bleb or sclerostomy site is indicated if the less-aggressive techniques fail to reverse the hypotony and the shallow or flat anterior chamber. Customizing the revision to the appearance of the bleb is essential.

BLEB TOO LARGE. If the bleb is large, extending around the eye nasally or temporally, excision of a portion of the conjunctiva in the interpalpebral area followed by cryotherapy to the edges of the incised area can be performed to decrease the surface area of filtration, as Fellman and Feldman[11] describe. This technique can be performed with the use of retrobulbar anesthesia in the office or in the minor surgery suite, as follows:

1. Antibiotic drops are placed before, during, and after the procedure.
2. A speculum is placed, and Vannas scissors and toothless forceps are used to excise a circular area of conjunctiva approximately 4 to 5 mm in diameter.
3. The cryoprobe is used to place several spots along the edge of the conjunctiva in a short freeze–slow thaw technique.

One can expect a rise in IOP of 3 to 10 mm Hg a few weeks postoperatively.

If the conjunctiva covering the bleb is excessively thin and friable, it can be excised and healthy conjunctiva brought forward and sutured in place with 10-0 nylon on a vascular needle with a mattress or figure-of-eight suture. If there is not enough conjunctiva to advance, a large conjunctival graft from the inferior fornix or from the other eye is sutured over the bleb site. The conjunctival epithelium over the bleb must be removed, either mechanically with a blade, via cautery, or chemically with absolute alcohol, before the graft is sutured in place via a running or mattress suture. To create a watertight wound, small bites are taken in the graft with larger bites in the host, placing the graft on stretch, as described by Wise.[12]

At the time of conjunctival revision, if there is also an excessively large sclerostomy, adding more 10-0 nylon sutures to the scleral flap (thus decreasing aqueous outflow) is the treatment of choice. If the scleral flap is very thin or absent (which may occur if mitomycin was used), a donor scleral patch graft is used to cover the sclerostomy and secured with 10-0 nylon. Other materials may be used, such as pericardium, dura, and fascia lata.

CYCLODIALYSIS CLEFTS

Cyclodialysis clefts also cause inadequate resistance to outflow (Fig. 22–10). Such clefts may occur inadvertently following cataract surgery or may be created in a planned procedure for pressure control in a patient with little con-

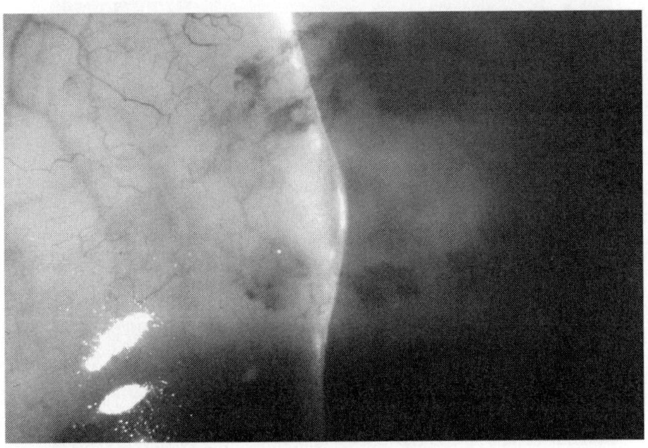

FIGURE 22–9. Blood in bleb 1 week after injection.

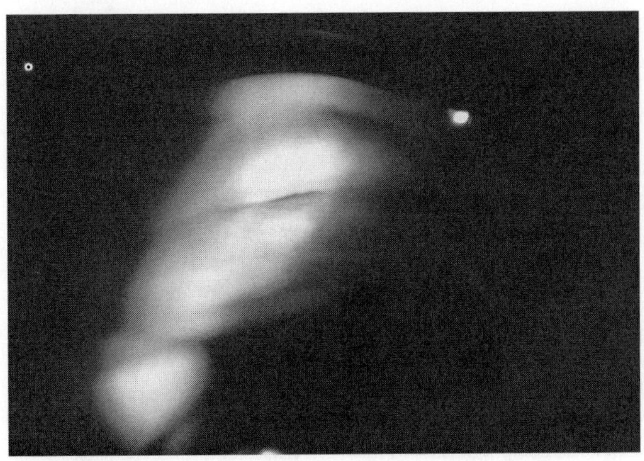

FIGURE 22–10. Gonioscopy of cyclodialysis cleft.

junctiva suitable for filtration surgery. In this condition, aqueous humor leaves the anterior chamber between the ciliary body and the sclera and is absorbed from the suprachoroidal space. A cleft may be difficult to diagnose because with a soft eye (low IOP), office gonioscopy leads to corneal striae, making the view of the angle difficult. If an inadvertent cleft is suspected, bringing the patient to the operating room and filling the eye with a viscoelastic agent allows better gonioscopic visualization of the angle and of the cleft.

Pharmacologic dilation of the pupil may close the cleft, particularly if it is not too large. This event is often accompanied by a temporary pressure spike, which the patient notes as pain. The pressure spike can be treated with glaucoma medications that decrease aqueous production. If the cleft persists, it may be treated with (1) argon laser application to the cleft walls with large spot size and low energy or (2) surgical closure with an 8-0 Vicryl mattress suture.[13]

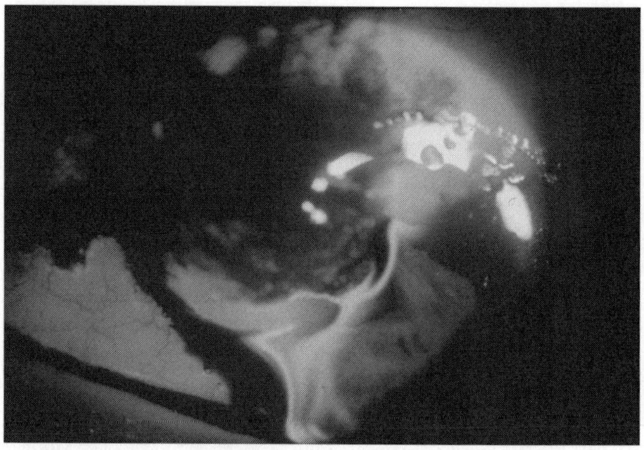

FIGURE 22–12. Fluorescein test of conjunctival buttonhole.

CONJUNCTIVAL BUTTONHOLES OR WOUND LEAKS

Conjunctival buttonholes or wound leaks commonly cause hypotony and a flat or shallow anterior chamber because of inadequate resistance to outflow (Fig. 22–11). They can occur early postoperatively secondary to inadequate closure of the conjunctival wound or an inadvertent buttonhole. A conjunctival buttonhole can also occur late postoperatively, particularly if antimetabolites, which create a thin, friable bleb, were used.

The clinical features of buttonhole are (1) low IOP, (2) shallow or flat anterior chamber, and (3) low bleb. The site of leakage is identified with Seidel's test,[14] which is performed by painting the bleb and conjunctival wound with a fluorescein strip. Under the cobalt blue light at the slit lamp, the fluorescein dye self-quenches at high concentration. As the aqueous dilutes it, the dye fluoresces to yellow in areas where the aqueous is egressing (Fig. 22–12). Minimal pressure applied to the globe may be necessary to push fluid through a hole if the chamber is flat, as there is little aqueous available for flow.

Treatment depends on the size of the hole. A small hole may close spontaneously if aqueous flow is reduced and antimetabolites have not been used. Reducing aqueous production with medications, such as beta-blockers, alpha-agonists, and carbonic anhydrase inhibitors, along with patching to prevent blinking, decreases the flow through the hole, which allows healing to occur.

Unfortunately, in some patients, conjunctival buttonholes can recur. If the first treatment measures are unsuccessful, a monofilament 10-0 nylon suture on a tapered vascular needle is used to suture the hole in a purse-string fashion.

A wound leak is treated similarly.[15] The goal is to treat the leak as quickly as possible to prevent bleb failure from permanent scarring of the conjunctiva to the sclera. In many cases, the hole can be sutured at the slit lamp with topical anesthesia and a lid speculum. If the patient is unable to cooperate, this procedure can be performed in a minor surgery suite. In either case, topical antibiotics are recommended to prevent infection. In general, if conservative, noninvasive procedures do not allow the wound to close within a week, suturing is required to help maintain the bleb.

Inadequate Aqueous Production

Inadequate aqueous production is another mechanism by which hypotony resulting in a shallow or flat anterior chamber can be seen. Serous choroidal effusions occur frequently in patients with hypotony (Figs. 22–13 and

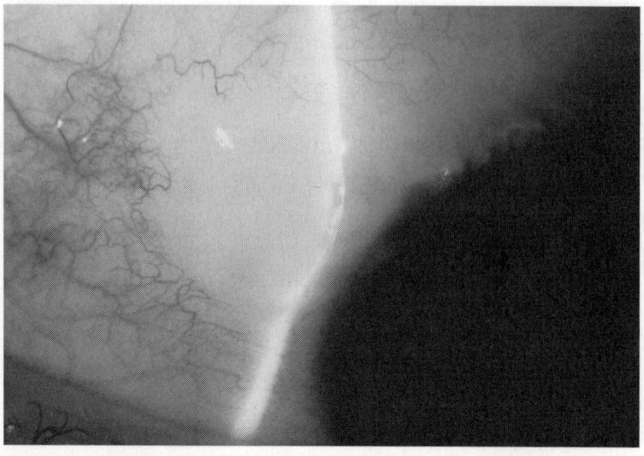

FIGURE 22–11. Conjunctival buttonhole.

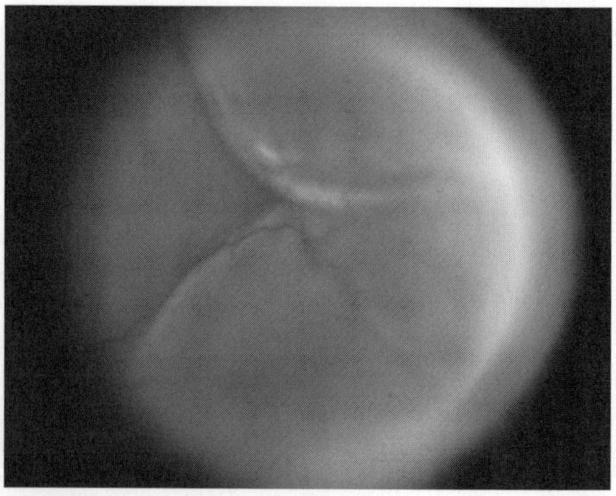

FIGURE 22–13. Choroidal detachment in a hypotonous patient.

22–14). However, they may be the inciting or perpetuating cause in ciliary body shutdown.

CILIARY BODY SHUTDOWN

Ciliary body shutdown and aqueous hyposecretion is the most common cause of inadequate aqueous production. This occurs most frequently in patients who have debilitating diseases, such as hypertension, diabetes, and cardiovascular disease, or have undergone previous cyclodestructive procedures. It also occurs in patients with severe ocular diseases, such as uveitic or neovascular glaucoma, which cause a breakdown of the blood-aqueous barrier. Aqueous production must drop to less than 10% of normal to cause hypotony.[16]

Decreased aqueous production can also occur as a result of or can be perpetuated by the cycle of choroidal effusion and hypotony. The exact relationship between the two is poorly understood. However, it has been shown that drainage of the suprachoroidal fluid alone can reverse hypotony. Therefore, one can conclude that the ciliary body detachment leads to aqueous hyposecretion by some as yet unexplained mechanism. In many patients, aqueous flare is present, leading to the conclusion that a breakdown of the blood-aqueous barrier may be responsible for the aqueous hyposecretion.

A monkey model has been created to further delineate the cause of this aqueous hyposecretion. Injection of silicone oil into the suprachoroidal space, creating large choroidal detachments in the monkeys, did not cause a decrease in IOP. However, if lactated Ringer's solution or autologous serum was injected into the suprachoroidal space, IOP decreased. It was concluded from these studies that uveoscleral outflow is enhanced and that perhaps the hyposecretion is due to concurrent iridocyclitis.[16] What is certain is that this cycle continues until it is broken either spontaneously or by surgical intervention.

To help break the cycle, patients are advised to increase fluid intake and to keep active. Although there is no proof that these activities affect aqueous production, they give patients a sense of participating in their recovery. However, patients should be warned that doing anything strenuous could lead to a suprachoroidal hemorrhage. Strenuous activities include (1) placing the head below the knees, (2) straining at stool, (3) lifting more than 5 lb, and (4) sexual intercourse. Topical corticosteroids, as well as oral corticosteroids if the patient can tolerate them, can be used to stimulate the ciliary body to produce aqueous by eliminating the iridocyclitis, which may be aiding in aqueous shutdown. Observation and noninvasive therapy are continued until (1) the bleb begins to fail clinically, (2) the choroidal detachments become so large that they touch ("kissing choroidals"), or (3) the anterior chamber is flat with the lens touching the cornea. The latter two indications are easy to diagnose; however, what constitutes a failing bleb is more difficult. Criteria for a failing bleb include decreasing height of the bleb, loss of microcysts, increasing injection of the conjunctiva, and thickening of the conjunctiva.

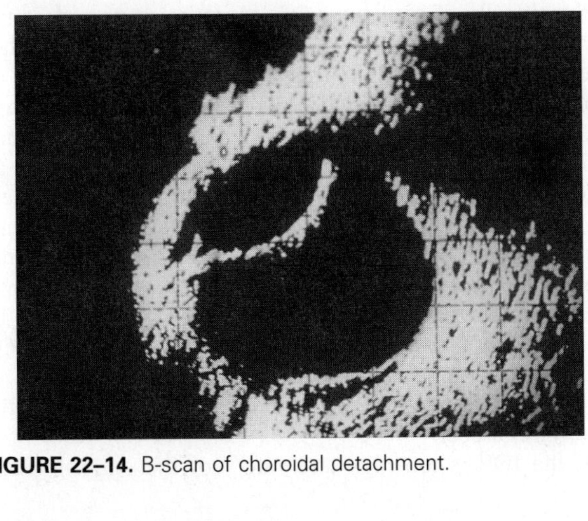

FIGURE 22–14. B-scan of choroidal detachment.

Surgical treatment involves drainage of the choroidal effusions with anterior chamber reformation, typically performed as an outpatient procedure.[17, 18] Retrobulbar anesthesia is usually sufficient. However, if there is a concern about increased risk of retrobulbar hemorrhage, one may consider general anesthesia; massive retrobulbar hemorrhage could be catastrophic. The procedure is performed as follows:

1. A circumferential conjunctival incision is created in the inferior temporal region of the eye, approximately 4 mm long and 3 mm posterior to the limbus in phakic patients.
2. Cautery is used to eliminate the scleral and episcleral vessels.
3. A supersharp blade or a No. 67 Beaver blade is used to slowly dissect a 2 to 3 mm circumferential scleral incision 3 mm posterior to the limbus just to the level of the suprachoroidal space.
4. Once this space is opened, a large amount of yellowish fluid is spontaneously released.
5. Careful massage of the eye expresses any loculated fluid that did not spontaneously drain.
6. A paracentesis is created with a 25-gauge butterfly needle connected to a bottle of BSS (500 mL) and is used to continuously fill the anterior chamber. This creates pressure in the eye, aiding in the expression of the suprachoroidal fluid; it is impossible to express all the fluid, however.
7. The indirect ophthalmoscope allows visualization of the choroidal effusions and ensures that they are significantly reduced.
8. The scleral incision is closed with 8-0 Vicryl, as is the conjunctiva, in a running fashion.
9. The anterior chamber is filled with a viscoelastic agent to a pressure of about 25 mm Hg to prevent hypotony and to facilitate reabsorption of remaining fluid.

This procedure may be required more than once if there is recurrent choroidal effusion and shallowing of the anterior segment with decreasing height of the bleb.

PREVIOUS CYCLODESTRUCTIVE SURGERY

Previous cyclodestructive procedures, such as Nd:YAG or diode cyclophotocoagulation or cyclocryotherapy, can cause decreased aqueous production. With both procedures, the ciliary body is destroyed by either photodisruption or freezing the epithelium. Patients undergoing this procedure typically are elderly and aphakic, with poor vision and a history of unsuccessful glaucoma filtering surgery. The complication rate for cyclocryotherapy is higher than that for cyclophotocoagulation. Vision loss can occur in 50% of patients undergoing cyclocryotherapy,[19] and phthisis in 12% to 22%. For cyclophotocoagulation, vision loss is seen in 10% to 40% of patients, and phthisis in less than 10%.[20] To prevent hypotony, the physician can try to treat only 270 degrees, allowing one quadrant to remain untreated and to produce aqueous. Aggressive corticosteroid treatment following the procedure minimizes inflammation, thereby decreasing one cause of ciliary body shutdown, which may help prevent serous choroidal effusion formation and thus decrease the risk of chronic hypotony.

UVEITIS

Inadequate aqueous production can also result from intraocular inflammation, or uveitis. The inflammation results in a breakdown of the blood-aqueous barrier, which decreases aqueous formation. This usually resolves with corticosteroid treatment at the underlying inflammation.

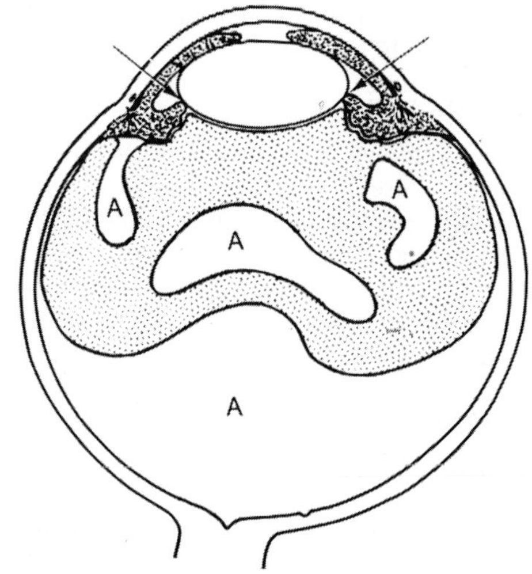

FIGURE 22–15. Schematic of aqueous misdirection demonstrating the flow of aqueous in the vitreous cavity. A, aqueous humor.

CAUSES OF A POSTOPERATIVELY SHALLOW CHAMBER WITH HIGH IOP

Occasionally, a physician encounters the unusual situation in which the anterior chamber is shallowed and yet, surprisingly, the IOP is increased. Four conditions can lead to this situation: aqueous misdirection, angle closure, plateau iris syndrome, and suprachoroidal hemorrhage. It is important to distinguish among these causes because the therapies are very different.

AQUEOUS MISDIRECTION

In aqueous misdirection, also known as malignant glaucoma or ciliary-block glaucoma, the patient presents with high pressures, a low bleb, and a shallow anterior chamber. After filtering surgery, the IOP may not be initially increased because there is filtration, but with progressive posterior pressure, tissue (iris, lens, hyaloid) occludes the sclerostomy, and the IOP increases considerably. This condition can be easily confused with angle-closure glaucoma. The two are clinically differentiated by the depth of the central anterior chamber and the presence or absence of a patent peripheral iridotomy. In contrast to angle-closure glaucoma, the central as well as peripheral chamber is shallowed in malignant glaucoma, and a peripheral iridotomy does not improve the condition.

Patients particularly at risk are those with previous angle closure attacks and nanophthalmos. Classic malignant glaucoma occurs in 0.6% to 4% of cases after surgical intervention for angle-closure glaucoma.[21] However, this rare complication can occur following any type of anterior segment surgery or potentially even in the absence of surgery. Postoperative aqueous misdirection usually occurs shortly after surgery but can be delayed for months or even years. Development of aqueous misdirection can also occur upon cessation of mydriatic agents or instillation of miotic drops. Treatment for aqueous misdirection is difficult because of its poor response to medical therapy.

Several pathophysiologic mechanisms promote the development of aqueous misdirection. In all forms, the underlying condition is a blockage of normal aqueous humor flow into the anterior chamber (Fig. 22–15).[22] Fluid is diverted and trapped posteriorly in the vitreous cavity via increased permeability in the anterior hyaloid face, which acts as a one-way valve preventing the escape of the fluid back into the posterior chamber. The aqueous humor subsequently pools within and behind the vitreous, causing a forward shift of the iris-lens diaphragm, thereby shallowing the anterior chamber, blocking the trabecular meshwork, preventing aqueous outflow, and raising the IOP. Studies suggest that the initiating factor is blockage of aqueous humor that occurs when the peripheral lens and anterior ciliary body processes come into contact, thereby creating what is termed ciliary block.[23] Blockage can also occur in aphakic patients, with the block being between the vitreous face and the ciliary body processes.

Management consists initially of conservative medical treatment followed by more aggressive surgical treatment.[24] Cycloplegic agents can ameliorate the condition by tightening the lens zonules, causing the iris-lens diaphragm to be pulled posteriorly in an attempt to break the ciliary block. Hyperosmotic and aqueous suppressant agents dehydrate the vitreous, reducing its forward pressure on the iris-lens diaphragm to thus allow posterior movement of the diaphragm to break the ciliary block. Miotics could precipitate the event by stimulating the circular muscle of the ciliary body, loosening the zonules and allowing forward movement of lens-iris diaphragm.

Specifically, if aqueous misdirection is suspected, initial treatment should consist of: atropine 1% four times a day, phenylephrine 2.5% four times a day, a beta-blocker, an alpha-agonist, acetazolamide 250 mg four times a day, and mannitol 1 to 2 g/kg IV over 30 minutes every 12 hours. This treatment can be potentially life-threatening in an elderly patient. One must be vigilant for the development of hypovolemia, expansion of the intravascular volume, hypokalemia, congestive heart failure, and subdural hematoma, which can occur with the use of hyperosmotic agents. Medical treatment should be continued as long as the situation is improving, that is, if the patient has a lower IOP and a deeper anterior chamber. The duration of treatment is determined by the IOP value and the shallowness of the anterior chamber.

If the IOP is too high and safety of the optic nerve is

compromised or if the chamber is flat, surgery is indicated. The aims of surgery are (1) to re-establish normal flow by correcting the anterior blockage of aqueous egress and (2) to drain the accumulated aqueous from the posterior segment. The type of surgery depends on the site of the block; in all procedures, however, the anterior hyaloid face must somehow be disrupted. If the patient is phakic, vitrectomy, lensectomy, or both are indicated; if the patient is pseudophakic or aphakic, rupture of the anterior hyaloid face by laser is indicated. This latter maneuver can be achieved with the Nd:YAG laser using the same settings used for posterior capsulotomy; if laser treatment is unsuccessful, vitrectomy is indicated.

ANGLE-CLOSURE GLAUCOMA

Angle-closure glaucoma is another condition in which the anterior chamber is shallowed with increased IOP. This condition must be excluded before the diagnosis of aqueous misdirection or plateau iris syndrome can be definitively made. Primary angle closure usually occurs in phakic patients; however, angle closure can occur following anterior segment surgery if posterior synechiae form between the iris and the lens or the iris and the vitreous, causing complete seclusion of the pupil, or pupillary block. Angle closure can also occur in the postoperative patient whose peripheral iridectomy is not patent or is only of partial thickness. Pupillary block is also seen in the patient with an anterior chamber lens and in an aphakic patient with an intact anterior hyaloid face and no patent iridotomy.

Clinically, the anterior chamber is shallowed more peripherally than centrally (the iris may have a bowed appearance, i.e., iris bombé) (Fig. 22–16). This picture is unlike that of aqueous misdirection, in which the peripheral as well as central anterior chamber is shallowed and the IOP is elevated.

Predisposing factors for angle closure include hyperopia, advancing age, and family history. The mechanism responsible is block of aqueous flow between the iris and the lens, obstructing the normal flow of aqueous from the posterior chamber into the anterior chamber, resulting in pupillary block. Fluid accumulates in the posterior chamber, causing forward bowing of the peripheral iris, occlusion of the trabecular meshwork, and sclerostomy, if present, leading to an increased IOP. Patient symptoms, which vary according to the level of the IOP, include severe pain, nausea, vomiting, decreased vision, and colored halos. Examination reveals a red eye, corneal edema, a mid-dilated pupil, closed angle (noted on gonioscopy), and very high IOP.

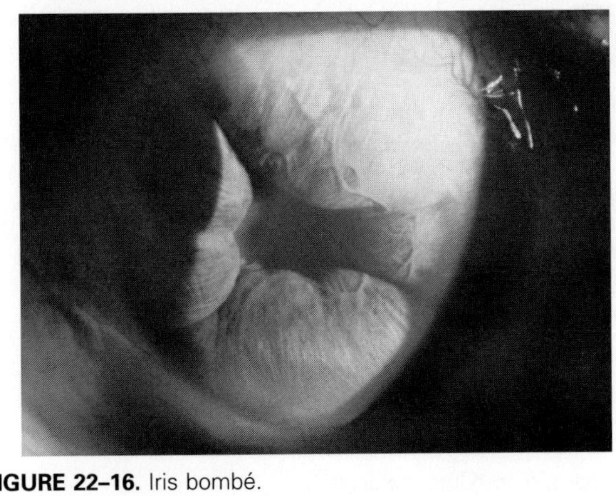

FIGURE 22–16. Iris bombé.

Initially, the patient is treated with medications to suppress aqueous production and low-dose pilocarpine to constrict the pupil, in hopes of breaking the pupillary block. Aqueous suppressants include a beta-blocker, an alpha-agonist, and a carbonic anhydrase inhibitor.

Indentation gonioscopy can also be used to mechanically break the pupillary block. This procedure is accomplished with the four-mirror gonioscopy lens, which is used to intermittently indent the central cornea and deepen the peripheral angle, under direct observation, in order to break the pupillary block.[25] Once the acute attack is broken (confirmed gonioscopically), a peripheral iridotomy (PI) is performed to prevent future attacks.

A PI can be created with the argon or Nd:YAG laser or through surgical incision. The procedure is indicated for the treatment of pupillary block; one must remember, however, that there are other causes of nonpupillary block angle closure for which an iridotomy is not indicated (e.g., neovascular glaucoma). A PI is appropriate in the contralateral eye of a patient who suffered acute primary angle closure in one eye. Less clear is its use in the asymptomatic patient with "occludable" angles. In general, if synechial or appositional angle closure (reversible with compression gonioscopy) cannot be excluded, a prophylactic PI should be performed in the presence of relative pupillary block.

The technique for *laser iridotomy* includes the use of a contact lens (Abraham lens) that helps stabilize the globe and improve visualization. The Abraham lens contains an iridotomy button that magnifies the area of interest and reduces the diameter of the laser spot by two, thus increasing the power density by a factor of four. Both laser treatment and incisional iridotomy are performed as outpatient procedures.

With laser iridotomy, only topical anesthesia is required. The Nd:YAG laser is the preferred technique in most instances because of its higher rate of success and lower rate of closure compared with the argon laser. Suggested settings are an offset of 0 in phakic eyes and a power of 6 mJ, with 3 pulses per burst. Usually one to six bursts will penetrate the iris. The argon laser can be useful for performing peripheral iridotomy, particularly in a patient with rubeosis, because it possesses cauterization capability, unlike the Nd:YAG laser. The settings are 50 μm, 500 to 1000 mW at 0.2 to 0.1 second. Approximately 100 spots are necessary to penetrate the iris.

Potential complications of laser peripheral iridotomy include inflammation, hemorrhage, lenticular damage, failure to penetrate the iris stroma, and elevated IOP. Hemorrhage is much more common with the Nd:YAG laser and can usually be controlled by direct compression of the globe with the laser contact lens. Pressure should be applied until the bleeding has stopped as verified by direct visualization. Once the contact lens is removed, a second examination should be immediately performed to ensure cessation of hemorrhaging. The most common complication is a postoperative IOP rise. This can be successfully prevented with the use of many of the available topical IOP-lowering agents. Alpha-adrenergic agents are probably the agents of choice, but it is important to use a drug that the patient is not already using for chronic therapy. Postoperative intraocular inflammation is generally treated with topical corticosteroids for 4 to 7 days.

Surgical iridectomy is indicated when a laser iridotomy cannot be performed because of a cloudy cornea or lack of patient cooperation. This operation is performed as an outpatient procedure with the use of topical or retrobulbar anesthesia. A small full-thickness corneal incision is created at the 12 o'clock position. The iris is pulled through the incision and amputated. One 10-0 nylon suture closes the corneal wound. Postoperative antibiotics and corticosteroids are used.

If the block does recur, it is of paramount importance to confirm that the iridotomy is patent. If the anterior lens capsule can be visualized through the iridotomy, it is truly patent. If the patient has uveitic disease, multiple peripheral iridotomies may be necessary because of loculation resulting from synechiae.

Following iridotomy, whether surgical or laser, gonioscopy must be performed to ensure that the angle is open. The IOP can be low without opening of the angle, as a result of aqueous shutdown from medications and inflammation and not of resolution of the pupillary block, which is essential to cure this condition. If the peripheral iridotomy appears patent, as demonstrated by direct visualization of the anterior lens capsule, but the angle did not open, two conditions should be considered: (1) the peripheral iridotomy is not patent or is not large enough or (2) the patient has plateau iris syndrome. Postoperatively, the patient's pupil should be dilated to prevent synechiae to the lens and to ascertain that the iridotomy is sufficient to prevent pupillary block and maintain a low pressure following dilation, as well as to allow examination of the posterior segment.

Pupillary block can also occur following surgery. It can be seen after placement of an anterior chamber intraocular lens, causing a pupillary block with the lens occluding the pupil; it is therefore important to perform a peripheral iridectomy at the time of lens insertion. Pupillary block can also occur following posterior chamber intraocular lens placement if the iris and intraocular lens form a 360-degree synechia. In this case, a peripheral iridotomy is curative. Silicone oil can also cause pupillary block after retinal detachment surgery. In this case, the peripheral iridotomy should be performed inferiorly because the silicone oil will float superiorly, allowing aqueous flow inferiorly.

PLATEAU IRIS SYNDROME

Once patency of the iridotomy is confirmed by direct visualization of the lens capsule in a patient in whom the angle remains occluded, the diagnosis of plateau iris syndrome must be considered.[26] This rare condition occurs most commonly in women between 30 and 50 years old who (1) are less hyperopic than their counterparts with angle closure and (2) have a family history of angle closure. In this condition, the natural iris configuration is such that it crowds the angle, and with dilation, the iris obstructs the trabecular meshwork. Plateau iris results from a large or anteriorly positioned ciliary process that is holding up the peripheral iris and maintaining apposition to the trabecular meshwork. Therefore, increased IOP results not from pupillary block but rather from an anatomic abnormality of the peripheral iris. Ultrasound biomicroscopy is the best way other than gonioscopy to demonstrate this unusual anatomy (Fig. 22–17).

Peripheral iridotomy does not solve the problem of plateau iris syndrome. Treatment requires pulling the thickened plateau iris away from the angle with either medications or laser iridoplasty. Miotics are the drug of choice. If the patient is intolerant of medication, an argon laser iridoplasty can be performed. This is performed as an outpatient procedure with topical anesthesia and pretreatment with an alpha-agonist to prevent a post-laser pressure spike. Settings are 0.1 to 0.5 sec, 100 to 200 μm, with 200 to 500 mW of energy.[27] Approximately 40 spots are placed circumferentially in the peripheral iris with the aid of a gonioscopy lens. The end-point is iris contraction with no pigment or tissue release. If pressure control remains

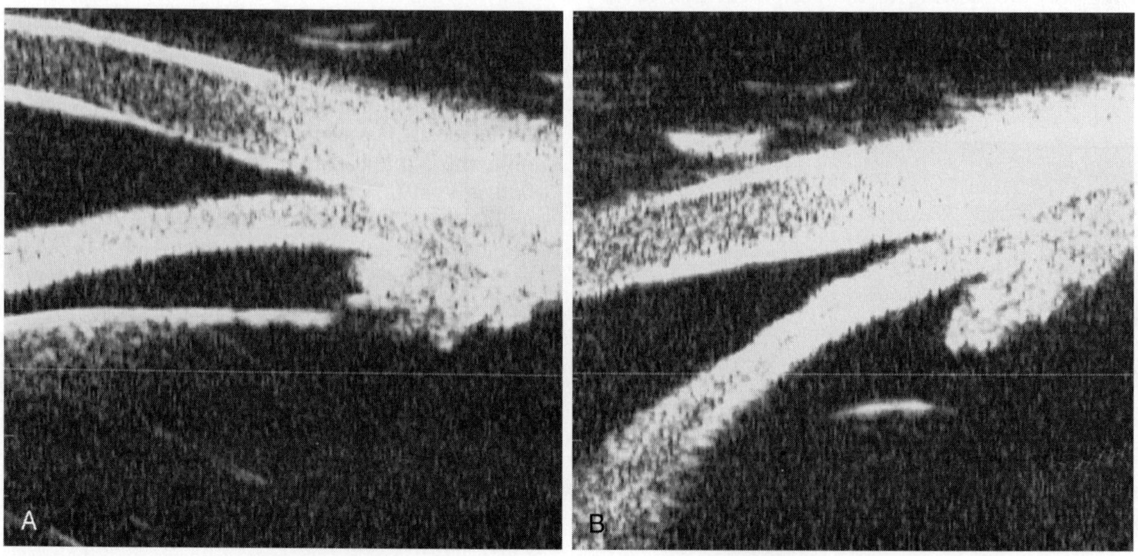

FIGURE 22–17. Ultrasound biomicroscopy of a plateau iris showing its abnormal approach into the angle.

problematic and the optic nerve is damaged, glaucoma filtering surgery is recommended.

HEMORRHAGE

Suprachoroidal hemorrhage, or hemorrhagic choroidal effusion, can present problems similar to those seen with patients who have serous choroidal effusions. Unlike serous choroidal effusions, however, suprachoroidal hemorrhages are often painful. The patient presents with a shallow chamber and normal to elevated IOP. The choroidals are large, dark, posterior segment masses that may become visible through the pupil or may be seen with indirect ophthalmoscopy (Fig. 22–18).

Suprachoroidal hemorrhages can occur at any time during surgery or postoperatively[28] and do so in approximately 2% of eyes undergoing glaucoma surgery.[29] Risk factors for their development include hypotony, advanced age, systemic vascular disease, aphakia, high myopia, prior vitrectomy, preoperative elevation of IOP, vascular abnormalities, previous cyclodestructive procedure, and postoperative straining (e.g., Valsalva maneuver).[30]

Drainage is indicated for reasons similar to those for the use of drainage of serous choroidal effusions. If the hemorrhagic choroidal effusions are large and touching, cause unbearable pain, or cause loss of the bleb or a flat anterior chamber, drainage is performed as described for serous choroidal effusions. The only difference is that a reddish brown fluid emerges rather than a clear, yellowish fluid. It is prudent to wait 4 to 5 days to enable the clot to liquefy, allowing easier blood drainage. Spontaneous reabsorption of the hemorrhage, if small, can also occur.

CAUSES OF A POSTOPERATIVELY NORMAL CHAMBER WITH HIGH IOP

The most common late complication of glaucoma filtering surgery is scarring of the sclerostomy,[31] which leads to either failure of the bleb secondary to episcleral fibrosis or encapsulation of the bleb. Although collagen production is the basic underlying mechanism for both conditions, the cause of inadequate filtration and the clinical appearance differ.

The *failed bleb* appears flat and thick, and the anterior chamber is of normal depth. Failure most commonly results from occlusion of the external ostia of the sclerostomy with scarring between the conjunctiva and Tenon's capsule by episcleral tissue (Fig. 22–19).[32] Antimetabolites, 5-fluorouracil (5-FU) and mitomycin C, are used to prevent scarring, with relatively good success.[33] Risk factors for scarring include (1) young age, (2) African ancestry, (3) previous surgery, (4) aphakia, and (5) uveitic, traumatic, or neovascular glaucoma.

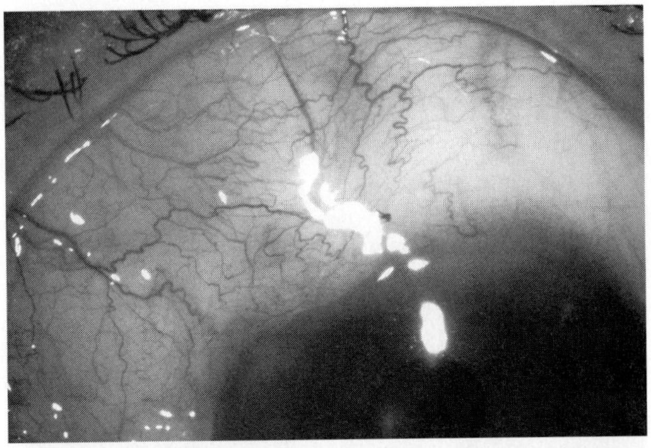

FIGURE 22–19. Failed bleb. Note the low height with conjunctival injection.

If flow can be maintained through the sclerostomy, the opening will not close. The most common cause of early postoperative (within the first 1 to 3 days) absence of a bleb is too much overlap of the scleral flap with inadequate flow of aqueous. Another common cause is occlusion of the sclerostomy by fibrin and blood. Applying mild external pressure under direct visualization to force fluid through the sclerostomy will dislodge the debris and enlarge the bleb to prevent permanent closure by scar tissue (Fig. 22–20).[34]

If that maneuver fails and subsequently the bleb flattens again with elevated pressure, suture lysis may be indicated. This procedure is performed with the use of a Hoskins laser suture lens, which allows one to visualize the suture through the conjunctiva (Figs. 22–21 and 22–22). The argon laser, set at 500 mW for 0.05 sec with a spot size of 50 μm, is used to cut the suture with one or two applications. Suture lysis works best if performed no sooner than the third postoperative day and within 2 weeks after a 5-FU

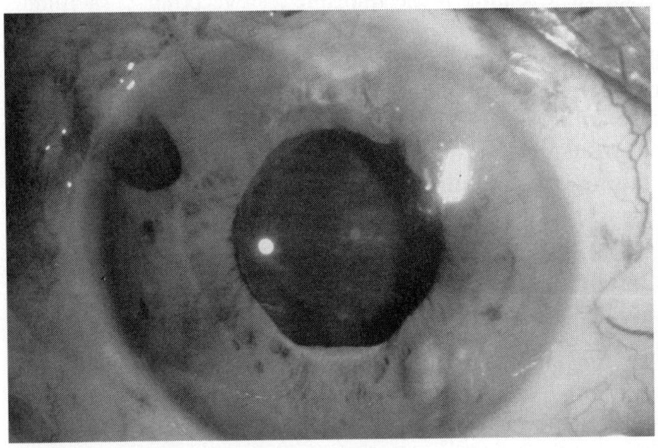

FIGURE 22–18. Hemorrhagic choroidal detachment viewed through the pupil.

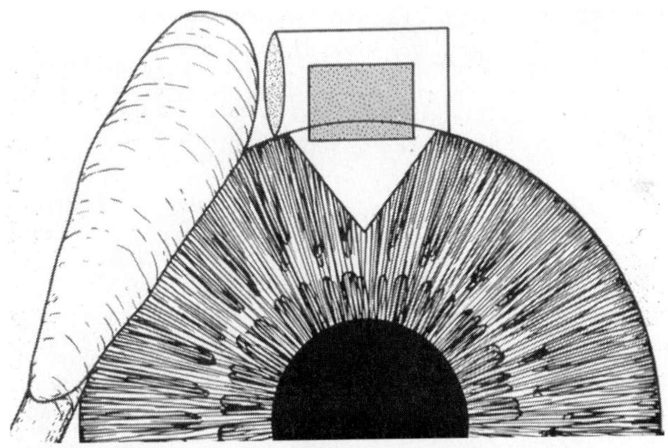

FIGURE 22–20. Schematic diagram of the method of scleral compression under direct visualization to ensure flow.

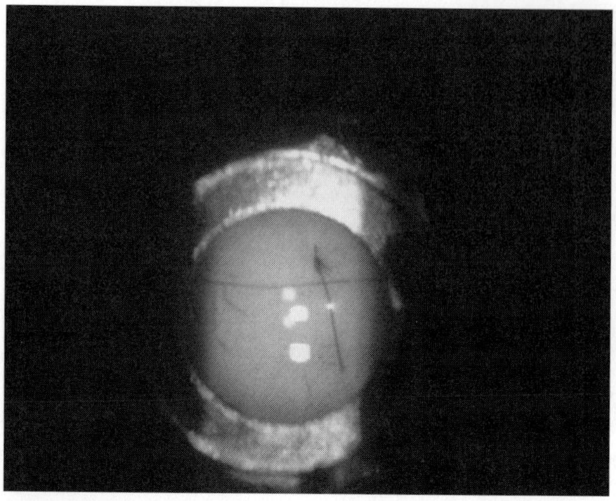

FIGURE 22–21. Scleral flap suture viewed through a Hoskins lens.

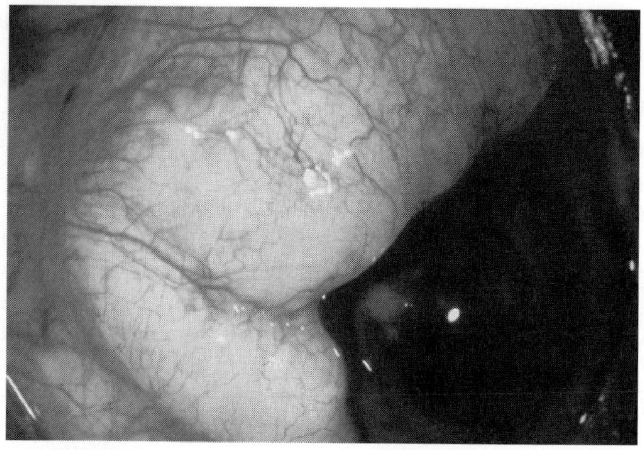

FIGURE 22–23. Encapsulated bleb. Note its thickened, "igloo-like" appearance.

trabeculectomy or within 1 month following a mitomycin C trabeculectomy. The reason is that at 2 weeks or a month postoperatively, respectively, the scar tissue is established and is not conducive to manipulation.

If bleb failure is unavoidable secondary to occlusion of the external sclerostomy by scar tissue, initial treatment includes reintroducing medical treatment or needling (discussed later). Surgical intervention should be postponed if possible for at least 6 months; at that time, options include (1) repeating the trabeculectomy with more postoperative 5-FU injections or mitomycin C, (2) placing a tube shunt, and (3) performing a cyclodestructive procedure.

In contrast to the flat, thick, failed bleb, the *encapsulated bleb* has a high and taut appearance (like an igloo) (Fig. 22–23). Patients with this condition have anterior chambers of normal depth. At initial evaluation, one might expect the pressure to be low because of the large size of the bleb; however, applanation tonometry demonstrates the opposite. Closer evaluation shows that the bleb has few microcysts and is firm.

Encapsulation can occur in up to 28% of patients undergoing glaucoma filtering surgery and typically occurs during the first 8 weeks after surgery.[35] Risk factors include previous argon laser trabeculoplasty, anterior uveitis, prolonged perioperative use of β-blockers and parasympathomimetic agents, previous encapsulated bleb, and preoperative corticosteroid injection over the fistula.

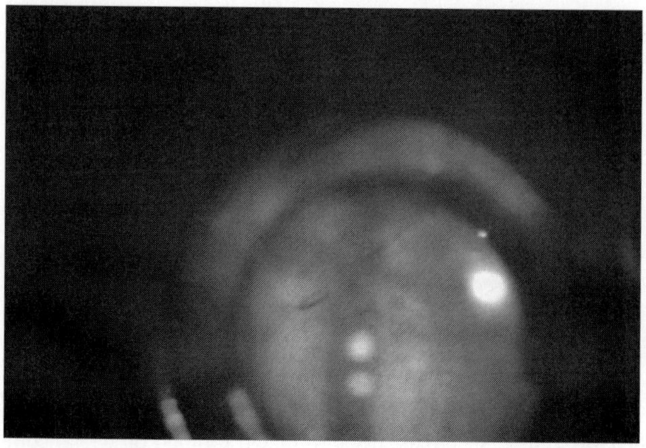

FIGURE 22–22. Cut suture viewed through a Hoskins lens.

The encapsulated bleb is composed of dense, compacted collagen tissue that creates a dome-like structure over the sclerostomy in direct communication with the anterior chamber. The thickened bleb wall prevents aqueous from exiting through the conjunctiva, resulting in the elevated pressure. Histopathologically, the encapsulation is composed of dense subconjunctival connective tissue sheets, few cells, and a noncellular lining.[36] Encapsulated blebs can create problems with high IOP and corneal dellen formation, leading to ocular discomfort.

Treatment options include observation, antiglaucoma medications, needling, and surgical revision. In some patients, the scar tissue thins spontaneously, and the pressure drops 8 to 12 weeks postoperatively. There are reports that aqueous egress itself promotes compaction of scar tissue and encapsulation. Therefore, with antiglaucoma medications, a temporary decrease in aqueous flow can lead to thinning of the encapsulated wall.[37]

If noninvasive measures fail, impaling or needling of the bleb with a 30-gauge needle has been advocated as having some success.[38] This technique is performed at the slit lamp with a lid speculum in place. The needle is passed into the encapsulated bleb from an entry site as distant as possible. Multiple passes are made into the encapsulation, with great care taken not to penetrate the overlying conjunctiva. Creating these multiple "sieve points" facilitates a drop in the IOP. However, many patients undergoing this procedure require medical augmentation or surgical revision for permanent IOP control.[39] Because of patient discomfort, surgical revision may also be required if the encapsulation is so large that it protrudes from the eye, causing corneal dellen.

HIGH IOP RESULTING FROM UNWANTED SUBSTANCES IN THE ANTERIOR CHAMBER

Any inappropriate substance in the anterior chamber can obstruct aqueous outflow through the trabecular meshwork and lead to an increase in IOP. This situation can occur in the patient who has undergone surgery or experienced trauma, or in some instances it can occur spontaneously.

TABLE 22–2. SUBSTANCES IN THE ANTERIOR CHAMBER THAT CAN CAUSE HIGH INTRAOCULAR PRESSURE

Blood (hyphema)
White blood cells (hypopyon, blebitis, endophthalmitis)
Pigment (pigmentary glaucoma, melanoma, uveitis-glaucoma-hyphema syndrome)
Vitreous
Fibrin
Lens components (cortex, denatured protein, and viscoelastic agents)
Intraocular gases and silicone oil

Treatment requires removal of the substance, with medications as necessary or observation for spontaneous resolution. Table 22–2 lists the various substances that commonly are found in the anterior chamber and lead to elevated IOP.

Hyphema

Hyphema (blood in the anterior chamber) can be seen after surgery or trauma (Fig. 22–24). The source of the blood may be the iris, ciliary body, or a scleral blood vessel. If the hyphema is small, observation alone is usually the treatment of choice. In a day or two, the blood either exits through the trabecular meshwork or, if glaucoma surgery was performed, flows out through the sclerostomy.

Rebleeding can also occur, at a reported incidence of 3.5% to 38%. Factors that lead to rebleeding are ocular hypotony, hypertension, aspirin use, and black race.[40] Rebleeds are a dreaded occurrence because they are likely to be more severe and to lead to complications such as glaucoma, corneal blood staining, and vitreous hemorrhage. Topical corticosteroids and dilating drops are used to prevent posterior synechiae and help clear the blood and its accompanying inflammation.

Increased IOP is related to the amount of hemorrhage in the anterior chamber. One study found elevated pressure in 13.5% of eyes with less than 50% hyphema, 27% of eyes with greater than 50% hyphema, and 52% with total hyphema.[41] Rebleeds lead to an even higher incidence of elevated pressure. Complete, or "eight-ball," hyphema has a 100% incidence of increased IOP. An "eight-ball" hyphema includes not only a 100% blood clot in the anterior chamber but also a clot in the posterior chamber. This results in a "collar-button" clot configuration that can cause papillary block. The treatment for this condition is the same as that for hyphemas described previously. Patients with this condition usually require surgery for resolution.

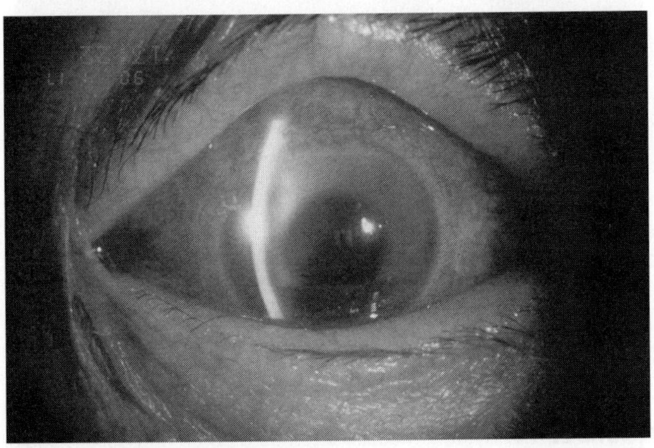

FIGURE 22–24. Hyphema; red blood cells in the anterior chamber.

The most common cause of the increased IOP resulting from hyphema is mechanical obstruction of the trabecular meshwork by red blood cells and blood products. Pupillary block may also occur if there is a large blood clot. Elevated pressure may also result from a poorly functioning traumatized trabecular meshwork. Bleb failure can occur via one of several mechanisms:

1. Fibroblastic precursor cells in the blood lead to excessive growth factors or scar formation, occluding the sclerostomy.
2. The blood can visually obscure the sutures in the flap, preventing suture lysis.
3. The blood can thicken the bleb wall, decreasing the flow of aqueous through the bleb.

Treatment is aimed at eliminating the blood clot. Tissue plasminogen activator (TPA) injected intracamerally can be used to dissolve the clot.[42, 43] Approximately 15 μL of a 1 mg/mL solution of lyophilized recombinant TPA in distilled water is injected into the anterior chamber. The clot usually disperses within 30 minutes. Potential complications include rebleeding and infection. If the treatment is unsuccessful, an anterior chamber washout may be indicated.

The risk of corneal blood staining increases if the hyphema persists with an increase in IOP. Classically, the cornea is opaque and rust-colored in appearance, with the discoloration occurring first in the posterior cornea. Once this complication appears, it can take years to resolve. If the amount of the hyphema is greater than 50% with IOP higher than 30 mm Hg for a prolonged period, an anterior chamber washout is indicated to prevent corneal blood staining.

If the hyphema develops several months after the anterior segment surgery, gonioscopy is needed to find the source of hemorrhage; most likely it is a small vessel near the sclerostomy or wound. This vessel can be ablated with the argon laser,[44] which is set for medium spot size with low energy and duration, just enough to cauterize the vessel.

Hypopyon

White blood cell–related causes of high IOP include hypopyon and endophthalmitis or blebitis. Hypopyon is an accumulation of white blood cells in the anterior chamber that can occur as a response to an infectious agent or a sterile condition associated with a systemic inflammatory disorder (Fig. 22–25).

Endophthalmitis immediately following surgery is rare, occurring in less than 0.1% of cases.[45] Its risk can be reduced with preoperative antibiotics and 1 drop of povidone-iodine solution preceding the surgery.[46, 47] The IOP increase in affected patients is secondary to blockage of the trabecular meshwork by the white blood cells and fibrin.

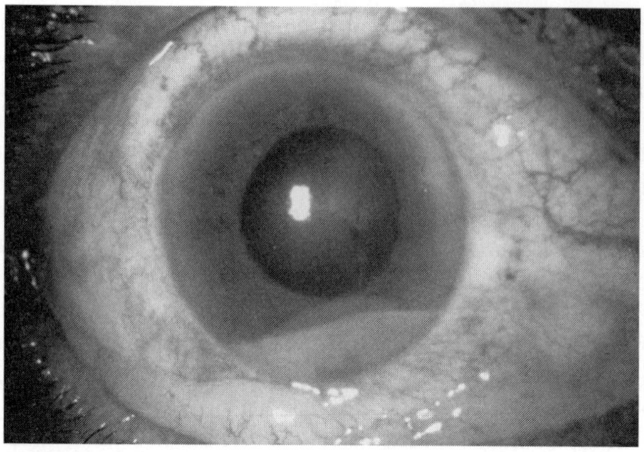

FIGURE 22–25. Hypopyon.

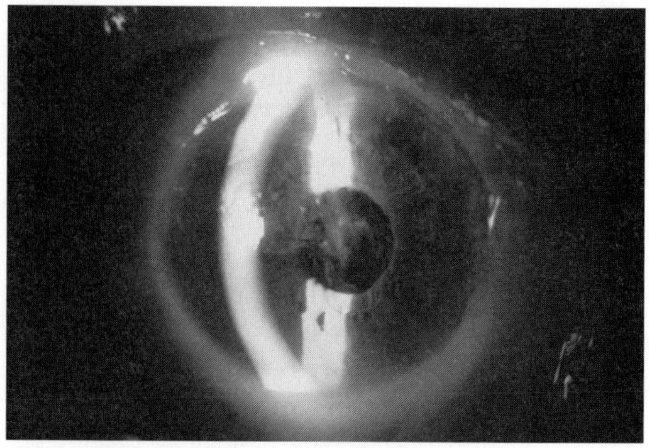

FIGURE 22–26. Vitreous to sclerostomy.

Pigment Plugging

Pigmentary glaucoma or pigment shedding in patients with ocular melanoma following trauma or surgery can cause an increase in IOP secondary to pigment plugging of the trabecular meshwork. See detailed discussion in Chapter 14.

Uveitis-Glaucoma-Hyphema Syndrome

Uveitis-glaucoma-hyphema (UGH) syndrome is another cause of blood and inflammatory cells in the anterior chamber.[48, 49] Although classically described as occurring after the implantation of anterior chamber intraocular lenses, now, most commonly, this condition occurs after cataract surgery in which a posterior chamber intraocular lens has been placed. The lens rubs against the ciliary body and posterior iris, causing pigment dispersion, uveitis, and, occasionally, blood in the anterior chamber if a ciliary vessel is damaged. Both the uveitis and the hyphema lead to IOP problems secondary to trabecular meshwork obstruction. This diagnosis is made clinically; the intraocular lens haptics are usually in the sulcus, and pigment chafing is noted as transillumination defects in the iris along the course of the haptics. UGH syndrome resolves with removal of the intraocular lens and placement of the new lens in the capsular bag.

Vitreous

Vitreous in the anterior chamber can be detrimental for IOP control. In the patient without glaucoma, vitreous loss during cataract surgery can occlude the trabecular meshwork, causing elevation of IOP. To prevent this complication, complete removal of the vitreous from the anterior chamber at the time of surgery is indicated. In the patient with glaucoma filtering surgery, vitreous can occlude the sclerostomy (following trabeculectomy) or the tube (following shunt placement) (Fig. 22–26).

This complication is best treated by prevention. Patients at risk for vitreous loss include those with large eyes and thin sclera, high myopia, pseudoexfoliation glaucoma, and aphakia. If the patient is aphakic or pseudophakic, care must be taken during surgery to prevent rupture of the anterior hyaloid face. A viscoelastic agent can be used to help keep the vitreous from coming forward and becoming incarcerated in the wound. If vitreous is present in the anterior chamber, a substantial vitrectomy is indicated, preferably from a pars plana approach. Vitreous that remains in the wound will occlude the sclerostomy, leading to filtration failure, and could create traction to the posterior pole, causing cystoid macular edema (Fig. 22–27) and possible retinal detachment.

Endophthalmitis or Blebitis

Endophthalmitis or blebitis can also occur years after a glaucoma filtering procedure. It has been reported in up to 1.5% of patients with filtration surgery.[47] The thinner the bleb, the greater the risk for development of endophthalmitis.[48] Bacteria enter the eye through the thin wall of the bleb, the most common bacteria being *Streptococcus*. Clinically, affected patients present with severe pain, a red eye, pus-fluid level in the bleb, intraocular inflammation (hypopyon), and decreased vision (Fig. 22–28).

Treatment depends on the presence and amount of anterior chamber and vitreous involvement. If the infection is limited to the bleb, topical fluoroquinolone and fortified cefazolin, 50 mg/mL, alternating every 30 minutes are usually sufficient to resolve the infection. As soon as the infection clears, topical corticosteroids should be initiated to prevent failure of the bleb. If the anterior chamber is

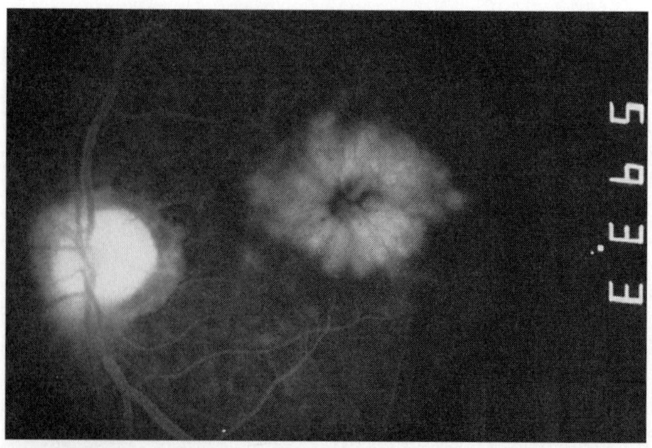

FIGURE 22–27. Cystoid macular edema noted on fluorescein angiogram.

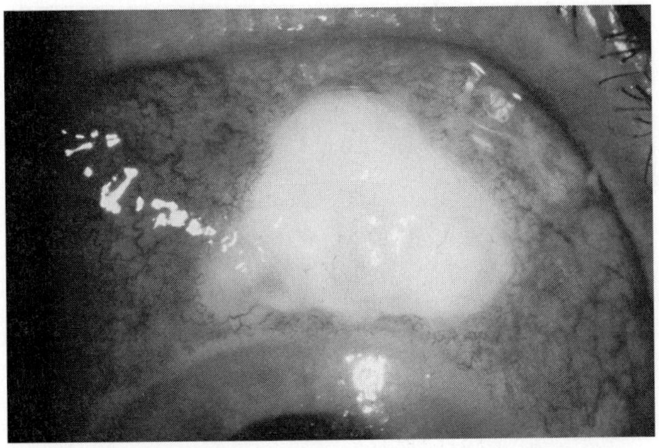

FIGURE 22–28. Blebitis. Note the infection in the filtering bleb.

involved, the eye is treated as for endophthalmitis. Anterior chamber and vitreous tap is performed with intravitreal injection of vancomycin, 1 mg/mL in 0.1 mL, and amikacin, 0.25 mg/ml in 0.1 mL, similar to the recommendation of the Endophthalmitis Vitrectomy Study.[50–52] In general, the earlier the treatment is initiated and the less virulent the bacteria, the better the visual outcome as well as the filter outcome. It is important to warn all patients with filtering blebs that they should immediately seek evaluation for any eye redness.

Fibrin

Fibrin can contribute to a sterile hypopyon (Fig. 22–29). This condition can occur after glaucoma filtering surgery, any anterior segment surgery or laser procedure, or spontaneously. It appears most commonly in patients with diabetes or an underlying systemic or ocular inflammatory disorder. The mechanism for the increase in IOP is similar to that for any unwanted substance in the anterior chamber: It clogs the trabecular meshwork. The underlying inflammatory disorder can also affect the function of the trabecular meshwork. In affected patients, endophthalmitis should always be considered and ruled out. Once infection is ruled out, topical and, if indicated, subconjunctival corticosteroids are used.

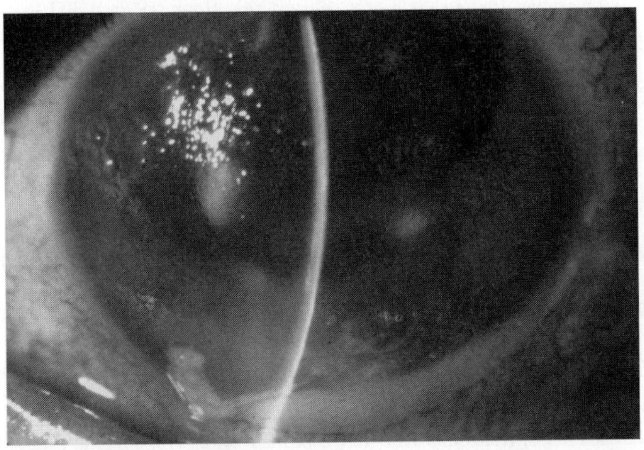

FIGURE 22–29. Fibrin hypopyon with sterile inflammatory products.

Cataract Components

Components of cataract, such as cortex, denatured lenticular protein, and viscoelastic agents, can all elevate the IOP by obstructing the trabecular meshwork. This situation usually occurs within the first few days after cataract surgery. In most cases, anti-inflammatory agents, glaucoma medications, and time resolve the problem. If not, surgical intervention may be indicated to remove the offending agent.

Intraocular Gas or Silicone Oil

Expansile intraocular gas and silicone oil are two other substances in the anterior chamber that could lead to increased IOP. As intraocular gas expands, the IOP increases, sometimes days after surgery. In many cases, antiglaucoma medications are sufficient to treat the temporary pressure spike.

Silicone oil can increase the IOP via two mechanisms. The first is direct obstruction of the trabecular meshwork by the large oil molecules. This situation is usually successfully treated with antiglaucoma medications. If the increase in IOP does not resolve and the integrity of the optic nerve is at risk, removal of the oil is indicated. The second mechanism is angle closure, which occurs via pupillary block at the oil interface with the pupillary margin. This condition is treated and prevented by placing a peripheral iridotomy inferiorly because the oil floats up. Should IOP not be controlled, this is a difficult situation because one needs silicone oil for its tamponading effects on the retina, and one typically is unable to perform filtering procedures with silicone oil present, as the silicone oil will exit through the filter.

Posterior Chamber

The posterior chamber is a small area bounded by the iris, lens, and zonules. It contains the ciliary body, which produces aqueous humor. Medications in particular can have significant effects on the posterior chamber, which in turn affects the anterior chamber.

Medications such as pilocarpine and atropine can affect the pupil and anterior chamber. The parasympathomimetic agent pilocarpine causes constriction of the pupil by its cholinergic effect on the iris sphincter muscle. It also contracts the ciliary muscle, causing forward movement of the iris-lens diaphragm, which in turn shallows the anterior chamber. Therefore, this agent should not be used in patients with aqueous misdirection. It does, however, reduce IOP in angle closure by reducing the pupillary block and relieving the crowded angle. In plateau iris syndrome, pilocarpine aids in relieving the crowded angle. In open-angle glaucoma, its effect of lowering intraocular pressure is mediated through increasing trabecular outflow of aqueous.

Atropine, an anticholinergic agent, has the opposite effect. It paralyzes both the iris sphincter and the ciliary muscle, resulting in pupillary dilation and posterior movement of the iris-lens diaphragm. The pupillary dilation is beneficial in postoperative patients because it prevents adhesions of the pupil to the lens. The relaxation of the ciliary muscle is beneficial in (1) deepening the anterior chamber after surgery, (2) preventing flattening of the chamber, and (3) relieving pain associated with postoperative inflammation. Atropine is useful in treating patients with aqueous misdirection: It pulls the lens back by tightening the zonules and may possibly break the ciliary block. This agent is also thought to stabilize the blood-aqueous barrier.

Iris and Pupil

The iris and pupil are two other anatomical structures that should be evaluated in any patient who has glaucoma or is to undergo surgery. Peripheral iridectomy (making a hole in the peripheral iris) is commonly performed with conventional glaucoma filtering surgery. It is created to prevent iris plugging of the sclerostomy and is also used to prevent or resolve angle-closure glaucoma. This is especially important in the patient with a shallow or flat anterior chamber secondary to hypotony.

The iridectomy itself can create problems for the patient, however. If it is too big, it can be a cosmetic problem, especially in a blue-eyed patient because it is more obvious (Fig. 22–30). There can also be a problem with glare if the iridectomy is so large that the upper lid does not cover it; a McCannel suture can reduce the size if the patient complains of unbearable glare. If the peripheral iridectomy is too small or imperforate, the iris may occlude the sclerostomy, causing failure of the surgery (Fig. 22–31).

Pupillary block may also occur if the too small laser iridotomy and the pupil become occluded, preventing the flow of aqueous from the posterior chamber into the anterior chamber. The too small iridotomy can be enlarged with the argon or Nd:YAG laser.

Lens

Lens problems after glaucoma filtering surgery are usually minimal. In the phakic eye, care must be taken to prevent lenticular penetration while creating the paracentesis, iridectomy, or sclerostomy. If penetration does occur, cataract extraction is indicated.

After surgery in patients with uveitis or diabetes, pupillary adhesions to the lens can occur, creating iris bombé with subsequent angle closure. Using cycloplegic agents to move the pupil can prevent this. If one is unable to break the synechiae, the treatment in these patients is peripheral iridotomy with the argon or Nd:YAG laser.

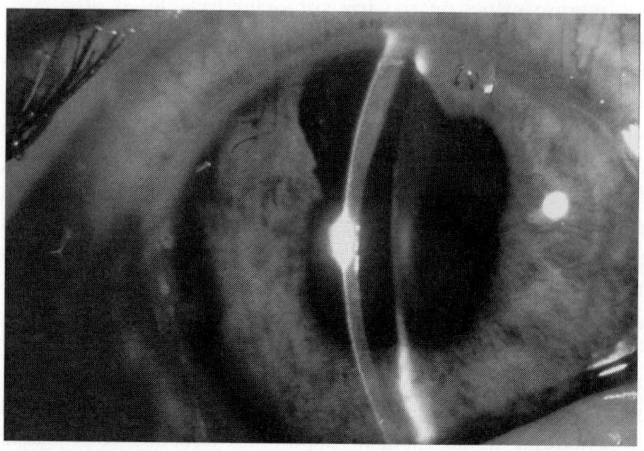

FIGURE 22–30. Large peripheral iridectomy.

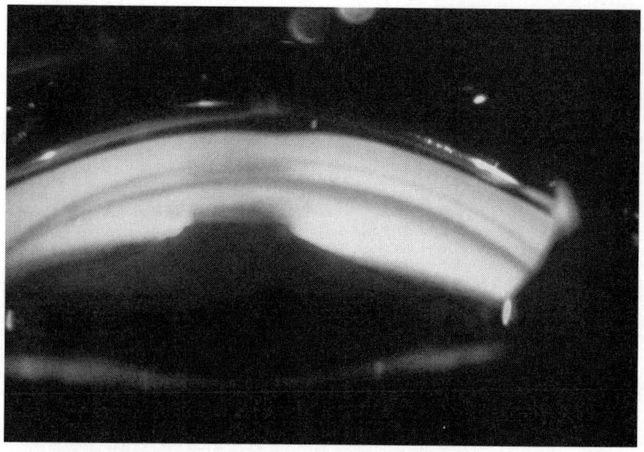

FIGURE 22–31. Gonioscopic view of iris plugging the sclerostomy.

Following glaucoma surgery, one may also note an increased progression to cataract formation, and it is important to warn patients that cataract extraction may become necessary earlier than if the glaucoma surgery were not performed.

SUMMARY

The biggest challenge for the ophthalmologist consists of the evaluation and treatment of the anterior and posterior chambers following surgery. By understanding the possible outcomes and subsequent treatments of glaucoma filtering surgery, the physician can avoid unnecessary worry and delays in resolving postoperative obstacles. Winston Churchill said it best: "Success is going from failure to failure without loss of enthusiasm." Good luck!

REFERENCES

1. Ritch R, Shield MB, Krupin T: Pressure dependent outflow. *In* The Glaucomas, 2nd ed. St. Louis, Mosby-Year Book, 1996, p 307.
2. Spaeth G: Glaucoma surgery. *In* Ophthalmic surgery: Principles and Practice. Philadelphia, WB Saunders, 1990, pp 335, 336
3. Starita RJ, Fellman RL, Spaeth GL, et al: Effect of varying size of scleral flap and corneal block on trabeculectomy. Ophthalmol Surg 1985;15:484.
4. Gehring R, Ciccarelli EC: Trichloroacetic acid treatment of filtering blebs following cataract extraction. Am J Ophthalmol 1972;74:622.
5. Yanuzzi LA, Theodore RH: Cryotherapy of postcataract blebs. Am J Ophthalmol 1973;76:622.
6. Lynch MG, Roesch M, Brown RH: Remodeling filtering blebs with the Nd:YAG laser. Ophthalmology 1996;103:1700.
7. Wise JD: Treatment of chronic postfiltration hypotony by intrableb injection of autologous blood. Arch Ophthalmol 1993;111:827.
8. Leen MM, Moster MR, Katz J, et al: Management of overfiltering and leaking blebs with autologous blood injection. Arch Ophthalmol 1995;113:1050.
9. Clinch TE, Kauffman HE: Repair of inadvertent conjunctival filtering blebs with a scleral flap. Arch Ophthalmol 1992;110:1652.

10. Cohen JD, Shaffer RN, Hetherington J Jr, et al: Revision of filtration surgery. Arch Ophthalmol 1977;95:1612.
11. Fellman R, Feldman R: Verbal communication 1997.
12. Wise JB: Mitomycin-compatible suture technique for fornix-based conjunctival flaps in glaucoma filtration surgery. Arch Ophthalmol 1993; 111:992.
13. Maumenee AE, Stark WJ: Management of persistent hypotony after planned or inadvertent cyclodialysis. Am J Ophthalmol 1971;71:320.
14. Romanchuk KG: Seidel's test using 10% fluorescein. Can J Ophthalmol 1979; 14:253.
15. Palmer RM, Burgoyne CF: Applications for a corneal mattress suture in anterior limbal wound repairs. Ophthalmic Surg 1994;25:726.
16. Bellows AR, Chylack JR, Hutchinson BT: Choroidal detachment: Clinical manifestation, therapy and mechanism of formation. Ophthalmology 1981;88:1107.
17. Katz LJ: Ciliochoroidal detachment. Ophthalmic Surg 1987;18:1775.
18. Stewart RJ, Kimbrough RL: A method of managing flat anterior chamber following trabeculectomy. Ophthalmic Surg 1980;11:382.
19. Brindley G, Shields MD: Value and limitations of cyclocryotherapy. Graefes Arch Clin Ophthalmol 1996;24:545.
20. Wright MM, Grajewski AL, Feuer WJ: Nd:YAG cyclophotocoagulation: Outcome of treatment for uncontrolled glaucoma. Ophthalmic Surg 1991;22:279.
21. Luntz MH, Rosenblatt M: Malignant glaucoma. Surv Ophthalmol 1987;32:73.
22. Shaffer RN, Hoskins HD: Ciliary block glaucoma. Ophthalmology 1978;85:215.
23. Trope G, Pavlin CJ, Bau A, et al: Malignant glaucoma. Clinical and ultrasound biomicroscopic characteristics. Ophthalmology 1994;101:1030.
24. Epstein DL, Steinert RF, Puliafito CA: Neodymium-YAG laser therapy to the anterior hyaloid in aphakic malignant (ciliovitreal block) glaucoma. Am J Ophthalmol 1984;98:137.
25. Anderson DR: Corneal indentation to relieve acute angle-closure glaucoma. Am J Ophthalmol 1979;88:1091.
26. Wand M, et al: Plateau iris syndrome. Trans Am Acad Ophthalmol Otolaryngol 1971;83:122.
27. Ritch R: Argon laser peripheral iridoplasty: An overview. J Glaucoma 1992;1:206.
28. Welch JC, Spaeth GL, Benson WE: Massive suprachoroidal hemorrhage: Follow-up and outcome of 30 cases. Ophthalmology 1988;95:1202.
29. Givens K, Shields MB: Suprachoroidal hemorrhage after glaucoma filtering surgery. Am J Ophthalmol 1987;103:689.
30. Liebmann JM, Ritch R: Complications of glaucoma filtering surgery. *In* The Glaucomas. St. Louis, CV Mosby 1996, p 1707.
31. Costa VP, Spaeth GL, Eiferman RA, et al: Wound healing modulation in glaucoma filtration surgery. Ophthalmic Surg 1993; 24:152.
32. Skuta GL, Parrish RK II: Wound healing in glaucoma filtering surgery. Surv Ophthalmol 1987;32:149.
33. Skuta GL: Antifibrotic agents in glaucoma filtering surgery. Int Ophthalmol Clin 1993;33:165.
34. Traverso CE, Greenidge KC, Spaeth GL, et al: Focal pressure: A new method to encourage filtration after trabeculectomy. Ophthalmic Surg 1984;15:62.
35. Richter CU, Singleton BJ, Bellows AR, et al: The development of encapsulated filtering blebs. Ophthalmology 1988;95:1163.
36. Addicks Em, Quigley HA, Green WR, et al: Histologic characteristics of filtering blebs in glaucomatous eyes. Arch Ophthalmol 1983;101:795.
37. Scott DR, Quigley HA: Medical management of a high bleb phase after trabeculectomies. Ophthalmology 1988;95:1169.
38. Shin DH, Juzych MS, Khatana AK, et al: Needling revision of failed filtering blebs with adjunctive 5-fluorouracil. Ophthalmic Surg 1993;24:242.
39. Pederson JE, Smith SG: Surgical management of encapsulated filtering blebs. Ophthalmology 1985;92:955.
40. Spoor TC, Kwitko GM, O'Grady JM, et al: Traumatic hyphema in an urban population. Am J Ophthalmol 1990; 109:23.
41. Cole WH: Traumatic hyphema: An analysis of 235 cases. South Med J 1968:61:813.
42. Tripathi RC, Tripathi BJ, Park JK, et al: Intracameral tissue plasminogen activator for resolution of fibrin clots after glaucoma filtering procedures. Am J Ophthalmol 1991:111:247.
43. Ortiz JR, Wakler SD, McManus PE, et al: Filtering bleb thrombolysis with tissue plasminogen activator. Am J Ophthalmol 1988;106:624.
44. Wilensky JT: Late hyphema after filtering surgery for glaucoma. Ophthalmic Surg 1983;14:227.
45. Katz LJ, Cantor LB, Spaeth GL: Complications of surgery in glaucoma: Early and late bacterial endophthalmitis following glaucoma filtering surgery. Ophthalmology 1985;92:959.
46. Apt L, Isenberg SJ, Yoshimori R, et al: Outpatient topical use of povidone-iodine in preparing the eye for surgery. Ophthalmology 1989;96:289.
47. Freedman J, Gupta M, Bunke A: Endophthalmitis after trabeculectomy. Arch Ophthalmol 1978;96:1017.
48. Aonuma H, Matsushita H, Nakajima K, et al: Uveitis-glaucoma-hyphema syndrome after posterior chamber intraocular lens implantation. Jpn J Ophthalmol 1997;41:98.
49. Magararal LE, Goldberg RE, Uram M, et al: Recurrent microhyphema in the pseudophakic eye. Ophthalmology 1983;90:1231.
50. Endophthalmitis Vitrectomy Study Group: Results of the endophthalmitis vitrectomy study: A randomized trial of immediate vitrectomy and of intravenous antibiotics for the treatment of postoperative bacterial endophthalmitis. Arch Ophthalmol 1995;113:1479.
51. Parke DW, Brinton GS: Endophthalmitis. *In* Tabbara KF (ed): Infections of the Eye. Boston, Little, Brown and Company, 1986, p 565.
52. Forster RK (ed): Endophthalmitis vitrectomy study. Arch Ophthalmol 1995;113:1555.

CHAPTER 23

Combined Cataract and Glaucoma Surgery

WELDON HAW, ROMMEL BAUTISTA,
and KULDEV SINGH

Cataract and glaucoma very commonly coexist in our patients. This chapter, by Weldon Haw, Rommel Bautista, and Kuldev Singh, addresses the complex question of how to surgically approach such cases. (Other implications of the two conditions are discussed in Chapter 15.) They begin with the initial decision as to the procedure to be performed: cataract extraction alone, glaucoma filtration surgery alone, or a combined procedure. The techniques for each of these procedures are described, with emphasis on those aspects that are most pertinent in patients with both cataract and glaucoma. In addition, the technique for single-site combined surgery is described in detail, including modifications often needed, such as management of the small pupil and the use of adjunctive antimetabolites. Next, these authors address the most common coexisting ocular disease, most commonly pseudoexfoliation. This chapter offers a rational approach to the common dilemma of the patient with coexisting cataracts and glaucoma.

Background

Both glaucoma and cataract are important causes of worldwide visual morbidity, and the two conditions commonly coexist in the same patient. An estimated 2 million Americans are afflicted with glaucoma, the incidence increasing with every decade of life to nearly 15% of the population more than 80 years of age.[1] The prevalence of visually significant cataracts is estimated to be 50% in individuals aged 65 to 74 years and to increase to 70% in those older than 75 years.[2] Thus, although coexistence of the two disorders may be rarely associated with a common etiology, the relationship between them is usually a simple matter of demographics—both conditions occur more commonly with increasing age. Given such high prevalences, the ophthalmic surgeon must be knowledgeable about current approaches to the evaluation, decision-making, and management for coexisting glaucoma and cataract.

Indications and Decisions

In patients with coexisting cataract and glaucoma, the determination to proceed with surgical intervention should encompass a detailed consideration of both the extent of glaucomatous damage and the status of the cataract. Particular attention should be given to the degree of lenticular opacity, visual impairment or symptoms experienced by the patient, the patient's visual needs and expectations, and concurrent disease that may affect postoperative visual function. The status of glaucomatous damage should also be evaluated with respect to the appearance of the optic nerve, visual field deficits, and the level of anticipated intraocular pressure (IOP) control needed to prevent progression. Last, the individual surgeon's experience and expertise should also be taken into account. Once the decision is made to proceed with surgical intervention, there are three basic therapeutic options to choose from:

- □ Cataract extraction alone
- □ Glaucoma filtering surgery alone with subsequent cataract extraction (two-stage approach)
- □ Combined cataract and glaucoma surgery

CATARACT EXTRACTION ALONE

With the advent of new surgical techniques and instrumentation, cataract extraction with posterior chamber intraocular lens (IOL) implantation have become a surgical intervention yielding increasingly efficacious, predictable, and safe outcomes. Despite the unique challenges of performing cataract extraction in a patient with glaucoma, the surgical results can be similarly successful. Thus, cataract extraction without filtration surgery is the ideal approach for treating patients with a visually significant cataract and mild glaucoma. In particular, the glaucomatous deficit should be minimal and the IOP should be acceptable and achieved with well-tolerated, simplified, low-dose glaucoma medication regimen.

In the 1970s, some ophthalmologists demonstrated an improvement in medical control of glaucoma with cataract extraction.[3–5] In 1971, Bigger and Becker[5] reported that 56% of eyes (in a surgical population of 100 eyes) that had glaucoma and underwent intracapsular cataract extraction (ICCE) demonstrated improvement, as evidenced by changes in mean IOP, medication use or both. Similar findings were reported in the same year by Randolph and colleagues,[3] who studied the effect of routine cataract extraction (then ICCE) on both controlled and uncontrolled glaucoma. In their series representing 166 cataract extractions, these investigators concluded that cataract extraction alone controlled primary open-angle glaucoma in 69.2% of eyes. By study definition, "controlled" meant that the patient did not have to use IOP-lowering medications for at least 2 years postoperatively. In 30.8% of the eyes, medical but not surgical therapy was subsequently necessary. In their discussion, Randolph and colleagues[3] speculated on two plausible explanations for the observed phenomenon. One was postoperative hypotony, which may last for 6 months, and the other was the physical deepening of the anterior chamber after cataract surgery. The researchers postulated that perhaps this chamber deepening helped facilitate trabecular meshwork functioning. One can propose the same hypothesis for modern-day phacoemulsification in patients with glaucoma.[6]

Improvement in IOP after cataract extraction is an unreliable postoperative outcome, however. Cataract extraction may, in fact, lead to progression of glaucomatous damage in a subset of patients who have compromised, glaucomatous optic nerves and who experience significant postoperative IOP spikes. Compared with controls, patients with glaucoma undergoing cataract extraction more commonly experience a significant elevation in IOP within the early postoperative period.[7]

This observation was clearly demonstrated in a 1996 study by Barak and associates[7] of early postoperative IOP patterns. The study involved IOP determinations in groups of glaucomatous and nonglaucomatous eyes undergoing routine extracapsular cataract extraction (ECCE) with posterior chamber IOL implantation. Applanation tonometry was then performed every 4 hours for 24 hours postoperatively. Study results revealed that glaucomatous eyes experienced more significant IOP elevations after cataract surgery than nonglaucomatous eyes. The significance of such data lies in the fact that IOP checks are usually performed only once on the first postoperative day and that early IOP rise (usually 6–12 hours after surgery) may go undetected. This study may imply serious consequences for compromised glaucomatous eyes with poor tolerance for IOP spikes. In such high-risk patients (i. e., those with glaucoma undergoing cataract surgery), there appears to be a clear and valid need for prophylactic treatment in the form of IOP-lowering medications or even laser trabeculoplasty.[8] From a surgical standpoint, it may be wise to consider combined glaucoma and cataract surgery.

Compared with the combined and two-stage approaches, cataract surgery alone offers several advantages. It not only is a technically simpler surgical intervention but also is less often associated with complications and more commonly results in rapid visual rehabilitation. In addition, long-term postoperative IOP may occasionally improve from preoperative levels with ECCE.[9, 61]

In any event, because the possibility of future trabeculectomy can never be completely excluded in any patient with glaucoma, care should be taken to preserve the maximal amount of conjunctiva during the cataract extraction. Doing so will optimize the chances of successful trabeculectomy if it becomes necessary. Small-incision surgery, clear cornea phacoemulsification, and the development of antimetabolites[10] can be expected to optimize successful filtration surgery in pseudophakic and aphakic eyes with glaucoma.

GLAUCOMA FILTERING SURGERY ALONE WITH SUBSEQUENT CATARACT EXTRACTION (TWO-STAGE PROCEDURE)

Under conditions of advanced glaucomatous damage or severe and uncontrolled glaucoma despite maximal medical management, the control of IOP is the primary concern. The visual concerns specific to the cataract become secondary to the possibility of progressive and irreversible glaucomatous disability and, thus, are managed at a later date. Immediate reduction of IOP is necessary, so the procedure with the maximal probability of success, trabeculectomy alone, is preferred.

The two-stage approach is also a viable consideration in patients with severe glaucoma and multiple risk factors for filtration failure namely, (1) neovascular or inflammatory glaucoma, (2) prior intraocular surgery, and (3) being young or of African heritage.[11] In addition, the two-stage approach may be particularly useful in patients with compromised visual function resulting from miotic therapy. In such patients, postoperative discontinuation of the miotic therapy may allow sufficient visual function despite the cataract, precluding cataract surgery.

When the two-stage approach is indicated, filtration surgery is performed several months prior to cataract extraction. The filtration procedure may involve trabeculectomy with or without use of antimetabolites or implantation of a shunt. It is advisable to perform trabeculectomy in the superonasal quadrant. A superonasal filtration bleb will not interfere with cataract extraction through either a clear cornea or inferotemporal approach.

The two-stage approach nevertheless has multiple shortcomings. The patient undergoes two surgical procedures with all the associated complications, including a longer recovery period, more frequent follow-up visits, and often poorer vision between filtration surgery and cataract extraction. In addition, subsequent cataract extraction may incite ocular inflammation, subconjunctival fibroblast proliferation, and scarring, enhancing the possibility of future filtration failure.

In view of those concerns, it is not surprising that the likelihood of long-term IOP control with two-stage procedures has been questioned.[12, 13] However, with the evolution of small-incision cataract surgery and the use of antimetabolites with trabeculectomy, the success of combined cataract and glaucoma surgery has dramatically improved. For these reasons, many surgeons perform combined surgery in patients for whom, historically, two-stage procedures were indicated. The basis for this decision has been supported with various studies that have described similar efficacy rates for combined procedures, isolated filtration surgery, and two-stage cataract and glaucoma surgery.[14, 62]

Hefetz and associates[62] attempted to make a comparison between combined and sequential (two-stage) procedures by using IOP control and visual outcome as determinants. The postoperative results in approximately 50 subjects divided into surgical groups (sequential surgery and combined surgery) suggested no significant difference in success rates as far as IOP and final visual acuity were concerned. Thus, as the success of combined procedures continues to evolve, the indications for two-stage procedures versus combined procedures will also change.

COMBINED CATARACT AND GLAUCOMA SURGERY

Cataract extraction combined with glaucoma filtration surgery has many advantages. It limits the patient's exposure to possible complications from two procedures, affords rapid restoration of vision in a single procedure, and often prevents postoperative IOP spikes. In addition, less cumulative follow-up time is required than for the two-stage approach. However, combined procedures are technically more difficult than cataract or glaucoma surgery alone and are associated with a slightly higher risk of early postoperative complications, including persistent inflammation, hypotony, shallow anterior chamber, and hyphema.[15] Additionally, some investigators have suggested that long-term IOP control may not be as reliable with combined procedures as with two-stage intervention.[16, 17, 63]

In a 1997 study conducted at Yale University, Park and associates[63] concluded that IOP control was less effective in patients undergoing phacoemulsification with separate-site superior trabeculectomy than in those undergoing trabeculectomy alone. Although long-term IOP control was noted to be less successful in the combined procedures group, these researchers maintained that combined glaucoma and cataract surgery remains an effective procedure for lowering IOP and reducing long-term antiglaucoma medication requirements and is certainly appropriate in selected patients.

Combined cataract and glaucoma surgery should be carefully evaluated and performed only in appropriate situations. It can be considered in patients in whom cataract extraction is indicated and one of the following conditions exists: (1) uncontrolled glaucoma, (2) intolerable, significant, medication-induced side effects, (3) advanced glaucomatous damage such that any transient postoperative IOP elevation may result in progressive visual field loss and (4) borderline glaucoma with infeasibility of two operations or doubt about long-term medication compliance.

Ritch and associates[18] suggest that prior to combined surgery, laser trabeculoplasty be considered. If glaucomatous damage is mild, successful laser trabeculoplasty may temporarily preclude the need for combined surgery and may allow the ophthalmologist to proceed with cataract extraction alone. In patients with moderate to severe glaucomatous damage, however, a combined procedure may still be indicated, because performing laser trabeculoplasty prior to cataract extraction does not reliably predict early or long-term postoperative IOP control. In all cases, the decision should be individualized for the patient's clinical status.

The standard approach to combined surgery historically involved either ICCE or ECCE in conjunction with filtration surgery.[19, 20, 64–67] This approach has yielded varying results in terms of IOP control compared with trabeculectomy alone.[14] The continued refinement in small-incision cataract techniques and the increasing use of antimetabolites in combined surgical intervention have made long-term IOP control an expectation rather than a rarity.

Although some preliminary studies comparing ECCE with phacoemulsification in combined procedures have failed to demonstrate a difference in glaucoma control with short-term followup,[22, 23] bleb formation is more often seen in conjunction with phacoemulsification than with ECCE.[23] This observation may be predictive of a longer duration of IOP control with phacotrabeculectomy.[22] Indeed, some studies have demonstrated better long-term IOP control after combined procedures using phacoemulsification.[23]

Additional advantages of combined surgery utilizing phacoemulsification over ECCE are (1) smaller incision size, resulting in less conjunctival trauma, (2) less deleterious astigmatic consequences, (3) accelerated visual rehabilitation, (4) reduced need for pupillary enlargement techniques, and (5) fewer complications (hyphema, fibrinous iritis, choroidal detachment, hypotony, and posterior capsular opacification).[24] Multiple studies have reinforced the safety and efficacy of phacoemulsification in combined procedures.[25, 68] Wedrich and colleagues,[68] in a series of 49 eyes with a mean follow-up of 31.5 months, found that functional long-term results of same-site phacoemulsification and trabeculectomy were excellent. Their data showed that IOP control was achieved in all eyes, 80% of eyes required no medications postoperatively, and 16% required fewer medications. In 78%, a final visual acuity of 20/40 or better was achieved, consistent with the results achieved by combined procedures using the ECCE technique.

Continuing advances in the surgical approach to combined procedures have led to the development of temporal clear cornea phacoemulsification combined with separate-incision trabeculectomy.[18, 26] The risks and benefits of this two-site combined technique relative to single-site surgery is under investigation.

Technique

PREOPERATIVE CONSIDERATIONS

Before proceeding with any surgical intervention, the surgeon should perform a detailed preoperative examination. If cataract extraction is anticipated, the examination should include an evaluation of postoperative visual acuity potential. Macular function undisrupted by media opacity may be estimated by near visual acuity through the pinhole and the Potential Acuity Meter (PAM). The PAM may be particularly useful in patients with mild to moderate glaucomatous damage and visual acuity better than 20/60.[27] Use of perifoveal thresholds from automated perimetry in conjunction with PAM provides reliable estimates of postoperative visual acuity as better than 20/40 in 90% of cases.[28] However, it is not significantly better than chance alone in predicting vision less than 20/40.[28]

External ocular examination and slit-lamp biomicroscopy are essential components of the preoperative evaluation. They allow an assessment of coexisting ocular disease that may alter the intraoperative or postoperative course. Conjunctival and eyelid infections, entropion, ectropion, and trichiasis should be identified and appropriately managed prior to surgery. Slit-lamp biomicroscopy of the anterior segment may reveal endothelial guttae, which may increase the chance of corneal decompensation and the need for large amount of a viscoelastic agent to protect the compromised endothelium. Phacodonesis may indicate the presence of loose lens zonules, increasing the chance of intraoperative vitreous loss. Pseudoexfoliative material alerts the surgeon to the higher risk of intraoperative zonular disruption and poor pupillary dilation. Iris neovascularization indicates underlying ocular disease that may influence the success and complication rates for a combined procedure (Table 23–1).

Preoperative gonioscopy should also be performed. The preoperative presence of angle closure may indicate a greater likelihood of postoperative IOP elevation or the rare complication of malignant glaucoma. The position of angle neovascularization and peripheral anterior synechiae should be noted in case anterior chamber IOL placement is required, because irritation of these areas may lead to a chronic iritis or a uveitis-glaucoma-hyphema (UGH) syndrome.

Pupillary dilation during the preoperative evaluation not only maximizes the surgeon's evaluation of the fundus and optic nerve but also allows the surgeon to assess whether iris surgery will be required intraoperatively. This issue is particularly important in the case of the rigid and immobile pupils more common in eyes affected with pseudoexfoliation syndrome and eyes that have undergone long-term miotic therapy. Dilation should be performed at least 2 days prior to the operation in order to avoid fatigue of the dilating mechanism, which would result in poor intraoperative dilation.

TABLE 23–1. EXAMPLES OF SLIT-LAMP EXAMINATION FINDINGS AND THEIR POSSIBLE SURGICAL COMPLICATIONS

Finding	Surgical Complication
Corneal guttae	Corneal decompensation
Phacodonesis	Loose zonules, vitreous loss
Pseudoexfoliation material	Zonular disruption, vitreous loss, poor pupillary dilation
Iris neovascularization	Intraoperative bleed

The patient's medications should also be reviewed. Particular attention should be given to medications that may (1) affect intraoperative pupillary dilation (if cataract extraction is to be performed) or (2) increase anterior segment–conjunctival hyperemia, which may exacerbate ocular surface bleeding or inflammation. Strong miotics, such as echothiophate iodide, may contribute to significant inflammation in the phakic eye as well as limit pupillary dilation and should be discontinued at least 2 weeks prior to surgery. Pilocarpine and carbachol should be stopped at least 1 day prior to surgery to allow maximal pupillary dilation. Epinephrine-like drugs, such as dipivefrin, may increase anterior segment hyperemia and should be discontinued 1 to 2 weeks prior to surgery.

For eyes in which progression of glaucomatous damage during this preoperative drug holiday is a concern, other topical medications or oral carbonic anhydrase inhibitors may be used. The medical risks of discontinuing systemic medications that increase bleeding, such as aspirin, nonsteroidal anti-inflammatory drugs, and anticoagulants (warfarin sodium [Coumadin]), should be evaluated in consultation with the patient's internist.

ANESTHESIA

Most surgeons prefer monitored anesthesia care in concert with peribulbar or retrobulbar injection. The three most commonly used injectable anesthetics are lidocaine, bupivacaine, and mepivacaine. With regard to lid akinesia, they have similar onset time (less than 6 minutes) but different durations of action. Bupivacaine has the longest duration (up to 6 hours), and lidocaine the shortest (15–30 minutes).[29] Thus, a commonly used mixture consists of a 1:1 mix of 2% lidocaine (Xylocaine) with epinephrine and 0.75% bupivacaine (Marcaine) along with 150 units of hyaluronidase (Wydase). Hyaluronidase produces a more rapid anesthetic effect by increasing the speed of diffusion of the anesthetic in the retrobulbar space.[30]

CATARACT SURGERY ALONE

In the select population undergoing cataract surgery alone, glaucoma filtration surgery is unanticipated but can never be completely excluded as a future possibility. Thus, the possibility that conjunctival scarring might preclude future successful filtration surgery must always be kept in mind. When the decision is made to proceed with cataract extraction alone in a patient who also has glaucoma, minimizing postoperative conjunctival mechanical trauma and inflammation becomes significant. This issue is especially important if the cataract surgery is to be performed at the superior limbal conjunctiva, which may be the site of choice for future trabeculectomy. With small-incision limbal cataract techniques in the superonasal or superotemporal quadrants or the temporal clear cornea approach, enough superior conjunctiva can generally be preserved to allow for future trabeculectomy.

As described earlier, particular attention should be given to minimizing postoperative IOP spikes, which may theoretically predispose a compromised glaucomatous optic nerve to further damage. Fortunately, patients with coexisting glaucoma and cataract in whom cataract extraction alone is indicated typically have minimal glaucomatous damage and their IOP is well controlled with medical therapy. Thus, preoperative laser trabeculoplasty may not be necessary.

Patients with glaucoma who are undergoing cataract extraction may pose numerous surgical challenges for the ophthalmologist. Small pupil techniques and other special surgical circumstances specific to cataract extraction in patients with glaucoma are described later. Other than keeping in mind the specific importance of maximizing conjunctival preservation, managing the preoperative medication regimen (addressed earlier), maximizing preoperative IOP control, and dealing with a small pupil and other special surgical circumstances, the surgeon can perform small-incision or temporal clear cornea phacoemulsification in association with posterior chamber IOL insertion in the standard manner. A detailed description of the technique of standard small-incision or temporal clear cornea phacoemulsification with posterior chamber IOL implantation is beyond the scope of this chapter.

COMBINED CATARACT AND GLAUCOMA SURGERY PERFORMED AT A SINGLE SITE

Combined surgery has made the evolution from cataract extraction, in conjunction with full-thickness filtration procedures or cyclodialysis, to the current "guarded" filtration techniques involving a scleral flap. The previous standard for combined surgery at a single incision site involved ECCE and filtration surgery. However, many surgeons have made the transition to combined surgery using phacoemulsification techniques. The success and safety of combined procedures with filtration, phacoemulsification, and IOL implantation have been well established.[31–34]

BRIDLE SUTURE

A bridle suture is rarely needed for a fornix-based approach. However, if a limbus-based approach is anticipated, a partial-thickness corneal bridle suture is important in achieving adequate conjunctival exposure (Fig. 23–1). A 6-0, 7-0, or 8-0 silk or polyglactin (Vicryl) suture is placed in the cornea just anterior to the superior limbal site where the planned trabeculectomy flap will be located. This placement avoids the conjunctival injury and subconjunctival hemorrhage seen with rectus muscle bridle sutures. The globe is then rotated inferiorly to provide adequate superior exposure. The traction suture is usually kept in place throughout the duration of the procedure.

CONJUNCTIVAL FLAP

A fornix-based or limbus-based conjunctival flap may then be carefully isolated with blunt dissection. A fornix-based flap is technically easier to perform, allows shorter operating time, and may improve visualization of the anterior chamber during phacoemulsification. There is a theoretical risk of greater bleb leakage with the fornix-based flap. However, studies have demonstrated that with the exception of higher incidence of posterior capsular rupture with limbus-based flaps, the safety and effectiveness of both types of conjunctival flaps appear to be quite similar in combined phacoemulsification, IOL implantation, and filtration procedures, even with the use of mitomycin C (MMC).[36, 37]

The surgeon constructs a fornix-based conjunctival flap (Fig. 23–2) by performing a 5.0- to 6.0-mm limbal peritomy and then isolating Tenon's fascia. Once Tenon's fascia is free, conjunctival manipulation can be restricted. Tenon's fascia should be handled with nontoothed forceps to prevent additional injury. With blunt dissection, sub–Tenon's space is exposed. Gentle diathermy may be required to achieve adequate hemostasis.

In contrast, the surgeon constructs a limbus-based flap (Fig. 23–3) by incising the conjunctiva as far superiorly as

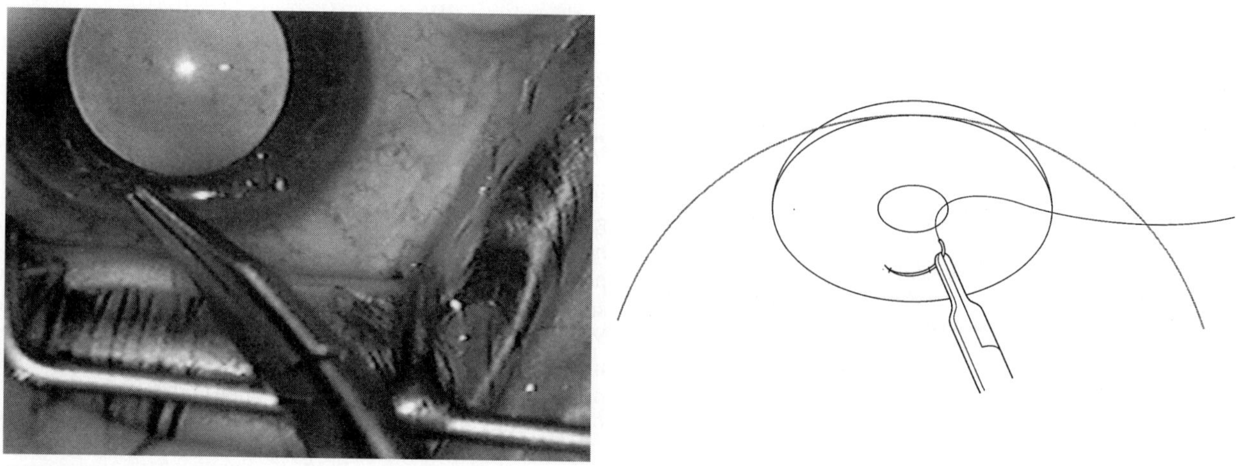

FIGURE 23–1. Bridle suture

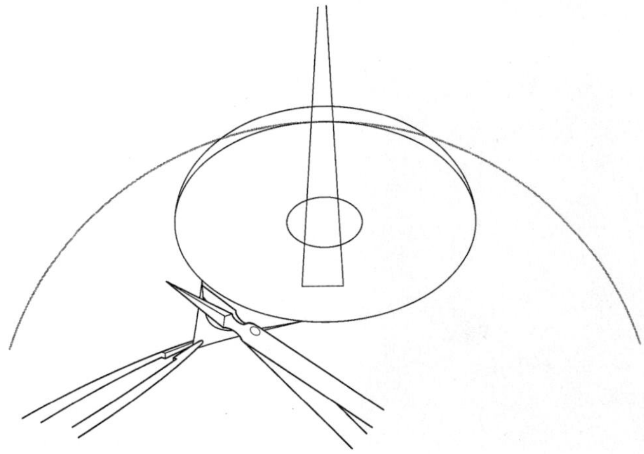

FIGURE 23–2. Fornix-based conjunctival flap

possible. The incision should involve approximately 2 "clock hours" and should be at least 8 mm posterior to the limbus. Adequate exposure is facilitated by inferior rotation of the globe with the corneal bridle suture. Blunt dissection within the sub–Tenon's space can be carried anteriorly to the limbus. As with the fornix-based flap, nontoothed forceps are used to handle Tenon's fascia (avoiding manual manipulation of conjunctiva).

HEMOSTASIS

Diathermy is applied gently over hemorrhaging blood vessels. Excessive burning or charring is avoided. A sponge (Weck-Cel, Bristol-Myers Squibb, New York, NY) is used to remove any coagulum deposited during the hemostatic process.

SCLERAL FLAP

A partial-thickness scleral flap measuring 3.5 mm horizontally and 2.5 mm vertically on either side is created (Fig. 23–4). A longer incision (6.0 mm vs. 3.0 mm) may result in poorer early postoperative visual acuity but does not make a significant difference in final visual acuity or IOP control.[38] Any shape flap, rectangular, triangular, or semicircular, may be used, its choice depending on surgeon preference. The scleral flap is isolated by directing the dissection anteriorly with a No. 69 Beaver blade or similar instrument. A 0.12 forcep can be used to carefully grasp the end of the scleral flap to facilitate dissection. The flap is carried anteriorly to just within clear cornea.

APPLICATION OF ANTIMETABOLITES

If intraoperative 5-fluorouracil (5-FU) or MMC is to be applied, a sponge (Weck-Cel) soaked in 0.2 to 0.5 mg/mL MMC or 50 mg/mL 5-FU may be placed over or under the scleral flap (with the conjunctiva–Tenon's fascial flap also reflected over the sponge) for approximately 1 to 5 minutes (Fig. 23–5). This is followed by aggressive rinsing of both the flap and the antimetabolite-contaminated instruments.

LIMBAL PARACENTESIS

A limbal paracentesis may be safely performed after all antimetabolite has been irrigated (Fig. 23–6). A No. 75 Beaver blade, Alcon SuperSharp 15-degree blade (Alcon, Fort Worth, TX), or similar blade is used to complete a

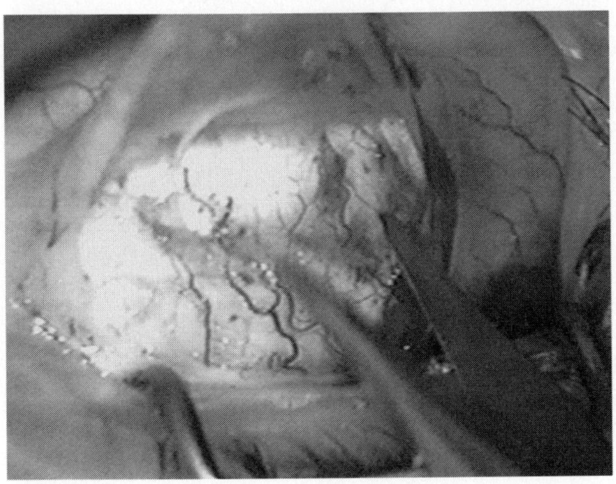

FIGURE 23–3. Limbus-based conjunctival flap

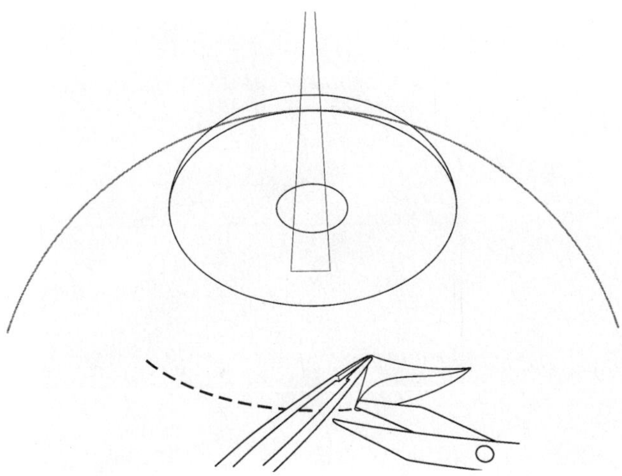

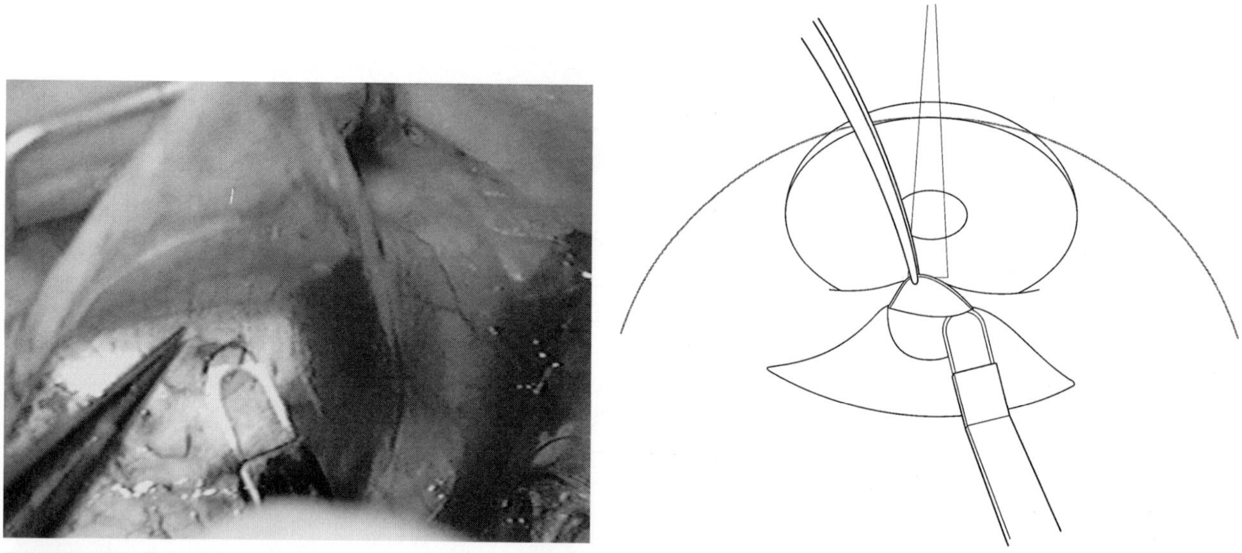

FIGURE 23–4. Scleral flap

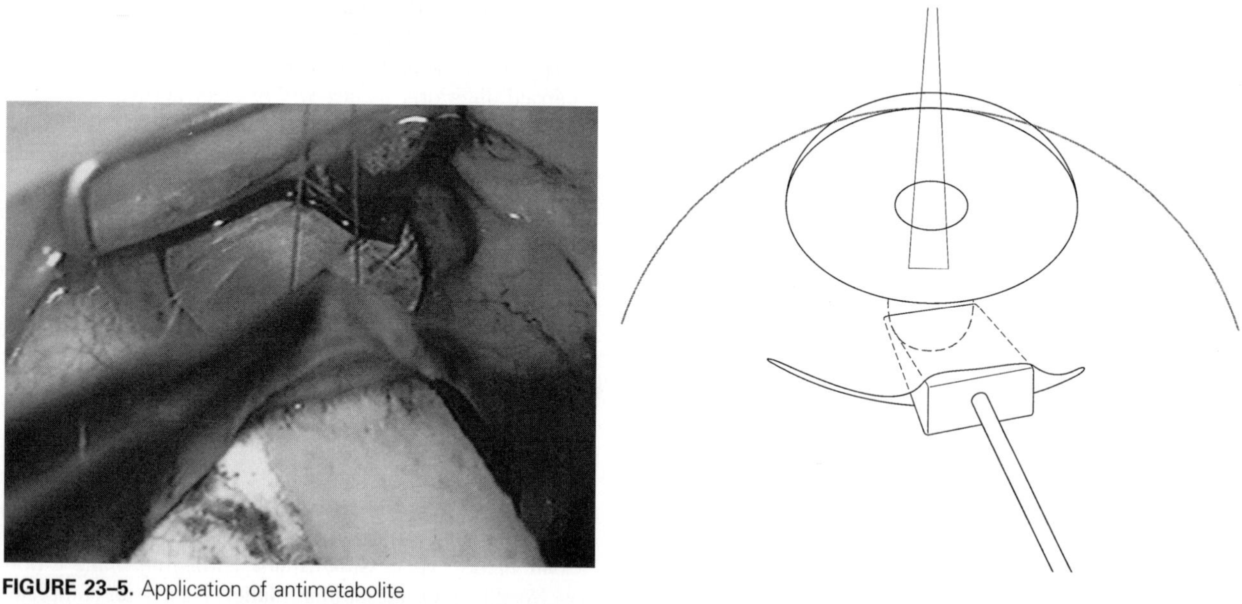

FIGURE 23–5. Application of antimetabolite

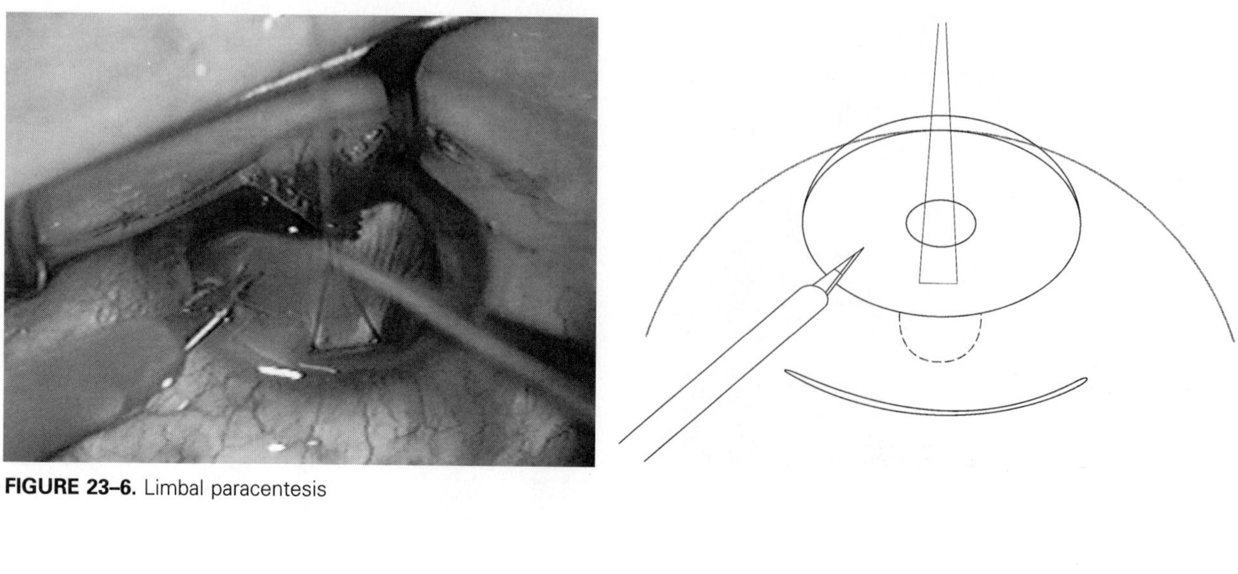

FIGURE 23–6. Limbal paracentesis

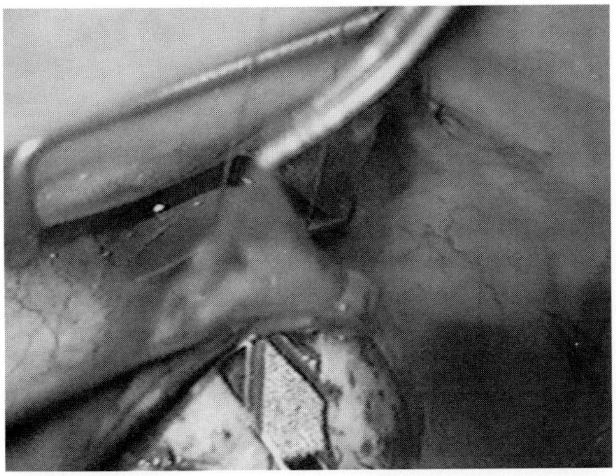

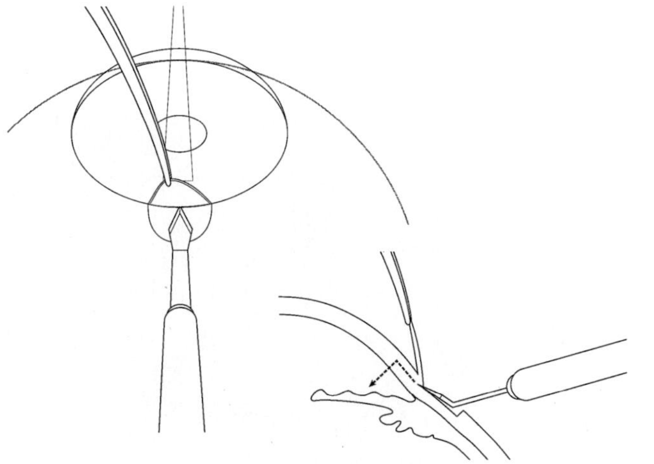

FIGURE 23–7. Entry into anterior chamber through the scleral tunnel

limbal paracentesis at the "1:30" position for a right-handed surgeon or the "10:30" position for a left-handed surgeon. A paracentesis allows insertion of a second instrument during cataract extraction, reformation of the anterior chamber, and inflation of the bleb to test for leakage at the conclusion of the operation.

ANTERIOR CHAMBER ENTRY

Following injection of viscoelastic fluid into the anterior chamber through the paracentesis, a 3.0-mm keratome may be used to enter the anterior chamber through the anterior-most aspect of the scleral tunnel (Fig. 23–7). Keeping the keratome perpendicular to the iris plane limits stripping of Descemet's membrane and traumatic dissection into the corneal stroma.

TECHNIQUES FOR SMALL PUPILS

Pupillary enlargement techniques (discussed later) may be performed as needed.

CAPSULOTOMY AND HYDRODISSECTION

A continuous-tear capsulotomy 5 to 6 mm in diameter is performed with the use of a cystotome or Utrata capsulorhexis forceps (Fig. 23–8). Hydrodissection and hydrodelineation may be performed, as in a typical cataract extraction, with the injection of balanced salt solution via a 27-gauge cannula (Fig. 23–9).

PHACOEMULSIFICATION

The surgeon then performs phacoemulsification by grooving the nucleus and removing pieces as either quadrants or smaller segments, as in "phaco-chop" techniques (Fig. 23–10). Phacoemulsification of the small pupil is discussed in more detail later. The epinucleus is removed, and cortical clean-up is performed using a standard automated irrigation and aspiration system (Fig. 23–11).

INSERTION OF THE INTRAOCULAR LENS

Additional viscoelastic fluid is injected within the anterior chamber and into the capsular bag. A blunt-tipped keratome may then be used to enlarge the incision to an appropriate length, and a foldable posterior chamber IOL is inserted into the inflated posterior capsular bag through the scleral tunnel incision (Fig. 23–12). Alternately, a polymethyl-methacrylate (PMMA) nonfoldable lens can be in-

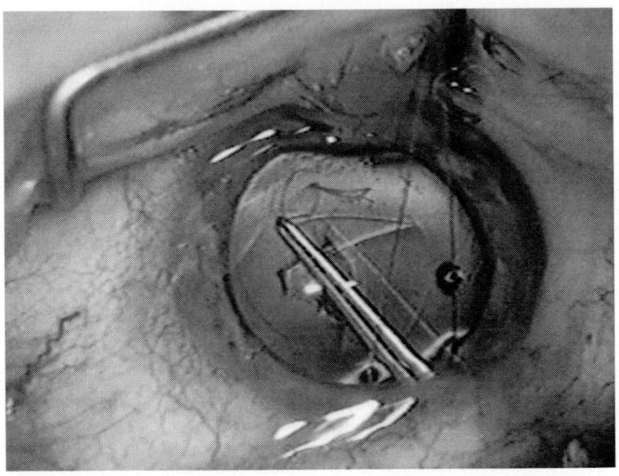

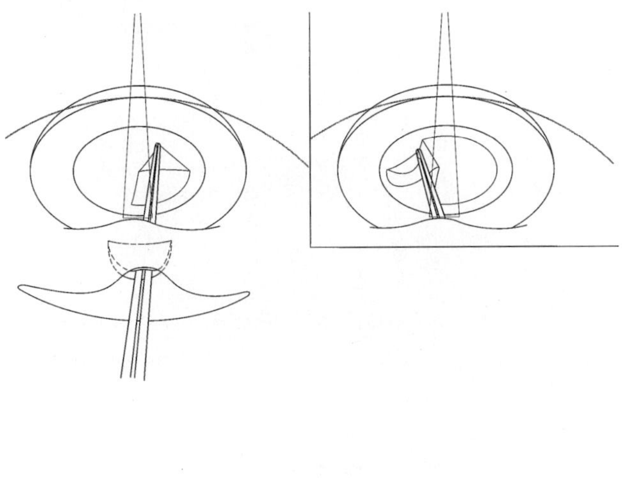

FIGURE 23–8. Capsulotomy

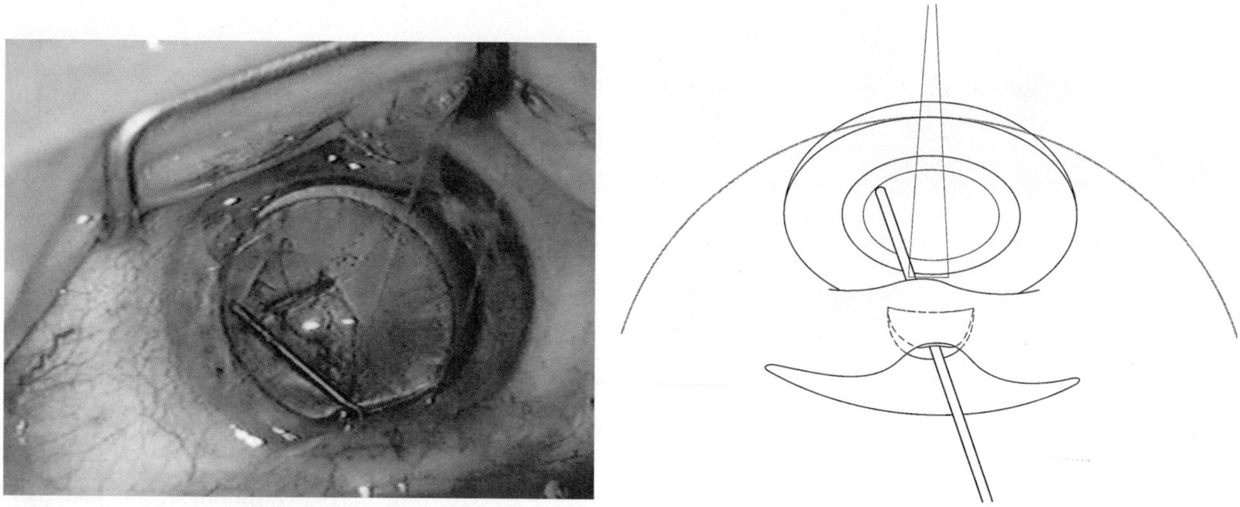

FIGURE 23–9. Hydrodissection

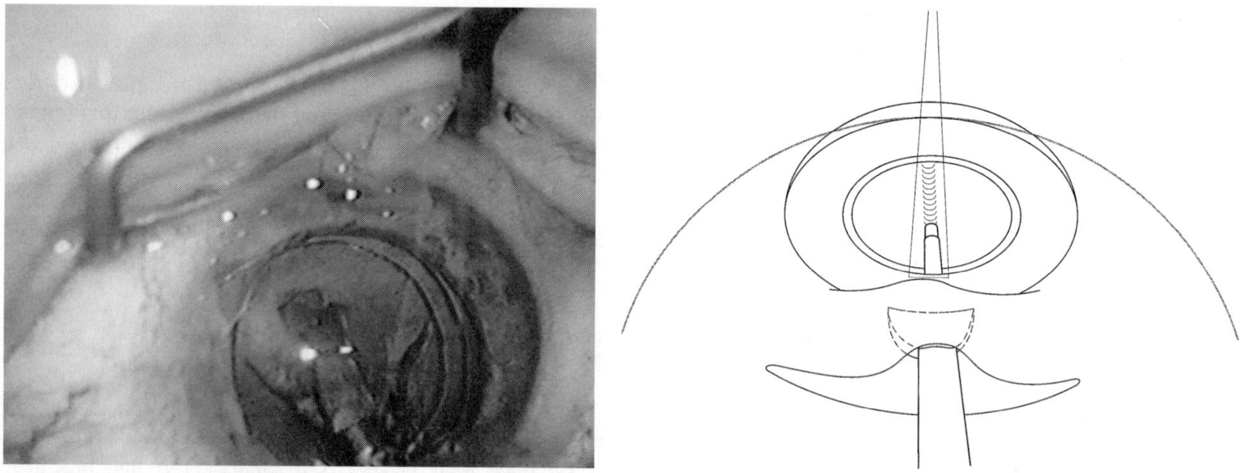

FIGURE 23–10. Phacoemulsification: grooving the nucleus

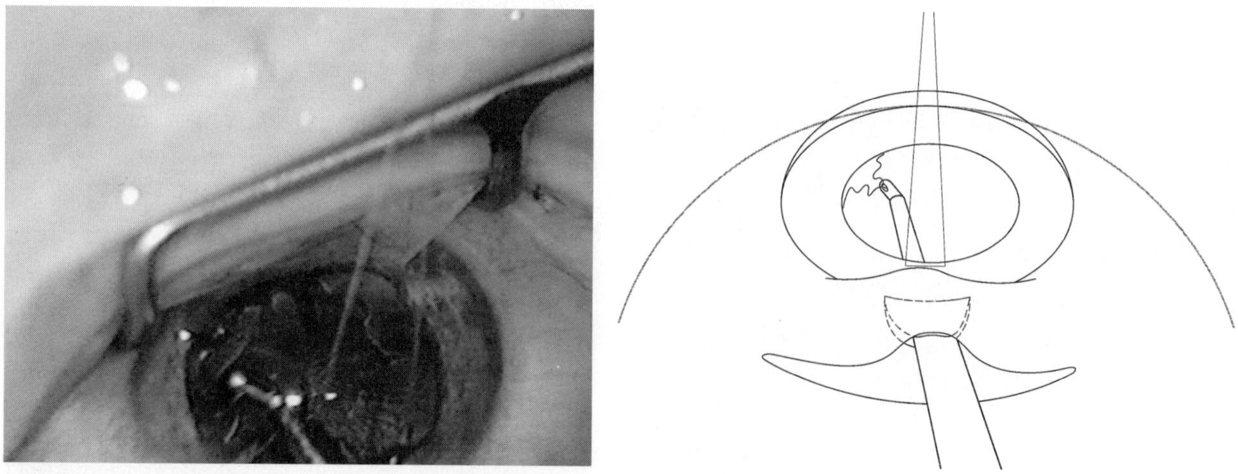

FIGURE 23–11. Phacoemulsification: cortical clean-up

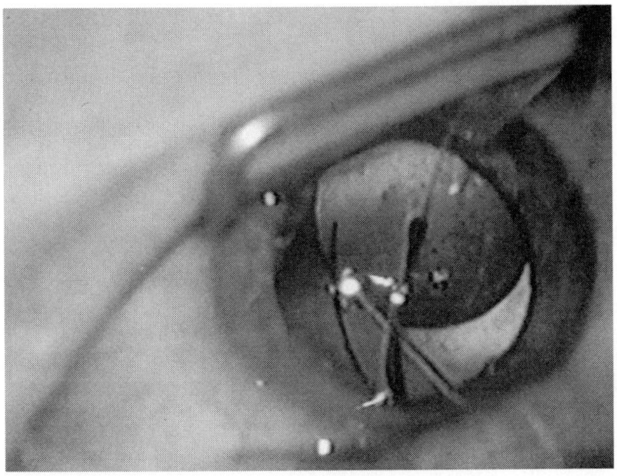

FIGURE 23–12. Insertion of intraocular lens

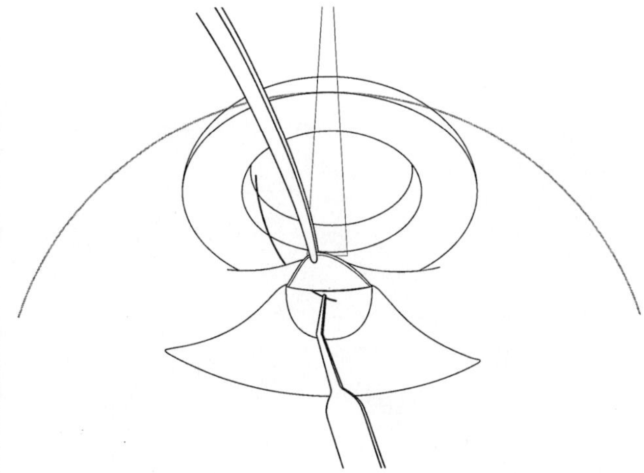

serted through a larger (5.0–7.0 mm) incision. Viscoelastic fluid is aspirated from the eye, and a miotic agent may be injected into the anterior chamber.

SCLERECTOMY

Up to this point, unless a trabeculectomy flap has already been fashioned, the procedure has resembled a typical phacoemulsification procedure. However, following IOL insertion, 0.12 forceps are used to grasp the flap. Using a Kelly-Descemet punch, the surgeon excises a segmental block of corneoscleral tissue measuring approximately 2.0 by 1.5 mm in order to create a trabecular fistula. (Fig. 23–13). This block of tissue may instead be removed prior to insertion of the IOL.

IRIDECTOMY

With an assistant retracting the scleral flap, the surgeon performs a broad-based peripheral iridectomy by withdrawing the peripheral iris with nontoothed forceps and excising a segment with Vannas scissors (Fig. 23–14). There are no rewards for performing an exceedingly small iridectomy.

CLOSURE OF THE SCLERAL FLAP

The flap is sutured firmly in place with multiple interrupted 10-0 nylon sutures (Fig. 23–15). The number of sutures may be adjusted according to the amount of filtration and the depth of the anterior chamber. Filtration may be assessed intraoperatively by injection of balanced salt solution through the paracentesis site and observation of flow from the scleral flap. If an intraoperative antimetabolite was used, firm closure is advisable to prevent hypotony. Postoperative suture lysis may always be performed if filtration is inadequate.

CLOSURE OF THE CONJUNCTIVAL FLAP

If a fornix-based flap is used, it is pulled firmly over the cornea with sutures securing the flap (Fig. 23–16). A limbus-based conjunctival flap can be closed with a running 8-0 or 9-0 polyglactin (Vicryl) suture on a noncutting blood vessel (BV) needle. The surgeon can achieve watertight closure safely by passing the noncutting needle through the underside of the incised end of conjunctiva, then from external to internal, and then from internal to external. This process is repeated in 0.5-mm steps until all conjunctiva is

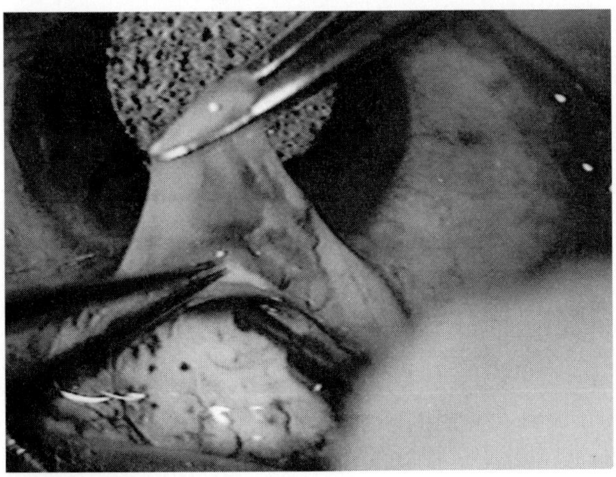

FIGURE 23–13. Sclerectomy

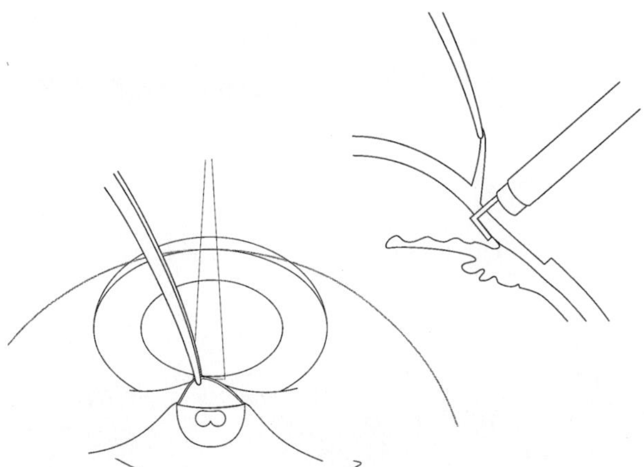

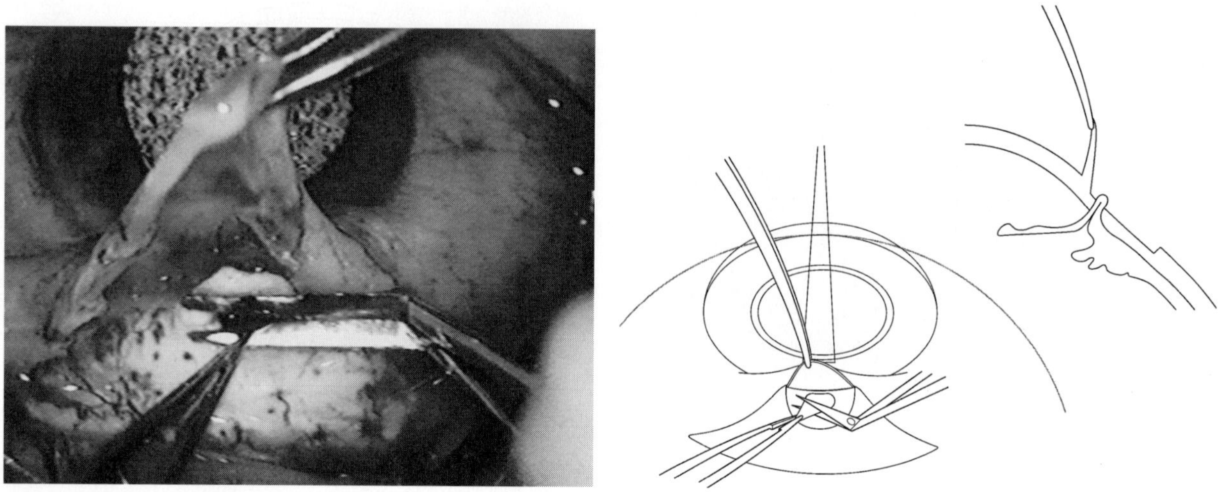

FIGURE 23–14. Iridectomy

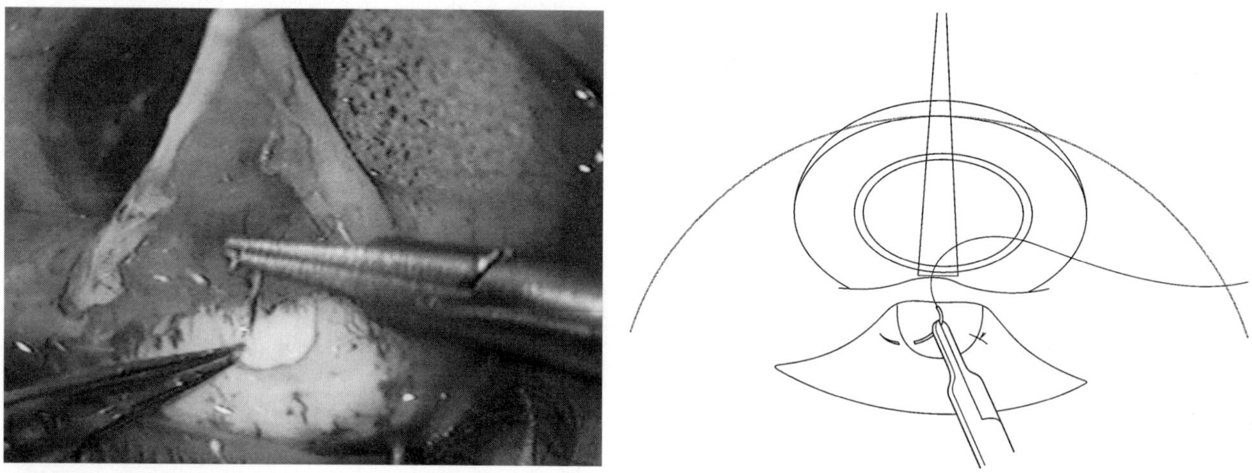

FIGURE 23–15. Closure of scleral flap

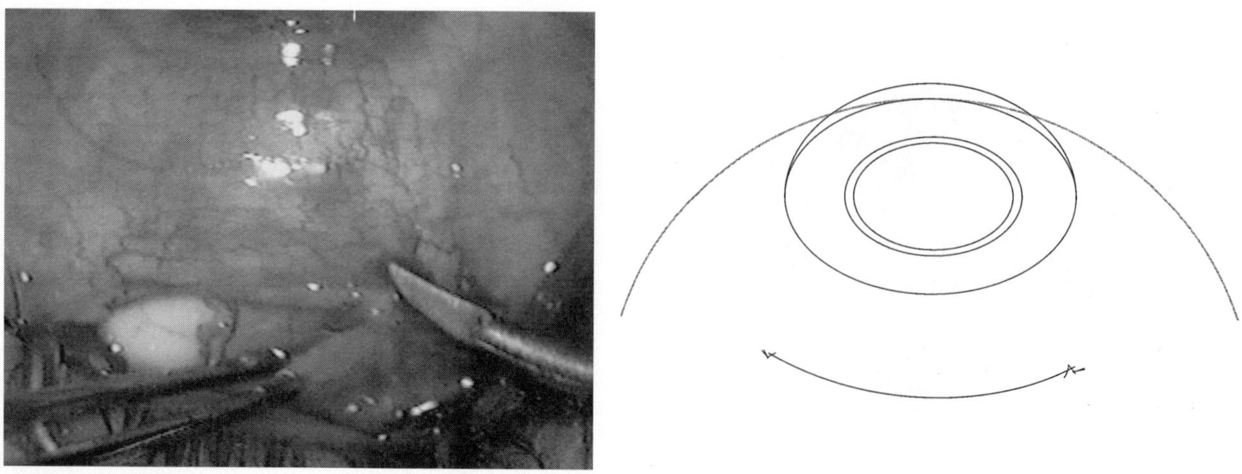

FIGURE 23–16. Closure of limbus-based conjunctival flap

secured. Taking a bite of posterior Tenon's fascia on alternating passes of the suture is recommended. Balanced salt solution is once again injected into the anterior chamber from the limbal paracentesis. The bleb is confirmed, the anterior chamber depth assessed, and a fluorescein strip applied to ensure a negative Seidel's test result. Leaks may be closed with 10-0 nylon on a BV needle.

SUBCONJUNCTIVAL INJECTIONS, OINTMENT, PATCHING

Cefazolin, 50 mg/0.5 mL, and dexamethasone, 2.0 mg/0.5 mL may be administered in the subconjunctival space in the area least likely to undergo subsequent trabeculectomy, the inferonasal quadrant. Polysporin ointment, a patch, and a shield are applied.

COMBINED CATARACT AND GLAUCOMA SURGERY AT A SEPARATE SITE

Multiple techniques have been proposed to refine combined cataract and glaucoma surgery. These methods may involve incision at two separate sites.[39, 41] Combined surgery with clear cornea phacoemulsification may be performed with the use of topical anesthesia and without sutures.[40, 69, 70] This two-site approach has potential advantages over combined surgery through a single incision. Reduced manipulation of the conjunctival and scleral flaps may limit postoperative flap inflammation and enhance long-term success of filtration. Without the bleeding, bulky conjunctival, and scleral flaps of a single-incision combined procedure, phacoemulsification may be more easily performed with a shorter tunnel and better visibility. In addition, separating the incision sites isolates flap suture lysis from the cataract wound incision.

Weitzman and Caprioli[41] describe a technique involving temporal clear cornea phacoemulsification combined with separate-incision superior trabeculectomy. Sitting at the side of the patient's head closer to the operated eye, the surgeon introduces a limbal paracentesis at the "12-o'clock" position, followed by a temporal clear cornea stab entrance with a 3.2 mm diamond keratome. This is followed by capsulorrhexis, hydrodissection, one-hand phacoemulsification, cortical clean-up, insertion of a foldable silicone or acrylic IOL within the capsular bag, and placement of a single 10-0 nylon suture to close the temporal wound. After the temporal clear cornea cataract extraction and IOL insertion, the surgeon moves to the top of the patient's head to complete the superior trabeculectomy in the typical fashion.

The choice of an acrylic or silicone IOL remains with the surgeon. To date, there has been no clear differentiation between these lenses with regard to postoperative visual acuity and complications.

COMBINED CATARACT EXTRACTION AND ENDOSCOPIC CILIARY PROCESS PHOTOCOAGULATION

This option is mentioned briefly because it is currently being evaluated in a select group of university-based ophthalmologic institutions. The procedure typically involves phacoemulsification, IOL implantation, and endoscopic laser photocoagulation of the ciliary processes. Uram[42] has demonstrated improved visual acuity, a 57% decrease in IOP, and minimal complications (transient vitreous hemorrhage) with a mean follow-up of 19.2 months for the procedure. Although the safety and efficacy of this approach in comparison with standard methods of combined surgery remains to be determined, preliminary results are encouraging.

POSTOPERATIVE CARE

Following a combined procedure, topical antibiotics and topical corticosteroids should be prescribed. An aggressive topical corticosteroid regimen, such as prednisolone acetate 1% every 4 hours or even every 2 hours, may be given. The corticosteroid drops may be gradually tapered according to clinical status over 3 to 4 months. Rapid tapering of topical corticosteroids is a common cause of delayed failure of trabeculectomy whether or not combined with cataract surgery.

Aqueous suppressants, such as β-blockers or carbonic anhydrase inhibitors, are ideally avoided to maximize postoperative aqueous production and thereby optimize bleb inflation and longevity. A shallow bleb associated with an unsatisfactory IOP may require further postoperative adjuncts, such as digital pressure, laser suture lysis, or 5-FU injections, often in combination with bleb needling (see later).

Laser Suture Lysis

Laser suture lysis is a safe and effective method of enhancing filtration through a tightly sutured scleral flap. Typically, it is not performed in the first to third postoperative days, when fibrin and residual viscoelastic fluid may artifactually elevate the IOP even though adequate filtration is indeed present. However, if the surgeon decides that postoperative IOP is not as expected, suture lysis may be performed as early as the first postoperative day although it is generally performed within the first 7 days.

When suture lysis is indicated, topical proparacaine 0.5% is given. A Zeiss gonioprism or a Hoskins lens is then placed on the bleb and drawn gently toward the wound. This maneuver allows visualization of the sutures through the compressed conjunctiva. Because the maneuver may precipitate a wound leak in the early postoperative period, particularly with fornix-based conjunctival flaps, care should be taken to avoid unnecessary trauma. Argon green (514 -nm) laser is then used to apply a 400 mW, 0.1 sec, 50-μ burst to the suture. The power can be increased if the desired result is not seen. It should be remembered that laser suture lysis not only affects the IOP but may also lead to alterations in postoperative astigmatism. The release of preplaced sutures provides the same benefits and risks as suture lysis.

Digital Pressure

Digital pressure, an alternative to irreversible laser suture lysis, can be useful in managing transient causes of elevated IOP in the early postoperative period. With the patient looking down, firm pressure is applied through the upper lid for 10 seconds. After 10 seconds of rest, the maneuver is repeated. The patient with a shallow bleb and high IOP may be instructed to perform digital pressure several times a day. This two-step process may be performed in sets of three repeated four to six times per day. Generally, digital pressure should be performed only by the patient's ophthalmologist in the early and middle postoperative period (first 2 months).

Adjunctive Antimetabolite Therapy

Glaucoma filtration surgery may fail as a result of internal obstruction of the sclerectomy with fibrin, iris, vitreous, or a fibrovascular membrane. More commonly, however, an external obstruction is present. The most common causes of external obstructions (in order of decreasing frequency) are (1) fibrosis involving the subconjunctival–sub-Tenon's space, (2) an episcleral cap overlying the edges of the trabeculectomy flap, (3) encapsulated filtration bleb. External obstruction may be more common with combined procedures, which may entail greater traumatic manipulation of the flap as well as increased postoperative inflammation. Antimetabolites are used with growing frequency to disrupt particular steps of wound healing, thereby increasing the efficacy of filtration surgery.[43–50] The two primary antimetabolites currently being used by glaucoma surgeons are MMC and 5-FU.

MITOMYCIN C

MMC is an antineoplastic antibiotic isolated from *Streptomyces caespitosus*. Its cytotoxic activity precludes its use as an anti-infective agent. This agent's mechanism of action is similar to that of the alkylating agents. It not only causes cross-linking of DNA but also, in high concentrations, may inhibit synthesis of RNA and protein. MMC has been used with growing frequency in combined ophthalmologic procedures. Protocols typically involve the intraoperative application of a sponge (Weck-Cel) soaked in 0.2 to 0.5 mg/mL of MMC to the exposed flap for 1 to 5 minutes.

Various investigators have demonstrated the efficacy of MMC in combined procedures involving both ECCE[48] and phacoemulsification.[51–55, 71–77] One study failed to demonstrate an advantage to using MMC as an adjunctive to combined procedures.[52] This large clinical trial involving 174 consecutive patients with primary open-angle glaucoma demonstrated no statistically significant difference at 2 years in postoperative IOP, number of medications, or visual acuity outcome between patients undergoing primary glaucoma triple procedure (PGTP) with adjunctive and those having PGTP without MMC.[53] In this same study, however, black race, diabetes, preoperative IOP greater than or equal to 20 mm Hg, and preoperative need for more than two medications were found to be significant independent prognostic factors for filtration failure after PGTP without adjunctive MMC but not after PGTP with adjunctive MMC.[53] Thus, although generalized use of MMC in combined procedures may not be indicated, this agent may be useful in selected patients in whom filtration surgery failure is likely without MMC. Although more studies must be performed to further evaluate the risk factors of filtration failure in combined procedures, one may speculate that the factors will be similar to those identified for filtration failure in patients undergoing filtration surgery alone.

MMC offers the advantage of a single intraoperative application, but in combined procedures utilizing ECCE or phacoemulsification, its use has been associated with symptomatic hypotony (4%), endothelial toxicity (1%), and wound instability (1%).[54] Transient wound leaks, superficial punctate keratitis, persistent hypotony, and a slight decrease in endothelial cell count have also been demonstrated with combined MMC procedures using MMC and phacoemulsification.[55, 77] However, the incidence of complications will continue to diminish with further refinements in MMC protocols and the use of small-incision surgery.

5-FLUOROURACIL

A fluorinated pyrimidine antagonist, 5-FU is an antimetabolite that interferes with DNA synthesis by inhibiting the enzyme thymidylate synthetase as well as interfering with RNA processing. In addition to its effects in decreasing fibroblast proliferation through this mechanism, 5-FU may disrupt fibroblast migration by means of its intracelluar metabolite, 5-fluorouracil, an inhibitor of fibroblast contraction.

5-FU may be administered intraoperatively or postoperatively. Intraoperative application of 5-FU may be less potent than similar application of MMC and may require additional postoperative injections. However, unlike intraoperative MMC, intraoperative 5-FU may not be associated with a high rate of hypotony, bleb avascularity, and corneal enclothelial toxicity.

Postoperative 5-FU may be given via subconjunctival injection every day or every other day for a week or longer.[49] Multiple protocols have been adapted for the administration of postoperative 5-FU.[56–60] Its dosage may be titrated for the individual patient and the clinical appearance of the bleb. Most protocols, however, involve the use of individual 5.0-mg subconjunctival injections (0.1 mL of a 50.0 mg/mL solution) administered between postoperative days 1 and 14. Typically, 7 to 10 injections may be required, with a variable mean total dosage (34.4–87 mg).[56–59] Unfortunately, these protocols, which expose the patient to multiple subconjunctival injections, require fastidious postoperative cooperation and compliance as well as a cornea free of underlying disease.

The efficacy of 5-FU in combined procedures is less convincing than that of MMC. Although some studies have found that postoperative subconjunctival injections of 5-FU in combined surgery improve the 1-year success rate for IOP control,[78] other large, prospective clinical trials have failed to support this finding.[79, 80, 86] Perhaps additional studies to refine 5-FU protocols and assess risk factors for filtration failure in combined procedures will unequivocally resolve this issue.

INDICATIONS FOR ANTIMETABOLITE THERAPY

Currently, there is a paucity of large, well-controlled studies evaluating risk factors for filtration failure after combined procedures.[53] One can speculate however, that these risk factors are not significantly different from those predicting poor prognosis in filtration surgery alone, which are (1) patients who are young[81] or of African American background, (2) the diagnosis of neovascular or inflammatory glaucoma, (3) conjunctival cicatrization due to prior intraocular surgery (i.e., scleral buckling procedure),[82] (4) prior failed filtration surgery, (5) aphakia,[83] (6) glaucoma requiring extremely low IOP for continued optic nerve health, and (7) the desire for long-term IOP control following combined surgery.[84] With the refinement of adjunctive antimetabolite protocols, many glaucoma surgeons now use antimetabolites in virtually all of their patients undergoing combined cataract and glaucoma surgery.

INTRAOPERATIVE CONSIDERATIONS IN ANTIMETABOLITE USE

When using intraoperative antimetabolites, the surgeon must take precautions to avoid overfiltration, hypotony, and all associated complications. Overfiltration from adjunctive antimetabolite use may occur in the presence of a loosely sutured trabeculectomy flap. It may also occur in areas of conjunctival compromise, such as buttonholes, which may heal slowly in the presence of antimetabolites.

Multiple surgical techniques can be employed to avoid overfiltration complications. The surgeon must (1) take care to avoid compromising the conjunctiva, (2) perform a limbus-based conjunctival flap to isolate the fibrovascular healing response from the area overlying the scleral flap, and (3) consider dissection of a thicker conjunctiva–Tenon's flap by dissecting between Tenon's capsule and episclera (not between conjunctiva and Tenon's capsule). Lower concentration of drug, shorter exposure to the antimetabolite with aggressive irrigation, and rinsing of all intraoperative instruments contaminated with the antimetabolite are also important ways to avoid antimetabolite-induced complications.

Special Considerations

An ophthalmic surgeon may be confronted with various circumstances specific to surgical intervention in an eye with coexisting glaucoma and cataract. The surgeon must be prepared to handle the miotic and immobile pupil and the challenges of an eye with pseudoexfoliation syndrome.

TECHNIQUES FOR MANAGING THE SMALL PUPIL

The patient with glaucoma who is undergoing cataract extraction may have a small pupil as a result of (1) long-term miotic therapy, (2) posterior synechiae, (3) pseudoexfoliation syndrome, or (4) simply, senile miosis, which is present in elderly patients. Senile miosis has been reported to occur secondary to hyalinization and sclerosis of both the blood vessels and stroma of the iris as well as preferential atrophy of the dilator muscle over the sphincter.[85] Whatever the etiology, a miotic pupil may make capsulorrhexis and lens extraction significantly more difficult. Historically, it has been estimated that as many as 42.5% of patients with glaucoma who are undergoing cataract extraction require sphincterotomy.[86] With the increasing use of glaucoma medications other than the miotics, this proportion is probably decreasing.

If the diameter of the pupil is inadequate to perform cataract extraction, multiple maneuvers to enlarge the pupil are available to the surgeon. The use of viscoelastic agents, nonincisional pupilloplasty, and iris retractors in small pupil phacoemulsification have virtually eliminated the need for sector iridotomies or sphincterotomies. Although a 4- to 5-mm pupil may be manageable for the surgeon experienced in phacoemulsification, the final size of the pupil prior to the procedure ultimately depends on the surgeon's technical expertise. Novice surgeons should aim for a pupil size larger than 5 mm.

Viscoelastic Agents

The initial attempt to enlarge the pupil should involve the use of a viscoelastic agent. In the majority of patients with glaucoma, the small pupil is secondary to senile miosis or drug-related hyalinization of the pupil. In these cases, the viscoelastic cannula can be placed in the middle of the pupil. As the viscoelastic agent is injected, it may push the pupillary margin peripherally and thereby facilitate phacoemulsification. Hyaluronate sodium (Healon GV), a long-chain hyaluronic acid, has been touted to have greater ability to displace the iris because of its high molecular weight and viscosity.

If posterior synechiae are limiting pupillary dilation, the cannula can be placed in an adjacent area of the iris unaffected by the synechiae. Viscoelastic injection in this area raises the iris off the lens and allows the cannula to be placed below the iris without damaging the lens capsule. The cannula can then be swept around the pupil to break remaining synechiae. This method is ideal for synechiae in the inferior 270 degrees. For superior synechiae, the surgeon (1) passes the viscoelastic cannula through a limbal paracentesis and directs it superiorly or (2) grasps the superior iris through the scleral tunnel incision with non-toothed forceps and gently pulls it superiorly until the synechiae are disengaged.

In the rare instance of 360 degrees of posterior synechiae, a superior peripheral iridectomy may be followed by injection of the viscoelastic agent into the posterior chamber via the iridectomy. The superior synechiae may be broken by the sweeping cannula. The inferior synechiae are then broken as previously described.

Nonsurgical Pupilloplasty

Various instruments can be used to mechanically enlarge the pupil by creating many small sphincter tears. After disengaging any posterior synechiae and adding viscoelastic agent to the anterior chamber but prior to capsulorrhexis, the surgeon inserts a single Graether collar button into the anterior chamber to engage the inferior pupillary border. The pupillary margin is then pushed inferiorly to the iris root. This process is repeated superiorly, nasally, and temporally. In general, this method is sufficient for small pupils resulting from posterior synechiae and miotic therapy. In the majority of cases of senile miosis, however, more vigorous stretching with two Graether collar buttons engaged 180 degrees apart is required. Stretching the pupil in the horizontal meridian and the vertical meridian usually achieves a sufficiently enlarged pupil. Alternatively, a Grieshaber pupil-dilating instrument may be used.

After mechanical stretching of the pupil, pigment and blood released during the process should be evacuated from the anterior chamber. Then the surgeon may proceed with the capsulorrhexis.

Iris Retractors

If viscoelastic agents and nonsurgical pupilloplasty do not yield an adequately dilated pupil, the employment of iris retractors may be considered. Monofilament nylon retractors, such as those designed by DeJuan and Hickingbotham,[87] are available. In such instances, four additional limbal corneal incisions are made, ideally, supratemporally, supranasally, inferotemporally, and inferonasally. These incisions should be oriented posteriorly toward the pupillary margin (not parallel to the iris plane) and should be self-sealing. The surgeon then passes retractors through the incisions by using a straight, locking needle holder to grasp each retractor halfway down the shaft and parallel to the long axis. The hook is inserted parallel to the iris and then rotated inferiorly 90 degrees to engage the pupil. The process is repeated for the other limbal sites. A 0.2-mm forceps can then be used to slide the polymeric silicone (Silastic) sleeve of the iris retractor down the shaft to enlarge the pupil. Iris prolapse may be minimized if the phacoemulsification entry site is straddled by the superior limbal retractor sites. To remove the retractors, the surgeon slides the hook of the iris retractor toward the center of the pupil, disengages the iris, and pulls the retractor through the paracentesis site while applying counterpressure on the limbus.

Surgical Pupilloplasty

Various techniques to surgically enlarge the pupil have been described. They include extending a midperipheral iridectomy to the pupillary aperture and sector iridectomy. For ECCE, a superior sector iridectomy in conjunction with multiple inferior sphincterotomies has been described. However, less traumatic methods have evolved with small-incision phacoemulsification. One such method is described by Fine,[88] who proposes making multiple, small, partial-thickness sphincterotomies at the pupillary margin with Rapasso scissors. The circumferentially intact iris muscle allows sparing of the constriction-dilation mechanism in response to typical pharmacologic agents. Following the sphincterotomies, injection of additional viscoelastic agent into the anterior chamber or further mechanical stretching of the iris can additionally dilate the pupil. Upon completion of cataract extraction and IOL placement, the iris should be repositioned and then both pharmacologically and mechanically constricted.

Phacoemulsification with the Small Pupil

If all of the previously described methods fail to enlarge a small pupil, endolenticular phacoemulsification may still be performed safely. When performing a continuous capsulorrhexis, the surgeon should not extend the capsulorrhexis out of visualization or under the iris. Making the initial tear more centrally allows the continuous capsulotomy to be carefully extended to the pupillary margin. If a tear extends under the iris, tearing in that direction is discontinued.

During hydrodissection and hydrodelineation, an adequate red reflex and fluid wave may be difficult to appreciate through the small pupil. However, this difficulty should not preclude vigorous irrigation under the capsule, which is essential for facilitating successful phacoemulsification. A J cannula may be used to assist hydrodissection and delineation of the superior lens. Some surgeons recommend fracturing the nucleus into multiple segments and then bringing each segment into the pupillary axis for emulsification.[89]

The small pupil limits exposure of the peripheral nucleus. Thus, the first central groove tends to be deep but short, and additional force is needed to split the nucleus along the groove. Rotating the nucleus 180 degrees enables the phacoemulsification tip to engage the inferior edge while a spatula engages the superior edge of the groove. This maneuver ensures sufficient force to fracture the nucleus along the shortened groove. Phacoemulsification of nuclear segments is followed by another 180-degree rotation so that the process can be repeated. Once all four quarters are created, the surgeon uses the phacoemulsification tip to engage each quarter, drawing it centrally for safe phacoemulsification within the mid-pupil along the iris plane.[90]

During the phacoemulsification, inadvertent chafing and aspiration of the iris may be limited by reducing the flow and vacuum settings giving the surgeon more time to react to prevent iris damage. Furthermore, sliding the sleeve over the distal metallic phacoemulsifier tip limits iris exposure to the tip.

COMBINED SURGERY IN AN EYE WITH PSEUDOEXFOLIATION SYNDROME

Pseudoexfoliation syndrome offers multiple surgical challenges in a patient undergoing combined cataract and glaucoma procedures. The risk of cataract surgery in such a patient is well documented.[35, 59, 91–95] Complications may result from zonular weakness and limited pupillary dilation. A weak zonular apparatus may predispose an affected eye to a higher incidence of zonular dialysis, capsular rupture, phacodonesis, lens decentration, and vitreous complications.

Limited mydriasis during cataract extraction, estimated to occur in 46.8% of eyes affected with pseudoexfolication sydrome,[59] may also be a significant intraoperative problem. Techniques for small pupils (discussed earlier) may be of dramatic assistance in dealing with it. Improvements in phacoemulsification technology and IOLs, as well as new capsular supporting rings may also improve the safety of cataract extraction in patients with pseudoexfoliation syndrome.

The patient with pseudoexfoliation syndrome may experience more significant postoperative inflammation, which results from alterations in the blood-aqueous barrier. Postoperative inflammation may be reduced by the use of

TABLE 23–2. COMPLICATIONS OF COMBINED CATARACT AND GLAUCOMA SURGERY

Intraoperative
- Anesthesia administration
- Retrobulbar hemorrhage
- Conjunctival buttonhole
- Bleb leaks
- Descemet's membrane detachment
- Hyphema
- Shallow anterior chamber
- Choroidal hemorrhage
- Vitreous loss

Early postoperative
- Hypotony
- IOP elevation
- Conjunctival defect
- Excessive filtration
- Choroidal detachment
- Uveitis
- Hyphema
- Dellen formation
- Loss of central island ("snuff-out")

Late postoperative
- Filtration failure
- Leaking filtration bleb
- Endophthalmitis
- Spontaneous hyphema
- Hypotony
- Posterior subcapsular opacification
- Ciliochoroidal detachment
- Staphyloma
- Ptosis
- Sympathetic ophthalmia

surface-modified IOLs and aggressive postoperative anti-inflammatory management with short-term topical, subconjunctival, or systemic corticosteroids.

Complications of Combined Cataract and Glaucoma Surgery

In general, the potential complications arising from combined cataract extraction, IOL insertion, and filtration procedures are an accumulation of the complications of each procedure. They may arise during the intraoperative, early postoperative, or late postoperative phase. Table 23–2 lists the possible complications at different phases of the procedure.

SUMMARY

Glaucoma and cataract are common causes of visual morbidity in the elderly population. We have discussed current concepts of evaluation, decision-making, indications, and management for the patient with coexisting cataract and glaucoma. The techniques and special considerations specific to the three basic surgical approaches—cataract extraction alone, glaucoma filtering surgery alone with subsequent cataract extraction (two-stage), and combined cataract and glaucoma surgery—have been reviewed. In all cases, however, the general principles reviewed in this section are intended to be applied on an individual basis, because each patient represents a unique and heterogeneous circumstance encompassing multiple variables and different expectations. As the refinement in small-incision techniques and antimetabolite protocols evolve, the approach to the patient with coexisting glaucoma and cataract will also change. In view of these developments, we expect the future to continue to brighten for the patient with coexisting glaucoma and cataract.

REFERENCES

1. American Academy of Ophthalmology: Glaucoma. Basic and Clinical Science Course, San Francisco, CA, American Academy of Ophthalmology, section 10. 1995–1996.
2. American Academy of Ophthalmology: Basic and Clinical Science Course. American Academy of Ophthalmology, section 11. 1995–1996.
3. Randolph ME, Maumenee AE, Iliff CE: Cataract extraction in glaucomatous eyes. Am J Ophthalmol 1971;71:328.
4. Palimeris G, Chimondou E, Magouritsas N: Cataract extraction in chronic simple glaucoma. Ophthalmic Surg 1974;5:62.
5. Bigger JF, Becker B: Cataracts and primary open angle glaucoma: The effect of uncomplicated cataract extraction on glaucoma control. Trans Am Acad Ophthalmol Otolaryngol 1971;75:260.
6. Yalvac I, Airaksinen PJ, Tuulonen A: Phacoemulsification with and without trabeculectomy in patients with glaucoma. Ophthalmic Surg Lasers 1997;28:469–475.
7. Barak A, Desatnik H, Ma-Naim T: Early postoperative intraocular pressure pattern in glaucomatous and nonglaucomatous patients. J Cat Refr Surg 1996;22:607.
8. Brown SVL, Thomas JV, Budenz DL: Effect of cataract surgery on intraocular pressure reduction obtained with laser trabeculoplasty. Am J Ophthalmol 1985;100:373.
9. Drolsum L, Haaskjold E: Extracapsular cataract extraction in eyes previously operated for glaucoma. Acta Ophthalmol Copenh 1994;72:273.
10. Fluorouracil Filtering Surgery Study Group: Three-year follow-up of the Fluorouracil Filtering Surgery Study. Am J Ophthalmol 1993;115:82.
11. Schuman JS: Surgical management of coexisting cataract and glaucoma. Ophthalmic Surg Lasers 1996;27:45.
12. Shields MB: Another reevaluation of combined cataract and glaucoma surgery. Am J Ophthalmol 1993;115:806.
13. Naveh N, Kottass R, Glovinsky J, et al: The long-term effect on intraocular pressure of a procedure combining trabeculectomy and cataract surgery, as compared with trabeculectomy alone. Ophthalmic Surg 1990;21:339.
14. Yu CB, Chong NH, Caesar RH, et al: Long-term results of combined cataract and glaucoma surgery versus trabeculectomy alone in low risk patients. J Cataract Refract Surg 1996;22:352.
15. McCartney DI, Memmen JE, Stark WJ: The efficacy and safety of combined trabeculectomy, cataract extraction and intraocular lens implantation. Ophthalmology 1988;95:754.
16. Murchison JF, Shields MB: An evaluation of three surgical approaches for coexisting cataract and glaucoma. Ophthalmic Surg 1989;20:393.
17. Caprioli J, Park HJ, Weitzman M: Temporal corneal phacoemulsification combined with superior trabeculectomy: A controlled study. Trans Ophthalmol Soc 1996;94:451.
18. Ritch R, Shields MB, Krupin T: The Glaucomas: Glaucoma Therapy, 2nd ed, vol 3. St. Louis, Mosby–Year Book, 1996.
19. Percival SPB: Glaucoma triple procedure of extracapsular cataract extraction, posterior chamber lens implantation, and trabeculectomy. Br J Ophthalmol 1985;69:99.
20. Yu CB, Chong NH, Caesar RH, et al: Long-term results of combined cataract and glaucoma surgery versus trabeculectomy alone in low-risk patients. J Cataract Refract Surg 1996;22:352.
21. Menezo J, Maldonado M, Munoz G, Cisneros A: Combined procedure for glaucoma and cataract: A retrospective study. J Cataract Refract Surg 1994;20:498.

22. Stewart W, Crinkley C, Carlson A: Results of combined phacoemulsification and trabeculectomy in patients with elevated preoperative intraocular pressures. J Glaucoma 1995;4:164.
23. Stewart W, Crinkley C, Carlson A: Results of trabeculectomy combined with phacoemulsification versus trabeculectomy combined with extracapsular cataract extraction in patients with advanced glaucoma. Ophthalmic Surg 1994;25:621.
24. Wishart PK, Austin MW: Combined cataract extraction and trabeculectomy: Phacoemulsification compared with extracapsular technique. Ophthalmic Surg 1993;24:814.
25. Mamalis N, Lohner S, Rand AN, Crandall AS: Combined phacoemulsification, intraocular lens implantation, and trabeculectomy. J Cataract Refract Surg 1996;22:467.
26. Weitzman M, Caprioli J: Temporal corneal phacoemulsification combined with separate incision superior trabecuoltomy. Ophthalmic Surg 1995;26:271.
27. Asbell PA, Chiang B, Amin A, et al: Retinal acuity evaluation with the potential acuity meter in glaucoma patients. Ophthalmology 1985;92:764.
28. Stewart WC, Connor AB, Hunt HH: Prediction of postoperative visual acuity in patients with total glaucomatous cupping using the potential acuity meter and automated perimetry. Ophthalmic Surg 1993;24:730.
29. Parrish RK, Spaeth GL, Poryzees EM, Hargens CW: Evaluation of local anesthesia agents using a new force sensitive lid speculum. Ophthalmic Surg 1983;14:575.
30. Atkinson WS: The use of hyaluronidase with local anesthesia in opthahlmology: A preliminary report. Arch Ophthalmol 1949; 42:628.
31. Parker JS, Gollamudi S, Joh G, Stark WJ: Combined trabeculectomy, cataract extraction and foldable lens implantation. J Cataract Refract Surg 1992;18:582.
32. Pasquale LR, Smith SJ: Outcome of phacoemulsification combined with a Pearce trabeculectomy in patients with glaucoma. J Cataract Refract Surg 1992;18:301.
33. Gregg FM: Phacoemulsification and modified trabeculectomy for managing combined cataracts and glaucoma. J Cataract Refract Surg 1992;18:362.
34. Wedrich A, Menapace R, Radax U: Combined small incision cataract surgery and trabeculectomy: Techniques and results. Int Ophthalmol 1992;16:409.
35. Drolsum L, Haaskjold E, Davanger M: Pseudoexfoliation syndrome and extracapsular cataract extraction. Acta Ophthalmol 1993;71:765.
36. Berestka JS, Brown SVL: Limbus- versus fornix-based conjunctival flaps in combined phacoemulsification and mitomycin C trabeculectomy surgery. Ophthalmology 1997;104:187.
37. Stewart WC, Crinkley CM, Carlson AN: Fornix vs. limbus-based flaps in combined phacoemulsification and trabeculectomy. Doc Ophthalmol 1994;88:141.
38. Lyle WA, Jin JC: Comparison of a 3 and 6 mm incision in combined phacoemulsification and trabeculectomy. Am J Ophthalmol 1991;111:189.
39. Gillies WE, Brooks AM: The results of combined cataract extraction and trabeculectomy using separate incisions. Aust N Z J Ophthalmol 1992;20:239.
40. Bloomberg LB: Modified trabeculectomy/trabeculotomy with no stitch cataract surgery. J Cataract Refract Surg 1996;22:4.
41. Weitzman M, Caprioli J: Temporal corneal phacoemulsification combined with separate-incision superior trabeculectomy. Ophthalmic Surg 1995;26:271.
42. Uram M: Combined phacoemulsification, endoscopic cilary process photocoagulation, and intraocular lens implantation in glaucoma management. Ophthalmic Surg 1995;26:346.
43. Palmer SS: Mitomycin as adjunct chemotherapy with trabeculectomy. Ophthalmology 1991;98:317.
44. Skuta GL, Beeson CC, Higginbotham EJ: Intraoperative mitomycin versus postoperative 5-fluorouracil in high risk glaucoma filtering surgery. Ophthalmology 1992;99:438.
45. Kitazawa Y, Kawase K, Matsushita H, Minobe M: Trabeculectomy, with mitomycin: A comparative study with fluorouracil. Arch Ophthalmol 1991;109:1693.
46. Lanigan L, Sturmer J, Baez KA, et al: Single intraoperative applications of 5-fluorouracil during filtration surgery: Early results. Br J Ophthalmol 1994;78:33.
47. Chen C, Huang H, Bair J, Lee C: Trabeculectomy with simultaneous topical application of mitomycin C in refractory glaucoma. J Ocular Pharmacol 1990;6:175.
48. Joos KM, Bueche MJ, Palmberg PF, et al: One year follow-up results of combined mitomycin-C trabeculectomy and extracapsular cataract extraction. Ophthalmology 1995;102:76.
49. Krug JH, Melamed S: Adjunctive use of delayed and adjustable low dose 5-fluorouracil in refractory glaucoma. Am J Ophthalmol 1990;109:412.
50. Heuer DK, Gressel MG, Parrish RK, et al: Trabeculectomy in aphakic eyes. Ophthalmology 1984;91:1045.
51. Carlson DW, Alward WL, Barad JP, et al: A randomized study of mitomycin augmentation in combined phacoemulsification and trabeculectomy. Ophthalmology 1997;104:4.
52. Shin DH, Simone PA, Song MS, et al: Adjunctive subconjunctival mitomycin C in glaucoma triple procedure. Ophthalmology 1995;102:1550.
53. Shin DH, Hughes BA, Song MS, et al: Primary glaucoma triple procedure with or without adjunctive mitomycin: Prognostic factors for filtration failure. Ophthalmology 1996;103:1925.
54. Joos K, Bueche M, Palmberg P, et al: One-year follow up results of combined mitomycin C trabeculectomy and extracapsular cataract extraction. Ophthalmology 1995;102:76.
55. Ruderman JM, Fundingsland B, Meyer MA: Combined phacoemulsification and trabeculectomy with mitomycin-C. J Cataract Refract Surg 1996;22:1085.
56. Nakano Y, Araie M, Shirato S: Effect of postoperative subconjunctival 5-fluorouracil injections on the surgical outcome of trabeculectomy in the Japanese. Graefes Arch Clin Exp Ophthalmol 1989;227:569.
57. Watanabe J, Iwata K, Sawaguchi S, Nanba K: Trabeculectomy with 5-fluorouracil. Acta Ophthalmol (Copenh) 1991;69:455.
58. Araie M, Shoji N, Shirato S, et al: Postoperative subconjunctival 5-fluorouracil injections and success probability of trabeculectomy in Japanese: Results of 5-year follow-up. Jpn J Ophthalmol 1992;36:158.
59. Drolsum L, Haaskjold E, Davanger M: Pseudoexfoliation syndrome and extracapsular cataract extraction. Acta Ophthalmol 1993;71:771.
60. Fluorouracil Filtering Surgery Study Group: Five year follow-up of the fluorouracil filtering surgery study. Am J Ophthalmol 1996;121:4.
61. McGuigan LJ, Gottsch J, Stark WJ: Extracapsular cataract extraction and posterior chamber lens implantation in eyes with preexisting glaucoma. Arch Ophthalmol 1986;104:1301.
62. Hefetz L, Ashkenazi I, Orpaz D, Naveh N: Comparison of intraocular pressure control and visual outcome after a triple procedure versus a sequential trabeculectomy and cataract surgery. Ann Ophthalmol Glaucoma 1994;26:238.
63. Park HJ, Weitzman M, Caprioli J: Temporal corneal phacoemulsification combined with superior trabeculectomy: A retrospective case-control study. Arch Ophthalmol 1997;115:318.
64. Jay JL: Extracapsular lens extraction and posterior chamber intraocular lens insertion combined with trabeculectomy. Br J Ophthalmol 1985;69:487.
65. Simmons ST, Litoff D, Nichols DA, et al: Extracapsular cataract extraction and posterior chamber intraocular lens implanation combined with trabeculectomy in patients with glaucoma. Am J Ophthalmol 1987;104:465.
66. Shields MB: Combined cataract extraction and guarded sclerectomy: Reevaluation in the extracapsular area. Ophthalmology 1986;93:366.
67. Savage JA, Thomas JV, Belcher CD III, Simmons RJ: Extracapsular cataract extraction and posterior chamber intraocular lens implantation in glaucomatous eyes. Ophthalmology 1985;92:1506.
68. Wedrich A, Menapace R, Radax U, Papapanos P: Long-term results of combined trabeculectomy and small incision cataract surgery. J Cataract Refract Surg 1995;21:49.
69. Gous PN, Roux P: Preliminary report of sutureless phacotrabeculectomy through a modified self-sealing scleral tunnel incision. J Cataract Refract Surgery 1995;21:160.
70. Dinsmore SC: Drop, then decide approach to topical anesthesia. J Cataract Refract Surg 1995;21:666.
71. Lederer CM Jr: Combined cataract extraction with intraocular lens implant and mitomycin-C augmented trabeculectomy. Ophthalmology 1996;103:1025.
72. Munden PM, Alward WL: Combined phacoemulsification, posterior

chamber intraocular lens implantation, and trabeculectomy with mitomycin C. Am Ophthalmol 1995;119:20.
73. Cohen JS, Greff LJ, Novack GD, Wind BE: A placebo-controlled, double-masked evaluation of mitomycin C in combined glaucoma and cataract procedures. Ophthalmology 1996;103:1934.
74. Wand M: Combined phacoemulsification, intraocular lens implant, and trabeculectomy with intraoperative mitomycin-C: comparison between 3.2mm and 6.0mm incisions. J Glaucoma 1996;5:201.
75. Lederer CM Jr: Combined cataract extraction with intraocular lens implant and mitomycin-augmented trabeculectomy. Ophthalmology 1996;103:1025.
76. Belyea DA, Dan JA, Lieberman MF, Stamper RL: Midterm follow-up results of combined phacoemulsification, lens implantation and mitomycin-C trabeculectomy procedure. J Glaucoma 1997;6:90.
77. Cohen JS, Greff LJ, Novack GD, Wind BE: A placebo-controlled, double-masked evaluation of mitomycin C in combined glaucoma and cataract procedures. Ophthalmology 1996;103:1934.
78. Hurvitz M: 5-FU supplemented phacoemulsification, posterior chamber intraocular lens implantation, and trabeculectomy. Ophthalmic Surg 1993;24:674.
79. O'Grady JM, Juzych MS, Shin DH, et al. Trabeculectomy phacoemulsification, posterior chamber intraocular lens implantation with and without 5-fluorouracil. Am J Ophthalmol 1993;116:594.
80. Wong PC, Runderman JM, Krupin T, et al: 5-Fluorouracil after primary combined filtration surgery. Am J Ophthalmol 1994; 117:149.
81. Gressel MG, Heuer DK, Parrish RKI: Trabeculectomy in young patients. Ophthalmology 1984;91:1242.
82. Rockwood EJ, Parrish RK, Heuer DK, et al: Glaucoma filtration surgery with 5-fluorouracil. Ophthalmology 1987;94:1071.
83. Heuer DK, Gressel MG, Parrish RK, et al: Trabeculectomy in aphakic eyes. Ophthalmology 1984;91:1045.
84. Joos KM, Bueche MJ, Palmberg PF, et al: One year follow-up results of combined mitomycin C trabeculectomy and extracapsular cataract extraction. Ophthalmology 1995;102:76.
85. Duke: System of Ophthalmology. St. Louis, CV Mosby, 1966; p 668.
86. Cole MD, Brown R, Ridgwae AE: Role of sphincterotomy in extracapsular cataract surgery. Br J Ophthalmol 1986;70:692.
87. DeJuan E Jr, Hickingbotham D: Flexible iris retractor (letter). Am J Ophthalmol 1991;111:776.
88. Fine IH. Pupilloplasty. *In* Koch PS, Davison JA (eds): Textbook of Advanced Phacoemulsification Techniques. Thorofare, NJ, Slack, 1991.
89. Gimbel HV: Nucleofractis phacoemulsification through a small pupil. Can J Ophthalmol 1992;27:115.
90. Nelson DB, Donnenfeld ED: Small pupil phacoemulsification and trabeculectomy. Int Ophthalmol Clin 1994;34:131.
91. Skuta GL, Parrish RK, Hodapp E, et al: Zonular dialysis during extracapsular cataract extraction in pseudoexfoliation syndrome. Arch Ophthalmol 1987;105:632.
92. Carpel EF: Pupillary dilation in eyes with pseudoexfoliation syndrome. Am J Ophthalmol 1988;105:692.
93. Zetterstrom C, Olivestedt G, Lundvall A: Exfoliation syndrome and extracapsular cataract extraction with implantation of posterior chamber lens. Acta Ophthalmol (Copenh) 1992;70:85.
94. Kuchle M, Nguyen NX, Horn F, Nauman GOH: Quantitative assessment of aqueous flare and aqueous "cells" in pseudoexfoliation syndrome. Acta Ophthalmol (Copenh) 1992;70:201.
95. Zetterstrom C, Lundvall A, Olivestedt G: Exfoliation syndrome and heparin surface modified intraocular lenses. Acta Ophthalmol (Copenh) 1992;70:91.

CHAPTER 24

Vitreous and Retina

TONY REALINI and ROBERT D. FECHTNER

As can be seen in Chapters 4, 5, and 16, examinations of the vitreous, retina, and optic nerve play a vital role in the care of patients with glaucoma. Tony Realini and Rob Fechtner reinforce that impression in this chapter. They review the common posterior segment findings associated with glaucoma, putting particular emphasis on the implications for treatment. These are neovascular glaucoma, intraocular hemorrhages (hyphema, ghost cell glaucoma, hemolytic glaucoma, and hemosiderotic glaucoma), retinopathy of prematurity, and posterior segment tumors. There follows a section dealing with glaucoma associated with posterior segment surgery. This subject was also included in Chapter 16 because it can be a cause of glaucoma as well as a result of a combined surgical approach involving the posterior and anterior segments. The primary focus in this chapter is the implications for glaucoma intervention. The authors then present the potential complications of glaucoma medical therapy, including latanoprost, epinephrine, and miotics. The final portion of the chapter is devoted to complications of glaucoma filtering surgery and their treatment: choroidal effusion and hemorrhage, decompression retinopathy, and hypotony maculopathy. This chapter gives the reader the confidence to correctly identify and treat these posterior segment findings.

In an earlier chapter, we looked to the posterior segment for clues to the etiology of elevated intraocular pressure. Those same clues, coupled with careful examination of the entire globe, can be useful guides in the development of a therapeutic plan. In this chapter, we consider several conditions with posterior segment findings and posterior segment complications of glaucoma intervention; for each, we describe the pertinent findings that can help guide treatment decisions and discuss how the response to treatment can aid in further treatment decision-making.

In the first section, neovascular glaucoma, intraocular hemorrhage, retinopathy of prematurity, posterior segment neoplasia, and the effects of posterior segment surgery are discussed. Each discussion is also condensed into an easy-to-read decision tree or flow chart. The reader should beware, especially in glaucoma management, that the "cookbook approach" to patient care is fraught with peril. The flow charts are meant to serve as guides, not as recipes. Each patient must be fully examined and all findings accounted for in the formulation of diagnostic and management decisions.

In the later sections of the chapter, we discuss posterior segment findings that result from complications of glaucoma medical therapy and surgery and their management.

Conditions with Posterior Segment Findings

NEOVASCULAR GLAUCOMA

The management of eyes with neovascular glaucoma (NVG) represents perhaps the greatest challenge facing today's glaucomatologist; in part because of the disease's unrelenting aggressiveness, and also because multiple interventions are often required to control the disease, each step becoming technically more difficult in an eye with multiple previous surgical procedures.

Successful management of NVG depends on early diagnosis. As discussed in Chapter 16, historical risk factors for development of NVG must be elicited (concurrent diabetes, recent central retinal vein occlusion, and other processes resulting in posterior segment ischemia) and a thorough examination must be performed. In general, when NVG is suspected, evaluation of the anterior segment confirms its presence and inspection of the posterior segment often provides clues to its cause.

CLINICAL FEATURES

Careful inspection of the anterior segment for neovascularization should begin at the pupil margin (or at the edges of a peripheral iridectomy) under high magnification, the examiner looking for tiny vascular tufts. Frequently, these fall in close proximity to—and resemble—pigment clumps at the pupil edge; awareness of this occurrence may help increase examiner sensitivity in detecting early neovascularization. On the anterior iris surface, rubeotic vessels are initially thin and wispy; in a blue eye, they may resemble normal iris vessels, and in brown eyes, they may be very hard to find. These vessels grow in caliber over time, and florid neovascularization is impossible to overlook.

Gonioscopy should be performed for any patient at risk for neovascularization. Even in the absence of iris neovascularization (or in the presence of subtle new iris vessels that are easily overlooked), angle neovascularization can be present. In fact, angle neovascularization may be present out of proportion to the extent of iris neovascularization. Pathologic neovascularization can often be differentiated from physiologic angle vascularity by the appearance of the vessel patterns: Nonpathologic vessels rarely reach Schwalbe's line, whereas pathologic vessels frequently arborize to form fronds that may grow to or even cross Schwalbe's line.

Similar to the evolution of iris neovascularization, angle neovascularization follows a progressive course. Early in NVG, the angle may appear normal or nearly so (with a few wispy vessels crossing the angle), but commonly, a transparent (and thus gonioscopically invisible) fibrovascular membrane has already traversed the angle, obstructing outflow and causing elevation of IOP. Over time, this membrane contracts, synechially scarring the angle shut permanently. Recognizing and treating an eye with angle neovascularization while the angle is still open may prevent synechial angle closure.

A detailed examination of the posterior segment is fundamental to determining the cause of and developing a treatment plan for NVG. Although the fundus changes in diabetes, central retinal vein occlusion, and carotid artery occlusive disease should be apparent, the ophthalmologist should keep in mind that many other diseases of the posterior segment can induce ocular neovascularization (see Table 16–1). It must be realized that NVG is never idiopathic. The disease always occurs secondary to ocular ischemia, usually of the posterior segment but not always; for instance, NVG can follow three-muscle strabismus surgery if anterior segment ischemia develops.

THERAPEUTIC CONSIDERATIONS

In the setting of posterior segment ischemia, the goal of therapy is to reduce the mass of viable retina within the eye. Two theories explain this nonintuitive goal:

1. Reducing retinal mass decreases the disparity between compromised blood supply and hypoxic retina, perhaps improving the blood-to-retina ratio and reducing the release of angiogenesis factor.
2. Ablating hypoxic retina is thought to reduce the amount of tissue available to release angiogenesis factor. This angiogenesis factor (as yet unidentified, although vascular endothelial growth factor is the leading candidate) is thought to stimulate neovascularization in various ocular tissues, including retina, iris, and angle.

The approach to management in eyes with NVG depends on the clarity of the ocular media, and occasionally, treatment is modified according to the visual potential of the eye (Fig. 24–1). In eyes with favorable visual potential, the first step is to employ retinal ablation in an effort to induce regression of the neovascularization. If the ocular media affords an adequate view of the posterior segment, panretinal photocoagulation is the treatment of choice. (Of note, heavier treatment may be required to cause regression of anterior segment neovascularization than for posterior segment neovascularization.) In the circumstance of favorable visual potential in the presence of opacities of the media (corneal edema, cataract, vitreous hemorrhage) precluding adequate view of the posterior segment, a combined anterior and posterior segment approach may be indicated to remove the cataract or vitreous hemorrhage, perform intraoperative retinal laser ablation, and place a tube shunt for IOP control that can often be placed through the pars plana. If there is less visual potential, transscleral retinal cryoablation should be carried out.

For retinal cryoablation, we prefer to use a transconjunctival approach. We use a retina probe and apply three rows with six applications in each row (18 spots) in each of two inferior quadrants. A single freeze-thaw at $-80°$ C for 15 seconds is used. This can be performed at the same session as cyclocryotherapy if the IOP is uncontrolled. Again, we use a transconjunctival approach, initially in the two inferior quadrants, sparing the superior portion of the globe should filtration be considered in the future. Using the glaucoma probe, we apply three spots in each quadrant with parameters of $-80°$ C for 60 seconds.

Given the rapidly progressive course of NVG, treatment should be performed as soon as possible, preferably within 24 to 48 hours. A reduction in IOP following retinal ablation is most likely in an eye with an open angle; a pressure response is unlikely following retinal ablation if synechial angle closure has already occurred. Staged treatment should be avoided, if possible, in the interest of providing a full treatment as quickly as possible. During the wait for an IOP-lowering response, judicious use of topical and oral antiglaucoma medications is advised. Acetazolamide often works well and is well-tolerated for short periods. Some agents should probably be avoided because of their theoretical ability to further close the angle (miotics) or induce inflammation (prostaglandin analog).

Careful and intense follow-up is mandatory for assess-

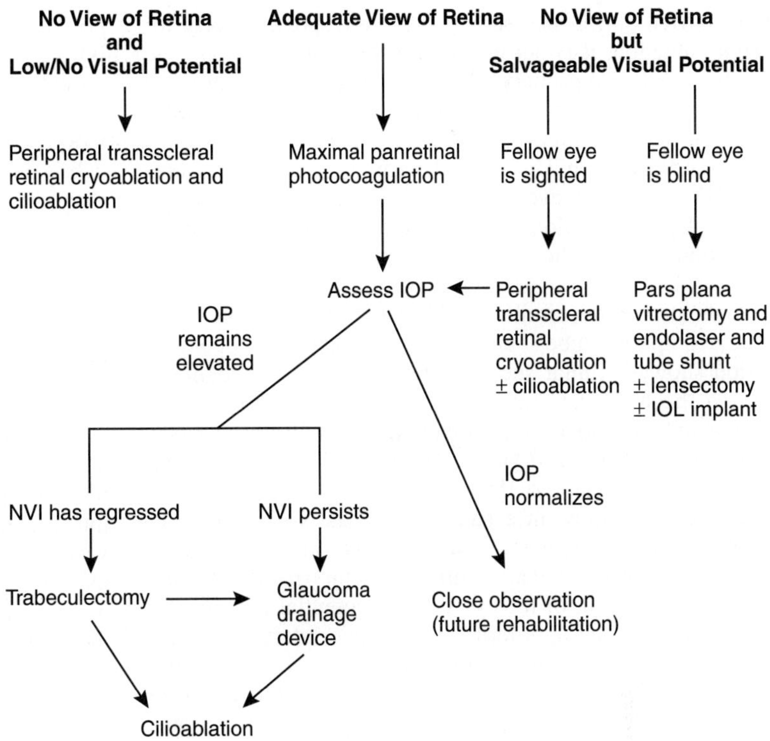

FIGURE 24–1. Management of neovascular glaucoma. IOL, intraocular lens; IOP, intraocular pressure; NVI, neovascularization of the iris.

ment of treatment effect and for decision-making about further treatment. Response to retinal ablation is variable and usually rapid. Regression of anterior segment neovascularization can be apparent within days. Whether this is accompanied by an IOP-lowering response depends on the stage of the disease at the time of intervention. If treatment is given before the angle is involved, or if only a few wispy vessels are present in the angle, pressure may return to normal. If, on the other hand, the angle has already been synechially scarred shut by contraction of the fibrovascular membrane, retinal ablation may lead to regression of iris neovascularization but is unlikely to reverse the anatomic disease of the angle or to lower IOP. In the setting of complete 360-degree synechial angle closure with attendant highly elevated IOP, retinal ablation may have a diminished effect even on iris neovascularization, perhaps because the angiogenesis factor is potentiated in the absence of any route for its egress from the eye.

If an initial IOP-lowering response occurs, the patient should be followed closely for signs of renewed neovascular proliferation. If they are seen, additional retinal ablation should be attempted. If retinal ablation has no effect on IOP (initially or with subsequent treatments), medical management alone is unlikely to provide adequate pressure control, and surgical options should be considered.

In the absence of compelling data favoring one procedure over another, often the surgical management of NVG varies among ophthalmologists, depending in part on their facility with glaucoma filtering procedures. Most would agree that in an eye with favorable visual potential, incisional filtering procedures are preferred over cilioablative procedures. But which incisional procedure should be undertaken?

Historically, trabeculectomy alone for NVG has provided 67% to 77% success in controlling IOP,[1, 2] and the advent of antimetabolite augmentation is anticipated to improve the outcome of this procedure. One study of trabeculectomy with 5-fluorouracil (5-FU) in eyes with NVG resulted in adequate pressure control in 68% of eyes at 3 years.[3] Data have not yet been reported for trabeculectomy with mitomycin C in the setting of NVG, but for many surgeons, trabeculectomy with mitomycin C is now the first step in the surgical management of NVG. We favor the use of mitomycin C in trabeculectomy for eyes with NVG. Assuming that the "evil" humor that has induced anterior segment neovascularization will now flow through our sclerostomy, aggressive use of antifibrotic agents is intuitive.

For others, tube shunt placement is the first line of therapy (the second line for those electing trabeculectomy first). Numerous drainage implant devices are available and have shown reasonable success in eyes with NVG. The Molteno implant has been shown to control pressure in 47% to 83% of eyes in various studies,[4, 5] although this device is less effective for NVG than for other types of glaucoma.[6] The Krupin-Denver valve demonstrated success in 67% of eyes in two studies.[7, 8] The newer Krupin valve controlled pressure in 77% of eyes.[9] Results with the Baerveldt implant have shown success at 12 and 18 months of 79% and 56%, respectively.[10]

The success rates for trabeculectomy with antimetabolites and tube shunt procedures are comparable. The incisional procedure of choice thus becomes even less obvious. We base the choice of procedure on the eye's response to retinal ablation. If there is substantial neovascular regression after retinal ablation, trabeculectomy with mitomycin

C is carried out. Conversely, if the eye responds poorly to retinal ablation, it is our experience that trabeculectomy is likely to fail, and primary tube shunt surgery is performed.

Eventually, however, many eyes with NVG eventually must be treated with cilioablation, by either photocoagulation or cryoablation. Cyclocryotherapy can control pressure in 34% to 63% of eyes,[11, 12] but with attendant hypotony, loss of light perception, and phthisis in significant numbers of patients. Cyclophotocoagulation has demonstrated success in 43% to 72% of eyes in various studies,[13–17] with complication rates similar to those for cryoablation. One study comparing tube shunt surgery with cyclophotocoagulation showed similar success rates for the two modalities during the first year, but more favorable success rates for tube shunts 3 years postoperatively (57% vs. 29% success), with less hypotony and vision loss in the group that underwent tube shunt surgery.[18]

Not uncommonly, in a patient who has NVG, no view of the posterior segment is afforded because of corneal edema, cataract, or dense vitreous hemorrhage. In this setting, assessment of the eye's visual potential is valuable in determining the appropriate therapeutic intervention. In the patient with concurrent ocular disease such as diabetic retinal detachment, ischemic central retinal vein occlusion, end-stage glaucomatous optic neuropathy, or other vision-limiting process, the goal of surgery is to lower the pressure, prevent discomfort, and preserve the globe for cosmesis. Such patients are perhaps best treated with a combination of primary cilioablation with simultaneous transscleral retinal cryoablation in an effort to both lower the pressure and halt the neovascular proliferative process.

Less commonly, the view of the posterior segment precludes panretinal photocoagulation but the ophthalmologist believes that the eye has potentially salvageable vision. This is often the case in monocular patients whose first eye previously lost vision from similar (or, occasionally, unrelated) disease. For NVG in the monocular patient, heroic measures are often called for. In such cases, a multiprocedure operation is often planned between the retina and glaucoma specialists, consisting of lensectomy (possibly with implantation of an intraocular lens), pars plana vitrectomy with endoscopic laser photocoagulation of the retina, and, finally, placement of a tube shunt in the anterior chamber or through the pars plana. This aggressive combination procedure may improve both vision and pressure control in a patient otherwise doomed to permanent, irreversible blindness.

For end-stage or absolutely uncontrolled NVG, in eyes with little or no visual potential and intractable pain, retrobulbar alcohol injection is a final management step, the only goal of which is to provide comfort.

This discussion is summarized in algorithm format in Figure 24–1.

INTRAOCULAR HEMORRHAGE
(See also Chapter 12)

Intraocular hemorrhage is a broad term covering many pathologic processes of multiple causes. Free blood can gain access to the anterior or posterior segment as a result of ocular trauma, surgery, or even spontaneously from pathologic neovascularization. Regardless of etiology, the presence of free blood in the eye can result in elevated IOP, often high enough to threaten optic nerve fibers or retinal circulation. The final common effect of blood in the eye is a reduction in aqueous outflow by (1) fresh red blood cells (RBCs) in the setting of hyphema, (2) hemolytic debris in ghost cell glaucoma following vitreous hemorrhage, (3) RBC-laden macrophages in hemolytic glaucoma, or (4) rarely, direct trabecular endothelial toxicity and subsequent dysfunction from iron deposits in hemosiderotic glaucoma.

Hyphema

CLINICAL FEATURES

Free blood can gain access to the anterior chamber in a number of ways. Most commonly, this occurrence follows blunt or penetrating ocular trauma but may result from intraocular surgery or even spontaneous bleeding from neovascularization (in NVG or juvenile xanthogranuloma, for instance). Any eye harboring a hyphema deserves a complete ophthalmologic history and examination to determine the cause and to identify any coincident disease. This approach is especially important in the setting of trauma, in which subsequent vision loss is almost always due to concurrent ocular disease and almost never to the presence of blood in the anterior chamber.

Although many hyphemas resolve without complication, acute IOP elevations are not uncommon and may predispose to poor outcome if not recognized and managed appropriately. The mechanism of IOP elevation in the setting of hyphema is physical plugging of trabecular outflow channels by RBCs. This can be especially dramatic in patients with sickle cell disease, in whom the RBCs sickle in the relative hypoxia of the anterior chamber, becoming less deformable and thus more effective as trabecular corks. Given that these patients have a higher risk for elevated pressure as well as the potential for compromised posterior segment blood flow, they should be followed very closely, because they are at high risk for posterior segment complications of elevated IOP (for instance, optic nerve damage or retinal vascular occlusion).

THERAPEUTIC CONSIDERATIONS

Perhaps not intuitively, there is little relationship between the size of the hyphema and the extent of the pressure rise. This is because although the settled hyphema is blocking only the inferior aspect of the meshwork, the floating RBCs are plugging all of the outflow channels 360 degrees around the angle. Therefore, even small hyphemas can manifest as markedly elevated IOP.

The management of IOP spikes in the setting of hyphema is most commonly medical rather than surgical, given the self-limited nature of the disease. Aqueous suppression is the first step, and two or more agents may be necessary. β-blockers, α-adrenergic agonists, and topical carbonic anhydrase inhibitors (CAIs) are often effective. Prostaglandin analogues offer the theoretical benefit of bypassing the obstructed trabecular channels and routing fluid through the uveoscleral outflow pathway. Miotic agents should be avoided because of their tendency to weaken the blood-ocular barrier and promote inflammation in eyes already at great risk for inflammation. Additionally, systemic CAIs should also be avoided, as they can induce systemic acidosis, which in turn promotes sickling of RBCs in patients predisposed to it. A hemoglobinopathy screen should be obtained routinely for patients at risk for sickle cell disease; if a systemic CAI is required for a sickle cell–positive patient, methazolamide is less likely to induce systemic acidosis than acetazolamide.

In the vast majority of cases, medical management alone adequately controls IOP until the blood clears the trabecular channels and IOP normalizes. Occasionally, however, IOP reaches intolerably high levels or remains elevated for a prolonged period (or both), and surgical intervention is required. This situation is commonly seen in the setting of total (so-called eight-ball) hyphema and in eyes with secondary hemorrhage (rebleeding). Suggested guidelines for surgical intervention based on extent and duration of IOP have been proposed, but we prefer to evaluate each patient's risk-benefit profile individually.

If we believe that IOP is too high and poses a threat to the eye (in terms of optic nerve damage, compromise of retinal circulation, or promotion of corneal blood staining), a surgical procedure is indicated. The most commonly performed procedure is the anterior chamber washout, in which the free-floating RBCs are evacuated from the eye by gentle irrigation through one or two limbal paracenteses. A chamber maintainer can be placed in one paracentesis and an evacuation cannula in the other. No attempt should be made to evacuate any clotted blood or to peel the clot, because (1) the clot probably plays only a minor role in IOP elevation and (2) manipulation of the clot could precipitate rebleeding. The goal of a washout procedure is to reduce the reservoir of RBCs in the anterior chamber waiting to plug the trabecular outflow channels. An acute drop in IOP following anterior chamber washout should not be expected; the remaining intratrabecular RBCs must be given time to clear the outflow channels. Occasionally, if a large residual clot is present after the washout, the operation may not successfully lower IOP, for as the clot dissolves, additional RBCs continue to plug the trabecular outflow channels.

For a marked IOP rise, or if anterior chamber washout fails to improve IOP, an acute pressure-lowering intervention is often required. In this case, coupling a small trabeculectomy with an anterior chamber washout is appropriate. Some ophthalmologists choose not to use antimetabolites, recognizing the usually self-limited nature of the disease. Others argue that RBCs, fibrin, and other substrates may cause early failure of the filter, especially if the blood has been in the eye long enough to promote formation of peripheral anterior synechiae and chronic angle-closure glaucoma; thus, these surgeons use antimetabolites. Blood patching is a well-recognized method to reduce filtration through a bleb; one doesn't want to risk losing the filter before its usefulness has expired. Intraoperative 5-FU with postoperative subconjunctival injections if needed might be a better choice than mitomycin because the former can be adjusted according to the clinical response. We also find a peripheral iridectomy to have value in the setting of an "eight-ball" hyphema, which commonly has an element of pupillary block, due to the collar button shape of the actual clot filling both the anterior and posterior chambers.

A tube shunt is rarely necessary, given that traumatic hyphemas eventually resolve (for chronic nonclearing hyphema associated with NVG, treatment should be aimed at the neovascular component, as discussed previously). If a tube shunt is to be placed, we are aware of no data to support the use of any particular implant over the others.

Ghost Cell Glaucoma

Despite its eerie name, managing ghost cell glaucoma need not be a frightening experience. Ghost cell glaucoma should be considered as the cause of elevated IOP in any eye satisfying these two conditions:

- Recent or remote vitreous hemorrhage
- Disrupted hyaloid face

CLINICAL FEATURES

Ghost cells are the empty degenerated husks of RBCs, consisting of little more than rigid cell membranes. Their characteristic semitransparent tan or khaki coloration, best seen under high magnification on slit-lamp examination as they float through the anterior chamber, gives rise to their name. These cells devolve from the RBCs of vitreous hemorrhage, resting in the vitreous until they have degenerated, then passing through the disrupted anterior hyaloid face to gain access to the anterior chamber. Once in the aqueous, they are drawn into the trabecular outflow channels, where their rigid, poorly deformable cell membranes render them effective trabecular plugs. As an aid to diagnosis, an anterior chamber tap can recover ghost cells, which when stained with methyl violet appear as degenerated RBCs with characteristic Heinz bodies within.

Ghost cell glaucoma usually lags behind the occurrence of vitreous hemorrhage, as the cells need time to degenerate within the vitreous reservoir. Once the pressure rises, it may stay elevated for a prolonged period, because a significant reservoir of ghost cells may be stored in the vitreous cavity, especially in large vitreous hemorrhages. As a result, the management of ghost cell glaucoma is likely to be more extensive than that for hyphema. In fact, so many ghost cells may spill into the anterior chamber that a pseudohypopyon—resembling a true hypopyon even in color until closer inspection—may result. There have even been case reports of a so-called candy-cane hypopyon, in which chronic recurrent vitreous hemorrhage alternately spills fresh RBCs and ghost cells into the anterior chamber so rapidly that they cannot clear, and they settle—in layers—in the inferior chamber angle.

THERAPEUTIC CONSIDERATIONS

Because ghost cell glaucoma is often self-limited, the initial management of elevated IOP in the setting of ghost cells is with topical medications. Aqueous suppression is effective, although more than one agent may be necessary. Unlike in hyphema, systemic CAIs are not contraindicated, but miotic agents should still be avoided to prevent inflammation in an eye filled with blood. Maximally tolerated medical therapy (MTMT) should be attempted before any surgical intervention, and might consist of a β-blocker, a topical (or systemic) CAI, a prostaglandin analogue, and an α-adrenergic agonist.

If the IOP is not adequately controlled with MTMT, surgical intervention is often required. Unlike with hyphema, an anterior chamber washout is ineffective because it does not eliminate the reservoir of degenerated RBCs in the vitreous cavity. Instead, a posterior chamber washout—commonly called *vitrectomy*—is indicated. This procedure can be performed through an anterior approach and coupled with trabeculectomy; this approach is challenging, however, because limited visibility of the posterior segment often prevents the extensive vitrectomy that is required to remove the ghost cell reservoir. Perhaps a better choice is the pars plana approach performed by the vitreoretinal surgeon, in combination with a trabeculectomy. The debate about the use of antimetabolites is identical to that already described for hyphema, and we favor use of antimetabolites in this setting.

The risk of trabeculectomy failure is higher in eyes with ghost cell glaucoma than in eyes without ghost cells. Ghost cells are by their nature debris, which can incite a granulomatous response in an effort to remove the debris. This inflammatory reaction can jeopardize the outcome of filtration surgery, which occasionally fails even when performed with adjunctive antimetabolite therapy. If such a failure occurs and IOP is still unacceptably high, the placement of a tube shunt should be considered. As already mentioned, no data favor choice of a particular drainage device over the others. Because eyes with ghost cell glaucoma often have concurrent or pre-existing vitreoretinal disease and may have scleral buckling elements in place, the reader is referred to the later discussion of the surgical placement of tube shunts in eyes with pre-existing scleral buckles.

Hemolytic Glaucoma

CLINICAL FEATURES

The eye's natural response to the presence of free blood is to send macrophages to consume and digest the RBCs. Because a degenerating RBC consists of little more than a lipid cell membrane, a diet consisting primarily of these cells results in the so-called lipid-laden macrophage, a golden phagocyte easily detectable on histologic evaluation of aqueous fluid. These large cells float freely in the aqueous and are drawn into and block the trabecular outflow channels, leading to an increase in IOP. These cells can be seen as red-brown cells floating in the anterior chamber under high magnification on slit-lamp examination and can also be seen as pigmented deposits in the inferior chamber angle on gonioscopy.

THERAPEUTIC CONSIDERATIONS

Medical management alone usually suffices to control the majority of cases of hemolytic glaucoma, as the disease is self-limited and tends to clear fairly rapidly. Medication choices are identical to those appropriate in the management of ghost cell glaucoma.

If MTMT fails to achieve IOP control, the first surgical step might be an anterior chamber tap, which can reduce the macrophage load within the anterior chamber as well as the physical volume of the anterior chamber, resulting in an acute pressure drop. Histologic analysis of the aspirate can also confirm the diagnosis once macrophages filled with golden-brown pigment are observed. If a more long-term solution is needed, vitrectomy is indicated because vitreous hemorrhage is the source of the RBCs upon which the macrophages are feeding. Trabeculectomy can be performed coincidentally with vitrectomy or can follow vitrectomy. Alternatively, trabeculectomy alone may be indicated if the RBC reservoir is thought to be exhausted, but an acute pressure spike demands intervention. Tube shunt surgery is rarely indicated but may benefit the occasional patient.

Hemosiderotic Glaucoma

A third form of blood-related glaucoma following vitreous hemorrhage is hemosiderotic glaucoma. As with ghost cell glaucoma, manifestation of hemosiderotic glaucoma lags behind the occurrence of vitreous hemorrhage. As the intravitreal RBCs degenerate, hemoglobin is released into the eye. Once dispersed into the vitreous and aqueous, hemoglobin is phagocytosed by trabecular endothelial cells. Further metabolism of hemoglobin within trabecular cells results in liberation of intracellular iron, which has a direct toxic effect on trabecular cells (as well as many other eye tissues). This toxicity ultimately results in decreased aqueous outflow, which may manifest as elevated IOP years after the initial vitreous hemorrhage.

CLINICAL FEATURES

Hemosiderotic glaucoma can be diagnosed only in an eye with a history of old vitreous hemorrhage. Usually, vitreous findings are still present. The trabecular meshwork may be moderately to heavily pigmented. A definitive diagnosis may be possible only with histologic confirmation by iron stain of the trabecular meshwork, using tissue obtained at the time of trabeculectomy, but only if the diagnosis is considered and the tissue submitted for the appropriate techniques.

THERAPEUTIC CONSIDERATIONS

The management of hemosiderotic glaucoma is problematic because by the time the IOP becomes elevated, irreversible damage has been done to the trabecular endothelial cells and often to other tissues of the eyes as well, especially the retina. MTMT can be attempted, but the glaucoma is often intractable. Surgical intervention (trabeculectomy or tube shunt surgery) can be undertaken if visual acuity remains viable, but in most cases, the original insult destroys not only the trabeculum but also other vital ocular tissues, and less invasive management is appropriate. Cilioablation can be of benefit in these eyes, although intractable pain in blind eyes often requires enucleation.

The discussion on glaucomas associated with intraocular hemorrhage is summarized in algorithm format in Figure 24–2.

RETINOPATHY OF PREMATURITY

The incidence of retinopathy of prematurity (ROP) is on the rise, not through any shortcomings in ophthalmic research, but rather because of the advances in neonatology that provide better survival odds for progressively more premature infants. The incidence of ocular complications associated with ROP is also on the rise, including second-

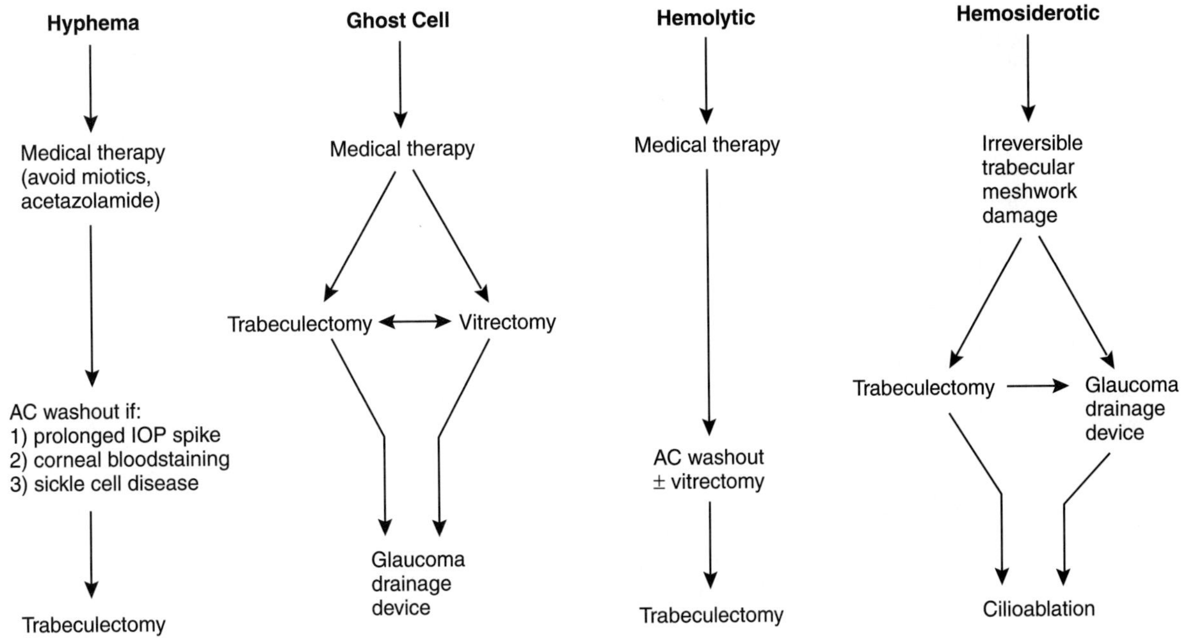

FIGURE 24–2. Management of glaucomas associated with intraocular hemorrhages. AC, anterior chamber; IOP, intraocular pressure.

ary glaucoma. Successful management of glaucoma in eyes with ROP requires a thorough knowledge of the mechanisms that may be at play in raising IOP.

The pathophysiology of ROP is not yet fully understood, but the leading theory is that the proliferation of retinal vessels in response to the hypoxic call for vascularization coming from the avascular peripheral retina somehow becomes disordered, and the classic fibrovascular proliferative process described by the ROP staging system ensues.

This pathophysiologic process is reminiscent of the cascade leading to NVG in eyes with posterior segment ischemia. Indeed, NVG can cause angle-closure glaucoma in eyes with ROP. Most often, this is seen in the setting of stage V ROP with total retinal detachment. Management of NVG has been discussed previously.

CLINICAL FEATURES

The clinical features of ROP are well described elsewhere and are not repeated here. A few important clinical findings affect therapeutic decisions. In eyes with severe ROP and glaucoma with poor visual prognosis, a cilioablative procedure is most often appropriate (see later). The following discussion applies to eyes in which there is potential for useful vision. In the setting of elevated IOP and a closed angle in an eye with ROP, pupillary block, nonpupillary block, and ciliary block mechanisms may be at play. As in eyes without ROP, the clinical distinction among these diagnoses can often be made by examining the iris configuration (e.g., iris bombé in pupillary block) and chamber configuration (e.g., central shallowing favors nonpupillary block or ciliary block).

THERAPEUTIC CONSIDERATIONS

The initial management of these individual disorders in the presence of ROP is no different from that in eyes without ROP. For pupillary block, a laser peripheral iridotomy or surgical peripheral iridectomy is advocated, although this procedure often does not completely break the attack, as pupillary block and nonpupillary block mechanisms tend to be at work simultaneously in many cases. Given the uncooperative nature of most children, examination and treatment with the patient under anesthesia may be necessary. Indirect ophthalmoscopic delivery of diode laser energy can be used for both anterior segment laser procedures (peripheral iridotomy) and posterior segment retinal ablation and can be performed on a conscious or sedated infant.

For eyes with nonpupillary block glaucoma, or for eyes that did not show response to peripheral iridotomy or iridectomy, therapy with mydriatic-cycloplegic agents should be attempted. Similarly, the initial management of eyes with ciliary block glaucoma is a course of mydriatic-cycloplegic therapy, followed (if that is unsuccessful) by laser or surgical disruption of the anterior vitreous face, followed (if that is unsuccessful) by full mechanical vitrectomy.

Once these initial steps have been taken to break the attack of angle-closure glaucoma, the eye should be carefully re-evaluated to assess angle status and determine any effect on IOP. If the angle has opened and the IOP has normalized, no further glaucoma-directed intervention is required, although careful follow-up is mandated. If the angle closure attack has been ongoing for an extended time, synechial closure of the chamber angle may have occurred; the angle will not open nor will the IOP drop in response to the therapies previously described. Alternatively, the angle may open, but the trabecular meshwork endothelial cells may have suffered significant damage, and the IOP may not drop despite the opening of the angle.

At this point, the management of angle-closure glaucoma becomes surgical, and the choice of surgical procedures depends on the visual prognosis of the eye. In eyes with poor visual potential (e.g., eyes with stage IVB or stage V ROP in which reattachment surgery has failed or that are not candidates for reattachment surgery), the appropriate

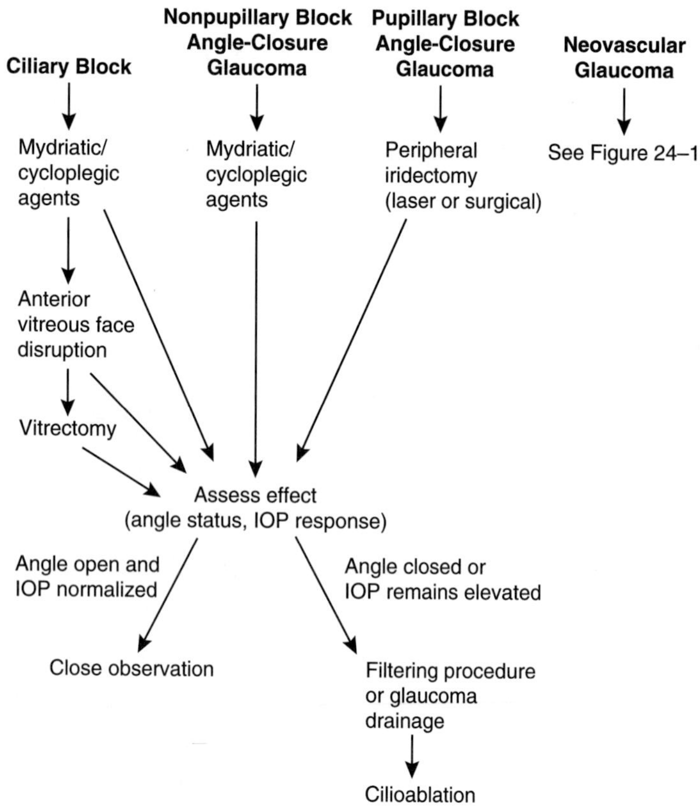

FIGURE 24–3. Management of glaucomas associated with retinopathy of prematurity. IOP, intraocular pressure.

treatment for chronic angle-closure or combined mechanism glaucoma is cilioablation. For eyes enjoying the potential for useful vision, a filtering procedure may be warranted. Among the procedures available are goniotomy, trabeculotomy, trabeculectomy, and tube shunt surgery. Goniotomy is often not a viable choice, given that corneal clouding often obscures the necessary view. Although little comparative data exist, we prefer trabeculectomy or tube shunt surgery for older children.

Not infrequently, a heroic approach is called for in infants who have lost the potential for useful vision in one eye and are in danger of losing the fellow eye to complications ensuing from ROP. In these eyes, a combination procedure—performed by both the vitreoretinal team and the glaucoma team—is warranted; it often consists of pars plana vitrectomy and lensectomy with liberal endoscopic laser treatment, retinal reattachment surgery (scleral buckle), or both, as well as a filtering procedure. Ideally, a tube shunt would be placed, but this option requires an eye and orbit large enough to accept such a device. Later enlargement of the globe may necessitate revision of the tube shunt.

This discussion is summarized in algorithm format in Figure 24–3.

GLAUCOMAS ASSOCIATED WITH POSTERIOR SEGMENT NEOPLASIA

Glaucoma, through a variety of mechanisms, can result from intraocular tumors. This discussion is general rather than specific because the management of glaucoma in eyes with posterior segment neoplasms is secondary in importance to management of the neoplasm itself. Often, enucleation is required, which cures the glaucoma.

CLINICAL FEATURES

As summarized in Table 24–1, posterior segment neoplasms can be primary or secondary. Among the common primary lesions are choroidal melanoma and retinoblastoma, which can lead to coincident glaucoma by (1) induc-

TABLE 24–1. MECHANISMS OF INTRAOCULAR PRESSURE (IOP) ELEVATION ASSOCIATED WITH POSTERIOR SEGMENT NEOPLASIA

Neoplasm	Mechanism of IOP Elevation
PRIMARY NEOPLASMS	

Posterior uveal melanoma	Neovascular glaucoma
	Outflow obstruction
	  Direct tumor invasion
	  Melanin-laden macrophages
	Angle-closure glaucoma

Retinoblastoma	Neovascular glaucoma
	Outflow obstruction
	  Necrotic tumor cells
	  Inflammatory cells
	Angle-closure glaucoma

Hemangioma	Increased episcleral venous pressure
METASTATIC NEOPLASMS	
Solid (lung, breast, kidney, rectum)	Neovascular glaucoma Angle-closure glaucoma

Other (leukemia, reticulum-cell sarcoma)	Outflow obstruction
	  Tumor cells
	  Inflammatory cells

ing angiogenesis and ultimately NVG, (2) from microscopic obstruction of trabecular outflow channels (by tumor debris, inflammatory debris, or direct tumorous infiltration), and (3) by angle closure secondary to the effect of the expansile posterior segment mass pushing the lens-iris diaphragm forward.

Of the metastatic lesions, solid tumors from lung, breast, kidney, and rectum are most common. In addition to inducing NVG, these tumors can grow large enough in the posterior segment to shift the lens-iris diaphragm forward and close the angle, raising IOP. Nonsolid tumors such as lymphoma and reticulum-cell sarcoma can mimic uveitis and can cause a uveitic glaucoma syndrome as well, plugging trabecular outflow channels with tumor cells and secondary inflammatory cells.

THERAPEUTIC CONSIDERATIONS

As stated previously, the management of glaucomas due to neoplasms must be undertaken with appropriate perspective for the long-term prognosis of the eye. Medical therapy should be instituted initially. Controversy exists regarding what role, if any, filtration surgery or tube shunt implantation should play in the management of glaucomas associated with primary intraocular neoplasia; theoretically, facilitating the egress of aqueous might also facilitate extraocular and intravascular seeding of floating tumor cells, leading to otherwise unexpected distant metastases. (Presumably, for an eye with a metastatic lesion, the tumor is already disseminated.) Similarly, if neoplasia should arise in an eye that has previously been filtered, a careful search for ocular surface metastases in the region of the filtering bleb—as well as distant metastases—should be undertaken.

Perhaps a better alternative for the patient with intractable glaucoma for whom MTMT has failed is to consider cilioablation. Obviously, for eyes with poor visual potential or uncontrollable lethal tumors, enucleation is recommended and obviates glaucoma management. It is advisable to work closely with an oncologist to assess the overall health status of the patient. Ocular tumors remain relatively rare, and it is often helpful to involve a specialist experienced in these diseases if one is available.

GLAUCOMA FOLLOWING POSTERIOR SEGMENT SURGERY

Elevated IOP is a common complication of vitreoretinal surgery. Most often the pressure rise is self-limited and of mild to moderate degree and poses little or no threat to the optic nerve. On occasion, however, the magnitude or duration of the pressure spike is great enough to endanger the optic nerve or even the retinal circulation, necessitating intervention. The most common vitreoretinal procedures associated with postoperative elevation of IOP are scleral buckling surgery, pars plana vitrectomy with placement of retinal tamponading agents (expansile gases or silicone oil), and panretinal photocoagulation. This discussion of the management of glaucomas associated with posterior segment surgery is summarized in algorithm format in Figure 24–4.

Scleral Buckling Surgery

Eyes with retinal detachment are at risk for glaucomatous pressure elevation stemming from the placement of a scleral encircling band. Although tightly secured buckles increase the risk of postoperative glaucoma, even appropriately placed buckling elements can induce pressure elevations, mediated by closure of the anterior chamber angle with subsequent reduction in outflow.

CLINICAL FEATURES

The etiologic first step in the development of postoperative glaucoma after scleral buckling surgery is impedance of flow through the vortex veins, presumably by mechanical compression of the vessels by the encircling band. Restriction of venous drainage from the eye leads to proximal congestion of ocular tissues, most notably in the ciliary body. In response to the reduced venous drainage, the plentiful vessels of the ciliary body increase in caliber, resulting in an overall enlargement of the ciliary body. The swelling of the ciliary body has been likened to the unfolding of a fan hinged at the scleral spur and prevented from opening posteriorly by the vitreous; the only direction for expansion is anterior, and as the ciliary body swells and rotates anteriorly, the anterior chamber depth is compromised.

Indeed, transient shallowing of the anterior chamber with elevation of IOP has been reported in 4% to 7% of eyes undergoing scleral buckling surgery.[19] Most cases of angle shallowing are self-limited, however, and frank angle-closure glaucoma is uncommon. When angle closure does occur, it is not mediated by pupillary block with an associated iris bombé configuration. Instead, as described previously, there is anterior rotation of the ciliary body with narrowing and eventual closure of the peripheral chamber angle, blocking the flow of aqueous through the trabecular outflow pathway.

THERAPEUTIC CONSIDERATIONS

MEDICAL THERAPY. The initial management of elevated IOP after scleral buckling surgery should be chosen with the self-limited nature of the process in mind. Aqueous suppressants are effective, and at least in theory, prostaglandin analogues might be useful in enhancing nontrabecular outflow. Epinephrine compounds are not likely to potentiate outflow through a closed angle, and miotics, such as pilocarpine, are not recommended because of their ability to enhance anterior rotation of the ciliary body, worsening angle closure. Conversely, cycloplegic agents should be used when attempting to rotate the ciliary body lens complex posteriorly.

There is often a role for oral or intravenous hyperosmotic agents in the short-term management of postoperative pressure spikes. Not only are the hyperosmotic agents effective in reducing IOP but also their ability to draw extravascular fluid into the intravascular space in part reverses the ongoing pathophysiologic process that initiated the pressure spike. Thus, to some extent, these agents treat the cause of the glaucoma.

SURGICAL THERAPY. In the majority of cases, medical management alone helps blunt the IOP spike until spontaneous resolution occurs. Occasionally, however, the pres-

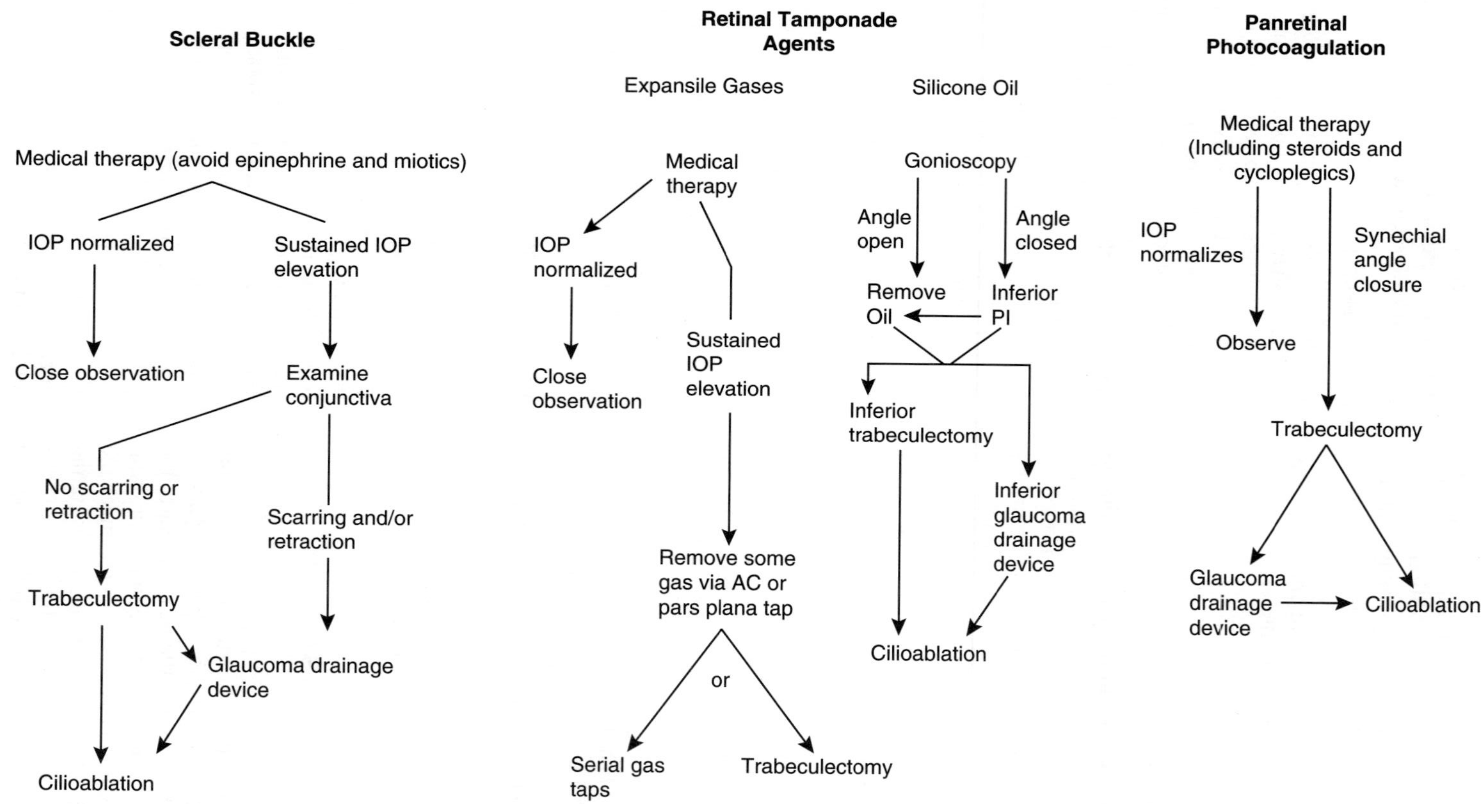

FIGURE 24–4. Management of glaucomas associated with posterior segment surgery. IOP, intraocular pressure; PI, peripheral iridotomy.

sure spike is of significant magnitude or duration that MTMT is ineffective or otherwise unacceptable, and surgical intervention must be considered. This is especially true in cases of persistent shallowing of the anterior chamber, with subsequent development of peripheral anterior synechiae and eventual chronic synechial angle closure. Thus, compression gonioscopy becomes an important diagnostic test in the preoperative assessment of these eyes.

The surgical procedures most commonly performed in this setting are trabeculectomy (with or without antimetabolites) and placement of a tube shunt. The choice of procedure is often based on the status of the conjunctiva, as there is no data to support the superiority of one procedure over another.

Scleral buckling surgery invariably includes a full 360-degree peritomy, which is often closed in less than meticulous fashion. In the choice between trabeculectomy and tube shunt implantation, the conjunctiva's location (degree of recession, if any) and mobility (extent of scarring to underlying tissue, if any) should be assessed. Recession and scarring make both procedures technically more difficult to perform; in the setting of unfavorable conjunctiva, however, trabeculectomy has a lower success rate than tube shunt implantation (in which case the bleb is posterior to the damaged region of conjunctiva). Additionally, trabeculectomy is more likely than tube shunt surgery to fail in an eye that has been recently operated (Fig. 24–5).

If the conjunctiva permits (and this is a rare instance), trabeculectomy is the procedure of choice. Both limbus-based and fornix-based conjunctival flap approaches have their advocates. The limbus-based flap has the advantage of a tighter, more leakproof closure. However, in the setting of prior scleral buckling surgery and conjunctival scarring, anterior dissection of the conjunctival flap from a posterior incision is often complicated by conjunctival buttonholing, which erases the advantage of tighter closure. A fornix-based flap has the advantage of a more limited dissection, reducing the risk of buttonholing the conjunctiva; this approach, however, is more difficult to close, and persistent leaks are common in the early postoperative period. These leaks usually heal spontaneously (or with application of a bandage contact lens) within the first week, however, and the added safety of the minimal dissection makes this the safer approach in the opinion of many glaucoma surgeons.

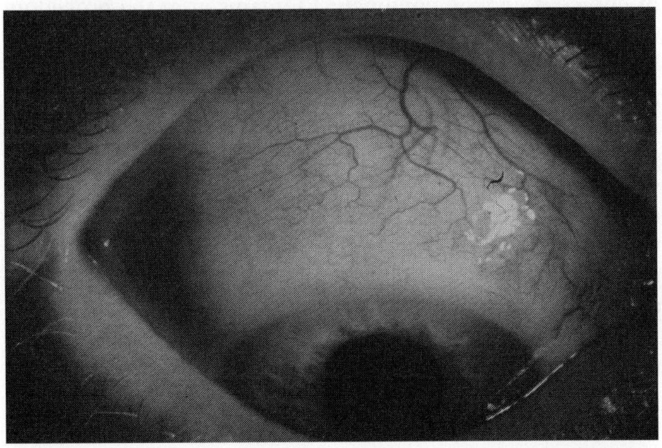

FIGURE 24–5. In this eye, there is extensive conjunctival scarring following a scleral buckle. (Courtesy of Lucian Del Priore, MD, PhD.)

The use of antimetabolites in trabeculectomy after scleral buckling surgery is worthy of discussion. Some surgeons acknowledge that the glaucoma following scleral buckling surgery usually resolves with time; thus, the filtering surgery is a temporary solution to a temporary problem. With this logic, antimetabolites are not used, and the filter is expected to fail in a short time (hopefully coincident with resolution of the glaucoma). Other surgeons approach this form of secondary glaucoma as they would any other glaucoma; they believe that antimetabolites are critical to the long-term success of a filter placed in conjunctiva with previous surgery.

In the absence of conclusive data, it is recommended that each patient be treated individually: Filtering procedures without antimetabolites may be appropriate if the surgeon believes strongly that the pressure spike is self-limited; antimetabolites are recommended for cases in which the pressure is likely to remain elevated for a protracted period. Although the use of antimetabolites is not without risk, all effort should be made to avoid necessitating a subsequent filtering procedure if the first procedure fails and the pressure rise fails to resolve.

In the setting of severely scarred conjunctiva, the likelihood of achieving successful filtration with trabeculectomy surgery is less than ideal, even with the use of antimetabolites. In these cases, it is advisable to consider tube shunt surgery. Although the latter procedure may be technically as difficult as, or more than, trabeculectomy, the surgeon can change the scarred anterior conjunctiva into an asset by directly covering the tube and preventing erosion and tube exposure. Implant choices include suturing tubing to the buckle to create a Shocket-like device to take advantage of the fibrous capsule associated with the scleral buckling element. An Ahmed valve, by virtue of its small size, may be of benefit as well in a cramped quadrant. We have successfully sutured a Baerveldt implant over a buckle. If necessary (and if approved by the vitreoretinal surgeon), a segment of the buckling element may be removed (if the retina is attached and healed) to make room for the drainage device.

As in all forms of glaucoma, the end-stage management of glaucoma after scleral buckling surgery takes the form of cilioablation. Given the risk of hypotony and related vision loss, this procedure is usually reserved for eyes in which trabeculectomy or tube-shunt surgery has failed or that have poor visual potential (for instance, eyes in which the buckling surgery failed and that are not candidates for additional reattachment procedures). In these cases, cyclophotoablation or cyclocryoablation is indicated. There is no data to support the choice of one ablative device over another in the setting of prior scleral buckling surgery.

Use of Retinal Tamponade Agents

SILICONE OIL

As an adjuvant to pars plana vitrectomy for a number of posterior segment diseases, silicone oil has become widely used to provide retinal tamponade. Silicone oil is capable of producing both an open-angle and a closed-angle glaucoma.

CLINICAL FEATURES. Ideally, silicone oil placed in the vitreous cavity would remain there; in more than half of eyes receiving silicone oil, however, the presence of emulsified oil can be demonstrated gonioscopically in the superior anterior chamber angle (oil floats in water). The mechanism of open-angle glaucoma in this setting is likely secondary to microbubbles of silicone oil obstructing the trabecular outflow channels. In addition, there may a direct toxic effect of silicone oil on the trabecular meshwork cells. Emulsified oil is visible in the anterior chamber on slit-lamp biomicroscopic examination.

The cohesive nature of the silicone oil mass within the hydrophilic fluid of the eye contributes to angle closure in some eyes. Surface tension holds the large cohesive bubble of silicone oil together as a single free-floating mass in the posterior segment, and this mass is capable of occluding the pupil and causing pupillary block, especially in aphakic patients. Clinically, the iris is bowed anteriorly, the silicone oil bubble is visible through the pupil, and the angle may not open with compression gonioscopy.

THERAPEUTIC CONSIDERATIONS. The medical management of silicone oil–related open-angle glaucoma is often unsuccessful; trabeculectomy and tube shunt surgery are also likely to fail because of obstruction of the new outflow pathway by the silicone oil, to say nothing of the loss of tamponade effect for which it was originally placed. Thus, the treatment of choice for open-angle glaucoma in eyes with silicone oil is removal of the oil. Obviously, the surgeon must make this decision in conjunction with the vitreoretinal specialist, after determining whether the glaucoma or the posterior segment disease poses the bigger threat to long-term visual prognosis.

Pupillary block is easily avoided if a peripheral iridectomy is performed in the inferior iris at the time of silicone oil infusion. Occasionally, a peripheral iridectomy placed at the time of surgery closes owing to fibrin accumulation or retroiridal proliferation of fibrovascular tissue (especially in proliferative vitreoretinopathy, an indication for the use of silicone oil). Such a closure can usually be reopened with the Nd:YAG laser, breaking pupillary block. If pupillary block cannot be broken (i.e., a peripheral iridotomy or iridectomy cannot be placed), the silicone oil should be removed. This decision must be made in consultation with the vitreoretinal surgeon.

Incisional surgery may be indicated if open-angle or angle-closure glaucoma secondary to silicone oil becomes chronic and unresponsive to medical therapy. If removal is not contraindicated, the silicone oil should first be removed from the eye to improve the probability of successful filtering surgery. If the oil can be removed, a traditional superior approach can be undertaken. Alternatively, if the eye requires both the retention of silicone oil and surgical pressure control, an inferior trabeculectomy or inferior tube shunt implantation should be considered. Otherwise contraindicated by the high rate of associated infectious endophthalmitis, an inferior approach is indicated in eyes with resident silicone oil because the very real likelihood of surgical failure from a superior approach outweighs even the risk of postoperative endophthalmitis. For end-stage glaucoma in eyes with poor visual potential or otherwise uncontrolled glaucoma in eyes with poor visual potential, cilioablation is an acceptable treatment choice.

EXPANSILE GASES

Sulfur hexafluoride (SF_6) and perfluoropropane (C_3F_8) are expansile gases commonly used in retinal reattachment procedures. Their slow resorption times (weeks) have won them favor with vitreoretinal surgeons, but their tendency to expand up to four-fold their original volume within 36 hours after injection has earned them disfavor with glaucoma specialists. Both open-angle and closed-angle forms of glaucoma have been reported with the use of expansile gases.

CLINICAL FEATURES. The surgical history and clinical examination should allow ready diagnosis of these conditions. Open-angle glaucoma can arise if the gas bubble has direct assess to the anterior chamber (common in aphakic patients). A gas bubble of adequate size within the anterior chamber can physically tamponade the trabecular meshwork, denying aqueous access to the outflow channels. Similarly, a bubble of adequate size in the posterior segment can (especially in aphakic eyes) occlude the pupil, causing pupillary block.

THERAPEUTIC CONSIDERATIONS. Peripheral iridectomy in the setting of angle closure is unlikely to break the attack if the entire posterior iris is apposed by the anterior aspect of the bubble. There is no potential route to bypass the pupil if the entire posterior iris surface is buttressed by gas.

Expansile gases all resorb eventually, and the management of elevated IOP in eyes with expansile gas bubbles should be planned accordingly. Aggressive aqueous suppression is fundamental; the combination of a β-blocker, a topical or oral CAI, and an α_2-agonist maximally suppresses aqueous production. Hyperosmotic agents may also be of benefit in the short term. Prostaglandin analogues may offer benefit by making use of alternate outflow pathways in the setting of angle-closure glaucoma. Pilocarpine should be avoided in the angle-closure form of the disease, owing to its potential to further shallow the chamber.

If temporizing with medical management is unsuccessful, a reasonable next step is to remove some of the gas via an anterior chamber or pars plana tap. This maneuver, performed in combination with constant prone positioning, may allow the lens-iris diaphragm to return to its posterior position and break the angle closure attack. Within the first few days after injection of an expansile gas, serial taps may be required during the expansile phase of the gas.

The surgical management of eyes with glaucoma related to expansile gases differs from that for silicone oil–filled eyes in that (1) the gas is not likely to permanently occlude sclerostomies or tubes and (2) the traditional superior approach can be undertaken. Trabeculectomy is the procedure of choice if enough conjunctiva remains after the procedure during which the gas was placed in the eye, and care must be taken not to allow egress of the gas bubble during the surgical procedure. Given the self-limited nature of the inciting disease, antimetabolites may not be necessary (as discussed previously for scleral buckling surgery). Tube shunt surgery is unlikely to be indicated because the glaucoma usually resolves coincident with progressive resorption of the gas bubble. If tube shunt surgery is to be undertaken, the tube may be stented with large-bore (3-0 or 4-0) polypropylene (Prolene) suture and externally ligated with polyglactin 910 (Vicryl) suture just posterior to the sclerotomy, to prevent egress of the gas.

PANRETINAL PHOTOCOAGULATION

Earlier in this chapter, panretinal photocoagulation was discussed as the "gold standard" in treatment for NVG.

Even panretinal photocoagulation therapy, however, is capable of increasing IOP through at least three separate mechanisms.

Of historical interest is the observation that primitive laser systems such as the xenon arc and ruby lasers could raise IOP by nearly 1000 mm Hg with each treatment application; this incredible pressure spike lasted less than half a millisecond, however, rendering it impressive but clinically irrelevant. Similarly, acute pressure rises (within 2 hours postoperatively) averaging 10 mm Hg have been noted in the presence of an open anterior chamber angle; this is an unexplained though self-limited process that has not been reported in association with a persistent pressure elevation.

CLINICAL FEATURES

Of more clinical relevance is the occurrence of angle-closure glaucoma after panretinal photocoagulation. Following argon laser photocoagulation, the incidence of transient shallowing of the anterior chamber has been reported to be 16%, and that of angle closure, 12%; dividing the treatment into multiple sessions reduced the incidence of chamber shallowing to 12% and eliminated the occurrence of angle closure.[20]

The mechanism by which angle closure occurs begins at the level of the retinal pigment epithelium, where light energy from the laser is converted to thermal energy. The resulting tissue injury induces intraocular inflammation, which in turn results in ciliochoroidal effusion. Expansion of the ciliary body is limited posteriorly by the vitreous gel, allowing only anterior displacement, which in turn narrows and often closes the angle. There may also be vitreous expansion by transudate from the choroid in response to inflammation, worsening the anterior shift of otherwise posterior structures. Angle-closure glaucoma in the absence of pupillary block results.

THERAPEUTIC CONSIDERATIONS

A sound treatment strategy must be based on the knowledge that photocoagulation-related angle closure is almost always self-limited. Thus, medical management is the mainstay of treatment. Because the pathophysiologic cascade is initiated by inflammation, topical steroids are recommended to control inflammation and speed resolution of the ciliochoroidal effusion. Additionally, cycloplegic agents may tighten the lens-iris diaphragm and promote deepening of the anterior chamber. In the meantime, treatment of IOP should be initiated. The appropriate medications are identical to those recommended in the medical management of glaucoma after scleral buckling surgery, discussed previously; of note, hyperosmotic agents are equally appropriate in this setting, for the same reasons.

In the vast majority of cases, angle-closure glaucoma following panretinal photocoagulation is self-limited, and supportive care facilitates resolution within a few days.

Complications of Medical Therapy

LATANOPROST

Much has been written about latanoprost, a prostaglandin analogue touted to reduce IOP by facilitating nontrabecular outflow through the ill-defined uveoscleral route. Initial reports billed latanoprost as the wonder drug for glaucoma therapy, and many glaucomatologists actually noted a decrease in surgical volume in the months following its 1995 release. This drug is a potent IOP-reducing agent. Its adverse extraocular and anterior segment effects include iris pigmentation,[21–23] eyelash growth, and anterior uveitis.[24] In the posterior segment, cystoid macular edema (CME)[25–28] has been associated with latanoprost use.

As a prostaglandin analogue, latanoprost has the potential to cause intraocular inflammation, which is a known risk factor for the development of macular edema. Macular edema in patients using latanoprost has been associated with, but not yet proved to be attributable to, use of the drug. Most reports are case reports or very small series.[25, 26] One larger series[27] has been reported—in which CME was seen in 2.1% of patients using latanoprost—but this study was retrospective in nature, and patients with CME were identified only if they presented to their ophthalmologist with symptoms suggestive of CME. Furthermore, no case of CME that improved upon cessation of latanoprost was rechallenged with the drug to establish causation.

In general, however, patients who experience CME while using latanoprost tend to be pseudophakic or aphakic. The onset of CME tends to occur soon after beginning latanoprost therapy but does not seem to be related to how long after surgery the therapy is started. CME often clears after cessation of latanoprost use, with at least partial if not complete recovery of visual acuity.

In one report, the effect of latanoprost given early after surgery to pseudophakic patients was observed.[28] There were increases in disruption of the blood-aqueous barrier (measured with a laser flare cell meter) and in the incidence of angiographically demonstrated CME formation. The magnitude of blood-aqueous disruption correlated with the incidence of CME. A nonsteroidal anti-inflammatory eyedrop (diclofenac) seemed to prevent these effects without interfering with IOP reduction.

EPINEPHRINE

Topical epinephrine therapy for glaucoma has been much more rigorously demonstrated to cause CME, especially in aphakic eyes. Several studies put the incidence at 10% to 20%.[29, 30] CME may occur years after the start of epinephrine therapy but resolves upon cessation of the drug in 80% of cases. Recognizing epinephrine as the cause of CME is important, for the macular changes may become permanent if the drug is not stopped promptly. The suspected mechanism by which epinephrine causes CME is through its stimulation of prostaglandin production within the eye, thus promoting inflammation, a risk factor for the development of CME. With the introduction of several new drugs, epinephrine is no longer commonly used.

PILOCARPINE AND OTHER MIOTIC AGENTS

The miotic agents are the oldest of the antiglaucoma medications, and although retinal detachment in patients receiving miotic therapy was reported as far back as 1877,[31] the causal relationship has not yet been proven. Presumably, contraction of the ciliary body exerts traction on the peripheral retina, predisposing to breaks, tears, and, ultimately, detachments. Retinal detachments in patients receiving miotic therapy usually occur in eyes with other risk factors for retinal detachment, such as lattice degeneration and high myopia. For most ophthalmologists, this fact is evidence that miotic agents potentiate detachments in predisposed patients; for others, the fact is proof that detachments in these eyes are unrelated to miotic therapy, because retinal detachments seldom occur in eyes that are being treated with miotic agents but have no other risk factors for detachment.

Although proof has not yet been established, most agree that miotic therapy in eyes at risk for detachment further increases the risk. To this end, a careful peripheral retinal examination is warranted before miotic therapy is given for glaucoma, to ensure the absence of factors predisposing to retinal detachment. As an aside, we find comfort in the fact that with so many newer antiglaucoma agents to choose from, we initiate miotic therapy only very rarely anymore.

Complications of Glaucoma Surgery

(See also Chapter 18)

The diagnosis and management of glaucoma often depends on careful observation of findings in the posterior segment (beyond the appearance of the optic nerve head). Conversely, therapy for glaucoma can create observable manifestations in the posterior segment. Indeed, glaucoma filtering surgery can have profound effects on the ocular posterior segment, in large part because of the IOP-dependent nature of the posterior uveal tract's structural anatomy. In this section, we discuss posterior segment findings that can occur after glaucoma filtering surgery, their significance and possible causes, clinical course, and treatment options.

CHOROIDAL EFFUSION

CLINICAL FEATURES

The choroid is a network of capillaries through which blood flows against very low resistance. One might imagine IOP and the sclera as bookends containing the posterior uveal tract and maintaining bidirectional external pressure on the potentially expansile choroid. If IOP is suddenly lowered below the intrachoroidal fluid pressure, the potential exists for the choroidal vasculature to leak. This leaked fluid collects in the suprachoroidal space and manifests clinically as a choroidal effusion.

Choroidal effusion is a painless and nearly ubiquitous postoperative finding after glaucoma filtering surgery. The typical clinical presentation is an eye with (1) low IOP (usually <6 mm Hg), (2) significant intraocular inflammation, and (3) a shallow anterior chamber. In a phakic or pseudophakic eye, the choroidal effusion produces a mass effect in the posterior segment, displacing the lens-iris diaphragm forward (hence the shallow anterior chamber) but not usually so far forward as to produce contact between the lens or iris (or vitreous) and the cornea. Careful evaluation of the posterior segment reveals a red-orange, dome-shaped elevated mass (or masses) in the peripheral choroid, thus confirming the diagnosis. Visual acuity can be compromised either through corneal edema or by physical blockage of the visual axis by the choroidal elevation. Larger choroidal effusions are visible through the pupil on slit-lamp examination or with the use of an indirect ophthalmoscope without a condensing lens (Fig. 24–6).

THERAPEUTIC CONSIDERATIONS

A thorough examination of the eye with choroidal effusion is mandated because treatment depends on clinical signs. Most choroidal effusions are small, are associated with minimal anterior segment shallowing, and resolve spontaneously as IOP rises slowly from hypotonous levels within the first postoperative week or two. These eyes should be treated with topical steroids (to reduce the associated inflammation) and cycloplegic agents (to tighten and rotate the lens-iris diaphragm posteriorly) and should only be observed as long as the eye remains stable. Often the chamber deepens before the choroidal effusion resolves. Small choroidal effusions that are difficult to observe can be detected with ultrasound biomicroscopy; they are unlikely to be clinically significant.

In rare cases, drainage of the suprachoroidal fluid is required. Individual surgeons vary in specifying a threshold for drainage. We rarely operate for this self-limited and spontaneously resolving condition; there are circumstances, however, that we believe are relative indications for drainage:

1. An effusion large enough to push the lens-iris diaphragm into contact with the cornea, resulting in decompensatory corneal edema. In this clinical setting, the bleb is often failing, the IOP is rising, and there is worsening inflammation (which may in turn be suppressing ciliary production of aqueous, prolonging the hypotony).
2. An effusion large enough to produce retinal apposition within the vitreous cavity (so-called kissing choroidals). In the presence of inflammation, retinal adhesions may develop. We have seen a rhegmatogenous retinal detachment arise from a tear at a

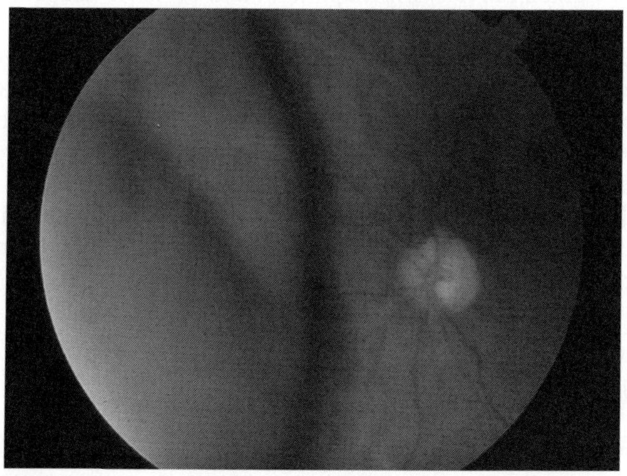

FIGURE 24–6. Postoperative choroidal effusion. (Courtesy of Lucian Del Priore, MD, PhD.)

retinal apposition site following spontaneous resolution of kissing choroidal effusions.

3. An effusion in the remaining eye of a monocular patient, to expedite visual recovery.

Surgical drainage is straightforward. First, the anterior chamber is re-formed with balanced salt solution (or with a viscoelastic agent, if necessary) through a limbal paracentesis. Ideally, a paracentesis was created at the time of trabeculectomy and can be used. Next, in the two inferior quadrants, sclerotomies are made 3.5 to 4 mm posterior to the limbus under small conjunctival peritomies, and suprachoroidal fluid is evacuated. Additional anterior chamber irrigation is carried out, and the sclerotomies are left open (under closed conjunctiva) to drain by gravity. A chamber maintainer is ideally suited for this procedure.

SUPRACHOROIDAL HEMORRHAGE

Suprachoroidal hemorrhage is possibly the most catastrophic complication of glaucoma filtering surgery. Unlike choroidal effusion, suprachoroidal hemorrhage is uncommon and is associated with several well-identified risk factors (Table 24–2), most commonly (1) advanced age, (2) systemic vascular disease (especially hypertension), and (3) hypotony. This event can occur intraoperatively (sometimes called an "expulsive hemorrhage") or postoperatively.

CLINICAL FEATURES

Clinically, suprachoroidal hemorrhage is a collection of free blood in the suprachoroidal space. It manifests as a raised elevation under the choroid and retina. Such an elevation may be small and focal or large and extensive, and typically has an irregular or lumpy surface contour, distinguishing it from choroidal effusion. Also different from effusion is the color of a suprachoroidal hemorrhage: dark orange or even brown. Also, a choroidal effusion usually extends from and involves ciliary body detachment, which is not routinely seen with suprachoroidal hemorrhage (Fig. 24–7).

THERAPEUTIC CONSIDERATIONS

The intraoperative suprachoroidal hemorrhage often occurs after surgical entry into an eye with markedly elevated

TABLE 24–2. RISK FACTORS ASSOCIATED WITH SUPRACHOROIDAL HEMORRHAGE

SYSTEMIC RISK FACTORS
Advancing age
Systemic vascular disease
Hypertension
Atherosclerosis
Bleeding disorders
OCULAR RISK FACTORS
Hypotony (especially after markedly elevated preoperative intraocular pressure)
Choroidal effusion
History of suprachoroidal hemorrhage in fellow eye
Aphakia or pseudophakia
High myopia
Previous vitrectomy
Intraocular vascular anomalies (e.g., hemangiomas)

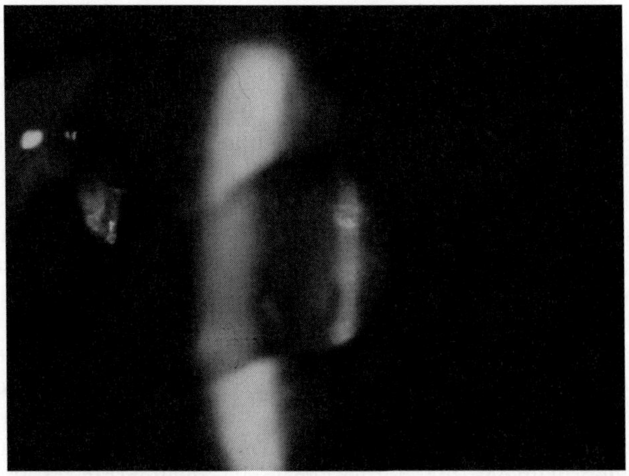

FIGURE 24–7. A postoperative suprachoroidal hemorrhage can be visualized through the pupil with the slit-lamp biomicroscope. (Courtesy of Lucian Del Priore, MD, PhD.)

preoperative IOP. The cascade of events commonly begins with the recognition of a dark mass expanding from within the posterior segment, often associated with loss of the red reflex. At the same time, the anesthesiologist comments on the elevated systemic blood pressure, the patient complains of severe ocular pain, and the anterior chamber shallows as the eye becomes rock-hard.

The level-headed, mentally prepared surgeon does not panic. Prompt, appropriate action can improve the outcome. The eye is immediately closed by tamponade of the wound with a finger until it can be sutured shut. In a guarded trabeculectomy, the flap should immediately be positioned firmly in its bed before intraocular contents extrude. The flap should be sutured tightly. The anterior chamber is reformed if this can easily be accomplished, although vigorous attempts to reform the chamber may result in further extrusion of contents. Intravenous acetazolamide and mannitol are administered to lower IOP and stabilize the eye. A dilated fundus examination may then be carried out while the patient remains on the operating table, and if a large suprachoroidal hemorrhage is present, the surgeon may elect to drain the hemorrhage from the suprachoroidal space immediately, as described previously. Alternatively, drainage may be deferred, and in fact, it may not be necessary. We prefer to delay drainage. If the uvea and retina have not been expelled through the wound prior to closure, the visual prognosis is reasonable.

More commonly, suprachoroidal hemorrhage occurs in the postoperative period, and again is characterized by the sudden onset of severe pain and markedly diminished visual acuity, often in the setting of postoperative hypotony. There may be a history of the Valsalva maneuver immediately prior to the onset of symptoms (often a sneeze or a cough, or straining at passage of stool). Patients give a characteristic history of sudden onset of pain in and around the eye, often in association with a rapid decrease in vision. One of our patients had a suprachoroidal hemorrhage while sitting in the examining room. Examination of the posterior segment reveals a "lumpy-bumpy" dark mass that may be either low-lying or quite elevated. B-scan ultrasonography should also be performed to evaluate for potential retinal detachment, retinal apposition, and vitreous hemorrhage.

Limited suprachoroidal hemorrhages without intractable pain or vitreoretinal disorder can often be conservatively managed and frequently resolve spontaneously. The decision to intervene surgically must be made with the knowledge that the hemorrhage will clot rapidly (hence the "lumpy-bumpy" appearance), and fibrinolytic clot liquefaction will occur within 7 to 14 days, thus facilitating evacuation of the hemorrhage at that time. Surgical drainage of the suprachoroidal space should be reserved for eyes with severe pain, extended retinal apposition or retinal detachment, vitreous hemorrhage, or profound hypotony.

Surgical drainage of the suprachoroidal space should be accompanied by re-formation of the anterior chamber and inflation of the bleb. Additionally, vitrectomy with instillation of an expansile gas can provide a tamponade that reapproximates the normal anatomic relationship of the posterior uveal tract with adjacent ocular structures and reduces the probability of rebleeding. After the procedure, all potential Valsalva maneuvers should be avoided, and to this end, cough suppressants and stool softeners should be prescribed liberally.

Suprachoroidal hemorrhage can be a catastrophic event following glaucoma surgery, but attentive evaluation and management can offer the hope for a reasonable visual recovery. The key step in management is to recognize the onset of suprachoroidal hemorrhage immediately and to respond appropriately. The eye should be closed immediately if the event occurs or is suspected intraoperatively. The eye should be carefully examined to determine the extent of the hemorrhage. If drainage is indicated, intravitreal gas should be considered in the surgical plan. And if the fellow eye later is to undergo glaucoma filtration surgery, the surgeon should approach the procedure mentally prepared for history to repeat itself.

OCULAR DECOMPRESSION RETINOPATHY

CLINICAL FEATURES

Ocular decompression retinopathy is a complication seen in the early postoperative period following glaucoma filtration surgery usually in eyes with markedly elevated preoperative IOP. The disease is characterized by scattered preretinal, superficial, and deep intraretinal hemorrhages throughout the retinal posterior pole and periphery, some of which have white centers suggestive of fibrin (Fig. 24–8). Disc edema can also be seen. The disorder does not appear to have an age preference, having been described in patients from 13 to 83 years of age. The hemorrhages resolve without visual sequelae if they do not involve the macula. The disorder is significant not so much for its threat to vision but for its dramatic appearance and the implications regarding alterations in ocular hemodynamics in glaucomatous eyes.

Two mechanisms have been proposed to explain this disease, one of which is vascular and the other mechanical. The vascular theory proposes that in eyes with chronically elevated IOP, retinal autoregulation is invoked to maintain perfusion. When there is a sudden reduction of IOP to zero (upon surgical entry into the eye), the retinal vascular bed is subjected to a sudden unopposed increase in blood flow, which may overwhelm the bed's autoregulatory capacity and create focal leaks. These leaks contain both blood and protein; hence, the white-centered hemorrhages seen clinically. The mechanical theory suggests that sudden IOP reduction allows the posteriorly displaced lamina cribrosa to shift forward, compromising axonal transport and leading to axonal and thus disc swelling, which can partially occlude the central retinal vein; thus, the disease may be a mild variant of central retinal vein occlusion.

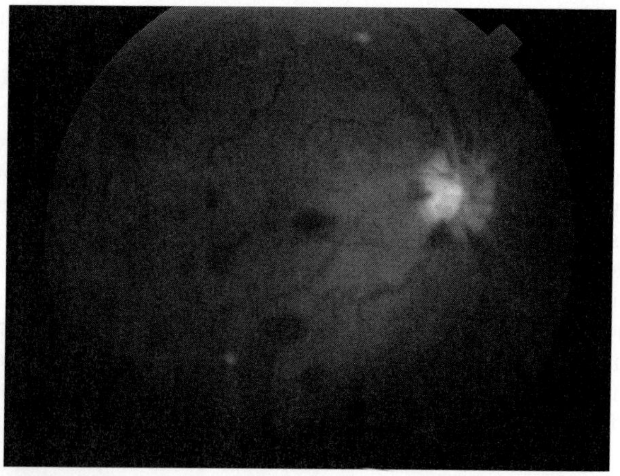

FIGURE 24–8. Multiple hemorrhages, some with white centers, are present in this eye with decompression retinopathy.

THERAPEUTIC CONSIDERATIONS

Eyes with markedly elevated preoperative IOP are at risk for ocular decompression retinopathy. Preoperative lowering of IOP or slow intraoperative reduction of IOP might possibly prevent this event. Although the clinical appearance of ocular decompression retinopathy is dramatic, the disorder is self-limited and usually is not visually significant. No intervention is required. Further understanding of this disorder may provide insight into the etiology of other ocular vascular events.

HYPOTONY MACULOPATHY

Surgical complications are like onions—they often unfold in layers and they bring tears to our eyes. When obtaining informed consent for glaucoma surgery, we routinely tell our patients that the new drain might not work as well as we want it to or that it might work too well. Certainly, hypotony is a well-recognized and often vexing complication of glaucoma filtering surgery. Also, hypotony is often not an end-point, but rather a springboard to further complications, among them hypotony maculopathy. The adjunctive use of antimetabolites in glaucoma surgery has made clinically significant hypotony a more common event.

CLINICAL FEATURES

Hypotony maculopathy appears to be most common in young patients. In myopic patients, it has a distinct clinical appearance, occurring in the setting of postoperative hypotony—usually with IOP of less than 6 mm Hg—and being associated with choroidal and retinal folds through the macular region (Fig. 24–9). In the presence of hypotony, the normally elastic sclera contracts against reduced

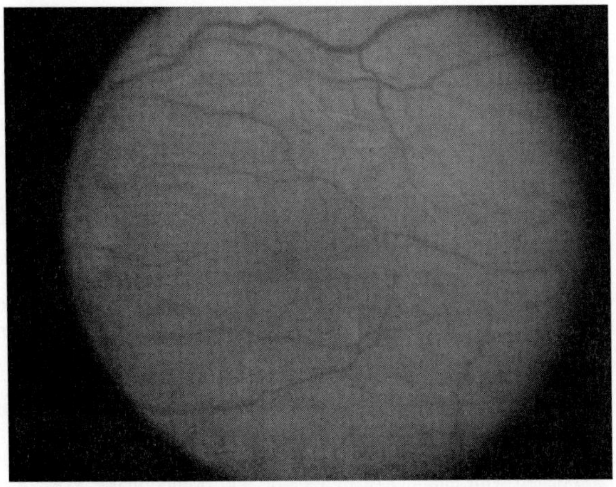

FIGURE 24–9. Hypotony maculopathy has developed after glaucoma surgery. (Courtesy of Reay Brown, MD.)

intraocular resistance, producing wrinkles in the posterior pole.

THERAPEUTIC CONSIDERATIONS

The successful preservation of visual acuity in hypotonous eyes depends on recognition and appropriate management of the consequences of hypotony. Clearly, in any case of postoperative hyoptony, the first step is to determine the cause of the abnormally low pressure. Seidel's test should be performed to rule out a wound leak of the conjunctival bleb. Overfiltration, characterized by a large intact bleb and a shallow chamber in the setting of hypotony, should also be ruled out. Significant inflammation can suppress aqueous production at the ciliary body and should be treated with aggressive topical steroids. Careful gonioscopy (which can be challenging in the hypotonous eye) may reveal a cyclodialysis cleft. Similarly, retinal detachment or choroidal detachment can promote increased uveoscleral outflow. Early intervention for hypotony can prevent the development of hypotony maculopathy.

The goal of treatment in hypotony maculopathy is to restore the IOP to a level that re-establishes normal hemodynamics and biomechanics within the posterior segment. Ideally, once the cause of hypotony is determined, appropriate steps are taken and the pressure is corrected promptly. Once IOP is appropriately normalized, hypotony maculopathy generally resolves. Resolution is more likely to occur if hypotony is reversed sooner rather than later; we have seen at least one case, however, in which visual acuity lingered at the "counting fingers" level for 3 months owing to hypotony maculopathy but improved to 20/30 when the hypotony was reversed. As a general recommendation, we would intervene if hypotony has not responded to conservative measures within 4 weeks.

The association between use of antimetabolites (mostly mitomycin C but also 5-FU) and hypotony maculopathy has been noted but not yet explained. Certainly, hypotony is more common after glaucoma filtering operations that have been augmented with antimetabolite therapy than after those that have not. Also, macular wrinkling occurs more often in hypotonous eyes that have been treated with mitomycin C than in those that have not been treated. Despite these implication, however, it is unlikely that mitomycin causes the disease, because there has never been a report of this clinical presentation in a nonhypotonous eye treated with mitomycin C.

Hypotony maculopathy can occur in the setting of postoperative hypotony following glaucoma filtering surgery. The etiology is unclear, but young patients with myopia are especially at risk. Identifying the cause of and correcting the hypotony usually leads to resolution of the macular changes, with visual outcomes being best if the maculopathy is corrected within days to weeks, rather than months.

SUMMARY

Glaucoma can arise as a manifestation of various ocular conditions afflicting the posterior segment, and careful examination of this region of the globe can provide both etiologic and therapeutic information. Neovascular glaucoma is most often explained by vascular findings in the fundus; similarly, glaucomas associated with retinopathy of prematurity, posterior segment neoplasia, and intraocular hemorrhage can be better understood and managed with the use of information derived from the posterior segment. Algorithms provided in this chapter are meant to serve as suggestions, not recipes. Every patient must be managed differently, because every tissue responds differently to different treatment modalities.

To make this point clearer, we have also discussed posterior segment tissue reactions to glaucoma interventions. In simplest terms, the eye does not appreciate sudden and dramatic reductions in IOP; although high IOP is dangerous to the eye, low IOP is no less noxious and no better tolerated. In the planning of glaucoma interventions, the "Goldilocks principle" always applies: "Not too high, not too low, . . . just right."

In this chapter, we have attempted to demonstrate that the posterior chamber can be a source both of clues to the cause of elevated IOP and of complications resulting from glaucoma therapies. This discussion underscores our fervent belief that glaucoma is a disease of the entire eye, not just a simple matter of too much pressure. Providing quality glaucoma care requires careful and comprehensive assessment of the entire globe and, often, the entire systemic medical status of the patient. Only after such an assessment can an appropriate treatment plan be derived.

REFERENCES

1. Allen RC, Bellows AR, Hutchinson BJ, Murphy SD: Filtration surgery in the treatment of neovascular glaucoma. Ophthalmology 1982;89:1181.
2. Fernandez-Vigo J, Castro J, Cordido M: Treatment of diabetic neovascular glaucoma by panretinal ablation and trabeculectomy. Acta Ophthalmol 1988;66:612.
3. Rockwood EJ, Parrish RK 2nd, Heuer DK, et al: Glaucoma filtering surgery with 5-fluorouracil. Ophthalmology 1987;94:1071.
4. Minckler DS, Heuer DK, Hasty B, et al: Clinical experience with the single plate Molteno implant in complicated glaucomas. Ophthalmology 1988;95:1181.
5. Molteno ACB, Haddad PJ: The visual outcome in cases of neovascular glaucoma. Aust N Z J Ophthalmol 1985;13:329.

6. Mills RP, Reynolds A, Edmond MJ, et al: Long-term survival of Molteno glaucoma drainage devices. Ophthalmology 1996;103:299.
7. Krupin T, Kaufman P, Mandell AI, et al: Long-term results of valve implants in filtering surgery for eyes with neovascular glaucoma. Am J Ophthalmol 1983;95:775.
8. Forestier F, Salvanet-Bouccara A: An evaluation of the Krupin-Denver valve implant in glaucoma. Glaucoma 1986;8:92.
9. Krupin T, Ritch R, Camras CB, et al: A long Krupin-Denver valve implant attached to a 180-degree scleral explant for glaucoma surgery. Ophthalmology 1988;95:1174.
10. Sidoti PA, Dunphy TR, Baerveldt G, et al: Experience with the Baerveldt glaucoma implant in treating neovascular glaucoma. Ophthalmology 1995;102:1107.
11. Krupin T, Mitchell KB, Becker B: Cyclocryotherapy in neovascular glaucoma. Am J Ophthalmol 1978;86:24.
12. Feibel RM, Bigger JF: Rubeosis iridis and neovascular glaucoma. Am J Ophthalmol 1972;74:862.
13. Dickens CJ, Nguyen N, Mora JS, et al: Long-term results of noncontact transscleral neodymium:YAG cyclophotocoagulation. Ophthalmology 1995;102:1777.
14. Trope GE, Ma S: Mid-term effects of neodymium:YAG transscleral cyclocoagulation in glaucoma. Ophthalmology 1990;97:73.
15. Schuman JS, Puliafito CA, Allingham RR, et al: Contact transscleral continuous wave neodymium:YAG laser cyclophotocoagulation. Ophthalmology 1990;97:571.
16. Brancato R, Giovanni L, Trabucchi G, Pietroni G: Contact transscleral cyclophotocoagulation with Nd:YAG laser in uncontrolled glaucoma. Ophthalmic Surg 1989;20:547.
17. Devenyi RG, Trope GE, Hunter WH, Badeeb O: Neodymium:YAG transscleral cyclocoagulation in human eyes. Ophthalmology 1987; 94:1519.
18. Eid TE, Katz LJ, Spaeth GL, Augsburger JJ: Tube-shunt surgery vs. neodymium:YAG cyclophotocoagulation in the management of neovascular glaucoma. Ophthalmology 1997;104:1692.
19. Sebestyen JG, Schepens CL, Rosenthal ML: Retinal detachment and glaucoma. I: Tonometric and gonioscopic study of 160 cases. Arch Ophthalmol 1962;67:736.
20. Doft BH, Blankenship GW: Single versus multiple treatment sessions of argon laser panretinal photocoagulation for proliferative diabetic retinopathy. Ophthalmology 1982;89:77.
21. Alm A, Stjernschantz J: Effects on intraocular pressure and side effects of 0.005% latanoprost applied once daily, morning or evening. A comparison with timolol. Scandinavian latanoprost study group. Ophthalmology 1995;102:1743.
22. Camras CB: Comparison of latanoprost and timolol in patients with ocular hypertension and glaucoma: A six-month masked, multicenter trial in the United States. The United States latanoprost study group. Ophthalmology 1996;103:138.
23. Watson P, Stjernschantz J: A six-month, randomized, double-masked study comparing latanoprost with timolol in open-angle glaucoma and ocular hypertension. The latanoprost study group. Ophthalmology 1996;103:126.
24. Fechtner RD, Khouri AS, Zimmerman TJ, et al: Anterior uveitis associated with latanoprost. Am J Ophthalmol 1998;126:37.
25. Ayyala RS, Cruz DA, Margo CE, et al: Cystoid macular edema associated with latanoprost in aphakic and pseudophakic eyes. Am J Ophthalmol 1998;126:602.
26. Callanan D, Fellman RL, Savage JA: Latanoprost-associated cystoid macular edema. Am J Ophthalmol 1998;126:134.
27. Warwar RE, Bullock JD, Ballal D: Cystoid macular edema and anterior uveitis associated with latanoprost use: Experience and incidence in a retrospective review of 94 patients. Ophthalmology 1998; 105:263.
28. Miyake K, Ita I, Maekubo K, et al: Latanoprost accelerates disruption of the blood-aqueous barrier and the incidence of angiographic cystoid macular edema in early postoperative pseudophakias. Arch Ophthalmol 1999;117;34.
29. Kolker AE, Becker B: Epinephrine maculopathy. Arch Ophthalmol 1968;87:196.
30. Mackool RJ, Muldoon T, Fortier A, Nelson D: Epinephrine-induced cystoid macular edema in aphakic eyes. Arch Ophthalmol 1977; 95:791.
31. Pape LG, Forbes M: Retinal detachment and miotic therapy. Am J Ophthalmol 1978;85:558.

SECTION V

KEY GLAUCOMA MEASURES

CHAPTER 25

Intraocular Pressure

HENRY JAMPEL

The care of all patients with glaucoma requires synthesis. As was addressed in the section "Key Diagnostic Signs," the entire history and examination must be brought together to reliably determine the correct working diagnosis. The optimal treatment regimen can then be formulated. Today, the key measure we are able to modify with glaucoma therapy is intraocular pressure (IOP). Intraocular pressure remains a very important risk factor in the development of glaucoma, but it no longer holds the singular role of the past. In this chapter, Henry Jampel does a wonderful job of summarizing the key points involved in the interpretation of intraocular pressure. He then expands on the implications of IOP for examination techniques. Management principles involving the reduction of intraocular pressure are then addressed specifically according to the magnitude of IOP elevation. Implicit in this discussion is the determination of target pressure. This portion also includes the implications of IOP less than 8 mm Hg. Finally, special cases are addressed, including measurement in infants and children, asymmetric IOP, and asymmetry in ocular pulse amplitudes. This chapter presents a complete overview of the care process of the treatment of patients with glaucoma based on the one factor identified that treatment currently changes, intraocular pressure.

Why Measure Intraocular Pressure?

Every eye care practitioner recognizes that measurement of intraocular pressure (IOP) is an essential portion of the ocular physical examination. The American Academy of Ophthalmology lists IOP measurement as one of the required elements of its Preferred Practice Patterns for a comprehensive eye examination. Knowledge of the IOP in a patient's eyes is important for two reasons: (1) a high or low IOP can be a sign of ocular or systemic disease and (2) high or low IOP can damage the eye and cause vision loss. This chapter does not address the theory or technique of IOP measurement because these topics have been extensively covered elsewhere.[1–3] The chapter is intended to aid the reader in (1) interpreting the significance of an IOP measurement in the context of other historical and physical findings and (2) formulating a diagnosis and a therapeutic plan.

Cautions in the Interpretation of Intraocular Pressure Measurements

The results of any clinical measurement and all laboratory studies should be interpreted in the context of the accuracy of the instrument, the reproducibility of the measurement, and fluctuations in the actual value over time. All of these considerations are relevant to the measurement of IOP.

The IOP varies with the time of day[4] and from day to day.[5] These fluctuations are unlikely to be important in the consideration of the implications of an extremely high or low IOP measured on one occasion. They become important, however, in the evaluation of (1) IOP over time and (2) the effect of treatment to lower the IOP. All good clinical studies of IOP lowering take into account the variation in IOP from hour to hour.

Another source of variation in IOP measurement is the instrument used. The "gold standard" for IOP measurement is the Goldmann applanation tonometer. In the range of IOP measurements between 10 and 25 mm Hg, the TonoPen correlates quite well with the Goldmann tonometer.[6] Outside this range, the correlation is not as good. The pneumatonometer tends to read higher than the Goldmann applanation tonometer across the range of IOPs.[7] If an IOP measurement is surprisingly high or low with the use of one of these two instruments, it should be confirmed with the applanation tonometer if at all possible. However, some pathologic conditions of the cornea can lead to either an underestimation or an overestimation of the IOP with the applanation tonometer. A cornea that is thickened from edema gives a falsely low IOP reading, whereas a cornea thickened from an increased amount of collagen fibrils produces an artifactually high reading.[2]

A final source of variation is simply that occurring in the performance of more than one measurement in an eye at the same time. It is apparent from clinical studies in which the IOP is measured up to three times in the course of a minute that there can be considerable variation among measurements.

There are weak relationships between IOP and systemic hypertension or diabetes mellitus.[8,9] Although the presence of either of these diseases might alter one's approach to lowering the IOP, it has little bearing on the implications of a given IOP measurement. In striking contrast is the importance of the presence of sickle cell anemia or sickle cell trait in the interpretation of an IOP measurement, particularly in the presence of a traumatic hyphema (see later).[10]

Diagnostic Maneuvers Stimulated by an Intraocular Pressure Value

HISTORY (Table 25–1)

Much can be learned from a patient history about the origin and significance of an elevated or depressed IOP measurement. Sometimes the most fundamental and obvious of questions are all that are required. The following questions can yield information far greater than the effort required to ask them:

TABLE 25–1. QUESTIONS TO ASK A PATIENT RELEVANT TO INTRAOCULAR PRESSURE

What is the reason for your visit?
Do you have glaucoma, or has anyone ever told you that you have high eye pressure?
Did you take eyedrops or pills for your eyes today?
When was the last time you saw an eye physician?
Have you ever had any surgery on your eyes?
Have you ever been struck in the eye or had any serious eye injury?
Has anyone in your family taken eye drops or been told that they have glaucoma?

What is the reason for your visit?

Is this a routine eye examination, or does the patient have symptoms of a change in vision or pain? If the patient is symptomatic, what are the nature and duration of the symptoms?

Do you have glaucoma or has anyone ever told you that you have high eye pressure?

This simple question will often separate persons with from those without glaucoma.

Did you take eyedrops or pills for your eyes today?

This question is worth asking whether or not the answer to the second question is "Yes." If the answer to this question is "Yes," the patient should be asked exactly when medicines were taken and to producc the bottles if possible. If the patient does not have the medication, he or she should be asked the name of the medication or the color of the bottle cap. A yellow or blue bottle cap indicates that the medication is a β-blocker; purple, an adrenergic agent; green, a miotic; orange, topical carbonic anhydrase inhibitor. If the IOP is abnormally low, it is possible that the patient is taking medications that should have been discontinued, for instance, after glaucoma surgery.

If the answer to this question is "No," the patient should be asked whether eyedrops or pills were ever prescribed and, if so, why he or she has not taken the medication today. The physician may learn that the patient did not understand that treatment was intended to be long-term, could not tolerate some medications, or could not afford a medication.

Whether or not a patient has recently taken medications for IOP has implications for the therapy used to lower the IOP, if indicated. For a patient who has simply run out of medications, the reinitiation of medications may be sufficient to control the IOP. If the patient has run out of medications, the physician needs to determine why. If the cost of medications is a problem, the physician can arrange for the patient to participate in one of the several programs that pharmaceutical companies offer to patients who find the cost of medications a hardship or recommend a more economical strategy for lowering the IOP. If the problem seems to be a lack of understanding of the condition and the need for treatment, it is incumbent upon the physician to educate the patient.

The possibility should also be explored that the eyedrops a patient has been using were taken for some reason other than to lower the IOP. In particular, patients should be asked whether they are taking "steroid" eye drops, prednisone drops, or drops for allergy or itchy eyes. If the IOP is elevated, it is important to exclude the use of corticosteroids as a contributing factor.

When was the last time you saw an eye physician?

If the patient has never seen an eye physician, the answer will be "Never." Otherwise, this question should provide an idea about how recently the patient has seen an eye physician, lead to the identity of the physician, and indicate whether previous medical records might be of use.

Have you ever had any surgery on your eyes?

Elevation of IOP can be caused by recent or remote intraocular surgery. Although patients usually spontaneously volunteer this information, they may not. Fortunately, a careful physical examination usually resolves any confusion regarding previous surgery.

The one exception to this last statement is laser trabeculoplasty, because there are rarely any definitive physical signs that it has been performed and because patients can forget whether or not a laser treatment was performed and on which eye. Because the role of repeat laser trabeculoplasty is limited,[11] obtaining previous medical records concerning laser trabeculoplasty is important for the formulation of a therapeutic plan.

Have you ever been struck in the eye or had any serious eye injury?

Traumatic glaucoma may manifest immediately after an injury or months to years later, and is a common cause of unilateral elevation of IOP. Trauma is almost certainly a more common cause of elevated IOP among an ocular emergency room population than among an eye clinic population.

Does anyone in your family use eye drops for glaucoma or been told that they have glaucoma?

The presence of a history of glaucoma in a family member, particularly if the patient thinks that the family member lost vision or went blind from glaucoma, may lower the practitioner's threshold for initiating IOP-lowering therapy. It also provides an opportunity for the practitioner to stress the need for careful eye care for all family members.

PHYSICAL EXAMINATION (Table 25–2)

Visual Acuity and Refractive Error

The visual acuity and refractive error may provide clues about the effect of a given IOP on ocular structures and insight into the cause of an abnormal IOP. If the patient has an uncorrected visual acuity of 20/30 or better in each eye, it is unlikely that the eyes are either hyperopic enough to raise the risk of closed-angle glaucoma or myopic enough to raise the risk of pigment dispersion syndrome or chronic open-angle glaucoma.

If the visual acuity is decreased, one must consider the possibility that the eye has suffered enough glaucomatous optic nerve damage to result in the loss of central vision. This hypothesis can be confirmed by pupillary testing, ocular examination, and visual field evaluation.

Pupillary Response

The swinging flashlight test is performed to detect a relative afferent pupillary defect. Although the presence of an afferent pupillary defect does not correspond tightly with the degree of asymmetry in optic nerve damage,[12] the presence of an afferent pupillary defect in an eye in which glaucomatous damage is suspected strongly suggests that optic nerve damage is present. A full ocular examination will exclude other possible causes for the pupillary abnormality.

A mid-dilated and nonreactive pupil is characteristic of an eye with IOP elevation to the point where iris sphincter ischemia has occurred, as in an acute attack of angle-closure glaucoma. The pupil in an eye with extensive neovascularization of the iris is usually mid-dilated and nonreactive. A small nonreactive pupil suggests the use of a miotic agent, such as pilocarpine, or may be the result of posterior synechiae from inflammation or miotic use. A large nonreactive pupil suggests the use of a cycloplegic agent, either postoperative or for the treatment of inflammation.

TABLE 25–2. ESSENTIAL ASPECTS OF THE OCULAR EXAMINATION RELEVANT TO INTRAOCULAR PRESSURE

Visual acuity and refractive error
Pupillary response
Biomicroscopy
Gonioscopy
Examination of the optic disc and retina

Biomicroscopy

(See also Chapters 10–15)

The skin of the lids and face should be examined to exclude Sturge-Weber syndrome and nevus of Ota as related to an elevation of IOP.

The conjunctiva should be examined for injection, which may point to acute angle closure, inflammation, or neovascularization. The presence of a conjunctival incision for either cataract surgery or glaucoma surgery should be noted as well as the presence of a filtration bleb. The observation of markedly dilated veins suggests elevated episcleral venous pressure. Adrenochrome deposits signify the long-term use of epinephrine eyedrops. The presence of follicles may signify an allergy to topical antiglaucoma medications.

Corneal edema can occur either with a rapid rise in IOP or from a more modest and constant elevation of IOP in an eye with a compromised cornea. Corneal edema can account for varying amounts of visual acuity decline in an eye with elevated IOP. Corneal edema can impede the view of intraocular structures and prevent a definite diagnosis. The view can be improved by the application of glycerin ophthalmic solution. A large corneal diameter and the presence of parallel breaks in Descemet's membrane suggest a diagnosis of congenital glaucoma. The presence of pigment on the corneal endothelium denotes pigment dispersion of some sort, most commonly as part of the pigment dispersion syndrome or following intraocular surgery. Keratic precipitates signify past or current inflammation. A unilateral beaten-metal appearance of the corneal endothelium is characteristic of iridocorneal endothelial syndrome. Bilateral endothelial changes are present in posterior polymorphous corneal dystrophy.

The anterior chamber depth, both central and peripheral, can be estimated on slit-lamp examination. A peripheral anterior chamber depth less than a quarter of the corneal thickness suggests that a narrow anterior chamber angle may be found on gonioscopy (van Herick's rule). Evidence of a layered hyphema and circulating erythrocytes or ghost cells should be sought, as well as cell and flare signifying inflammation.

The iris should be carefully examined at both low and high magnification and with direct illumination and retroillumination. The pupillary margin should be examined at high magnification for the presence of posterior synechiae, ectropion uveae, new blood vessels, exfoliation material, and sphincter tears. New blood vessels should also be sought elsewhere on the iris. Transillumination should be performed to detect the presence of the midperipheral radial defects of pigment dispersion syndrome; the spontaneous iris holes that occur in Axenfeld-Rieger syndrome and the iridocorneal endothelial syndrome; iris defects due to surgery, such as laser iridotomies and surgical peripheral iridectomies; and iris defects, such as an iridodialysis, due to trauma. Segmental iris atrophy, a sign of previous IOP-related ischemia of the iris, should be noted. The contour of the midperipheral iris should be examined in eyes with a suspicion of pigment dispersion syndrome to determine whether there is midperipheral posterior bowing.

The crystalline lens may have exfoliation material on the anterior lens capsule in the characteristic pattern of a centrally involved disc, a clear surrounding annulus, and a peripherally involved area, or in any other pattern. The whitish sub–anterior basement membrane opacities known as glaucomflecken, if present, suggest a previous attack of angle-closure glaucoma. The lens may appear thickened and cataractous, providing the anatomic substrate for angle closure. The lens may be so cataractous that the capsule has become permeable to lens protein, resulting in lens protein–induced, or phakolytic, glaucoma.

The position of an intraocular lens within the eye may provide clues regarding the IOP. There may be cells in the anterior vitreous, signifying inflammation.

Gonioscopy

(See also Chapter 13)

Gonioscopy should be a part of all initial, complete, eye examinations. The following questions pertaining to the IOP should be addressed by gonioscopy:

- Is the anterior chamber angle open or closed?
- If the angle is closed, is this an acute attack of pupillary block glaucoma?
- If the angle is closed and this is not an attack of pupillary block, why is the angle closed?

Chronic narrow-angle glaucoma, uveitis, neovascularization, and previous flat anterior chamber secondary to surgery or trauma are some of the more common causes. If the angle is open, are any abnormalities present, such as hyperpigmentation, neovascularization, and angle recession characteristic of trauma? The finding of a surgical fistula may confirm that a trabeculectomy has been performed.

The question of whether or not the angle is closed can be a difficult one when gonioscopy is compromised by corneal edema, which is often the case in an emergency situation. The fellow eye should be examined with the gonioscope. If the fellow eye does not have a narrow angle, one should assume that the acute event in the affected eye is not pupillary block glaucoma until all other causes have been excluded.

Examination of the Optic Disc and Retina

(See also Chapter 16)

Once the pupillary response has been evaluated and the anterior segment and gonioscopic examinations have been completed, the pupils may be dilated for optimal examination of the optic nerves. The exception is in the eye with a potentially occludable angle, in which mydriasis might precipitate pupillary block. Examination of the optic nerve usually allows the practitioner to categorize the optic nerve as unlikely to be damaged, possibly damaged, almost certainly damaged, or definitely damaged. This categorization, along with the IOP level and other risk factors, determines whether a visual field test should be performed.

The detection of proliferative diabetic retinopathy raises the likelihood that an IOP elevation may be due to neovascularization of the anterior segment.

Principles of Management

DETERMINING WHETHER INTRAOCULAR PRESSURE SHOULD BE LOWERED

The IOP *should* be lowered under the following circumstances:

1. The magnitude of the IOP value represents a threat to the immediate health of the eye, regardless of the status of the optic nerve.

2. Glaucomatous optic nerve damage is present, and the IOP is statistically elevated. No single value separates elevated IOP from IOP that is not elevated. The minimum IOP value for inclusion of a subject in the Ocular Hypertension Treatment Study is 24 mm Hg; that for the Collaborative Initial Glaucoma Treatment Study is 20 mm Hg. The standard of care seems to be that if the IOP is 20 mm Hg or greater and glaucomatous optic nerve damage is present, by virtue of either disc appearance or visual field characteristics, the IOP should be lowered.

An exception to this standard is the patient in whom the rate of progression of damage is likely to be so slow that the risk of clinically significant damage during the patient's lifetime is extremely low. For example, a 90-year-old patient with IOP values around 25 mm Hg but with minimal visual field loss in only one eye is unlikely to go blind from glaucoma.

3. There is no definite glaucomatous optic nerve damage, but the likelihood of the development of optic nerve damage is substantial. There exists a wide variety of opinion as to what is an acceptable IOP in an eye in which there is no visual field loss and the optic nerve has no glaucomatous damage. Some physicians are uncomfortable merely observing such an eye if the IOP is 25 mm Hg, whereas others observe such eyes with IOP values of 30 mm Hg or higher. The Ocular Hypertension Treatment Study allows random assignment of eyes to observation with IOPs of 32 mm Hg or less.

The presence of a large cup, a nerve fiber layer defect, or both lowers the IOP value at which treatment is desirable, because these findings may signify that early damage has already occurred. Because the risk of developing significant damage is a function of how long the IOP is elevated as well as how high it is, the patient's age is an important factor in the decision to treat. A 40-year-old patient with normal visual fields and an IOP of 25 mm Hg is more likely to lose vision from glaucoma over the course of his or her life than the 90-year-old patient previously mentioned.

Many physicians adhere to the philosophy that the more non–IOP-related risk factors a patient has for the development of glaucoma damage, the lower the threshold for treatment. They therefore reduce the threshold IOP for beginning treatment if the patient is black, has a family history of glaucoma, or, perhaps is myopic or has diabetes.

The IOP *may* be lowered under the following circumstance:

Glaucomatous optic nerve damage is present, but the IOP is not statistically elevated. In at least one sixth of patients with glaucoma damage, IOP values do not exceed 20 mm Hg.[13] The Normal Tension Glaucoma Study randomized patients with IOPs in the normal range up to 24 mm Hg and who had glaucomatous optic nerve damage to either IOP-lowering therapy or observation. The study found that lowering the IOP by 30% in such patients greatly reduced the rate of progression of glaucoma damage.[14, 15] Therefore, there is a strong rationale for lowering IOP in persons with glaucomatous optic nerve damage and statistically normal IOP. The benefits of reducing the IOP to a very low value must be weighed against the side effects of the therapy necessary to achieve this goal.

Approaches to this problem have included (1) observe the eyes in question for the development of further damage and initiate treatment if progression is observed, (2) treat one eye but observe the other without therapy, and (3) treatment if indicated.

DETERMINING HOW FAST INTRAOCULAR PRESSURE MUST BE LOWERED

The rapidity of IOP lowering is in part dictated by the acuteness of the IOP rise. If the patient presents with the sudden onset of pain and blurred vision, the IOP rise has been recent. The IOP should be aggressively controlled because one cannot be sure that it is not still rising. If, however, the patient is asymptomatic and there is no corneal edema, the process is likely to be chronic and the IOP relatively stable.

For an IOP value of 40 mm Hg or less, the rapidity of IOP lowering is related to the extent of optic nerve damage. The more severe the damage, the more quickly one will want to achieve the target IOP.

DETERMINING WHETHER THE LOWERING OF THE INTRAOCULAR PRESSURE IS SUFFICIENT

Unfortunately, we have no means to determine prospectively whether the amount of IOP lowering that we have achieved is sufficient. If we could lower a patient's IOP and then observe reversible cupping or visual improvement, we could conclude that a safe target pressure has been met.[16] Such observations are not possible in the vast majority of patients today. Instead, we must observe a patient over time, concluding, if more damage occurs, that our target was not low enough. Conversely, we have no means of determining whether we have required too much IOP lowering in a patient who does not show any evidence of worsening; such a patient may be suffering from the side effects of unnecessary treatment.

DETERMINING WHETHER THE INTRAOCULAR PRESSURE NEEDS TO BE RAISED

If there are signs of anatomic distortion of the macula, visual function is impaired as a result of low IOP, or both, the IOP needs to be raised.

Implications of an Intraocular Pressure Value (Table 25–3)

In the following discussion, arbitrary categories of IOP have been defined. This should not be misconstrued as suggesting that there are abrupt transition points at which the significance of the IOP suddenly changes. All data indicate that the risks inherent in elevated IOP increase in a continuous fashion in the population as a whole. With regard to abnormally low IOP measurements, there is only a weak correlation between how an eye sees and its IOP. Some eyes appear to function normally at an IOP of 3 mm Hg; others show structural and functional changes at an

TABLE 25–3. IMPLICATIONS OF AN INTRAOCULAR PRESSURE (IOP) VALUE

IOP (mm Hg)	Significance	Diagnosis	Management
>40	Needs to be lowered	Consider neovascular, exfoliation, pigmentary, traumatic, uveitic and acute angle closure glaucomas	Time frame: Lower IOP within hours to days; panretinal photocoagulation for neovascular glaucoma; laser iridotomy for angle closure IOP need not be "normalized" if there is no optic nerve damage
25–40	Probably needs to be lowered, depending on optic nerve status and other risk factors	Dilated stereoscopic disc examination and visual field testing	Establish target IOP; if IOP higher than target, use medications, laser, or surgery to achieve target
8–24	IOP measurement has little significance on its own in an individual patient	Dilated stereoscopic disc examination to determine whether disc is normal; if disc is abnormal, obtain visual field test	Establish target pressure on basis of baseline IOP and optic nerve appearance and function Lower the IOP
<8	IOP is abnormally low May or may not be associated with poor vision	Look for wound leak, cyclodialysis cleft, traction on ciliary body, choroidal and retinal detachment, and systemic disease	Repair wound leak, cyclodialysis cleft, retinal detachment Drain choroidal detachment, treat inflammation

IOP of 9 mm Hg. The sections that follow, however, provide a "ballpark estimate" of what the physician and patient may expect for an eye with a given IOP.

An important question is whether the elevation or depression of the IOP is unilateral or bilateral. This issue is discussed in the section on asymmetric IOP.

INTRAOCULAR PRESSURE GREATER THAN 40 mm Hg

Significance

There is universal agreement that an IOP greater than 40 mm Hg is not normal. IOP greater than 40 mm Hg may develop (1) acutely, as in a case of acute angle-closure glaucoma or glaucoma associated with uveitis, (2) intermittently, as in some cases of pigment dispersion or glaucomatocyclitic crises, or (3) chronically, as in some cases of chronic open-angle glaucoma.

The presence of pain is helpful in determining whether the IOP elevation is acute or chronic. Acute elevation of IOP is often painful, perhaps because of the acute stretching of the globe and the stimulation of sensory pain fibers. Eyes in which the IOP has gradually risen tend not be painful. The rapid onset of pain suggests a rapid rise in IOP. This history should stimulate the examiner to look more carefully for evidence of some disorder other than chronic open-angle glaucoma.

It is common for patients with IOP greater than 40 mm Hg to report vision loss, which is often the presenting complaint. If the IOP has been greater than 40 mm Hg for some time, the patient may have vision loss from glaucomatous optic atrophy. If the IOP has risen recently, the patient may have corneal edema that reduces vision. If the blood supply to the optic and retina is compromised, the patient may notice transient obscurations of vision, particularly when changing positions.

One important concern about markedly elevated IOP is that it may result in a central retinal vein or artery occlusion. It stands to reason that an IOP that exceeds the systolic blood pressure within the central retinal artery or that is simply high enough to impede blood flow through the central retinal vein may cause ischemia, sluggish blood flow predisposing to thrombosis, or both. One study has provided further evidence for a relationship between elevated IOP and glaucoma and central retinal vein occlusion (CRVO), but in most of the patients in the study, IOP was well below 40 mm Hg.[17] If an extensive hyphema is present, the markedly elevated IOP increases the rapidity with which corneal blood-staining occurs.

If the IOP rapidly rises to even higher levels, temporary or permanent damage can be done to the iris sphincter muscle, resulting in a dilated and poorly reactive pupil. Furthermore, necrosis of the lens epithelial cells can produce anterior opacities in the lens (glaucomflecken).

An IOP greater than 40 mm Hg is highly likely to produce glaucomatous atrophy of the optic nerve if it persists. If one extrapolates data from models of IOP elevation in monkeys,[18] one could expect to detect glaucomatous optic atrophy after several months to a few years in humans. The relationship between risk of glaucomatous optic atrophy and IOP is not linear; damage probably occurs much more quickly at 50 mm Hg than at 40 mm Hg.[13]

Diagnosis

All the aspects of the history and physical examination described previously as well as visual field testing should be performed in patients with IOP greater than 40 mm Hg. Special attention should be given to what glaucoma medications, if any, the patient is currently taking and when the medications were taken, because in most instances, the physician will wish to lower the IOP over the course of hours to days.

Although primary open-angle glaucoma can produce IOP in this range, the likelihood of other diagnoses seems to increase as the IOP is higher and higher. Slit-lamp and gonioscopic examinations concentrating on signs of trauma, uveitis, neovascularization, exfoliation, and pigment dispersion have a high yield in this group of patients.

The presence of arterial pulsations at the optic disc should be noted. If there are spontaneous arterial pulsations, the IOP is between the systolic and diastolic blood pressures in the central retinal artery. This is a sign that the blood supply to the inner retina may be compromised. If there are no spontaneous arterial pulsations, the physician can raise the IOP in the eye with gentle pressure on the globe. If this maneuver brings out pulsations, presumably the IOP is less than diastolic, and the eye is at low risk for a vascular occlusion. If, however, there are no spontaneous arterial pulsations and they are not elicited by pressure on the globe, the IOP is greater than the systolic blood pressure in the central retinal artery, and the globe is hypoperfused.

Management

Eyes with IOP values of 40 mm Hg or greater should receive IOP-lowering therapy, because IOP elevations of this magnitude may be associated with CRVO and because the likelihood of glaucomatous optic neuropathy is extremely high.

Lowering the IOP is urgent when the value exceeds 50 mm Hg or if the central retinal artery is compromised. In cases of nonpupillary block glaucoma, the IOP should be lowered medically in the physician's office to a level at which the eye is not in immediate danger (generally between 30 and 40 mm Hg). For pupillary block glaucoma, iridotomy should be performed, either immediately or after medical lowering of the IOP. Close follow-up is necessary to ensure that dangerous IOP elevation does not recur.

If the IOP is between 40 and 50 mm Hg and the central retinal artery is not compromised, medical treatment can be initiated in the office and the patient sent home on treatment. The patient must be made aware that the IOP is potentially imminently sight-threatening, so that he or she will understand the necessity of keeping the follow-up visits. The first follow-up visit should generally be scheduled for less than 1 week after the first visit to make sure that the IOP has been adequately lowered.

INTRAOCULAR PRESSURE BETWEEN 25 AND 40 mm Hg

Significance

An IOP value between 25 and 40 mm Hg is unlikely to pose an immediate and permanent risk to vision. Exceptions to this statement include (1) the eye with a visual field defect imminently threatening fixation, (2) the eye with a hyphema in a patient with sickle cell disease, and (3) a patient experiencing an acute episode of IOP elevation.

In most eyes, however, an IOP in this range indicates the possibility that glaucomatous optic nerve damage has already occurred or will occur in the future. It is important to emphasize at this point that *glaucoma* is defined as an optic neuropathy that produces a characteristic optic nerve appearance and a characteristic defect in the field of vision and is generally not defined in terms of IOP.

IOP is the most important risk factor for the development of glaucomatous damage. The greater the IOP, the greater the likelihood that glaucomatous damage is present,[13] and the greater the chance that the glaucoma damage is more severe.[19] The rising risk of glaucomatous damage with increasing IOP is not a linear relationship; each increase in IOP of 1 mm Hg raises the risk of damage much more than the previous 1–mm Hg increase. This is a statistical concept, however, that applies to populations. For a given individual, the risk of glaucomatous damage from a given IOP is much harder to predict. There is marked individual variation in susceptibility to pressure-induced optic nerve damage.

The risk of sustaining glaucoma damage from a given IOP is probably influenced by other risk factors for glaucoma damage, such as race and family history. In addition, as discussed previously, one or even several, measurements of IOP provide only a rough idea of the IOP from hour to hour and day to day. It is quite possible that the mean IOP is not as important in glaucomatous damage as are other parameters, such as peak IOP.

For most eyes, measuring an IOP in this range should not cause panic or provoke rash therapeutic measures to lower the IOP. There is almost always time for a thorough eye examination and even close follow-up without therapy.

Diagnosis

All the aspects of the history and physical described previously should be performed for patients with IOP between 25 and 40 mm Hg. Because the prevalence of glaucomatous damage is approximately 8% at 25 mm Hg and increases with rising IOP, a full-threshold visual field examination is indicated in all patients with IOPs in this range.

Management

The extent of IOP lowering should be based on the risk for and the consequences of future damage. The greater the likelihood of future glaucomatous damage, the more the IOP should be reduced. As Anderson[20] has stated, "The likelihood of future damage is best predicted by the degree of damage already present and its rate of progression." Therefore, the more severe the pre-existing glaucomatous damage, the more the IOP should be lowered. The extent of damage not only is the best predictor of the likelihood of future damage but also determines the likely effect on the patient's useful visual function if he or she has progressive damage.[21] In an eye with a fovea-threatening visual field defect, one cannot afford to underestimate the amount of IOP-lowering necessary, because an underestimation could lead to a significant decrease in the eye's function.

Many researchers have advocated factoring in the side effects of IOP-lowering therapy in determining how much the IOP should be lowered. Taniguchi and Kitazawa[22] have suggested that the drug or the combination of drugs that will achieve the target IOP and will have no or negligible adverse effect should be identified for each glaucoma patient, considering the patient's ocular and systemic conditions. Hodapp and colleagues[21] have stated that "to determine a pressure goal, the risks and cost, including side effect cost, of treatment to lower pressure any given amount must be weighed against the risk of the pressure itself."

Although determining the appropriate amount by which to lower the IOP is distinct for each patient, one way of estimating the amount of IOP lowering desirable is to use the following equation:

$$\frac{\mathrm{IOP}^2}{100} - Z + Y \text{ mm Hg}$$

where Z is an optic nerve damage severity factor, and Y is a burden of therapy factor (Table 25–4).

INTRAOCULAR PRESSURE BETWEEN 8 AND 24 mm Hg

Significance

An IOP value between 8 and 24 mm Hg has no diagnostic significance. Many more persons with such values, even those with IOPs at the higher end of this range, do not have disease than do. The prevalence of glaucoma damage in the Baltimore Eye Survey was only 8.3% for IOP values of 22 to 24 mm Hg.[13] However, the risk of a person having glaucoma appears to increase with IOP at all levels of IOP, so the prevalence of glaucomatous damage may be as much as 12-fold greater at 24 mm Hg than at 15 mm Hg.[13]

Obtaining an IOP measurement in this range does have the value of providing confidence that there is no imminent threat to visual function solely from the IOP. There is the great danger, however, that finding an IOP in the "normal" range, the practitioner will conclude that glaucoma cannot

TABLE 25–4. GRADING OF DAMAGE AND BURDEN OF THERAPY

Value of Z and Y (mm Hg)	Z, Optic Nerve Damage	Y, Burden of Therapy
0	Normal disc, normal visual field	No effect upon patient's QOL
1	Abnormal disc, normal visual field	Small effect
2	Visual field loss not threatening fixation	Moderate effect
3	Visual field loss threatening or involving fixation	Large effect

From Jampel HD: Target pressure in glaucoma therapy. J Glaucoma 1997;6:133–138.
QOL, quality of life.

be present and will not perform a complete ophthalmologic examination with sufficient diligence. The proportion of patients with glaucoma who have a one-time IOP measurement of 24 mm Hg or less is approximately 75%, and the proportion of those who have a one-time IOP measurement of 20 mm Hg or less is approximately 50%.[13] One of the problems with using IOP as the only tool for screening for glaucoma is that the patients participating in the screening may believe that they do not have glaucoma simply because their IOP values were within the normal range.

Because an IOP between 8 and 24 mm Hg has little diagnostic value, the physician must rely solely on the history, physical examination, and, perhaps perimetry to determine whether glaucoma is present or whether the patient is at high risk for the development of the disease.

Diagnosis

All the aspects of the history and physical described earlier should be performed for the patient with an IOP between 8 and 24 mm Hg. The main diagnostic decision is whether or not a visual field test should be performed, and there is no absolute answer to this question. One reasonable approach would be that if there are no history or physical findings suggesting that glaucoma is present, a visual field test is not indicated. If, on the other hand, there are substantial risk factors,, such as a positive family history, a history of chronic corticosteroid use, pigment dispersion, or optic nerves that appear abnormal, a visual field test should be obtained. Because the prevalence of glaucomatous damage is much higher at the upper end of this IOP range than at the lower, fewer historical or physical risk factors for the presence of damage need to be present to justify the performance of a visual field test.

The decision to order a visual field test for a patient with an IOP in this range should take into account the fact that many patients without glaucomatous damage have an abnormal visual field test the first time that they are tested. Therefore, the decision to perform a visual field test may at times be a decision to perform two or three such tests to confirm the normality of the patient's visual fields.

Management

The basic principles underlying the management of eyes with IOP values between 25 and 40 mm Hg apply for eyes with IOP values between 8 and 24 mm Hg. Although factors other than IOP may play an increasingly greater role in the development of optic nerve damage in eyes with lower IOP, intraocular pressure stills appears to play a role in pathogenesis.[23] One study even suggests that an IOP value in the "low teens" is better than IOP in the "high teens" in eyes without any evidence of glaucoma.[24] Furthermore, although definite proof is still lacking, the results of several studies demonstrating that eyes with glaucoma in which IOPs are in the "low teens" do better, in terms of vision preservation, than those in which IOP values are in the "high teens"[25, 26] suggest that IOP lowering is beneficial in this range.

There are some differences in management of eyes with glaucoma damage in this IOP range: First, the need to lower the IOP is rarely urgent; there is usually ample time to establish the patient's IOP pattern and to determine, through several visual field tests, the extent of glaucoma damage. Second, it may be difficult to obtain a substantial decrease in the IOP with medication or laser treatment, particularly if the IOP is 15 mm Hg or below to begin with. Third, because the absolute amount of IOP lowering in this range is less than if the IOP were 40 mm Hg to begin with, it is more difficult to sort out a therapeutic lowering of IOP from imprecision in measurement and IOP fluctuation. For example, is a drop from 15 mm Hg to 13 mm Hg really a reduction in IOP?

INTRAOCULAR PRESSURE LESS THAN 8 mm Hg

Significance

The number of normal eyes with IOP of 8 mm Hg or less is very small, in part because the episcleral venous pressure is normally 8 to 9 mm Hg.[27] Under normal circumstances, the IOP is always at least as great as the episcleral venous pressure. Abnormally low IOP can affect vision through several mechanisms, including alteration of the refractive error, macular edema, and hypotony maculopathy. In some of these problems, there may be a greater chance for reversal if the hypotony is detected and treated as early as possible. Therefore, finding an IOP this low warrants a systematic search for a cause.

Diagnosis

HISTORY

Knowledge of the common elements in the differential diagnosis of hypotony aids in the selection of diagnostic features on which to concentrate. A history of intraocular surgery is a key finding, whether the surgery was intended to lower the IOP (glaucoma surgery) or not (cataract surgery). Most cases of hypotony after intraocular surgery are self-limited, and often nothing more than observation is required. One exception is the hypotony that can occur from epiciliary proliferation following vitrectomy for proliferative vitreoretinopathy.[28] Ciliodestructive procedures, particularly cyclocryotherapy, have been associated with hypotony. If the patient with hypotony has not undergone eye surgery, a history of trauma should be sought. For example, a posterior scleral rupture from blunt trauma can produce hypotony.

Other historical factors relevant to an eye with hypotony include the use of IOP-lowering drugs, such as alpha-adrenergic agonists and prostaglandin analogs, that can lower the IOP below episcleral venous pressure. The use of β-blockers even in the fellow eye of an eye that has undergone filtration surgery has been associated with hypotony.[29, 30] Because acute anterior uveitis can produce hypotony, a history of ocular inflammation is germane, as is a history of photopsia and floaters, because retinal detachment may produce low IOP. Hypotony has also been associated with myotonic dystrophy, dehydration, uremia, and carotid artery disease.

One should not forget that phthisis is preceded by a period of hypotony and that hypotony and phthisis are the final pathway for some severely diseased eyes.

PHYSICAL EXAMINATION

SLIT-LAMP BIOMICROSCOPY. If the hypotonous eye has undergone a filtration procedure, a large filtration bleb may be sufficient to explain the low IOP. A label of ultrafiltration is used for this condition, and efforts to change the situation are made only if vision is threatened. If a conjunctival bleb is visible for a prolonged period after cataract surgery, a permanent passageway from the anterior chamber to the subconjunctival space has been created. As with the overfiltering glaucoma bleb, this situation generally does not require therapy if the vision is good.

One exception to this rule is if there is a bleb leak, that is, a free communication between the subconjunctival space and the tear film. This entity can sometimes be diagnosed under conditions of standard white light but is most easily diagnosed with a Seidel's test. A concentrated solution of 2% fluorescein, or a fluorescent strip, is placed in the vicinity of the putative leak. Under blue illumination, with or without digital pressure on the globe, a stream of brilliant yellow is seen emanating from the leak. Wound leaks are undesirable because of the presumed increased risk of endophthalmitis and so, in general, should be treated.

Slit-lamp biomicroscopy is also used to determine (1) the depth of the anterior chamber and (2) whether anterior uveitis is present. In addition, pigment in the anterior vitreous, which can be seen on slit-lamp examination, is a sign of a retinal break.

GONIOSCOPY. Gonioscopy is useful for the detection of a cyclodialysis cleft. A cyclodialysis is the separation of the ciliary body from its insertion to the scleral spur. Cyclodialysis clefts may occur as a result of trauma or may be formed inadvertently at the time of cataract and glaucoma surgery or intentionally at the time of glaucoma surgery or combined cataract and glaucoma surgery.

OPHTHALMOSCOPY. Indirect ophthalmoscopy is used to detect choroidal detachment and retinal breaks with or without retinal detachment. Examination of the macula with a slit-lamp beam and either a hand-held lens or a contact lens is performed to determine whether there are folds in the macula characteristic of hypotony maculopathy or macular edema.

ULTRASOUND. If the media are opaque, B-scan ultrasonography can provide visualization of choroidal and retinal detachment. Ultrasonic biomicroscopy can be used to detect a cyclodialysis cleft and ciliary body detachment.

Management

If there is no leak across the conjunctiva, there are no signs of anatomic distortion of the macula, and visual function is not impaired, observation is all that is required. When treatment is required, it is directed toward the underlying abnormality. Wound leaks of the conjunctiva and sclera can be repaired, cyclodialysis clefts closed, suprachoroidal fluid drained, retinal detachments repaired, and inflammation treated.

Special Cases

ELEVATED INTRAOCULAR PRESSURE IN THE SETTING OF TRAUMATIC HYPHEMA

IOP should be followed carefully in all patients with a traumatic hyphema. Read and Goldberg[31] have observed that in patients with normal hemoglobin, the risk of optic atrophy increases if the IOP is greater than 50 mm Hg for 5 days or greater than 35 mm Hg for 7 days.

Elevation of IOP is much more ominous in patients with sickle cell disease, sickle cell trait, or other hemoglobinopathies. There are several reports in the literature of retinal vein and artery occlusions in patients with sickle cell trait, even with only modest elevation of IOP.[32, 33] In addition, such patients are at greater risk of optic atrophy. Patients with hyphema and hemoglobinopathy should be hospitalized so that the IOP can be monitored several times a day. The recommendations of Deutsch and associates[10] from their study of 22 patients with sickle cell trait and hyphema were as follows: If the IOP remains greater than 25 mm Hg for 24 consecutive hours, or if it transiently and repeatedly exceeds 30 mm Hg, a paracentesis and anterior chamber washout should be performed. Alternative methods of effective IOP lowering may also be considered.

INFANTS AND CHILDREN

IOP measurement is not a standard part of a pediatric eye examination, because (1) abnormalities of IOP are unusual in infants and children and (2) IOP measurement can be difficult, and hence unreliable, in this age group. If the patient has a syndrome associated with elevated IOP, or if there are symptoms such as photophobia or signs such as corneal haze or a large optic disc cup, IOP measurement becomes mandatory.

The measurement of IOP in infants and children can be complicated by problems of cooperation. The best way to measure the IOP is without the use of systemic anesthetics. In the patient younger than 6 months, the IOP can generally be measured if the baby has just been fed and is resting in a parent's arms. Some older infants, toddlers, and preschool children can be coaxed into cooperating, but in many children, the IOP cannot be measured accurately while they are conscious. The development of the TonoPen has allowed the measurement of IOP in conscious children in whom it was not possible by other methods.

If the child needs to be anesthetized, intramuscular ketamine should be considered, because unlike the inhalation anesthetics, it does not lower the IOP.[34] When the patient is anesthetized, the rest of the eye examination, including gonioscopy and optic nerve evaluation, can be performed in a thorough fashion not always possible with the child conscious.

As in the adult, the IOP in a child should always be interpreted in the context of the entire ophthalmologic and patient examination. In most instances of glaucoma in childhood, however, the IOP is markedly elevated, and the decision that the IOP needs to be lowered is straightforward. It can be difficult, however, to establish a target pressure. This is because the amount of glaucoma damage, in the presence of reversible cupping of the optic nerve but without information about the visual fields, can be difficult to determine. Furthermore, proving that the target pressure has been consistently achieved is problematic if the child must be anesthetized for every measurement of the IOP.

ASYMMETRIC INTRAOCULAR PRESSURE

The measurement of a difference in IOP of more than 25% between a patient's two eyes should raise the possibility in the examiner's mind of something more than primary open-angle glaucoma. History and physical examination often yield an obvious explanation, such as glaucoma surgery in one eye and not the other, or a severe unilateral secondary glaucoma (e.g., neovascular). If they do not, the physician should devote extra effort to detecting a subtle secondary glaucoma, such as pigment dispersion, exfoliation, and traumatic glaucoma, as well as undiagnosed chronic angle-closure glaucoma. Another entity to be considered is unilateral carotid artery disease,[35] particularly if the IOP has suddenly decreased unilaterally and if the patient has a history of atherosclerosis. Often, no explanation is found for the asymmetric IOP measurements.

ASYMMETRY IN THE OCULAR PULSE AMPLITUDE

The IOP varies with each heartbeat, as blood is forced through the choroidal and retinal vasculature. The *ocular pulse amplitude* is the difference between the minimum and maximum IOP values during the cardiac cycle. This can be detected as the rhythmic pulsation of the mires of the applanation tonometer, or as the sine waveform of the tracing of the pneumatonometer. Although a large ocular pulse amplitude is associated with conditions such as carotid artery–cavernous sinus fistula, finding a difference in ocular pulse amplitude between a patient's two eyes is a much more sensitive and specific finding.[36] A difference in ocular pulse amplitude greater than 1.6 mm Hg was found in one study to be 100% sensitive and 93% specific for carotid artery–cavernous sinus fistula, with the increased amplitude in the affected eye.[36] Other causes of asymmetry in the ocular pulse amplitude are unilateral high myopia, choroidal hemangiomas and melanomas, unilateral ocular ischemic disease, and extremely elevated IOP.[36]

REFERENCES

1. Grant W, Schuman J: Tonometry and tonography. *In* Epstein D (ed): Chandler and Grant's Glaucoma. Baltimore, Williams & Wilkins, 1997, pp 41–45.
2. Schottenstein E: Intraocular pressure and tonometry. *In* Ritch R, Shields M, Krupin T (eds): The Glaucomas. St. Louis, Mosby–Year Book, 1996, p 414.
3. Shields M: Textbook of Glaucoma, 3rd ed. Baltimore, Williams & Wilkins, 1992, pp 59–74.
4. Wilensky JT, Gieser DK, Dietsche ML, et al: Individual variability in the diurnal intraocular pressure curve. Ophthalmology 1993;100:940–944.
5. Jensen AD, Maumenee AE: Home tonometry. Am J Ophthalmol 1973;76:929–932.
6. Frenkel R, Hong Y, Shin D: Comparison of the Tono-Pen to the Goldmann applanation tonometer. Arch Ophthalmol 1988;106:750–753.
7. Quigley H, Langham M: Comparative intraocular pressure measurements with the pneumatonograph and Goldmann tonometer. Am J Ophthalmol 1975;80:266–273.
8. Tielsch J, Katz J, Quigley H, et al: Diabetes, intraocular pressure, and primary open-angle glaucoma in the Baltimore Eye Survey. Ophthalmology 1995;102:48–53.
9. Tielsch J, Katz J, Sommer A, et al: Hypertension, perfusion pressure, and primary open angle glaucoma: A population-based assessment. Arch Ophthalmol 1995;113:216–221.
10. Deutsch TA, Weinreb RN, Goldberg MF: Indications for surgical management of hyphema in patients with sickle cell trait. Arch Ophthalmol 1984;102:566–569.
11. Jorizzo PA, Samples JR, Van BE: The effect of repeat argon laser trabeculoplasty. Am J Ophthalmol 1988;106:682–685.
12. Brown RH, Zilis JD, Lynch MG, Sanborn GE: The afferent pupillary defect in asymmetric glaucoma. Arch Ophthalmol 1987;105:1540–1543.
13. Sommer A, Tielsch JM, Katz J, et al: Relationship between intraocular pressure and primary open angle glaucoma among white and black Americans: The Baltimore Eye Survey. Arch Ophthalmol 1991;109:1090–1095.
14. Collaborative Normal-Tension Glaucoma Study Group: Comparison of glaucomatous progression between untreated patients with normal-tension glaucoma and patients with therapeutically reduced intraocular pressures. Am J Ophthamol 1998;126:487–497.
15. Collaborative Normal-Tension Glaucoma Study Group: The effectiveness of intraocular pressure reduction in the treatment of normal-tension glaucoma. Am J Ophthalmol 1998;126:498–505.
16. Katz LJ, Spaeth GL, Cantor LB, et al: Reversible optic disk cupping and visual field improvement in adults with glaucoma. Am J Ophthalmol 1989;107:485–492.
17. The Eye Disease Case-Control Study Group. Risk factors for central retinal vein occlusion. Arch Ophthalmol 1996;114:545–554.
18. Quigley HA, Hohman RM, Sanchez R, Addicks EM: Optic nerve head blood flow in chronic experimental glaucoma. Arch Ophthalmol 1985;103:956–962.
19. Quigley HA, Tielsch JM, Katz J, Sommer A: Rate of progression in open-angle glaucoma estimated from cross-sectional prevalence of visual field damage. Am J Ophthalmol 1996;122:355–363.
20. Anderson D: Glaucoma: The damage caused by pressure. Am J Ophthalmol 1989;108:485–495.
21. Hodapp E, Parish II RK, Anderson D: Clinical Decisions in Glaucoma. St. Louis, Mosby–Year Book, 1993.
22. Taniguchi T, Kitazawa Y: A risk-benefit assessment of drugs used in the management of glaucoma. Drug Saf 1994;11:68–74.
23. Cartwright MJ, Anderson DR: Correlation of asymmetric damage with asymmetric intraocular pressure in normal-tension glaucoma (low-tension glaucoma). Arch Ophthalmol 1988;106:898–900.
24. Varma R, Hilton SC, Tielsch JM, et al: Neural rim area declines with increased intraocular pressure in urban Americans. Arch Ophthalmol 1995;113:1001–1005.
25. Roth SM, Spaeth GL, Starita RJ, et al: The effects of postoperative corticosteroids on trabeculectomy and the clinical course of glaucoma: Five-year follow-up study. Ophthalmic Surg 1991;22:724–729.
26. Migdal C, Gregory W, Hitchings R: Long-term functional outcome after early surgery compared with laser and medicine in open-angle glaucoma. Ophthalmology 1994;101:1651–1656.
27. Asamoto A, Yablonski M: Physiology and measurement of episcleral venous pressure. *In* Ritch R, Shields M, Krupin T (eds): The Glaucomas, 3rd ed. St. Louis, Mosby–Year Book, 1996, p 352.
28. Zarbin MA, Michels RG, Green WR: Dissection of epiciliary tissue to treat chronic hypotony after surgery for retinal detachment with proliferative vitreoretinopathy. Retina 1991;11:208–213.
29. Burney EN, Quigley HA, Robin AL: Hypotony and choroidal detachment as late complications of trabeculectomy. Am J Ophthalmol 1987;103:685–688.
30. Vela MA, Campbell DG: Hypotony and ciliochoroidal detachment following pharmacologic aqueous suppressant therapy in previously filtered patients. Ophthalmology 1985;92:50–57.
31. Read J, Goldberg M: Comparison of medical treatment for traumatic hyphema. Trans Am Acad Ophthalmol Otolaryngol 1974;78:799–815.
32. Goldberg MF: Sickled erythrocytes, hyphema, and secondary glaucoma. I: The diagnosis and treatment of sickled erythrocytes in human hyphemas. Ophthalmic Surg 1979;10:17–31.

33. Wax MB, Ridley ME, Magargal LE: Reversal of retinal and optic disc ischemia in a patient with sickle cell trait and glaucoma secondary to traumatic hyphema. Ophthalmology 1982;89:845–851.
34. Quigley HA: Childhood glaucoma: Results with trabeculotomy and study of reversible cupping. Ophthalmology 1982;89:219–226.
35. Knox D: Ocular pressure studies in the diagnosis of carotid artery disease. Trans Am Ophthalmol Soc 1973;71:459–487.
36. Golnik KC, Miller NR: Diagnosis of cavernous sinus arteriovenous fistula by measurement of ocular pulse amplitude. Ophthalmology 1992;99:1146–1152.

CHAPTER 26

Visual Fields

RONALD FELLMAN

The current standard for definitively determining the presence of glaucomatous damage is visual field testing. Many aspects of perimetry are complex and confusing. They can diminish the physician's ability to interpret the result, and make patient care more difficult. In this chapter, Ron Fellman deciphers the standard achromatic Humphrey Field Analyzer visual field printout. He logically identifies the key areas of the field and makes sense out of the "apostilbs." In addition, he provides insight into how to clinically approach the field test statistics and interpretation so that the appropriate information is obtained to guide the determination of the status of the patient's glaucoma. As clinicians, we depend on the visual field as the major test to quantify the amount and possible progression of glaucomatous damage. In this chapter are the tools to facilitate this process.

The major goal of perimetry is to find and follow visual field defects, and achromatic techniques remain the "gold standard" for accomplishing this task. The classic method of achromatic perimetry tests short-, middle-, and long-wavelength–sensitive neural visual channels by projecting a white test object onto a white background. Other exciting perimetric modalities designed to isolate neural subchannels, which are beyond the scope of this discussion, are frequency doubling, motion, high-pass resolution, flicker, foveal, and chromatic field techniques (see also Chapter 5). A clearer understanding of achromatic perimetry serves as a building block for comprehending other field assessment techniques.

This chapter is intended to be a departure from the usual "apostilb," "isopter"-like textbook approach. A plethora of book chapters are dedicated to this cause, one even by the author, who urges their reading. This chapter presents the nine categories of the single field analysis (SFA) of the Humphrey Field Analyzer (HFA); Humphrey Instruments, San Leandro, CA) in order, from top to bottom, of the field printout (Fig. 26–1). My purpose is to define the critical sign or common pattern recognition (CPR) associated with this particular printout and to enlighten the reader about why it occurred. Every example has been gleaned from a busy glaucoma clinic visit. Practically all meaningful glaucoma clinic field visits revolve around this printout. Psychophysics is incorporated into the discussion when helpful to the explanation of the phenomena.

The visual field analysis is a diagnostic test highly dependent on physician acumen for interpretation. There are many "scotoma traps" along the perimetric way. This chapter is intended to help the reader avoid falling into them. The level of physician expertise is critical in integrating the final interpretation of the field data. The process of testing and the means of data expression continue to improve, a sign of current imperfection and technologic evolution. Physician knowledge of the physiologic, pathologic, and artifactual conditions that alter the visual field has a dramatic impact on the patient's quality of life. In order to understand early pathologic changes, the physician must be familiar with normal variations.

An apparently "statistically normal" visual field does not imply a disease-free state. Conversely, an apparently "abnormal" field may simply be due to a trivial artifact. This chapter is dedicated to explaining the difference. A *normal* reliable static field implies that differential light sensitivities at preselected retinal locations are within age-adjusted normal limits. An *abnormal* reliable static field implies that differential light sensitivities at preselected retinal locations are outside age-adjusted normal limits. The physician still has to determine whether an abnormal field is "pathologic" by ultimately correlating its findings

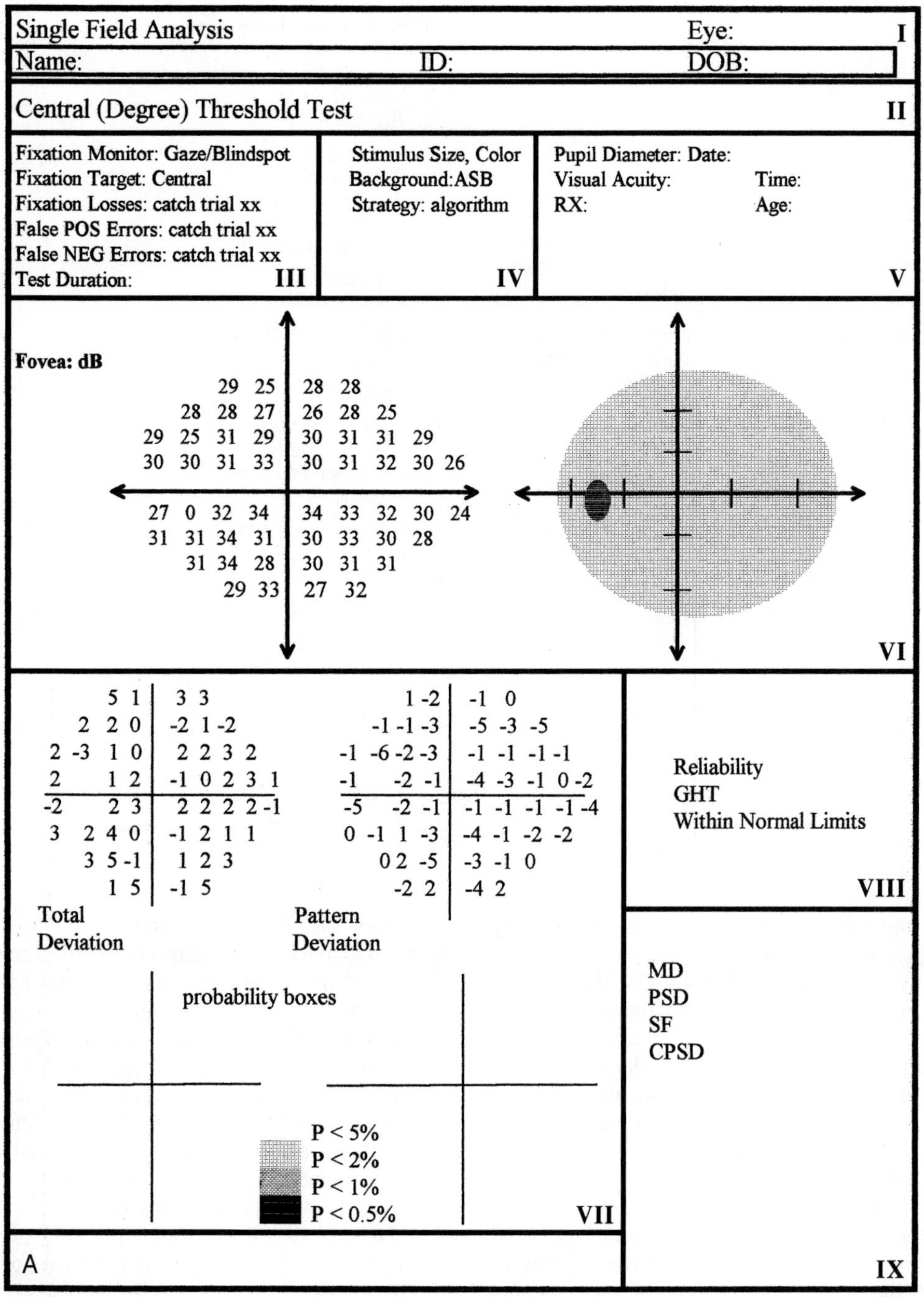

FIGURE 26–1. *A,* The single field analysis (SFA) is the flagship of visual field printouts and is the basis for this chapter. Each section is covered, demonstrating common and confusing clinical corollaries that plague the physician. The majority of physician decision and indecision regarding critical field signs comes from this printout. The typical occurrences and problems associated with each section are presented, in the order of the field printout, from top to bottom. Understanding how the data were generated is a special educational bonus.

Illustration continued on following page

Field Printout Data	Category
1. Patient name, eye, and ID 2. Patient date of birth	I: Patient Demographics
3. Type of threshold test	II: Degrees of Visual Field Tested
4. Fixation monitor: gaze/blind spot 5. Fixation losses 6. False POSitive errors 7. False NEGative errors 8. Test duration	III: Reliability Indices
9. Stimulus size 10. Stimulus color 11. Background luminance 12. Background color 13. Strategy: threshold algorithm	IV: Perimetric Test Parameters
14. Pupil diameter 15. Visual acuity 16. Refraction used for central field 17. Date 18. Time 19. Patient age	V: Patient Test Parameters
20. Fovea threshold 21. Numeric grid raw data plot 22. Corresponding gray scale with interpolation	VI: Threshold Data Points
23. Total deviation and probability plots 24. Pattern deviation and probability plots	VII: Probability of Deviation from Normal
25. Glaucoma hemifield test	VIII: Hemifield Test
26. Global indices: MD (mean deviation) 27. Global indices: PSD (pattern standard deviation) 28. Global indices: SF (short-term fluctuation) 29. Global indices: CPSD (corrected pattern standard deviation)	IX: Global Indices, Island of Vision Concept

B

FIGURE 26–1 *Continued. B,* Twenty-nine sections of data are represented on the SFA printout. They can be classified into 9 categories, as shown here. Typically, 5 questions are asked for each of 76 threshold points, and 10 points tested twice, averaging 400 to 450 questions. Therefore, close to 500 bits of information may be necessary to generate the SFA printout. For purposes of simplicity, it is assumed that the statistical software programs STATPAC I and STATPAC II are operational. For the SFA, STATPAC I provides probability plots and global indices, and STATPAC II the glaucoma hemifield test (GHT).

with the history and physical examination. An abnormality may simply be lens rim artifact.

If the reliability parameters are invalid and the data are suspect the physicians judgment is even more important. The statistical interpretation of the data obviously depends on how accurately the data were gathered. Decisions about the visual field must be made not by machine fiat but, ultimately, by a physician with experience of and grounded in the basics of psychophysics, perimetric algorithms, disease states, and field artifacts.

The interpretation of a visual field change may significantly affect the socioeconomic and visual fate of a patient. An incorrect identification of abnormality or worsening of disease may start the patient on a lifetime of antiglaucoma therapy with its attendant cost and risks. Incorrect decisions may lead to (1) false reassurance about an uncontrolled blinding disease, (2) needless worry about visual field artifacts, (3) harmful systemic side effects of antiglaucoma therapy, or even (4) blindness from a surgical procedure. It is incumbent upon the physician to learn as much as possible about perimetry and its interpretation in order to provide high-quality eye care.

Every attempt should be made to explain correctly, *document,* and *chart* all visual field findings, whether artifactual or pathologic. This discussion concentrates on the critical signs associated with interpretation of glaucomatous visual fields. All of the lessons in this chapter are gathered from clinical experience generated by correlation of clinical findings and field printouts. The emphasis is on clinical medicine, not just the psychophysics of differential light sensitivity. The basics of visual fields, such as threshold, retinal sensitivity, frequency of seeing curve, and spatial summation, are woven into the clinical interpretation. Readers interested in greater detail are referred to the large number of chapters and texts devoted to the visual field. The HFA is the most commonly used perimeter, and its single field analysis printout is the basis for this chapter. A discussion of all the available printouts is beyond the scope of this chapter and can be found in other sources.

Anatomy of the Single Field Analysis Printout

The SFA printout (see Fig. 26–1) includes the statistical support of STATPAC I and II software (Humphrey Instruments) and is the heart and soul of the perimeter output. The latest version of the perimeter, the HFA II, is the best from an ergonomic and space-saving standpoint. To have this analyzer without the additional benefit of the statistical software significantly reduces physician productivity. This discussion is structured according to how each section of the printout affects clinical decision making. The voluminous information contained in the SFA printout is the key to understanding visual fields. Without an understanding of the normal SFA, it is impossible to interpret the abnormal SFA, let alone identify pathologic changes due to glaucoma. The ability to truly understand normal facilitates the earliest recognition of disease. Therefore, attention is first directed at the basic information of the printout, at the same time pointing out day-to-day critical signs that are easily misconstrued. As previously mentioned, the printout can be divided into nine categories comprising 29 sections of data (see Fig. 26–1).

Category I: Patient Demographics

PATIENT NAME AND IDENTIFICATION

At first glance, the patient's name is a simple, straightforward entry that requires no further explanation. The patient's name should evoke all the global or supratentorial factors that go into the final field product. *Although the statistical interpretation of the data is objective, the raw data gathering is still subjective and constantly modulated by the patient's psyche*. The patient's name should remind the physician of the whole patient, not an isolated nerve undergoing testing.

The reliability parameters discussed later indicate the areas of localized weakness in test taking. More global systemic factors, however, are associated with patient performance. The most important is the criterion effect[1] (Fig. 26–2). The patient's criteria for responding "Yes" to a stimulus varies widely, depending on the circumstance. For example, a monocular individual with 20/70 visual acuity is far more likely to respond "Yes" to a test object if he or she has been instructed that this test is vital for continuing care rather than the instruction implying that the test is not very useful or important. The patient shifts willingness to respond "Yes" according to the circumstance. This is a very neglected area of perimetry because the perimeter and software are unable to report this phenomenon. The criterion effect, sensitivity, threshold, and decibels are all related. It is easiest to explain their relation with Traquair's concept of "island of vision in a sea of blindness" (Fig. 26–3). The island of vision and the frequency with which its landmarks are seen is related to the frequency of seeing curve (Fig. 26–4). It is amazing how these supratentorial factors alter field performance; and many other factors in the printout also apply. Patients are our best teachers when it comes to understanding this part of the field examination, but one must talk to patients to understand this phenomenon.

EYE TESTED

When the technician tests the correct eye but inadvertently enters the incorrect eye on the computer screen, an unusual pattern may occur. The HFA uses the Heijl-Krakau[2] method of fixation and therefore attempts to map the physiologic blind spot early in the test. With initial patient inattentiveness, two blind spots appear, one physiologic, the other an inattentive blind spot (Fig. 26–5). This method of fixation monitoring involves projecting bright stimuli periodically at the expected location of the physiologic blind spot.

PATIENT AGE

Psychophysical tests are always age dependent.[3] Visual sensitivity decreases with each decade of life mainly on a neural basis[4] (Fig. 26–6). Fortunately, the statistical packages used with the HFA (STATPAC I and STATPAC II) account for age-dependent retinal sensitivity by comparing each threshold value with age-adjusted normal values. Very young and older patients perform better with the faster algorithm test methods. For example, the Swedish Interactive Threshold Algorithm (SITA) is a newer, faster method of reaching threshold, decreasing patient anxiety, and alleviating field loss secondary to fatigue. It is designed to reduce test time without diminishing the quality of the data.

Category II: Type and Degrees of Field Tested

The degrees of field evaluated are often an overlooked part of perimetry. From a glaucoma viewpoint, there are three reasonable options for central threshold testing. Testing the peripheral field outside 30 degrees yields little additional information and is extremely fatiguing to the patient. Some physicians elect to test this area with kinetic automated perimetry, but this method also has many problems.[5]

CENTRAL 30-2 THRESHOLD TEST

Typically, five responses per test point are required in a 30-2 test to reach threshold for a full threshold algorithm, for a total of 350 to 450 questions asked for a normal field (Fig. 26–7). Disease states may require up to 750 test presentations, for a total of 20 minutes of field testing per eye, exhausting the patient. Fatigue becomes a major factor undermining the validity of the visual field result. Patients are resistant to future field examinations, and the added time is neither feasible nor worthwhile for the vast majority of patients. From a practical viewpoint, there is a tradeoff between degrees of field covered and reliable data. This dilemma led to the creation of the 24-2 threshold test.

CENTRAL 24-2 THRESHOLD TEST

The 24-2 test (Fig. 26–8) is by far the most popular field test for detecting and monitoring glaucoma. It tests 29% fewer retinal locations, significantly decreasing test time in a normal eye from 13 minutes to 8 minutes. With the new SITA algorithm, test time is even shorter; however, the detection rate for shallow scotomas may be slightly lower. Occasionally, patients demonstrate radial nerve fiber layer defects off the nasal side of the disc that require the 30-2 test for plotting. Otherwise, the 24-2 test is sufficient for

Text continued on page 428

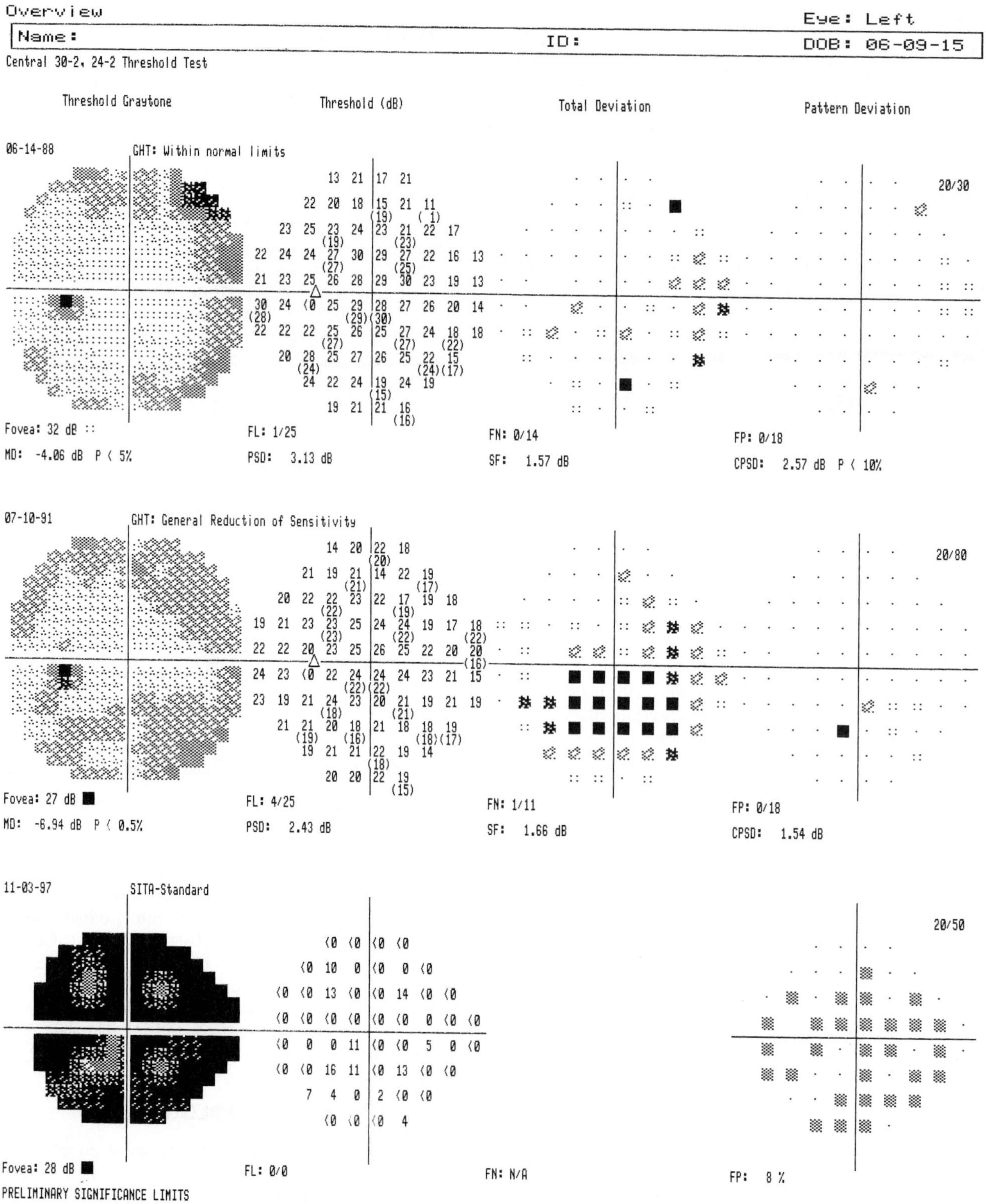

A

FIGURE 26–2. *See legend on opposite page.*

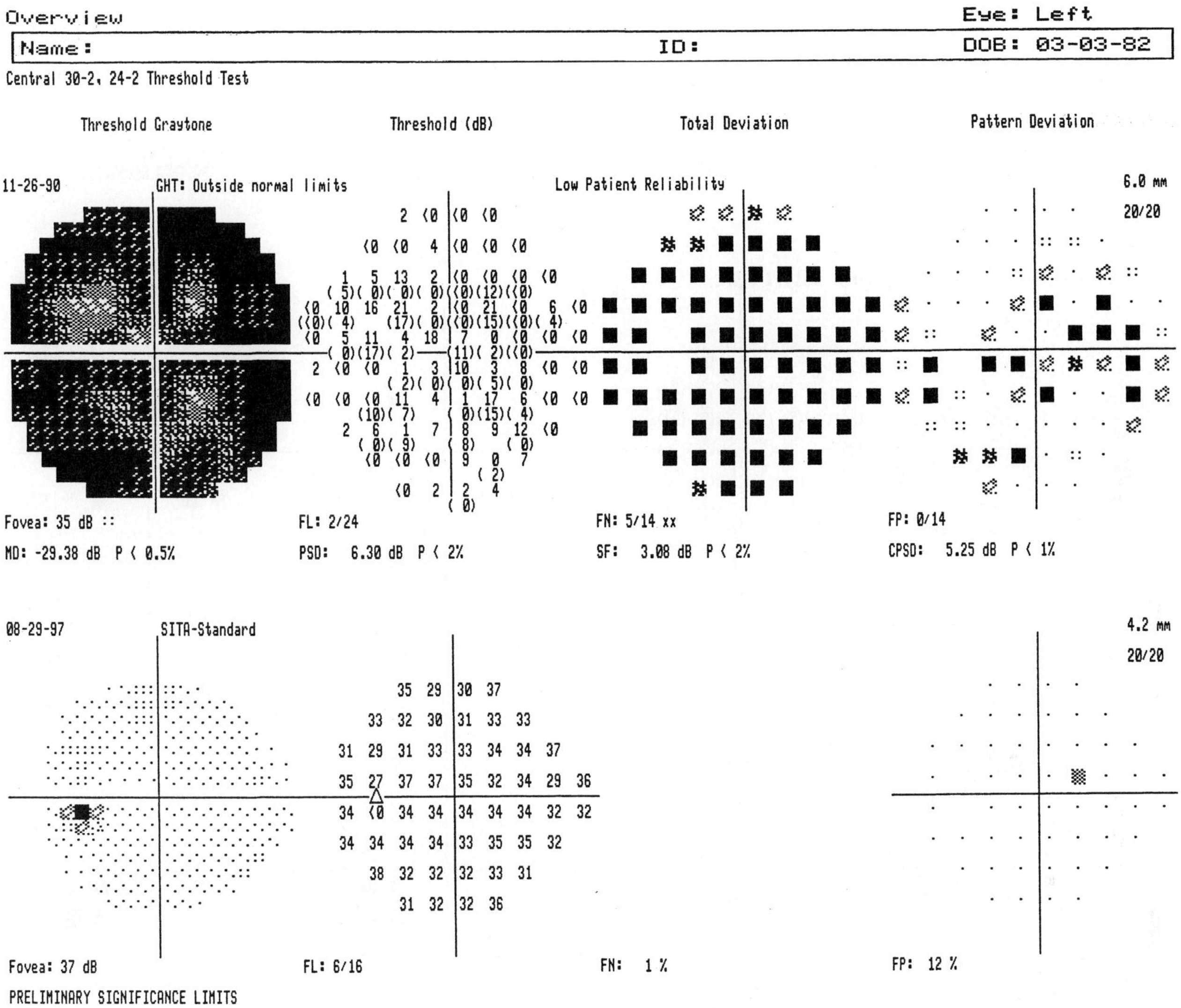

B

FIGURE 26–2. The *criterion effect* is a psychophysical term that describes the patient's willingness to respond to a test object. In other words, the patient changes his or her willingness or criterion to respond to the light stimulus. The most common clinical example of this phenomenon occurs with the cloverleaf pattern. The cloverleaf pattern is an unmistakable sign of global patient error, due to misunderstanding the test process, lack of attention, or altered mentation. The perimeter initiates the field test by checking threshold in the center of each quadrant, and then the region grows around this area. In the beginning of the field test, the central quadrant area is always mapped out first along with the physiologic blind spot. This may produce two unusual patterns, a white cloverleaf pattern on a black background or a black cloverleaf on a white background. This occurs most commonly with new patients or young patients, when there are language barriers between physician and patient, and during follow-up examinations of patients whose mental status has worsened. *A,* White cloverleaf on black background sign due to altered mental status. These three successive field analyses cover almost a decade of care for this patient. The first and second fields show mild loss but nothing like the last field, which shows severe damage. The last field is clearly abnormal, but is it ocular disease? Abnormal field findings must be documented in the chart, and appropriate action must be taken. This pattern is not a sign of optic nerve fiber disease but, unfortunately, of central nervous system (CNS) disease. The physician should learn to recognize the cloverleaf sign. *It is a sign of global amnesia after a successful start of the test, and may be an early sign of altered mentation.* The patient responds during the initial, region-growing portion of the test, then "phases out." This pattern is most common in patients with language barriers or altered mental status. In this case, between 6/14/88 and 11/03/97, the patient unfortunately developed Alzheimer's disease. Notice that the prior fields show mild reduction of sensitivity but are otherwise unremarkable. The optic nerve was unchanged, but there were significant CNS changes that altered mentation. This pattern is simply due to the order in which the perimeter seeks threshold at the various preselected retinal points. *B,* White cloverleaf on black background sign, due to patient's youth and to misunderstanding of test. This child with Sturge-Weber syndrome and secondary glaucoma took her first field test at age 8 years. She initially was attentive but then rapidly became uninterested. The cloverleaf pattern was recognized, and the test was repeated when she was 16 years old; results were found to be normal. Understanding the process of region growing clearly explains how this pattern occurs.

Illustration continued on following page

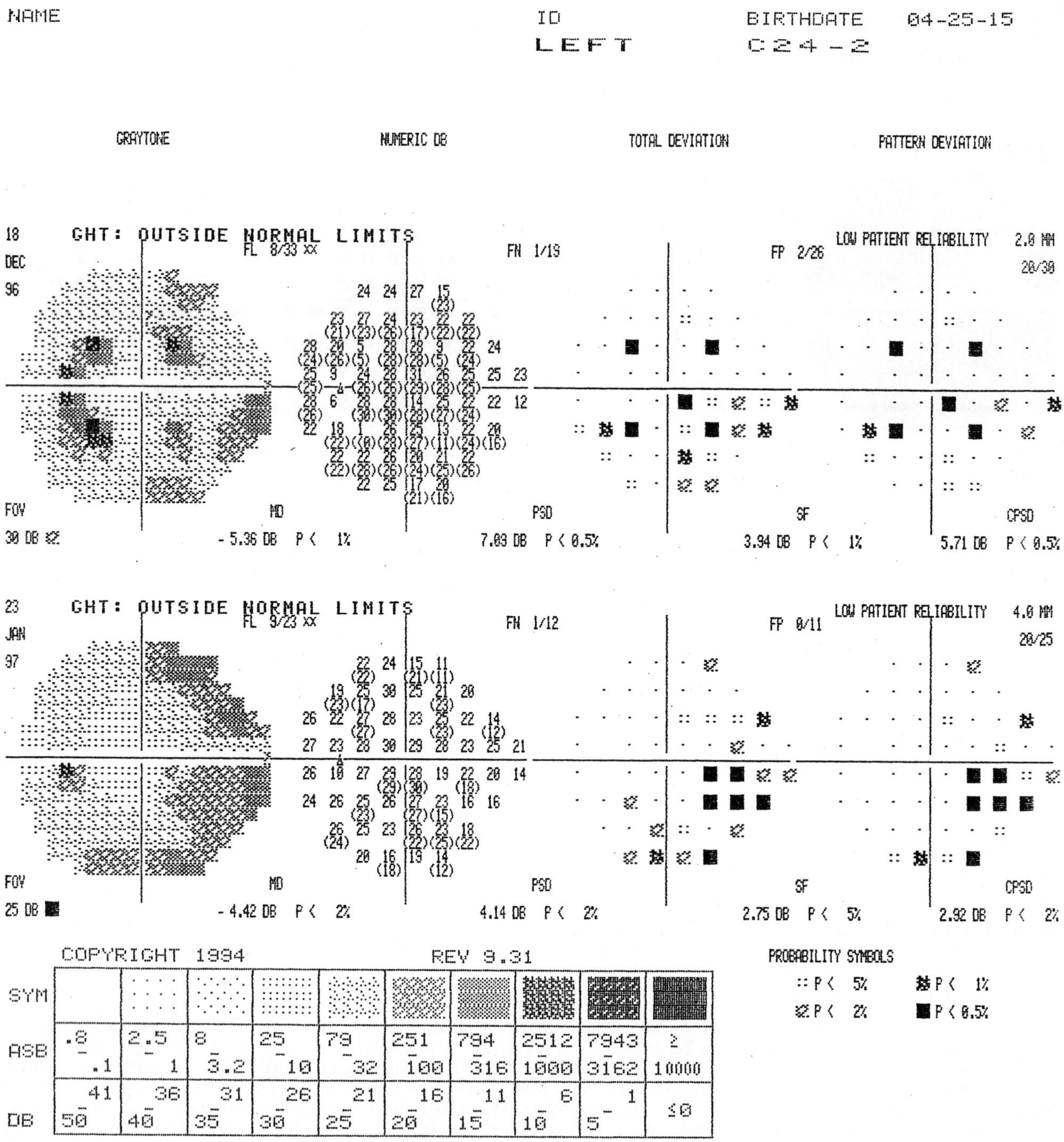

C

FIGURE 26–2 *Continued. C,* Black cloverleaf on white background sign due to anxiety and confusion (CPR-2). The corollary is that some patients are slow to learn the test and are unresponsive during the initial region-growing phase, but otherwise do a good job as the test progresses. These patients typically perform better for the fellow eye. This confusing pattern manifests as a mild four-quadrant scotoma. This 81-year-old new patient with intraocular pressure of 24 mm Hg and disc damage has the cloverleaf sign in his left eye. Both eyes were tested on 12/18/96, but the left eye was tested first. The patient better understood the test for the right eye and properly reached threshold at each point tested. The left eye field test was repeated 1 month later. The cloverleaf pattern is gone in this printout, and an inferior nasal step is present. Awareness of this pattern is critical in counseling patients and family members.

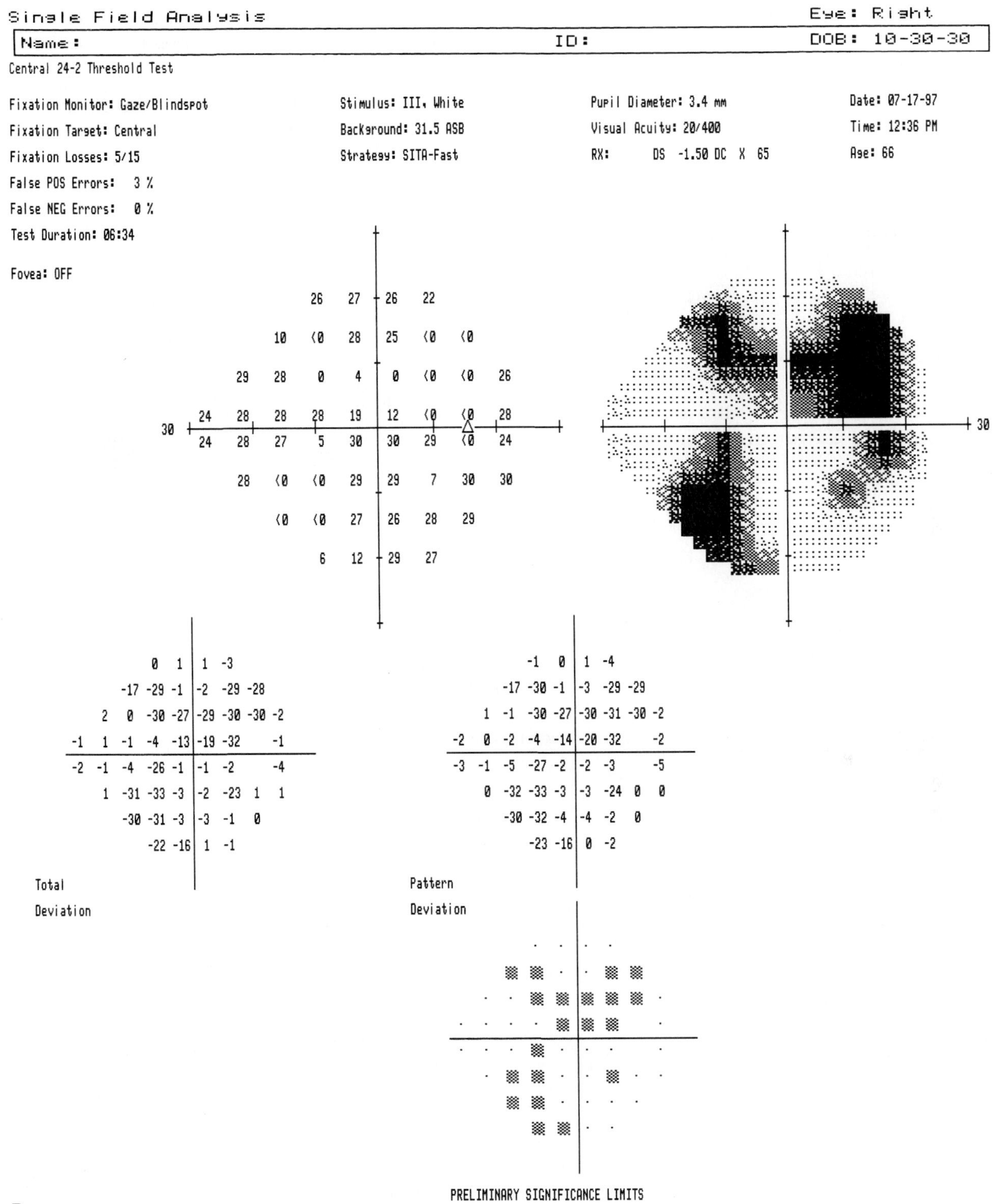

D

FIGURE 26–2 *Continued.* Black cloverleaf on white background sign due to a language barrier. The first field test from this patient, who was born in another country, revealed a significant cloverleaf pattern for the right eye test *(D).* The optic nerve did not correlate with this field.

Illustration continued on following page

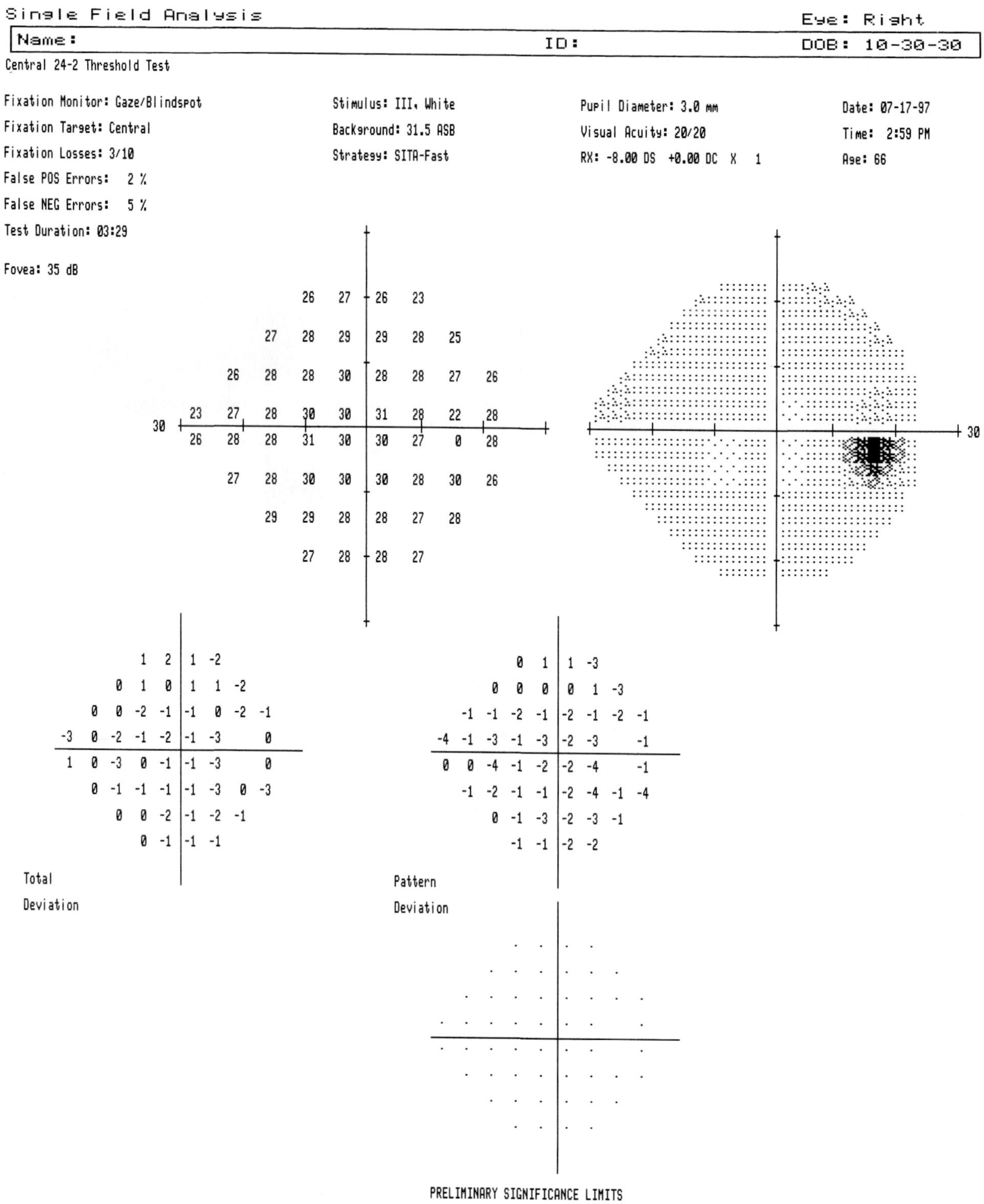

E

FIGURE 26–2 *Continued.* After further test explanations, the field test was *repeated 2 hours later (E)* and found to be normal. The physician should learn to recognize this field pattern; it is easy to spot, understand, and correct. The size of the cloverleaf pattern varies according to the initial period of confusion.

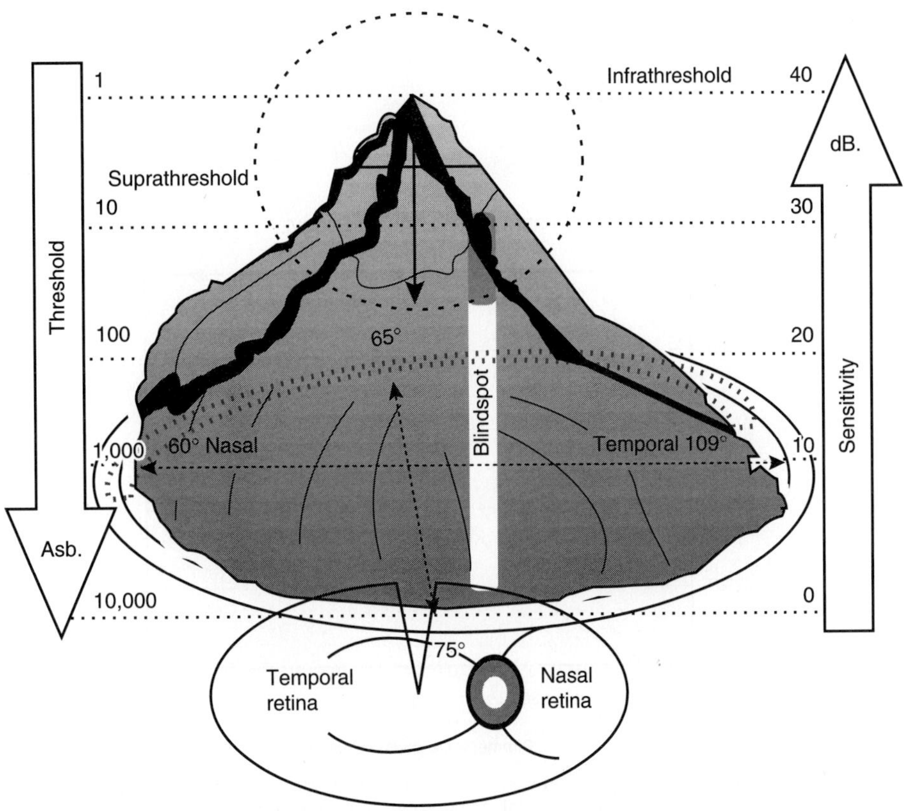

FIGURE 26–3. The "island of vision in a sea of blindness." This concept was romantically coined by Traquair decades ago and remains a valuable and time-honored graphic tool. The normal visual field has a specific conceptual "island shape." Note that the island is not flat, which would imply equal sensitivity throughout the field. Instead, the neurophysiologic expression of retinal sensitivity mandates a gradient slope of visual sensitivity, greatest at fixation and tapering off as the peripheral limits at "sea level" are reached. At the bottom of the illustration is the *funduscopic view* of the retina. The neuroanatomic connections of the retina and optic pathways dictate the variable light sense and boundaries noted in degrees. It takes practice to translate the decibel (db) data from the single-field analysis into the island concept, but this is a useful exercise. Should you accept this assignment, in fact, you will not self destruct but will be utilizing that often neglected "artsy" part of your brain. The ability to make this transformation facilitates the necessary understanding of the difference in sensitivity and threshold, decibels and apostilbs (Asb.), and frequency of seeing. Without these elemental basics, future perimetric thoughts may be infrathreshold.

The beauty of the island concept is that visual sensitivity is greatest at the zenith, best expressed by decibels, a relative logarithmic scale. Note the decibel scale on the right with 0 dB at sea level and 40 dB at the peak of fixation with their reciprocal apostilb values on the left, 10,000 Asb at sea level, 1 Asb at fixation. Sensitivity increases as one climbs the island; thus, the amount of light necessary to see the test stimulus is less, along with threshold. This is obviously confusing, because less is better in a pure sense but confusing from a diagnostic sense. To simplify matters, the light sense is recorded in absolute units, apostilbs, but reported in relative units, decibels. Therefore, the brightest white light on the HFA is 10,000 Asb, which correlates with 0 dB, and conversely, one of the dimmest stimuli is 1 Asb, equal to 40 dB. Consequently, threshold and sensitivity are the reciprocal of each other. One decibel is a change equivalent to 0.1 log unit. A decrease of 1 dB (20 dB to 19 dB) represents a 25% increase in projected light, and an increase of 1 dB (19 dB to 20 dB) is equivalent to a 20% decrease in projected light.

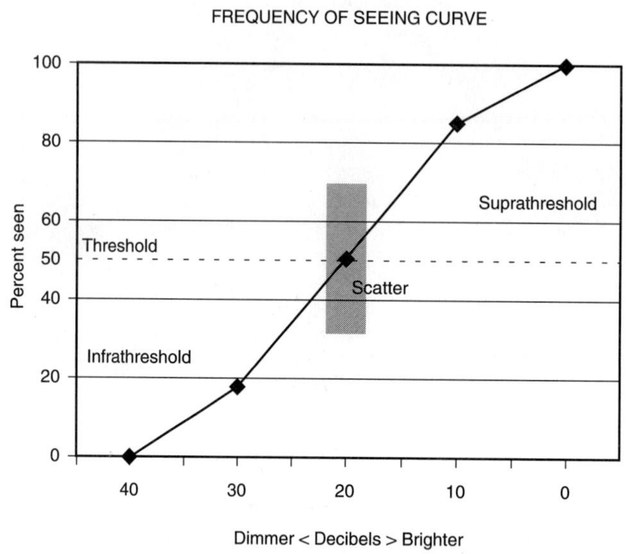

FIGURE 26–4. The frequency of seeing curve. The generation of this perimetric curve is the essence of psychophysics. *Threshold* is typically defined as a stimulus value having a 50% probability of being seen. In this example, 20 dB is the threshold value. The perimeter algorithm is designed to seek this number accurately and rapidly. The typical field threshold value, normal or abnormal, is supposed to represent this probability. In psychometric terms, threshold intensity is just bright enough to be seen 5 out of 10 times. *Suprathreshold* implies a stimulus intensity brighter than threshold, and *infrathreshold,* a stimulus intensity dimmer than threshold. Most of the screening field tests are suprathreshold and are usually brighter than projected threshold by 6 dB.

Patients may skew the data by altering their criteria for responding. Waiting to respond until the stimulus is excessive flattens the island of vision and makes the field look worse. If one were to change the criterion for threshold to "I want to see the light 9 out of 10 times," a 90% chance of seeing the light, imagine how bright it would have to be so one misses it only 1 time out of 10; this would make the field look worse. The corollary is seeing a stimulus so dim that it normally only has a 10% chance of being seen, but instead is seen 50% of the time, a superhuman feat that would make the field appear much better than expected. It is to be hoped that the patient's criterion for responding remains relatively stable for all tests.

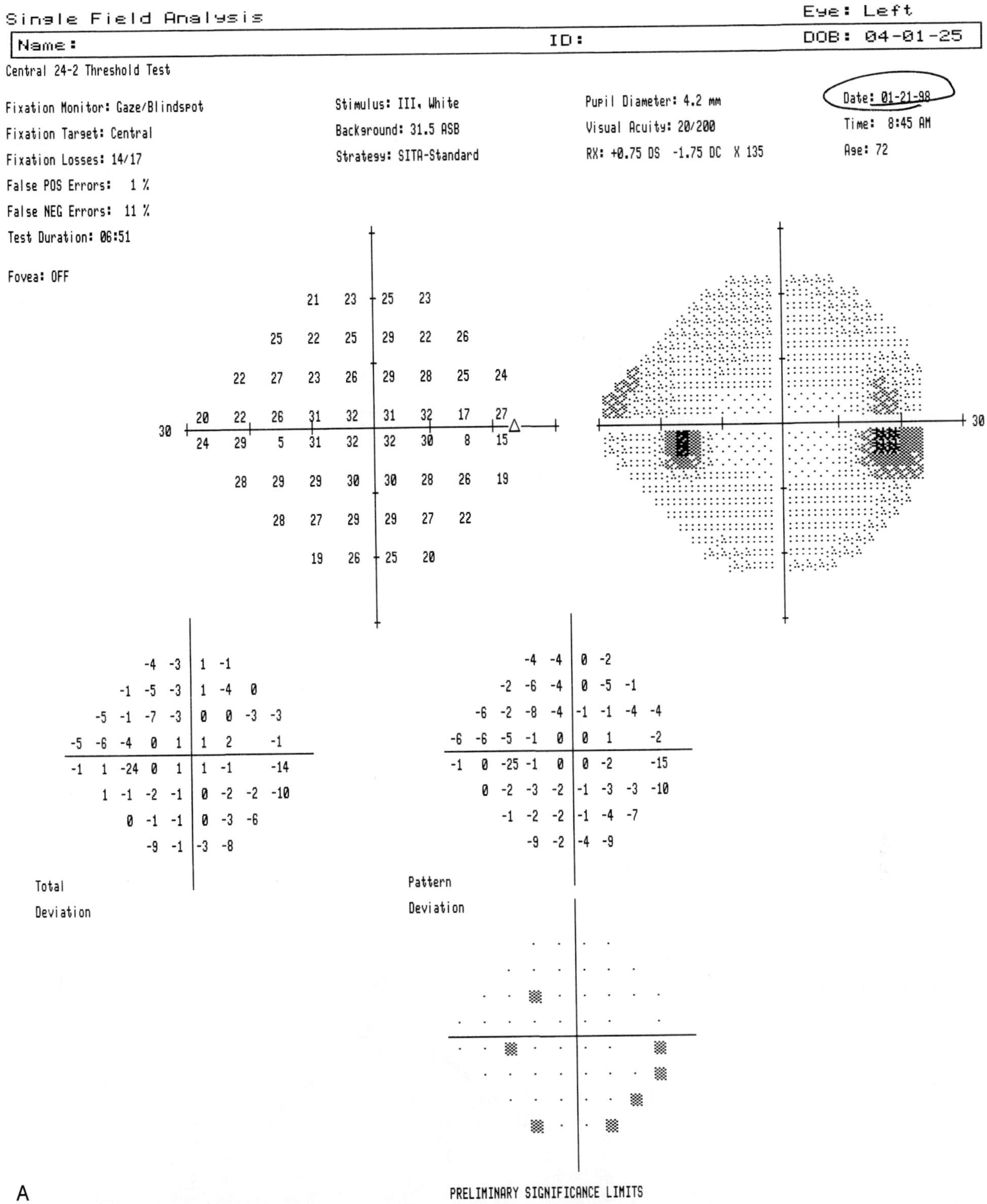

A

FIGURE 26–5. The dual blind spot syndrome. When the technician selects the correct eye to test but inadvertently selects the fellow eye on the computer screen, confusion abounds. This 72-year-old monocular patient with 20/25 visual acuity and early primary open-angle glaucoma underwent multiple perimetric exams in his left eye. Both the patient and the technician recognized that the test results were different. At the end of the test, the technician realized that the wrong eye was entered into the computer, marked through Right eye, and wrote "Left" on the printout *(A)*. The physician was notified. Acuity was entered as 20/200 but is 20/20; tough day for the technician! The patient also noted that the test went differently. Note the high fixation losses. During the beginning of the test, the blind spot is mapped out, temporal to fixation, because the perimeter "thinks" the right eye is being tested. Probably because of the initial confusion, a blind spot was mapped temporally, and another blind spot showed up "nasally." The "nasal" blind spot is truly the patient's physiologic blind spot.

Illustration continued on following page

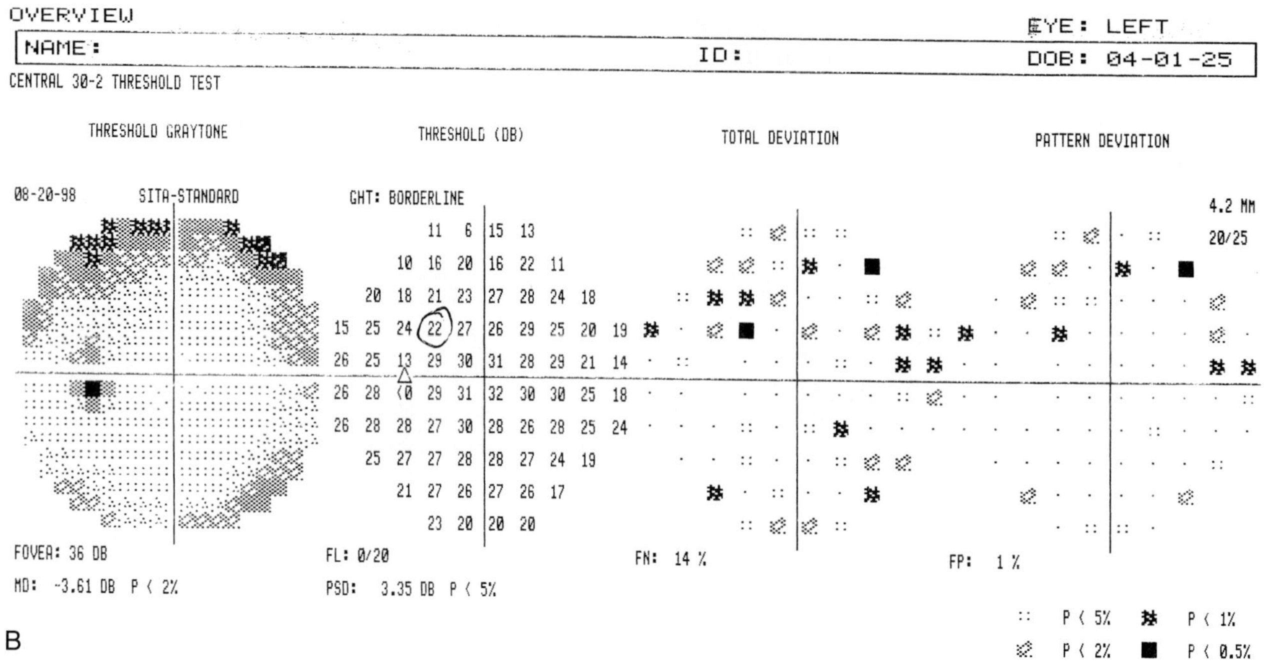

B

FIGURE 26–5 *Continued. B,* The field test was repeated the same day and appeared essentially normal.

FIGURE 26–6. Effects of aging on the "island of vision": an 80-year-old "island." Sensitivity decreases markedly with age, starting at 20 years or earlier. Age influences the upper half of the visual field to a larger extent than the lower half, with an average decrease in the visual field of 0.58 decibels (dB) to 0.8 dB per decade. The island of vision tends to steepen with advancing age, and variation increases with eccentricity. Obviously, the patient's mental status and attention span significantly affect field performance. Asb, apostilbs.

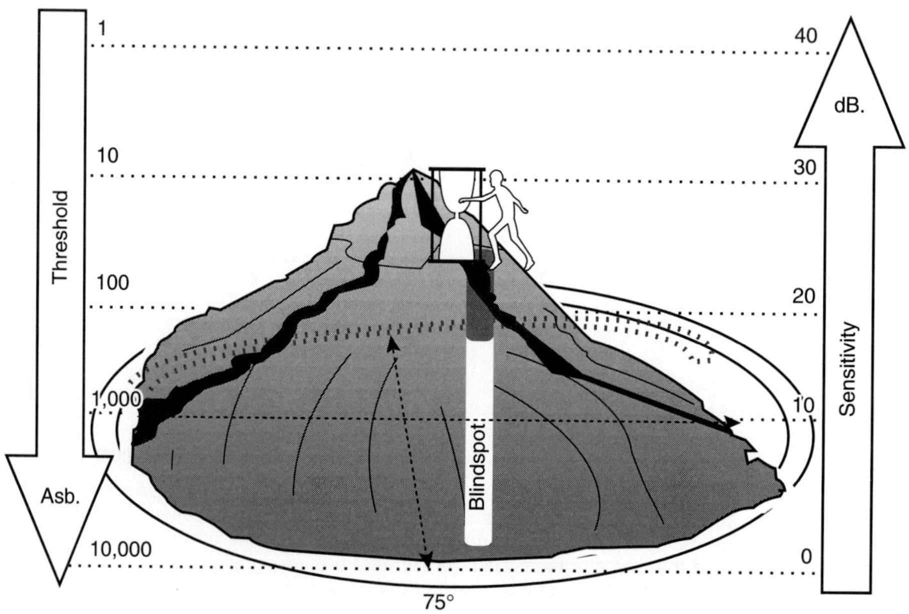

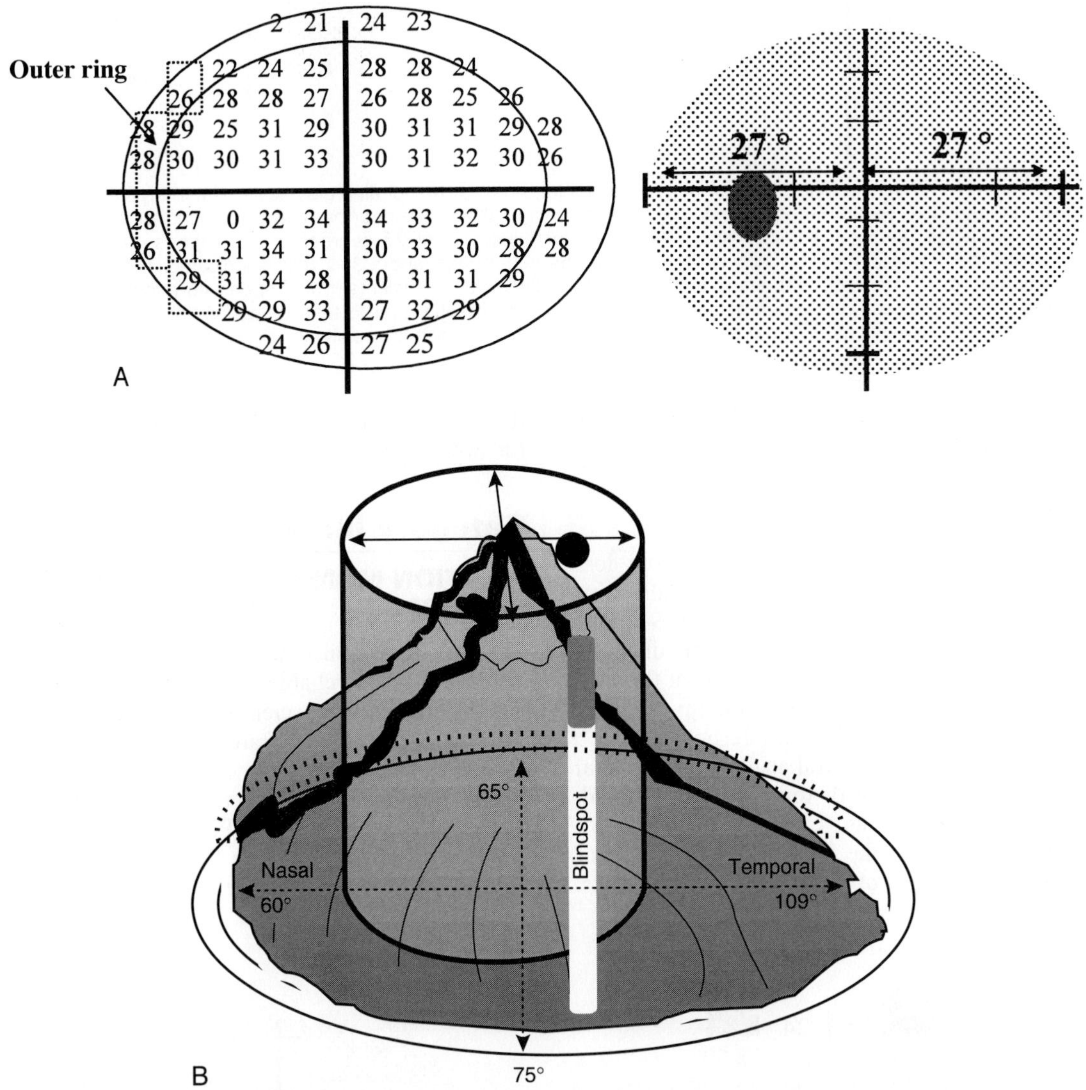

FIGURE 26–7. *A,* Central 30-2 threshold test. *Left,* numeric raw data plot; *right,* corresponding gray scale with interpolation. This 76-point 6-degree test grid covers 54 degrees along both the horizontal and vertical meridia. From fixation, the test extends 27 degrees horizontally and vertically. The 30-1 HFA test truly extends 30 degrees from fixation along both the horizontal and vertical meridia. However, this particular grid pattern is more likely to miss the physiologic blind spot. For testing patients with glaucoma, the 30-2 test is preferable because testing is centered on either side of the horizontal raphe, enhancing detection of the superior and inferior nerve fiber bundles. The minimally increased yield from testing the outer ring is severely offset by the additional time needed. The temporal six spots (in *dotted box*) are an especially low yield area for detection and follow-up of glaucoma and alone require an average of 30 additional unnecessary presentations. The principle of deleting low yield points for the sake of time led to the 24-2 test. All except two points, on either side of the nasal 27 degrees, were eliminated from the outer ring to form the 24-2 test. *B,* "Island of vision" and its relation to the central 30-2 test area. The cylindrical region denotes the actual area tested for a typical glaucoma program. This area has the greatest yield for time spent.

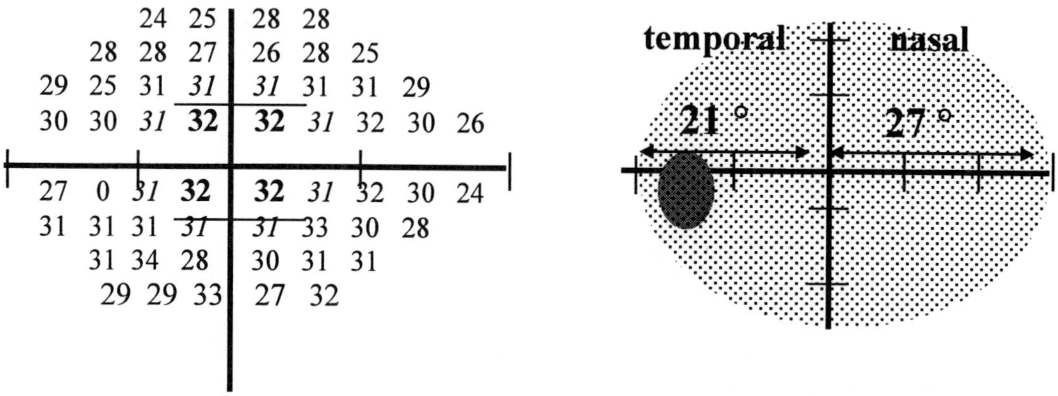

FIGURE 26–8. Central 24-2 threshold test. *Left,* numeric raw data plot; *right,* corresponding gray scale with interpolation. The test consists of 54 points with the standard square 6-degree grid. The nasal portion of the field along the horizontal meridian tests out to 27 degrees, as in the 30-2 test, but the temporal, superior, and inferior portion reduces from 27 degrees to 21 degrees, saving valuable time and energy. Occasionally, the physician may suspect damage outside the tested area, and a 30-2 test is indicated. The time necessary to test the peripheral field outside 30 degrees with static techniques is hardly worth it. Patients would spend 45 minutes per eye if the entire field were evaluated with a standard static perimetric algorithm. Some physicians prefer to test the peripheral field with kinetic techniques in addition to a central static examination. From a practical viewpoint, this approach is usually not clinically necessary.

coverage because it still extends out to 27 degrees along the all-important nasal horizontal raphe.

10-2 THRESHOLD TEST

When the 24-2 or 30-2 field demonstrates marked loss centrally and the patient still has reasonable central acuity, the 10-2 analysis is extremely useful (Fig. 26–9). This technique is much more valuable and yields significantly more data than testing of blind peripheral areas of the field with a larger grid. In the appropriate situation, this problem can be eliminated with the central 10-2 threshold test.

This test is very underused. Central acuity is most useful to patients, and closer mapping of this area is warranted, especially in monocular patients (Figs. 26–10 to 26–12). The critical point is to tailor the field test to the shape of the patient's remaining island of vision and the complaints. It is a poor habit to order the same type of field analysis for every patient.

Category III: Reliability Indices

FIXATION MONITOR, GAZE, AND BLINDSPOT

Category III is concerned with field reliability. Fixation is "everything" to reliable perimetric data. Monitoring fixation is an evolving science. The HFA monitors fixation with two systems, an infrared tracker and the Heijl-Krakau (blind spot check) system.

The infrared gaze tracker system presents information that is still investigational. For example, at the bottom of the SFA printout in Figure 26–12A is the record of the HFA II variable gaze tracker system. Upward deflections

Text continued on page 435

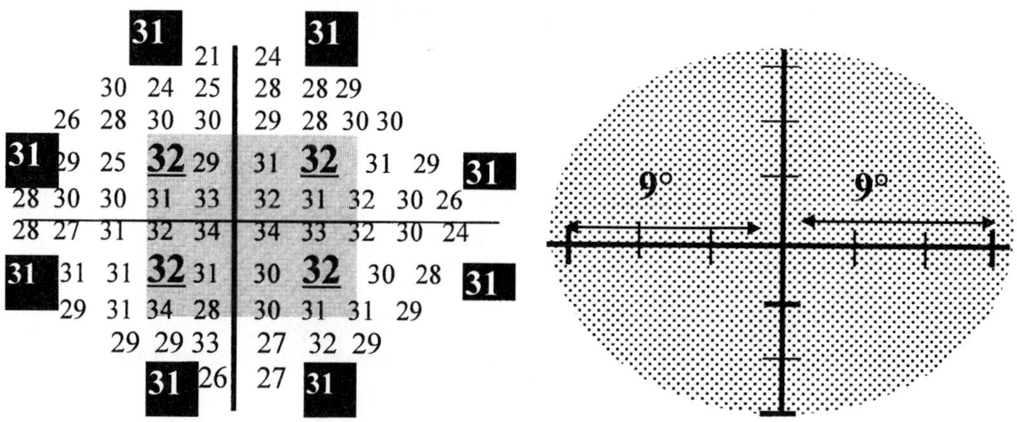

FIGURE 26–9. Central 10-2 threshold test. *Left,* numeric raw data plot; *right,* corresponding gray scale with interpolation. This is a 68-point 2-degree grid that concentrates on the central 10 degrees (actually 9 degrees) of the visual field. The field extends 9 degrees from fixation along the horizontal and vertical meridia. Essentially, 68 data points cover an area normally covered by 12 points on a 24-2 test. The increase in data is extremely useful in patients with tunnel vision. Threshold testing completely blind areas of the field is a major socioeconomic drain. The four decibel values underlined and in bold correspond to the points tested on the 24-2 test shown in Figure 26–8, also in bold. The numbers in black boxes (31 dB) correspond to the points tested in the 24-2 test but are just barely outside the test range for the 10-2 test. The corresponding figures are italicized in Figure 26–8. Only 4.6 test size III objects can fit side by side between the test locations of the 2-degree grid, (.43° × 4.6 = 2°). Compare this to 14 size III stimuli between the test locations of the 6-degree grid. One can see how easy it is to miss small scotomas.

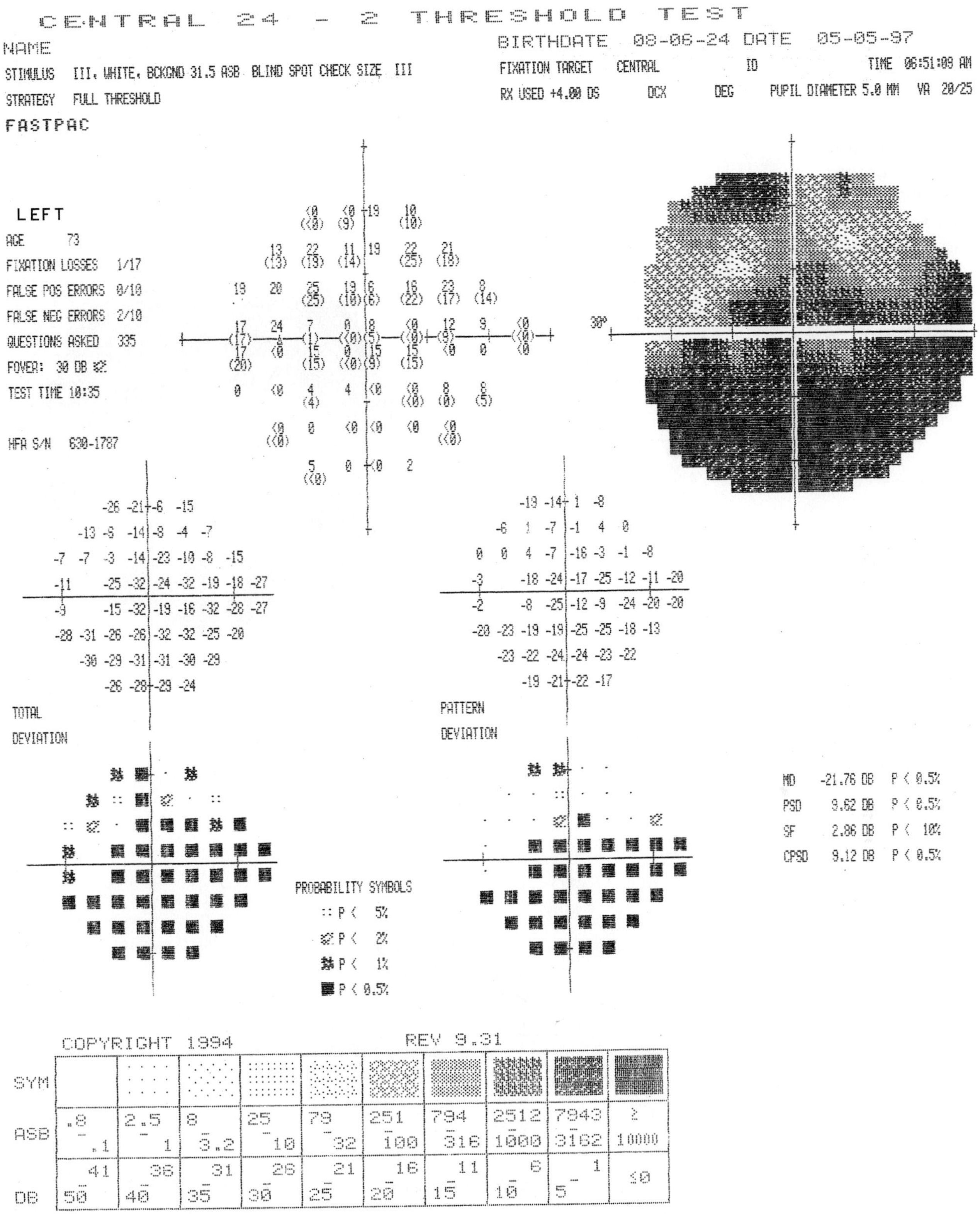

A

FIGURE 26–10. Comparison of central 24-2 and 10-2 threshold tests in a 73-year-old monocular patient with glaucoma. *A,* The 24-2 field reveals severe end-stage glaucoma damage in this patient's left eye, which has 20/25 visual acuity. The central sensitivity of this test does not accurately reflect the excellent visual acuity. The four closest points to the center are all 4.2 degrees away from fixation. The point inferonasal to fixation yields 15 dB, repeat 9 dB. The central 10 degrees of the 24-2 field test has only 4 test points, as noted in Figure 26–4.

Illustration continued on following page

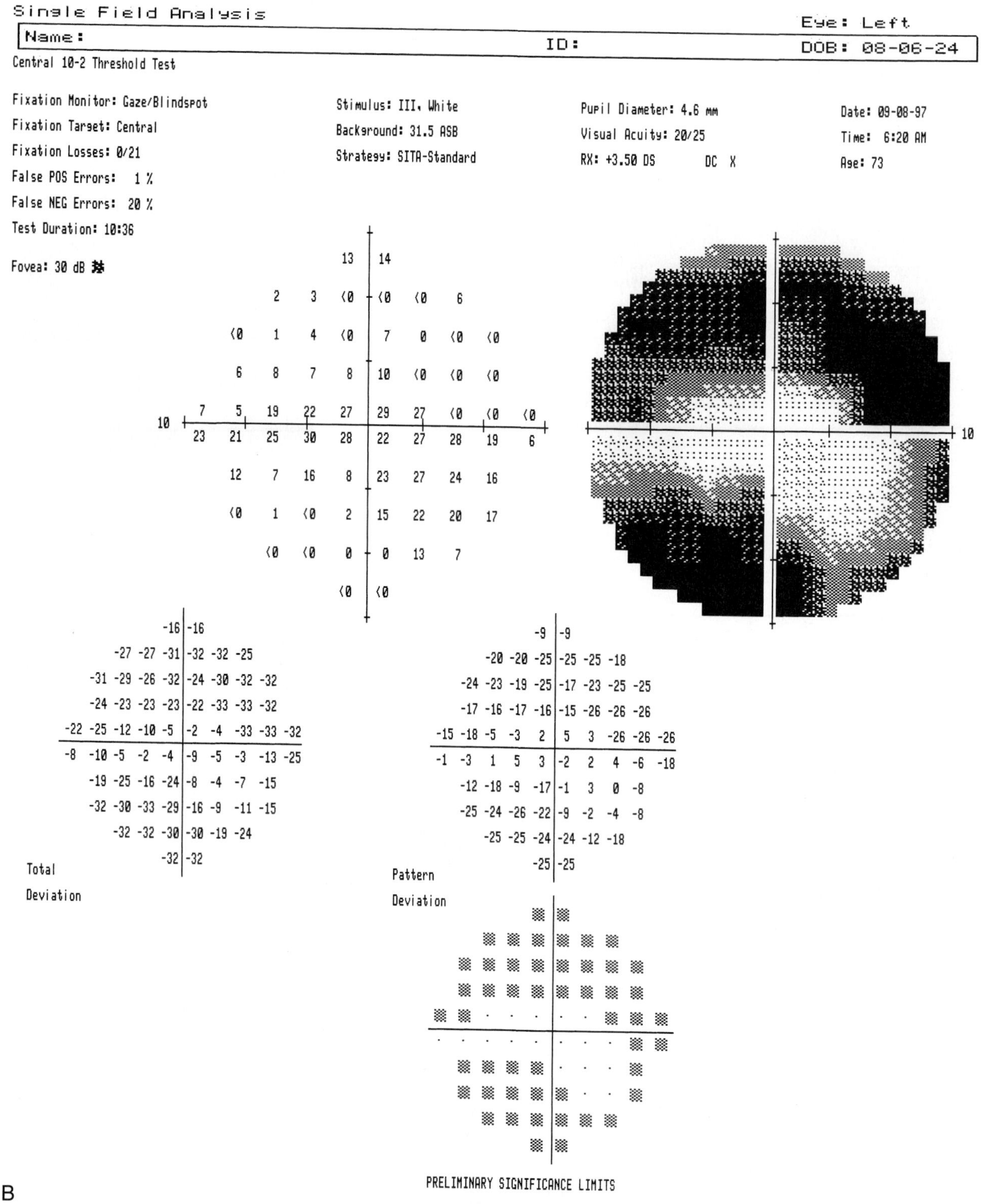

B

FIGURE 26–10 *Continued. B,* The 68-point 10-2 field test demonstrates an important tiny central island of sensitivity that was completely missed on the larger grid examination. The four closest points to fixation with this test are all 1.4 degrees away from fixation, considerably closer than the 4.2 degrees identified with the larger 24-2 grid. Close comparison of the fields demonstrates that in the superotemporal quadrant, where 0 dB was detected at 4.2 degrees from fixation, an area of vision was detected in between this area and fixation at 27 dB! Without the 10-2 test, this area of vital retinal sensitivity could go completely blind, the patient would complain of continued loss, but the physician would remain unaware of the problem.

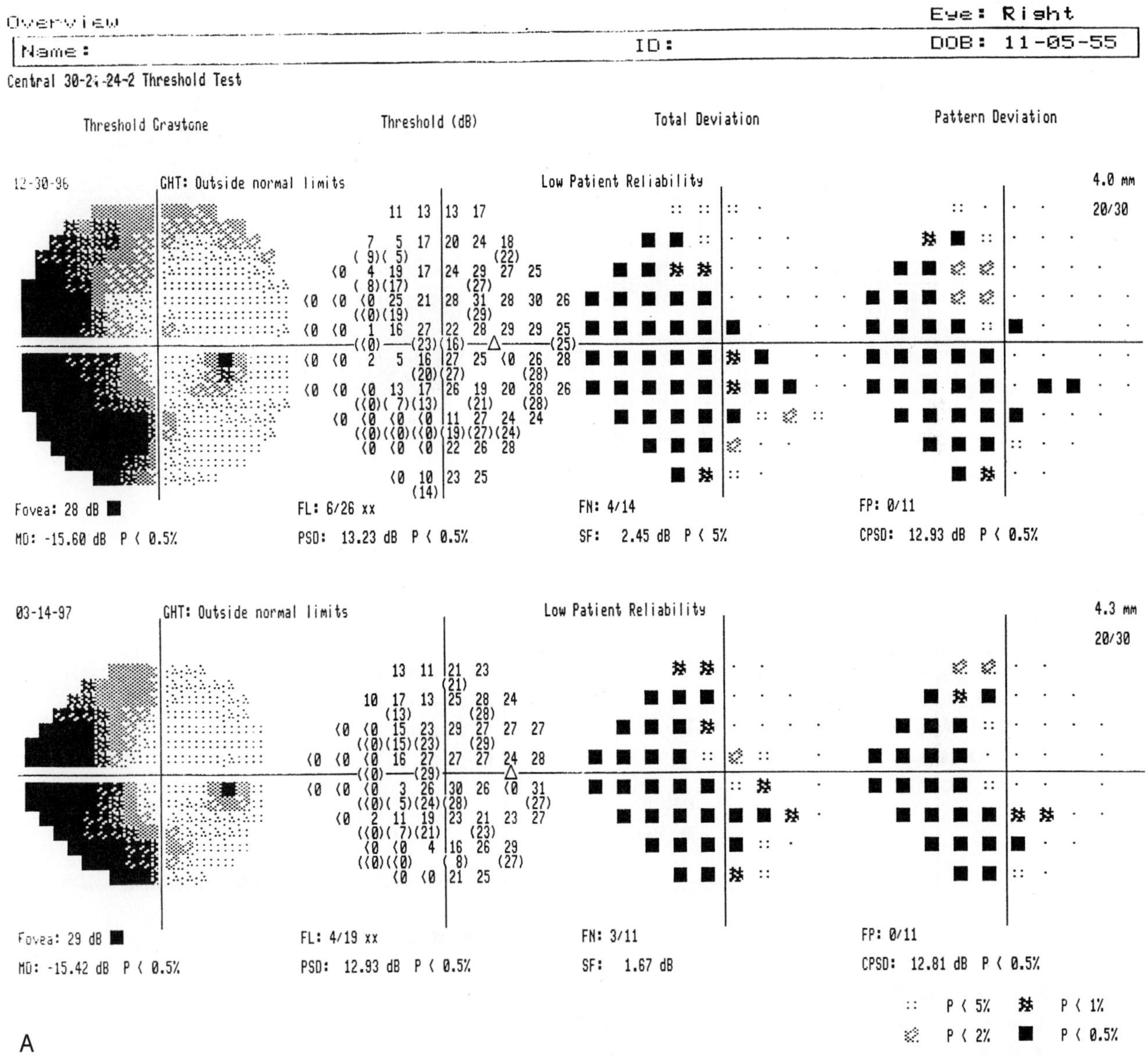

A

FIGURE 26–11. Comparison of central 24-2 and 10-2 threshold tests in a 42-year-old monocular patient with glaucoma. *A,* This patient has extensive nasal field loss as detected on the 24-2 test. Patient complaints of decreased central vision were out of proportion to the apparent excellent central sensitivities of 27 dB to 30 dB.

Illustration continued on following page

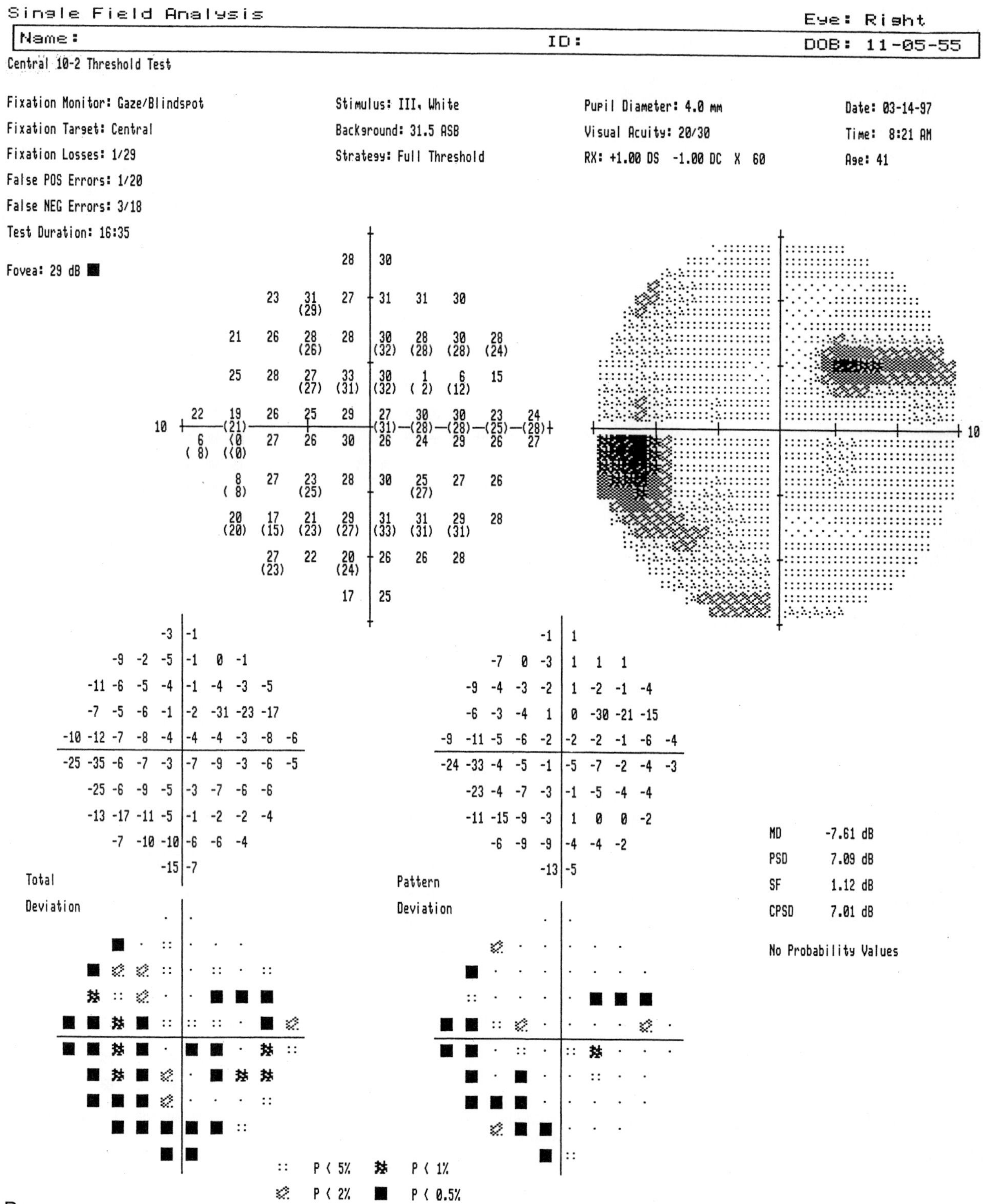

B

FIGURE 26–11 *Continued. B,* A 10-2 microgrid demonstrated a small superotemporal 4- to 5-degree scotoma 1.4 degrees from fixation that was previously undetected. Both 3/14/97 field tests were performed the same day, a few minutes apart. The gray scale is misleading because it interpolates and makes up sensitivity in between test points. In actuality, there may be microscotomas between apparently normal test points.

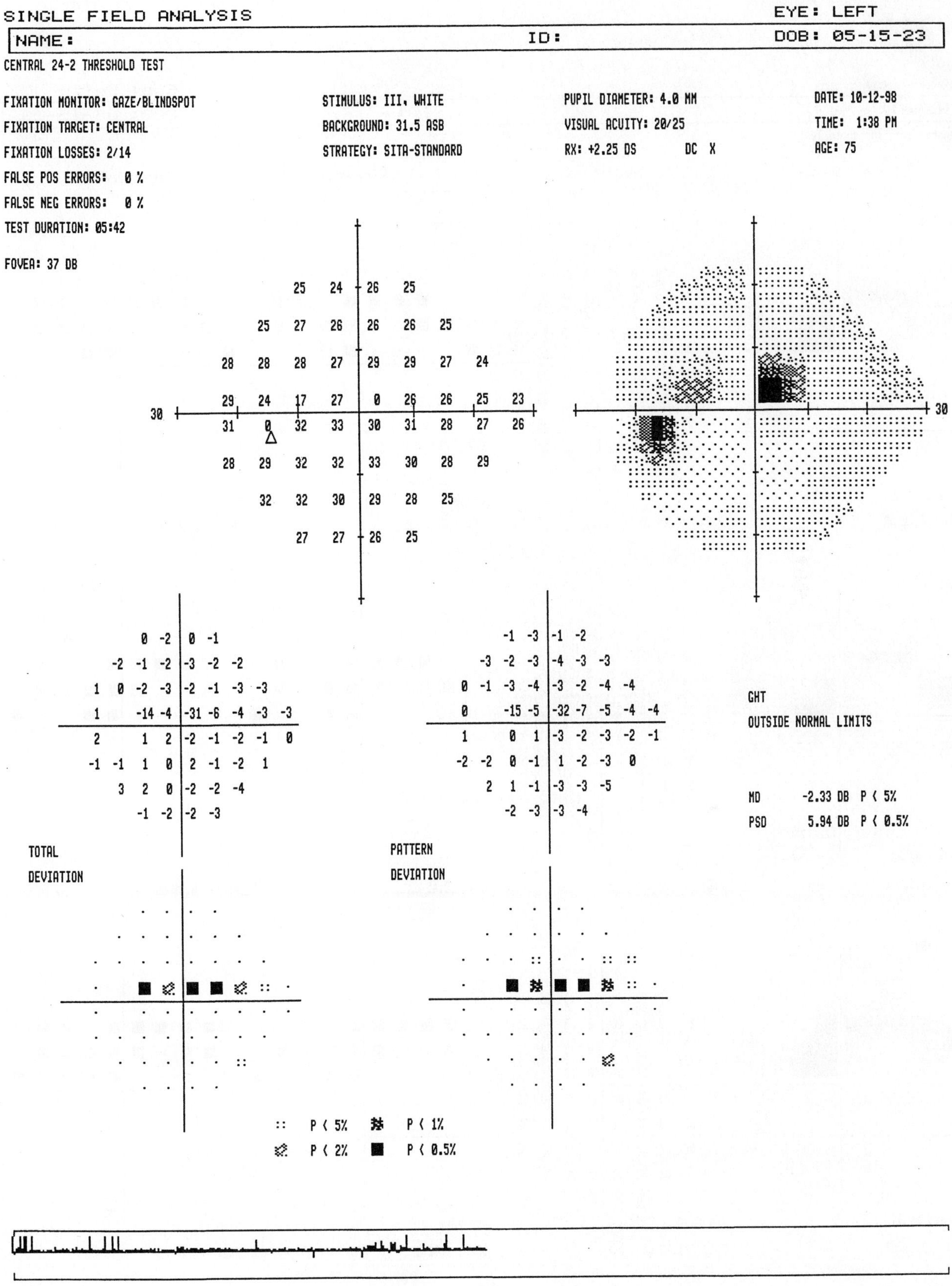

A

FIGURE 26–12. Comparison of central 24-2 and 10-2 threshold tests. *A,* Note the dense superonasal scotoma found on the 24-2 test. This monocular patient always had significant complaints about reading.

Illustration continued on following page

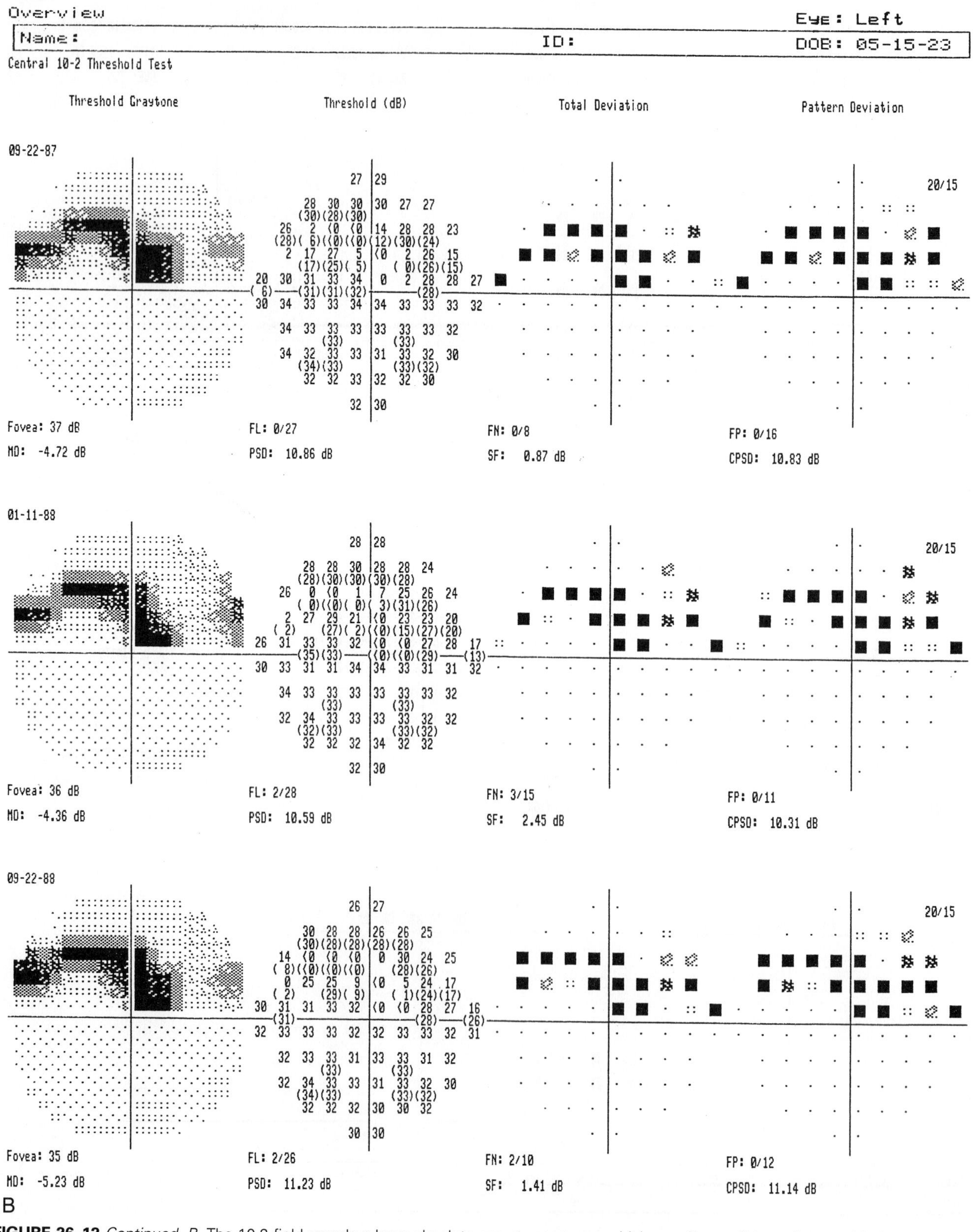

FIGURE 26–12 *Continued. B,* The 10-2 field reveals a large absolute arcuate scotoma, which was impossible to detect with the larger grid.

in the tracing indicate occasional deviations of gaze. The downward defection is probably a blink.

The blind spot system maps out the physiologic blind spot at the beginning of the test and then intermittently presents multiple bright size III stimuli into the blind spot. The data are recorded as a fraction of stimuli seen over stimuli presented and are recorded as fixation losses (Fig. 26–13). A double-x sign (xx) posted next to the fraction implies excessive eye movement during the test; the data are suspect and should be interpreted with caution.

The greater the fixation loss, the better the field looks, because the patient changes fixation and looks directly at the new spot presented. Patients with poor fixation yield highly suspect data. If repeated testing continues to show this problem, both the patient and physician rapidly reach a point at which field analysis is not useful and should be discounted. The critical sign is to recognize the effect of poor fixation on the field printout.

FALSE-POSITIVE ERRORS

False-positive errors are another index of test reliability (Fig. 26–14). The parameter is flagged with a double-x sign (xx) if deemed to be unreliable. A high false-positive rate is the signal of a "button-happy" patient, who basically is pressing the machine's clicker every few seconds, responding to auditory and visual cues. This behavior has a dramatic effect on field sensitivity, producing a totally unreliable field. It also generates a "whiteout" effect on the gray scale, another visual clue to field unreliability. If the STATPAC II software was used for the test, the report "Abnormally high sensitivity" printed in the glaucoma hemifield test (GHT) area is further evidence of an unreliable test. The most common cause of high fixation loss and false-positive responses is patient apprehension. Proper counseling may result in readable fields in the future for some patients; for others, static perimetry may not be useful.

FALSE-NEGATIVE ERROR RATE

A high false-negative error rate tends to make the visual field seem worse. In a same-session retest of a completed threshold location, failure to see a one log unit brighter test stimulus is a false-negative error. This should not be confused with short-term fluctuation, in which a single test location undergoes threshold determination twice. With the advent of shorter test times, this error rate will probably decrease. Thresholds decline the longer the test goes on, and fatigue typically accounts for this phenomenon.

TEST DURATION

Test duration mainly depends on the algorithm used to reach threshold and the area covered. Algorithms are discussed in the strategy section (Category IV). The newer algorithms significantly reduce test duration. Test duration simply records the time required to complete the test. Figure 26–15 is a good example of a reduction in test time due only to changing from a 30-2 to 24-2 test strategy.

Category IV: Perimetric Test Parameters

STIMULUS SIZE

Traditionally, a size III stimulus is used to probe the visual field and is the default stimulus size for most perimeters. For patients with advanced glaucoma, increasing test object size is more effective than decreasing background bowl luminance to uncover previously blind areas. Patients become very frustrated when they are unable to see the majority of presentations. An excessively dark gray scale printout should prompt the physician to increase test object size for the next field test[6] (Fig. 26–16). Designated as numerals 0 and I through V, the test stimulus, its size (mm^2), and angular degrees are clarified in Table 26–1. The standard geometric increase in test object size is obtained by multiplying the former test object's area by 4. Test-retest variability is excessive with a size I stimulus, and small scotomas may be obliterated by a size V stimulus. A size III stimulus, with an area of 4 mm^2 and angular degrees of 0.43, is a good compromise. When large areas of the field are blind to a size III stimulus, a 16-fold increase in area with a size V stimulus (1.72 angular degrees) allows recruitment of less damaged surrounding receptive fields.[7] The critical point here is that the size V stimulus is typically underused. Nineteen size III stimuli cover the same area occupied by a single size V stimulus.

STIMULUS COLOR, BACKGROUND LUMINANCE, AND BACKGROUND COLOR

The use of chromatic perimetry is gaining momentum. The most popular chromatic field is the blue-on-yellow examination, which isolates a small subset of ganglion cells of the short-wavelength–sensitive cone system. Many investigators believe that isolation of this system is more sensitive in the detection of early glaucoma than the standard white-on-white examination. Unfortunately, this test also results in a larger range of normal values, with the potential for high false-positive and false-negative findings. Obviously, decibel (dB) values vary according to color of the test object, background color, and luminance. Discussion of these variables is beyond the scope of this chapter. The standard white background luminance in the Goldmann perimeter and Humphrey Analyzer is 31.5 apostilbs (Asb).

TABLE 26–1. PARAMETERS FOR STIMULI USED IN PERIMETRIC TESTING

	Test Stimulus					
	0	*I*	*II*	*III*	*IV*	*V*
Size (mm^2)	1/16	1/4	1	4	16	64
Degrees*	0.0054	0.108	0.216	0.431	0.9862	1.724

*Angular degrees measures at the pupil.

Text continued on page 447

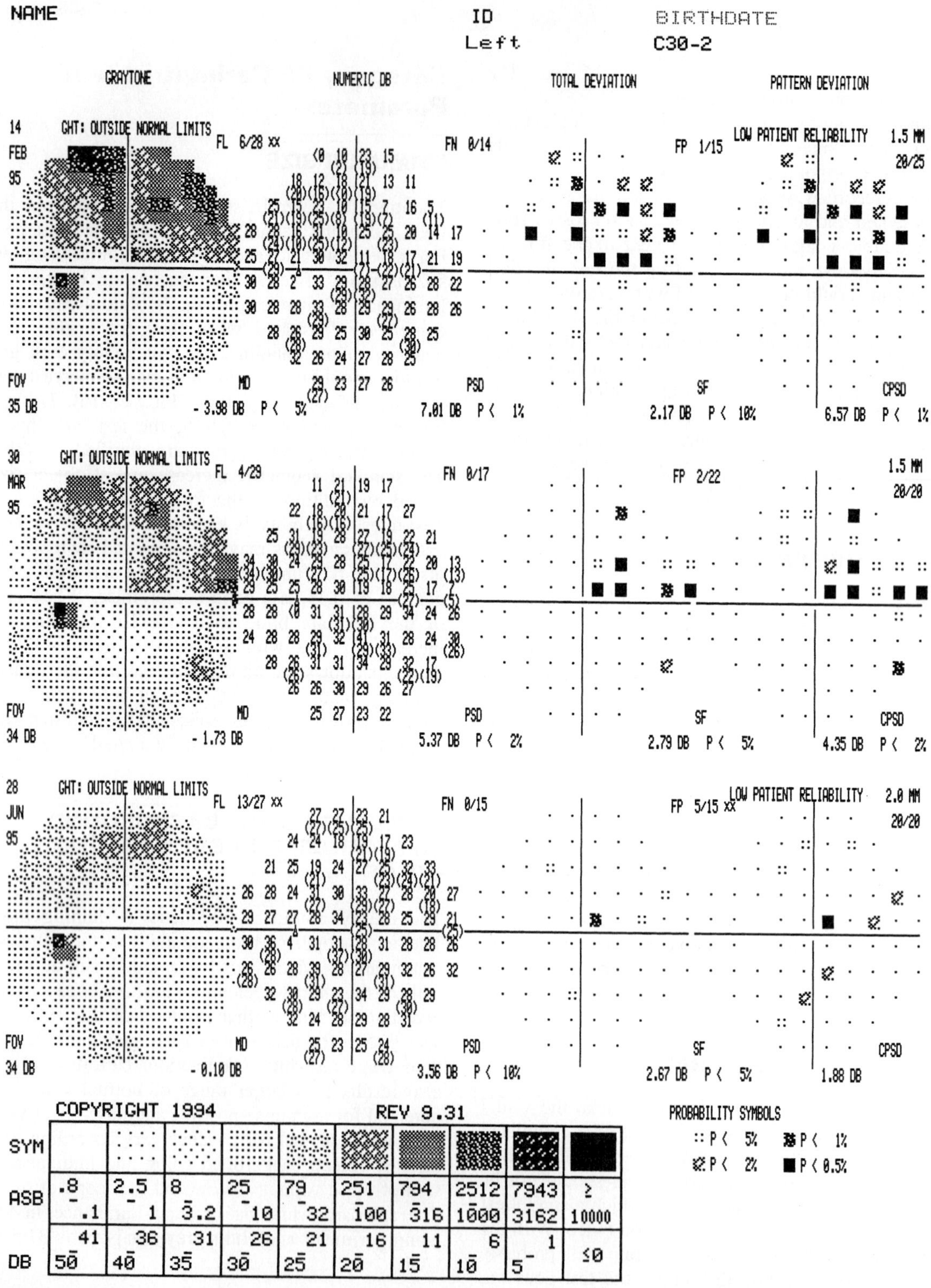

FIGURE 26–13. The effect of excessive fixation loss on field sensitivity: the "scotoma disappearing act." Without good fixation, it is impossible to accurately map the normal gradient of a visual field. The eye to be tested must constantly fixate on a light or other target positioned directly ahead. Near the beginning of the field test, the area of the physiologic blind spot is determined. One method of monitoring fixation is to periodically probe the patient's physiologic blind spot with a predetermined test object (size III), and express the number seen as a fraction of the total. The probe is never seen with excellent fixation, is rarely seen with moderate fixation, and is always seen with poor fixation. Excessive fixation loss, greater than 33%, may invalidate the field because the patient tends to shift fixation toward the object of regard. Because visual sensitivity is maximal at fixation, the continued shifts invalidate the normal gradient of sensitivity; this always makes the field look better than expected. When previous scotomas disappear for unknown reasons, the most likely cause is excess fixation loss.

In this example of three successive field tests, sensitivity appears best on the last field, where 13 of 27 blind spot checks were seen *(arrow)*. The March 1995 field demonstrates a nasal step that mysteriously disappears 3 months later. The normal blind spot is 5 × 7 degrees, a huge area to hide (a 0.43-degree size III test object). Sixteen size III stimuli can be stacked inside the vertical portion of the physiologic blind spot. One can imagine the degree of fixation shift that must occur to have a red flag on fixation shifts. This indicates large fixation shifts that tend to "play hide and seek" with scotoma. The patient learns where the pathologic blind spot is located and shifts fixation into that area to look for the test presentation. This obviously moves the physiologic blind spot out of the area previously mapped out at the beginning of the test. Subsequent visual fields may appear worse as a result of improved fixation.

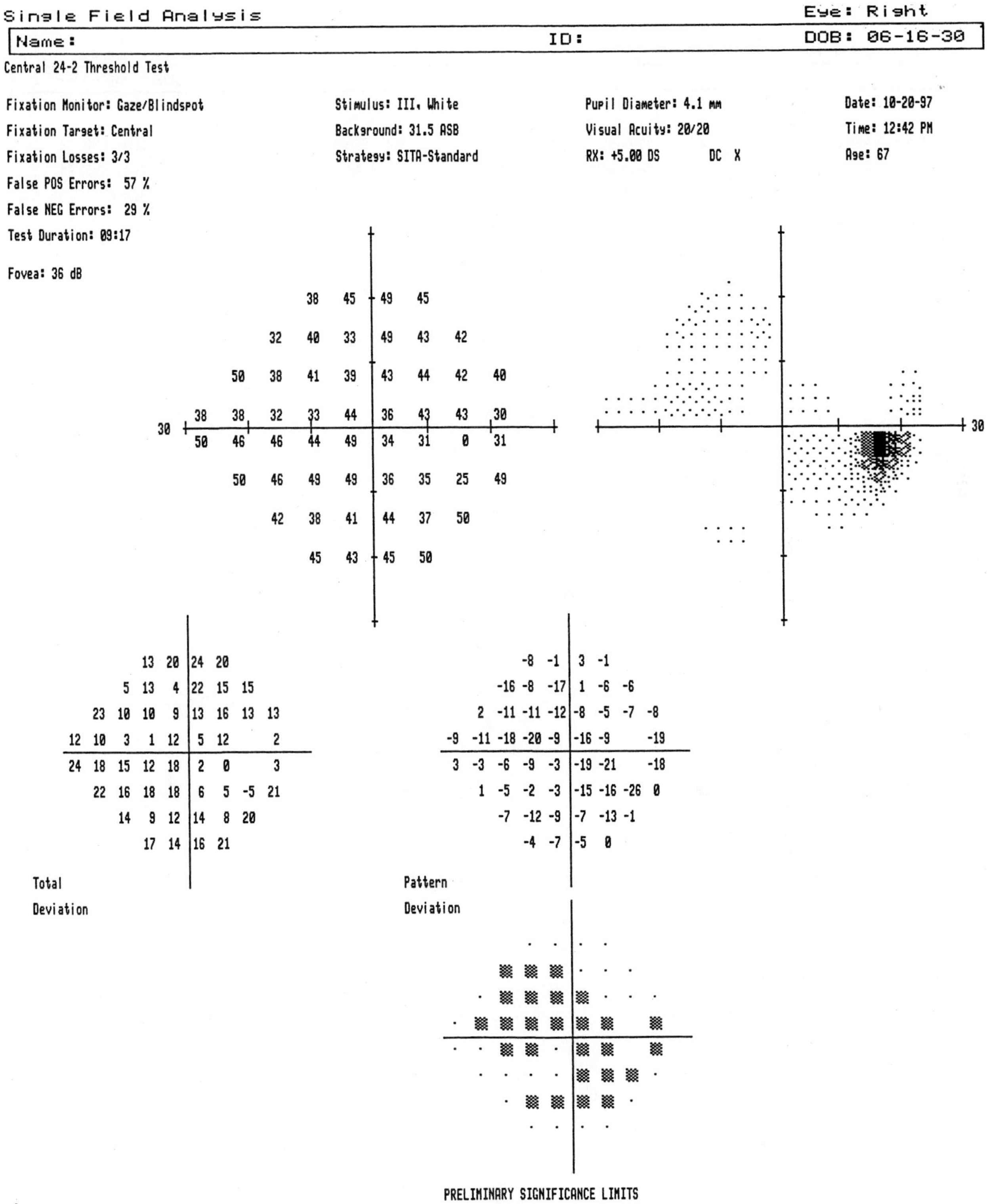

A

FIGURE 26–14. False-positive error rate. Visual field whiteout due to high false-positive error rate. A moderate fixation loss in itself does not result in a totally invalid field if the false-positive rate is acceptable. A false-positive error occurs when an auditory cue of test presentation is given but no test object is presented. If the patient responds during that "empty presentation," a false-positive error is recorded. A very high false-positive error rate indicates intentional button punching, or the "happy clicker" syndrome. Such a patient believes he or she can outguess the machine by responding to every auditory cue, clicking whether he or she can see the stimulus or not; this syndrome produces a "superhuman" field. Such a pattern occurs innocently, when the patient simply does not understand how to take the test, as in the analysis shown in *A* and *B*. This new patient's right eye was tested first *(A),* demonstrating a partial whiteout syndrome; additional instructions given immediately prior to the left eye test *(B)* results in a normal field.

Illustration continued on following page

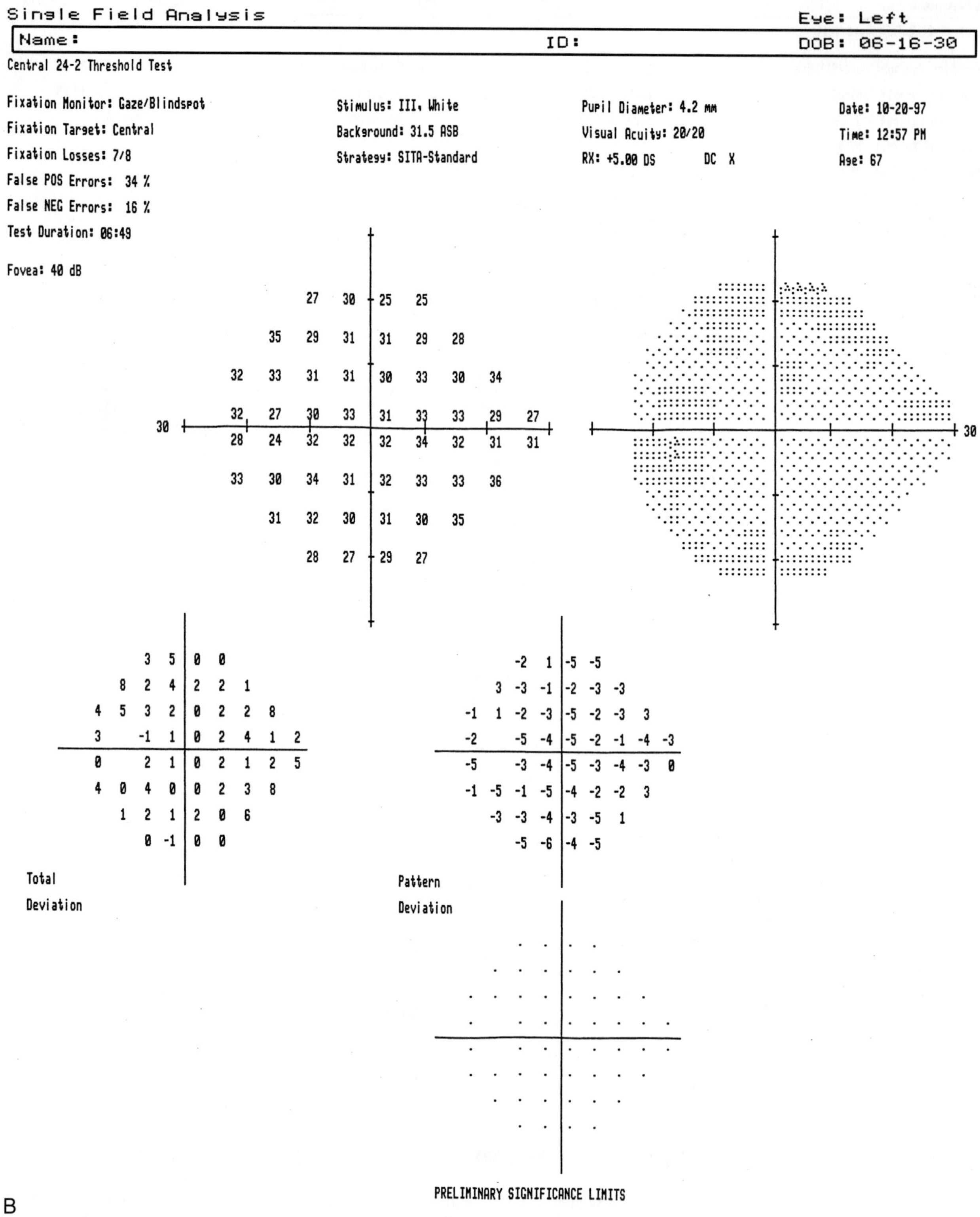

B

FIGURE 26–14 *Continued*

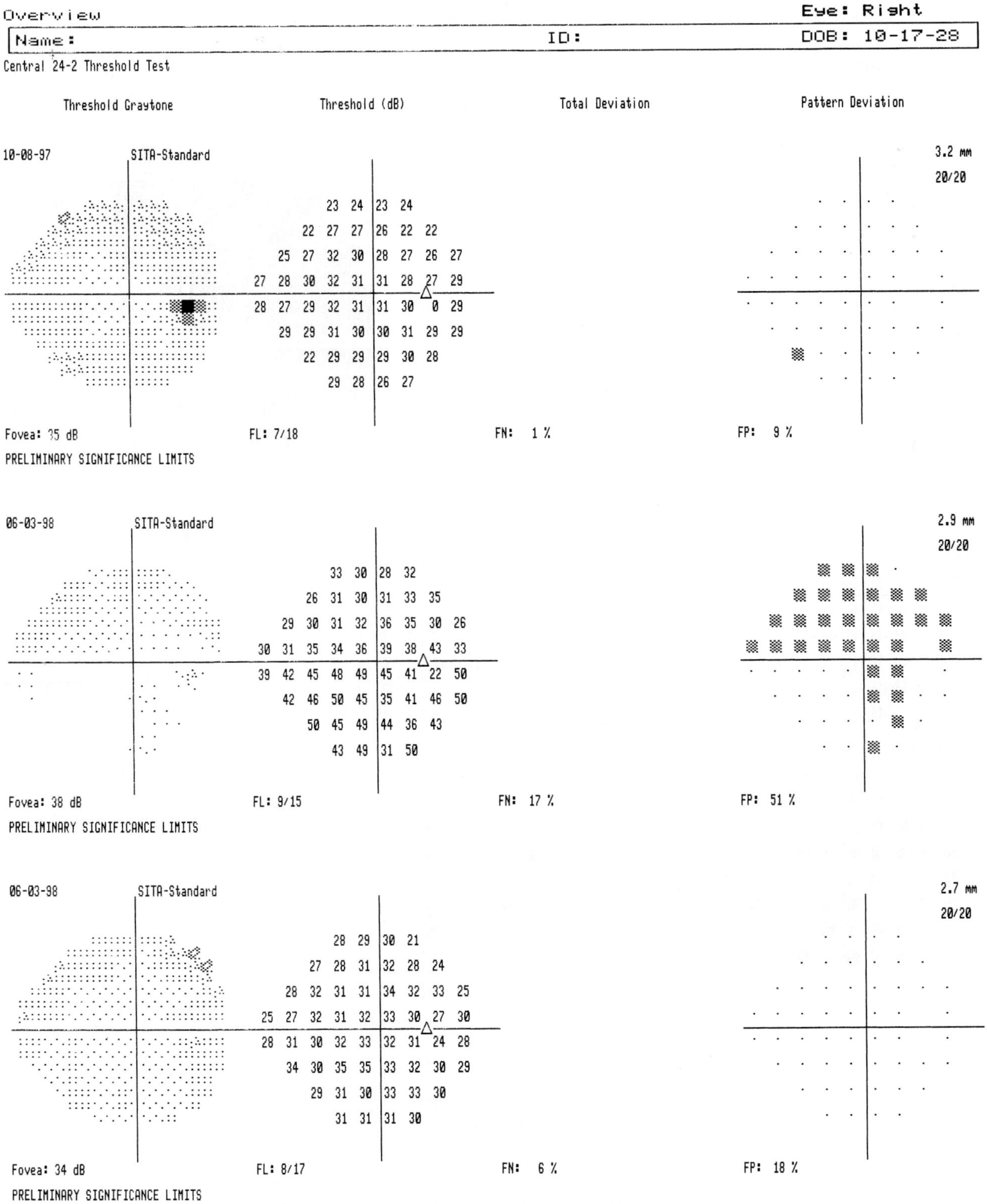

C

FIGURE 26–14 *Continued. C,* A similar situation occurs when a patient actually forgets how to take the test. This 71-year-old patient produced a reliable 10/08/97 field with a 9% false-positive rate *(arrow).* He was distracted, lost concentration, and states he "phased out" during the first 6/03/98 field test, scoring a 51% false-positive rate *(arrow).* The test was immediately repeated, with only an 18% false-positive rate and reasonable data. Notice that the fixation losses are not significantly different but that the false-positive rate has a huge effect on threshold.

Illustration continued on following page

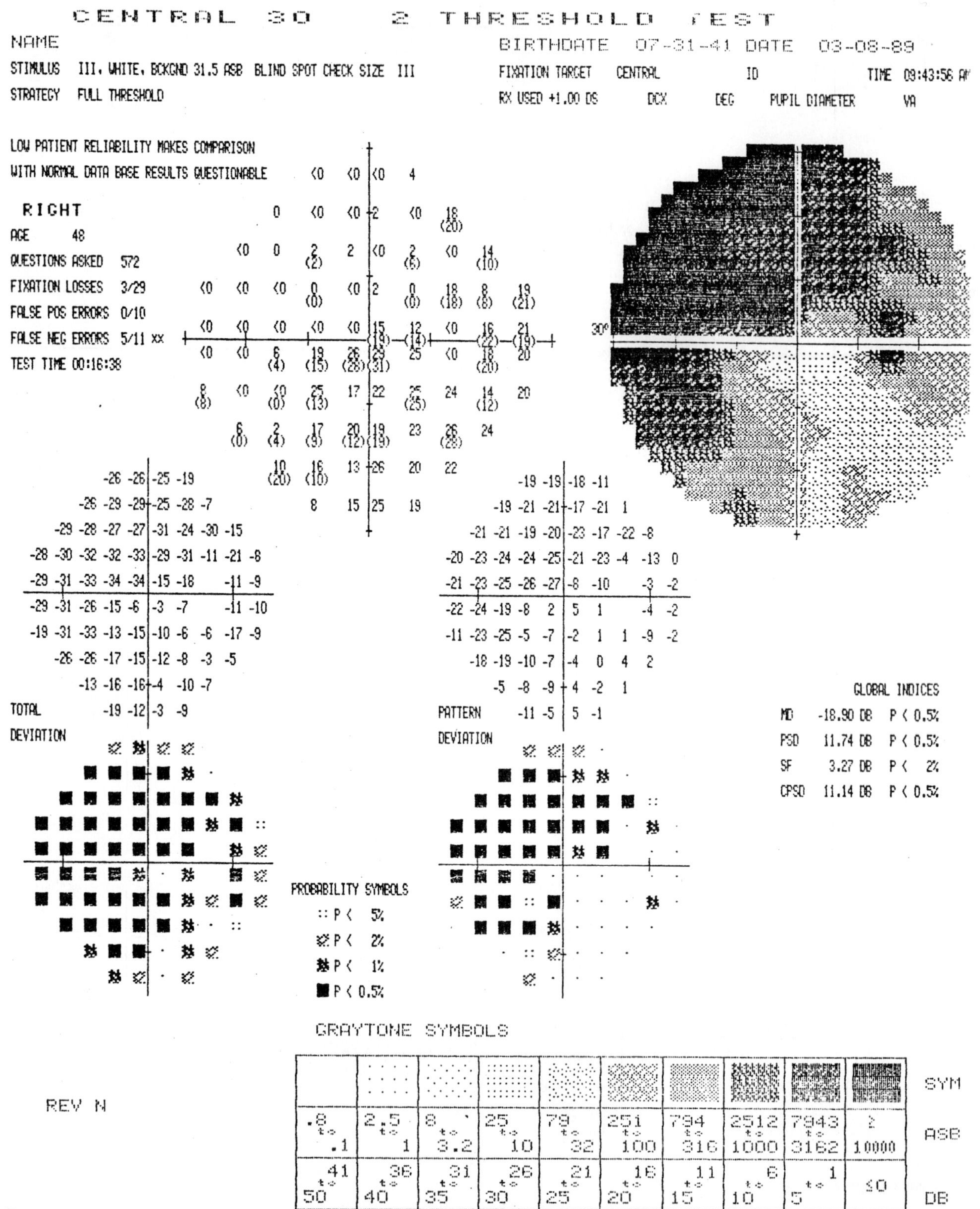

D

FIGURE 26–14 *Continued. D* and *E* are dramatic examples of how large scotomas may disappear with severe test taking deficiencies as exemplified by high false-positive rates and high fixation losses *(arrowhead).* These field loss printouts are from the test of a young, apprehensive patient with pigmentary glaucoma. The March 1989 field test *(D)* reveals a dense superior arcuate scotoma and absolute inferior nasal step.

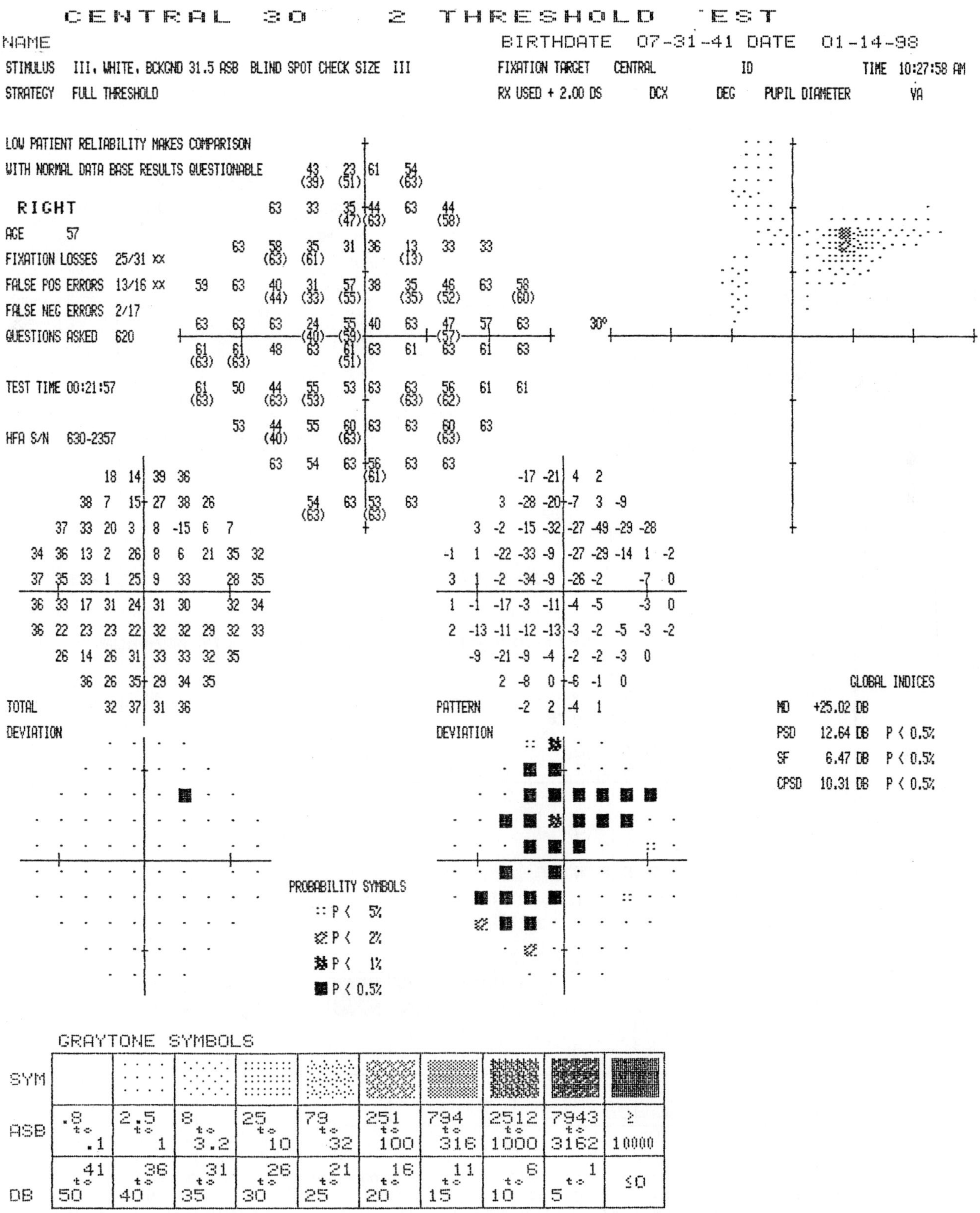

E

FIGURE 26–14 *Continued.* The January 1998 field test *(E)* reveals the gray scale whiteout with a superhuman field. This scotoma "disappearing act" is due to a clicking of the response button at every auditory cue. The patient knew that surgery was indicated if the field appeared to have worsened.

Illustration continued on following page

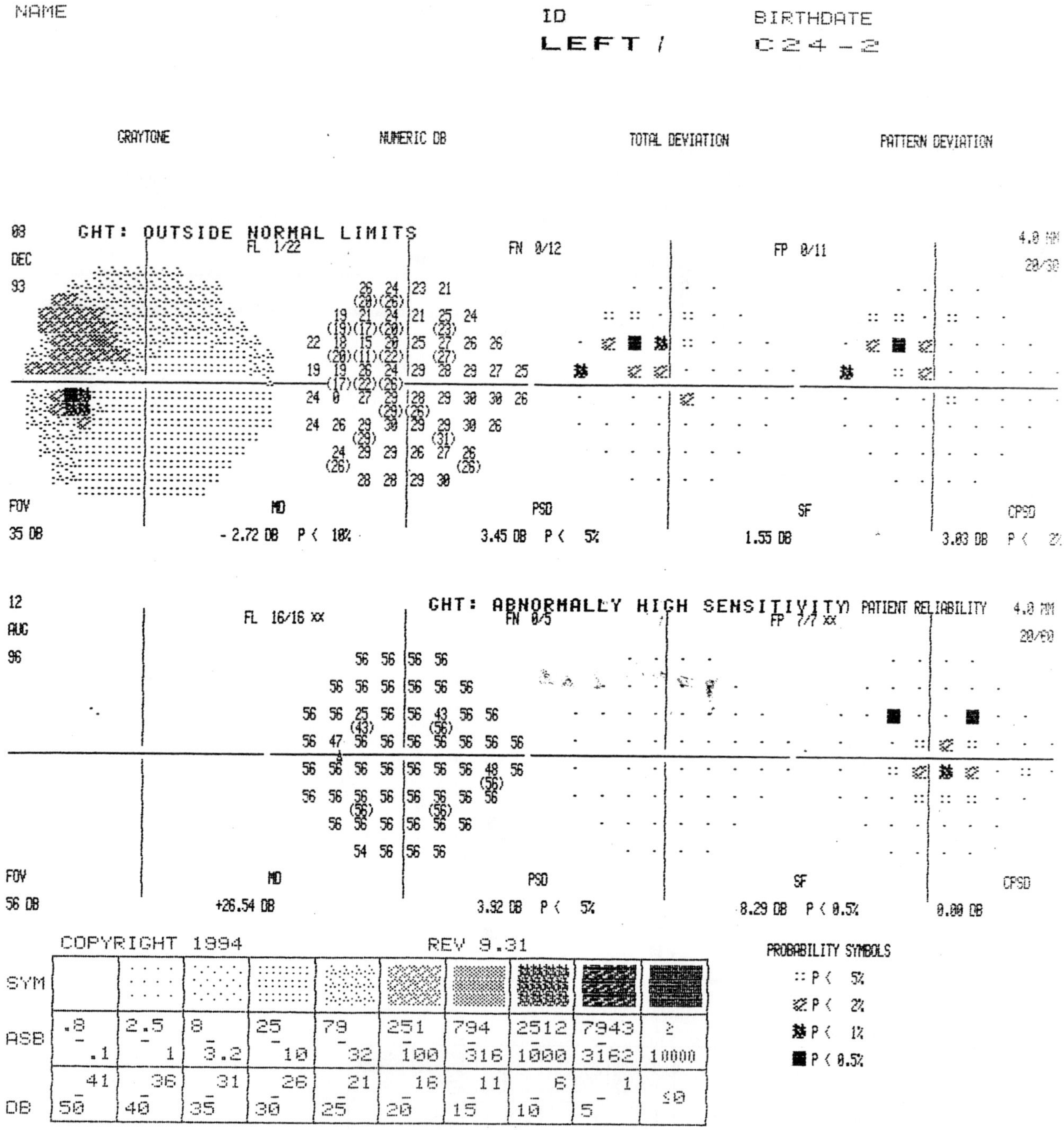

F

FIGURE 26–14 *Continued. F,* Another example of "whiteout"; however, this time the prior field was normal. In this example, the glaucoma hemifield test from STATPAC II was operational, indicating an abnormally high sensitivity. This additional software is helpful in pointing out invalid superhuman fields due to poor test taking, including high false-positive rates. These fields are totally worthless, and because of subtle mental status changes in this patient, future attempts will be futile. I call this the 56-decibel syndrome; the patient scored so well that he never has to take the test again. These test-taking discrepancies should be noted on the patient's chart, documenting the futility of future test procedures.

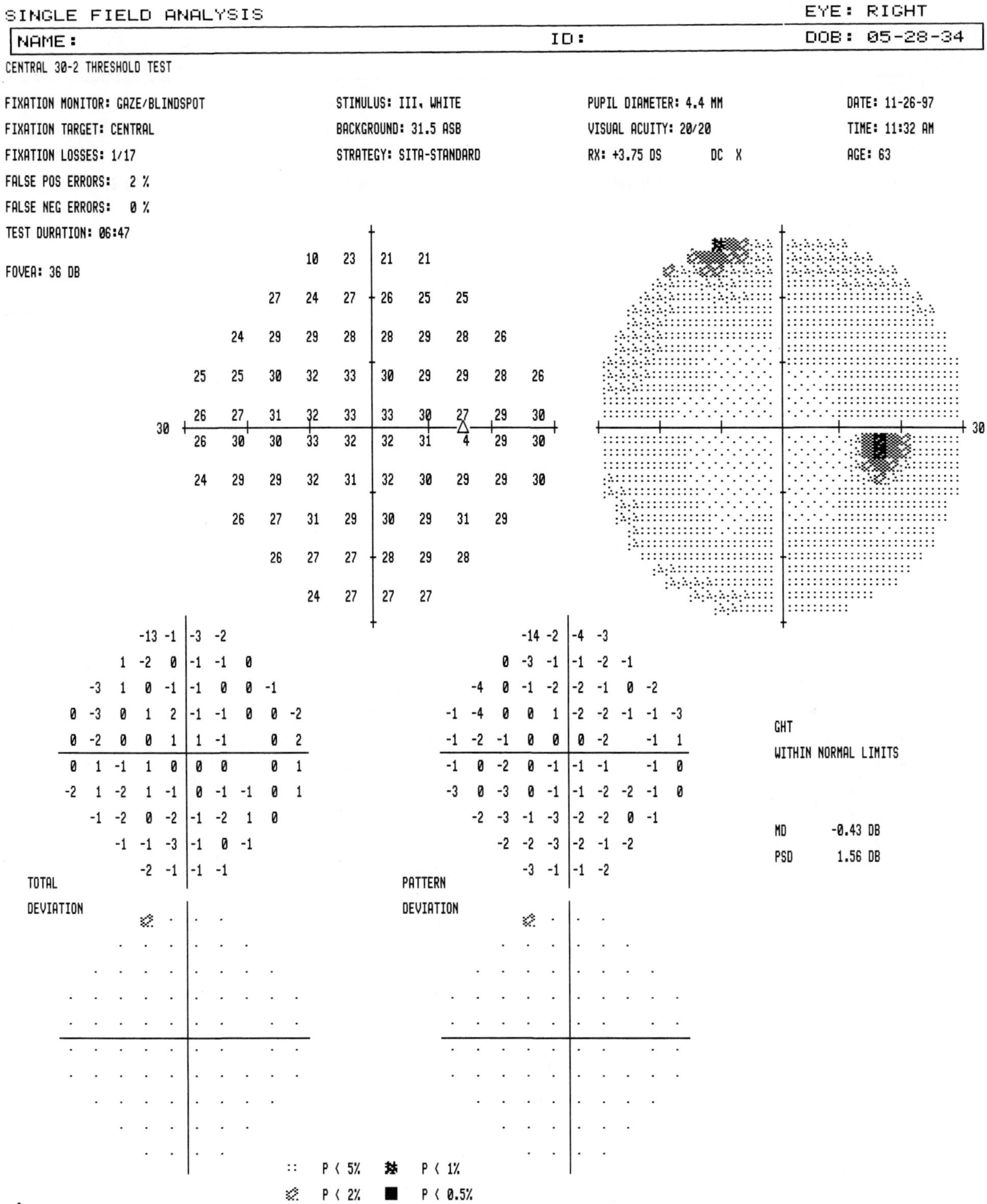

A

FIGURE 26–15. Comparison of test duration for 30-2 *(A)* and 24-2 *(B)* programs. Changing from the 76-point 30-2 program to the 54-point 24-2 program results in considerable time savings. If the physician correlates the field data with the rest of the ocular examination, it is rare for any progression with the 24-2 test to be missed. Notice the "clean data," as seen in Category III findings. The test is incredibly reliable and easy to read. Test duration is 6 minutes, 47 seconds for the 30-2 test and 4 minutes, 39 seconds for the 24-2 test *(arrow)*. A 29% reduction in test locations results in roughly a 31% time savings. Patients rarely complain about a test that takes less than 5 minutes. Patients who do complain get reminded of the 30-minute Goldmann test and the 20-minute full threshold test (time per eye).

Illustration continued on following page

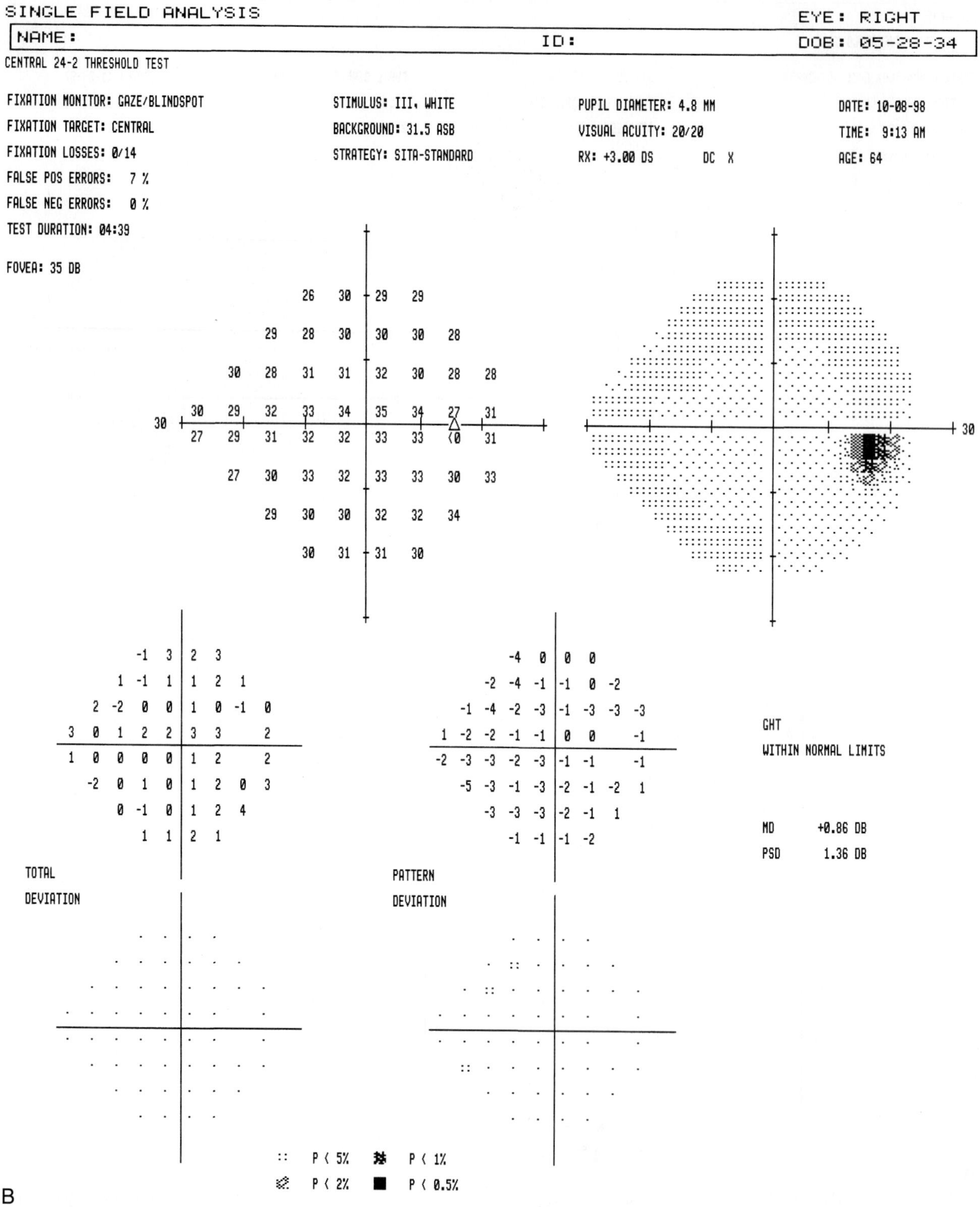

B

FIGURE 26–15 *Continued*

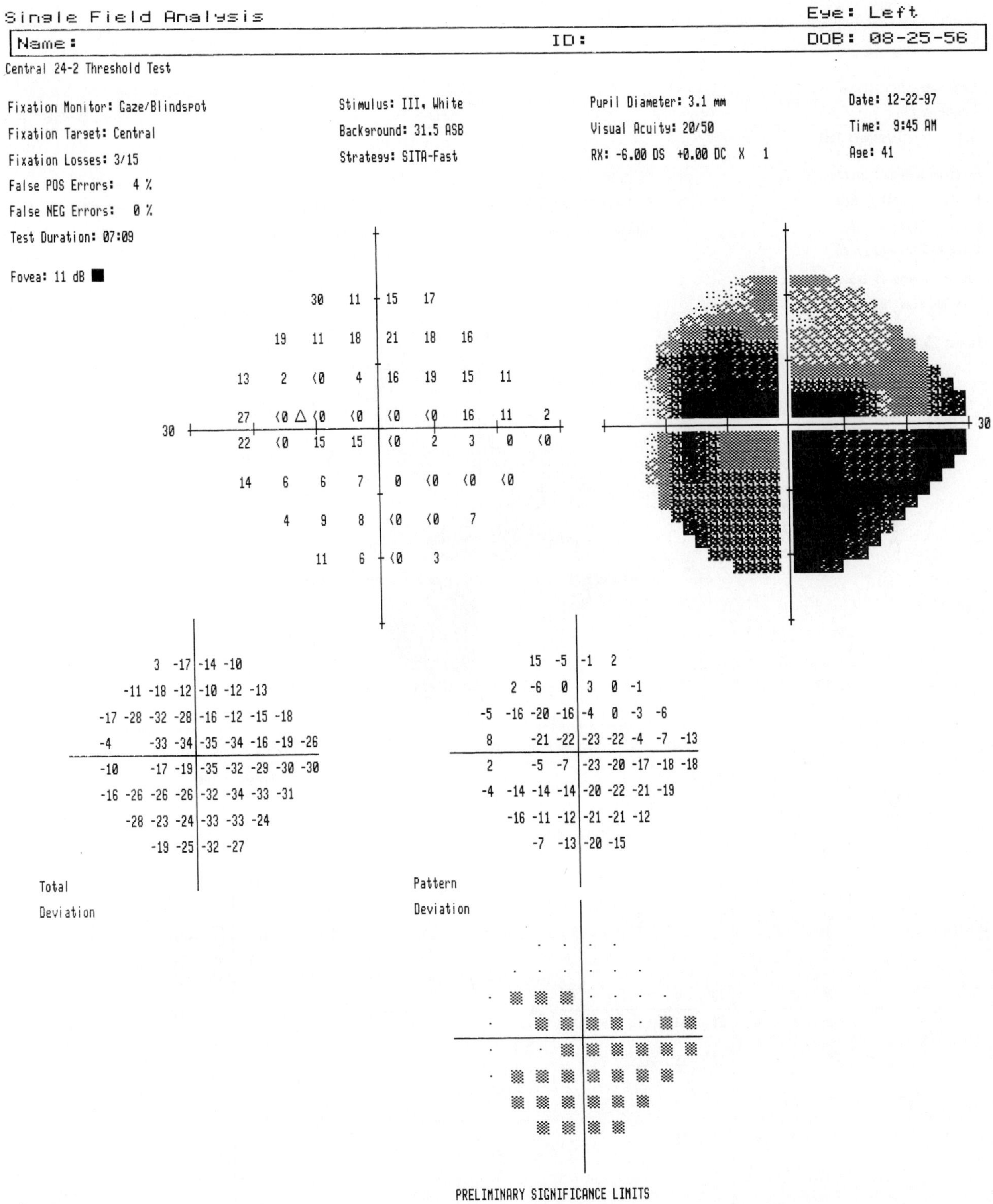

A

FIGURE 26–16. The clinical importance of stimulus size and spatial summation. Spatial summation is the ability to recognize a change in threshold when the test object area is increased or decreased while all other test variables are kept constant. This concept is clinically useful in uncovering previously blind areas of the field. In normal eyes, summation increases with increasing retinal eccentricity, and one would expect an average of 5 dB to 8 dB of improved sensitivity when a change is made from a size III to a size V stimulus. However, pathologic summation may occur in diseased field areas as seen in this example. The bottom line is: changing to a larger stimulus uncovers a much larger portion of useful field to follow. Therefore, the areas with 0 dB, which implies inability to see 10,000 Asb test object, require a larger stimulus in order to record areas of still useful vision. Patients with advanced field damage are better served with a larger test object, typically a size V. Notice that in *A* (size III stimulus *[arrowhead]*), the inferonasal quadrant is blind.

Illustration continued on following page

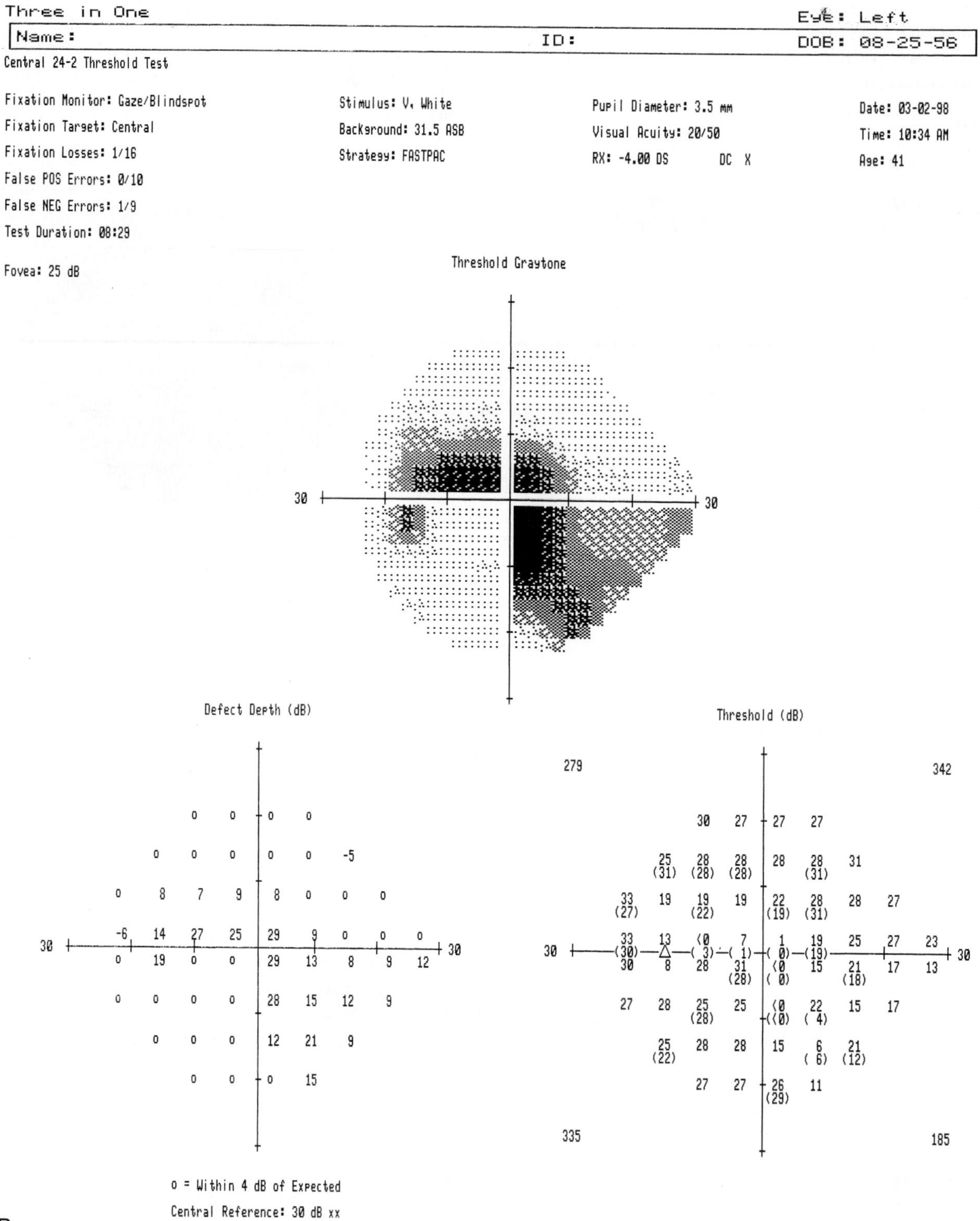

B

FIGURE 26–16 *Continued.* Changing to a size V stimulus *(arrowhead) (B)* allows better mapping of the deepest part of the scotoma and reveals clinically useful adjacent vision. In addition, the patient appreciates an easier, more "user-friendly" test.

STRATEGY

The strategy used to seek retinal threshold affects the measured threshold. The SITA algorithm is rapidly becoming the most popular algorithm owing to its accuracy and ability to determine threshold quickly (Fig. 26–17). If a change is made to a new algorithm and scotoma appear different, the field analysis should be repeated prior to intervention. If necessary, a new baseline should be obtained and then the patient's status should be monitored. When a change is made to the newer SITA algorithm, the most recent field analysis should appear slightly better because of less fatigue. A worsening field is significant, requiring explanation. If the status is in doubt, the test should be repeated. Statistical and numeric differences in printout with the use of the SITA include lack of short-term fluctuations (SF), corrected pattern standard deviation (CPSD), and the actual number of presentations for false-positive and false-negative error rates.

Category V: Patient Test Parameters

Patient test parameters obviously have a huge effect on field sensitivity. Correction of refractive error creates the most problems for data in this category.

PUPIL DIAMETER

A pupil diameter of less than 2.4 mm decreases the resolving power of the eye, affecting form and light sense. A decrease in pupil diameter from 4.75 to 1.5 mm causes a 10-fold (1 log unit) reduction in the amount of light arriving at the retina. Pupillary constriction causes a uniform reduction in field sensitivity. A constant pupil size is necessary in order to make valid comparisons for serial visual fields. The field may commonly appear worse after the addition of miotics or better following filtration surgery, when miotics are discontinued (Fig. 26–18). Pupil size should always be recorded and reviewed by the physician if there is a field change.

VISUAL ACUITY

Visual acuity has an impact on selection of field parameters. If acuity is less than 20/60 because of glaucoma, a larger test object, such as a size V stimulus, is helpful. If visual acuity is decreased owing to macular disease, the remaining nerve fiber bundles may test well with a standard size III stimulus. As the maculopathy progresses, the patient may fixate eccentrically, shifting peripheral scotomas. With macular disease, fixation may be spotty but still good enough for useful field data to be obtained. Macular disease is very common in the patient age group with glaucoma, and useful data may still be obtained with a size III stimulus (Fig. 26–19).

REFRACTION

Inability to accurately focus the test object stimulus on the retina results in reduced contrast sensitivity with loss of retinal sensitivity, especially in the central 30 degrees, where focus is most critical. If light from the test object is poorly focused on the retina, a refractive scotoma may result. This is very apparent with posterior staphyloma. It is embarrassing to diagnose or treat glaucoma according to detection of pseudoscotomas of refractive or lens rim origin (Figs. 26–20 to 26–22). These artifactual defects fit especially well into the fundamentals of common pattern recognition.

Refractive scotomas should be eliminated with proper refraction and appropriate head and lens positioning. Refractive scotomas occur most commonly in contact lens wearers; when the contact is left off and lens correction used, particularly with large corrections (Fig. 26–23). Astigmatism greater than 1.5 diopters should be added to the correction. Perimetry should routinely be performed with accurate distance refraction combined with age-adjusted near correction. The new perimeters automatically calculate the correct add after the distance correction is entered, and the technician makes the necessary change.

Lens and lens rim holder artifacts remain the bane of visual field analysis because they interfere with or falsely indicate pathologic scotomas. The sources of error are (1) obstruction of field by the lens holder, (2) incorrect head positioning, and (3) using the wrong type of lens. Effects of the wrong dioptric power and high-power artifacts have already been discussed.

The examiner should always inspect the perimeter to determine the position of the lens holder. In the older models, the lens holder is positioned laterally, and nasal and temporal lens rim artifacts are more common (Fig. 26–24). In the newer nodels, the holder is located inferiorly, creating a different set of problems.

Lens rim artifacts tend to occur in the analysis of patients with hyperopia because of spherical aberration or obstruction of the periphery which may result from poor head positioning with regard to the lens holder (Fig. 26–25). Patients, especially the elderly, have difficulty staying in exactly the same position during the test; they tend to drift away from the corrective lenses. Even with the newer model perimeters, which are programmed to intermittently reposition the patient's head, improper head positioning is a common source of error. The technician is still crucial in generating reliable information during visual field analysis and should be present in the room during the test. These artifacts are more common with higher-plus lenses.

Rarely, the wrong type of lens is used. If the technician uses the wide metal rim lens that is typically used for trial frame refractions, an incredibly large ring scotoma is created, as shown in Figure 26–26. Such an appearance on an SFA printout should prompt suspicion of this error.

Category VI: Threshold Data Points

FOVEA

The fixation monitoring system requires the subject to fixate on a light-emitting diode, precluding the ability to obtain threshold directly at fixation. The patient must shift fixation away from the standard fixation light into the center of a diamond-shaped area, where normal bowl luminance allows accurate threshold determination.

Text continued on page 464

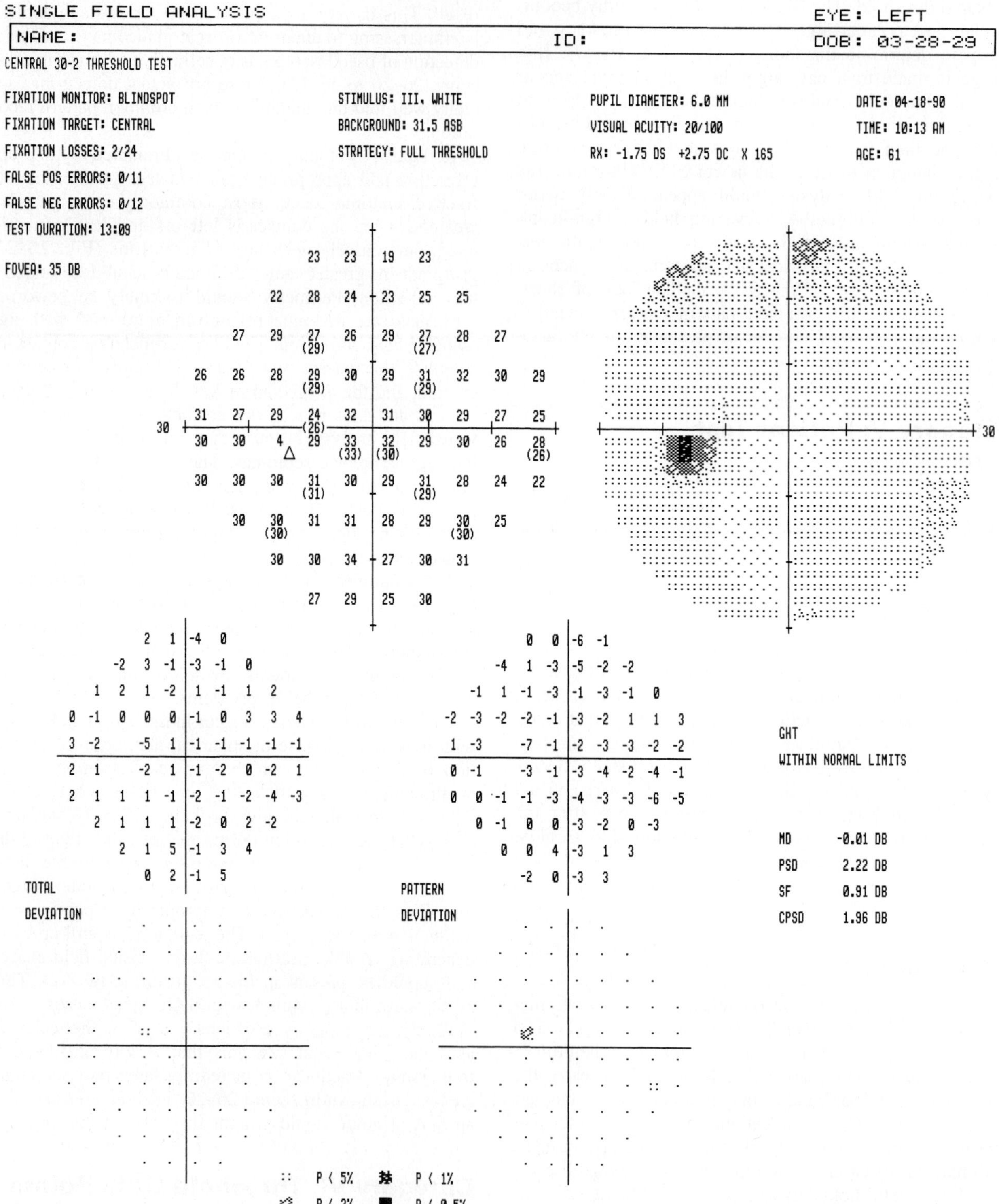

A

FIGURE 26–17. Threshold strategy: SITA versus full threshold. *SITA* stands for Swedish Interactive Threshold Algorithm, but the *S* could stand for "streamlined." Notice that in *A*, the full threshold test took 13 minutes, 9 seconds *(arrowhead)*. This is a typical test duration for a 30-2 field obtained in the early 1990s. The reliability indices are excellent.

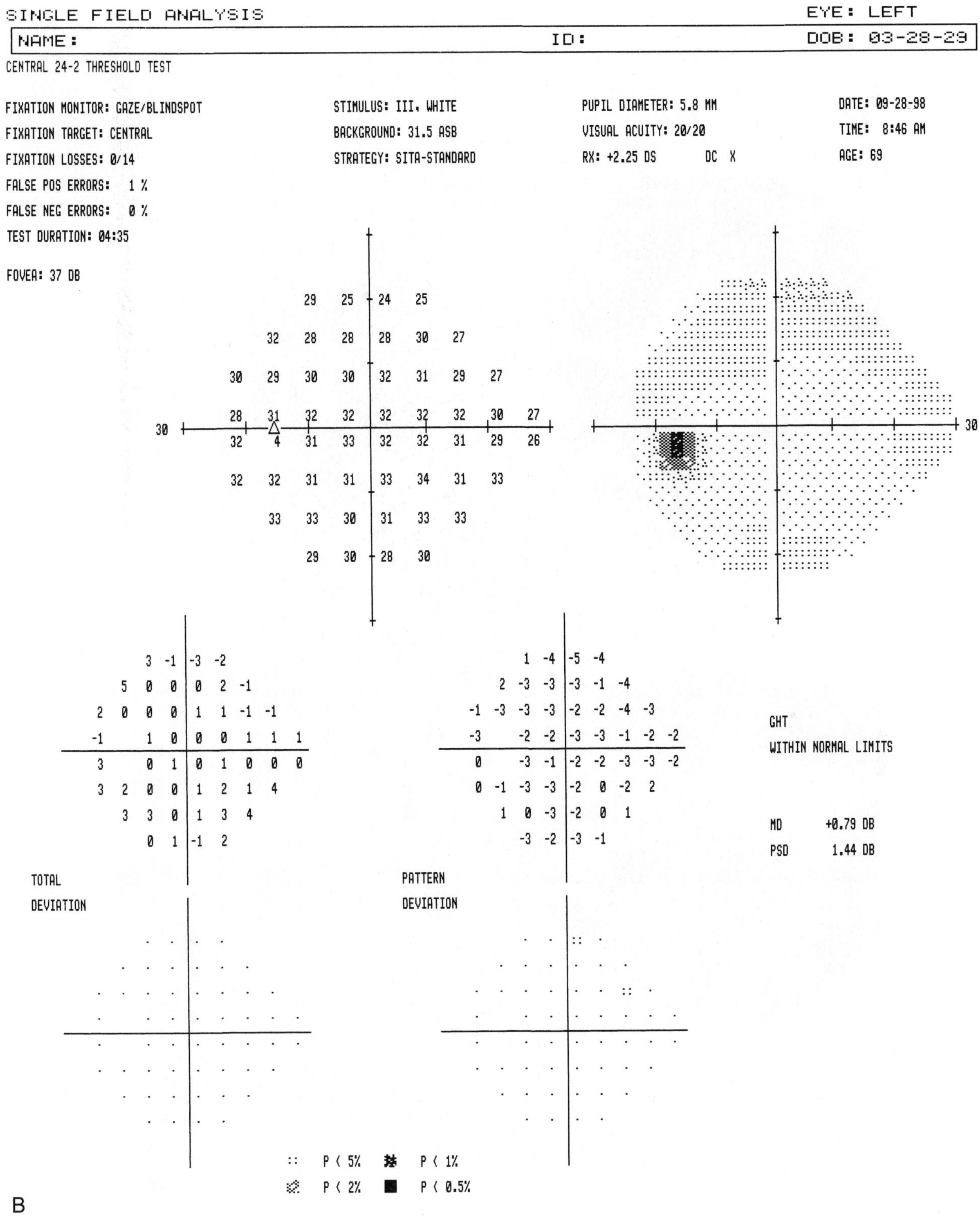

B

FIGURE 26–17 *Continued. B* shows the streamlined field of the late 1990s. The test is a 24-2 with a duration of 4 minutes, 35 seconds *(arrowhead)* cutting 8.5 minutes off the test. Both eyes could be tested in the time it used to take for one eye. With the current changes in health care and the need to evaluate more and more patients, this algorithm is gaining popularity. At this time, data are still lacking about the exact correlation of the SITA with previous algorithms. Clinically, the transition is easy.

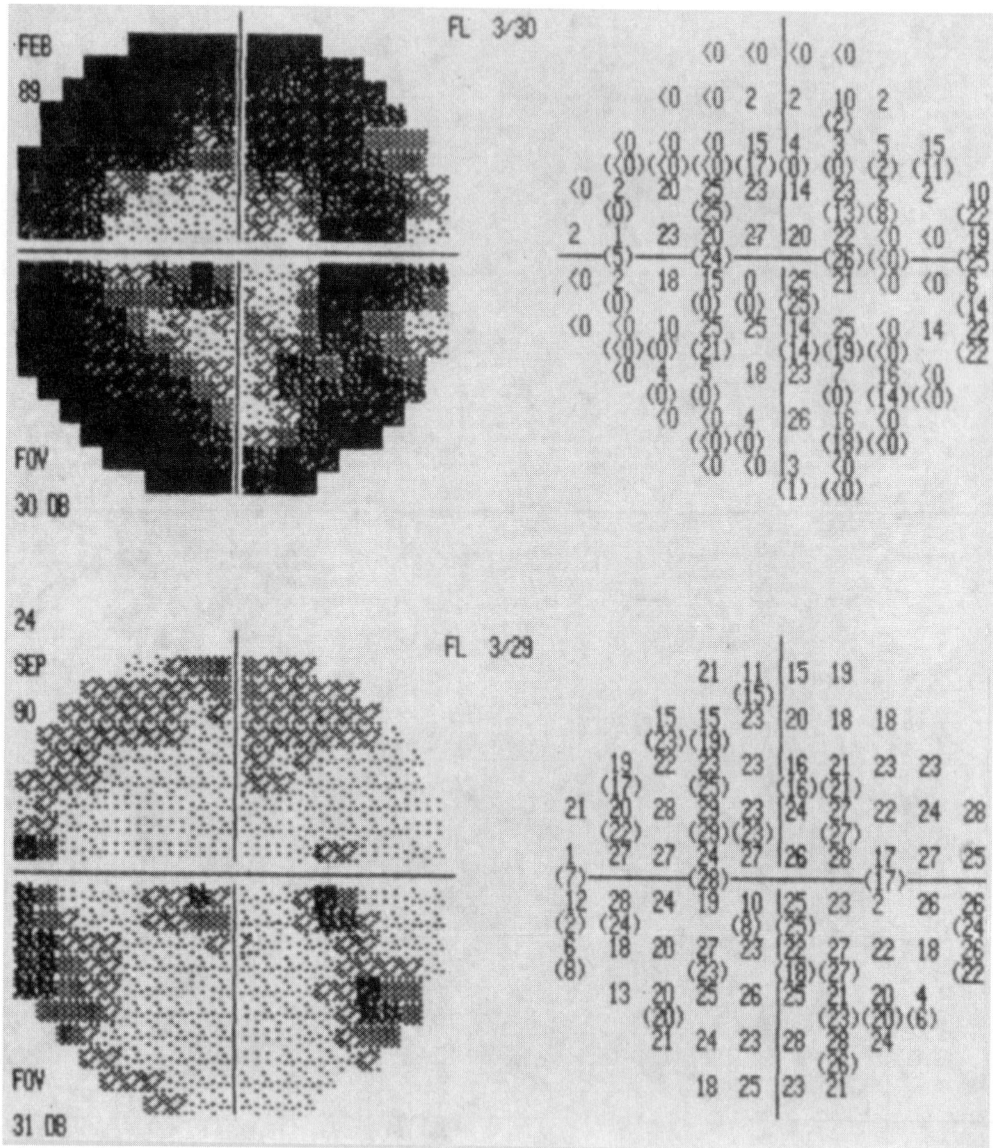

FIGURE 26–18. The effect of pupil size on field performance. The two most common traps with regard to pupil size involve the addition or cessation of miotic drug therapy. Field improvement after filtering surgery may be purely due to a larger pupil after miotics are discontinued as seen in this patient that demonstrates a marked improvement in the September 1990 postoperative field compared to the previous field while on miotics. More importantly, if a miotic agent is added to the therapy, the next field test may appear worse. If this occurs, tell the patient to discontinue miotic therapy for 24 hours prior to the next field test. This is a reasonable compromise. Dilating the pupil every time a field is obtained could eventually lead to problems that occur after office hours are over.

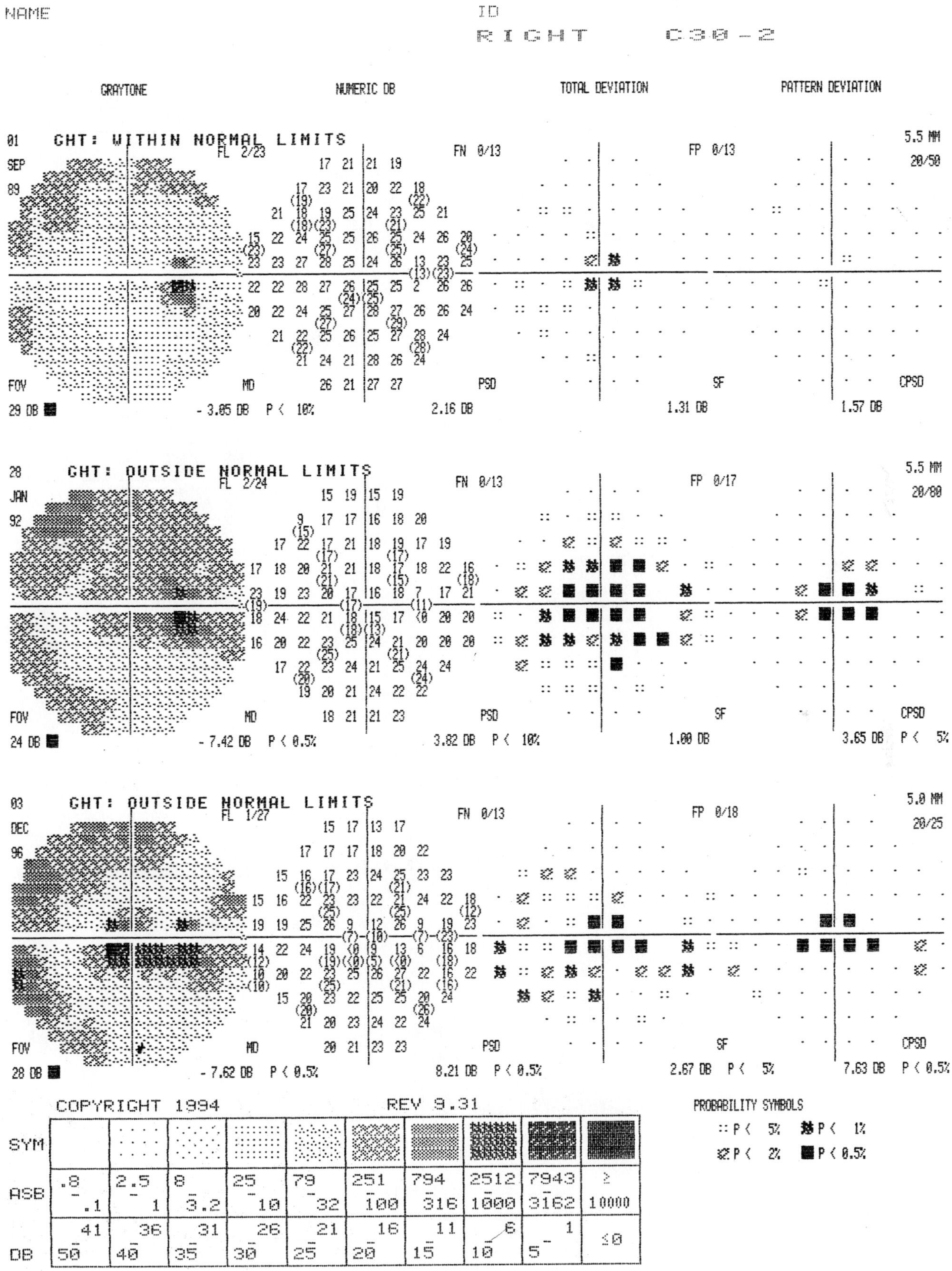

A

FIGURE 26–19. Advancing central scotoma secondary to macular disease in a patient with glaucoma. This 85-year-old patient has primary open-angle glaucoma and advancing macular disease. *A,* The 1989 field shows a mild decrease in central sensitivity with a foveal threshold of 29 dB.

Illustration continued on following page

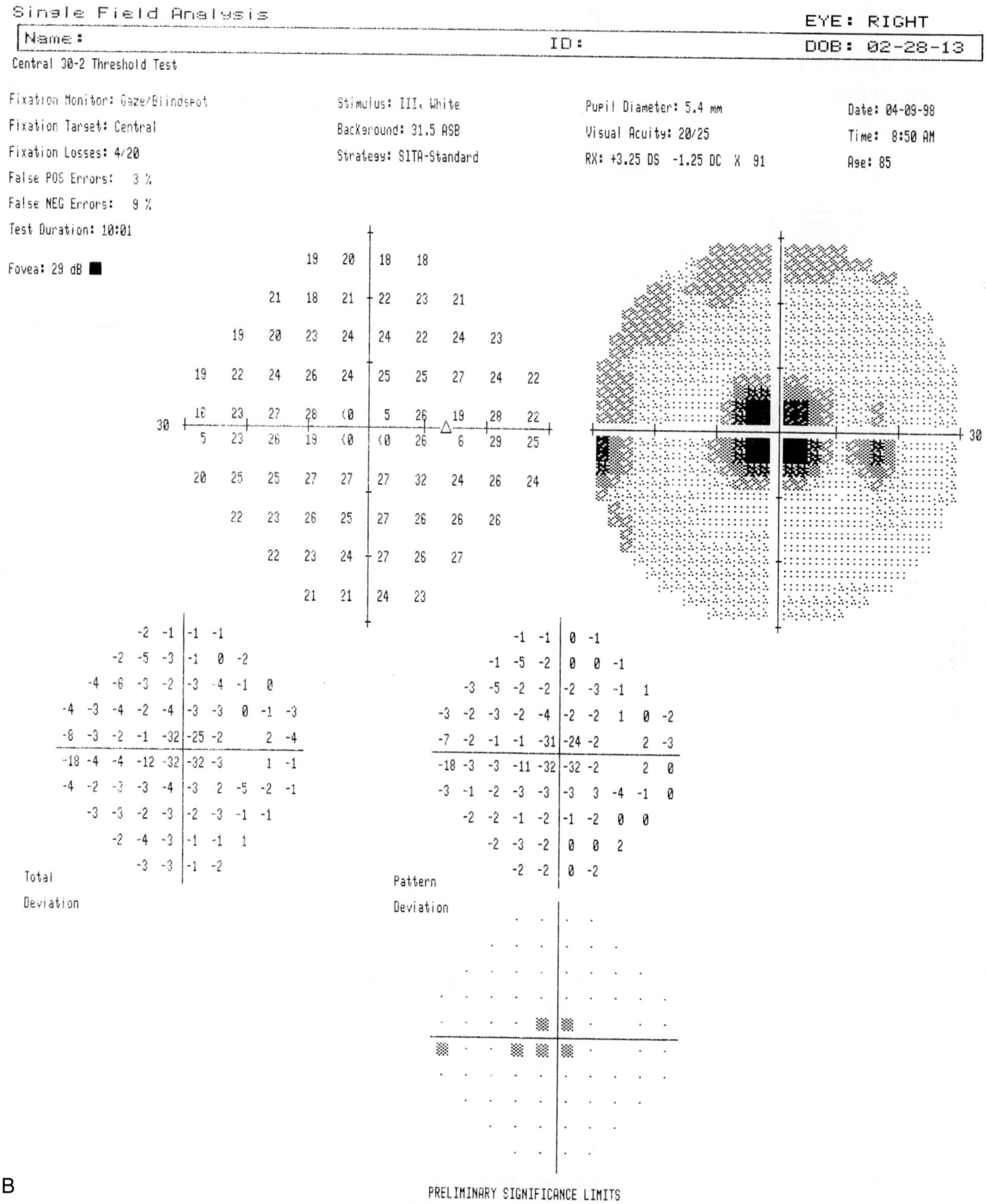

B

FIGURE 26–19 *Continued. B,* Nine years later, the central sensitivity remains 29 dB, and visual acuity is 20/25, probably the result of one micro-island of sensitivity with much worse retinal sensitivity surrounding fixation. However, the ability to test the field for glaucoma has been reliable. This is a common macular pattern without any respect for either the horizontal or vertical midline, a critical sign that it is likely to be retinal and not glaucomatous in origin.

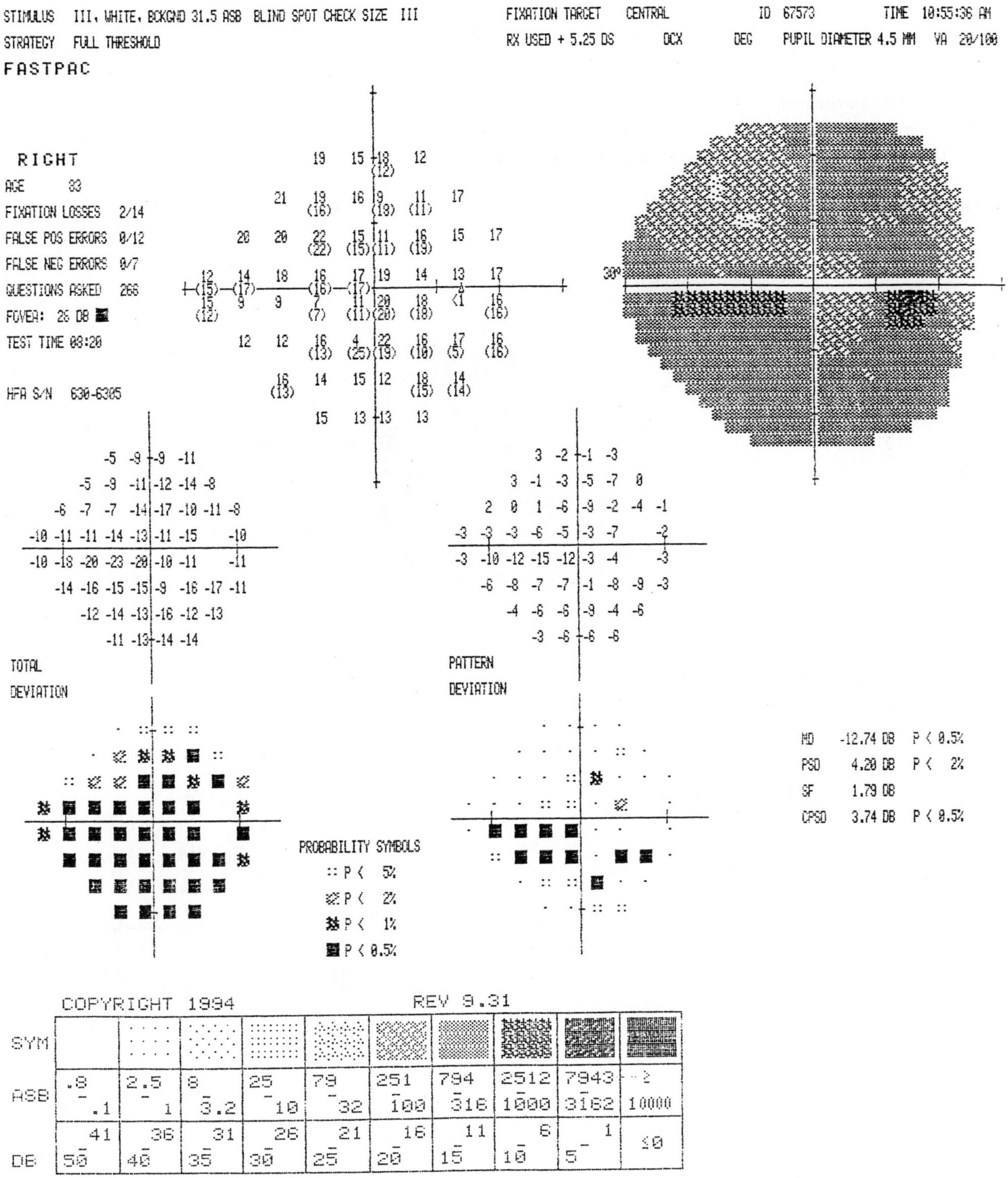

A

FIGURE 26–20. Refractive scotoma/improper spectacle correction. This 82-year-old patient with pseudophakia and glaucoma had difficulty with postoperative refractions following cataract surgery and was treated with a +2.25-diopter correction with 20/100 vision. *A,* The field reveals a generalized reduction in sensitivity with a nasal step.

Illustration continued on following page

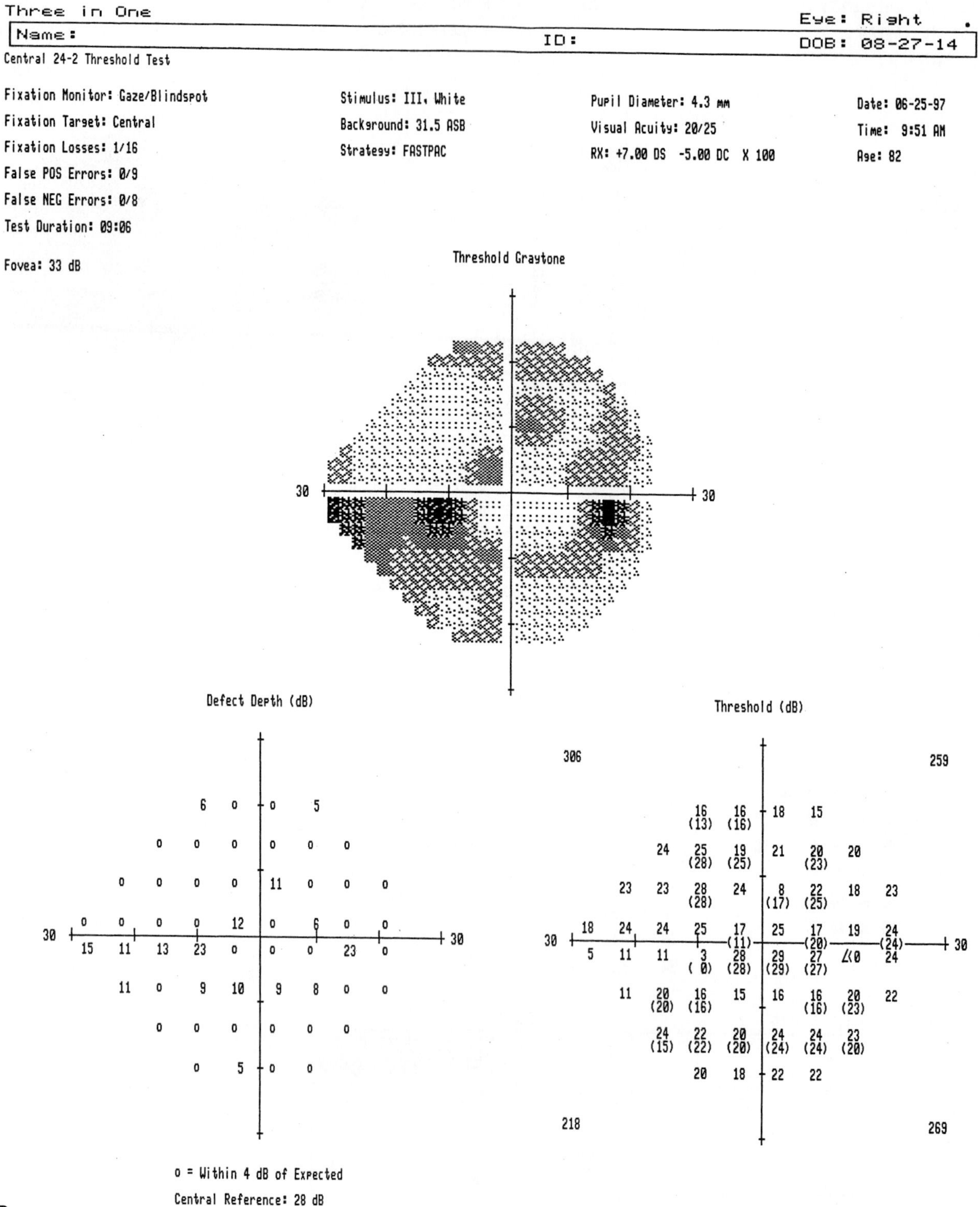

B

FIGURE 26–20 *Continued. B,* Proper correction with a +7.00 −5.00 at 100-degrees results in significant improvement in acuity (20/25) and retinal sensitivity. Failure to detect excessive astigmatism severely affected the quality of the projected retinal image and consequently the field.

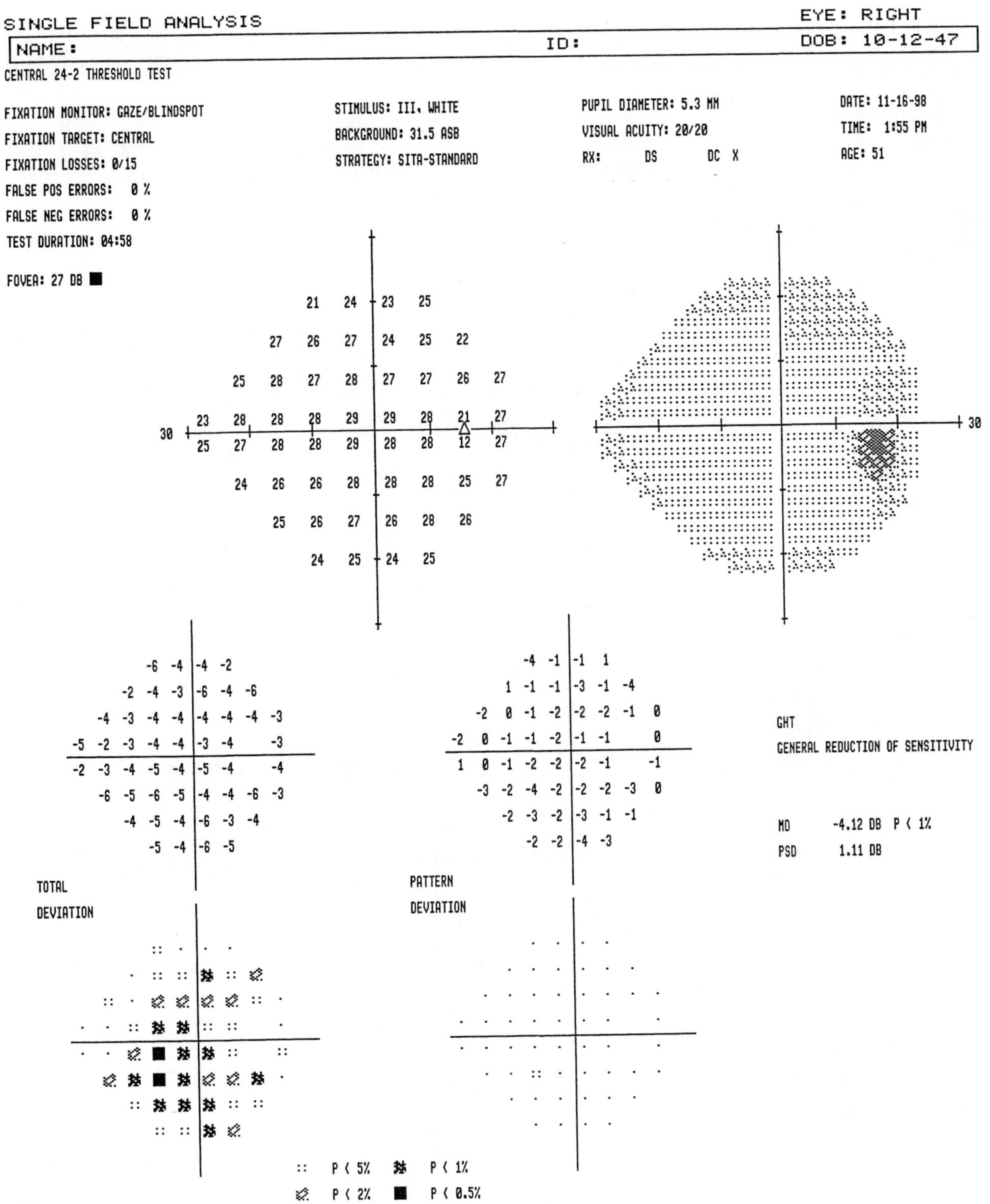

C

FIGURE 26–20 *Continued.* In another patient, these fields reflect the typical decibel drop when a +3.00 add is forgotten. These fields are from the same day. *C,* The appropriate add was left off creating central depression.

Illustration continued on following page

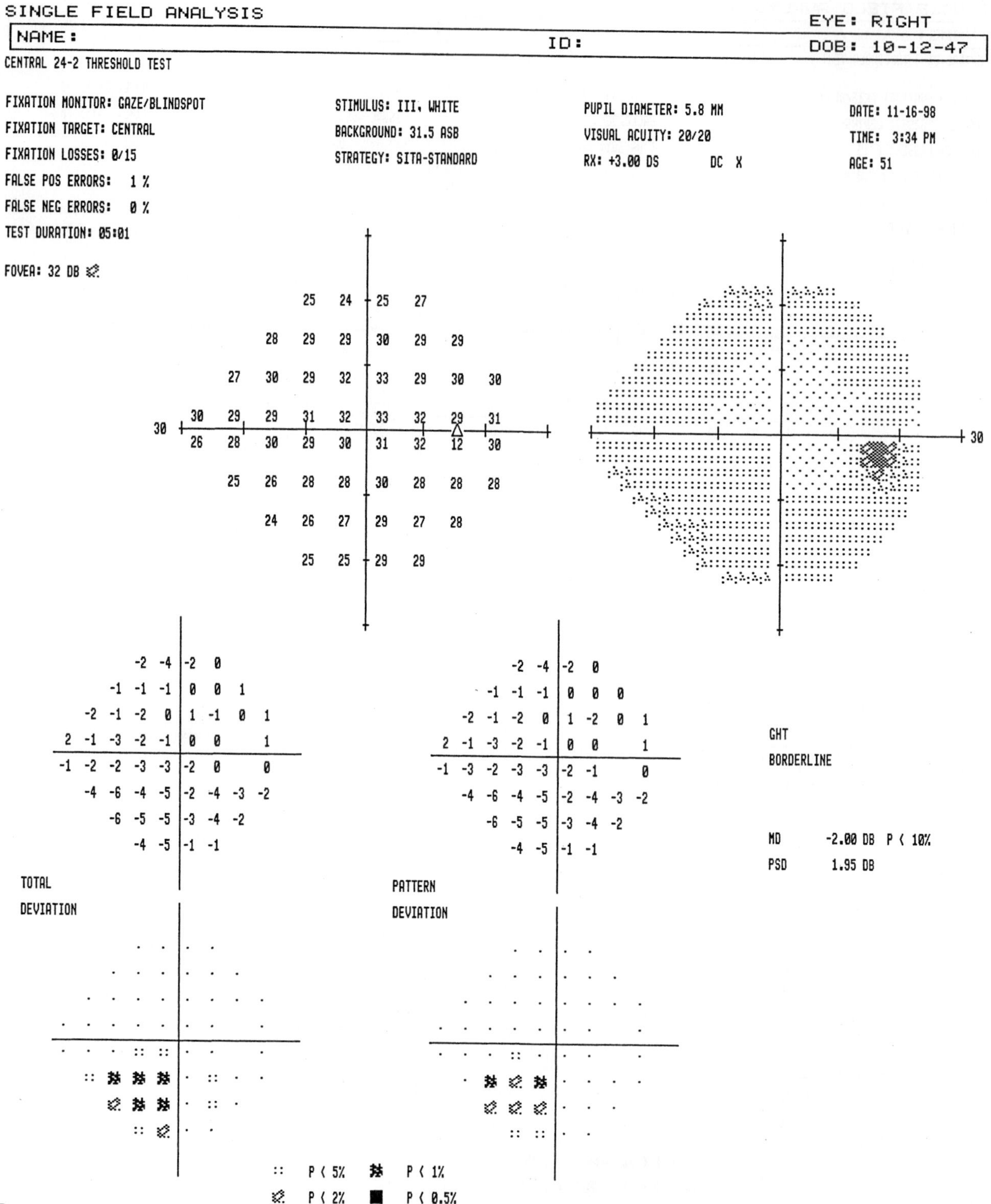

D

FIGURE 26–20 *Continued. D,* An hour and a half later, the field was repeated with improvement. Central foveal threshold improved from 27 to 33 dB. These are common errors that continue to plague everyone involved in perimetry.

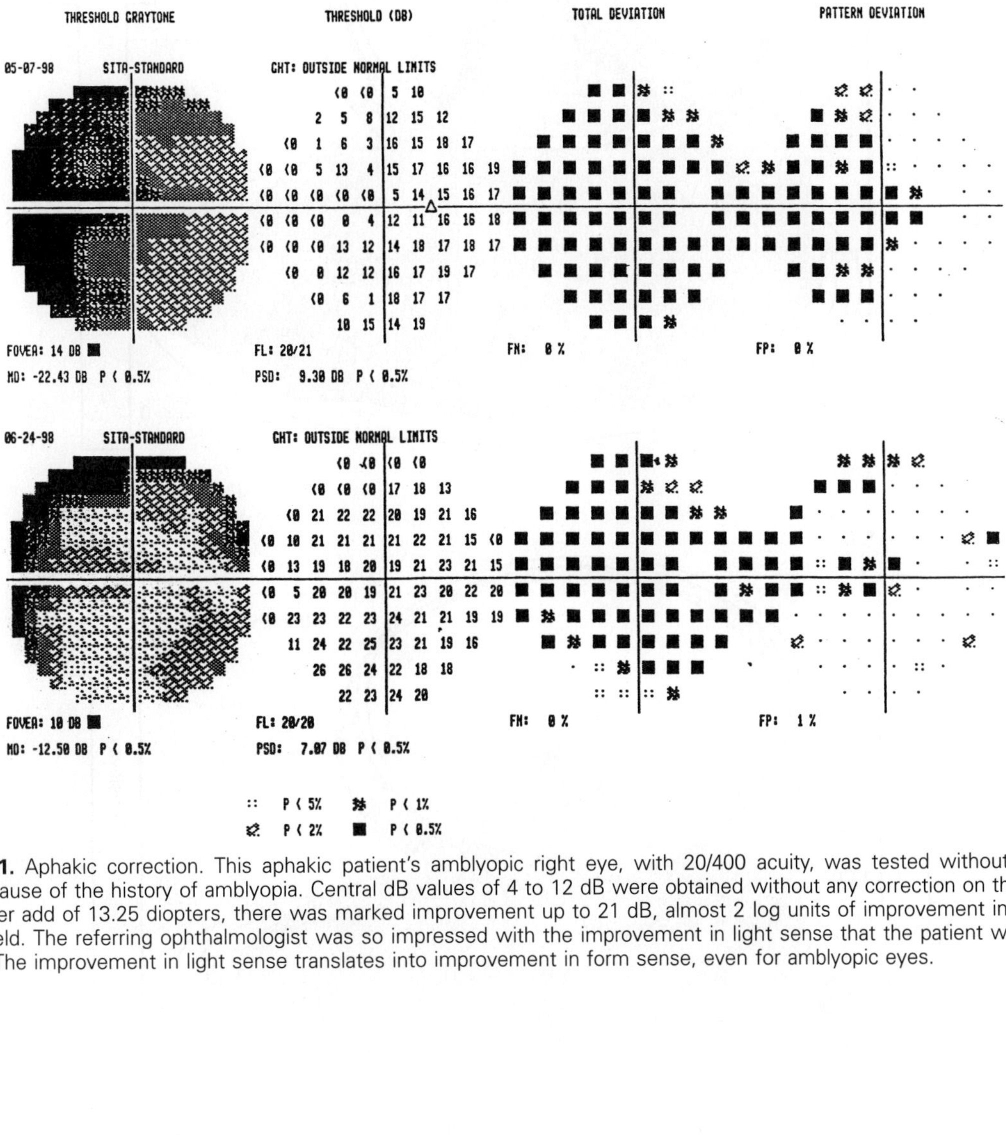

FIGURE 26–21. Aphakic correction. This aphakic patient's amblyopic right eye, with 20/400 acuity, was tested without any spectacle correction because of the history of amblyopia. Central dB values of 4 to 12 dB were obtained without any correction on the 5/07/98 field. With the proper add of 13.25 diopters, there was marked improvement up to 21 dB, almost 2 log units of improvement in light sense for the 6/24/98 field. The referring ophthalmologist was so impressed with the improvement in light sense that the patient was fitted with a contact lens. The improvement in light sense translates into improvement in form sense, even for amblyopic eyes.

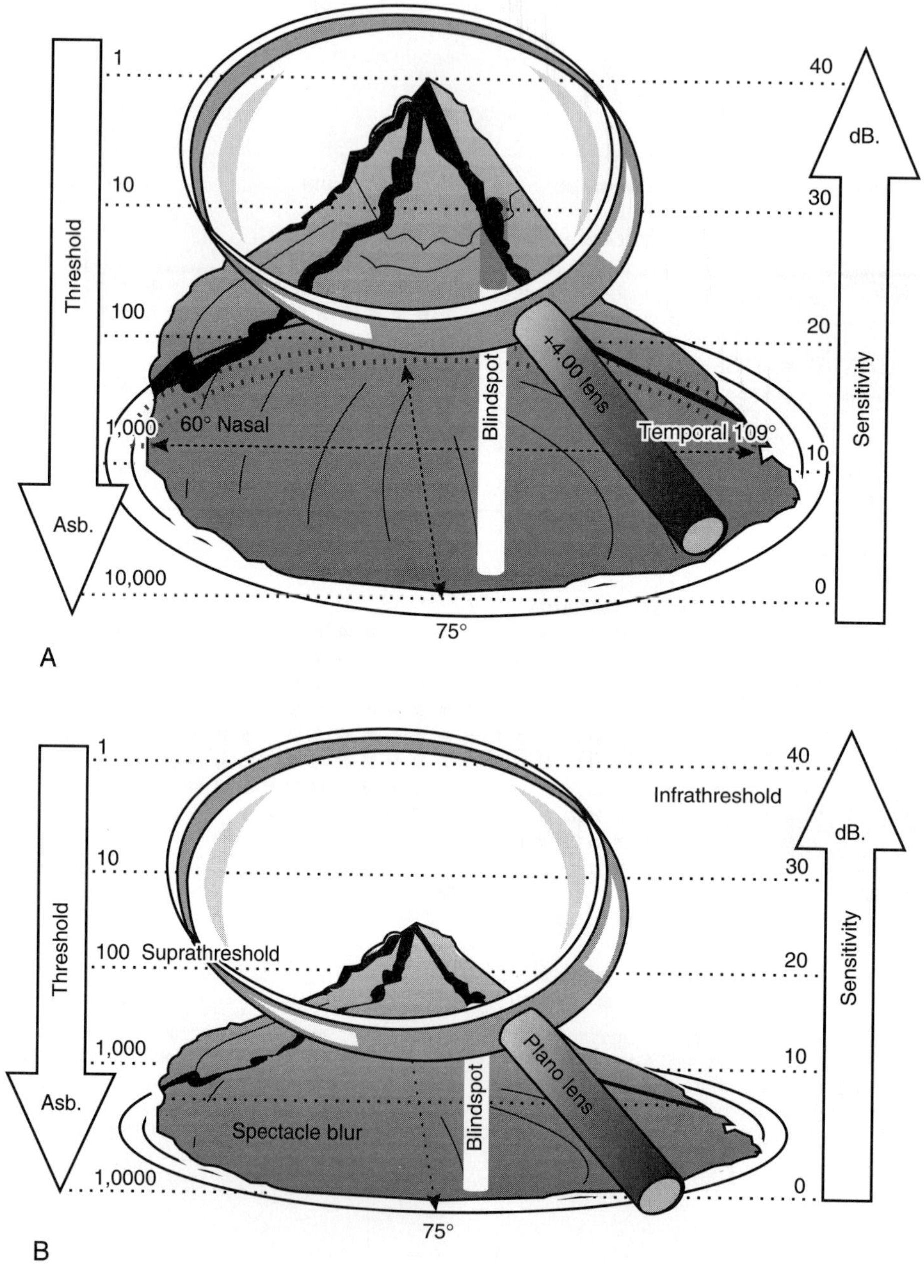

FIGURE 26–22. The effect of inaccurate spectacle correction on the "island of vision in a sea of blindness." *A,* The focused "island." *B,* The depressed "island." dB, decibel; Asb, apostilbs.

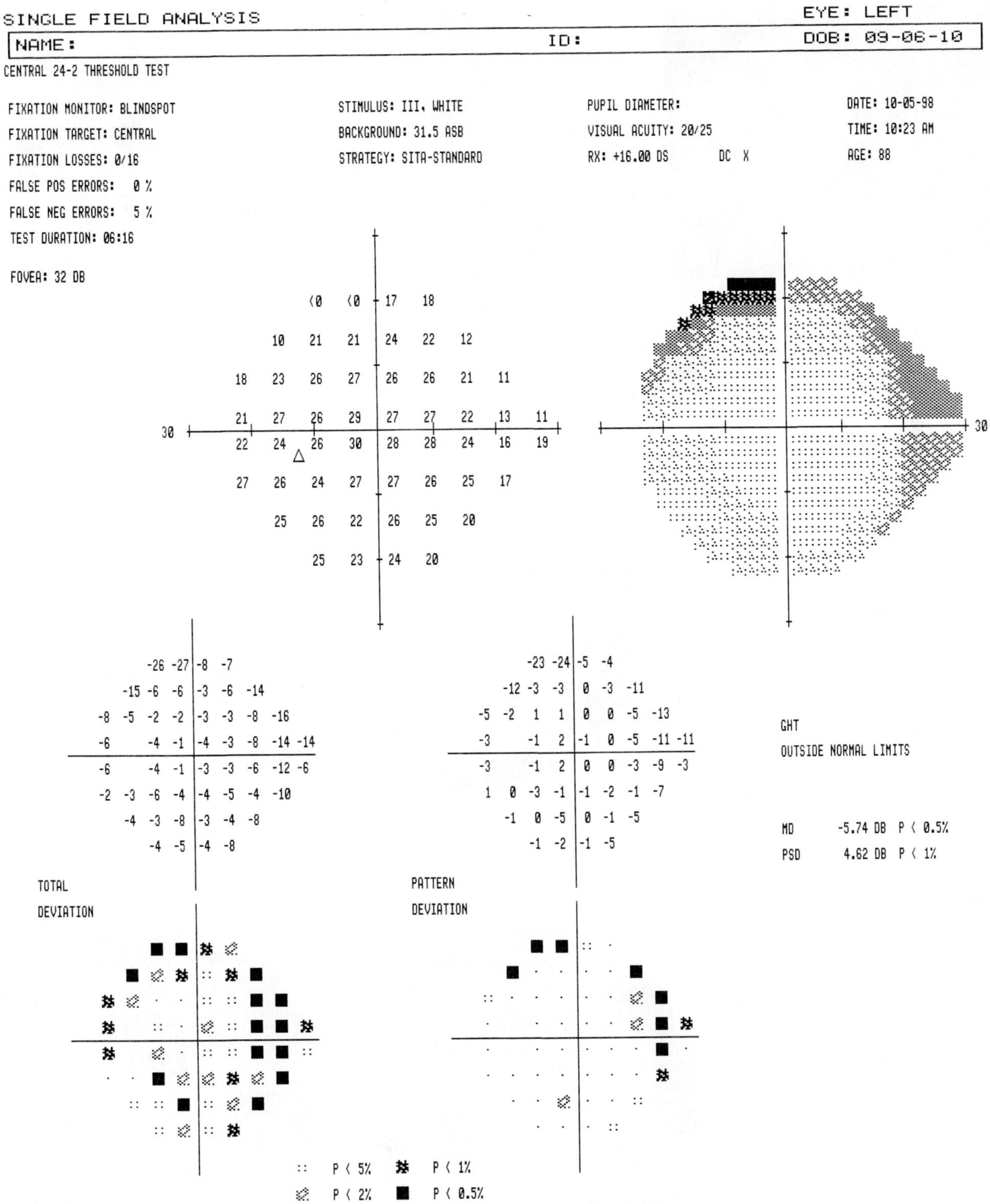

FIGURE 26–23. Chromatic and spherical aberration with "jack-in-the-box" scotoma. Significant chromatic or spherical aberration may occur in the periphery of the lens if the corrective lens power is high. The slightest malalignment is exaggerated owing to higher power and causes peripheral field erosion. This 88-year-old patient has a healthy nerve but suspicion of glaucoma remains because of elevated IOP. The peripheral depression in the left eye is likely artifactual owing to the +16 diopter lens.

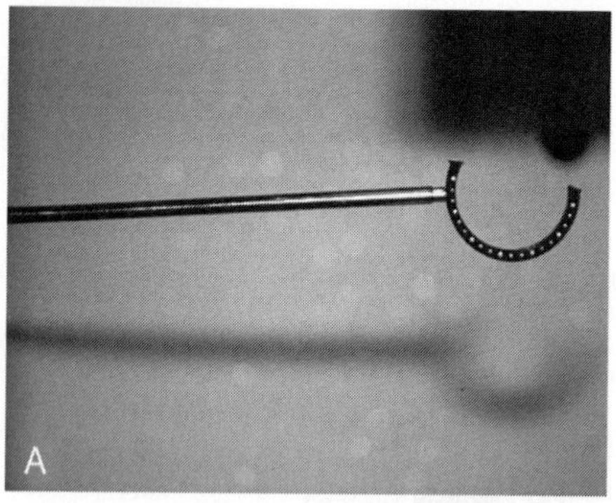

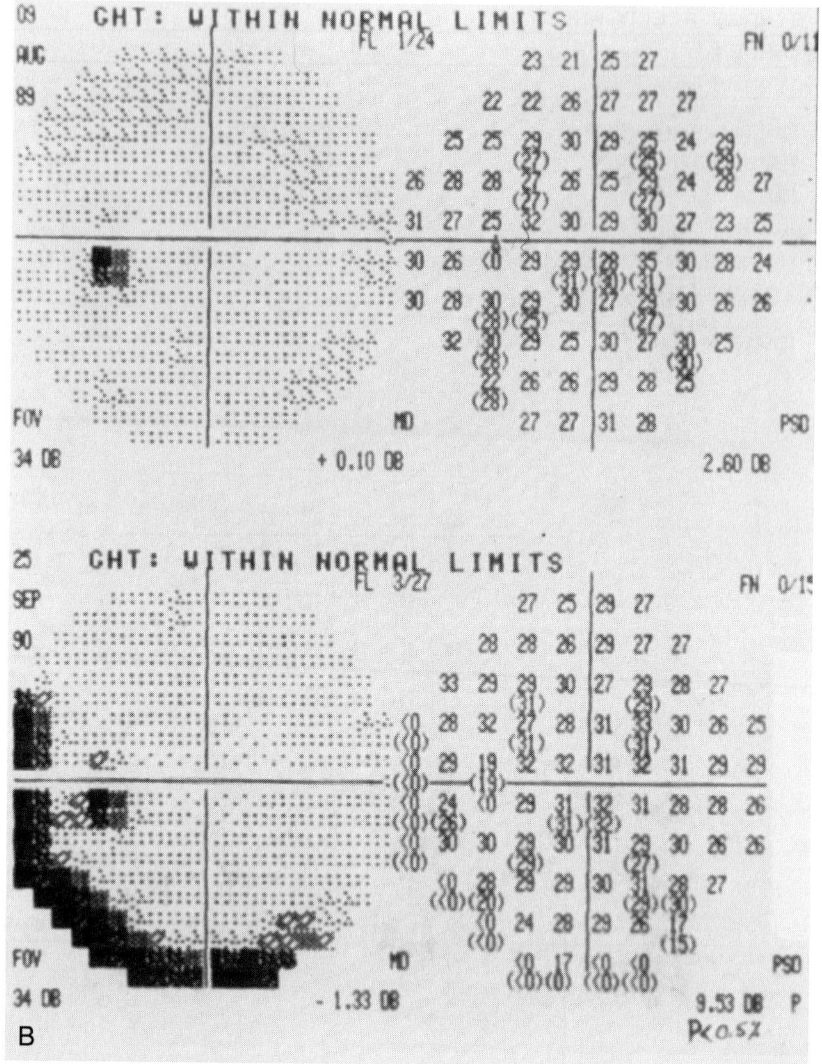

FIGURE 26–24. *A,* The lens holder in the Humphrey Field Analyzer. *B,* A follow-up left eye field test revealing a temporal absolute defect. One can readily correlate the defect with the lens holder rim.

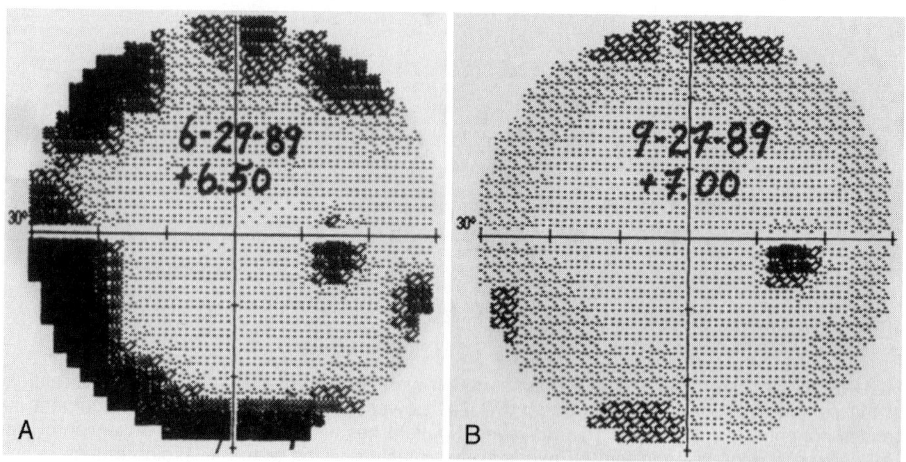

FIGURE 26–25. Lens holder artifact. *A,* During this test, either the eye was not perfectly centered or the patient tilted the head back. *B,* With more careful attention to alignment throughout the entire field, the lens holder artifact disappears.

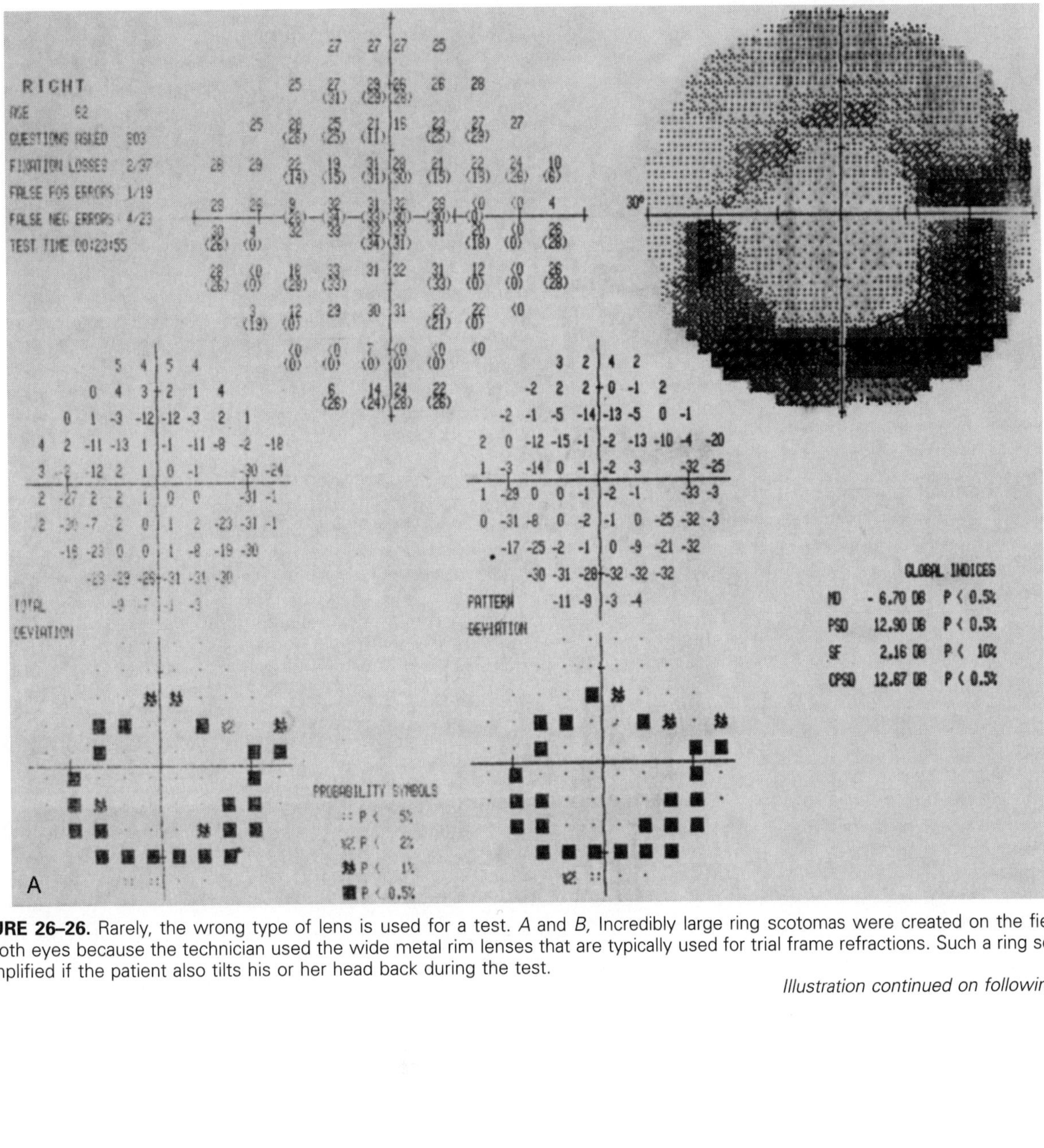

FIGURE 26–26. Rarely, the wrong type of lens is used for a test. *A* and *B*, Incredibly large ring scotomas were created on the field test for both eyes because the technician used the wide metal rim lenses that are typically used for trial frame refractions. Such a ring scotoma is amplified if the patient also tilts his or her head back during the test.

Illustration continued on following page

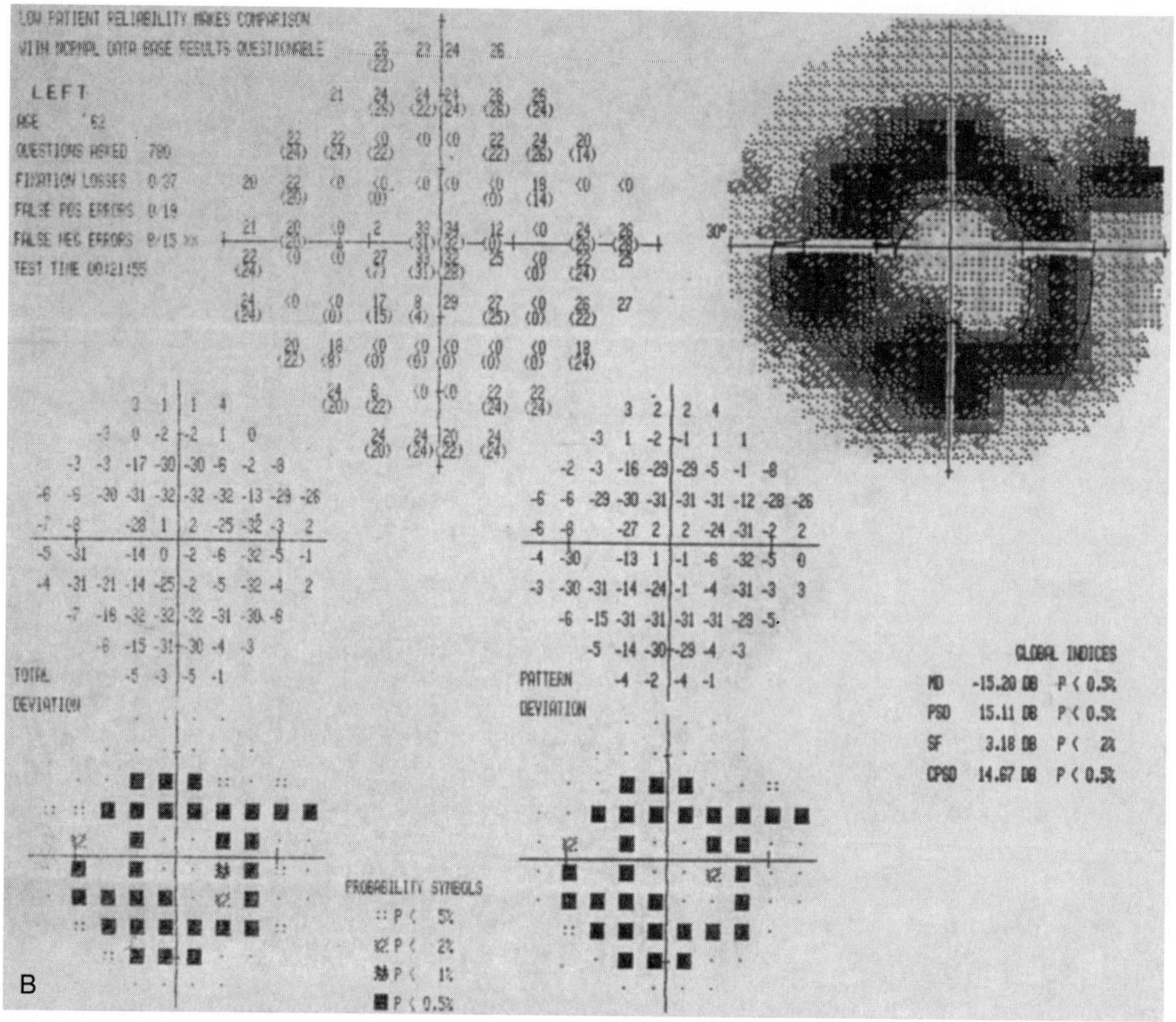

FIGURE 26–26 *Continued*

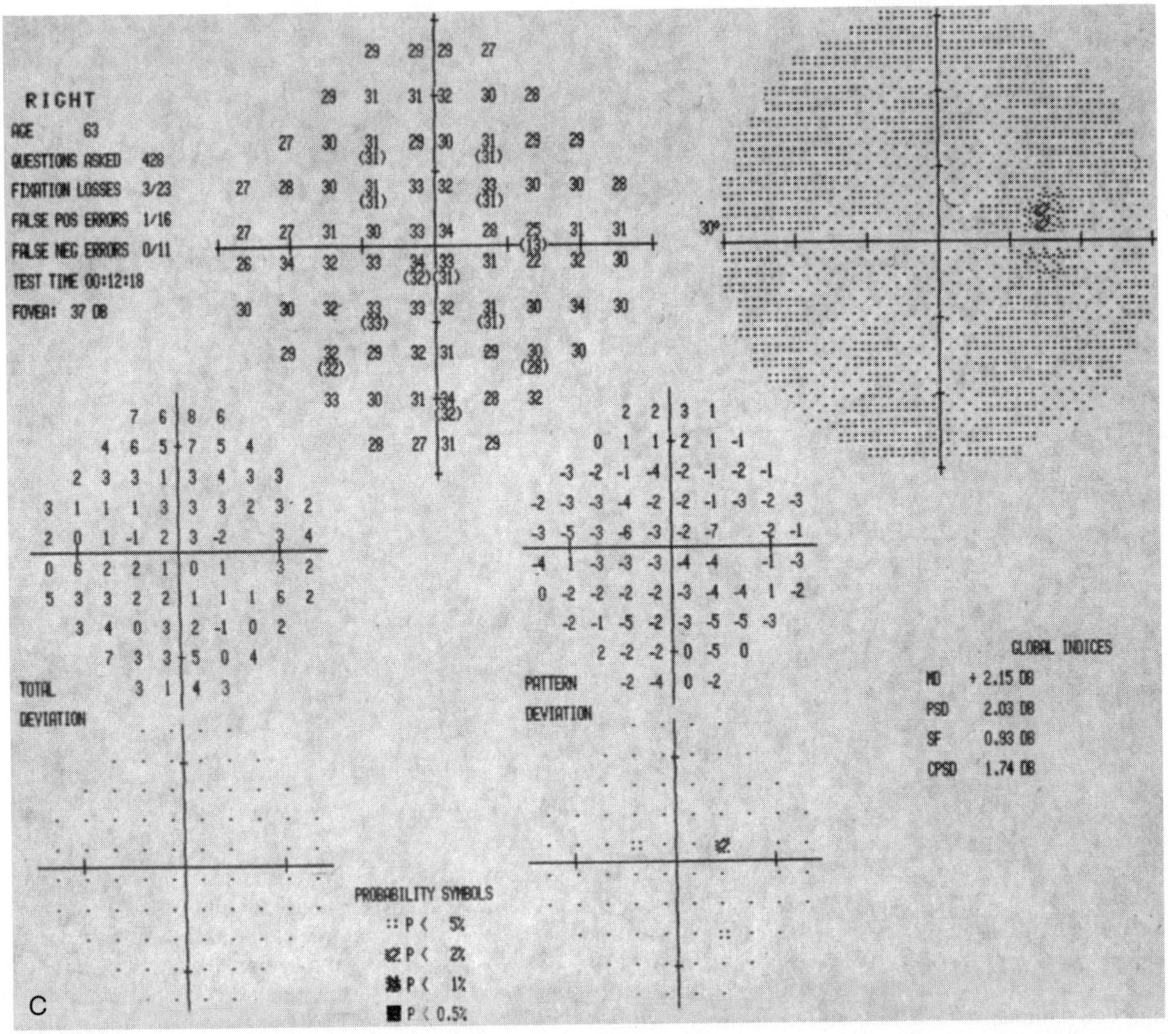

FIGURE 26–26 *Continued. C* and *D,* After the lenses were replaced with the proper wire-rim lenses, the scotomas "disappeared." In this case, the appearance of the optic nerves did not correlate with the ring scotomas. Such a finding should prompt the physician to turn into a detective and solve any field discrepancies.

Illustration continued on following page

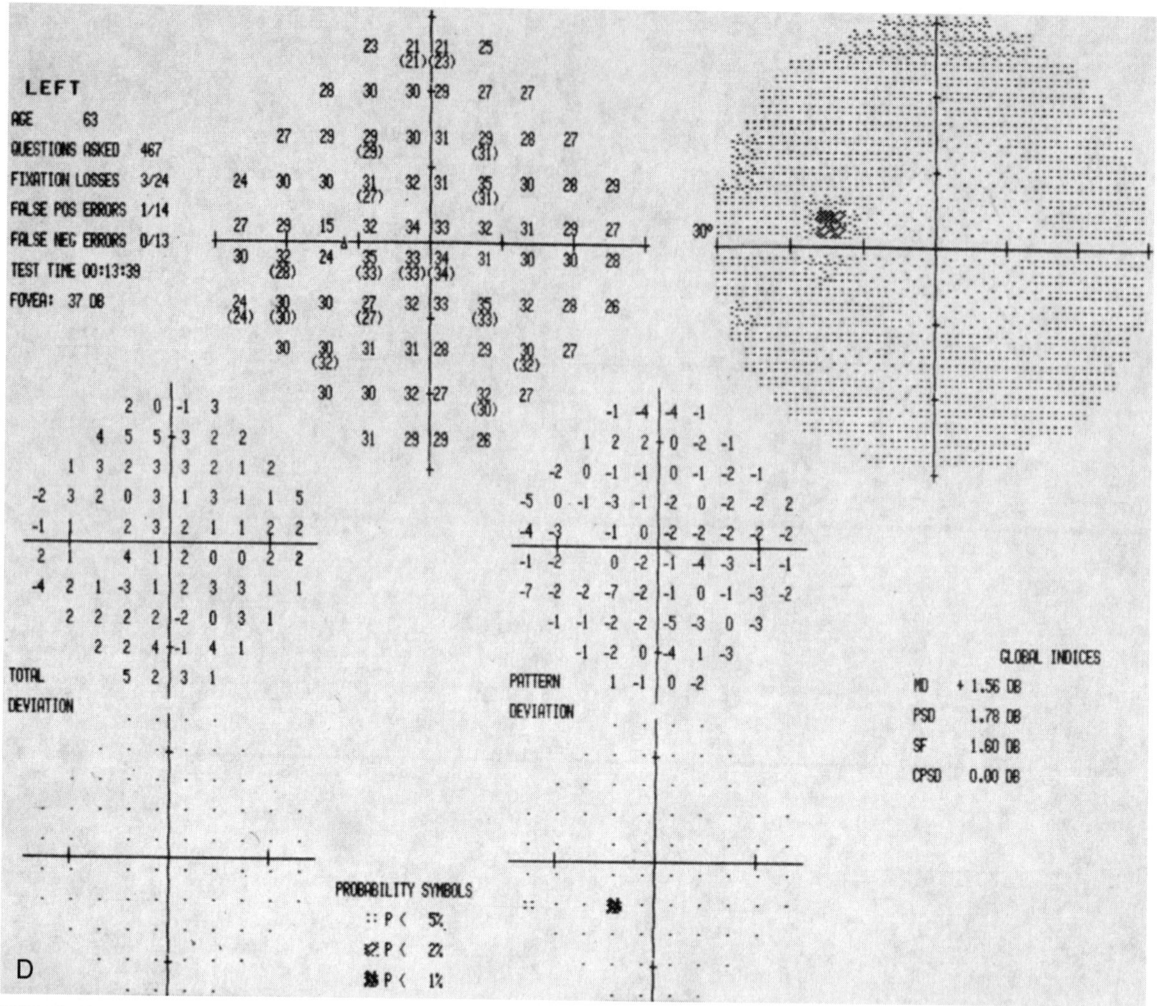

FIGURE 26–26 *Continued*

NUMERIC PRINTOUT

The 6-degree grid decibel printout is the core for all data analysis. The decibel value is a relative scale established by assigning a 0 dB value to the perimeter's brightest light, 10,000 Asb. The decibel values used by different manufacturers may not be comparable owing to differences in background luminance and test object intensity. With threshold strategies, a threshold value for each retinal location is reported. In addition, how much each value deviates from age-adjusted normal ranges is reported. However, the physician is left wondering whether the deviation is significant. Many physicians read the fields with only threshold printouts, which is the only option if STATPAC software is not available. Without the use of STATPAC software, the physician must decide whether a 7 dB loss of vision is normal variability or a change to worry about. To further complicate matters, when the field is retested at a later date to check for disease progression, the 7 dB loss now may be 10 dB. Is that a significant change? STATPAC II software addresses whether the field change is significant by comparing it to the values obtained from a group of medically stable patients with glaucoma.

GRAY SCALE

This black and white graduated scale interpolation between threshold points is useful to demonstrate field defects to patients. Areas of reduced sensitivity appear darker than adjacent lighter areas representing more normal sensitivity. If grossly abnormal, the black defects are readily apparent to both physician and patient; however, singular early defects are easy to miss if only the gray scale is examined. Gross inaccuracies result from evaluating only the raw data and gray scale.

STATPAC AND STATPAC II SOFTWARE

STATPAC software produces several analyses: single field analysis, overview, change analysis, and GHT. The SFA and overview are the most important, especially the SFA. The bottom half of the SFA printout represents the statistical software results. STATPAC is a statistical analysis software program that facilitates interpretation of the field test. Differences from normal are quantified and presented in both numeric and graphic forms.

Category VII: Probability of Deviation from Normal

The SFA allows the physician to separate normal from abnormal. Correlation with ocular pathology is then necessary to determine disease. The probability plots, GHT, and global indices facilitate this interpretation.

TOTAL DEVIATION NUMERIC PRINTOUT

Total deviation is a point-by-point difference in decibels between age-adjusted normal threshold values and the patient's threshold values:

Total deviation = age-adjusted threshold − patient's threshold

Obviously, if the patient's age is entered incorrectly, these data are suspect.

TOTAL DEVIATION PROBABILITY PLOT

A diagnostic test that immediately points out deviation from normal is a significant improvement in glaucoma care, and probability plots easily provide this service. The probability plot indicates abnormal areas of the field, especially when they reach the 0.5% significance level, denoted by a black box; this implies less than 0.5% of normals have this defect (1 in 200). A cluster or progression of black boxes is a significant critical sign that requires documentation on the patient's chart as well as an explanation.

The *P* value does not signify that the field is pathologic; it indicates how much the field deviates from age-adjusted normal values. The physician must analyze the statistical deviation and determine whether it is of clinical significance. An abnormal probability plot is important because the algorithm has already taken into account typical artifacts gathered from age-adjusted normal control subjects (Fig. 26–27).

PATTERN DEVIATION (PD) NUMERIC PRINTOUT

It is not unusual to observe a generalized depression of the visual field that may mask underlying, deeper scotomas. PD adjusts for the generalized depression and seeks out a localized scotoma. This is most helpful in patients with generalized depression from cataracts or miosis. However, in patients with uniform concentric cupping due to elevated IOP, a generalized loss of retinal sensitivity may be the first sign of glaucomatous visual field loss. The physician must make the final clinical correlation.

PATTERN DEVIATION PROBABILITY PLOT

The pattern deviation plot is similar to the total deviation plot. It denotes significant areas with the probability boxes. It is helpful to look at the plots side by side, first the total deviation plot to look for defects, then the pattern deviation plot to see whether there is a specific *localized* defect in the field.

Category VIII: Glaucoma Hemifield Test

The GHT is part of the STATPAC II software program. The GHT result is printed on the SFA, change probability analysis, and the overview. The GHT was designed to judge whether a single test could show evidence of glaucomatous field loss (Fig. 26–28). Sensitivity is 92%, and specificity 87%, for detecting field loss with the GHT.[9] This implies that the GHT will miss 8% of glaucoma cases and overcall the disease in 13% of patients tested. The GHT evaluates five nerve fiber layer distribution zones in the superior field and compares them with their mirror-image inferior zones. Probability maps determine the comparison and print five possible messages:

Outside Normal Limits: At least one mirror zone has a value that exceeds that in 99% of the normal population or the values in both zones of a mirror pair exceed those found in 99.5% of normal individuals.

Borderline: At least one mirror zone has a value that exceeds that in 97% of the normal population.

General reduction of sensitivity: "Outside normal limits" conditions have not been met but the best part of the field is depressed to an extent that occurs in fewer than 0.5% of the normal population.

Abnormally high sensitivity: The best part of the field has a sensitivity higher than that found in 99.5% of the population.

Within normal limits: The preceding conditions are not met.

The only two messages that can appear simultaneously are "borderline" and "general reduction of sensitivity."

Category IX: Global Indices

The global indices (GI) are located beneath the gray scale on the printout. The educated field observer can merely look at these numbers and envision the shape and abnormalities of the patient's visual field. This information, in conjunction with the patient's clinical history and physical findings, can lead to a rapid diagnosis. Attached to global indices are statistical interpretations of their significance. To fully appreciate the global indices, the physician must have a global concept of the "island of vision," as explained earlier in the chapter.

MEAN DEVIATION

Mean deviation (MD) is the average elevation or depression of the patient's overall field compared with those in age-adjusted normal subjects (Fig. 26–29). The change in threshold at each point is summed and then is divided by the total number of points. MD is usually an index of diffuse change, but a high MD may also occur with deep localized scotomas.

For example, it will become apparent that a significant pattern standard deviation (PSD) defect with an insignificant MD implies a dense localized scotoma (Fig. 26–30; Table 26–2). Quite the opposite is the case for a significant MD and insignificant PSD; the field has an overall depression, not a dense localized defect. Physicians recognize

Text continued on page 472

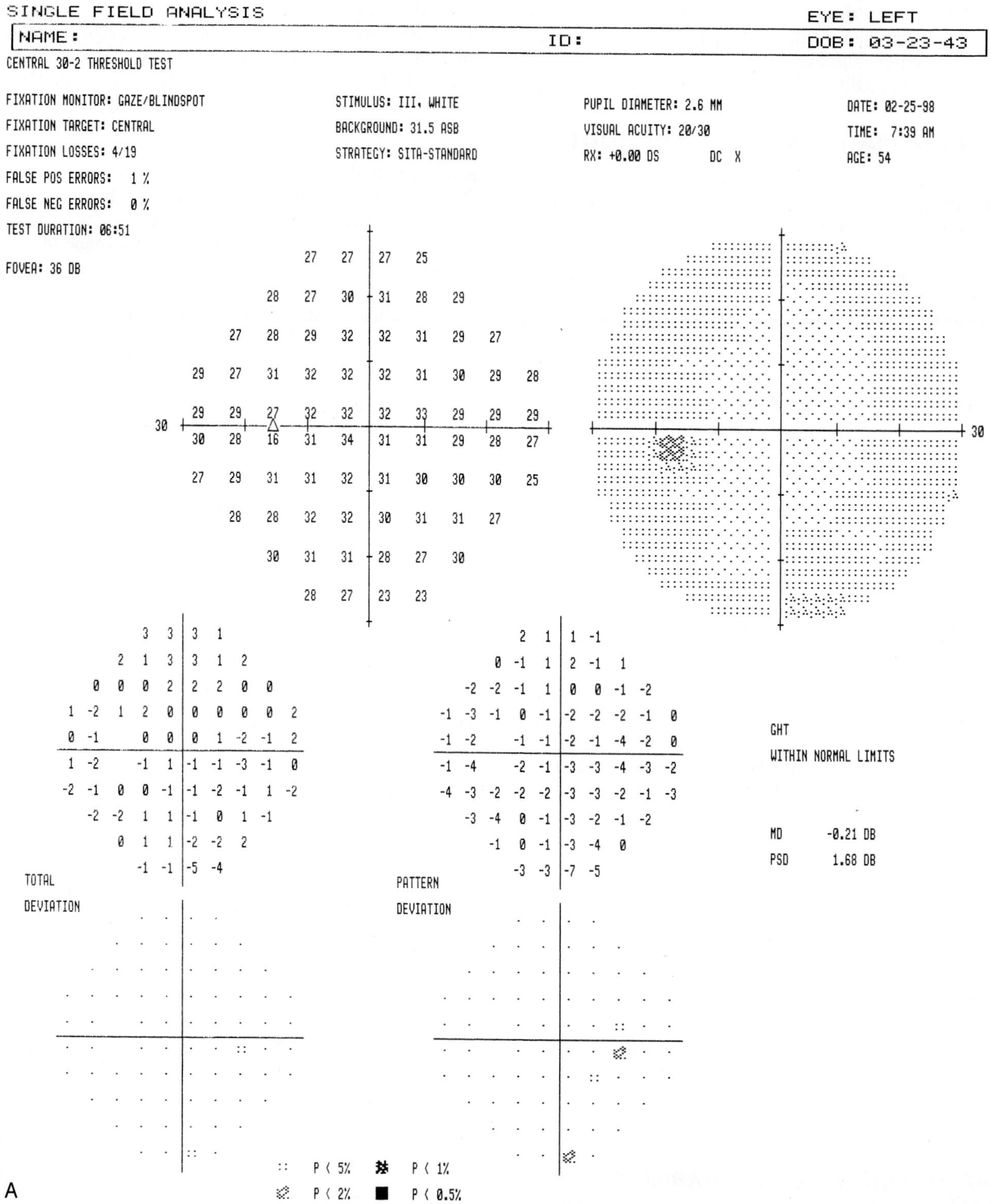

A

FIGURE 26–27. Total and pattern deviation with probability boxes. *A,* The left eye of this 55-year-old patient with low-tension glaucoma is a "clean sweep." The gray scale, probability plots, glaucoma hemifield test (GHT), and global indices are all normal and correlate with the optic nerve.

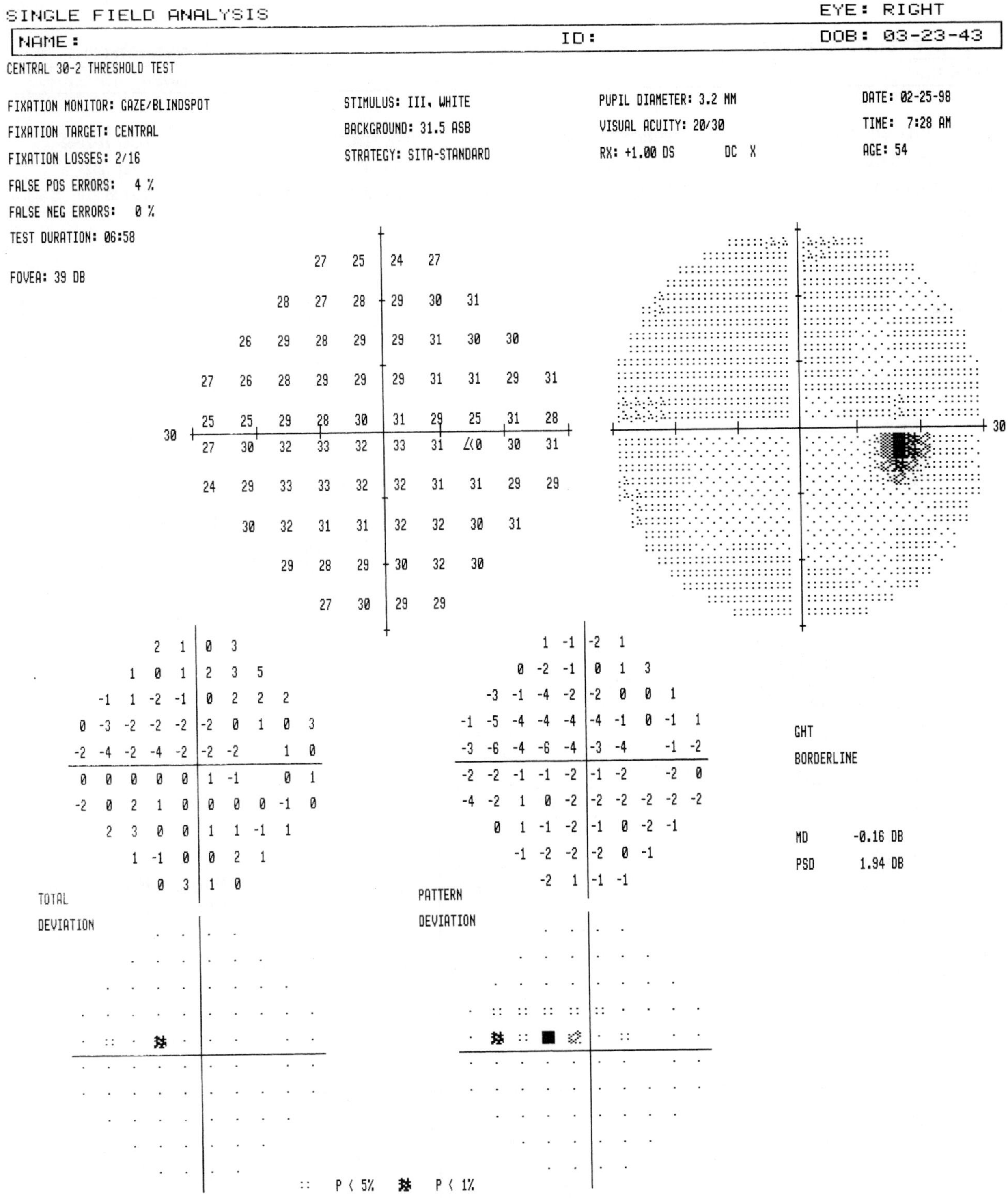

B

FIGURE 26–27 *Continued. B,* The gray scale of the right eye appears normal; however, the total deviation and pattern deviation plots appear abnormal along with the GHT. The global indices are not statistically significant. The gray scale of the right eye is unimpressive, but the optic nerve clearly shows inferior damage. The pattern deviation probability plot is an expression of localized field loss and is clearly abnormal in the superior nasal quadrant. In addition, it is important to compare with the fellow eye. The cluster of dark boxes is highly significant, especially in conjunction with the "borderline" GHT reading. This finding is a very early nasal step defect, although the optic nerve shows considerable inferior damage.

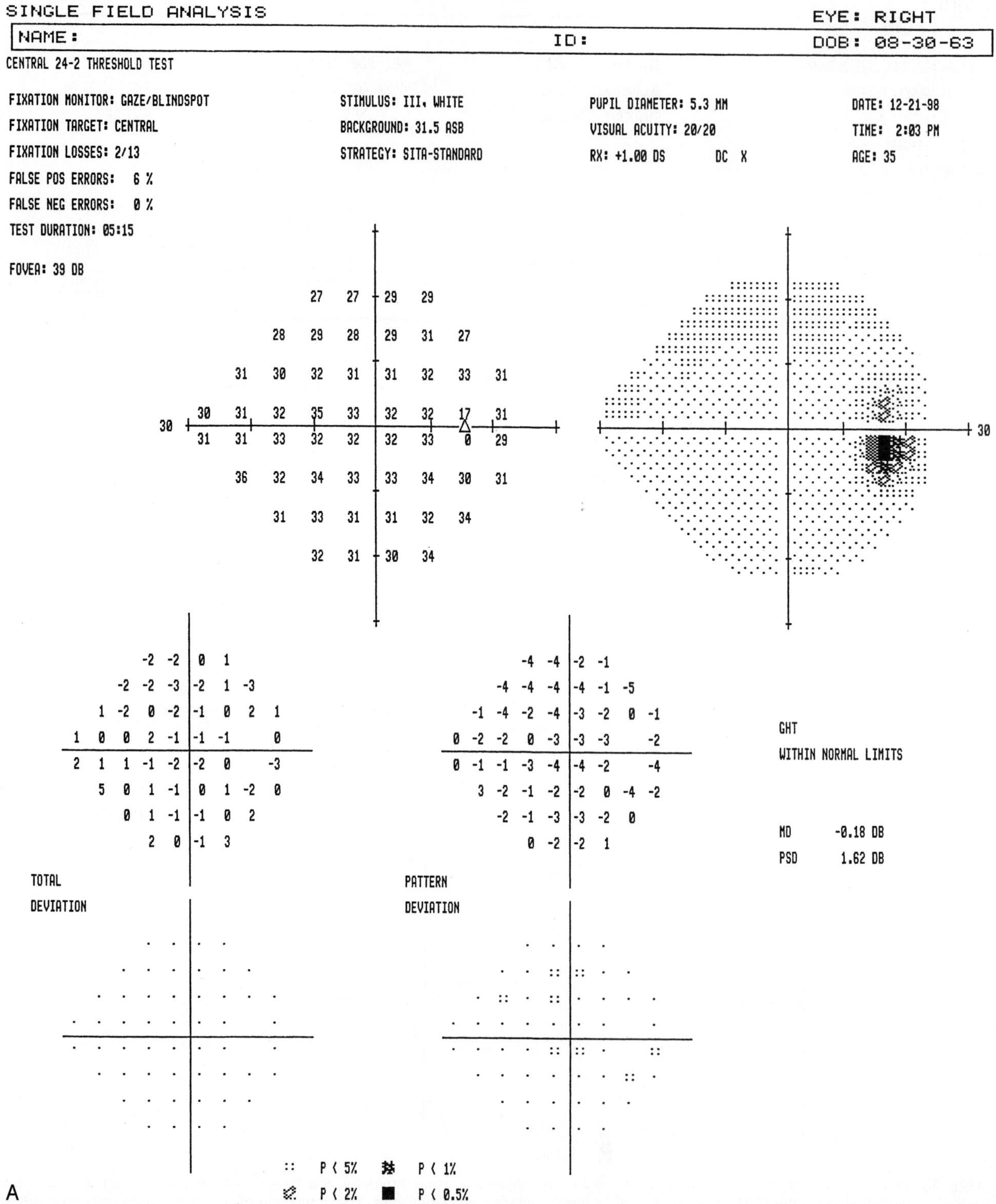

A

FIGURE 26–28. Glaucoma Hemifield Test (GHT). The GHT, part of STATPAC II, is a mirror-image analysis of the nerve fiber layer patterns above and below the horizontal raphe. This 35-year-old patient has intraocular pressures up to 40 mm Hg in the left eye with asymmetric cupping, 0.2 cup-to-disc ratio O.D., and 0.5 cup-to-disk ratio O.S. The right eye field *(A)* is reliable and completely normal.

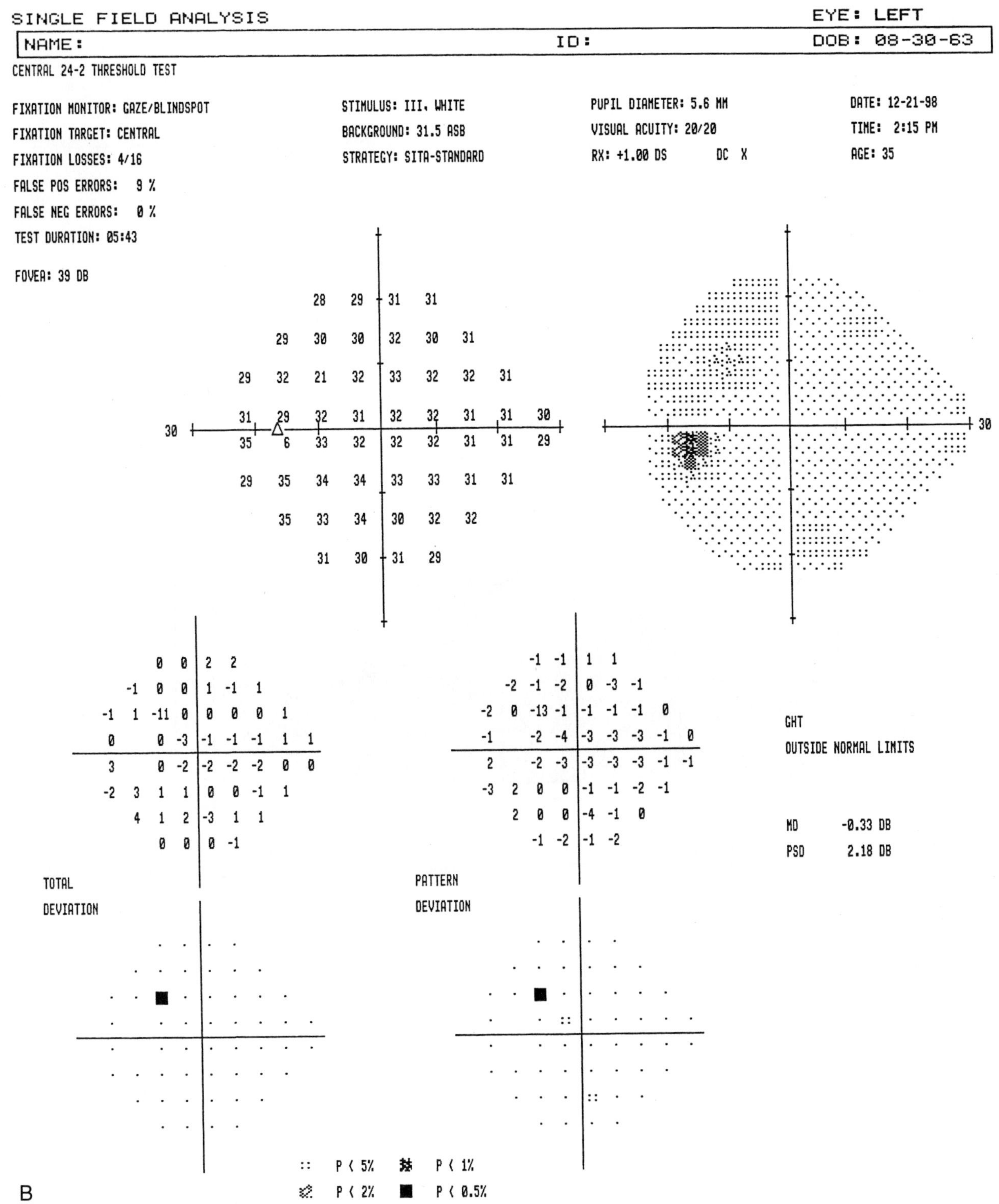

FIGURE 26–28 *Continued.* The left eye field *(B)* is reliable and abnormal. The gray scale is uneventful, but the probability plots indicate that the 11 dB loss above the blind spot is highly significant. The GHT in the right eye is normal, but the left eye GHT is "outside normal limits *(arrowhead).*" This finding correlated highly with the appearance of the optic nerve, and antiglaucoma therapy was initiated. The GHT reading is especially important in early glaucoma, before the "island of vision" is destroyed and the global indices are affected. The global indices are a reflection of what is happening to the entire island of vision, but if only one "tree" is down (i.e., in the very early stages of glaucomatous damage), the island does not look very different.

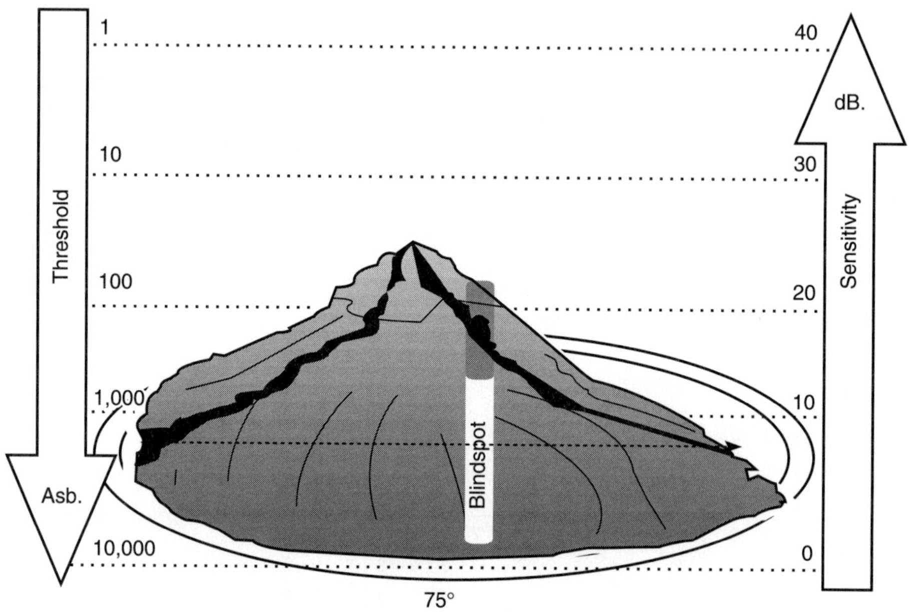

FIGURE 26–29. Generalized depression of the "island of vision." This is the typical loss associated with cataract, miosis, or early diffuse loss. One would expect the mean deviation to be significant but the pattern standard deviation to be insignificant. dB, decibels; Asb, apostilbs.

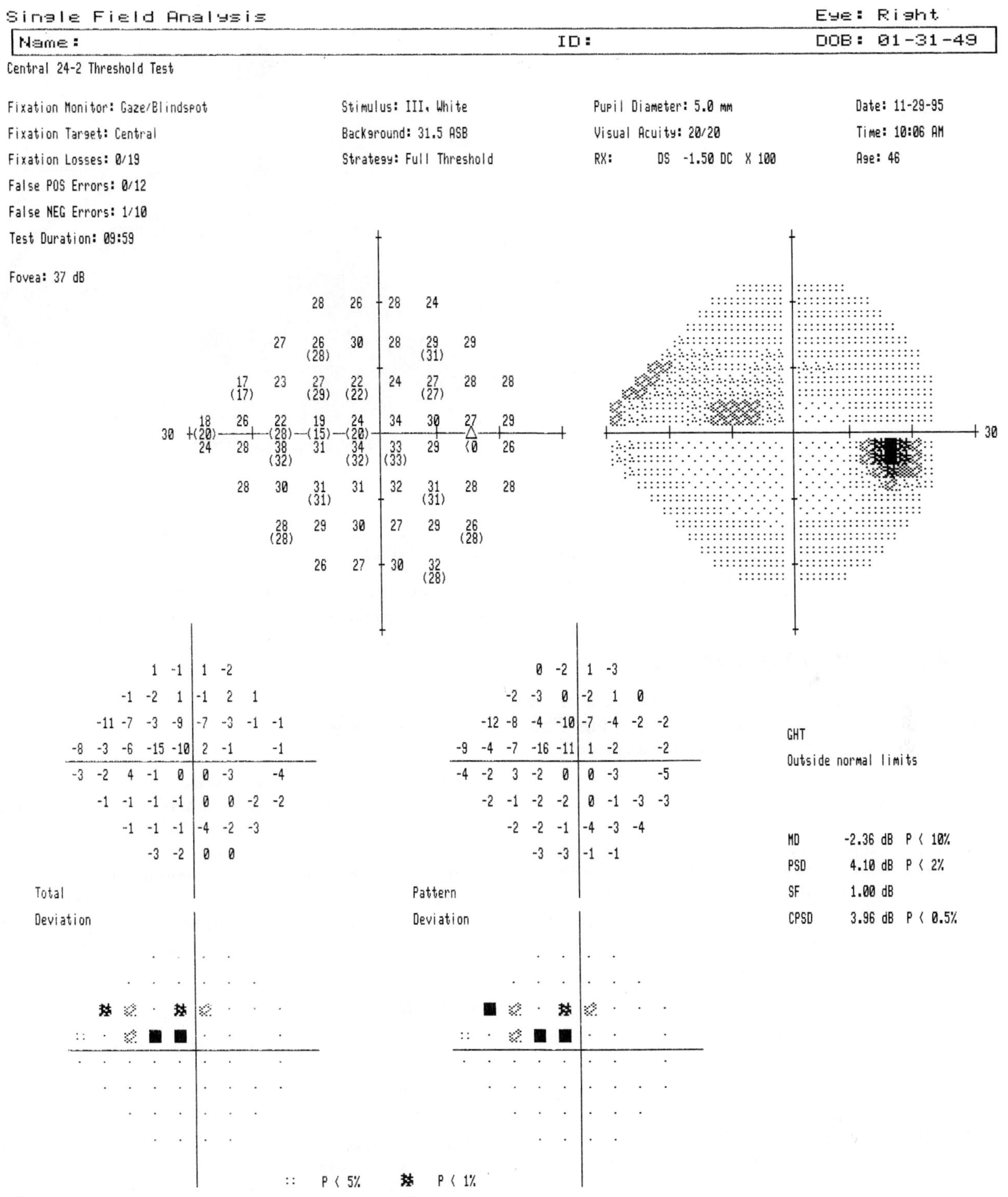

A

FIGURE 26–30. Localized loss of the "island of vision." *A,* A localized scotoma as seen in this reliable single field analysis printout activates the global indices into the statistical significance range mainly for the pattern standard deviation (PSD) at 2%, but the mean deviation (MD) value is only 10%. This finding implies vision loss in a localized fashion. Correcting for short-term field fluctuation makes the localized defect even more significant at 0.5%. The glaucoma hemifield test (GHT) is outside normal limits, and the probability plots are abnormal.

Illustration continued on following page

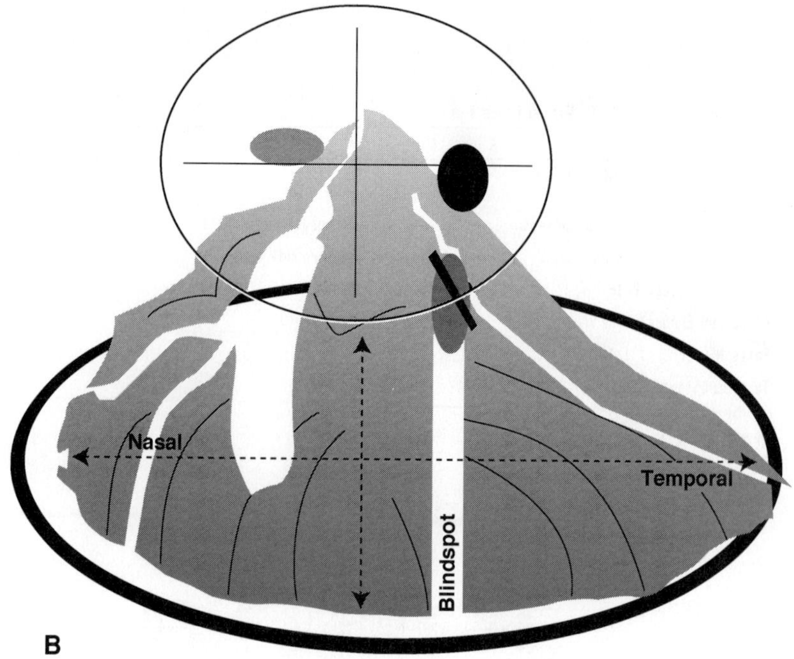

FIGURE 26–30 *Continued. B* illustrates these findings on the "island of vision."

that different disease states alter the shape of the "island of vision" in various ways. After inspecting the shape of the pattern, the physician correlates this defect with the patient's clinical history and examination.

PATTERN STANDARD DEVIATION

Pattern standard deviation (PSD) is a measurement of the local non-uniformity of the "island of vision." A high PSD indicates an irregular island with a deep localized defect.

SHORT-TERM FLUCTUATION

Scatter is to kinetic perimetry as fluctuation is to static automated perimetry. Short-term fluctuation (SF) is a measurement of intratest variability determined by testing twice ten preselected locations; the differences between the paired values are squared, summed, and divided by 20 before the square root is extracted. SF is a measurement of variability in visual performance. Theoretically, if a measured point threshold is 20 dB and the SF is 1 dB, there is a 99% chance that the actual threshold is between 17 and 23 dB.

TABLE 26–2. APPEARANCE OF THE "ISLAND OF VISION" WITH VARIATIONS IN MEAN DEVIATION AND PATTERN STANDARD DEVIATION

Mean Deviation	**Pattern Standard Deviation**	
	Normal	*Abnormal*
Normal	Normal	Localized defect
Abnormal	Depressed	Deep localized defect, depressed, or both

CORRECTED PATTERN STANDARD DEVIATION

Corrected pattern standard deviation (CPSD) eliminates short-term fluctuation error as a cause of the local non-uniformity and gives a more accurate picture of localized defects.

SUMMARY

It should be obvious that myriad "scotoma traps" can interfere with the interpretation of the SFA printout. The nine categories of the printout contain an immense amount of information and serve as the foundation for the rest of the analyses. Recognition of these factors should strengthen the physician's interpretation of all other fields and provide additional knowledge to facilitate understanding of newer perimetric modalities.

REFERENCES

1. Tate GW Jr, Lynn JR: Principles of Quantitative Perimetry: Testing and Interpreting the Visual Field. New York, Grune & Stratton, 1977, pp 295–305.
2. Heijl A, Krakau CET: An automatic static perimeter: Design and pilot study. Acta Ophthalmol Copenh 1975;53:293–310.
3. Jaffe GJ, Alvarado JA, Juster RP: Age-related changes of the normal visual field. Arch Ophthalmol 1986;104:1021–1025.
4. Haas A, Flammer J, Schneider U: Influence of age on visual fields of normal subjects. Am J Ophthalmol 1986;101:199.
5. Lynn JR, Swanson WH, Fellman RL: Evaluation of automated kinetic perimetry (AKP) with the Humphrey Analyzer. *In* Mills RP, Heijl A (eds): Perimetry Update 1990/1991: Proceedings of the IXth International Perimetric Society Meeting, Malmo, Sweden, June 17–20, 1990. New York, Kugler Publications, 1991, pp 433–452.
6. Choplin NT, Sherwood MB, Spaeth GL: The effect of stimulus size on the measured threshold values in automated perimetry. Ophthalmology 1990;97:371–374.

7. Fellman RL, Lynn JR, Starita RJ, Swanson WH: Clinical importance of spatial summation in glaucoma. *In* Heijl A (ed): Perimetry Update 1988/1989. Proceedings of the VIIth International Perimetric Society Meeting. Berkeley, Kugler and Ghedini Publications, 1990, pp 313–324.
8. Donahue SP: Lens holder artifact simulating glaucomatous defect in automated perimetry. Arch Ophthalmol 1998;116:1681–1683.
9. Katz J, Sommer A, Gaasterland DE, Anderson DR: Comparison of analytic algorithms for detecting glaucomatous visual field loss. Arch Ophthalmol 1991;109:1684–1689.

CHAPTER 27

Optic Nerve Damage and Dysfunction in Glaucoma

USHA KURUMETY and ROHIT VARMA

The optic nerve represents the site of damage in glaucoma. Previous chapters have covered the anatomy and physiology of glaucoma as well as methods of assessment (see Chapters 4 and 5). Here, Usha Kurumety and Rohit Varma discuss the basis for the important link between glaucoma and the optic nerve, including the retinal ganglion cells and nerve fiber layer. They also provide additional information on the assessment and documentation of the optic nerve. The major part of this chapter describes the pathologic changes in the structure of the optic nerve associated with glaucoma: the changes that can be identified in both the nerve fiber layer and the optic nerve head itself. Because glaucoma is an optic neuropathy, careful examination of the optic nerve is vital to assess the presence of glaucomatous damage and determine whether stability of disease has been achieved with therapy.

Glaucoma is an optic neuropathy, the quintessential feature of which is a loss of retinal ganglion cells and their axons. Although numerous experimental and clinical studies over the years have furthered our knowledge of the disease, our understanding of the exact mechanism of the damage caused by glaucoma is incomplete.

This chapter (1) explores the pathophysiologic changes that occur in the retina and optic nerve with glaucoma, (2) discusses how the changes are clinically manifested, and (3) describes how these manifestations are useful in diagnosing and managing the disease. A variety of methods are available to qualitatively and quantitatively assess the changes that occur in the optic nerve and retinal nerve fiber layer. The chapter also compares the performance of these various methods in evaluating glaucomatous damage. Although the pathophysiology of the damage is unknown, early detection and quantification of this damage to retinal ganglion cell axons can help in the diagnosis and management of glaucoma.

Pathophysiology

The essential pathologic process in glaucoma is the loss of retinal ganglion cell axons. Glaucoma causes a degeneration of the ganglion cell and the retinal nerve fiber layers. Although this degeneration is related to intraocular pressure (IOP), the exact mechanism is not clear. Both mechanical and vascular theories have been proposed to explain the relationship between the glaucomatous damage and an increase in IOP. This chapter discusses the disorder that occurs in the retina, optic nerve, and lamina cribrosa and how this disorder relates to glaucomatous damage.

GANGLION CELL LAYER

The retinal ganglion cells are subdivided into two main functional groups, the large M cells and the small P cells. Histologic studies on human eyes and monkey eyes have suggested that larger ganglion cells are selectively damaged in early glaucoma (Fig. 27–1).[1–3] These studies support the concept that large ganglion cells are inherently more susceptible to damage. Two possible reasons for this increased susceptibility to damage are: (1) ganglion cells with larger axon diameters are more susceptible to elevated intraocular pressure and (2) such larger optic nerve fibers are more likely to be found in areas with less connective

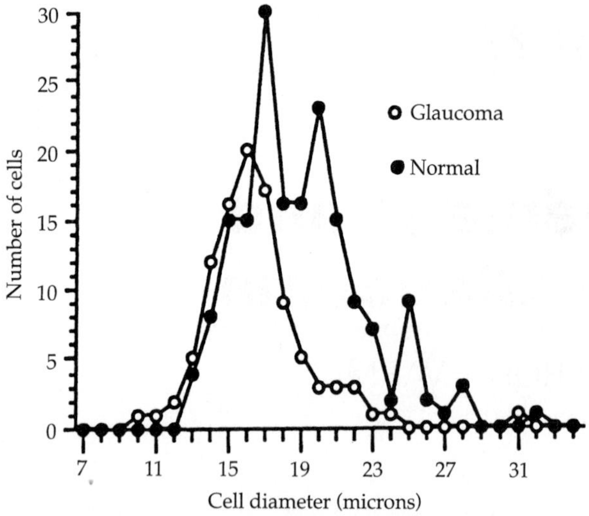

FIGURE 27–1. Frequency distribution of various sizes of ganglion cells in a *glaucoma* patient with glaucoma in whom 50% of normal density remained. The normal distribution is also presented. Both measurements were obtained 27 degrees superior to the fovea. There are fewer larger ganglion cells compared with the normal distribution. (From Quigley HA, Dunkelberger GR, Green WR: Retinal ganglion cell atrophy correlated with automated perimetry in human eyes with glaucoma. Am J Ophthalmol 1995;107:453.)

tissue support and thus are more likely to be prone to damage from increased IOP.

Compared with the retinas of normal eyes, the retinas of glaucomatous eyes have 20% to 50% fewer ganglion cells with selective loss of larger cells in certain areas. Some clinical evidence also supports the concept of early loss of the larger ganglion cells. In both monkey and human eyes, abnormalities in contrast sensitivity and pattern electroretinography point toward decreased responsiveness to fast-flicker testing, which is a function of the larger ganglion cells.[4]

Quigley and colleagues,[2] however, noted a loss of both small and large cells, without selectivity, in two of the six glaucomatous eyes they studied (Fig. 27–2). This lack of selectivity or preferential loss of large ganglion cells could imply that selective loss may be a phenomenon of early glaucomatous damage and that, with continued damage, both large and small cells are lost. In addition, there may also be a subset of small and large ganglion cells that are more susceptible to IOP-related damage. Although much of the evidence to date points toward the preferential loss of larger ganglion cells, there appear to be some discrepancies. Further investigation is necessary to determine which ganglion cell types are most sensitive to glaucomatous damage, and in what order these cells degenerate.

Clinicopathologic correlation studies have revealed that a loss of ganglion cells is associated with a reduction in retinal sensitivity in corresponding areas.[5] Studies comparing manual visual field results in glaucomatous eyes with the number of remaining optic nerve fibers have indicated that 25% to 50% of all ganglion cells died before reproducible field loss was detected on the Goldmann perimeter.[2, 6] A later comparison using automated perimetry revealed that a 5-dB loss in sensitivity at an average point occurs when 20% of the ganglion cells are gone, and a 10-dB decrease occurs after 40% of the retinal ganglion cells are lost in the corresponding area. Within the central 12 degrees, however, where there is a greater density of ganglion cells, a 5-dB loss in retinal sensitivity corresponds to a 50% loss of ganglion cells. The number of cells per square millimeter is ten times higher in the central 4 degrees than it is in the area 24 degrees from the fovea, resulting in a greater overlap of function in the stimulated area. This greater overlap in the central region implies that a larger number of ganglion cells must be lost before retinal sensitivity is affected.[2]

RETINAL NERVE FIBER LAYER

The nerve fiber layer (NFL) is composed of ganglion cell axons as well as the supporting neuroglia and astrocytes. In the retina, the ganglion cell axons are spread out in a thin layer that projects to the optic disc by systematic stratification (Fig. 27–3). The striations seen in the retinal NFL are glial tissue boundaries of axon bundles formed by Müller's cell processes.[7] When viewed by ophthalmoscopy or photography, the silvery striations correspond to individual axon bundles, and the dark striations to the intervening glial tissue (Fig. 27–4). The glial tissue provides support to the ganglion cell axons and maintains the appropriate environment for signal conduction by axons and axoplasmic flow. Because the axons are spread out in a thin layer, even minor losses of axons can be observed in the retinal NFL when appropriate techniques are used.

In 1972, Hoyt and Newman[8] first described slit- and wedge-shaped retinal NFL defects as the earliest observable changes in glaucoma. Since then, many investigators have evaluated the NFL and have correlated changes in its appearance and thickness with the progression of glaucoma. Nerve fiber layer atrophy can be visualized as a loss of its striate pattern. With glaucoma, NFL atrophy usually begins in the superior or inferior arcuate regions. Thinning of the NFL leads to greater visibility of the retinal vessels.

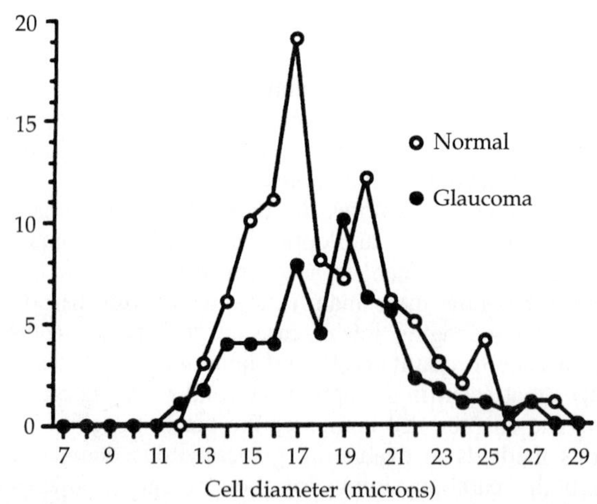

FIGURE 27–2. Frequency distribution of ganglion cell size in a patient with glaucoma with 50% of normal ganglion cell density. The normal distribution is also presented. Both measurements were obtained 27 degrees from the fovea. There are fewer small and large ganglion cells compared with the normal distribution. (From Quigley HA, Dunkelberger GR, Green WR: Retinal ganglion cell atrophy correlated with automated perimetry in human eyes with glaucoma. Am J Ophthalmol 1989;107:453.)

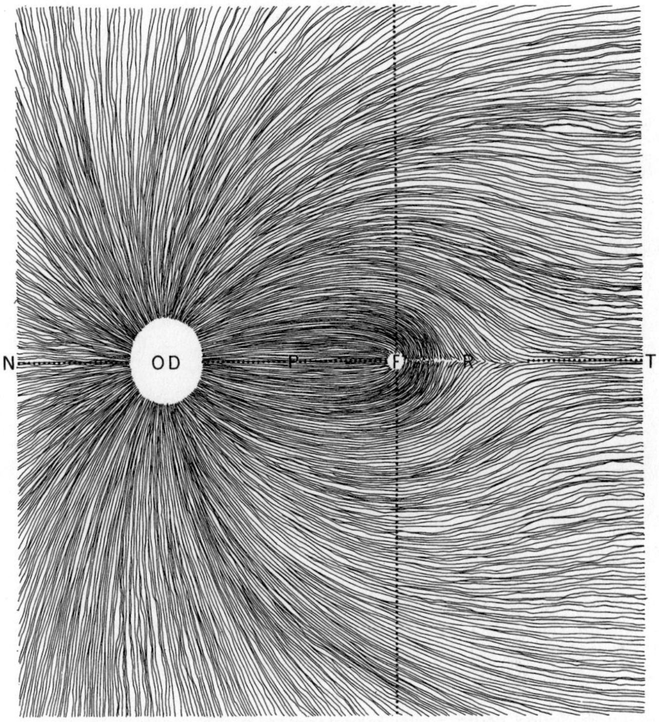

FIGURE 27–3. Schematic representation of the projection pattern of retinal ganglion cell axons from the retina to the optic disc (OD). The axons from ganglion cells in the nasal macula form the papillomacular bundle (P). The horizontal raphe (R) is temporal to the fovea (F). N, Nasal; T, temporal. (From Hogan MJ, Alvarado JA, Weddell JE: Histology of the Human Eye. Philadelphia, WB Saunders, 1971.)

Diffuse thinning of the NFL is seen as a loss of the normal retinal striate pattern overlying the second order vessels.[9] Localized defects beginning near the disc margin can fan out toward the retinal periphery and become diffuse. With progressive loss of the NFL, the superior and inferior arcuate regions lose their striate pattern, and the only striations that remain are those of the papillomacular bundle. In end-stage glaucoma, no striations are present, not even in the papillomacular bundle.

OPTIC NERVE

The optic nerve can be regarded as a bulk representation of the ganglion cell axons in the eye. The rim of the optic disc is formed by axons converging from the retina to the scleral canal. As discussed previously, the essential pathologic process in glaucoma is the loss of ganglion cell axons. As axons are lost, the amount of neural tissue in the neural rim decreases, resulting in alterations in the appearance of the neural rim and the configuration of the optic cup. The changes in the prelaminar portion of the optic nerve are considered characteristic of glaucomatous optic nerve damage. These structural changes are presumably preceded by changes in axonal transport.

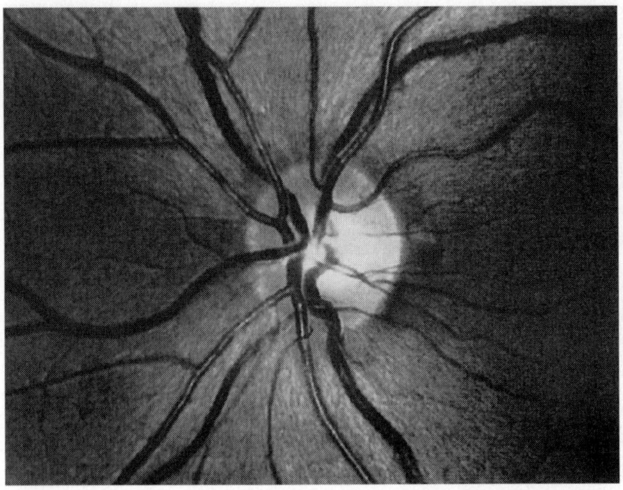

FIGURE 27–4. Photograph of retinal nerve fiber layers in a normal human subject showing striations. The silvery striations are axon bundles, whereas the dark striations correspond to intervening glial tissue. (Courtesy Victor Bruce.) (From Ritch R, Shields MB, Krupin T (eds): The Glaucomas. St. Louis, Mosby–Year Book, 1996.)

In experimental glaucoma in primate eyes, both orthograde and retrograde axonal transport are markedly obstructed around collagen beams in the lamina cribrosa.[10–12] Injection of horseradish peroxidase into the lateral geniculate body of primate eyes has shown that even a minimal elevation of pressure produced a blockage of retrograde transport in the lamina cribrosa within 24 hours of the onset of pressure elevation (Fig. 27–5).[10] In monkeys, blockage of orthograde transport in the lamina cribrosa has been shown despite a marked elevation of arterial oxygen pressure (Po_2) and the apparent integrity of capillary circulation in the lamina cribrosa.[12] Radioisotope studies in primates have shown that the temporal quadrants of the lamina cribrosa are the most likely location of transport blockage (Fig. 27–6).[12]

Although controversy persists as to the relative role of mechanical and vascular factors in the pathogenesis of glaucomatous damage,[13] alterations in axonal transport noted in experimental studies may be explained by mechanically induced injury. With aging, however, vascular disease and compromised perfusion may play an important role. In either case, alterations of axonal transport in the optic nerve head are an important part of the cascade of events provoked by elevation of IOP that lead to axonal injury and ganglion cell death.

Glaucomatous changes evident in the prelaminar portion

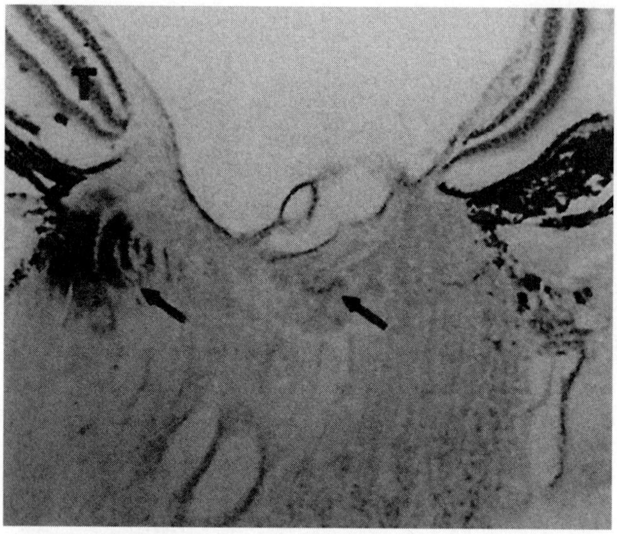

FIGURE 27–5. Section (adjacent to that shown in Fig 27–6) reacted for horseradish peroxidase (HRP) after lateral geniculate body injection of HRP 24 hours previously. The dark material represents HRP reaction product accumulated at the level of the lamina cribrosa in the temporal and central portion *(arrows)* of the optic nerve head. This represents blockage of retrograde transport. (From Minckler DS, Bunt AH, Johanson GW: Orthograde and retrograde axoplasmic transport during acute ocular hypertension in the monkey. Invest Ophthalmol Vis Sci 1977;16–426.)

of the optic nerve illustrate compression and loss of prelaminar tissue with enlargement of the optic cup (Figs. 27–7 to 27–10). The loss of these axons occurs initially in the superior and inferior quadrants of the nerve head,[14, 15] where there is a relative lack of laminar support compared

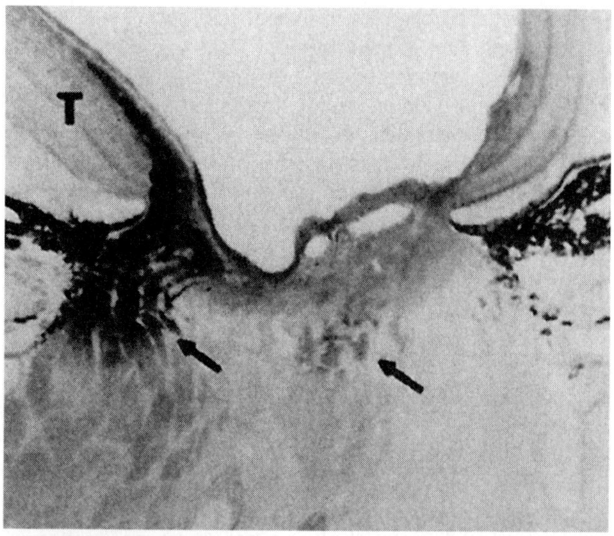

FIGURE 27–6. Autoradiograph of the optic nerve head of a monkey with intraocular pressure maintained at 50 mmHg for 23 hours and enucleated 24 hours after intravitreal ^{3}H-leucine injection. There is marked accumulation of isotope at the level of the lamina cribrosa in the temporal portion of the disc (T) and in the nerve fiber layer and some accumulation in the central portion *(arrows)* of the disc. This represents blockage of orthograde transport. (From Minckler DS, Bunt AH, Johanson GW: Orthograde and retrograde axoplasmic transport during acute ocular hypertension in the monkey. Invest Ophthalmol Vis Sci 1977;16:426.)

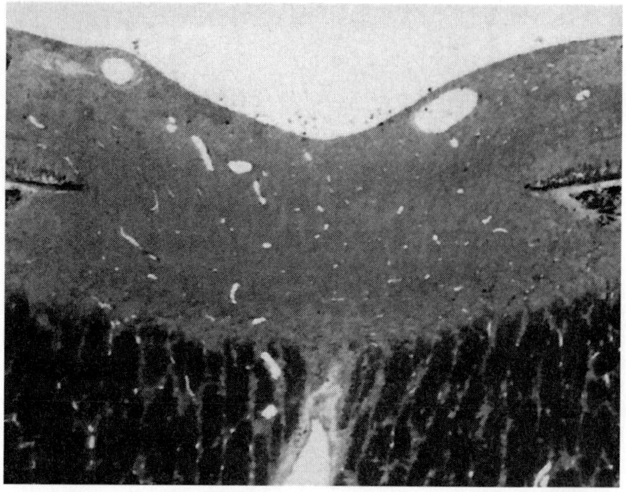

FIGURE 27–7. Normal optic nerve head. The vitreous cavity is above, and the dark myelinated retrobulbar nerve is below. (From Quigley HA: Blood vessels of the glaucomatous optic disc in experimental primate and human eyes. Invest Ophthalmol Vis Sci 1984;25:918.)

with the nasal and temporal quadrants (Fig. 27–11). It is thought that axons traveling through the superior and inferior quadrants of the nerve head are more susceptible to pressure-induced damage.

Studies have shown a quantitative correlation between cupping of the optic disc, increasing loss of neural rim tissue, and increasing loss of axons in primate eyes.[16, 17] In primates with experimental glaucoma, an increase in the cup-to-disc ratio of 0.1 corresponds to a loss of approximately 120,000, or 10% of, the optic nerve fibers.[15]

LAMINA CRIBROSA

The lamina cribrosa is a sieve-like extension of the sclera with openings in its superficial surface to allow the exit of

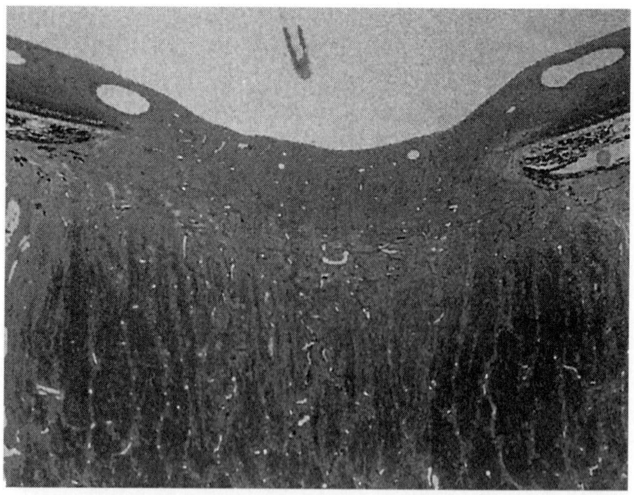

FIGURE 27–8. Compression and loss of prelaminar tissue with enlargement of the optic cup following development of elevated intraocular pressure. (From Quigley HA: Blood vessels of the glaucomatous optic disc in experimental primate and human eyes. Invest Ophthalmol Vis Sci 1984;25:918.)

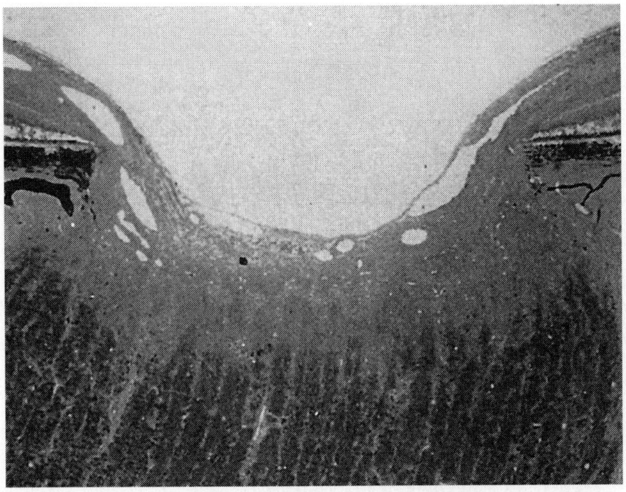

FIGURE 27–9. Moderate loss of tissue and compression of nerve head. (From Quigley HA: Blood vessels of the glaucomatous optic disc in experimental primate and human eyes. Invest Ophthalmol Vis Sci 1984;25:918.)

axon bundles from the eye. Its collagenous beams are not of uniform size and thickness; therefore, they provide variable amounts of support to the nerve bundles that transit the lamina cribrosa.

Numerous changes occur in the lamina cribrosa with elevated IOP. Examination of postmortem eyes with glaucoma has shown that early changes in the lamina cribrosa include outward movement and vertical compression of the laminar sheets. Compression of laminar sheets presumably leads to kinking of the optic nerve axons, causing optic nerve damage. The larger laminar pore size in the superior and inferior regions of the lamina cribrosa presumably provides weak support, thereby contributing to the greater damage of the optic nerve axons in these regions than in the nasal and temporal quadrants of the lamina cribrosa.[18, 19]

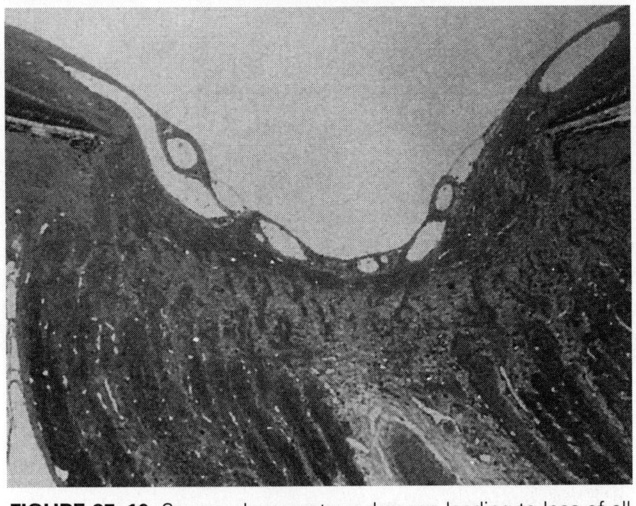

FIGURE 27–10. Severe glaucomatous damage leading to loss of all axonal tissue and consequently a large optic cup (× 40, paraphenylenediamine staining). (From Quigley HA: Blood vessels of the glaucomatous optic disc in experimental primate and human eyes. Invest Ophthalmol Vis Sci 1984;25:918.)

Thus, preferential early damage to these axons leads to development of the typical arcuate and paracentral visual field loss seen in glaucoma.

Methods of Documenting Changes in Optic Nerve and Retinal Nerve Fiber Layers

The invention of the ophthalmoscope made it possible to examine the interior of the eye and document changes of the optic nerve that occur in glaucoma. Available techniques for imaging and measuring the optic disc and retinal nerve fiber layer are discussed in Chapter 5. This section analyzes the qualitative, clinical techniques for evaluation of the optic disc and retinal NFL by ophthalmoscopy and photography as well the quantitative techniques, such as image analyzers and retinal nerve fiber layer analyzers.

Methods of measuring optic nerve characteristics range from those that are entirely observer dependent to those that are mostly instrument dependent. All methods involving instruments, however, require some observer input. For example, in computerized image analysis, an observer must provide the landmarks of the optic disc margin with which the image analyzer aligns its measures.

DIRECT OPHTHALMOSCOPY

Direct ophthalmoscopy is the oldest and probably the most widely used technique to evaluate the optic disc in glaucoma. Through dilated pupils, it is possible to see the retinal NFL with the use of a white or green light, but a better view may be obtained with other techniques discussed later. The ophthalmoscope is relatively inexpensive, portable, and simple to use. Although it can be difficult to obtain an image with hazy media, the direct ophthalmoscope is an excellent instrument for screening large numbers of people for optic nerve disease when bulkier and more expensive instruments are not available. It may also be useful in determining the size and color of the optic nerve head. The major disadvantage of the ophthalmoscope is the lack of stereopsis, because three-dimensional viewing of the optic nerve is critical for the evaluation of glaucoma.

INDIRECT OPHTHALMOSCOPY

Standard indirect ophthalmoscopy with a head-mounted biomicroscope provides only a 3× magnification of the fundus, which is not adequate for the detailed evaluation of the optic nerve and retinal NFL required in glaucoma. Also, the exaggerated axial magnification relative to the angular magnification distorts the three-dimensional appearance of the optic disc.[20] For these reasons, indirect ophthalmoscopy is not recommended for careful examination of the optic nerve and retinal NFL in glaucoma.

SLIT-LAMP TECHNIQUES

The slit-lamp may be combined with a variety of lenses to provide an excellent image of the optic nerve head and

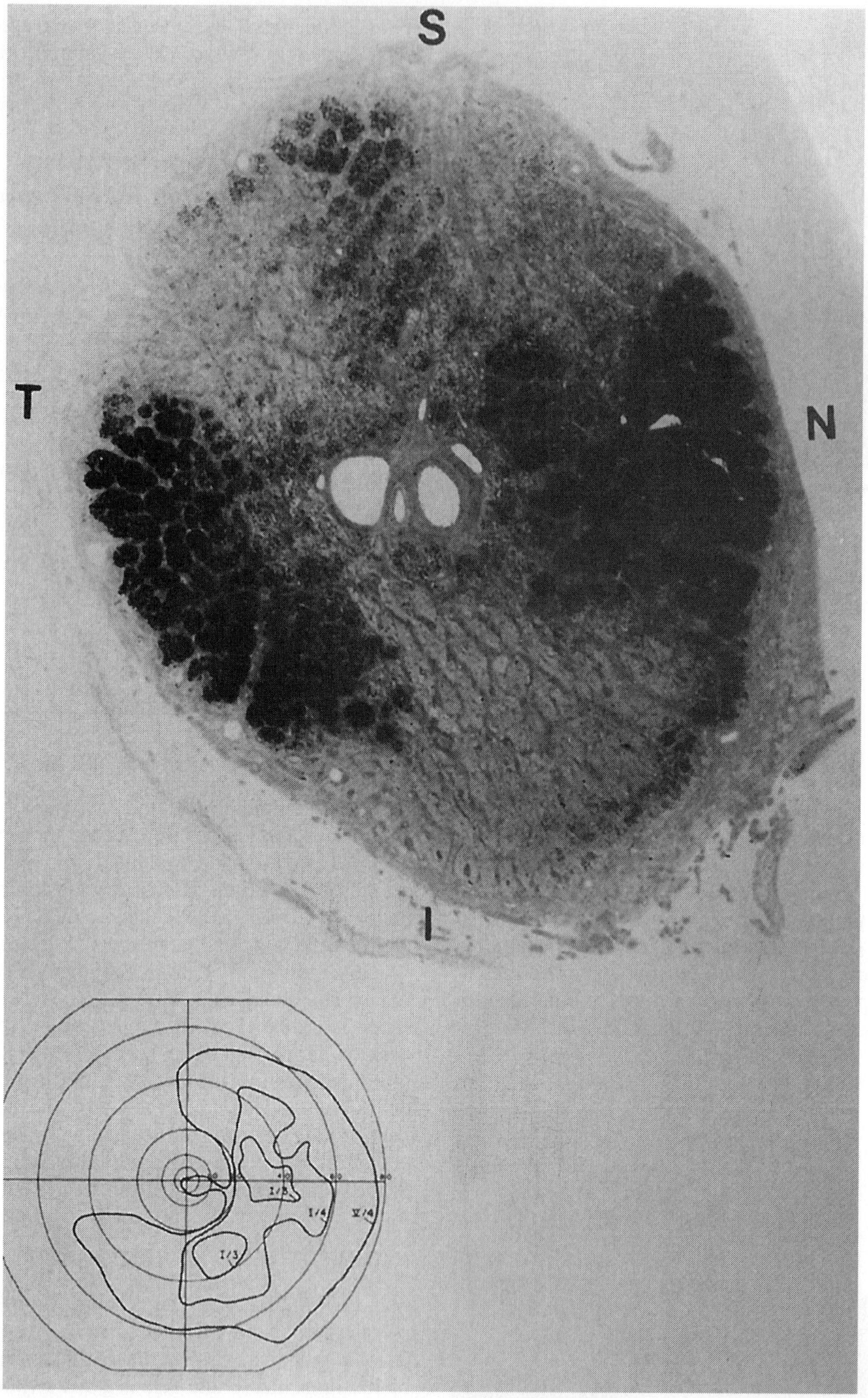

FIGURE 27–11. Cross-section of the optic nerve demonstrating preferential damage to the superior (S) and inferior (I) quadrants with its associated visual field. Intact myelinated axons are present in the dark areas nasally (N) and temporally (T) (x40, paraphenylenediamine staining). (Quigley HA, Green WR: The histology of human glaucoma cupping and optic nerve damage: clinicopathologic correlation in 21 eyes. Ophthalmology 1979;86:1803.)

retinal NFL. Evaluation of the retinal NFL requires the addition of a red-free filter. The Goldmann three-mirrored contact lens, the slit-lamp–mounted Hruby lens, and the hand-held 60-, 78-, and 90-diopter lenses may all be combined with the slit-lamp to view the optic nerve and NFL.

The Goldmann lens produces a virtual, upright image with minimal magnification that can be increased to 16× or higher with the optics of the slit-lamp. This technique probably provides the best view of the disc compared with the other lens systems. The Goldmann lens, however, is somewhat cumbersome to use because it requires contact with the cornea and use of a viscous coupling material that can make subsequent examination or photography of the fundus difficult.

The Hruby lens eliminates the need for corneal contact and, therefore, is more convenient to use. However, the lens has a small field of view, making it difficult to obtain a good-quality, stereoscopic image of the disc.[21]

The use of the hand-held lens with the slit-lamp is another convenient way of evaluating the optic nerve. The lenses convert the slit-lamp into an indirect ophthalmoscope and produce excellent stereopsis. The 78- and 90-diopter lenses are the most widely used. This technique requires patient cooperation and a fairly well-dilated pupil. The 78-diopter lens provides more magnification and detail, whereas the 90-diopter lens has a wider field of view and can often be used even in the patient with a smaller pupil.

When combined with a red-free filter, binocular slit lamp ophthalmoscopy is very useful in evaluating the NFL. Overall, the slit-lamp combined with hand-held lenses provides the most ideal stereoscopic view of the optic disc and retinal NFL although it is also limited by hazy media.

OPTIC DISC AND RETINAL NERVE FIBER LAYER EVALUATION AND PHOTOGRAPHY

Documented description of the optic disc is critical in the management of patients with glaucoma. Drawings have proved less than satisfactory because of both interobserver and intraobserver variability.[22, 23] Optic disc photography is an indispensable adjunct to the clinical evaluation of, the establishment of a baseline for, and the documentation of changes in the optic nerve.

Optic disc photographs should be obtained during initial examination as a baseline. Guidelines developed by the 1996 American Academy of Ophthalmology Preferred Practice Pattern for Primary Open Angle Glaucoma recommend that optic nerve evaluation and recording should be performed every 6 to 18 months in a patient in whom the target IOP has been achieved and who does not demonstrate progression of damage. A patient who has progression of damage or in whom the target IOP has not been achieved should be evaluated every 1 to 6 months, depending on the severity of disease, the rate of progression, the extent to which the IOP exceeds the target value, and the number and strength of other risk factors for damage to the optic nerve.

Stereoscopic photography is preferred over monoscopic images for recording the appearance of the disc. With the use of a green or blue filter and a relatively high-contrast, fine-grain, black-and-white film, the retinal NFL can also be photographed. Nerve fiber layer photography is especially helpful in detecting diffuse nerve fiber loss that can be difficult to see on slit-lamp examination.

Several studies using optic disc photographs have shown that agreement between repeated measurements by a single observer (intraobserver agreement) is excellent.[22–24] However, it has also been shown that interobserver agreement is lower than intraobserver agreement for both optic nerve and NFL assessments. For example, for the vertical cup-to-disc ratio, an intraobserver disagreement among experts of 0.2 disc diameter or more was seen in only 4% to 5% of the discs studied. For the same parameter, interobserver disagreement among experts of 0.2 disc diameter or more was seen in 19% of the discs studied. Such a level of interobserver disagreement limits the clinical usefulness of optic disc photographs.[25]

OPTIC NERVE HEAD ANALYZERS

Image analyzers allow us to quantitatively measure the optic nerve and retinal NFL. Quantitative means of measuring the optic nerve and retinal NFL enable us to objectively document the status of the optic nerve and NFL and to share meaningful information with other examiners. Traditionally used techniques for evaluating the optic nerve are subjective and have been shown to have wide variation not only between observers but also between examinations by the same observer.[22, 23]

Computerized image analysis systems can potentially improve our ability to diagnose and manage glaucoma. In order for these systems to be clinically useful, they must first provide accurate and reproducible quantitative information about the optic nerve and the retinal NFL. In addition, characteristics of the "normal" optic nerve and retinal NFL and their relation to age, race, refraction, and IOP must be understood. This understanding of the normal characteristics is mandatory before we can apply this technology meaningfully to the diagnosis and management of glaucoma. Once this information is obtained with reproducibility and accuracy, image analyzers can be very powerful tools that can improve our ability to diagnose and manage glaucoma.

Several image analyzers are currently in use and have been discussed in Chapter 5. Image analyzers include the Topcon image analyzer, the Glaucoma-scope, and the confocal scanning laser ophthalmoscope (CSLO). Despite their unique characteristics, these devices all consist of essential features: an acquisition device, an analysis station, and a storage device.[26] The acquisition device is by far the most important part of the system, because the quality of results provided by the analysis is directly related to, and limited by, the quality of the images initially acquired. Some acquisition devices use simultaneous stereoscopic optics, and others use confocal optics.

Image analyzers using simultaneous stereoscopic optics preceded the CSLO. The earlier image analyzers were a necessary first step, but variability and lack of resolution, as well as high cost, have limited the enthusiasm for them.[27] Also, these imaging systems require a 4- to 5-mm or greater pupil size, which may be difficult to attain in some patients with glaucoma. Cataracts and other media opacities can significantly degrade the quality of the image and compromise the value of the image analysis.

The CSLO goes beyond the traditional optic nerve head analyzers, and it has overcome many of the limitations of previous systems. The CSLO requires minimal depth of focus; therefore, it provides better images with a reduced need for pupil dilation and clear media. This system provides real-time images of the fundus that can be evaluated at the time of the patient visit (Fig. 27–12). Compared with the earlier image analyzers, axial resolution is better with the CSLO, and the variability is reduced.[28]

Currently, the CSLO is considered the state-of-the-art

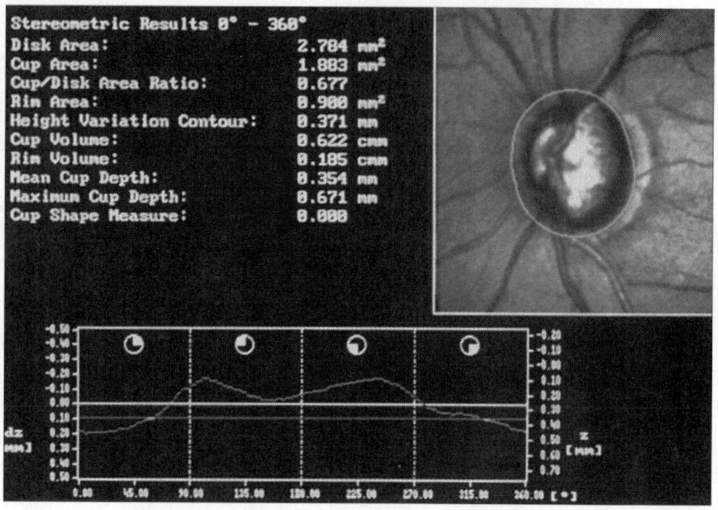

FIGURE 27–12. Printed report for confocal scanning laser ophthalmoscopy. The report includes a confocal scanning laser ophthalmoscopy image that shows marked cupping, especially superiorly, and thinning of the neuroretinal rim, a battery of optic nerve head parameters, which include cup, disc, and rim areas and volumes, and a mean height contour line at the disc margin. (From Zangwill L, de Souza Lima M, Weinreb RN: Confocal scanning laser ophthalmoscopy to detect glaucomatous optic neuropathy. *In* Schuman JS [ed]: Imaging in Glaucoma. Thorofare, NJ, Slack, Inc, 1997.)

instrument for optic nerve head assessment. In their present state, however, CSLOs are expensive and difficult to use. Even with an experienced operator, it can take 2 to 5 minutes or longer to adjust the instrument and properly position the patient before an image can be obtained. Eye movements, even a blink, can degrade the image series.[28] To date, there is no standardized method for outlining the disc margin, which defines many topographic optic nerve parameters; therefore, it is almost impossible to compare data obtained with different CSLOs.

The CSLO has been shown to produce images with greater accuracy and reproducibility compared with the earlier generations of image analyzers. Further study of "normal" optic nerve heads is necessary to establish a reference from which a deviation can be detected. Confocal scanning laser ophthalmoscopy shows promise for improving our ability to detect glaucomatous damage to and changes in the optic nerve. Continued study is needed to understand the role of this technique in clinical decision-making.

RETINAL NERVE FIBER ANALYZERS

Retinal nerve fiber analysis is useful in detecting early glaucoma. Clinical NFL examination and NFL photography are difficult techniques that are both subjective and qualitative. Two different technologies are currently employed to obtain objective, quantitative NFL measurements: polarimetry and optical coherence tomography. These technologies use different approaches to provide objective, quantitative information about the NFL.

Polarimetry utilizes the birefringent properties of the

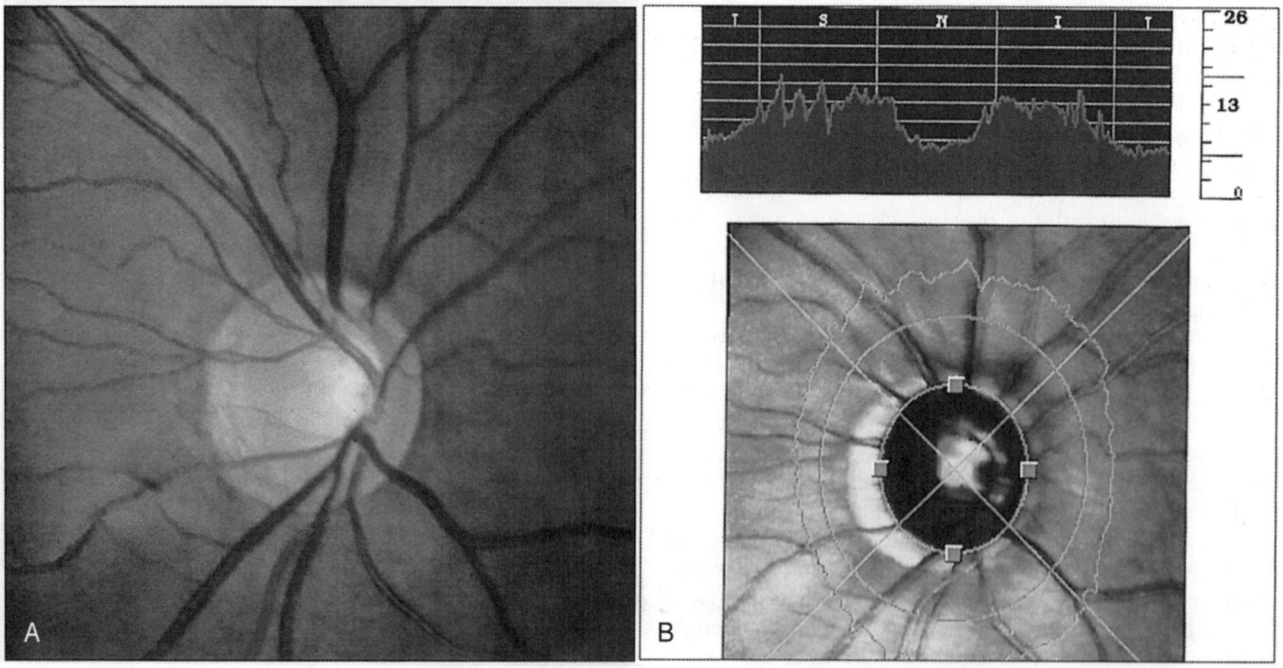

FIGURE 27–13. *A*, Normal optic disc. *B*, Retardation (NFA II) appears as a double-hump pattern with the possibility of diffuse loss (1995). (From Schuman JS [ed]: Imaging in Glaucoma. Thorofare, NJ, Slack, Inc, 1997.)

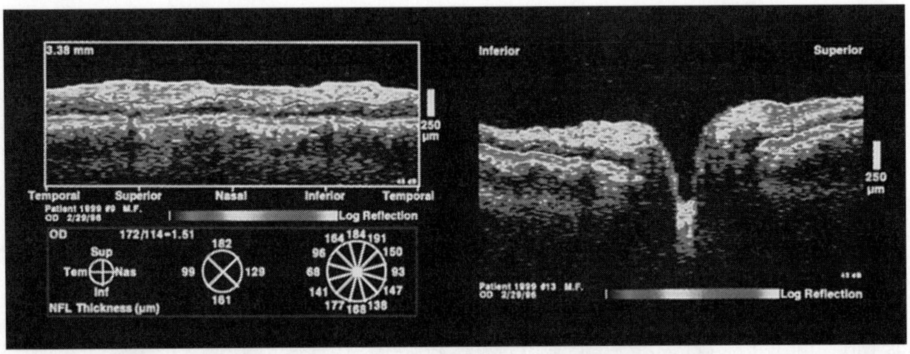

FIGURE 27–14. Optical coherence tomography. Circular scan at 3.4 mm around the optic nerve head. Note the thicker nerve fiber layer superiorly and inferiorly. Borders of the retina and nerve fiber layer are designed by a computer algorithm that calculates threshold reflectivity. Retinal thickness equals the distance between the posterior (posteriormost *blue line*) and anterior retinal border *(white line)*. Nerve fiber layer thickness is equal to the distance between the white and anterior blue lines. (From Yanoff M, Duker JS (eds): Ophthalmology. St. Louis, Mosby, 1999.)

NFL. It employs a CSLO to shine a polarized light into the eye and measures the change in rotation of this light as it exits the eye.[29, 55] With the scanning laser polarimeter, retardation maps of the NFL can be obtained (Fig. 27–13). Measurements obtained from retardation do not have magnification errors, and a reference plane is not required. Retardation provides a relative measure of the NFL thickness, not an absolute measure. Although the examination is easy to perform through an undilated pupil, the equipment is expensive and requires compensation for other polarizing media, such as the cornea. This instrument shows promise, but longitudinal studies are needed to determine whether the quantitative measurements it provides will improve our ability to detect glaucoma and monitor its progression.

Optical coherence tomography (OCT) uses an interferometer with low coherence light to produce 10-μm resolution, two-dimensional, cross-sectional images of the retina, from which quantitative NFL thickness measurements are made (Fig. 27–14).[30] The OCT allows the clinician to visually evaluate the NFL for areas of local abnormalities, such as focal defects and sectoral thinning (Fig. 27–15). The potential utility of OCT as a diagnostic tool in glaucoma is extremely high. OCT is new technology. To date, large-scale normative data for comparison and evaluation do not exist. Longitudinal studies examining NFL loss in glaucomatous and normal eyes are currently under way. This information will help to establish patterns of NFL damage in glaucoma. OCT is a promising new technology that provides a useful parameter for the detection and follow-up of very early glaucomatous abnormalities.

Glaucomatous Changes of the Retina and Optic Nerve

Glaucomatous damage is manifested in the retinal NFL and the optic nerve head. With glaucoma, the appearance of the NFL and the optic disc changes in characteristic ways. Some changes are more characteristic of glaucoma than others, but no feature is pathognomonic of glaucoma. These changes are helpful to various extents for the diagnosis and management of glaucoma. Unfortunately, there is no "gold standard" or single fundamental criterion for defining optic nerve damage. Many studies have been conducted to assess glaucomatous optic nerve damage with the use of a variety of optic disc characteristics and clinical methods. The results of these studies do not draw a clear conclusion as to which parameter or which method of measurement provides the most accurate measure of glaucomatous optic nerve damage.[25]

The following discussion describes some of the changes seen in the retina and optic nerve head and how they relate to glaucoma.

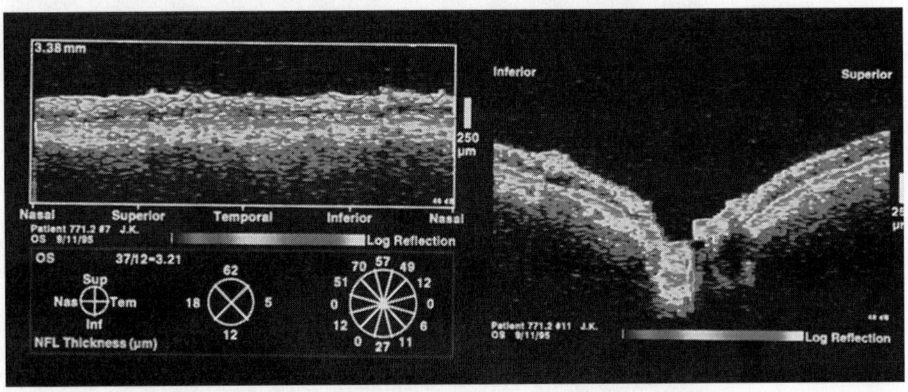

FIGURE 27–15. A patient who has advanced primary open-angle glaucoma. Note severe and generalized thinning of nerve fiber layer. (From Yanoff M, Duker JS [eds]: Ophthalmology. St. Louis, Mosby, 1999.)

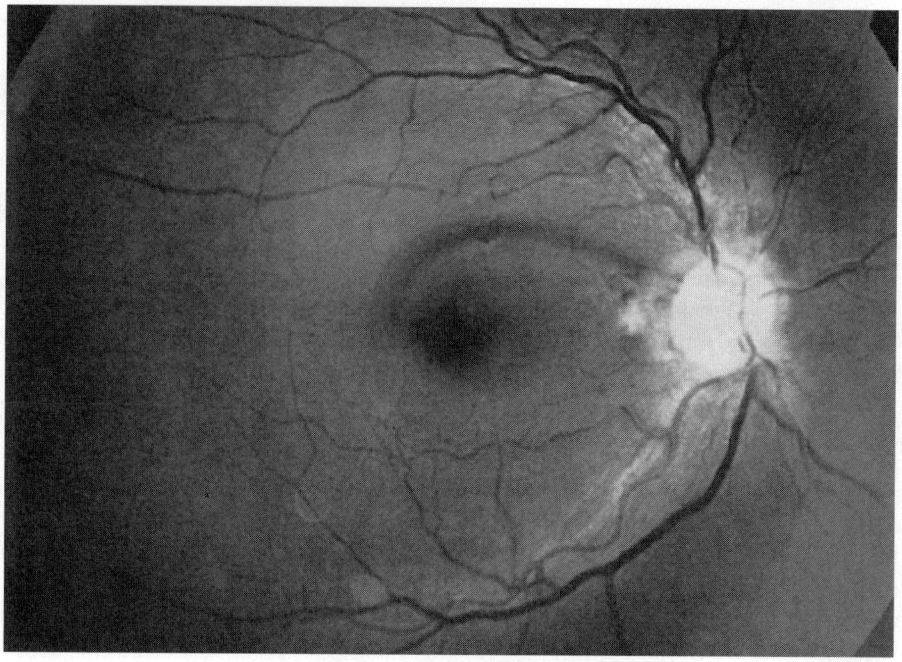

FIGURE 27–16. A dense but strictly localized superior nerve fiber layer defect next to the papillomacular bundle. (From Ritch R, Shields MB, Krupin T (eds): The Glaucomas. St. Louis, Mosby–Year Book, 1996.)

RETINAL NERVE FIBER LAYER

Examination of the retinal NFL can be very helpful in the early detection of glaucoma.[25] Retinal NFL abnormalities, which are reported to be the first observable changes of glaucomatous optic nerve damage, may precede detectable visual field damage by as much as 6 years.[31] Retinal NFL defects have been used to predict visual field loss with average specificity and sensitivity of 80% and 94%, respectively.[35]

Many patterns of NFL atrophy are associated with glaucoma. These defects can be separated by appearance into three groups: (1) slit-like defects, (2) wedge-shaped defects, and (3) diffuse or generalized NFL loss.

Slit-Like Defects

Slit-like defects are often difficult to distinguish from the dark striations that correspond to the intervening glial tissues in a healthy NFL that are rarely wider than a retinal vessel and do not come to the margin of the disc. In many cases, slit-like defects are probably not a sign of abnormality. However, there are many such defects, and if they extend to the disc margin, they are likely to be abnormal (Fig. 27–16). At this stage, abnormalities of the optic disc and visual field are usually not present. Close follow-up is required to detect a possible progression of the findings or the development of a visual field defect that would confirm the diagnosis of glaucoma.

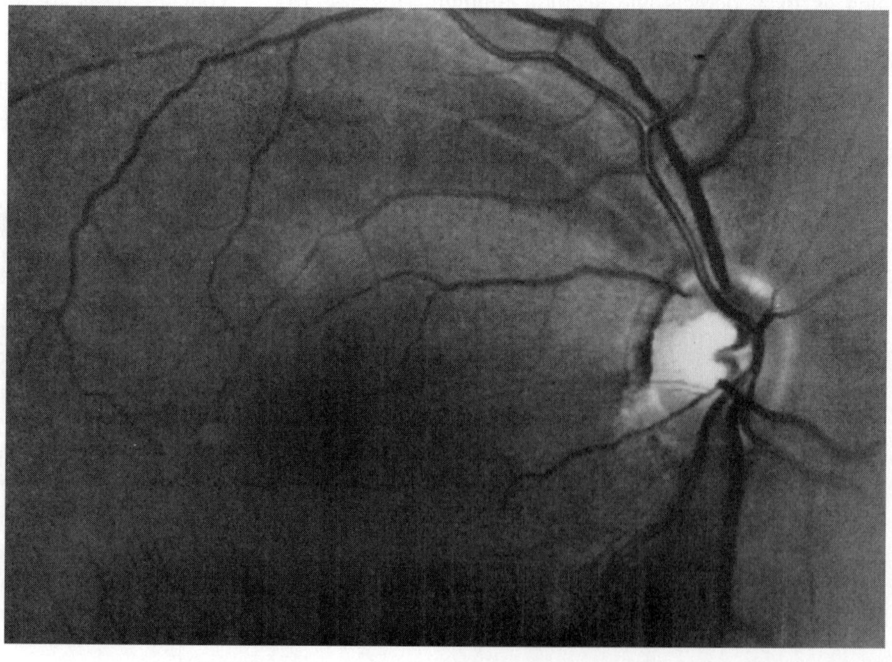

FIGURE 27–17. A wide, localized, wedge-shaped defect in the superior temporal nerve fiber bundle area with a few axon bundles remaining in the defective area. Visual fields showed a mild, relative abnormality in the inferonasal visual field. There are no apparent optic disc changes. (From Ritch R, Shields MB, Krupin T (eds): The Glaucomas. St. Louis, Mosby–Year Book, 1996.)

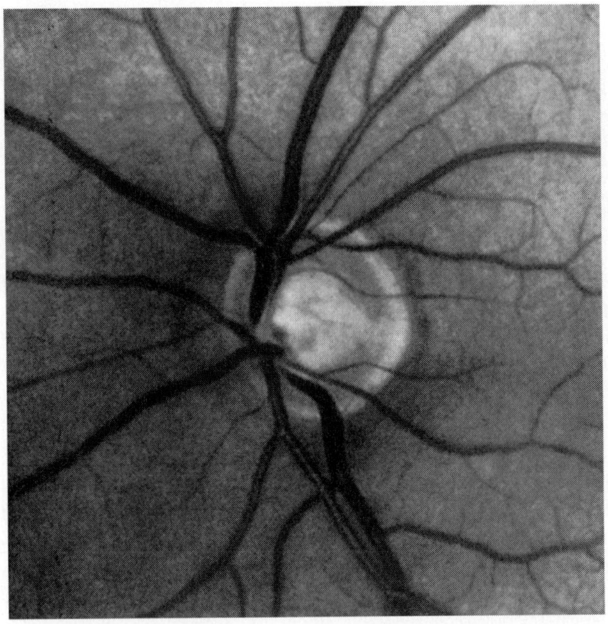

FIGURE 27–18. Marked diffuse thinning of the retinal nerve fiber layer in association with a concentrically enlarged optic cup. Note good visibility of vessels, including small capillaries. Atrophy of the retinal nerve fiber layer has unmasked the mottled appearance of the retinal pigment epithelium. (From Ritch R, Shields MB, Krupin T (eds): The Glaucomas. St. Louis, Mosby–Year Book, 1996.)

Wedge-Shaped Defects

The easiest to detect, wedge-shaped defects are most commonly found in the superior and inferior arcuate regions. They appear as well-outlined, dark, wedge-shaped areas in the brightly striated pattern of the surrounding healthy NFL (Fig. 27–17). Some eyes may have multiple local NFL defects separated by relatively normal areas.

Diffuse or Generalized NFL Loss

Diffuse or generalized NFL loss is the most common abnormality, but it is also the most difficult to detect (Fig. 27–18). The frequency of purely diffuse damage in the literature varies from 49% to 94%.[32, 33] This large variation may be due to different photographic techniques, or it may be that localized defects are easier to detect. With progression of glaucoma, the separation of NFL defects into localized or diffuse types may become difficult. It is not uncommon to see localized damage with diffuse atrophy.

OPTIC NERVE

Typical glaucomatous changes of the optic nerve include alterations in the size, configuration, and color of the optic disc, cup, and neural rim. Peripapillary atrophic changes and alterations in the blood vessels on the surface of the disc and peripapillary retina are also typical of glaucomatous damage.[57] All of these changes signify loss of ganglion cell axons in the prelaminar portion of the optic nerve.

The cup-to-disc ratio has been the most commonly used method of qualitative evaluation of the optic nerve head. In one study, a 65% to 95% rate for sensitivity and specificity was attained when cup-to-disc ratios were used to assess for the presence of visual field defects.[25] If rim-to-disc measurements are used in place of cup-disc ratios, slightly higher sensitivity and specificity are found.[25]

The size and shape of the optic disc have been the subject of numerous histologic and clinical studies. The data from most of these studies are summarized in Table 27–1. The optic disc is approximately 12% larger in blacks than in whites.[34] Similarly, the disc diameter is also larger in blacks. Data from the Baltimore Eye Survey suggest that men's optic discs may be 3% larger than women's.[56] However, these differences do not appear to be of any clinical significance. In addition, no age-related or refractive error–related differences in size of the optic disc were noted in the Baltimore Eye Survey. The asymmetry in optic disc size between the right and left eyes of normal black and white persons is less than 1 mm^2 in 99% of cases.[34]

TABLE 27–1. STUDIES ON OPTIC DISC PARAMETERS

Author	Type of Study	No. of Eyes	Race	Age (yr)	Disc Area (mm^2)	Disc Diameter (mm)
Ogden et al. (1988)	Histologic	12	N/A	22–74*	2.54	1.80
Jonas et al. (1988)	Histologic	107	W	20–80*	2.60	1.82
Quigley et al. (1990)	Histologic	24	B	65 ± 14†	2.75	1.87
Quigley et al. (1990)	Histologic	36	W	67 ± 14†	2.48	1.78
Franceschetti, Bock (1950)	Clinical	100	N/A	N/A	2.06	1.62
Britton et al. (1987)	Clinical	113	N/A	51 ± 17†	2.10	1.61
Caprioli, Miller (1987)	Clinical	38	N/A	36 ± 12†	1.70	1.47
Jonas et al. (1988)	Clinical	457	W	43 ± 20†	2.69	1.84
Chi et al. (1989)	Clinical	58	B	30 ± 4†	2.15	1.65
Chi et al. (1989)	Clinical	59	W	27 ± 4†	1.73	1.48
Funk et al. (1989)	Clinical	194	N/A	42 ± 20†	2.13	1.64
Tsai et al. (1992)	Clinical	41	W	27 ± 6†	1.84	1.53
Tsai et al. (1992)	Clinical	40	W	69 ± 8†	1.67	1.46
Varma et al. (1994)	Clinical	2903	B	40–80+*	2.94	1.93
Varma et al. (1994)	Clinical	3475	W	40–80+*	2.63	1.83

*Range.
†Mean ± standard deviation.
B, black; N/A, data not available; W, white.
From Ritch R, Shields MB, Krupin T (eds): The Glaucomas, 2nd ed, vol 1. St. Louis, Mosby–Year Book, 1996.

ENLARGEMENT OF THE OPTIC CUP

Glaucoma is associated with an increase in the absolute size of the optic cup and in the cup-to-disc ratio.[21] The optic cup enlarges in glaucoma as a result of loss of retinal nerve fibers. The cup is more likely to enlarge vertically than horizontally because early nerve fiber loss typically occurs at the superior and inferior poles of the optic disc. In the normal optic cup, the vertical diameter rarely is noticeably larger than the horizontal diameter.[35]

ASYMMETRY OF CUP SIZE

In the absence of a congenital anomaly of the optic nerve or a significant degree of anisometropia, the optic cup of each eye in a normal individual should be similar. In the Framingham study, an asymmetry of the cup-to-disc ratio of greater than 0.1 was found in less than 7% of the population.[36] Asymmetry between the two optic cups is a common finding, however, in patients with glaucoma.[35]

ALTERATION OF THE LAMINA CRIBROSA

Normally, the sieve-like openings of the lamina cribrosa are not well seen because they are obscured by the overlying nerve fibers. As the nerve fibers are lost in glaucoma, the openings are seen more easily; this process is called *baring of the lamina* or the *laminar dot sign* (Fig. 27–19).

Backward bowing and compaction of the lamina cribrosa are also prominent features of glaucoma (Figs. 27–20 to 27–22).[36] Backward bowing is visible as an increase in the apparent depth of the cup (see Fig. 27–10). The lamina cribrosa often appears more bowed at the superior and inferior poles than centrally, producing an hourglass appearance.

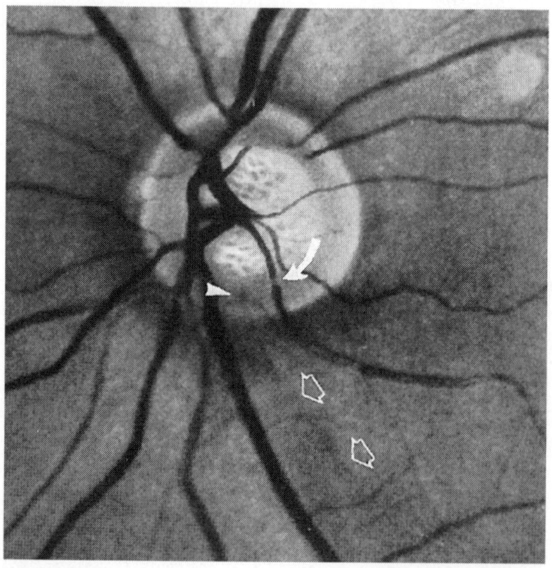

FIGURE 27–19. Baring of the lamina cribrosa. Openings in the lamina cribrosa are easily visible in areas where neural tissue has been lost. This is called the laminar dot sign. Small remnants of an optic disc hemorrhage are seen on the neuroretinal rim at the six o'clock position *(arrowhead)*. There is a narrowing of the inferotemporal artery *(closed arrow)* next to the hemorrhage, a possible sign of localized vasospasm. A wedge-shaped nerve fiber layer defect extends from the optic disc hemorrhage *(open arrows)*. (From Ritch R, Shields MB, Krupin T (eds): The Glaucomas. St. Louis, Mosby–Year Book, 1996.)

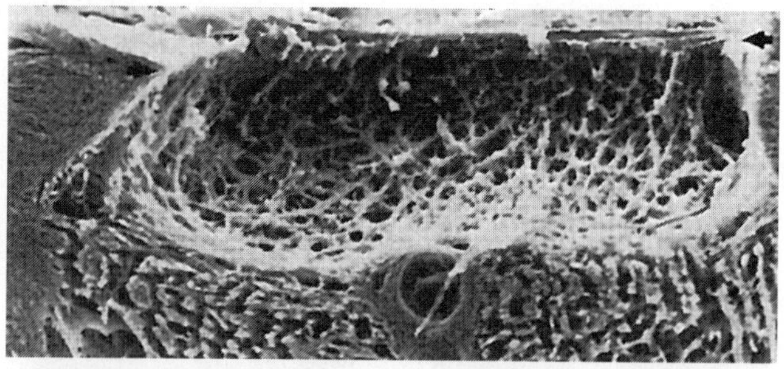

FIGURE 27–20. Moderately severe glaucomatous damage. (From Quigley HA, Addicks EM: Regional differences in the structure of the lamina cribrosa and their relation to glaucomatous optic nerve damage. Arch Ophthalmol 1981;99:137.)

LOSS OF NEURAL RIM

Neural rim loss can occur in either a localized or a diffuse pattern. In an individual patient, either or both patterns may occur. With generalized rim loss, concentric thinning of the rim occurs in all quadrants of the disc. This generalized expansion of the optic cup was found to be the most common type of progressive optic disc change in glaucoma (Fig. 27–23).[37] Concentric thinning of the neural rim is also common in childhood glaucoma.

Focal expansion of the cup can produce notching (Fig. 27–24), which appears as well-defined areas of thinning or complete loss of the rim in an area. Notching occurs more commonly in the lower pole than in the upper pole.[38, 39] Localized notching may sometimes be so deep as to resemble a congenital pit. These defects have been termed *pseudopits* or *acquired pits* of the optic nerve. They may represent an area of focal laminar insufficiency.[26]

It is unclear why some patients show localized loss of neural tissue but others show either diffuse loss of fibers or a combination of the two patterns. Some researchers have found focal fiber loss to be more common in eyes with moderate to low IOP and diffuse rim loss more common in eyes with high IOP.[21] Others have thought that

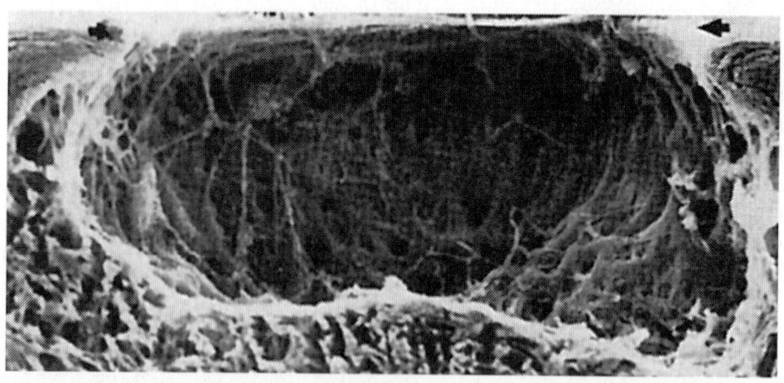

FIGURE 27–21. Blind glaucomatous eye. The lamina cribrosa illustrates posterior bowing along the floor and outward bowing along the margin (×80). (From Quigley HA, Addicks EM: Regional differences in the structure of the lamina cribrosa and their relation to glaucomatous optic nerve damage. Arch Ophthalmol 1981;99:137.)

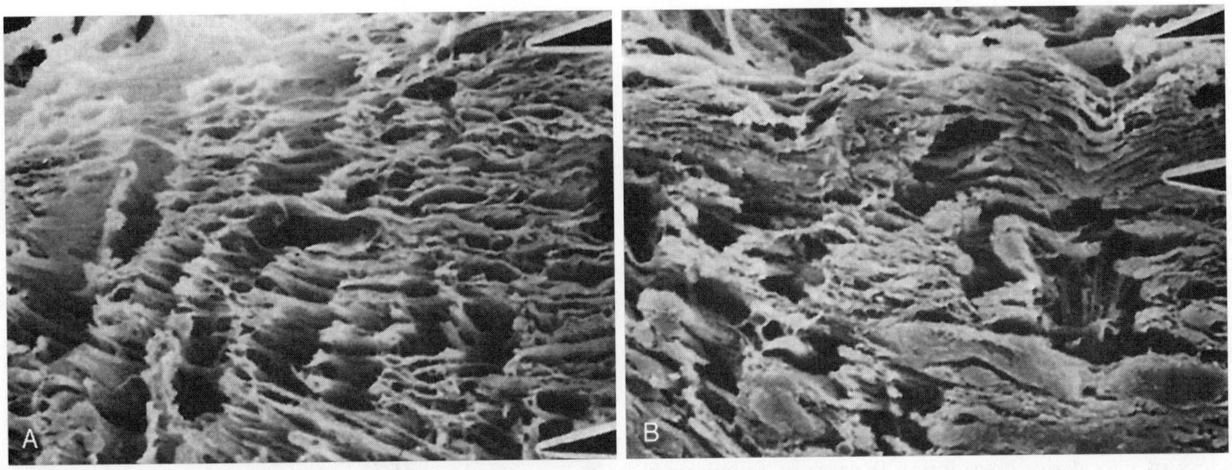

FIGURE 27–22. Trypsin digest preparations of the laminar sheets demonstrating vertical compression of the laminar sheets in glaucomatous optic nerve damage. *A*, Normal eye. *B*, Severe optic nerve damage (×85). (From Quigley HA, Hohman RM, Addicks EM, et al: Morphologic changes in the lamina cribrosa correlated with neural loss in open-angle glaucoma. Am J Ophthalmol 1983;95:673.)

these two patterns of optic nerve damage occur successively during disease progression, initial diffuse fiber loss being followed by small, focal fiber losses.[37] Quigley and associates,[40] however, presented histologic evidence that damage starts with focal nerve fiber loss and is later followed by diffuse loss.

PALLOR OF THE OPTIC DISC

Cupping and pallor are both manifestations of glaucomatous loss of retinal nerve fibers and neural rim. Cupping can be thought of as the change in the three-dimensional contour of the optic disc. Pallor represents a change in color resulting from the thinning of neural tissue and the consequent change in tissue composition and transparency. Thinning of the rim decreases the total number of capillaries, allowing more white light to reflect back from the collagenous portion of the nerve head.[21]

In normal eyes, the area of pallor increases with age, and the maximum color contrast generally coincides with the area of cupping. In early glaucomatous eyes, however,

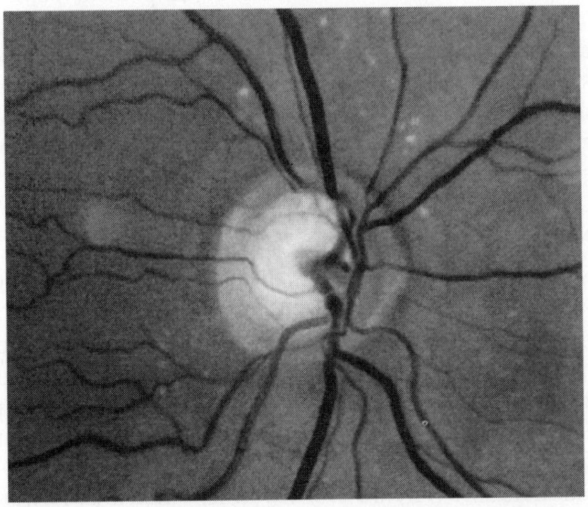

FIGURE 27–23. Generalized enlargement of the cup resulting from concentric loss of the neural rim in a patient with glaucoma. The central cup and the area of pallor are large. The neural rim is uniformly thin and does not demonstrate areas of focal narrowing. This disc also demonstrates baring of the circumlinear vessels. Both superiorly and inferiorly, the neuroretinal rim has receded, leaving the circumlinear vessels behind and rendering the laminar pores visible. (From Ritch K, Shields MB, Krupin T (eds): The Glaucomas. St. Louis, Mosby–Year Book, 1996.)

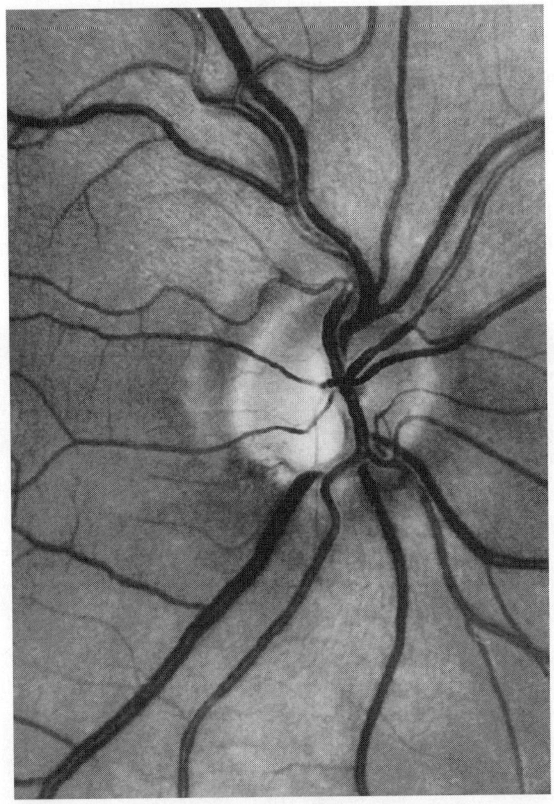

FIGURE 27–24. Localized notching of the neural rim between the six o'clock and seven o'clock positions. There is a deep localized notch reaching to the edge of the optic disc. The retinal nerve fiber layer corresponding to this area is thinned (compare with corresponding area superiorly). At the eight o'clock position, there are remnants of an optic disc hemorrhage. (From Ritch R, Shields MB, Krupin T (eds): The Glaucomas. St. Louis, Mosby–Year Book, 1996.)

the area of pallor tends to be smaller than the area of cupping.[21] The area of total disc pallor has been positively correlated with the extent of visual field loss as measured by Goldmann perimetry.[26]

PERIPAPILLARY ATROPHY

Acquired peripapillary atrophy has been correlated with localized optic nerve damage[41] and visual field defects in glaucomatous eyes.[42] It has been shown to be moderately predictive of visual field loss.[26] Some researchers have suggested that a crescent of atrophy may mark a sector that is anatomically weak and therefore susceptible to glaucomatous damage.[41] Others, however, found only a weak correlation between the degree of peripapillary atrophy and the loss of neural rim area during 9 years of follow-up.[43] It is unclear at this point whether the presence or absence of peripapillary atrophy influences the rate of neural rim change in glaucoma.

VASCULAR CHANGES ON THE DISC

As the optic cup enlarges in glaucoma, the normal course and pattern of the retinal vessels on the disc may alter. Characteristic changes are (1) nasalization of vessels, (2) bayonetting of vessels, (3) baring of circumlinear vessels, (4) narrowing of retinal vessels, (5) the presence of collateral vessels on the disc, and (6) disc hemorrhages.

Nasalization

Nasalization of vessels is thought to be a sign of glaucomatous cupping (Fig. 27–25). The retinal vessels normally enter the eye along the nasal border of the cup. If the cup is large, the vessels appear to be displaced nasally as a result of the normal anatomic configuration.[26, 44, 45] Nasal displacement of the major retinal vessel branches has been shown with progressive cupping.[4] Nasalization of the vessels is not specific for glaucoma, unless a change in displacement is documented.[21]

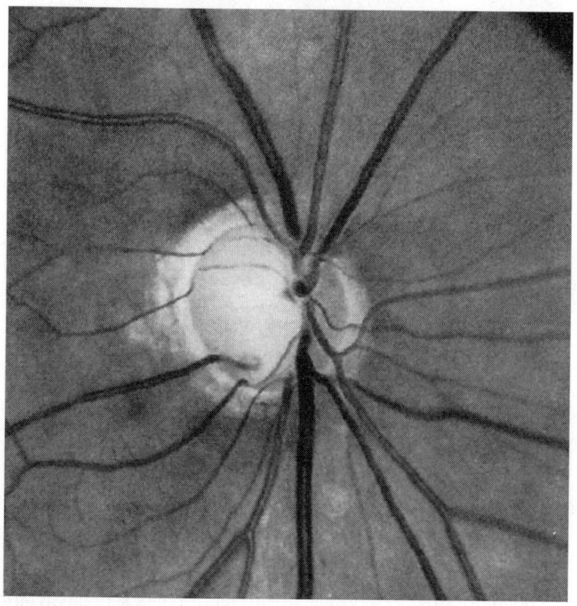

FIGURE 27–25. Nasalization and bayonetting of vessels in an optic disc with advanced cupping. (From Ritch R, Shields MB, Krupin T (eds): The Glaucomas. St. Louis, Mosby–Year Book, 1996.)

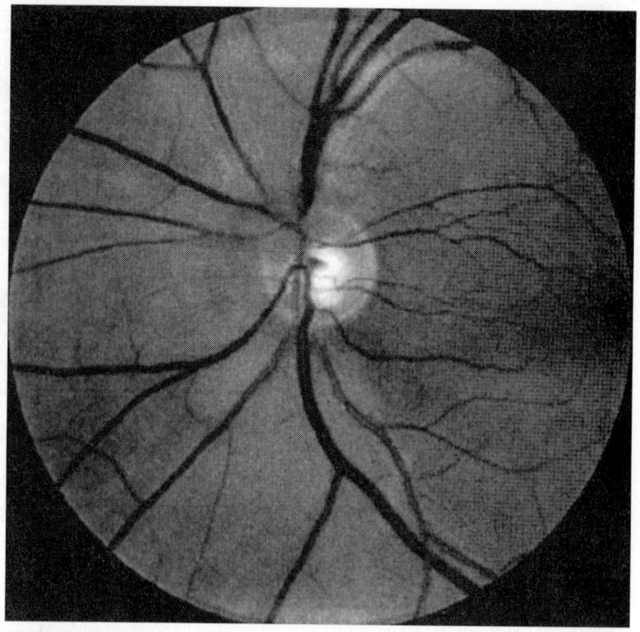

FIGURE 27–26. An optic disc with inferior localized rim loss and baring of the circumlinear vessel. There is an area of cupping and pallor between the remaining neural rim and the circumlinear vessel. (From Ritch R, Shields MB, Krupin T (eds): The Glaucomas. St. Louis, Mosby–Year Book, 1996.)

Bayonetting

Bayonetting of vessels occurs from a lack of support of the retinal vessels as they cross the cup margin (see Fig. 27–25). In areas where the neural rim is absent or very thin, a retinal vessel must make a sharp bend before it passes the overhanging edge of the cup. This process has been termed "bayonetting" because the sharp bend in the vessel resembles the sharp bend made by a bayonet at the end of a rifle. Bayonetting of vessels is rarely seen in normal discs, even in the presence of a large physiologic cup.[26, 45]

Baring

Circumlinear vessels are small branches of the central retinal artery or vein that follow a curved path along the margin of the optic cup. These vessels are bared if the cup enlarges and the cup margin recedes from the vessels near it to expose an area of pallor (Fig. 27–26). This sign is not specific for glaucoma and may be seen in eyes with large physiologic cups.[21] Baring of circumlinear vessel predicts visual field loss only 40% of the time.[26] There is, however, some evidence that a bared circumlinear vessel in a patient with a normal visual field is associated with a greater risk of subsequent field loss.[46]

Narrowing

Narrowing of retinal vessels has been documented in glaucoma. It has been suggested that the retinal vessel diameter

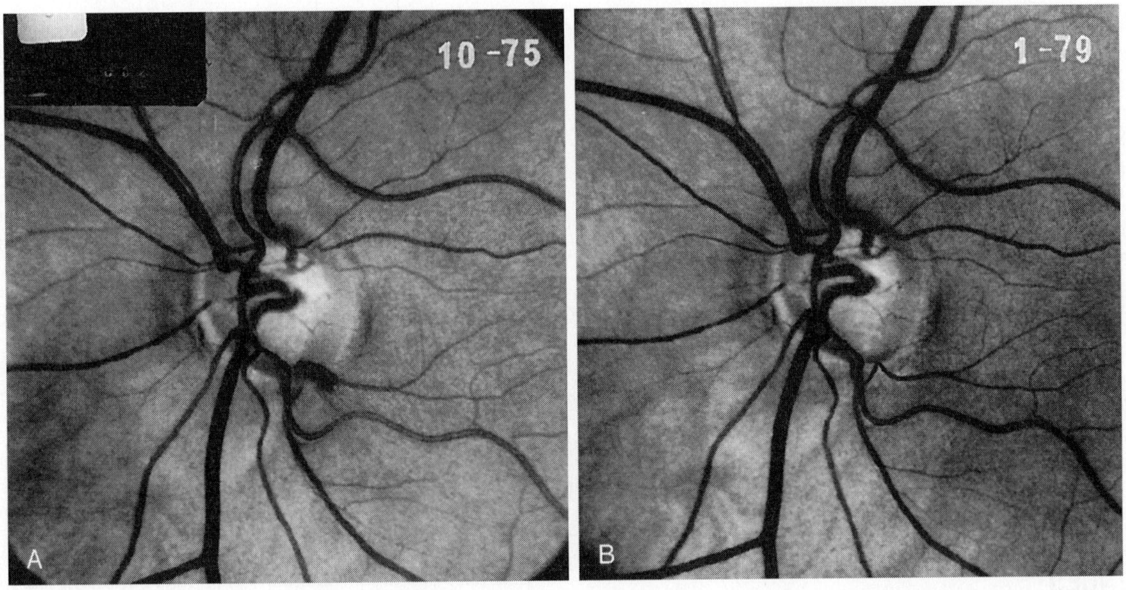

FIGURE 27–27. *A*, An optic disc hemorrhage at the five o'clock position in October 1975. The hemorrhage has developed at a previously damaged location. *B*, In January 1979, all of the neural tissue at that location has disappeared, and the optic disc is excavated all the way to the edge of the disc. (From Ritch R, Shields MB, Krupin T (eds): The Glaucomas. St. Louis, Mosby–Year Book, 1996.)

decreases as a result of the reduction in the ganglion cell population in the retina. It has also been suggested that the narrowest vessels occur in association with areas of greatest neural rim and nerve fiber loss.[47–49]

Collateral Vessels

Collateral vessels on the optic nerve head may result from vascular occlusion and have been associated with glaucoma. In one study, collateral vessels were noted in 3% of eyes with glaucoma and ocular hypertension.[50] Collateral vessels develop as a result of ischemia and, therefore, are associated with other conditions, such as proliferative diabetic retinopathy, vein occlusions, meningiomas, and intraocular tumors. This finding indicates disturbed circulation at the optic nerve head and may be associated with progression of glaucoma.

Disc Hemorrhages

Hemorrhages on the optic disc are a common finding in patients with glaucoma and may be a risk factor for future progressive damage. They appear as splinter- or flame-shaped hemorrhages that assume the shape of the superficial NFL on the optic disc surface (Fig. 27–27). Disc hemorrhages are usually found in the inferotemporal sector of the optic nerve head and correlate with the finding that glaucomatous visual field defects are more common in the superior than in the inferior visual field.[51] Optic disc hemorrhages are often associated with neural rim notching at the site of the bleeding and have been reported to predict the site of a retinal NFL defect.[52]

The etiology of disc hemorrhages is unclear. Some investigators believe disc hemorrhages in glaucoma are evidence that ischemia plays a role in glaucomatous optic nerve damage, but others advocate a mechanical obstruction. A vascular origin similar to a vein occlusion has also been proposed to explain the etiology of disc hemorrhages.

The prognostic significance of disc hemorrhages in glaucoma is also controversial. Some researchers have reported that the presence of a disc hemorrhage is a significant risk factor for the progression of optic nerve damage.[53] Tuulonen and associates,[54] however, found no statistically significant differences between patients with and without optic disc hemorrhages in a comparison of the rate of change of optic disc cupping and pallor. Although the exact implication of disc hemorrhages is not known, an isolated disc hemorrhage is a sign of an active pathologic process at the disc that may herald early glaucomatous optic nerve damage.

Diagnostic Value of Optic Disc and Nerve Fiber Layer Change

The utility of various disc parameters to predict for glaucomatous nerve damage has been evaluated in selected populations. Although the relative value of the various measurements can be estimated, their performance in large, more general populations remains to be evaluated. The optic disc characteristics that best measure glaucomatous nerve damage are NFL defects, the ratio of neuroretinal rim area to disc area, and the vertical cup-to-disc ratio.

SUMMARY

Numerous specific anatomic and physiologic changes in the retina and optic nerve are characteristic of glaucoma. However, the exact mechanism and pathogenesis of these changes remain to be clarified. Neither mechanical compression of the axons nor the compromise of the optic nerve vasculature can explain all the changes in glaucoma. These glaucomatous changes, as manifested in the retina and optic nerve, can improve our ability to diagnose and manage patients with glaucoma.

No one characteristic change in the retina or optic

nerve is diagnostic of glaucoma. Evaluation of multiple characteristics, however, may improve our ability to detect and follow glaucomatous changes. The information gathered from evaluations of the retina and optic nerve must be included in the overall clinical picture and used in conjunction with the patient's history, IOP, and visual field changes.

Although numerous methods are currently available to qualitatively and quantitatively assess changes in the optic nerve and retinal NFL, the technology is rapidly changing and improving. The technology for these evaluations will continue to improve as our understanding of what distinguishes pathologic glaucomatous change of the optic disc from normal variation also improves. Insight into the pathogenesis and causes of this blinding disease will continue to evolve rapidly as new investigative tools are developed.

REFERENCES

1. Quigley HA, Dunkelberger GR, Green WR: Chronic human glaucoma causing selectively greater loss of large optic nerve fibers. Ophthalmology 1988;95:357.
2. Quigley HA, Dunkelberger GR, Green WR: Retinal ganglion cell atrophy correlated with automated perimetry in human eyes with glaucoma. Am J Ophthalmol 1989;107:453.
3. Quigley HA, Sanchez RM, Dunkelberger GR, et al: Chronic glaucoma selectively damages large optic nerve fibers. Invest Ophthalmol Vis Sci 1987;28:913.
4. Tyler CW: Specific deficits of flicker sensitivity in glaucoma and ocular hypertension. Invest Ophthalmol Vis Sci 1981;20:204.
5. Varma R, Minckler DS: Anatomy and pathophysiology of the retina and optic nerve. *In* Ritch R, Shields MB, Krupin T (eds): The Glaucomas, 2nd ed, vol I. St. Louis, Mosby–Year Book, 1996, p 139.
6. Quigley HA, Addicks EM, Green WR: Optic nerve damage in human glaucoma. III: Quantitative correlation of nerve fiber loss and visual field defect in glaucoma, ischemic neuropathy, papilledema, and toxic neuropathy. Arch Ophthalmol 1982;100:135.
7. Radius RL, Anderson DR: The histology of retinal nerve fiber layer bundles and bundle defects. Arch Ophthalmol 1979;97:948.
8. Hoyt WF, Newman NM: The earliest observable defect in glaucoma? Lancet 1972;1:692.
9. Quigley HA: Examination of the retinal nerve fiber layer in the recognition of early glaucoma damage. Trans Am Ophthalmol Soc 1986;84:920.
10. Anderson DR, Hendrickson A: Effect of intraocular pressure on rapid axoplasmic transport in monkey optic nerve. Invest Ophthalmol 1974;13:771.
11. Minckler DS, Bunt AH, Johanson GW: Orthograde and retrograde axoplasmic transport during acute ocular hypertension in the monkey. Invest Ophthalmol Vis Sci 1977;16:426.
12. Quigley H, Anderson DR: The dynamics and location of axonal transport blockade by acute intraocular pressure elevation in primate optic nerve. Invest Ophthalmol 1976;15:606.
13. Yablonski ME, Asamoto A: Hypothesis concerning the pathophysiology of optic nerve damage in glaucoma. J Glaucoma 1993;2:119.
14. Quigley HA, Green WR: The histology of human glaucoma cupping and optic nerve damage: Clinicopathologic correlation in 21 eyes. Ophthalmology 1979;86:1803.
15. Radius RL, Anderson DR: The course of axons through the retina and optic nerve head. Arch Ophthalmol 1979;97:1154.
16. Jonas JB, Gusek GC, Naumann GOH: Optic disc, cup and neuroretinal rim size, configuration, and correlations in normal eyes. Invest Ophthalmol Vis Sci 1988;29:1151.
17. Varma R, Quigley HA, Pease ME: Changes in optic disc characteristics and the number of nerve fibers in experimental glaucoma. Am J Ophthalmol 1992;114:554.
18. Quigley HA, Addicks EM: Regional differences in the structure of the lamina cribrosa and their relation to glaucomatous optic nerve damage. Arch Ophthalmol 1981;99:137.
19. Radius RL, Gonzales M: Anatomy of the lamina cribrosa in human eyes. Arch Ophthalmol 1981;99:2159.
20. Shields MB, Tiedeman JS: Binocular ophthalmoscopic techniques for evaluation of the optic nerve head. *In* Varma R, Spaeth GL (eds): The Optic Nerve in Glaucoma. Philadelphia, JB Lippincott, 1993.
21. Airaksinen PJ, Tuulonen A, Werner EB: Clinical evaluation of the optic disc and retinal nerve fiber layer. *In* Ritch R, Shields MB, Krupin T (eds): The Glaucomas, 2nd ed, vol I. St. Louis, Mosby–Year Book, 1996, p 617.
22. Lichter PR: Variability of expert observers in evaluating the optic disc. Trans Am Ophthalmol Soc 1976;74:532.
23. Tielsch JM, Katz J, Quigley HA, et al: Intraobserver and interobserver agreement in measurement of optic disc characteristics. Ophthalmology 1988;95:350.
24. Varma R, Steinmann WC, Scott IU: Expert agreement in evaluating the optic disc for glaucoma. Ophthalmology 1992;99:215.
25. Steinmann WC, Varma R: An analysis of various methods of optic nerve evaluation. *In* Varma R, Spaeth GL (eds): The Optic Nerve in Glaucoma. Philadelphia, JB Lippincott, 1993, p 325.
26. Spaeth GL: Development of glaucomatous changes of the optic nerve. *In* Varma R, Spaeth GL (eds): The Optic Nerve in Glaucoma. Philadelphia, JB Lippincott, 1993.
27. Schuman JS: Introduction: What do I need imaging for? *In* Schuman JS (ed): Imaging in Glaucoma. Thorofare, NJ, Slack, Inc, 1996.
28. Zangwill L, de Souza Lima M, Weinreb RN: Confocal scanning laser ophthalmoscopy to detect glaucomatous optic neuropathy. *In* Schuman JS (ed): Imaging in Glaucoma. Thorofare, NJ, Slack, Inc, 1996.
29. Varma R: Image analyzers: Introduction. *In* Varma R, Spaeth GL (eds): The Optic Nerve in Glaucoma. Philadelphia, JB Lippincott Co, 1993, p 209.
30. Schuman JS: Optical coherence tomography for imaging and quantitation of nerve fiber layer thickness. *In* Schuman JS (ed): Imaging in Glaucoma. Thorofare, NJ, Slack, Inc, 1996.
31. Sommer A, Quigley HA, Robin AL, et al: Evaluation of nerve fiber layer assessment. Arch Ophthalmol 1984;102:1766.
32. Lachenmayr BJ, Drance SM, Airaksinen PJ: Diffuse nerve fiber loss and central visual function in glaucoma. J Glaucoma 1992;1:32.
33. Quigley HA, Reacher M, Katz J, et al: Quantitative grading of nerve fiber layer photographs. Ophthalmology 1993;100:1800.
34. Varma R, Tielsch JM, Quigley HA, et al: Race-, age-, gender-, and refractive error-related differences in the normal optic disc. Arch Ophthalmol 1994;112:1068.
35. Jonas JB, Gusek GC, Naumann GOH: Optic disc morphometry in chronic primary open angle glaucoma. I: Morphometric intrapapillary characteristics. Graefes Arch Clin Exp Ophthalmol 1988;226:522.
36. Quigley HA, Hohman RM, Addicks EM, et al: Morphologic changes in the lamina cribrosa correlated with neural loss in open-angle glaucoma. Am J Ophthalmol 1983;95:673.
37. Pederson JE, Anderson DR: The mode of progressive disc cupping in ocular hypertension and glaucoma. Arch Ophthalmol 1980;98:490.
38. Hitchings RA, Spaeth GL: The optic disc in glaucoma. I: Classification. Br J Ophthalmol 1976;60:778.
39. Iwata K: Topographical analysis of the genesis of glaucomatous cupping. Glaucoma 1979;1:16.
40. Quigley HA, Miller NR, George T: Clinical evaluation of nerve fiber layer atrophy as an indicator of glaucomatous optic nerve damage. Arch Ophthalmol 1980;98:1564.
41. Kasner O, Feuer WJ, Anderson DR: Possibly reduced prevalence of peripapillary crescents in ocular hypertension. Can J Ophthalmol 1989;24:211.
42. Heijl A, Samander C: Peripapillary atrophy and glaucomatous visual field defects. *In* Heijl A, Greve EL (eds): Sixth International Visual Field Symposium. Dordrecht, Netherlands, W Junk, 1985.
43. Airaksinen PJ, Juvala PA, Tuulonen A, et al: Change of peripapillary atrophy in glaucoma. *In* Krieglstein GK (ed): Glaucoma Update III. Berlin, Springer-Verlag 1987, p 97.
44. Hitchings RA, Genio C, Anderton S, et al: An optic disc grid: Its evaluation in reproducibility studies on the cup/disc ratio. Br J Ophthalmol 1983;67:356.
45. Katz LJ: Optic disc drawings. *In* Varma R, Spaeth GL (eds): The Optic Nerve in Glaucoma. Philadelphia, JB Lippincott, 1993, p 147.
46. Kasner O, Balazsi AG: Glaucomatous optic nerve atrophy: The circumlinear vessel revisited. Can J Ophthalmol 1991;26:264.
47. Jonas JB, Fernandez MC, Naumann GOH: Parapapillary atrophy and

retinal vessel diameter in nonglaucomatous optic nerve damage. Invest Ophthalmol Vis Sci 1991;32:2942.
48. Jonas JB, Naumann GOH: Parapapillary retinal vessel diameter in normal and glaucoma eyes. II: Correlations. Invest Ophthalmol Vis Sci 1989;30:1604.
49. Jonas JB, Nguyen XN, Naumann GOH: Parapapillary retinal vessel diameter in normal and glaucoma eyes. I: Morphometric data. Invest Ophthalmol Vis Sci 1989;30:1599.
50. Tuulonen A: Asymptomatic miniocclusions of the optic disc veins in glaucoma. Arch Ophthalmol 1989;107:1475.
51. Nicholas SP, Werner EB: Location of early glaucomatous visual field defects. Can J Ophthalmol 1980;15:131.
52. Airaksinen PJ, Mustonen E, Alando HI: Optic disc hemorrhages precede retinal nerve fiber layer defects in ocular hypertension. Acta Ophthalmol (Copenh) 1981;59:627.
53. Drance SM, Schulzer M, Thomas B, et al: Multivariate analysis in glaucoma: Use of discriminant analysis in predicting glaucomatous visual field damage. Arch Ophthalmol 1981;99:1019.
54. Tuulonen A, Takamoto T, Wu DC, et al: Optic disk cupping and pallor measurements of patients with a disk hemorrhage. Am J Ophthalmol 1987;103:505.
55. De Souza Lima M, Zangwill L, Weinreb RN: Scanning laser polarimetry to assess the nerve fiber layer. *In* Schuman JS (ed): Imaging in Glaucoma. Thorofare, NJ, Slack, Inc, 1996.
56. Tielsch JM, Katz J, Singh K, et al: A population-based evaluation of glaucoma screening: The Baltimore Eye Survey. Am J Epidemiol 1991;134:1102.
57. Varma R, Spaeth GL, Hanau C, et al: Positional changes in the vasculature of the optic disc in glaucoma. Am J Ophthalmol 1987;104:457.

Index

Note: Page numbers in *italics* refer to illustrations; page numbers followed by t refer to tables.

ISBN 0-7216-7272-8

90038

9 780721 672724